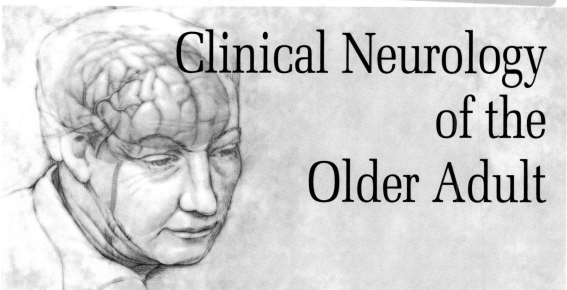

Clinical Neurology
of the
Older Adult

SECOND EDITION

Edited by

Joseph I. Sirven, MD
Associate Professor
Department of Neurology
College of Medicine, Neurology
Phoenix, Arizona

Barbara L. Malamut, PhD
Adjunct Professor
Institute for Graduate Clinical Psychology
Widener University
Chester, Pennsylvania

 Wolters Kluwer | Lippincott Williams & Wilkins
Health
Philadelphia • Baltimore • New York • London
Buenos Aires • Hong Kong • Sydney • Tokyo

Acquisitions Editor: Frances R. DeStefano
Managing Editor: Leanne McMillan
Project Manager: Jennifer Harper
Manufacturing Coordinator: Kathleen Brown
Marketing Manager: Kimberly Schonberger
Art Director: Risa Clow
Production Services: GGS Book Services

© 2008 by LIPPINCOTT WILLIAMS & WILKINS, a WOLTERS KLUWER business
530 Walnut Street
Philadelphia, PA 19106 USA
LWW.com

First edition © 2002 by Lippincott Williams & Wilkins

Printed in the USA

Library of Congress Cataloging-in-Publication Data

Clinical neurology of the older adult / edited by Joseph I. Sirven, Barbara L. Malamut.—2nd ed.
      p. ; cm.
   Includes bibliographical references and index.
   ISBN-13: 978-0-7817-6947-1 (hardcover)
   ISBN-10: 0-7817-6947-7 (hardcover)
   1. Geriatric neurology. I. Sirven, Joseph I. II. Malamut, Barbara L.
   [DNLM: 1. Nervous System Diseases. 2. Aged. WL 140 C6407 2008]
   RC346.C543 2008
   618.97'68—dc22

                                                                              2007035908

Care has been taken to confirm the accuracy of the information presented and to describe generally accepted practices. However, the authors, editors, and publisher are not responsible for errors or omissions or for any consequences from application of the information in this book and make no warranty, expressed or implied, with respect to the currency, completeness, or accuracy of the contents of the publication. Application of the information in a particular situation remains the professional responsibility of the practitioner.

The authors, editors, and publisher have exerted every effort to ensure that drug selection and dosage set forth in this text are in accordance with current recommendations and practice at the time of publication. However, in view of ongoing research, changes in government regulations, and the constant flow of information relating to drug therapy and drug reactions, the reader is urged to check the package insert for each drug for any change in indications and dosage and for added warnings and precautions. This is particularly important when the recommended agent is a new or infrequently employed drug.

Some drugs and medical devices presented in the publication have Food and Drug Administration (FDA) clearance for limited use in restricted research settings. It is the responsibility of the health care provider to ascertain the FDA status of each drug or device planned for use in their clinical practice.

To purchase additional copies of this book, call our customer service department at (800) 638-3030 or fax orders to (301) 223-2320. International customers should call (301) 223-2300.

Visit Lippincott Williams & Wilkins on the Internet: at LWW.com. Lippincott Williams & Wilkins customer service representatives are available from 8:30 am to 6 pm, EST.

10 9 8 7 6 5 4 3 2 1

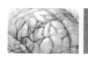

CONTENTS

SECTION III

SPECIFIC NEUROLOGICAL CONDITIONS AFFECTING THE OLDER ADULT **241**

SECTION IV

PSYCHOSOCIAL ISSUES IN THE OLDER ADULT 541

CONTRIBUTORS

Neil B. Alexander, MD
Professor
Department of Internal Medicine, Division of
    Geriatric Medicine
University of Michigan
Ann Arbor, Michigan

Director
Geriatric Research, Education, and Clinical Center
    (GRECC)
VA Ann Arbor Health Care System
Ann Arbor, Michigan

Alice P. Armbruster, MA, CCC-SLP
Clinical Instructor and Student Intern Supervisor
Speech-Language Pathology, Department of
    Neurology
Mayo School of Health Sciences Arizona
Scottsdale, Arizona

Lead Staff Speech-Language Pathologist
Speech-Language Pathology, Department of Neurology
Mayo Clinic Arizona
Phoenix, Arizona

Alon Y. Avidan, MD, MPH
Associate Professor
Director, UCLA Neurology Clinic
Associate Director, Sleep Disorders Center
Department of Neurology
University of California, Los Angeles
Los Angeles, California

Mayurkumar D. Bhakta, MD
Cardiology Fellow
Department of Cardiology
The Mayo Clinic School of Graduate Medical
    Education
Scottsdale, Arizona

Kevin M. Biglan, MD, MPH
Assistant Professor
Department of Neurology
University of Rochester School of Medicine
    and Dentistry
Rochester, New York

Jennifer J. Bortz, PhD, ABPP/ABCN
Assistant Professor
Department of Psychiatry and Psychology
Mayo Clinic Hospital
Scottsdale, Arizona

David J. Capobianco, MD
Associate Professor
Department of Neurology
Mayo Clinic Jacksonville
Jacksonville, Florida

Richard J. Caselli, MD
Professor
Department of Neurology
Mayo Clinic College of Medicine
Scottsdale, Arizona

Chair
Department of Neurology
Mayo Clinic Arizona
Scottsdale, Arizona

Julio A. Chalela, MD
Associate Professor of Neurology and
    Neurosurgery
Department of Neurology and
    Neurosurgery
Medical University of South Carolina
Charleston, South Carolina

James C. Cloyd, PharmD
Professor and Lawrence C. Weaver Endowed
    Chair-Orphan Drug Development
Director, Center for Orphan Drug Research
Experimental and Clinical Pharmacology,
    College of Pharmacy
University of Minnesota
Minneapolis, Minnesota

Jeannine M. Conway, PharmD
Assistant Professor
College of Pharmacy
University of Minnesota
Minneapolis, Minnesota

John R. Corboy, MD
Professor
Department of Neurology
University of Colorado School of
    Medicine
Aurora, Colorado

Staff Physician
Department of Neurology
University of Colorado Hospital
Aurora, Colorado

Nabila A. Dahodwala, MD
Fellow
Robert Wood Johnson Clinical Scholars Program
University of Pennsylvania
Philadelphia, Pennsylvania
Fellow
PADRECC
Philadelphia VA Hospital
Philadelphia, Pennsylvania

H. Gordon Deen, Jr., MD
Professor
Department of Neurosurgery
Mayo Clinic College of Medicine
Rochester, Minnesota

Consultant
Department of Neurosurgery
Mayo Clinic Jacksonville
Jacksonville, Florida

David W. Dodick, MD
Professor of Neurology
Department of Neurology
Mayo Clinic Arizona
Phoenix, Arizona

Joseph F. Drazkowski, MD
Assistant Professor of Neurology
Department of Neurology
Mayo Clinic Arizona
Phoenix, Arizona

Director, EEG Laboratory
Department of Neurology
Mayo Clinic Arizona
Phoenix, Arizona

Jeffrey S. Durmer, MD, PhD
Adjunct Professor
College of Health and Human Sciences
Georgia State University
Atlanta, Georgia

Medical Director and Chief Medical Officer
Fusion Sleep, Program in Sleep Medicine
Suwanee, Georgia

James M. Ellison, MD, MPH
Associate Professor of Psychiatry
Harvard Medical School
Boston, Massachusetts

Clinical Director
Geriatric Psychiatry Program
McLean Hospital
Belmont, Massachusetts

Adam E. Flanders, MD
Professor of Radiology and Rehabilitation Medicine
Department of Radiology

Thomas Jefferson University Hospital
Philadelphia, Pennsylvania

Laura A. Flashman, PhD
Associate Professor
Department of Psychiatry
Dartmouth Medical School
Hanover, New Hampshire

Director, Neuropsychology Postdoctoral Fellowship
Department of Psychiatry
Dartmouth Hitchcock Medical Center
Lebanon, New Hampshire

Rod Foroozan, MD
Assistant Professor
Department of Ophthalmology
Baylor College of Medicine
Houston, Texas

Deborah W. Frazer, PhD
Independent Practice and Consultant in Geropsychology
Philadelphia, Pennsylvania

Elliot M. Frohman, MD, PhD
Professor
Director, MS Program
Department of Neurology and Ophthalmology
University of Texas, Southwestern Medical Center
Dallas, Texas

Brent P. Goodman, MD
Instructor in Neurology
Department of Neurology
Mayo Clinic College of Medicine
Scottsdale, Arizona

Consultant in Neurology
EMG Laboratory Co-Director
Department of Neurology
Mayo Clinic Arizona
Scottsdale, Arizona

Gary L. Gottlieb, MD, MBA
Professor of Psychiatry
Harvard Medical School
Boston, Massachusetts

President
Brigham and Women's Hospital
Boston, Massachusetts

Julie E. Hammack, MD
Assistant Professor
Department of Neurology
Mayo Clinic, Minnesota
Rochester, Minnesota

Susan L. Hickenbottom, MD, MS
Adjunct Associate Professor
Department of Neurology
University of Michigan
Ann Arbor, Michigan

Director, Stroke Program
St. Joseph Mercy Health System
Ann Arbor, Michigan

Reginald T. Ho, MD
Clinical Assistant Professor
Department of Medicine
Thomas Jefferson University Hospital
Philadelphia, Pennsylvania

Charlene R. Hoffman Snyder, MSN, NP-BC
Instructor
Department of Neurology
Mayo Clinic College of Medicine
Scottsdale, Arizona

Michael D. Hollander, MD
Radiology Associates of Roanoke
Department of Radiology
Lewis-Gale Hospital
Salem, Virginia

Howard I. Hurtig, MD
Frank and Gwladys Elliott Professor and
    Vice-Chair
Department of Neurology
University of Pennsylvania
Philadelphia, Pennsylvania

Chief of Neurology
Department of Neurology
Pennsylvania Hospital
Philadelphia, Pennsylvania

Bryan D. James, M Bioethics
Research Coordinator
Department of Medicine
University of Pennsylvania
Institute on Aging
Philadelphia, Pennsylvania

Jason H.T. Karlawish, MD
Associate Professor
Department of Medicine
University of Pennsylvania
Philadelphia, Pennsylvania

Scott E. Kasner, MD
Associate Professor
Department of Neurology
University of Pennsylvania
Philadelphia, Pennsylvania

Director
Comprehensive Stroke Center
University of Pennsylvania Health System
Philadelphia, Pennsylvania

Edmund Y. Ko, MD
Resident
Department of Urology
Mayo Clinic Arizona
Phoenix, Arizona

Joyce Liporace, MD
Clinical Associate Professor
Department of Neurology
Thomas Jefferson University
Jefferson Hospital for Neuroscience
Philadelphia, Pennsylvania

Director, Women and Epilepsy Program
Center for Neuroscience
Riddle Memorial Hospital
Media, Pennsylvania

Barbara L. Malamut, PhD
Adjunct Professor
Institute for Graduate Clinical Psychology
Widener University
Chester, Pennsylvania

Elliott L. Mancall, MD
Emeritus Professor
Department of Neurology
Jefferson Medical College
Philadelphia, Pennsylvania

Attending
Department of Neurology
Thomas Jefferson University Hospital
Philadelphia, Pennsylvania

Karen T. McNett, MNS, CCC-SLP
Clinical Instructor and Student Internship Supervisor
Speech-Language Pathology, Department of Neurology
Mayo School of Health Sciences Arizona
Scottsdale, Arizona

Supervisor of Speech-Language Pathology Department
Speech-Language Pathology, Department of Neurology
Mayo Clinic Arizona
Phoenix, Arizona

Mark L. Moster, MD
Professor
Department of Neurology
Thomas Jefferson University School of Medicine
Philadelphia, Pennsylvania

Chair
Division of Neuro-ophthalmology
Albert Einstein Medical Center
Philadelphia, Pennsylvania

Maria A. Nagel, MD
Instructor
Department of Neurology
University of Colorado Health Sciences Center
Denver, Colorado

Maromi Nei, MD
Assistant Professor
Department of Neurology
Jefferson Medical College
Philadelphia, Pennsylvania

Attending Physician
Department of Neurology
Thomas Jefferson University Hospital
Philadelphia, Pennsylvania

David E. Newman-Toker, MD, PhD
Assistant Professor
Department of Neurology and Otolaryngology
The Johns Hopkins University School of Medicine
Baltimore, Maryland

Active Staff
Department of Neurology
The Johns Hopkins Hospital
Baltimore, Maryland

Katerine H. Noe, MD, PhD
Instructor
Department of Neurology
Mayo Clinic Arizona
Phoenix, Arizona

Donald E. Novicki, MD
Professor of Urology
Department of Urology
Mayo Clinic College of Medicine
Scottsdale, Arizona

Judith R. O'Jile, PhD
Assistant Professor
Department of Psychiatry and Human Behavior
University of Mississippi Medical Center
Jackson, Mississippi

Director, Neuropsychology Laboratory
Department of Psychiatry and Human Behavior
University of Mississippi Health System
Jackson, Mississippi

Benjamin J. Osborne, MD
Assistant Professor
Department of Neurology and Ophthalmology
Georgetown University
Washington, District of Columbia

Assistant Professor
Department of Neurology and Ophthalmology
Georgetown Hospital
Washington, District of Columbia

Julie L. Pickholtz, PhD
Clinical Neuropsychologist
Stroke and Neurological Disorders Program
Moss Rehabilitation Hospital
Elkins Park, Pennsylvania

Rita A. Reichard, MD
Staff Physician
Department of Medicine
Abington Memorial Hospital
Abington, Pennsylvania

Henry J. Riordan, PhD
Vice President and Global Lead
Department of Medical and Scientific Affairs
i3 Research
West Chester, Pennsylvania

Adjunct Professor
Department of Neurology
Thomas Jefferson
Philadelphia, Pennsylvania

Karen L. Roos, MD
John and Nancy Nelson Professor of Neurology
Indiana University School of Medicine
Indianapolis, Indiana

Mark A. Ross, MD
Associate Professor
Department of Neurology
College of Medicine, Mayo Clinic
Rochester, Minnesota

Consultant
Department of Neurology
Mayo Clinic Hospital
Phoenix, Arizona

Laurie M. Ryan, PhD
Program Director, Alzheimer's Disease Clinical Trials
Neuroscience and Neuropsychology of Aging Program
National Institute on Aging
Bethesda, Maryland

Andrew J. Saykin, PsyD
Professor of Radiology
Department of Radiology
Indiana University School of Medicine
Indianapolis, Indiana

Director
IU Center for Neurology
Indiana University School of Medicine
Indianapolis, Indiana

Enrique Noé Sebastián, MD, PhD
Assistant Neurologist
Brain Injury Rehabilitation Unit
Hospital NISA Valencia Al Mar
Valencia, Spain

Stacie Segebart, DPT, CSCS
Outpatient Rehabilitation Services
Department of Rehabilitation Services
Mayo Clinic Hospital
Phoenix, Arizona

Janaka K. Seneviratne, MBBS, FRACP (Australia)
Neurophysiologist, Neurologist
Neuromuscular Division, Department of Neurology
Monash Medical Centre
Melbourne, Australia

Vicki L. Shanker, MD
Attending Neurologist
Department of Neurology
Beth Israel Medical Center
New York, New York

Tanya Simuni, MD
Director, Parkinson's Disease and Movement
    Disorders Center
Associate Professor of Neurology
Department of Neurology
Northwestern University
Chicago, Illinois

Director, Parkinson's Disease and Movement
    Disorders Center
Associate Professor of Neurology
Department of Neurology
Northwestern Memorial Hospital
Chicago, Illinois

Joseph I. Sirven, MD
Associate Professor
Department of Neurology
College of Medicine, Neurology
Mayo Clinic Hospital
Phoenix, Arizona

Benn E. Smith, MD
Associate Professor of Neurology
Department of Neurology
Mayo Clinic College of Medicine
Scottsdale, Arizona

David Solomon, MD, PhD
Assistant Professor
Neurology and Otolaryngology
John Hopkins University School of Medicine
Baltimore, Maryland

Assistant Professor
Department of Neurology and Otolaryngology
Johns Hopkins Hospital
Baltimore, Maryland

Joshua R. Steinerman, MD
Postdoctoral Clinical Fellow
Neurological Institute
Columbia University Medical Center
New York, New York

Yaakov Stern, PhD
Professor of Clinical Neuropsychology
Department of Neurology, Psychiatry, and Psychology
Columbia University College of Physicians and Surgeons
New York, New York

David A. Thomas, DO, PhD
Chief
Department of Neurology
Riddle Memorial Hospital
Media, Pennsylvania

Sneha S. Vaish, MD
Department of Urology
Mayo Clinic College of Medicine
Scottsdale, Arizona

Eelco F.M. Wijdicks, MD, PhD
Professor of Neurology
Chair Division for Critical Care Neurology
Mayo Clinic College of Medicine
Rochester, Minnesota

Kathryn Willcox, BS
Research Coordinator
Center for Neuroscience
Riddle Memorial Hospital
Media, Pennsylvania

Dean M. Wingerchuk, MD, MSc, FRCP(C)
Associate Professor
Neurology
Mayo Clinic Arizona
Scottsdale, Arizona

Bryan K. Woodruff, MD
Assistant Professor
Department of Neurology
Mayo Clinic Arizona
Scottsdale, Arizona

Assistant Professor
Department of Neurology
Mayo Clinic Hospital
Phoenix, Arizona

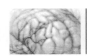

PREFACE

In 2002, we published the first edition of Clinical Neurology of the Older Adult. Since that time, the number of elderly adults has steadily increased making aging an even greater public health concern for physicians and other health practitioners alike. Along with the rising number of elderly people, there has been a rapid growth of scientific, medical and neuropsychological advances that have improved our knowledge of neurological disorders and in some cases, considerably altered diagnosis and treatment practices. Because neurological disorders account for a significant majority of diseases afflicting older adults, a book focusing strictly on this age group is no longer a novelty, but rather it is essential.

Neurological illnesses in older adults are a major cause of disability and dependence and account for a disproportionate number of patients treated in neurological outpatient and hospital settings. With the expected growth in the aging population, there is an ever increasing demand for information regarding the course of normal aging, its impact on the nervous system, ways to maintain wellness, and diseases that impact the elderly and their management. In both medical and psychological settings, it has become abundantly clear that the approach to diagnosis and treatment of disorders in the aged can be quite different and markedly more complicated than in a younger adult. It is not uncommon for the older patient to have a complex array of neurological and medical problems so that the usual treatment for one illness is prohibited due to complications from a second disease. Furthermore, older patients often take multiple medications; each with its own side effects and the interactions of the drugs can lead to various adverse reactions that can resemble a new disorder. Therefore, an essential understanding of the many facets of neurological illness is needed to make accurate diagnosis, implement a well-integrated treatment plan, and ultimately lead to improved quality of life and other favorable health outcomes. In 2002, we found that there were few books that surveyed the field of geriatric neurology. This continues to be the case at the time of this publication in 2008.

The purpose of this book has not changed from the first edition. It is intended to serve as a practical guide to all physicians, psychologists, medical students, and others who serve the geriatric population. It reflects the multidisciplinary nature of geriatric neurology by including chapters on the neurology and neuropsychology of various diseases such as Parkinson's disease and dementia, as well as important psychosocial and ethical considerations that confront most clinicians in their day-to-day practice. In this second edition we have updated all new diagnostic and treatment options for various neurological problems since the printing of the first edition. We have incorporated genomics where appropriate; particularly, for the issues of the varying dementias. Changes in neuroimaging techniques and their applications are also reflected in many chapters in the new edition of this book. We have created a chapter on driving which is an emotional touchstone issue for most individuals and an important concept for physician, family, and public health concern. Lastly, we have increased coverage of physical and speech therapy both of which are cornerstones of therapy for issues such as stroke and trauma.

The scope of the book is broad to include the most prevalent categories of neurologic illness in the peripheral and central nervous systems affecting the elderly. In the first section, diagnostic tests commonly used in the elderly are discussed. The second section includes common neurological problems based on signs and symptoms such as mood or gait disorders. The third section discusses specific disease entities such as epilepsy or dementia and the fourth section involves psychosocial issues. As noted by the popularity of the first edition, we have continued to approach the topics in geriatric neurology from the two viewpoints of signs and symptoms and disease specific states. We have found this format to be a useful tool to clinicians because a disease can be referenced based on the symptoms it presents or looked up by the disease entity itself. The medication charts and diagnostic algorithms have been updated and are provided so that beneficial information can be quickly obtained. It is out hope that the second edition of Clinical Neurology of the Older Adult will be of even greater assistance to all practitioners in helping their patients enjoy healthy, productive lives as they age.

Joseph I. Sirven
Barbara L. Malamut

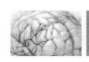

ACKNOWLEDGMENTS

The preparation of this text reflects research findings as well as day-to-day clinical issues in treating the elderly patient. In this regard, we thank all of our patients for providing an invaluable resource by teaching us many life lessons. We thank our families: Joan, Larry, and Robby. Without their support and understanding, this book would never have come to fruition. A special acknowledgment is made to Ellen, a medical librarian, who relentlessly tracked down many of the medical and psychological journals referenced in this book. Lastly, we thank all of the contributors who enthusiastically agreed to update their chapters, despite their busy schedules.

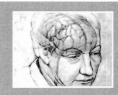

INTRODUCTION: WHAT MAKES THE OLDER ADULT UNIQUE?

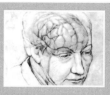

CHAPTER 1

Gerontology and Neurology

Rita A. Reichard

INTRODUCTION

Our population is aging. In July 2003, there were 35.9 million people in the United States over the age of 65. In 2030, it is expected that this number will double (1).

There are various concerns associated with this growth, one of which is appropriate health care for this group of people. This chapter will serve as an overview of the field of geriatric medicine, a field of medicine specifically devoted to the care of the elderly patient. Traditionally, the age at which geriatric medicine begins is 65. However, as we will see, geriatrics is defined by more than just an age criterion.

HISTORICAL BACKGROUND

The field of geriatric medicine is a relatively young specialty. The term "geriatrics" was first described in clinical medicine in 1909 by Ignatz L. Nascher (2).

Dr. Nascher recognized that there was a need to distinguish care for those who were over the age of 65. As the years passed, specific training for those interested in serving the geriatric population became available. In 1968, the first fellowship training program was developed at the City Hospital Center in Queens, NY. The fellowship training accepted those who had completed a residency in either Internal Medicine or Family Practice and required candidates to complete 2 years of training. In 1981, there were 36 geriatric medicine programs (2). Currently, there are over 100 training programs in the United States.

In 1988, a certification exam was established by the American Board of Family Practice and the American Board of Internal Medicine. Until 1994, fellowship training was not required to take the exam. Those with "substantial clinical experience" could get certified in geriatric medicine. Beginning in 1994, a fellowship was required to take the certification exam. In 1995, partially as a response to try to attract more physicians to the field of geriatrics, the fellowship length was changed to 1 year.

WHAT IS A GERIATRICIAN?

Although 65 is the arbitrary age used to define geriatrics, people who should see a geriatrician are often those who are more frail and debilitated. The typical "geriatric patient" is one who presents with multiple, chronic health conditions that are impairing his ability at a physical, emotional, social, and economic level. These health conditions are generally progressive in nature over time. However, how these chronic health conditions affect a person is variable. The way in which disability is evaluated is by using functional assessment tools. A person is evaluated for his ability to perform activities of daily living (ADL). These are activities we need to do every day and include such items as walking, toileting, and feeding oneself. A person is also evaluated for his ability to do instrumental activities of daily living (IADL). These include activities such as driving, medication management, and financial management. The inability to properly perform IADL can affect a person's ability to remain independent in the community.

Geriatricians use the baseline functional assessments and the patient's goals as a guide to help decide which disabilities are most bothersome and should be addressed. Multiple persons become involved, and the goal in a treatment plan is to try and maximize independence as much as possible for as long as possible. The geriatrician can be viewed as the "team leader" who helps involve other health practitioners from various disciplines, such as nursing, social work, physical therapy, and medicine subspecialties such as neurology, to help maximize independence.

The functional assessment is also important to help decide appropriate options for diagnosis and treatment of medical conditions. Let us consider two 75-year-old patients with arthritis, Parkinson's disease, and congestive heart failure. One patient may be very independent, living at home, and managing all of his ADL without difficulty. This person may be one in whom screening for cancers and aggressive treatment of other medical issues are warranted. On the other hand, the other 75-year-old patient may be so functionally impaired that he needs to live in a nursing facility. This person may benefit from more of a palliative approach to his health care. In other words, a look at the whole person really defines the approach to each individual medical issue.

The geriatrician is considered to be more of an expert in distinguishing normal aging from a disease process, which may help guide decisions about whether an intervention is warranted in the evaluation of a symptom. In addition, the geriatrician is more comfortable with the evaluation and management of "geriatric syndromes." These diseases, which are not a normal part of aging, are more prevalent in the older population and more readily identified and treated by one who primarily cares for the older patient. These syndromes include dementia, depression, falls, pressure ulcers, chronic pain, and delirium. Many of these syndromes may coexist in the same patient. Many of these disease processes involve the nervous system, and the geriatrician understands the importance of being able to adequately perform a physical exam of this organ system.

As already discussed, the health conditions that are managed by geriatricians tend to be progressive over time. Eventually, these conditions often impair function so much that remaining in the community is no longer an option. Geriatricians are regularly involved in taking care of people in assisted living and nursing home environments. Both at home and in facilities, the geriatrician is dealing with people in the final stages of diseases. Addressing and managing end-of-life-care issues becomes an important role of the geriatrician at this time of life.

Being a geriatrician involves more than clinical responsibilities. Geriatricians are often asked to assume administrative responsibilities at assisted living and nursing homes in the role of medical director. The geriatrician can bring his expertise to help define appropriate policies and procedures at these facilities. He also is intricately involved in ensuring that quality medical care is being provided to all at the facility.

A geriatrician may also have the role of educator. Many geriatricians are affiliated with academic institutions and are involved in teaching the principles of geriatric medicine to residents and fellows. There is also a need for education of peers. The majority of geriatric medicine will be practiced by internists and family practitioners, not by geriatricians who have been through fellowship training. Geriatricians should be sharing their knowledge with their colleagues through formal educational seminars and at an individual level.

In sum, knowledge of the best way to care for the older person is essential as our population is living longer. Understanding the principles of maximizing independence and trying to ensure quality of life are inherent in the practice of geriatric medicine.

The role of the geriatrician is to be available to provide medical knowledge, leadership, and education to both the lay public and all disciplines involved in the care of the older adult to try to attain these goals.

REFERENCES

1. He W, Sengupta M, Velkoff V, DeBarros K. US Census Bureau, Current Population Reports P23–209, 65+ in the United States: 2005. Washington, DC: US Government Printing Office; 2005.
2. Warshaw G, Bragg E. The training of geriatricians in the United States: three decades of progress. *J Am Geriatr Soc.* 2003;51(suppl):S338–S345.

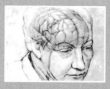

CHAPTER 2

Neurological Examination of the Older Adult

Joseph I. Sirven and Elliott L. Mancall

The neurologic examination, for the most part, is an exercise in detailed observation, consisting of two tasks: (a) localizing the part of the nervous system that is malfunctioning, and (b) identifying the cause for that malfunction. Every aspect of the patient's behavior, including the way he or she sits, speaks, and responds, tells the physician about nervous system function. However, in older adults, the parameters of a normal neurologic examination require redefining, and the results from a neurologic examination must be considered within the context of known age-related changes. Thus, findings in older patients that suggest pathology may not be pertinent if such findings occur frequently at advanced ages. Table 2-1 describes the normal morphologic and physiologic changes in the aging nervous system.

In his seminal papers on the neurologic changes in the aged, Critchley (2,3) identified several changes that occur in the neurologic examination. These were subsequently confirmed by other reviews (1,4). Changes tend to affect the visual, auditory, olfactory, motor, and sensory nervous systems. The most consistent of the neurologic signs of aging are shown in Table 2-2.

MENTAL STATUS EXAMINATION

Changes in mental status functioning that occur with aging may be apparent on formal standardized tests of mental status, but they are difficult to detect clinically. Older patients are generally alert and have normal levels of consciousness. It is abnormal for an older patient not to maintain orientation to time, place, and situation. Judgment is expected to be normal, and calculations and thought content are equally unaffected unless a pathologic process is present. Remote and recent memory is usually normal; however, the speed of processing and retrieving information slows. Thus, when abnormalities of speech or language are noted, an underlying brain lesion must be considered. For a detailed discussion regarding mental functioning, see Chapter 6.

CRANIAL NERVE CHANGES

Cranial nerve abnormalities are rarely associated with normal aging, yet important exceptions are seen. Changes in hearing, particularly progressive hearing loss (presbycusis), especially for high tones, are commonly observed, as is a decline in speech discrimination. These changes are secondary to a reduction in the number of hair cells in the organ of Corti. Similarly, olfaction generally declines symmetrically with age; the key to a pathologic process is finding asymmetric loss. Changes in visual acuity are almost always related to abnormalities in the eye and do not reflect changes in visual neural circuits. Pathologic conditions (e.g., cataracts, glaucoma, and other

Table 2-1. *Age-Related Nervous System Changes*

Neuroanatomic Location	Change
Anterior horn cells, sensory ganglion	Decline of 25%
Brain weight	Weight decline of 233 g from third decade to sixth to seventh decade
Hippocampus	Neuronal loss and gliosis by 27%
Neuronal cytoplasm	Increased accumulation of lipofuscin granules
Nerve roots	Accumulation of amyloid
Blood vessels and flow	Hyalinization of the walls of small blood vessels
	Cerebral flow declines with age with an increase in cerebrovascular resistance
Neurotransmitters	Decline in the concentrations of acetylcholine, norepinephrine, dopamine, and gamma-aminobutyric acid
Muscles and peripheral nerves	Skeletal muscle fiber loss with concomitant atrophy
	Myelin changes occur with a decrease in conduction velocity
	Loss of motor and sensory axons

Table 2-2. *Age-Related Changes in the Neurologic Examination*

Modality	Change
Auditory	Perceptive hearing loss for higher tones
Gait	Attitude of general flexion Decreased fluidity of movement
Motor	Diminished reaction time Impaired agility and coordination Reduced muscle bulk and power
Ophthalmic	Decreased pupillary size Delayed pupillary reaction to light and accommodation Diminished upward gaze
Olfactory	Diminishment in olfaction
Reflexes	Reduced or absent ankle reflex
Sensory	Impairment of vibratory sensation, but preservation of proprioception

causes) must be sought in patients complaining of diminished vision and not be attributed to normal aging. Aging does not cause a change in the appearance of the retina. Thus, funduscopic changes should be considered abnormal, and consideration should be given to systemic causes such as diabetes.

Older adults have smaller pupils than those seen in younger adults as well as sluggish light and accommodation reactions. These changes, which occur symmetrically, result from aging changes in the muscles of the sphincter pupillae. Thus, unilateral abnormalities need to be investigated. The aged also have abnormalities in eye movement, including restriction of upward gaze, failure to dissociate head movements from eye movements, and gaze nystagmus, which is generally associated with medications. For a more detailed discussion on the visual changes associated with aging, see Chapter 12.

MOTOR EXAMINATION

Muscle tone can alter with aging, with rigidity and paratonia (increased tone) being the most common manifestation. The increased tone can cause diminished agility. Motor strength is well preserved except for a mild reduction in muscle power, especially proximally, with advancing age. The reduction in power is related to a decrease in the number of muscle fibers and the bulk of each fiber. The strength of handgrip lessens 20% to 30% from age 20 onward,

with an equal decline on both sides of the body, but this is only apparent if an older adult is compared with a younger adult.

Aging is also associated with a decline in coordination when older adults are compared with young controls. This change is almost undetectable, but caution should be taken in assuming that ataxia is secondary to aging as well. Action tremors often occur in older adults. However, tremor should not be considered a normal sign of aging but rather a symptom aggravated by age that can be treated. Motor reaction time is decreased with older age. Common functions (e.g., donning trousers, rising from a chair, or climbing stairs) can require more time for an older adult compared with a younger individual. A decrease in coordination occurs, with a possible increase of dysmetria on finger-to-nose testing, as well as dysdiadochokinesia. At times, a mild, unexplained ataxia is encountered.

Gait can slow with age, and signs such as a reduced arm swing and a stooped posture are present. A shuffling gait should not be considered a normal sign of aging. If slowness is extreme with regard to these functions, then extrapyramidal pathology should be considered (i.e., Parkinson's disease). Although aged patients may have gaits that appear unsteady, they do not necessarily have repeated falls or trouble with tandem walking. For further information regarding gait and movements disorders, see Chapters 9 and 22, respectively.

REFLEXES

Deep tendon reflexes are generally preserved in the elderly, and their absence or asymmetry usually indicates disease. Loss of ankle jerks is considered common and may be a consequence of the inelasticity of the Achilles tendon rather than a result of changes within the nerve or the reflex arc. In most instances, however, loss of a reflex is considered a sign of disease rather than a normal consequence of aging. Snout, glabellar (inability to inhibit blinking), and palmomental reflexes are a frequent finding in the elderly. However, the suck and grasp reflex are indicative of frontal lobe disease. Superficial reflexes (e.g., the abdominal responses) are frequently not obtainable. Flexor plantar responses can be difficult to attain because of withdrawal, but a positive response must be regarded as indicating a lesion in the corticospinal tract.

THE SENSORY EXAMINATION

One of the most common manifestations of aging seen on the neurologic examination is change in sensation. Impairment or loss of vibratory sense in the toes and ankles is a well-known finding, with a decrease in function of 50% to 60% in the feet of

Table 2-3. *Age-Related Changes in Activities of Daily Living*

Function	No Difficulty (%)	With Difficulty, But Does Not Need Help (%)	Needs Help (%)
Getting in and out of bed	78	21	1
Sitting or standing from a chair	69	29	2
Continence	68	31	1
Eating, cutting food	96	4	0
Preparing own meals	92	1	7
Dressing	82	17	1
Climbing stairs	50	45	5
Shopping	83	9	8
Handling finances	88	8	4

From Katzman R, Terry R, eds. *The neurology of aging*, 1983, with permission.

persons over 80 years of age, whereas proprioception is well preserved. Thresholds for the perception of cutaneous stimuli increase with age but can be difficult to detect. The changes in cutaneous sensation correlate with a loss of sensory fibers on sural nerve biopsy, as well as reduced amplitude of sensory nerve action potentials and loss of dorsal root ganglion cells. Decreases in both two-point discrimination and stereognosis have been reported but are not well characterized in the context of the neurologic examination.

AUTONOMIC NERVOUS SYSTEM

Autonomic function is impaired with aging. Autonomic control of heart and peripheral vasculature may be impaired and lead to orthostatic hypotension. Orthostatic hypotension accounts for a small but significant number of falls by older patients. This hypotension may be related to dysfunction of several anatomic loci, including the hypothalamus, brainstem, spinal cord, or peripheral nerve. Temperature control mechanisms can also be reduced, with hypothermia or hyperthermia a possible consequence. For a more detailed discussion, see Chapter 8.

EFFECTS OF AGING ON THE ACTIVITIES OF DAILY LIVING IN THE HEALTHY ELDERLY

When multiple illnesses are superimposed on normal aging, physical reserves used to perform the complex motor activities required for daily living are compromised. Table 2-3 shows the result from the Bronx Aging Study, which consisted of healthy, ambulatory, community-living volunteers, aged 74 to 85 years, studied over time (5). The study helped to define the effects of normal aging with regard to activities of daily living. For the most part, function is well preserved, but clearly, decrements in motor strength take their toll

as evidenced by the difficulties in getting out of bed and climbing stairs.

It is the loss of functional ability that is most important to understand because this is what frequently leads to a request for neurologic, psychological, and psychiatric consultation. Detailed discussions of the normal changes of aging with respect to various aspects of the central and peripheral nervous system are found throughout this text.

SUMMARY

Health care practitioners who care for the older adult must first understand the neurologic changes that occur with age and how they affect function. The aging process in essentially healthy, disease-free persons is associated with decrements in many aspects of motor and sensory function. It is important to comprehend these changes and understand their impact on function in order to accurately diagnose, treat, and care for the older adult with neurologic disease.

REFERENCES

1. Benassi G, D'Alessandro RD, Gallassi R, et al. Neurological examination in subjects over 65 years: an epidemiological survey. *Neuroepidemiology*. 1990;9:27–38.
2. Critchley M. Neurological changes in the aged. *J Chronic Dis*. 1955;3:459–477.
3. Critchley M. The neurology of old age. *Lancet*. 1931;1:1119–1127.
4. Kokmen E, Bossemeyer RW, Barney J, et al. Neurological manifestations of aging. *J Gerontol*. 1977;32:411–419.
5. Wolfson LI, Katzman R. The neurologic consultation at age 80. In: Katzman R, Terry RD, eds. *The neurology of aging*. Philadelphia: FA Davis; 1983:221–244.

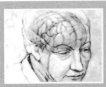

CHAPTER 3.1

Imaging of the Aging Brain

Michael D. Hollander and Adam E. Flanders

Over the past several decades, dramatic advances have been made in imaging of the neuroaxis. Today, computed tomography (CT), magnetic resonance imaging (MRI), single photon emission computed tomography (SPECT), and positron emission tomography (PET) are the primary imaging techniques currently being used to evaluate the brain. CT and MRI allow for an easy, safe, noninvasive way to study the brain. CT is limited by single-plane imaging and poor visualization of the temporal lobe and posterior fossa structures from skull base artifacts and diminished contrast resolution compared with MRI. MRI, on the other hand, is a multiplanar technique; therefore, the temporal lobe can be evaluated in the coronal plane with little or no artifact from the skull base. SPECT and PET imaging allow for a physiologic evaluation of the brain and for physiologic comparison of different regions of the brain. These two techniques require the intravenous injection of a radiopharmaceutical and give less information about the morphologic appearance of the brain. Therefore, for the complete evaluation of the aging brain, most studies suggest using both an imaging study and a nuclear medicine study to allow for a morphologic and functional assessment of the brain.

Various imaging pitfalls must be recognized when assessing the brain of the elderly, whether healthy or diseased (23). From the third decade of life to the beginning of the tenth decade, the weight of the average male brain declines from 1,394 to 1,161 g, a loss of 233 g, presumably caused by degeneration of neurons and replacement gliosis (4,18). This change is slow initially but accelerates with advancing age and is usually readily apparent by the seventh decade. Changes involve both the cerebrum and the cerebellum (59). The neuronal population in the neocortex is progressively depleted in the seventh, eighth, and ninth decades. The greatest loss appears to be among the small neurons of the second and fourth layers (external and internal granular laminae) in the frontal and superior temporal regions, approaching a 50% neuronal loss by the ninth decade. Neuronal loss and replacement gliosis, which represent the primary aging process, can occur in the absence of neurofibrillary changes associated with Alzheimer's disease (AD) and senile plaques (4,18).

IMAGING FINDINGS ASSOCIATED WITH NORMAL AGING

VENTRICULAR ENLARGEMENT

As the median and paramedian parts of the brain regress with age, the third ventricle slowly begins to widen (59). Yakovlev studied the growth and maturation of the nervous system and noted the regression of the median nuclei of the thalamus and widening of the third ventricle beginning by the fifth decade (59). In addition, he observed a progressive decrease in the size of the massa intermedia (59). In a different study, Morel and Wildi measured the ventricular volume in cadaveric specimens ranging in age from 55 to 99 years and noted an increase in the size of the ventricles up to the ninth decade (59). The ventricles were larger in the men than in the women, and the left lateral ventricle was usually larger than the right (59). In addition to the ventricles becoming larger, Knudson found that the temporal lobes, particularly the hippocampus, uncus, and parahippocampal and fusiform gyri, and area around the insula involute with age (59). The relationship between size of the lateral ventricles and age is more variable than that of the third ventricle (59). In contrast, only mild enlargement of the temporal horns of the lateral ventricles is observed with aging, and the left temporal horn is usually slightly larger than the right.

Multiple brain CT studies have been performed to distinguish normal age-related ventricular changes from pathologic states. Various measurements and ratios have been employed to establish normal metrics, including the Evans, frontal horn, bicaudate, and third ventricle–Sylvian fissure methods (Table 3-1). These studies all found progressive enlargement of the ventricles and cortical sulci (Fig. 3-1) with age. In fact, Nagata et al. reported that the cerebrospinal fluid (CSF)-to-brain ratio remains constant for the first six decades and then begins to change thereafter. One of the most reproducible measures used in these studies is the ratio of ventricular width to the corresponding width of the skull or brain.

SULCAL ENLARGEMENT

Enlargement of the superficial sulci, particularly in the frontal parasagittal region and in the parietal and temporal lobes, is a commonly described normal

Table 3-1. *Computed Tomography Ratios*

Evans: frontal horn span or internal diameter of skull (Gawler et al., 1976)
  <0.29 in patients <60 yr
  >0.50 obstructive hydrocephalus (LeMay, 1984)
Bicaudate: width of ventricles between caudate or internal diameter of skull (Pelicci, 1979)
  <0.17 normal
  >0.20 abnormal (Hahn and Rim, 1976)
Third ventricle: sum of distance lateral margin of third and Sylvian fissure/internal
  diameter of skull
  <0.59 demented patients (Brinkman et al., 1981)
Gray matter to white matter (normal values):
  1.13 (20 yr) 1.28 (50 yr) 1.55 (100 yr) (Miller et al., 1980)

feature of aging. The etiology for this observation may be related to a decrease in volume of subcortical structures rather than to a change in width of the cortex (59). Miller et al. (61) reported that the ratio of gray matter versus white matter was 1.13 at age 20, 1.28 at age 50, and 1.55 at age 100, which suggests that white matter atrophy exceeds that of gray matter. Most authors suggest that physiologic atrophy commences at the age of 50. However, CT studies on postmortem and living patients do show a wide variation in the CSF space size, ranging between 30% and 50% of the size of healthy young adults. Associated widening of the interhemispheric fissure, extending posteriorly to or beyond the callosomarginal sulci, has also been observed. Progressive widening of the sulci occurs in the frontal lobes and cerebellar vermis, beginning in the teenaged years (13). Widening of the superficial sulci seen with normal aging is often termed cortical atrophy by radiologists; however, in fact, this should more correctly be referred to as *gyral* or *superficial atrophy*. Sulcal enlargement in aging is diffuse; however, changes are best identified in specific locations after 50 years of age (12). Widening of the superficial cortical sulci is seen first in the frontal and parietal parasagittal regions (81). The anterior interhemispheric fissure and the CSF spaces around the cerebellar vermis also widen with age (37). The sulci around the central, precentral, postcentral, and superior frontal gyri widen later (49,82).

CEREBRAL WHITE MATTER

Studies have shown that white matter volume diminishes by 12% with normal aging and that this age-related change may contribute to the development of mild cognitive impairment (MCI) in the aged. MCI is now being proposed as a transitional stage between normal aging and dementia (30). Studies have shown that 30% to 80% of elderly individuals without neurologic deficits have focal abnormalities in the white matter (11). These foci are seen as areas of high signal in the periventricular, subcortical white matter, with capping of the lateral ventricular margins on T2-weighted images. On electron microscopy, these corresponding MRI changes feature atrophy of axons and myelin with associated gliosis, tortuous thickened vessels, and increased intracellular water (23). Some of these changes histologically are thought to be secondary to ectasia of the arterioles, with enlargement of the surrounding perivascular spaces (23). These findings were first described by Durand-Fardel in 1843 (28) and were termed état criblé. In addition, aging is associated with an increase in iron deposition specifically in the corpus striatum (2). This iron accumulation is thought to be related to a decrease in oligodendroglial function and dopamine production

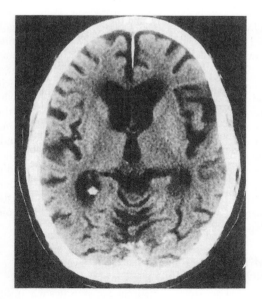

Figure 3-1. A 92-year-old man with atrophy. Noncontrast axial-computed tomography imaging demonstrates diffuse ventricular and sulcal widening.

and an increase in the free radical formation (2). Iron is also deposited in the walls of blood vessels. Iron is more easily visualized on T2-weighted images as focal regions of low signal secondary to field heterogeneity and magnetic susceptibility (25).

SKULL CHANGES WITH AGING

Finby and Kraft (59) found that most skull radiographs taken of the same individuals over time revealed an increase in the size of the cranial vault, facial bones, and paranasal sinuses and in the skull thickness, which is thought to be secondary to continuous resorption and regrowth of the skull and facial bones.

(1H) PROTON MAGNETIC RESONANCE SPECTROSCOPY

Magnetic resonance spectroscopy (MRS) is an MRI technique that permits noninvasive quantitative measurement of cerebral biochemical metabolites. MRS can be used to selectively "sample" a biochemical map of a selected volume of the brain (voxel) (77). The principle cerebral metabolites that are routinely measured with MRS are *N*-acetylaspartate (NAA), creatine and phosphocreatine (PCr/Cr), choline (Cho), myoinositol (mI), and glutamate plus glutamine (Glx). NAA is principally found within neurons and is a sensitive indicator of neuronal loss. Creatine is a byproduct of oxidative phosphorylation and the energy cycle associated with adenosine triphosphate (ATP) production; the concentration of this metabolite is very constant, and therefore, this value is often used as an internal reference standard. Myoinositol is a byproduct of glucose metabolism and is known to occur in elevated concentrations in diabetes and Alzheimer's disease. Choline (Cho) is abundant in the cell membrane, and elevation in this metabolite's concentration is reported in neoplasia and demyelination (72).

As seen in Table 3-2, the normal aging brain shows very small but definite changes in the MRS spectral signature as compared with a young adult. With aging, NAA has been shown to decrease in the occipital gray matter, the generalized concentration of choline is reported to elevate, and myoinositol (mI) is relatively reduced. Ross et al. (72) has shown that none of these changes exceed 10% of the normal young adult.

MOLECULAR NEUROIMAGING

The complex but close relationship between brain physiologic activity and brain blood flow is the basis for nuclear medicine imaging protocols for the brain. The development of scintillation multiprobe systems provided a technique to quantify regional cerebral blood flow (rCBF), or perfusion, within individual regions of the cortex and, ultimately, to compare the rCBF with regional brain function. Single photon

Table 3-2. *Magnetic Resonance Changes in Aging*

Age Range	NAA/Cr	Cho/Cr	ml/Cr
Gray matter			
16–25	1.40	0.56	0.60
26–37	1.36	0.61	0.60
40–78	1.26	0.60	0.59
White matter			
16–25	1.54	0.77	0.59
29–37	1.49	0.78	0.60
40–78	1.41	0.82	0.63

Cho, total choline; Cr, total creatine; ml, myoinositol; NAA, N-acetylaspartate.

From Ross BD, Bluml S, Cowan R, et al. In vivo MR spectroscopy of human dementia. *Neuroimaging Clin N Am.* 1998;8(4):809–822, with permission.

emission computed tomography (SPECT) and positron emission tomography (PET) have the ability to perform rapid three-dimensional physiologic imaging of the brain. This has become particularly important in geriatric brain imaging by helping to differentiate the various causes of dementia. For example, the reduction of metabolism and perfusion in the temporoparietal areas in the brain has become a biomarker for Alzheimer's disease (AD). Another potential use for PET biomarkers is to follow the response to drug or other treatments (39).

The radiopharmaceuticals that are in common use (1) to evaluate brain physiology by rCBF SPECT include ^{99m}Tc-hexamethyl propylene amine oxime (HMPAO; exametazime, Ceretec, Amersham Inc.), ^{123}I-inosine monophosphate (IMP; which is intermittently available), ^{133}Xe gas (General Electric Corp.), and ^{99m}Tc-ethyl cysteinate (ECD; Merck Du Pont Inc.).

The most commonly used radiopharmaceuticals for PET imaging (22) of the brain are ^{18}F-fluorodeoxyflucose (18F-FDG), which measures the cerebral metabolic rate for glucose (CMRGlc), and ^{15}O-H_2O, which measures rCBF. Two new compounds being used for imaging in the AD patient are fluorine-18–labelled FDDNP and the Pittsburgh compound B (carbon-11–labelled PIB). The [^{18}F]FDDNP labels both neurofibrillary tangles and beta-amyloid neuritis plaques, whereas [^{11}C]PIB only labels the amyloid deposits (83).

MOLECULAR IMAGING IN NORMAL AGING

Normal age-related atrophy can significantly influence qualitative and quantitative analyses of 18F-FDG-PET studies. The 18F-FDG-PET findings in a normally aging brain, as reported in the literature, have been inconsistent. A number of investigators have described diminished regional glucose metabolism (CMRGlc) in the temporal, parietal, somatosensory, and, especially, frontal regions. Others have described more prominent decreases in the frontal and somatosensory cortices in comparison with younger controls (15,51,87). When brain atrophy was not considered, mean CMRGlc values were lower in older patients, particularly in the frontal, parietal, and temporal regions. Also, women had significantly higher mean CMRGlc than men. Cerebrovascular risk factors in the population were also seen not to have any effect on CMRGlc (87).

VOLUMETRIC MRI

Volumetric MRI is a relatively new and increasingly important technique in the study of dementias, especially in the aid of diagnosis and to follow progression of disease (85). The availability of inexpensive powerful computing platforms provides methods for automatic volumetric analysis of three-dimensional datasets. Voxel-based morphometry involves a voxelwise statistical comparison of the local concentration of gray matter between two groups of subjects. It is used to assess patterns of atrophy (85).

PATHOLOGIC CONDITIONS

Most dementing illnesses are typically irreversible and progressive (31). Therefore, it is of the utmost importance to exclude reversible systemic causes such as infection, electrolyte or chemical imbalance, heart disease, or nutritional disorders that can mimic dementia. The major role of imaging is to detect treatable structural disorders such as hemorrhage, malignancy, posttraumatic lesions, infection, and hydrocephalus (57). CT and MRI have greatly improved our ability to detect these treatable conditions. In addition, physiologic imaging procedures (e.g., MRS, SPECT, and PET) are leading the advances in early diagnosis of debilitating diseases such as AD.

ALZHEIMER'S DISEASE (AD)

With more people living longer, the prevalence of AD has doubled since 1980 and will likely triple by the year 2050 (14). Although it is possible to make an accurate clinical diagnosis of dementia in most patients with severe disease, it is very difficult to differentiate between AD and other dementing disorders in patients with mild disease (80). With functional imaging studies such as SPECT and PET, it is believed to be possible to make an early diagnosis of AD and possibly help in elucidating the mechanisms underlying the disorder. AD is known to target specific brain regions, especially the cholinergic basal forebrain and medial temporal lobe structures including

the hippocampus, amygdala, and entorhinal cortex (14). The role of neuroimaging has been detection of early structural changes in the hippocampal formation and parahippocampal gyrus because memory loss is a prominent feature of AD. Table 3-3 summarizes the benefits and disadvantages of various imaging techniques.

Computed Tomography (CT) in AD

CT is diagnostically limited because of skull base artifacts and a limited view of the hippocampus. However, it has been shown that, when imaging is performed in an angulated fashion to optimize capture of the cross section of the temporal lobe, it is possible to measure the minimal width of the medial temporal lobe (MTL), which has been shown to be a useful marker for AD (63). The MTL in patients with AD is significantly lower than the MTL of patients with clinical depression. O'Brien et al. (63) showed that the mean MTL for patients with AD was 10.8 mm versus 14.0 mm for patients with depression.

Magnetic Resonance Imaging (MRI) in AD

The best visualization of the MTL is provided by MRI (Fig. 3-2). High-resolution imaging in the coronal plane, using a fluid-attenuated inversion recovery (FLAIR) sequence as well as a three-dimensional volume gradient echo sequence, is useful to image the temporal lobe, allowing for both morphologic and volumetric analysis to be done. Volumetric evaluation

Table 3-3. *Value of Imaging Techniques in Alzheimer's Disease*

CT	Of limited value (bone artifact inhibits evaluation of the medial temporal lobe)
MRI	Allows for volumetric measurements of the temporal lobe with significant reduction seen in Alzheimer's disease (AD) as compared with depression and other dementias
MRS	Myoinositol is elevated in AD and decreased in other dementias
SPECT	Bilateral hypoperfusion of the temporal and parietal lobes using HMPAO or inosine 5′-monophosphate
PET	Decrease in whole brain CMRGlc values, especially in the temporal and parietal lobes

CMAGlc, cerebral metabolic rate for glucose; CT, computed tomography; HMPAO, ^{99m}Tc-hexamethylpropyleneamine oxime; MRI, magnetic resonance imaging; MRS, magnetic resonance spectroscopy; PET, positron emission tomography; SPECT, single photon emission computed tomography.

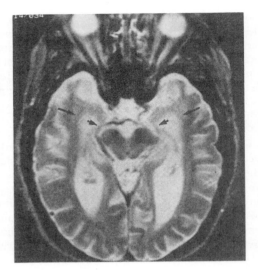

Figure 3-2. A 76-year-old man with Alzheimer's disease. Axial T2-weighted magnetic resonance imaging demonstrates bilateral hippocampal (*short arrows*) and temporal lobe atrophy with resulting compensatory widening of the temporal horns (*long arrows*).

of the temporal lobes can be performed and compared with normative data published by Bhatia et al. (7). In patients with AD, volumetric measurements reveal significantly lower measurements compared with a group of controls (47). A more recent study by Cuenod et al. (19) has shown that atrophy of the amygdala can occur earlier than hippocampal atrophy.

Magnetic Resonance Spectroscopy (MRS) in AD

Using proton (1H) MRS (58) in the evaluation of AD has shown a loss of NAA and an increase in myoinositol (mI) (Fig. 3-3) in the posterior cingulate region, which suggests a loss of neuronal content. The specific regions of the brain that show the largest and earliest reduction in NAA are the mesial temporal lobe, entorhinal cortex, hippocampus, and limbic system (44). The mean reduction in NAA is approximately 10% when compared to normal controls. Changes in mI concentration have been shown to occur earlier than the decrease in NAA, and these changes are most pronounced in the mesial temporal lobe (44). Myoinositol has been used to distinguish patients with AD from normal patients or patients with other causes of dementia. This elevation is thought to result secondary to an astrocytic reaction to the presence of neurofibrillary tangles. Elevation of choline (Cho) has been neither reproducible nor specific to AD (72). Ross et al. (72) have shown that MRS can distinguish AD with a specificity of 95%.

Volumetric Magnetic Resonance Imaging (MRI) in AD

This technique has become more important in the study of dementias. Voxel-based morphometry involves a voxel-wise statistical comparison of the local concentration of gray matter between two groups of subjects (85). The gray matter loss is not only seen in the medial temporal lobe, but also within the posterior cingulate, insula, temporoparietal association cortex, and prefrontal gyri. In addition, structures in the central gray matter are also involved (85).

Single Photon Emission Computed Tomography (SPECT) in AD

SPECT imaging is more widely available than PET and provides the equivalent diagnostic information (84). Several studies report that certain SPECT radiotracers (e.g., HMPAO or IMP) have high sensitivity (64% to 100%) and a similar specificity in the diagnosis of AD as the radiopharmaceuticals used in PET (16,38,60).

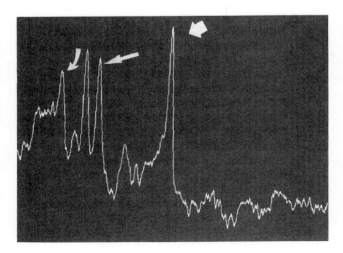

Figure 3-3. A 71-year-old woman with Alzheimer's disease. Magnetic resonance spectroscopy demonstrates decreased *N*-acetylaspartate (*short arrow*) and an increase in myoinositol (*curved arrow*) related to creatine (*long arrow*).

Many of these studies emphasize that bilateral hypoperfusion of the temporal and parietal lobes is the most common finding and, diagnostically, the most specific finding in AD. There is infrequent involvement of the frontal lobes, and when this finding is present, it is found in association with temporoparietal hypoperfusion and in advanced stages of the disease. In actual practice, however, almost 30% of patients will present with a unilateral posterior perfusion defect. When first seen, it is more commonly on the patient's left, whereas bilateral defects are often asymmetric. Frontal flow defects can appear later in the course of the disease (9,40,69,79). Some observers have related left posterior perfusion defects to short-term memory deficits and right posterior defects to visual spatial abnormalities, whereas a left frontal perfusion defect is often accompanied by a degree of aphasia (9,40,69,79). Typically, the primary sensorimotor cortex, visual cortex, subcortical structures, and cerebellar lobes are spared (84).

Positron Emission Tomography (PET) in AD

There is now ample evidence that the pattern of temporal and parietal hypometabolism and hypoperfusion is sensitive and specific for AD (39). Also, in patients with AD of varying severity, the magnitude and extent of hypometabolism on PET correlate with the severity of the dementia symptoms (Fig. 3-4) (27,32,43). Studies indicate no significant CMRGlc changes or only minor decreases in the parietal lobes with early AD. Moderately affected patients show significantly decreased metabolism in the midfrontal lobes, bilateral parietal lobes, and superior temporal regions. In patients with severe AD, the same regions are affected, but the hypometabolism is more pronounced. In all patients with AD, the parietal lobes show the greatest changes, with a 38% decrease in patients with moderate disease and a 53% decrease in patients with severe disease; other areas (sensorimotor and visual cortices, subcortical nuclei, brainstem, and cerebellum) have relatively preserved CMRGlc (1,53).

The temporoparietal perfusion abnormalities have been found to be the best discriminator between normal persons and Alzheimer patients. In mild AD, the sensitivity was 42%, whereas in moderate and severe disease, it was 56% and 79%, respectively (16). In assessing the sensitivity of FDG studies versus HMPAO studies to detect AD, it appears that FDG-PET may be a more sensitive tracer.

Whereas the bilateral temporoparietal hypoperfusion pattern on PET is highly predictive of AD, it is not pathognomonic for it (10,33–35,54,61). Therefore, in evaluating a patient with perfusion abnormalities in the temporoparietal regions, it is important to exclude stroke, and a comparison with MRI or CT studies is required. In patients with predominant frontal hypoperfusion, also consider Pick's disease, dementia of the frontal type, and progressive supranuclear palsy (PSP). PSP can be differentiated by clinical findings (e.g., parkinsonian symptoms and ocular findings). Also note that patients with Parkinson's disease with dementia have patterns that appear to be indistinguishable from those seen in AD patients. Other entities that can produce a similar pattern to that seen in AD include Creutzfeldt-Jakob disease, vascular dementia, dementia in association with Down's syndrome, carbon monoxide poisoning, and occasionally, normal pressure hydrocephalus (10).

A new PET tracer [18F]FDDNP targets the amyloid beta senile plaques and neurofibrillary tangles seen in AD. This tracer has the greatest accumulation in the areas of the brain most affected by plaque and tangles and, therefore, may prove to be more specific for AD (17).

VASCULAR DEMENTIA

Dementia secondary to vascular disease is the second most common type of dementia in the elderly. As the incidence of cerebrovascular disease increases in the general population, this etiology may soon become

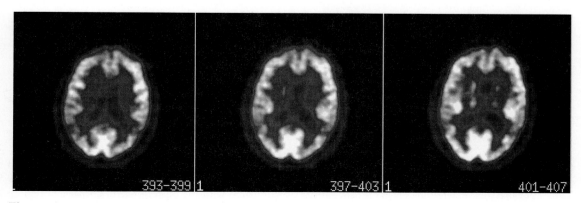

Figure 3-4. PET image of Alzheimer's disease.

the most common cause of dementia (48). There are many causes, including acute stroke, CADASIL (cerebral autosomal dominant arteriopathy with subcortical infarcts and leukoencephalopathy), and amyloid angiopathy.

Multi-infarct dementia (MID) is likely the most common cause of vascular dementia, characterized by separate episodes of infarction. In the presence of diffuse cerebral atrophy, multiple old and new cortical infarcts are seen on CT and MRI, with none involving an entire vascular territory.

This disease entity exists as a spectrum of imaging abnormalities, which, in its most severe form, results in subcortical hyperintensities similar to Binswanger microangiopathic leukoencephalopathy (24). There is relative sparing of the subcortical arcuate fibers in the peripheral white matter and associated lacunar infarctions in the basal ganglia, thalamus, and pons. In addition, abnormally decreased signal intensity is seen in the putamen secondary to iron deposition. SPECT or FDG-PET imaging demonstrates multiple scattered areas of hypoperfusion or hypometabolism throughout the brain (both gray and white matter) corresponding to areas of infarctions seen on CT or MRI (6,26). Often, involvement of the sensorimotor cortex is seen, which is almost invariably spared in AD.

BINSWANGER'S DISEASE

Binswanger disease is characterized by severe, bilaterally symmetric, confluent regions of increased signal intensity in the cerebral white matter, as seen on long

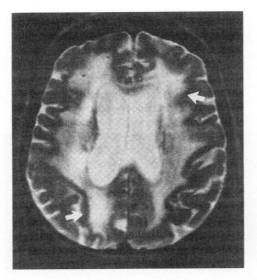

Figure 3-5. A 75-year-old woman with vascular dementia. Axial T2-weighted magnetic resonance imaging demonstrates marked, confluent hyperintensity in the periventricular white matter bilaterally that extends subcortically (*arrows*).

T2-weighted images (Fig. 3-5). The presence of a marked degree of periventricular white matter abnormality is thought to be secondary to atherosclerosis and arteriosclerosis of the cerebral vessels. In addition, small infarcts are seen in the basal ganglia and thalamus. The corpus callosum is not involved, and the cerebral cortex is preserved in contradistinction to MID.

The spectroscopic signature has not been characterized, but a decrease in NAA and mI with an elevated lactate would be expected. On SPECT, Binswanger demonstrates reductions in perfusion in the frontal lobe of the brain on the side of small infarcts in the dorsomedial part of the optic region and lower parts of the internal capsule (45). PET demonstrates ipsilateral reductions in hemisphere metabolism, especially in the frontal lobe in patients with single small infarcts in the optic region.

Patients with Binswanger's disease (or chronic progressive subcortical encephalopathy) have been found to have decreased rCBF and regional cerebral metabolism rate for oxygen on PET in the white matter and in the frontal, temporal, and parietal cortices, despite normal CT or MRI scans (3,86). The occipital cortex and striatum are less affected. It is suggested that the decrease in rCBF and regional cerebral metabolic rate for oxygen ($rCMRO_2$) in the white matter is caused by primary damage sites from ischemia, whereas similar decreases in the cortex likely represent disconnection between cortical and subcortical structures. Benson et al. (6) suggested that PET scanning could distinguish between AD and MID because, in AD, the primary motor and sensory cortices are spared, whereas in MID, multifocal asymmetric irregular areas of hypometabolism are seen.

AMYLOID ANGIOPATHY

Cerebral amyloid angiopathy results from the deposition of beta-amyloid in the media and adventitia of the vessels of the leptomeninges and the cortex of the brain (48). These patients suffer from multiple lobar hemorrhages of varying age. Therefore, MRI is particularly beneficial in establishing this diagnosis due to its exquisite sensitivity in the detection of hemorrhagic byproducts in the white matter from microhemorrhages in addition to microvascular demyelination in the periventricular and subcortical white matter (Fig. 3-6).

FRONTAL AND FRONTAL TEMPORAL DEMENTIA

Imaging features of frontal dementia include severe frontal atrophy with wide separation of the hemispheres. A pronounced reduction in cortical blood flow and metabolism is observed in the frontal regions compared with the posterior temporoparietal region; this is a differentiating feature from the pattern

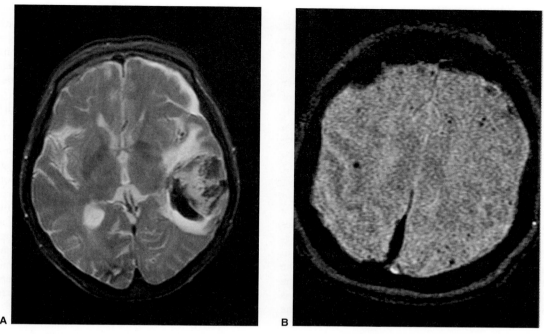

A   **B**

Figure 3-6. Cerebral amyloid angiopathy in a 75-year-old male. **A:** Axial T2-weighted image shows a large hemorrhage in the left temporal lobe. **B:** Axial gradient echo image in another patient shows multiple punctate low-signal intensity foci in both hemispheres indicative of previous microhemorrhages.

observed in AD (41,62). The medial temporal lobes are relatively spared in frontal temporal dementia (FTD). The absence of reduced perfusion in the posterior cingulate cortex is a diagnostic marker of FTD, and this feature distinguishes it from AD (29).

PICK'S DISEASE

The neuropathologic markers for Pick's disease are Pick's bodies, which are round cytoplasmic inclusions (64). Pick's disease is a neurodegenerative dementia with a predilection for the frontal and temporal lobes, where Pick's bodies are seen on histopathologic examination.

The imaging hallmarks of Pick's disease include frontal and temporal lobe atrophy. The parietal and occipital lobes are commonly spared. Osborne described the changes seen on MRI as markedly shrunken gyri, which have a knifelike appearance (Fig. 3-7) (64).

MRS samples obtained in the frontal lobes show a marked reduction in NAA (by as much as 30%), indicating neuronal loss, an increase in mI, and the presence of lactate. In contrast, MR spectra sampled in the frontal lobes of patients with AD show no evidence that lactate is present, and the NAA is not reduced to the same degree as seen in Pick's disease. mI is elevated in the frontal lobes in both diseases (72).

HMPAO-SPECT and FDG-PET images of patients with Pick's disease show hypoperfusion and

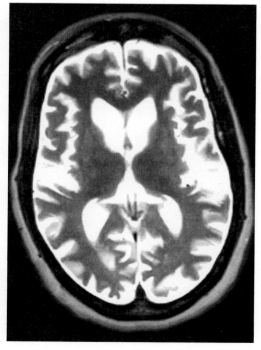

Figure 3-7. Pick's disease in a 56-year-old male with psychosis. Axial CT image shows striking frontal lobe atrophy with widening of the sulci and narrowing of the gyri.

hypometabolism, respectively, in the frontal and anterior temporal lobes bilaterally (10,46,74). The pattern of anterior hypometabolism is consistent with the findings on histopathologic examination. Although the pattern of anterior hypoperfusion or hypometabolism distinguishes Pick disease from other forms of dementia such as AD, it is not characteristic of any particular entity. Various disorders, including multiple system atrophy, PSP, nonspecific frontal gliosis, adult polyglucosan body disease (a storage disorder), neurosyphilis, and chronic alcohol-related dementia, can all demonstrate a similar pattern (10).

PARKINSON'S DISEASE (PD)

Parkinson's disease (PD) is generally thought of as a movement disorder; however, the disease also carries a cognitive component. The dementia in PD is characterized by attention deficits and impairment in executive function. PD specifically affects the dopaminergic system of the cerebrum, centered in the basal ganglia. The neuropathologic marker of PD is loss of the neuromelanin-containing neurons in the substantia nigra, the locus ceruleus, and the dorsal vagal nucleus (64). Approximately 25% of patients with PD have more severe symptoms and respond poorly to dopamine replacement; these patients are then grouped into the plus syndromes. This group of

related disorders includes Shy-Drager (SD) syndrome, PSP, and olivopontocerebellar degeneration (OPCD).

CT imaging has not been useful in the differential diagnosis of PD except that it can exclude other causes of dementia (e.g., normal pressure hydrocephalus or subcortical arteriosclerotic encephalopathy) (67). Imaging studies are nonspecific, showing generalized atrophy with large, supratentorial sulci and posterior fossa cisterns (64). MRI usually does not demonstrate any features that characterize PD; however, in some instances, narrowing of the pars compacta in the substantia nigra has been reported in patients with long-standing PD, whereas right/left asymmetry in the pars compacta may be seen early on in the disease (48). Patients with SD syndrome can demonstrate low signal in the putamen as seen on T2-weighted images. PSP is characterized by midbrain and tectal atrophy, whereas OPCD typically reveals atrophy of the pons and cerebellum, with an abnormal MR signal seen in the transverse pontine fibers and brachium pontis (the tiger sign) (Fig. 3-8).

Currently, MRS has not been proven useful in diagnosing PD or its related syndromes. However, severe dementia in PD can be indistinguishable from AD on PET images, with both showing significant bilateral parietal hypometabolism (68,73). Patients

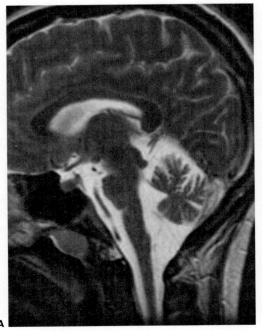 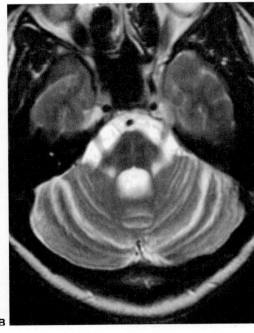

Figure 3-8. Olivopontocerebellar atrophy. **A:** Sagittal T2-weighted image shows marked atrophy of the brainstem and cerebellum. **B:** Axial T2-weighted image through the mid-pons level shows marked atrophy of the pons with increased signal noted centrally.

with PD dementia differed from those without dementia in that the former had hypometabolic perirolandic and angular gyrus regions (68). Patients with PD dementia did not have significantly different CMRGlc values compared with patients with AD, indicating that patients with PD and dementia may suffer from an underlying Alzheimer-type process. In fact, histopathologic studies have shown findings of true AD, in conjunction with findings of parkinsonism.

HUNTINGTON'S DISEASE (HD)

Huntington's disease (HD) is an autosomal dominant condition characterized by a movement disorder and a cause of presenile dementia. CT and MRI often show no changes early in the course of HD and subsequently reveal atrophy of the head of the caudate and frontal cortex in the later stages of the disease (Fig. 3-9) (76,78). PET studies have consistently revealed hypometabolism in the caudate nuclei and the putamen, which often precedes the atrophy seen on CT or MRI (52,55,71). It has been postulated that cortical changes in glucose metabolism, especially in the frontoparietal and temporo-occipital areas, may correlate with the severity of dementia in patients with HD (56).

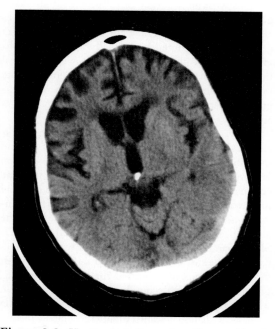

Figure 3-9. Huntington's disease in a 38-year-old male with a movement disorder. Axial T2-weighted image reveals widening of the anterior horns of the lateral ventricles secondary to caudate nucleus atrophy. There is generalized cerebral atrophy as well.

NORMAL PRESSURE HYDROCEPHALUS (NPH)

Normal pressure hydrocephalus (NPH) is a form of chronic communicating hydrocephalus that is characterized clinically by the classic triad of dementia, incontinence, and ataxia in conjunction with enlarged ventricles and normal CSF pressure (70). Imaging with CT and MRI often demonstrates ventricular enlargement that is out of proportion to the degree of sulcal enlargement, possibly with a prominent flow void at the level of the third ventricle or aqueduct of Sylvius (Fig. 3-10). Some investigators suggest that CSF flow patterns and velocity are important, not only in diagnosing this disease, but also in predicting the results of surgical intervention. Nonspecific changes in the cerebral white matter are also reported on imaging.

Suspected cases of NPH are often initially evaluated with radionuclide cisternogram, which is performed using a lumbar intrathecal injection of ^{111}In-diethylenetriamine pentaacetic acid (DTPA) (20). Head imaging is performed at 4, 24, and 48 hours in the anterior, left lateral, and posterior projections. In normal adults, tracer activity enters the basal cisterns and extends into the interhemispheric and sylvian fissures by 3 to 4 hours, with subsequent activity over the convexities by 24 hours. Under normal conditions, radionuclide does not enter the lateral ventricles. The "classic" diagnostic finding of NPH is early entry of pharmaceutical into the lateral ventricles, which persists at 24 and 48 hours with impairment of flow over the convexities of the brain (5,66). This procedure can support the diagnosis of NPH, but it cannot predict which patients would benefit from diversionary ventriculoperitoneal (VP) surgery (42). Other studies have shown that this pattern of radionuclide deposition is not specific for NPH (36).

OTHER ORGANIC CAUSES OF DEMENTIA WITH IMAGING MANIFESTATIONS

One to four percent of cases of dementia are caused by brain tumors. Most brain tumors are either metastatic or malignant primary tumors (Fig. 3-11) (31). CT is often the initial imaging modality used; however, MRI provides a more comprehensive evaluation of the size and extent of the lesion, including assessment for infiltration of adjacent structures and a more accurate assessment of peritumoral/vasogenic edema. Moreover, MRI is mandated for preoperative planning.

Although not routinely used for this application, MRS is sometimes used as a problem-solving tool in cases with atypical imaging features. The spectroscopic signature of primary cerebral neoplasia is elevation of choline and the presence of lipid and an associated reduction in the NAA concentration.

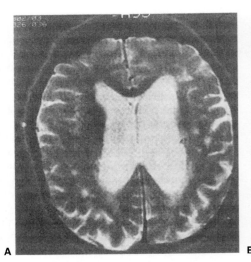
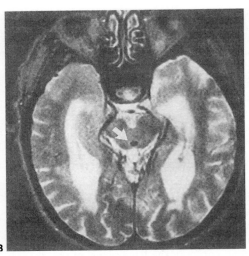

A   B

Figure 3-10. A: A 74-year-old man with normal pressure hydrocephalus. Axial T2-weighted magnetic resonance imaging (MRI) demonstrates marked widening of the lateral ventricles out of proportion to the sulcal widening. **B:** Axial T2-weighted MRI demonstrates widening of the temporal horns out of proportion to the sulcal widening of the temporal lobes. A prominent flow void from cerebrospinal fluid pulsation is seen within the aqueduct (*arrow*).

Similarly, thallium-201 (^{201}Tl) SPECT and FDG-PET are not used for primary diagnosis of brain neoplasms. Their main role is to help in the differentiation of low-grade (grades 1 and 2) from high-grade (grades 3 and 4) gliomas and thereby determine the prognosis in these patients. A thallium SPECT and FDG-PET index has often been used to

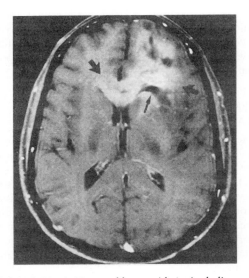

Figure 3-11. A 45-year-old man with a mixed oligoastrocytoma. Axial postcontrast T1-weighted magnetic resonance imaging demonstrates a heterogeneously enhancing lesion within the left frontal lobe crossing the corpus callosum (*large arrows*). Note some of the markedly hypointense signal representing calcification (*small arrow*).

distinguish low-grade from high-grade gliomas. The index compares tumor uptake normalized to the homologous contralateral hemisphere and corrected for tissue attenuation. With ^{201}Tl, a threshold index of 1.5 helps distinguish low-grade versus high-grade gliomas with an accuracy of 89%, with high-grade gliomas showing greater values (8,50). The studies also report that low-grade gliomas with an index greater than 1.5 acted biologically more like high-grade tumors, with decreased median patient survival time (8). Similarly, with FDG-PET, a tumor-to-white matter ratio of more than 1.5 was indicative of a high-grade tumor, with a sensitivity and specificity of 94% and 77%, respectively (21).

Conventional imaging techniques are often unreliable in distinguishing between recurrent glioma and radiation necrosis in patients who exhibit progression in symptoms after high-dose radiotherapy. In some circumstances, therapeutic doses of radiation can lead to necrosis of the irradiated brain. The associated clinical syndrome is usually one of progression of the already existing neurologic disability. Both ^{201}Tl-SPECT and FDG-PET have been shown to be effective in differentiating glioma from radiation necrosis (65,75). Regions of increased thallium uptake (i.e., greater than the scalp uptake) suggest active tumor, whereas regions of low to no uptake suggest radiation necrosis. Radiation is known to suppress glucose metabolism of tumor cells in tissue cultures. Therefore, PET has a proven utility in distinguishing areas of radiation necrosis, where the rate of glucose utilization is markedly reduced, from recurrent tumor, where the rate of glucose utilization is increased.

Chronic subdural hematomas have been reported to produce a subacute form of dementia. These usually form over a period of weeks to months after onset of an untreated subdural hematoma. The initial hematoma lyses, fragile internal membranes form, and serum may coalesce rather than resorb within the cavity. Subsequent relatively minor trauma can induce additional hemorrhage into the existing space, resulting in progressive enlargement and compression upon the adjacent cerebrum. On CT, an acute subdural hematoma is crescentic and hyperdense and will often span the convexity. Chronic subdural hematomas are of lower density on CT and are typically heterogeneous due to the mixture of chronic and acute components (Fig. 3-12). On MRI, the chronic subdural hematoma is often loculated and of a mixed signal intensity, differing from CSF.

The most common infectious agents that can produce a clinical syndrome of acute/subacute dementia are the human immunodeficiency virus (HIV) and progressive multifocal leukoencephalopathy (PML). The most frequent brain imaging findings associated with HIV infection are generalized atrophy and diffuse, confluent white matter abnormalities especially in the periventricular white matter, corpus callosum, and optic radiations (Fig. 3-13) (48).

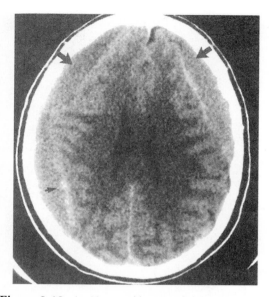

Figure 3-12. An 80-year-old man with bilateral subdural hematomas. Axial noncontrast computed tomography imaging demonstrates bilateral isohypodense subdural hematomas (*large arrows*) resulting in no significant midline shift. The hyperdense component represents more recent hemorrhage (*small arrow*).

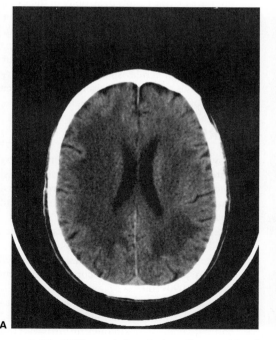

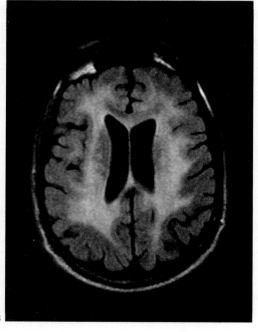

Figure 3-13. HIV encephalopathy in a 51-year-old male with progressive dementia. **A:** Axial CT image shows marked hypoattenuation of the cerebral white matter in both hemispheres indicative of demyelination. **B:** Axial FLAIR MRI image shows the abnormal hyperintensity of the central white matter bilaterally.

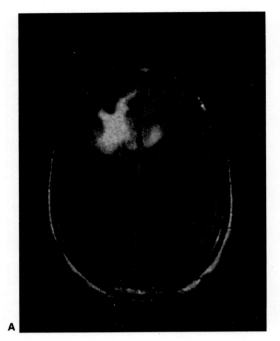
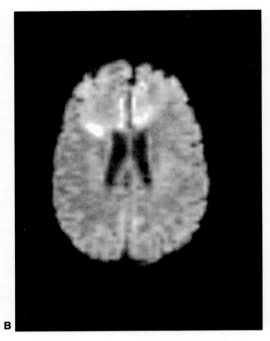

A   **B**

Figure 3-14. Progressive multifocal leukoencephalopathy in a 45-year-old immunocompromised female. **A:** Axial FLAIR MRI shows abnormal increased signal within the subcortical and central white matter of the frontal lobes with greater involvement on the right side. **B:** Axial trace diffusion-weighted image shows corresponding restrictive diffusion as faint areas of increased signal intensity. This additional finding is helpful in establishing this diagnosis.

Progressive multifocal leukoencephalopathy is an opportunistic infection that is associated with AIDS and specific malignancies. It is thought to be caused by a reaction to the Jamestown Canyon (JC) virus. The most common imaging findings on CT and MRI are a leukoencephalopathy involving the subcortical U fibers and scalloping at the gray-white junction. The lesions can be unilateral or bilateral, but typically, they are asymmetric without contrast enhancement (Fig. 3-14).

CONCLUSION

The primary role of imaging in the evaluation of dementia is to exclude any reversible or organic conditions that may mimic a primary dementia. There are many common imaging features associated with the various types of dementia. Distinguishing between these various conditions in addition to the changes associated with normal aging can be challenging. Recognition of several key imaging features can provide clues to the diagnosis. Whereas normal aging and Parkinson's disease result in generalized atrophy, the other diseases generally lead to more focal volume loss. AD results in atrophy of the MTLs (including the amygdala and hippocampus), Pick's disease results in atrophy of the frontal and temporal lobes, and

Huntington's disease results in atrophy of the caudate, putamen, and frontal cortex. Further evaluation with physiologic studies (e.g., SPECT and PET) may be necessary. In normal pressure hydrocephalus, the widened CSF spaces are not caused by atrophy but by poor resorbtion of cerebrospinal fluid at the convexities, which leads to diffuse widening of the ventricular system out of proportion to the sulci.

REFERENCES

1. Alavi A, Hirsch LJ. Studies of central nervous system disorders with single photon emission computed tomography and positron emission tomography: evolution over the past 2 decades. *Semin Nucl Med.* 1991;21:58–81.
2. Awad IA, Johnson PC, Spetzler RF, et al. Incidental subcortical lesions identified on magnetic resonance imaging in the elderly. II. Postmortem pathological correlations. *Stroke.* 1986;17:1090–1097.
3. Babikian V, Ropper A. Binswanger disease: a review. *Stroke.* 1987;18:2–12.
4. Ball MJ. Neuronal loss, neurofibrillary tangles and granulovacuolar degeneration in the hippocampus with aging and dementia. *Acta Neuropathol (Berl).* 1997;111:27.

5. Bannister R, Gilford E, Kocen R. Isotope encephalography in the diagnosis of dementia due to communicating hydrocephalus. *Lancet.* 1967;2:1014–1017.

6. Benson DF, Kuhl DE, Hawkins RA, et al. The fluorodeoxyglucose 18F scan in Alzheimer's disease and multi-infarct dementia. *Arch Neurol.* 1983;40:711–714.

7. Bhatia S, Bookheimer SY, Gaillard WD, et al. Measurement of whole temporal lobe and hippocampus for MR volumetry. Normative data. *Neurology.* 1993;43:2006–2010.

8. Black KL, Hawkins RA, Kim KT, et al. Use of thallium-201 SPECT to quantitate malignancy grade of gliomas. *J Neurosurg.* 1989;71:342–346.

9. Bonte FJ, Ross ED, Chehabi HH, et al. SPECT study of regional cerebral blood flow in Alzheimer's disease. *J Comput Assist Tomogr.* 1986;10:579–583.

10. Bonte FJ, Tintner R, Weiner MF, et al. Brain blood flow in the dementias: SPECT with histopathologic correlation. *Radiology.* 1993;186:361–365.

11. Bradley WG, Waluch V, Brant-Zawadzki M, et al. Patchy, periventricular white matter lesions in the elderly: a common observation during NMR imaging. *Noninvasive Medical Imaging.* 1984;1:35–41.

12. Brody H. Organization of cerebral cortex. Study of aging in human cortex. *J Comput Neurol.* 1955; 102:511–556.

13. Cala LA, Thickbroom GW, Black JL, et al. Brain density and cerebrospinal fluid space size: CT of normal volunteers. *Am J Neuroradiol.* 1982;2:41–47.

14. Caselli RJ, Beach T, Yaari R, et al. Alzheimer's disease a century later. *J Clin Psychiatry.* 2006;67:1784–1800.

15. Chawluk JB, Alavi A, Dann R, et al. Positron emission tomography in aging and dementia: effect of cerebral atrophy. *J Nucl Med.* 1987; 28:431–437.

16. Claus JJ, Harskamp VF, Bretler MMB, et al. The diagnostic value of SPECT with Tc-99m HMPAO in Alzheimer's disease: a population-based study. *Neurology.* 1994;44:454–461.

17. Coleman RE. Positron emission tomography diagnosis of Alzheimer's disease. *Neuroimaging Clin N Am.* 2005;15:837–846.

18. Critchley M. Neurologic changes in the aged. *J Chronic Dis.* 1956;3:459.

19. Cuenod CA, Denys A, Michot JL, et al. Amygdala atrophy in Alzheimer's disease. An in vivo magnetic resonance imaging study. *Arch Neurol.* 1993;50:941–945.

20. Datz FL, Patch CG, Arias JM, et al., eds. *Nuclear Medicine: A Teaching File.* St. Louis: CV Mosby; 1992:240–243.

21. Delbeke D, Meyerowitz C, Lapidus RL, et al. Optimal cutoff levels of F-18 fluorodeoxyglucose uptake in the differentiation of low-grade from high-grade brain tumors with PET. *Radiology.* 1995;195:47–52.

22. Diksic M, Reba RC, eds. *Radiopharmaceuticals and Brain Pathology Studied with PET and SPECT.* Boca Raton: CRC Press; 1991.

23. Drayer B. Imaging of the aging brain. Part I: Normal findings. *Radiology.* 1988;166:785–796.

24. Drayer B. Imaging of the aging brain. Part II: Pathologic conditions. *Radiology.* 1988;166: 797–806.

25. Drayer B, Burger P, Darwin R, et al. Magnetic resonance imaging of brain iron. *Am J Neuroradiol.* 1986;7:373–380.

26. Duara R, Barker W, Loewenstein D, et al. Sensitivity and specificity of positron emission tomography and magnetic resonance imaging studies in Alzheimer's disease and multi-infarct dementia. *Eur Neurol.* 1989;29:9–15.

27. Duara R, Grady C, Haxby J, et al. Positron emission tomography in Alzheimer's disease. *Neurology.* 1986;36:879–887.

28. Durand-Fardel M. *Traite du Ramollissement du Cerveau.* Paris: Bailliere; 1843.

29. Ebmeier KP, Donaghey C, Dougall NJ. Neuroimaging in dementia. *Int Rev Neurobiol.* 2005; 67:43–72.

30. Filley CM. White matter and behavioral neurology. *Ann NY Acad Sci.* 2005;1064:162–183.

31. Foster G, Scott D, Payne S. The use of CT scanning in dementia. A systematic review. *Int J Technol Assess Health Care.* 1999;15:406–425.

32. Frackowiak R, Poizilli C, Legg N, et al. Regional cerebral oxygen supply and utilization in dementia. A clinical and physiologic study with oxygen-15 and positron emission tomography. *Brain.* 1981; 104:753–788.

33. Friedland RP. "Normal"-pressure hydrocephalus and the saga of treatable dementia. *JAMA.* 1989;262:2577–2581.

34. Friedland RP. Positron emission tomography in dementia. *Semin Neurol.* 1989;9:338–344.

35. Friedland RP, Prusiner SB, Jagust WJ, et al. Bitemporal hypometabolism in Creutzfeldt-Jakob disease measured by positron emission tomography with 18F-2-fluorodeoxyglucose. *J Comput Assist Tomogr.* 1984;8:978–981.

36. Greenberg JO, Shenkin HA, Adam R. Idiopathic normal pressure hydrocephalus: a report of 73 patients. *J Neurol Neurosurg Psychiatry.* 1977; 40:336–341.

37. Haug G. Age and sex dependence of the size of normal ventricles on computed tomography. *Neuroradiology.* 1977;14:201–204.

38. Holman BL, Johnson KA, Gerada B, et al. The scintigraphic appearance of Alzheimer's disease: a prospective study using technitium-99m-HMPAO SPECT. *J Nucl Med.* 1992; 33:181–185.
39. Jagust W. Molecular neuroimaging in Alzheimer's disease. *NeuroRx.* 2004;1:206–212.
40. Jagust WJ, Budinger TF, Reed BR. The diagnosis of dementia with single photon emission computed tomography. *Arch Neurol.* 1987; 44:258–262.
41. Jagust WJ, Reed BR, Seab JP, et al. Clinical-physiological correlates of Alzheimer's disease and frontal lobe dementia. *Am J Physiol Imaging.* 1989;4:89–96.
42. James AE, DeBlanc HJ, DeLand FH, et al. Refinements in cerebrospinal fluid diversionary shunt evaluation by cisternography. *Am J Roentgenol Radium Ther Nucl Med.* 1972;115: 766–773.
43. Jamieson DG, Chawluck JB, Alavi A, et al. The effect of disease severity on local cerebral glucose metabolism in Alzheimer's disease. *J Cereb Blood Flow Metab.* 1987;7:S410.
44. Jones RS, Waldman AD. 1H-MRS evaluation of metabolism in Alzheimer's disease and vascular dementia. *Neurol Res.* 2004;26:488–495.
45. Kalashnikova LA, Gulevskaya TS, Kashina EM. Disorders of higher mental function due to single infarctions in the thalamus and in the area of the thalamofrontal tracts. *Neurosci Behav Physiol.* 1999;29:397–403.
46. Kamo H, Mcgeer R, Haroop R, et al. Positron emission tomography and histopathology in Pick's disease. *Neurology.* 1987;37:439.
47. Kesslak JP, Nalcioglu O, Cotman CW. Quantification of magnetic-resonance scans for hippocampal and parahippocampal atrophy in Alzheimer's disease. *Neurology.* 1991;41:51–54.
48. Keyserling H, Mukundan S. The role of conventional MR and CT in the work-up of dementia patients. *Neuroimaging Clin N Am.* 2005;15: 789–802.
49. Kido DK, LeMay M, Levinson AW, et al. Computed tomographic localization of the precentral gyrus. *Radiology.* 1980;135:373–377.
50. Kim KT, Black KL, Marciano D, et al. Thallium-201 SPECT imaging of brain tumors: methods and results. *J Nucl Med.* 1990;31:965–969.
51. Kuhl DE, Metter EJ, Reiger WH, et al. Effects of human aging on patterns of local cerebral glucose utilization determined by the 18-F fluorodeoxyglucose method. *J Cereb Blood Flow Metab.* 1987;7:411.
52. Kuhl DE, Phelps ME, Markham CH, et al. Cerebral metabolism and atrophy in Huntington's disease determined by 18-F-FDG and computed tomography scan. *Ann Neurol.* 1982;12:425–434.
53. Kushner M, Tobin M, Alavi A, et al. Cerebral glucose consumption in normal and pathological states using fluorine-FDG and PET. *J Nucl Med.* 1987;28:1667–1670.
54. Kuwabara Y, Ichiya Y, Otuska M, et al. Differential diagnosis of bilateral parietal abnormalities in I-123 IMP SPECT imaging. *Clin Nucl Med.* 1990;15:893–899.
55. Kuwert T, Lange HW, Langen KJ, et al. Cerebral glucose consumption measured by PET in patients with and without psychiatric symptoms of Huntington's disease. *Psychiatry Res.* 1989; 29:361–362.
56. Kuwert T, Lange HW, Langen KJ, et al. Cortical and subcortical consumption measured by PET in patients with Huntington's disease. *Brain.* 1990;113:1405–1423.
57. Larson EB, Reifler BV, Sumi SM, et al. Diagnostic tests in the evaluation of dementia: a prospective study of 200 elderly outpatients. *Arch Intern Med.* 1986;146:1917–1922.
58. Lazeyras F, Charles HC, Tupler LA, et al. Metabolic brain mapping in Alzheimer's disease using proton magnetic resonance spectroscopy. *Psychiatry Res.* 1998;82:95–106.
59. LeMay M. Radiologic changes of the aging brain and skull. *Am J Roentgenol.* 1984;143:383–389.
60. Messa C, Perani D, Luciganani G, et al. High-resolution technitiun-99m-HMPAO SPECT in patients with probable Alzheimer's disease: comparison with fluorine-18-FDG PET. *J Nucl Med.* 1994;35:210–216.
61. Miller BL, Cummings JL, Villaneuva-Meyer J, et al. Frontal lobe degeneration: clinical, neuropsychological, and SPECT characteristics. *Neurology.* 1991;41:1374–1382.
62. Neary D, Snowden JS, Northen B, et al. Dementia of the frontal lobe type. *J Neurol Neurosurg Psychiatry.* 1988;51:353–361.
63. O'Brien JT, Metcalfe S, Swann A, et al. Medial temporal lobe width on CT scanning in Alzheimer's disease: comparison with vascular dementia, depression and dementia with Lewy bodies. *Dement Geriatr Cogn Disord.* 2000;11:114–118.
64. Osborn A. *Diagnostic Neuroradiology.* Philadelphia: Mosby; 1994.
65. Patronas NJ, Chiro GD, Brooks RA, et al. Work in progress: fluorodeoxyglucose and positron emission tomography in the evaluation of radiation necrosis of the brain. *Radiology.* 1982;144:885–889.
66. Patten DH, Benson DF. Diagnosis of normal-pressure hydrocephalus by RISA cisternography. *J Nucl Med.* 1968;9:457–461.

67. Paulus W, Trenkwalder C. Imaging of nonmotor symptoms in Parkinson syndromes. *Clin Neurosci.* 1998;5:115–120.
68. Peppard RF, Martin WF, Clark CM, et al. Cortical glucose metabolism in Parkinson's and Alzheimer's disease. *J Neurosci Res.* 1990;27:561–568.
69. Perani D, DiPiero V, Vallar G, et al. Technetium-99m-HMPAO SPECT study of regional cerebral perfusion in early Alzheimer's disease. *J Nucl Med.* 1988;29:1507–1514.
70. Peterson RC, Modri B, Laws E. Surgical treatment of idiopathic hydrocephalus in elderly patients. *Neurology.* 1985;35:307–311.
71. Phelps ME, Mazziota JC, Wapenski J, et al. Cerebral glucose utilization and blood flow in Huntington's disease. *J Nucl Med.* 1985;26:47.
72. Ross BD, Bluml S, Cowan R, et al. In vivo MR spectroscopy of human dementia. *Neuroimaging Clin N Am.* 1998;8:809–822.
73. Rougemont D, Baron JC, Collard P, et al. Local cerebral glucose utilization in treated and untreated patients with Parkinson's disease. *J Neurol Neurosurg Psychiatry.* 1984;47:824–830.
74. Salmon E, Maquet P, Sadzot B, et al. Positron emission tomography in Alzheimer's and Pick's disease. *J Neurol.* 1988;235:S1.
75. Schwartz RB, Carvalho PA, Alexander E, et al. Radiation necrosis vs high-grade recurrent glioma: differentiation by using dual-isotope SPECT with 201Tl and 99mTc-HMPAO. *Am J Neuroradiol.* 1992;12:1187–1192.
76. Simmons JT, Pastakea B, Chase TN, et al. Magnetic resonance imaging in Huntington's disease. *Am J Neuroradiol.* 1986;7:25–28.
77. Soher BJ, Doraiswamy PM, Charles HC. A review of 1H MR spectroscopy findings in Alzheimer's disease. *Neuroimaging Clin N Am.* 2005;15:847–852.
78. Starkstein SE, Folstein SE, Brandt J, et al. Brain atrophy in Huntington's disease. A CT-scan study. *Neuroradiology.* 1989;31:156–159.
79. Testa HJ, Snowden JS, Neary D, et al. The use of Tc-99m HMPAO in the diagnosis of primary degenerative dementia. *J Cereb Blood Flow Metab.* 1988;8:S123–S126.
80. Tierney MC, Gisher RH, Lewis AJ, et al. The NINCDS-ADRDA Workgroup criteria for the clinical diagnosis of probable Alzheimer's disease. A clinical pathological study of 57 cases. *Neurology.* 1988;38:359–364.
81. Tomlinson BE, Blessed G, Roth M. Observations on the brains of non-demented old people. *J Neurol Sci.* 1968;7:331–356.
82. Valentine AR, Moseley IF, Kendall BE. White matter abnormality in cerebral atrophy: clinicoradiological correlations. *J Neurol Neurosurg Psychiatry.* 1980;43:139–142.
83. van der Flier WM, Scheltens P. Use of laboratory and imaging investigations in dementia. *J Neurol Neurosurg Psychiatry.* 2005;76(suppl V):v45–v52.
84. Warwick JM. Imaging of brain function using SPECT. *Metab Brain Dis.* 2004;19:113–123.
85. Whitwell JL, Jack CR. Comparisons between Alzheimer's disease, frontotemporal lobar degeneration, and normal aging with brain mapping. *Top Magn Reson Imaging.* 2005;16:409–425.
86. Yao H, Sadoshima S, Kuwabara Y, et al. Cerebral blood flow and oxygen metabolism in patients with vascular dementia of the Binswanger type. *Stroke.* 1990;21:1694–1699.
87. Yoshii F, Barker WW, Chang JY, et al. Sensitivity of cerebral glucose metabolism to age, gender, brain volume, brain atrophy, and cerebrovascular risk factors. *J Cereb Blood Flow Metab.* 1988;8:654–661.

SUGGESTED READING

Banna M. The ventriculo-cephalic ratio on computed tomography. *Can Assoc Radiol J.* 1977;28:208–210.
Bottino C, Almeida O. Can neuroimaging techniques identify individuals at risk of developing Alzheimer's disease? *Int Psychogeriatr.* 1997;9:389–403.
Brinkman SD, Sarwar M, Levin H, et al. Quantitative indexes of computed tomography in dementia and normal aging. *Radiology.* 1981;138:89–92.
Chase TN, Fedio P, Foster NL, et al. Weschler Adult Intelligence Scale performance. *Arch Neurol.* 1984;16:649–654.
Cutler NR, Haxby J, Duara R, et al. Clinical history, brain metabolism, and neurophysiological function in Alzheimer's disease. *Ann Neurol.* 1985;18:298–309.
De Leon MJ, George AE, Golomb J, et al. Frequency of hippocampal formation atrophy in normal aging and Alzheimer's disease. *Neurobiol Aging.* 1997;18:1–11.
Erkinjunitti T, Bowler J, DeCarli C. Imaging of static brain lesions in vascular dementia: implications for clinical trials. *Alzheimer Dis Assoc Disord.* 1999;13(suppl 3):581–590.
Faulstich ME. Brain imaging in dementia of the Alzheimer type. *Int J Neurosci.* 1991;57:39–49.
Fayad PB, Brass LM. Single photon emission computed tomography in cerebrovascular disease. *Stroke.* 1991;22:950–954.
Fieschi C, Argentino C, Lenzi GL, et al. Clinical and instrumental evaluation of patients with ischemic stroke during the first six hours. *J Neurol Neurosurg Psychiatry.* 1989;91:311–322.
Foster NL, Chase TN, Mansi L, et al. Cortical abnormalities in Alzheimer's disease. *Ann Neurol.* 1984;16:649–654.

Foundas A, Zipin D, Browning C. Age-related changes of the insular cortex and lateral ventricles: conventional MRI volumetric measures. *J Neuroimaging.* 1998;8:216–221.

Friedland RP, Budinger TF, Ganz E, et al. Regional cerebral metabolism in dementia of the Alzheimer's type. positron emission tomography with (18F) fluorodeoxyglucose. *J Comput Assist Tomogr.* 1983; 7:590–598.

Gawler J, duBoulay GH, Bull JHD, et al. Computerized tomography: a comparison with pneumoencephalography and ventriculography. *J Neurol Neurosurg Psychiatry.* 1976;39:203–211.

Golomb J, Kluger A, deLeon M, et al. Hippocampal formation size in normal human aging: a correlate of delayed secondary memory performance. *Learn Mem.* 1994;1:45–54.

Granado JM, Diaz F, Alday R. Evaluation of brain SPECT in the diagnosis and prognosis of normal pressure hydrocephalus syndrome. *Acta Neurochir.* 1991;112:88–91.

Hahn FJY, Rim K. Frontal ventricular dimensions on normal computed tomography. *Am J Roentgenol.* 1976;126:492–496.

Hanyu H, Imon Y, Sakurai H, et al. Regional differences in diffusion abnormality in cerebral white matter lesions in patients with vascular dementia of the Binswanger type and Alzheimer's disease. *Eur J Neurol.* 1999;6:195–203.

Haug G. Age and sex dependence of the size of normal ventricles on computed tomography. *Neuroradiology.* 1977;14:201–204.

Haxby JC, Grady CL, Koss E, et al. Heterogeneous anterior-posterior metabolic patterns in dementia of the Alzheimer's disease. *Neurology.* 1988;38: 1853–1863.

Hilker R, Thiel A, Geisen C, et al. Cerebral blood flow and glucose metabolism in multi-infarct-dementia related to primary antiphospholipid antibody syndrome. *Lupus.* 2000;9:311–316.

Jelic V, Nordberg A. Early diagnosis of Alzheimer's disease with positron emission tomography. *Alzheimer Dis Assoc Disord.* 2000;14(suppl 1):S109–S113.

Jobst KA, Hindley NJ, King E, et al. The diagnosis of Alzheimer's disease: a question of image? *J Clin Psychiatry.* 1994;55(suppl 11):22–31.

Katzman R, Saitoh T. Advances in Alzheimer's disease. *FASEB J.* 1991;5:278–286.

Khujneri R, De Sousa JA. Magnetic resonance imaging of the ageing brain. *East Afr Med J.* 1997; October:656–659.

Kinkel WR, Jacobs L, Polachini I, et al. Subcortical arteriosclerotic encephalopathy (Binswanger's disease). Computed tomographic, nuclear magnetic resonance, and clinical correlations. *Arch Neurol.* 1985;42:951–959.

Larseen A, Moonen M, Bergh AC, et al. Predictive value of quantitative cisternography in normal pressure hydrocephalus. *Acta Neurol Scand.* 1990;81:327–332.

Mann DMA, South PW. The topographic distribution of brain atrophy in frontal lobe dementia. *Acta Neuropathol.* 1993;85:334–340.

Moretti J, Defer G, Sinotti L, et al. "Luxury perfusion" with [Tc99m] HMPAO and [I-123] IMPSPECT imaging during the subacute phase of stroke. *Eur J Nucl Med.* 1990;16:17–22.

Nagy ZS, Hindley NJ, Braak H, et al. The progression of Alzheimer's disease from limbic regions to the neocortex: clinical, radiological and pathological relationships. *Dement Geriatr Cogn Disord.* 1999;10:115–120.

Pantono P, Baron JC, Samson Y, et al. Crossed cerebellar diaschisis. Further studies. *Brain.* 1986;109: 677–694.

Rhinehart DL, Cox LA, Long BW. MR spectroscopy of Alzheimer's disease. *Radiol Technol.* 1998;70:23–28.

Sandson TA, Daffner KR, Carvalho PA, et al. Frontal lobe dysfunction following infarction of the left-sided medial thalamus. *Arch Neurol.* 1991;48: 1300–1303.

Terry RD, Katzman R. Senile dementia of the Alzheimer type. *Ann Neurol.* 1983;14:497–506.

Van Gijn J. Leukoaraiosis and vascular dementia. *Neurology.* 1998;51(suppl 3):S3–S8.

Vermersch P, Leys D, Pruvo JP, et al. Parkinson's disease and basal ganglia calcifications: prevalence and clinico-radiological correlations. *Clin Neurol Neurosurg.* 1992;94:213–217.

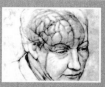

CHAPTER 3.2

Diagnostic Tests in the Older Adult: EEG

Joseph F. Drazkowski

Electroencephalography (EEG) is a diagnostic procedure that measures temporal changes in summated postsynaptic potentials from the superficial layers of the cerebral cortex. Currently, EEG is used principally in two major areas of clinical practice: seizure disorders and alterations in mental status. Technologists connect electrodes to the patient and record and store the EEG data. After the study is completed, physicians with specialized training interpret the stored data. In emergency situations, such as status epilepticus, the EEG may be viewed while it is being recorded. The technologist places a series of electrodes in symmetric locations according to the International 10-20 System on the scalp. The EEG signals are amplified and stored on a specialized digital recording device. A routine EEG is recorded for about 30 minutes but may be recorded for periods of days as required by the clinical situation. While the EEG is being recorded, the technologist documents the patient's behavioral state (i.e., awake, asleep) by asking the patient to perform certain tasks to judge the level of alertness. Hyperventilation and photic stimulation are performed by the patient during the recording if the patient is physically able to do so. These procedures, along with having the patient fall asleep during the EEG, are called "activation procedures" because they have the potential to provoke a seizure or abnormal EEG activity. The technologist observes and notes on the record any alteration in responsiveness, abnormal movements, seizure activity, or responses to noxious and auditory stimuli. If status epilepticus is found during the recording, a physician may administer antiepileptic drugs (AEDs) intravenously during the study to determine the effectiveness of therapy. An EEG may be recorded for a longer duration, either with concurrent video monitoring in the hospital in a specialized monitoring unit or in the ambulatory setting with a portable Holter-like recording device for up to several days. Video EEG recording is used to correlate electrographic activity with clinical behavioral features. Video EEG is especially useful in the classification of spells or in the surgical evaluation of a patient with medically refractory partial epilepsy. Ambulatory EEG is limited by the lack of video correlation with behaviors and is prone to technical artifacts.

NORMAL ELECTROENCEPHALOGRAM

The normal EEG remains relatively unchanged from adolescence until at least 80 years of age. In interpreting EEG studies, the reader must be familiar with changes that may be explained by age and behavioral state. EEG rhythms are divided into four normal-frequency bands: delta (<4 Hz), theta (4 to 7 Hz), alpha (8 to 13 Hz), and beta (>13 Hz). The normal EEG signals are low voltage in comparison to EMG and ECG with the average background activity ("alpha rhythm" or posterior dominant rhythm) being about 50 mV during the waking state. A mixture of faster and slower frequencies predominates over the more anterior head regions during the waking state. In people over 60 years of age, the EEG is not distinguishable from other normal adults; in people over 80 years of age, some slowing of this dominant posterior rhythm is considered normal, along with some increase in brief intermittent focal slowing in other areas.

Hyperventilation may provoke physiologic slowing of the background rhythm and further intermittent slowing in many normal subjects, but this is commonly absent in the elderly. Photic stimulation can evoke a repetitive, time-locked occipital rhythm (so-called photic driving response) with the same photic stimulus in normal subjects. Hyperventilation and photic stimulation are known to provoke seizures and abnormal epileptiform activity in prone individuals. Characteristic EEG features in the EEG background determine the various stages of non–rapid eye movement (REM) and REM sleep. In many patients with epilepsy, the

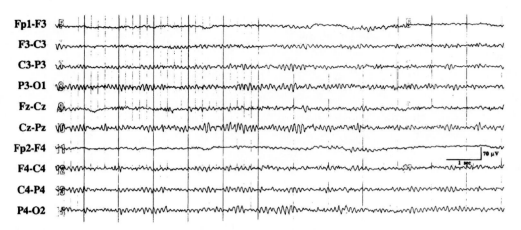

Figure 3-15. Well-regulated, symmetric, 8- to 9-Hz alpha activity in a normal 89-year-old man.

sleep-deprived and sleep EEGs may activate abnormalities and improve the diagnostic yield of the test.

NORMAL EEG CHANGES IN THE ELDERLY

Extensive literature describes normal EEG changes in the elderly. Some variation in what is considered normal exists, chiefly because of the care involved in case selection. Recent studies indicate that truly normal elderly people show remarkably well-formed EEG rhythms that cannot be distinguished from younger patients.

DOMINANT BACKGROUND FREQUENCY

Hubbard et al. (10) reported EEG findings in 10 centenarians. Seven of the 10 were living in the community and were considered generally healthy. Six of these seven had a background alpha frequency of

8 Hz or faster. In four separate studies of patients aged 60 to 80 years (3,7,11,21), the mean alpha frequency was approximately 9.5 Hz. Therefore, in healthy people 80 years old and older, an alpha frequency of 9 Hz should be expected (Fig. 3-15). After age 50, alpha frequency activity may appear in either temporal region, especially the left. It is often higher in voltage than occipital alpha and is considered to be normal. Fragments of this temporal alpha can appear as wicket spikes, which is an epileptiform variant seen in older adults and the elderly that will be discussed later.

INTERMITTENT FOCAL SLOWING

Intermittent focal slowing, especially in the left temporal region (Fig. 3-16), was considered a normal finding after mid-life (19). However, recent studies in which patients have been rigorously screened suggest that this finding, when present, should be infrequent. Katz and Horowitz (11) found intermittent focal slowing in 17% of 52 normal septuagenarians, but in

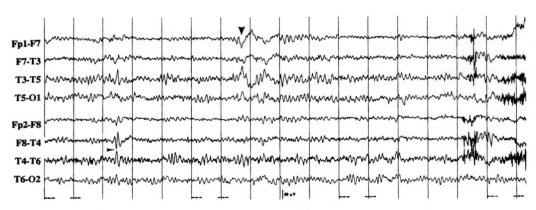

Figure 3-16. Sharply contoured left temporal slowing (*large arrowhead*) in a 73-year-old patient with new onset of partial seizures. The *narrow arrowhead* points to a higher amplitude alpha wave in the right temporal region (an isolated wicket spike) that is part of the normal background at this age and is not epileptiform.

no patient did it occupy more than 1% of the total record. Arenas et al. (3) found slowing in 18 (36%) of 50 subjects. Theta activity was present in all 18 subjects, but delta activity was present in only six (12%). The combined theta and delta activity occupied less than 1.8% of the total recording in all but one subject. Maximal temporal slowing was left-sided in 72% of these patients. Intermittent slowing was best displayed on the transverse bipolar montage.

Visser et al. (22) correlated EEG, neuroimaging, and neuropsychological data in 27 "normal" subjects aged 65 to 83 years (mean age, 78 years). Patients were divided into those with left frontotemporal slowing and those with normal EEGs. Patients with focal delta slowing demonstrated significantly decreased performance on verbal fluency tests and ventricular dilatation on head computed tomography. How frequent the intermittent focal slowing (delta waves) and the amount of focal delta slowing on the record determines whether the record is normal or abnormal.

Substantial variation exists among electroencephalographers interpreting focal slowing. Figure 3-16 is an example of a routine EEG in a 73-year-old patient with new-onset complex partial seizures. The normal phenomenon of sharply contoured alpha transient is seen in the third second in the right temporal region (arrowhead). The abnormal feature of this patient's EEG was the high-amplitude, sharply contoured slowing seen over the left temporal region, which is highlighted with the large arrowhead. No interictal epileptiform activity was seen on the record.

CHANGES IN SLEEP OR DROWSINESS

Katz and Horowitz (12) reported the abrupt onset of drowsiness or sleep in healthy normal septuagenarians with frontally dominant rhythmic delta activity of 1 to 4 Hz and 40 to 150 µV for at least 3 seconds at a time. This activity is indistinguishable from the pathologic

frontal intermittent rhythmic delta activity (FIRDA). Changes also occur in non-REM sleep and sleep cycles. In Stage II sleep, K-complexes and spindles of Stage II sleep are noted to be decreased in amplitude, number, and duration compared with younger adults (8). The delta activity of Stages III and IV is lower in voltage compared to younger people. Septuagenarians also spend less time in slow-wave sleep (13).

BENIGN EPILEPTIFORM VARIANTS

Two benign variants occur frequently in middle-aged and older people. Wicket spikes consist of monophasic, arciform, 6- to 8-Hz waves seen maximally in the temporal regions with a tendency to occur in brief trains of about 1 second (Fig. 3-17) (17). Although these wicket spikes occur in wakefulness, they are often masked by normal background activity. Occasionally, they appear singly when they retain the morphology of the individual waves in a train. Wicket spikes occur in a bitemporal, independent fashion, with approximately equal frequency over each hemisphere. Wicket spikes must be distinguished from anterior or middle temporal focal spikes. Wicket spikes have no correlation with epilepsy or any particular symptom complex, as opposed to anterior temporal spikes, which are correlated with seizures.

Subclinical rhythmic EEG discharge of adults (SREDA) (23) consists of repetitive, bilateral, temporoparietal theta discharges with abrupt onset and termination without any clinical accompaniment. SREDA is usually seen during waking in older adults and is a gradual change of frequency reaching 4 to 7 Hz and lasting 40 to 80 seconds before stopping. SREDA occurs in patients with diverse clinical complaints and is not associated with a clinical history of seizures. In some patients, it can be triggered by hyperventilation.

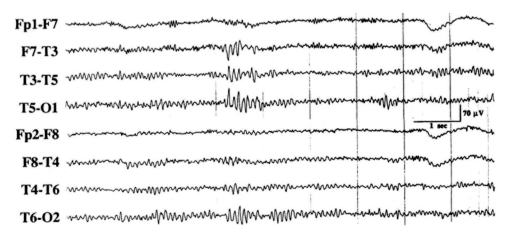

Figure 3-17. A 1-second train of left temporal wicket spikes from a middle-aged patient without a history of seizures.

EEG IN THE ELDERLY WITH EPILEPSY

DEFINITION OF INTERICTAL AND ICTAL ACTIVITY

Interictal epileptiform activity (IEA) consists of spikes, sharp waves, or spike-wave complexes. These discharges may be isolated or repeat in brief trains, can be either focal or generalized, and are not associated with an alteration in awareness or behavior.

Ictal activity usually consists of a rhythmic discharge that is distinct from the interictal pattern in at least duration (especially in the generalized epilepsies) but usually also in morphology and topography. An EEG may be diagnostic of a seizure when there is a rhythmic evolving pattern that may or may not be associated with a change in clinical behavior. If no change in clinical behavior occurs or the patient reports no clinical correlation, the event is termed a "subclinical" or "electrographic" seizure.

APPROACH TO EEG ANALYSIS

An orderly approach to the analysis of EEG activity is crucial. EEG analysis must always begin with an assessment of background activities that are judged against the age and behavioral state of the patient. Those transients that are potentially epileptiform must satisfy the following criteria: (a) they are of cerebral origin, not artifact; (b) they are abnormal for the age and the state of the patient, recognizing that many features that are normal at one age may be abnormal at another; and (c) they must have a significant epileptiform character (not a benign epileptiform normal variant).

INTERICTAL EEG

Although the interictal EEG findings in the appropriate clinical setting can be extremely useful in establishing a seizure diagnosis, the test has inherent limitations. Some normal members of the population can have abnormal EEGs, and patients with definite epilepsy have repeatedly normal studies. Of 1,824 EEG records from 308 patients with a reasonably certain diagnosis of epilepsy (average of six records per patient), 30% had consistently positive EEGs, 52% had some positive and some negative studies, and 17.5% had consistently negative EEGs. Only 8% of 79 patients with a follow-up of at least 1 year had consistently negative EEGs. Positive findings in the first examination were obtained in 55.5% of the patients. Generally, the type of seizure disorder was unrelated to positivity or negativity of the records. People with complex partial seizures of temporal lobe origin had persistently normal EEGs in only 2% of their tracings (1).

A clear relationship exists between the presence of IEA and the individual patient's seizure frequency. In the study by Ajmone-Marsan and Zivin (1), patients with one or more seizures per month had 60.2% positive records. Patients with less than one seizure per year had 37.6% positive records. EEG records were significantly more likely to be positive when obtained on the same day as a clinical seizure.

Interictal epileptiform activity rarely occurs in individuals who will never have a seizure. In the study by Zivin and Ajmone-Marsan (24) of 6,497 unselected, nonepileptic patients receiving EEG examinations, 142 (2.2%) had epileptiform discharges. With clinical and EEG follow-up ranging from a few months to more than 10 years, 20 of these patients (14.1%) ultimately developed seizures.

Relatively few data are found in the literature about the frequency of IEA in the elderly. Most of the relevant studies concern the presence of epileptiform activity in patients after stroke (9,16) and, therefore, are not representative of most elderly patients with unprovoked seizures seen in the outpatient setting. In a recently completed analysis of 125 ambulatory patients aged 60 years or older in whom a confident diagnosis of epilepsy was made by a board-certified neurologist, 70 of these patients had the onset of their epilepsy after age 60 (5). The waking background EEG in these 70 patients was normal in eight, showed generalized slowing in 13, and showed focal slowing with or without additional generalized slowing in 49. IEA was present on the first EEG in 35% of 55 patients (mean age, 65 years) with pre-existing epilepsy and 26% of 70 patients (mean age, 70 years) with seizure onset after age 60 years. No significant differences were seen in the frequency of IEA in patients with late-onset epilepsy in the seventh or eighth decade of life. Most IEA was focal. Of the 18 patients with onset of epilepsy after 60 years of age, IEA was generalized in three and focal in 15, most being of temporal lobe origin. Activation procedures of hyperventilation and photic stimulation produced little additional beneficial information. Patients with at least one seizure per month were significantly more likely to have IEA present ($p = 0.016$). No differences were found in the presence of IEA, depending on the underlying cause of the seizures. No correlation was found between the presence or absence of IEA and seizure type or use of AEDs. In 308 patients with epilepsy (1), the frequency of IEA on the first EEG in the first four decades of life was 77%, 60%, 56%, and 51%, respectively. In 51 patients aged 40 years or older, the frequency of IEA was 39%. Age-related epileptogenesis has been little studied (4). It is speculated that the decreased number and complexity of synaptic connections with age may contribute to less synchronized neuronal discharges and, therefore, less frequent IEA detected on scalp EEG.

DIAGNOSTIC CLOSED-CIRCUIT TELEVISION EEG

The clinical manifestations of epilepsy, which are more diverse in the elderly than in younger patients, are more easily confused with other common medical problems (e.g., cardiac arrhythmias, transient ischemic attacks, or dizziness). Elderly patients with epilepsy are more likely to be seen by primary care providers or specialists in other disciplines who may be unfamiliar with the fact that an EEG can be normal or show nonspecific abnormalities. A low rate of definitively abnormal EEGs in the elderly patient with epilepsy may lead to misdiagnosis.

Prolonged inpatient video EEG monitoring is an extremely useful diagnostic tool in all patients with possible epilepsy but is underused in the elderly. Only 1.4% of video EEG inpatient monitoring at a major epilepsy referral center was performed on elderly patients (14). This low utilization rate was recently confirmed at another referral center, which showed that only 4.6% of 976 admissions were performed on the elderly (6). Of these, eight patients were critically ill with known or suspected status epilepticus, and there were 18 patients whose primary reason for hospitalization was the monitoring itself. Of the 18 patients admitted for monitoring only, mean age was 69.5 years (range, 60 to 90 years). The mean length of stay was 4.3 days (range, 2 to 9 days). Five patients had complex partial seizures recorded. Three patients, all treated with AEDs, had no spells recorded, and no additional diagnostic information was gained from the admission. The other 10 patients, eight of whom had been treated with AEDs, were symptomatic during their admissions, leading to a change in diagnosis and stoppage of AEDs. Fifteen of the 18 elderly patients received a definitive diagnosis during admission. These results suggest that inpatient video EEG monitoring is useful in elderly patients with spells suspected of having epilepsy. Making a definitive diagnosis in this population has specific implications concerning treatment. Ruling out seizures will likely reduce the inappropriate use of AEDs in this susceptible population.

Even in those elderly people with epilepsy, the ictal semiology may change as one ages and is often different from the seizures that occurred at a younger age (14,20). The 20 patients in their report represented only 1.5% of all patients who had video EEG and led to a wide variety of diagnoses (sleep apnea in two, epilepsy in two, nonepileptic events of psychogenic origin in two, syncope in one, and was not diagnostic in two).

Epilepsy is common in the elderly and often presents differently than in younger individuals. With advanced age, an extensive differential diagnosis is part of the evaluation process. Video EEG is a valuable and underused diagnostic tool in this population.

Ictal activity recorded during long-term video EEG is generally similar to younger patients.

AMBULATORY EEG

Electroencephalograms can be recorded outside of the hospital environment with ambulatory EEG (AEEG), where EEG electrodes and a small recording device are attached to the patient. AEEG has the advantage of recording activity in an environment that reproduces daily life. Patients maintain a diary of their activities and any events that occur during the recording session. Especially in the elderly with a high incidence of cardiac abnormalities, a dedicated ECG rhythm strip is important to monitor in addition to the EEG during ambulatory recordings. AEEG recording devices have improved significantly in recent years and are comfortable for the patient to wear and usually well tolerated for several days. Some ambulatory equipment now allows for the use of concurrent video recording. Seizure and spike detection software is also available and may improve the sensitivity of the procedure.

EEG IN ENCEPHALOPATHIES AND DEMENTIA

Abnormalities on the EEG that manifest slower frequencies than expected for the age and behavioral state of the patient are termed "slow-wave abnormalities." Slowing on the EEG can be generalized or focal and intermittent or persistent (>80% of the EEG). Slow-wave abnormalities can be seen in patients with epilepsy and are considered nonspecific if no epileptiform activity is seen during the same recording. Focal slow-wave abnormalities imply a local disturbance of cortical and sometimes adjacent subcortical structures in the focal epilepsies but are also nonspecific because they may also be seen in a variety of unrelated conditions (e.g., stroke, brain tumors, severe migraine, trauma). Generalized, intermittent slowing occurs most commonly in diffuse encephalopathies. The slower the EEG frequency is on the recording correlates with the severity of the encephalopathy. Stuporous patients often show a moderate degree of slowing of background rhythms and brief intermittent trains of even slower waveforms. Noxious or auditory external stimulation of the patient may accelerate (activate) the background frequency. Comatose patients show a more marked and persistent degree of slowing that typically does not change or minimally changes with stimulation. Occasionally, comatose patients have EEG findings highly suggestive of a particular cause (Table 3-4). A combination of unreactive persistent delta rhythms

Table 3-4. *Electroencephalogram Findings of Patients with Dementia, Stupor, or Coma*

Diagnosis	EEG Findings
Stupor (i.e., renal or hepatic)	Moderate degree of background slowing with intermittent further slowing. Stimulation of the patient accelerates the background frequency.
Coma (i.e., posthypoxic-ischemic injury)	Marked and persistent slowing that does not react to stimulation.
Brain death	Isoelectric EEG.
Focal brain lesions	Focal slowing. Periodic lateralized epileptiform discharges (PLEDs), if acute.
Encephalitis	PLEDs or Bi-PLEDs; generalized or multifocal slowing.
Creutzfeldt-Jakob disease	Generalized periodic sharp wave complexes.
Alzheimer's disease	Mild to moderate generalized background slowing.

EEG, electroencephalogram.

with superimposed widespread beta activity suggests medication effect and should lead to a suspicion of overdose (barbiturates or benzodiazepines). In heavily sedated patients or patients who are paralyzed with neuromuscular blocking agents, EEG recordings are an extremely useful bedside measure of the integrity of brain function. The EEG is one of the confirmatory tests that can be useful in establishing brain death but is not required to make the diagnosis. EEG should be used to confirm brain death only when the clinical exam is unreliable. The EEG must meet multiple specific requirements to be interpreted as showing no cerebral activity (Table 3-5) (2).

In patients with well-defined focal brain lesions such as tumors or stroke, no indication exists for the routine use of EEG. A characteristic EEG pattern seen in severe focal encephalitis, such as a herpes simplex infection, or other acute focal brain lesions, such as stroke, is known as periodic lateralized epileptiform discharges (PLEDs). PLEDs are dramatic, high-amplitude, regularly recurring, sharp waves on a background of marked voltage and frequency attenuation between periodic discharges (Fig. 3-18).

Focal seizures, secondarily generalized tonic-clonic seizures, and signs of more generalized cerebral dysfunction with altered levels of alertness may all be seen. Typically, the EEG and behavioral features are transient, typically resolving over days to weeks. After resolution, a localization-related epilepsy with associated focal slowing and IEA may be seen.

The EEG has no particular utility in the investigation of patients with degenerative disorders of the nervous system with one notable exception. Patients with acute or subacute presentation of a dementing illness should have one or more EEG recordings performed to search for the generalized periodic sharp wave complexes (PSWCs) of Creutzfeldt-Jakob disease. This illness is characterized by rapidly progressive dementia, myoclonus, cerebellar ataxia, and visual dysfunction. The EEG may be useful in establishing a diagnosis in those suspected of having the illness. Typical features are the 1- to 2-Hz PSWCs, which may be present as early as 3 weeks after onset and have been seen in 88% of EEGs after the 12th week of illness (15). Myoclonic jerks often occur in association with the presence of PSWC, but no consistent temporal relationship exists between the jerks and the complexes.

Table 3-5. *EEG Criteria for Brain Death*

1. Minimum of 8 scalp electrodes
2. Interelectrode impedances of <10k ohms and >100 ohms
3. Test the integrity of the entire recording system
4. Interelectrode distances of >10 cm
5. Sensitivity of 2 μV/mm for >30 minutes of recording time
6. Appropriate filter settings
7. Use of additional monitors as needed (ECG, respirator, EMG monitors)
8. No reactivity to afferent stimulus
9. Performed by a qualified technologist
10. Repeat the EEG as needed

STATUS EPILEPTICUS

The elderly clearly have a higher incidence of epilepsy when compared to younger adults and adolescents. As noted previously, the semiology of seizures in the elderly can be confusing, leading to delay in treatment and misdiagnosis. This is highlighted in a recent study of elderly patients admitted to the hospital with an altered mental status (18). Patients had a variety of presenting symptoms and etiologies for their seizures. Given the extensive comorbidities in this age group and often subtle clinical manifestations, an extended time course to making the diagnosis was observed. The use of EEG was crucial to making the diagnosis. As with other age groups, the underlying cause and

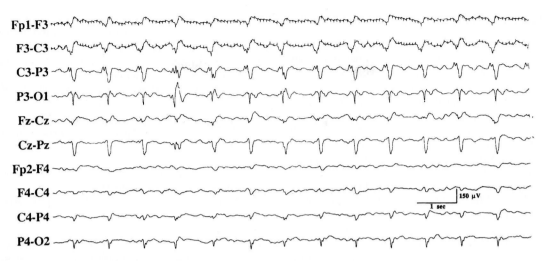

Figure 3-18. Periodic, lateralized epileptiform discharges arising from the left hemisphere with a posterior maximum after acute posterior cerebral territory ischemic infarction in an elderly patient.

length of nonconvulsive status epilepticus impacted morbidity and mortality. Convulsive status epilepticus generally does not present a diagnostic challenge to the health care practitioner. When the abnormal motor activity resolves, the patient often remains unresponsive for a variable length of time. If the recovery time is prolonged, determining the presence of ongoing subclinical electrographic activity presents an important challenge. Performing an emergent EEG should resolve the issue; a diffusely slow postictal pattern informs the evaluator that the seizure has resolved. Ongoing epileptiform activity on the EEG alerts the care team that more aggressive therapy is needed.

CONCLUSION

The EEG has a limited but important role as a diagnostic test in the older adult. It is a critically important study in people with known or suspected seizure disorders. Video EEG inpatient monitoring is underused and often provides a diagnosis in patients with challenging or undiagnosed seizure-like events. Using the EEG in the evaluation of acute encephalopathies, dementing illnesses, and status epilepticus where characteristic patterns may occur remains important and useful for health care providers.

GLOSSARY OF TERMS

Benign epileptiform variants: One of a number of EEG patterns that has epileptiform features but occurs in the normal population and has no known association with epilepsy.

Ictal: That which occurs during a seizure.

Ictal epileptiform activity: EEG feature of a rhythmic discharge that is distinct from the interictal pattern in at least duration (especially in the generalized epilepsies) but usually also in morphology and topography.

Interictal: The periods between seizures.

Interictal epileptiform activity: EEG feature of spikes, sharp waves, or spike-wave complexes that are isolated or repeat in brief trains, are either focal or generalized, and are not associated with an alteration in awareness or behavior.

Montage: In EEG, the manner in which electrodes are linked together to examine the EEG; hence, transverse bipolar when scalp electrodes are linked in chains going transversely across the scalp.

PLED: Periodic lateralized epileptiform discharges. EEG feature seen in acute focal insults to the brain. When bilateral and independent, known as BiPLED.

SREDA: Subclinical rhythmic electroencephalographic discharge of adults. A benign EEG phenomenon consisting of repetitive discharges of abrupt onset and termination without any clinical accompaniment. Superficially resembles an ictal EEG discharge.

Semiology: The behavioral manifestations and experiences of the patient during an epileptic seizure.

REFERENCES

1. Ajmone-Marsan C, Zivin LS. Factors related to the occurrence of typical paroxysmal abnormalities in the EEG records of epileptic patients. *Epilepsia.* 1970;11:361–381.
2. American Clinical Neurophysiology Society Guidelines. Minimum technical standards for EEG recording in suspected cerebral death. *J Clin Neurophysiol.* 1994;11:10–13.
3. Arenas AM, Brenner RP, Reynolds CF. Temporal slowing in the elderly revisited. *Am J Electroencephalogr Technol.* 1986;26:105–114.
4. Dichter MA, Weinberger LM. Epileptogenesis and the aging brain. In: Rown AJ, Ramsay RE, eds. *Seizures and epilepsy in the elderly.* Boston: Butterworth-Heinemann; 1997:21–27.
5. Drury I, Beydoun A. Interictal epileptiform activity in elderly patients with epilepsy. *Electroencephalogr Clin Neurophysiol.* 1998;106:369–373.
6. Drury I, Selwa LN, Schuh LA, et al. Value of inpatient diagnostic CCTV-EEG monitoring in the elderly. *Epilepsia.* 1999;40:1100–1102.
7. Giaquinto S, Nolfe G. The EEG in the normal elderly: a contribution to the interpretation of aging and dementia. *Electroencephalogr Clin Neurophysiol.* 1986;3:540–546.
8. Guazelli M, Feinberg I, Aminoff M, et al. Sleep spindles in normal elderly: comparison with young adult patterns and relation to nocturnal awakening, cognitive function and brain atrophy. *Electroencephalogr Clin Neurophysiol.* 1986;63:526–539.
9. Gupta SR, Naheedy MH, Elias D, et al. Post-infarction seizures: a clinical study. *Stroke.* 1998; 19:1477–1481.
10. Hubbard O, Sunde D, Goldensohn ES. The EEG in centenarians. *Electroencephalogr Clin Neurophysiol.* 1976;40:407–417.
11. Katz RI, Horowitz GR. Electroencephalogram in the septuagenarian: studies in a normal geriatric population. *J Am Geriatr Soc.* 1982;3:272–275.
12. Katz RI, Horowitz GR. Sleep-onset frontal rhythmic slowing in a normal geriatric population. *Electroenccephalogr Clin Neurophysiol.* 1983; 56:27P.
13. Katzmann R, Terry R. *The Neurology of Aging.* Philadelphia: FA Davis; 1983:1–249.
14. Lancman ME, O'Donovan C, Dinner D, et al. Usefulness of prolonged video-EEG monitoring in the elderly. *J Neurol Sci.* 1996;142:54–58.
15. Levy SR, Chiappa KH, Burke CJ, et al. Early evolution and evidence of electroencephalographic abnormality in Creutzfeldt-Jakob disease. *J Clin Neurophysiol.* 1986;3:1–21.
16. Luhdorf K, Jensen LK, Plesner AM. The value of EEG in the investigation of postapoplectic epilepsy. *Acta Neurol Scand.* 1986;74:279–283.
17. Reiher J, Lebel M. Wicket spikes: clinical correlates of a previously undescribed EEG pattern. *Can J Neurol Sci.* 1977;4:39–47.
18. Sheth R, Drazkowski J, Sirven JL, et al. Protracted ictal confusion in elderly patients. *Arch Neurol.* 2006;63:529–532.
19. Silverman AJ, Busse EW, Barnes RH. Studies in the processes of aging: electroencephalographic findings in 400 elderly subjects. *Electroencephalogr Clin Neurophysiol.* 1955;7:67–74.
20. Tinuper T. The altered presentation of seizures in the elderly. In: Rowan AJ, Ramsay RE, eds. *Seizures and epilepsy in the elderly.* Boston: Butterworth-Heinemann; 1997:123–127.
21. Torres F, Faoro A, Loewenson R, et al. The electroencephalogram of elderly subjects revisited. *Electroencephalogr Clin Neurophysiol.* 1983;56: 391–398.
22. Visser SL, Hooijer C, Jonker C, et al. Anterior temporal focal abnormalities in EEG in normal aged subjects: correlations with psychopathological and CT brain scan findings. *Electroencephalogr Clin Neurophysiol.* 1987;66:1–7.
23. Westmoreland BF, Klass DW. A distinctive rhythmic EEG discharge of adults. *Electroencephalogr Clin Neurophysiol.* 1981;51:186–191.
24. Zivin L, Ajmone-Marsan C. Incidence and prognostic significance of "epileptiform" activity in the EEG of non-epileptic subjects. *Brain.* 1968; 91:751–778.

SUGGESTED READING

Rowan AJ, Ramsay RE, eds. *Seizures and epilepsy in the elderly.* Boston: Butterworth-Heinemann; 1997.
Daly DD, Pedley TA, eds. *Current practice of clinical electroencephalography.* 2nd ed. New York: Raven Press; 1990.

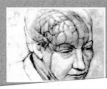

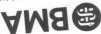
eedle
1 the
cted
ware
1 to
sues
and
.....are

..... will lessen the likelihood of false-positive and false-negative NCS and EMG tests.

NCS and EMG should be considered an extension of the neurologic examination. Primary reasons for referral to the EMG laboratory include pain, sensory loss, weakness, fatigue, and bulbar symptoms (such as diplopia, dysarthria, or dysphagia). These symptoms can be caused by neurologic and nonneurologic disorders. In the elder individual, particularly the medically complicated patient, EMG plays a critical role in establishing a diagnosis.

The roles of NCS and needle EMG are to confirm or refute neurologic disease, localize disease within the peripheral nervous system, characterize the nature of the disease, define disease severity, provide prognostic information, and assess response to treatment (Table 3-6). It is helpful to consider these roles when considering patient referral to the EMG laboratory and when performing electrodiagnostic testing.

Table 3-6. *Purpose of EMG*

1. Confirm presence of neurologic disorder
2. Localize process (to nerve, root, muscle, neuro-muscular junction, anterior horn cell)
3. Characterize the nature of the disorder
4. Determine severity
5. Provide prognostic information
6. Assess response to treatment

MOTOR AND SENSORY NERVE CONDUCTION STUDIES

NCSs involve the electrical stimulation of motor and sensory nerves in the limbs and face. When performing motor nerve conduction studies, a small recording electrode is placed over the endplate region of a muscle. Electrical stimulation is then performed at consistent sites proximally and distally, specific for the nerve being studied. Electrical stimulation is increased until a maximal electrical potential is generated—the motor compound muscle action potential (CMAP). The amplitude and configuration of the CMAP is noted at both proximal and distal sites of stimulation. The CMAP reflects the electrical summation of all muscle fibers stimulated by that nerve.

By calculating the quotient of distance and time between the proximal and distal CMAPs, the conduction velocity of that nerve can be calculated (recorded in meters per second). In addition, conduction time along the very distal part of the nerve is recorded by calculating the time from distal nerve stimulation to onset of CMAP generation. This is referred to as the distal latency (recorded in milliseconds). F-waves are electrical potentials that can be elicited by antidromic stimulation of motor nerves. Stimulation of F-waves involves propagation of an electrical impulse proximally to the anterior horn cells of that motor nerve, which in turn generate an electrical potential that travels orthodromically down the motor nerve to muscle endplate and is recorded as an F-wave potential. The time to generation of this F-wave potential is considered the F-wave latency. The primary utility of the F-wave latency is to provide an estimate of proximal conduction velocity (at the root or plexus level). The conduction velocity, distal latency, and F-wave latency provide an assessment of the speed of conduction along different segments of motor nerves.

Electrical potentials can also be elicited by stimulation of sensory nerves. These sensory nerve action potentials (SNAPs) are generated by either antidromic or orthodromic stimulation of sensory nerves and are recorded with small surface or ring electrodes. SNAP amplitude, conduction velocity, and distal latency for individual sensory nerves are collected and analyzed based on the same principles used for motor NCS. The SNAP represents the electrical potential of large, myelinated fibers. Small, unmyelinated or thinly myelinated fibers cannot be identified. This is clinically important in cases of suspected small-fiber neuropathy because NCS can be normal in these patients.

Repetitive stimulation of motor nerves is performed in patients with suspected neuromuscular transmission disorders, such as myasthenia gravis or the Lambert-Eaton myasthenic syndrome. The objective of repetitive nerve stimulation (RNS) is to stress the integrity (safety factor) of the neuromuscular junction. Repetitive stimulation of a motor nerve at a rate of 2 Hz is performed before and after exercise. The elicited electrical potentials are recorded and assessed for an abnormal decrease (decrement) or increase (increment) in amplitude and area.

NEEDLE ELECTROMYOGRAPHY

Needle EMG involves the insertion of a recording needle electrode into a skeletal muscle to assess the electrical activity of the muscle, both at rest and during voluntary activation. The electrical activity is displayed on a monitor and recorded over a loudspeaker to allow simultaneous visual and auditory assessment. During the needle examination, insertional activity and motor unit potentials (MUPs) are evaluated. When evaluating insertional activity, the patient is instructed to keep the muscle relaxed so that there is no volitional activation of MUPs. The needle is then passed through different areas of the muscle so that the resting electrical activity of that muscle can be assessed. Insertional activity is then graded as normal, increased, or decreased.

In normal persons, needle electrode insertion and movement elicits only a brief discharge that ends with or shortly after needle movement. However, a more prolonged discharge can occur when the needle is in the vicinity of the muscle endplate. This is referred to as endplate noise or endplate spikes; endplate noise and endplate spikes sound like a "seashell" and "fat on a frying pan," respectively. Endplate spikes and endplate noise are found in normal persons and in individuals with neuromuscular disease. Decreased insertional activity typically reflects a longstanding or even old (neurogenic or myopathic) process that has caused muscle atrophy and fibrosis.

Increased insertional activity can be seen with disorders affecting nerve or muscle. These abnormal electrical discharges can be stimulated by needle movement and often persist long after the needle has stopped moving. The nature of the increased insertional activity is characterized based on the firing rate, firing pattern, and configuration of the electrical discharges (Table 3-7). The most commonly seen abnormal discharges in the EMG laboratory are fibrillation potentials and fasciculation potentials. Fibrillations are an electrical potential of a denervated muscle fiber and are best appreciated by their regular rhythmic firing pattern. Fasciculation potentials are electrical potentials generated by an entire motor unit and typically occur sporadically and are nonrhythmic. Fasciculation potentials can be considered "benign" when they are not associated with fibrillation potentials or MUP changes.

The second portion of the needle examination involves collection and analysis of MUPs. MUPs are generated with voluntary activation of the muscle being examined. A single MUP is an electrical potential generated by the discharge of one motor unit. MUP characteristics assessed include duration, height, complexity, firing rate, and stability. All of these features are analyzed and used in determining whether a peripheral nervous system (PNS) disorder is present and, ultimately, whether the underlying process is a disease of nerve or muscle.

A reduction in the size of the MUP is generally observed in muscle disorders but can also be seen in neuromuscular junction disorders and in neurogenic

Table 3-7. *Insertional Activity*

Type of Discharge	Rhythm	Rate/Second	Appearance
Fibrillation	Regular	2–20	Spike or positive
Fasciculation	Irregular	0.01–10	Triphasic/polyphasic
Myotonic	Regular	20–80	Spike or positive
Complex–repetitive	Regular	5–80	Complex
Myokymia	Regular	10–60	Triphasic
Neuromyotonia	Regular	150–300	Triphasic
Endplate spike	Irregular	50–200	Spike
Cramp	Irregular	4–100	Triphasic

disorders affecting the nerve terminal. Large MUPs are seen in neurogenic disorders affecting anterior horn cells, nerve roots, or peripheral nerves. MUP recruitment is assessed by determining the number of activated MUPs and the firing rate of the MUPs at a given level of activation. In normal individuals, as the strength of muscle contraction increases, MUP firing rate increases, and additional MUPs are recruited. Reduced recruitment is seen in neurogenic disorders and is noted as a decrease in the number of MUPs and an increase in the firing rate of the activated MUPs. In myopathic disorders, rapid recruitment is seen, whereby increased numbers of MUPs are activated at a given level of contraction.

Single-fiber EMG is a highly specialized technique used primarily in the investigation of suspected neuromuscular transmission disorders (predominantly myasthenia gravis). Some institutions use a highly specialized single-fiber needle, but increasingly, a concentric needle is being used for single-fiber EMG studies (12). The recording and filtering characteristics of the single-fiber study are such that individual potentials from single muscle fibers are collected. Variation in muscle fiber firing times relative to each other is recorded and calculated as "jitter" and "blocking." Individuals with neuromuscular transmission disorders have increased jitter and may have blocking. Generally, single-fiber EMG is performed when RNS studies are normal. It is also important to understand that disorders other than neuromuscular junction disorders, such as neuropathy, radiculopathy, myopathy, or motor neuron disease, are associated with abnormal single-fiber EMG studies.

TECHNICAL CONSIDERATIONS

Recognition of potential technical issues is critical in the accurate performance and interpretation of NCS and EMG. Limb temperature is one such issue. Limb temperature is typically assessed using a surface thermometer. If the limb temperature is below the accepted range, the limb being studied is typically warmed with a heat pack, heat lamp, or warm water bath. Low limb temperatures can have a significant impact on NCS, resulting in distal latency prolongation and slowing of conduction velocities, and can result in falsely increased motor and sensory nerve amplitudes. Limb edema, which is not uncommon in the elderly patient, can result in falsely low (or even absent) motor and sensory responses. This is due to difficulties with appropriate electrode placement and in achieving supramaximal stimulation. Obesity can have similar effects on nerve conduction studies through similar mechanisms due to increased limb girth.

Recognition of anomalous innervation, particularly the Martin-Gruber anastomosis, is critically important when performing and interpreting NCS. Anomalous innervation is considered to be a normal variant, where motor fibers leave one motor nerve and join another motor nerve. Not surprisingly, this impacts motor NCS by creating a difference in the elicited motor CMAP between the proximal and distal sites of stimulation. The Martin-Gruber anastomosis is especially important to recognize because it can mimic an ulnar neuropathy to the unwary electromyographer. With this type of anomalous innervation, a small number of motor fibers from the median nerve join the ulnar nerve in the forearm. This causes the ulnar CMAP to be larger with stimulation at the wrist than at the elbow, suggesting that there is a drop in the amplitude of the ulnar potential across the elbow. This can lead to a spurious electrophysiologic diagnosis of an ulnar neuropathy at the elbow.

EFFECTS OF AGING ON NERVE CONDUCTION STUDIES AND NEEDLE ELECTROMYOGRAPHY

Physiologic changes in the peripheral nervous system occur with aging. These changes are often recognized at the time of neurologic examination. Manifestations such as loss of ankle deep tendon reflexes, reduction in vibration sense, and an increase in tactile threshold in the fingers and toes occur in the elderly (3,5,8). These findings are recognized as being "normal" in the elderly patient who has an otherwise normal neurologic examination. Not surprisingly, these physiologic changes can also be reflected in NCS and EMG studies in the elderly. The clinical and electrodiagnostic findings that occur with aging are due to recognized morphometric changes within the peripheral nervous system.

Degeneration and demyelination of myelinated fibers occur in the elderly. In a study of the morphometric changes of the sural sensory nerve with aging, a marked reduction in the density of myelinated fibers was noted (9). This is presumed to be primarily due to axonal degeneration, with secondary demyelination of peripheral motor and sensory nerves. Loss of anterior horn cells also occurs in the elderly (13). The mechanisms of axonal degeneration and anterior horn cell loss that occur with aging are unknown.

Motor and sensory NCSs change with age, paralleling the morphometric findings. Motor and sensory nerve conduction velocities decline by 1 to 2 m/s/decade (4). SNAP amplitudes also decline with age, and sensory distal latencies prolong with age. In many laboratories, an absent sural sensory response is recognized as being normal. For example, in our laboratory, routine sensory NCSs decline, on average, by 65% in normal male subjects 60 or older. Motor nerve distal latencies also increase in the elderly. Motor CMAP amplitudes decline with aging, although this decrease is much less marked than that seen with SNAPs.

In general, insertional activity as assessed by needle EMG does not change with aging. However, it has been recognized that the presence of isolated fibrillation potentials in foot muscles can be seen in a significant proportion of normal elderly individuals (2). Fibrillation potentials in foot muscles of younger patients may indicate a peripheral neuropathy or sacral radiculopathy. MUP characteristics change with aging. MUP duration, amplitude, and complexity all increase with aging (1). This is most likely due to axonal degeneration and loss of anterior horn cells, leading to remodeling of motor units.

NCS AND EMG IN DISEASE

MONONEUROPATHIES

Patients with mononeuropathies typically complain of extremity numbness, tingling, weakness, or pain. While the prevalence of mononeuropathies increases with age, so do other conditions such as arthritis, vascular disease, and limb edema, which can cause similar symptoms. NCS and needle EMG play an important role not only in establishing the presence of a mononeuropathy, but also in localizing the site of abnormality, determining severity, and establishing whether there is other subclinical peripheral nervous system disease (e.g., peripheral neuropathy).

Median and ulnar neuropathies are the most common mononeuropathies seen in clinical practice, typically because of entrapment at the wrist and elbow, respectively. In most cases, sensory NCS changes are most sensitive in individuals with an early or mild mononeuropathy. In patients with carpal tunnel syndrome, a prolongation in the distal latency of the median sensory nerve and a decrease in the median SNAP are typical abnormalities seen in early or mild disease. A decrease in the ulnar SNAP or a slow ulnar sensory nerve conduction velocity across the elbow is seen in patients with an early or mild ulnar neuropathy at the elbow. In patients with moderate or severe disease, the motor CMAPs may decrease, slow motor conduction velocities may be seen, and prolonged motor distal latencies become evident. Ultimately, it is the demonstration of focal slowing that allows the precise localization of a mononeuropathy. Distal latency prolongation with stimulation of a motor nerve at the wrist suggests localization to the wrist. Occasionally with motor NCS, a decrease in the motor CMAP with proximal stimulation can occur, suggesting conduction block. When this occurs, short

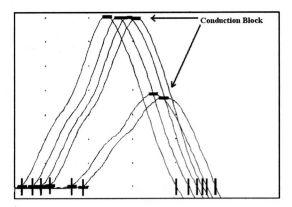

Figure 3-19. Conduction block involving ulnar nerve. Ulnar motor NCS in a patient with an ulnar neuropathy at the elbow. Study depicts short segmental stimulation ("inching") across the elbow. There is an approximate 50% drop in the motor potential amplitude, consistent with conduction block, across the elbow.

segmental stimulation ("inching") can precisely localize the site of conduction block. In clinical practice, this is most frequently demonstrated with an ulnar neuropathy at the elbow (Fig. 3-19).

Needle EMG is frequently normal in patients with mild or even moderately severe mononeuropathies. With more severe disease, needle EMG is expected to be abnormal in the distribution of the involved nerve, distal to the lesion, or site of entrapment. Fibrillation potentials or large MUPs can be seen. Typically, the most important role of needle EMG in the electrodiagnostic evaluation of suspected mononeuropathy is to exclude other disease, such as radiculopathy or plexopathy.

RADICULOPATHY AND PLEXOPATHY

The majority of individuals with radiculopathy or plexopathy have pain, and many have weakness and sensory loss. Localization of disease to nerve root or plexus is often difficult, even with thoughtful neurologic examination and electrodiagnostic testing. In the older adult, neuroimaging studies may not be helpful given the high prevalence of degenerative disc disease in even asymptomatic individuals (7). Patients with clinically suspected radiculopathy or plexopathy should be considered for NCS and EMG testing. The primary role of electrodiagnostic testing is to establish the presence or extent of disease, to localize the process to nerve root or plexus, and to determine whether the disease process is "active."

Most patients with radiculopathy have normal motor and sensory NCS (Table 3-8). Occasionally, low-amplitude motor CMAPs can be seen with severe or longstanding radiculopathy. Sensory NCS abnormalities suggest either an alternative localization

Table 3-8. *NCS and EMG Findings in Radiculopathy versus Plexopathy*

Electrodiagnostic Features	Radiculopathy	Plexopathy
Motor CMAP	Normal/decreased	Normal/decreased
SNAP amplitude	Normal	Decreased*
EMG paraspinal muscles	Frequently abnormal	Normal
EMG pattern	Abnormalities in root distribution	Abnormalities may be diffuse/patchy

*Often need to compare to unaffected/opposite limb.

(such as a plexopathy) or a secondary disease process. Sensory NCSs are typically abnormal in brachial or lumbosacral plexopathies because the disease process is distal to the cell body of the sensory nerve (the dorsal root ganglion).

Needle EMG can be abnormal in both radiculopathy and plexopathy. Signs of denervation, such as fibrillation potentials, and large MUPs are typical findings. Fibrillation potentials in paraspinal muscles suggest radiculopathy. The distribution of needle EMG abnormalities can be helpful. In most plexopathies, EMG abnormalities are diffuse or patchy. EMG abnormalities in the distribution of one nerve root would be far more typical of a radiculopathy, although in clinical practice, findings suggesting multiple cervical radiculopathies are frequently seen.

In patients with suspected radiculopathy, fibrillation potentials are typically interpreted as showing active disease. Large MUPs without fibrillation potentials suggest that reinnervation has occurred. In patients with acute neurogenic processes, fibrillation potentials typically do not appear for 2 to 3 weeks following the injury. However, with significant neurogenic processes causing weakness, reduced recruitment of MUPs can be seen on needle EMG immediately after nerve injury.

PERIPHERAL NEUROPATHY

Patients with peripheral neuropathy typically report symptoms of numbness, tingling, pain, or weakness. The primary role of electrodiagnostic testing in this setting is to determine whether the neuropathy is axonal or demyelinating, to define what modalities are involved, and to determine the anatomic pattern of peripheral nerve involvement.

Recognition of the limitations of EMG in the evaluation of peripheral neuropathy is also important. NCS and needle EMG evaluate only large-fiber nerve function. Small-fiber nerves, which are unmyelinated or thinly myelinated nerve fibers, cannot be assessed with routine NCS and needle EMG. In many cases, NCS and needle EMG are normal in patients with a small-fiber neuropathy. Such patients may need autonomic testing (which assesses small-fiber nerve function) or skin biopsy to establish a diagnosis.

In the majority of patients with peripheral neuropathy, sensory nerves are preferentially involved early in the disease course. Hence, sensory NCS may be the only abnormality in individuals with early or mild disease. Furthermore, in patients with a sensory neuropathy or sensory neuronopathy, abnormal sensory NCS may be the only abnormality seen with electrodiagnostic testing. Identification of the anatomic pattern of peripheral nerve disease is also important. For example, asymmetric, multifocal electrodiagnostic abnormalities suggest a mononeuritis multiplex pattern of peripheral nerve disease, which not infrequently is due to vasculitis.

Electrodiagnostic testing can predict whether a neuropathy is axonal or demyelinating. NCS features suggestive of demyelination include prolongation of distal latencies, prolongation of F-wave latencies, slowing of conduction velocities, and the presence of temporal dispersion or conduction block. Furthermore, the presence of temporal dispersion or conduction block suggests a noninherited (acquired) disorder. Low-amplitude motor and sensory NCSs are seen in axonal processes, with normal or only minor distal latency and conduction velocity abnormalities.

MYOPATHY

Patients with muscle disease present primarily with weakness and fatigue and, occasionally, with muscle pain. The role of electrodiagnostic testing in the patient with weakness is to confirm myopathy, exclude a disorder of neuromuscular transmission, and establish the distribution and severity of disease. In addition, electrodiagnostic testing plays an important role in determining whether a muscle biopsy should be performed and in selection of a muscle to biopsy. NCSs are typically normal in patients with myopathy. Repetitive nerve stimulation is normal in muscle disease and is helpful to exclude a neuromuscular transmission disorder.

Needle EMG is abnormal in myopathy. Fibrillation potentials are frequently seen. The presence of fibrillation potentials in muscle disease has been correlated with abnormal findings on muscle biopsy, including inflammation, fiber splitting, necrosis, and vacuolar change. Because fibrillation potentials can be seen in

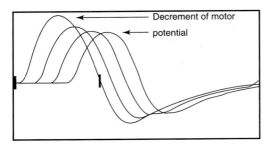

Figure 3-20. Decrement with repetitive nerve stimulation. Repetitive stimulation (2 Hz) of the accessory nerve in a patient with myasthenia gravis. There is a 25% decrease in the electrical potential with repetitive stimulation.

both neurogenic and myopathic disorders, MUP analysis ultimately provides the electrodiagnostic evidence of myopathy.

Small, polyphasic MUPs with rapid recruitment are seen on needle EMG. Although needle EMG abnormalities are not disease specific, the anatomic distribution of myopathic findings can suggest or predict certain diseases. For example, inclusion body myositis, the most common inflammatory myopathy in the elderly, has a predilection for early and prominent involvement of finger flexor and quadriceps muscles. Predominant myopathic changes in these muscles are predictive of inclusion body myositis in the elderly patient with weakness and myopathy on EMG. However, muscle biopsy is required to establish a diagnosis of specific myopathic disorders.

NEUROMUSCULAR JUNCTION DISORDERS

Patients with myasthenia gravis and the Lambert-Eaton myasthenic syndrome present with symptoms of fatigue and weakness. These symptoms are not uncommon in the elderly, particularly in the patient with multiple medical comorbidities. Some patients with myasthenia gravis present with bulbar symptoms. Patients with ocular myasthenia gravis present with ptosis and diplopia. Dysarthria, dysphagia, or difficulties with chewing, with little or no limb weakness, can occasionally occur in patients with generalized (bulbar) myasthenia gravis. Electrodiagnostic testing is required in these patients to establish the presence of a neuromuscular junction disorder.

NCSs are normal in myasthenia gravis. In neuromuscular transmission disorders, a decrement of the CMAP with repetitive stimulation is demonstrated (Fig. 3-20). A decrement on RNS is seen in 85% of patients with generalized myasthenia gravis and in 17% of patients with ocular myasthenia gravis (10). When RNS studies are normal in patients with suspected myasthenia gravis, single-fiber EMG is performed. Single-fiber EMG is the most sensitive technique in the diagnosis of myasthenia gravis, with a sensitivity of 92% (11).

In the Lambert-Eaton myasthenic syndrome, motor CMAP amplitudes may be reduced. RNS typically shows a decrement with baseline stimulation. Immediately following either brief exercise or high-frequency RNS, an increment or increase is seen in the amplitude of the motor potentials (Fig. 3-21). This is referred to as increment or facilitation.

Assessing response to treatment is an important role of electrodiagnostic testing in the patient with a neuromuscular junction disorder. Not infrequently, patients will report persistent or recurrent weakness or fatigue during or following treatment. RNS studies can establish whether such symptoms are due to an inadequate treatment response (by showing persistent decrement).

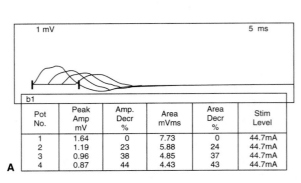

Pot No.	Peak Amp mV	Amp. Decr %	Area mVms	Area Decr %	Stim Level
1	1.64	0	7.73	0	44.7mA
2	1.19	23	5.88	24	44.7mA
3	0.96	38	4.85	37	44.7mA
4	0.87	44	4.43	43	44.7mA

A

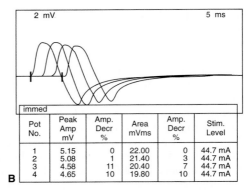

Pot No.	Peak Amp mV	Amp. Decr %	Area mVms	Amp. Decr %	Stim. Level
1	5.15	0	22.00	0	44.7 mA
2	5.08	1	21.40	3	44.7 mA
3	4.58	11	20.40	7	44.7 mA
4	4.65	10	19.80	10	44.7 mA

B

Figure 3-21. Increment with repetitive nerve stimulation in Lambert-Eaton myasthenic syndrome. Typical RNS findings in a patient with Lambert-Eaton myasthenic syndrome. **A:** Baseline 2-Hz stimulation of the ulnar nerve. Note the low-amplitude ulnar motor CMAP of 1.54 mV (normal >6 mV) and large decrement with RNS. **B:** A 234% increment in the ulnar CMAP following brief (10 seconds) exercise. Also note the repair of the decrement following exercise.

MOTOR NEURON DISEASE

Patients with motor neuron disease present with symptoms of weakness, fasciculations, and often muscle cramps. Patients with bulbar-onset motor neuron disease may present with dysarthria or dysphagia. The role of electrodiagnostic testing in suspected motor neuron disease is to exclude other neuromuscular disorders (such as multifocal motor neuropathy, myopathy, or polyradiculoneuropathy) and to establish the extent and severity of anterior horn cell disease.

NCSs are frequently abnormal in motor neuron disease. Motor CMAPs are often low amplitude, and motor distal latencies may be mildly prolonged. Motor conduction velocities and F-wave latencies are usually normal. Mild sensory NCS abnormalities are occasionally seen in patients with motor neuron disease. Patients may have an unrelated peripheral neuropathy due to some other cause (e.g., diabetic polyneuropathy). A small percentage of patients with true motor neuron disease may have mild sensory NCS abnormalities, possibly due to concomitant motor and sensory nerve degeneration (6). Severe sensory NCS abnormalities, conduction block or temporal dispersion of motor nerves, or marked slowing of motor conduction velocities should suggest an alternate diagnosis, such as a polyradiculoneuropathy or multifocal motor neuropathy.

Increased insertional activity, including fibrillation potentials and fasciculation potentials, is present on needle EMG. With activation, large motor unit potentials with reduced recruitment are seen. Needle EMG of muscles in bulbar, cervical, thoracic, and lumbosacral segments is examined to determine the extent and severity of disease.

REFERENCES

1. Bischoff C, Machetanz J, Conrad B. Is there an age-dependent continuous increase in the duration of the motor unit action potential? *Electroencephalogr Clin Neurophysiol.* 1991;81:304–311.

2. Boon AJ, Harper CM. Needle EMG of abductor hallucis and peroneus tertius in normal subjects. *Muscle Nerve.* 2003;27:752–756.

3. Critchley M. The neurology of old age. *Lancet.* 1931;i:1221–1230.

4. Dumitru D. *Electrodiagnostic Medicine.* Philadelphia: Hanley & Belfus; 1995.

5. Dyck PJ, Schultz PW, O'Brien PC. Quantitation of touch-pressure sensation. *Arch Neurol.* 1972; 26:465–473.

6. Dyck PJ, Stevens JC, Mulder DW. Frequency of nerve fiber degeneration of peripheral motor and sensory neurons in amyotrophic lateral sclerosis. *Neurology.* 1975;25:781–785.

7. Hitselberger WE, Witten RM. Abnormal myelograms in asymptomatic patients. *J Neurosurg.* 1968;28:204–206.

8. Howell TH. Senile deterioration of the central nervous system: a clinical study. BMJ. 1949;1:56–58.

9. Jacob JM, Love S. Qualitative and quantitative morphology of human sural nerve at different ages. *Brain.* 1985;108:897–924.

10. Oh SJ, Eslami N, Nishihara T, Sarala PK, Kuba T, Elmore RS, Sunwoo IN, Ro YI. Electrophysiological and clinical correlation in myasthenia gravis. *Ann Neurol.* 1982;12:348–354.

11. Oh SJ, Kim DE, Kuruoglu R, Bradley RJ, Dwyer D. Diagnostic sensitivity of the laboratory tests in myasthenia gravis. *Muscle Nerve.* 1992;15: 720–724.

12. Sarrigiannis PG, Kennett RP, Read S, Farrugia ME. Single-fiber EMG with a concentric needle electrode: validation in myasthenia gravis. *Muscle Nerve.* 2006;33:61–65.

13. Tomlinson BE, Irving D. The numbers of limb motor neurons in the human lumbosacral cord throughout life. *J Neurol Sci.* 1977;34: 213–219.

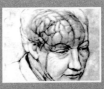

CHAPTER 4

Age-Related Changes in Pharmacokinetics, Drug Interactions, and Adverse Effects

James C. Cloyd and Jeannine M. Conway

Older adults (65 years of age or older) comprise 13% of the population and account for 35% of all prescription expenditures ($12.7 to $14.3 billion in 1991), and more than 69% of the elderly have more than one chronic medical condition (53,116). Community-dwelling older adults are reported to take, on average, 3.1 to 7.9 prescription and nonprescription medications, whereas nursing home residents have an average of 8.8 medication orders, with 32% of residents taking more than nine medications (23,119). Adults older than 65 are at double the risk for adverse drug reactions (ADRs) compared with younger adults, and they are more than seven times more likely to be hospitalized (10). Neuropsychiatric medications are among the most common causes of ADRs (10,65,111). Age alone does not appear to be a risk factor for ADRs, but older adults are at greater risk because they take a larger number of medications and have a greater number of medical problems (12,49,51). Alterations in pharmacokinetics and pharmacodynamics can also increase the ADR susceptibility in older adults, but no well-controlled studies

have evaluated their influence on ADRs (51). Problems associated with drug therapy in the elderly will likely become even more pronounced with the rapid rise in the population of the oldest old (≥85 years of age). Individuals ≥85 years old are projected to increase in number by 2050 to 5% of the U.S. population (124). Age-related changes in parameters necessitate a different approach to drug therapy in the elderly and place the older patient at greater risk for serious drug interactions and adverse events compared with younger adults. An understanding of the effects of advancing age on drug disposition and response and the mechanisms by which interactions occur permits the clinician to rationally prescribe and more effectively manage neuropsychiatric drug therapy in the older patient.

AGE-RELATED CHANGES IN PHYSIOLOGY: EFFECT ON PHARMACODYNAMICS AND PHARMACOKINETICS

The marked alterations in physiology that occur with advancing age affect both the pharmacokinetics and pharmacodynamics of drugs used to treat neuropsychiatric disorders. Changes in pharmacokinetics result in either higher or lower drug concentrations, depending on the variable contributions of absorption and elimination. Response, either beneficial or adverse, can be exaggerated or diminished even when the plasma drug concentration is unchanged. Physiologic changes affecting all aspects of drug disposition—absorption, distribution, metabolism, and elimination—occur as a person ages (Table 4-1). Aging also alters the number and function of central nervous system (CNS) receptors that determine the nature and intensity of response to drugs (103). Many diseases common to the elderly alter pharmacokinetics, pharmacodynamics, or both.

ABSORPTION

Drug absorption is influenced by several anatomic and physiologic factors, including gastric emptying, gastric and intestinal pH, quantity and quality of bile

Table 4-1. *Age-Related Changes in Physiology*

Absorption
Gastrointestinal blood flow	↓
Absorption	↔
Gastric pH	↓
Gastric emptying	↓
Intestinal motility	↓

Distribution
Lean body mass	↓
Body fat	↑
Plasma albumin	↓↔

Metabolism
Liver mass	↓
Hepatic blood flow	↓

Excretion
Kidney mass	↓
Renal blood flow	↓
Glomerular filtration	↓
Filtration fraction	↓

secretions, intestinal motility, condition and number of absorptive cells, enterocyte efflux, metabolizing enzymes, and intestinal blood flow (5,135). Absorption is also dependent on a drug's physical and chemical properties, such as release from the dosage form, dissolution, and lipophilicity (29).

No significant age-related change appears to exist in the anatomic features of the small intestine (73). Contrary to conventional wisdom, only a small percentage of the elderly (>70 years) have lost the ability to secrete acid due to chronic atrophic gastritis (54, 55). Pharmacotherapy with proton pump inhibitors results in an artificial achlorhydria, which may impact drug absorption. Gastric pH is important for drugs, including iron salts, ketoconazole, and ampicillin, that require an acidic pH for absorption (57). Gastric emptying can be decreased by half in 25% of the elderly greater than 70 years of age (27). Reduced motility will result in a longer residual time for medications and can affect absorption, depending on a drug's chemical properties. If a medication is rapidly absorbed because it readily dissolves and easily diffuses across luminal membranes into systemic circulation, changes in motility are unlikely to affect absorption. Drugs that are slowly absorbed because of poor aqueous solubility or decreased diffusion rate will exhibit increased bioavailability because of a longer resident time in the absorptive segment of the small intestine (29). Blood flow to the gastrointestinal tract is reduced with age; theoretically, this could result in decreased absorption of some drugs, but there is insufficient evidence to determine whether this is clinically important (5).

Until recently, it was assumed that the mechanism for drug absorption across the intestinal mucosa was passive diffusion. Active influx and efflux transport enzymes are now known to play a role in both the rate and extent of absorption. Gabapentin bioavailability is primarily mediated by an L-amino acid transport system that becomes saturated at clinically relevant doses (118). P-glycoprotein (P-gp), an efflux transporter located in intestinal enterocytes, pumps medications out of the cell and into the intestinal lumen, thereby decreasing drug absorption (129). P-gp is expressed in many tissues, including the adrenal cortex, brush border of the proximal renal tubule epithelium, pancreatic ductules, luminal surface of biliary hepatocytes, immunomodulation cells, blood–brain barrier, and the mucosa of the small and large intestines (69). P-gp is responsible for excreting 16% of an intravenous dose of digoxin into the gut lumen in mice, whereas only 2% of the dose was excreted in a P-gp knockout mouse (77). Certain drugs can either induce or inhibit P-gp, resulting in a decrease or increase in the bioavailability of the affected medication (34). Finally, drug absorption is affected by the presence of drug-metabolizing enzymes in the gastrointestinal mucosa. Cytochrome P450 (CYP) enzymes, which are located in intestinal enterocytes, can have a substantial impact on absorption (70). Midazolam, a CYP3A4 substrate, has a bioavailability of >90% following intramuscular administration but approximately 36% when given by mouth (96). The difference is largely attributable to metabolism in the gut wall. It is not known whether either the amount or function of P-gp or CYP enzymes in the gut changes with age.

Age-related changes in gastrointestinal physiology do not have a predictable effect on drug absorption. Most importantly, age-related changes in gastric function both within a patient and among patients may be highly variable. These unpredictable changes may alter the bioavailability of slowly absorbed drugs and should be considered when changes in response occur.

DISTRIBUTION

Drug distribution has two components: the extent to which the drug distributes throughout the body and the percentage bound to plasma proteins. Both are altered in old age. The distribution of a drug is partially dependent on its polarity. Highly polar compounds are hydrophilic and tend to distribute mainly into extracellular water. Lipophilic drugs tend to distribute mainly into tissue compartments, particularly muscle and fat. Age-related changes in body composition will alter volume of distribution (Vd). The percentage of body fat increases and lean body mass decreases with age (24,31,113). This shift in body composition may cause an increase in the Vd for lipophilic drugs and a decrease in the Vd for hydrophilic drugs.

Distribution volume is the key parameter in calculating loading doses, as is shown in the following equation: Loading dose = (Concentration desired—baseline concentration) * wt in kg * Vd (L/kg).

Distribution volume is usually determined from studies in younger adults. The elderly may have an unexpected response to a medication because their Vd deviates from the average younger adult values, resulting in a subtherapeutic or toxic plasma drug concentration.

Advancing age affects the extent to which CNS drugs bind to plasma proteins. Medications may bind to albumin, alpha$_1$-acid glycoprotein, globulins, and lipoproteins. Some drugs (e.g., zonisamide and topiramate) may also bind to erythrocytes (38,60,91). In the older adult, albumin, on average, declines slightly with age (11,44). Other conditions common in the elderly such as renal insufficiency, rheumatoid arthritis, and malnutrition also reduce albumin concentrations (44,128). In contrast, alpha$_1$-acid glycoprotein, which binds alkaline drugs, increases with age, and further elevations can occur from conditions such as stroke, heart failure, infection, trauma, myocardial infarction, arthritis, surgery, and chronic obstructive pulmonary disease (128).

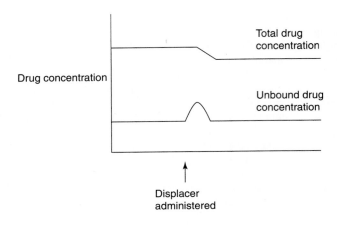

Figure 4-1. Effect of changes in protein binding and clearance on total concentration and unbound concentrations.

Only drugs protein-bound by 80% or more are significantly affected by alterations in plasma proteins. Most disruptions in binding are clinically unimportant but can cause a misinterpretation of drug concentrations. As shown in Figure 4-1, a decrease in protein binding results in lower total, but not unbound, concentrations for low hepatic extraction drugs. This occurs because only unbound drug in plasma diffuses into the hepatocyte or renal cell, where it is either metabolized or excreted. At steady-state, the dose and the clearance of unbound drug determine the unbound concentration in plasma. Drug freed from protein-binding sites (e.g., because of decreased albumin) becomes available for elimination. Because neither daily dose nor unbound clearance changes, unbound drug concentrations remain the same. Alterations in plasma proteins can complicate interpretation of laboratory values of highly bound drugs such as phenytoin (PHT). PHT is normally 90% bound to albumin. At a total PHT concentration of 15 mg/mL, the unbound concentration is 1.5 mg/L. This relationship can change over time as an elderly patient experiences a decline in plasma albumin. In such a patient, binding can decline to 80%, resulting in a total concentration of 7.5 mg/L, whereas the unbound concentration remains at 1.5 mg/L. In this situation, an increase in dose is not indicated.

METABOLISM

The two most important age-related physiologic changes that occur in the liver are decreased mass and reduced blood flow (Fig. 4-2). Wynne et al. (134) examined changes in liver mass (as assessed by ultrasound) and liver blood flow (indocyanine green clearance) with respect to age in men. Sixty-five patients were divided into three groups (<40, 40 to 64, and >65 years), with 20 patients over the age of 65. A 21% decrease in liver volume (in relation to body weight) was observed in the elderly male population. A 28% reduction in liver blood flow was also observed. The

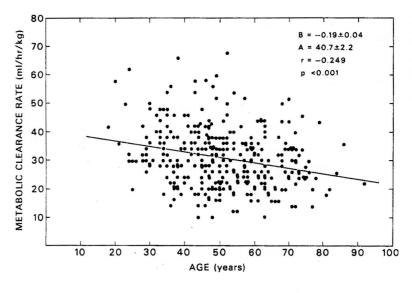

Figure 4-2. Effect of advancing age on antipyrine clearance. (From Vestal RE, Norris AH, Tobin JD, et al. Antipyrine metabolism in man: influence of age, alcohol, caffeine, and smoking. *Clin Pharmacol Ther.* 1975;18 (4):425–432.)

impact of advancing age on drug metabolism has been primarily studied in healthy, ambulatory subjects aged 65 to 75 years. No information is found regarding hepatic changes in the oldest old (≥85 years) or in frail older patients. Both groups are likely to have diminished drug-metabolizing capacity relative to younger, healthier elderly adults.

Hepatic metabolism is divided into two phases. Phase I consists of oxidative, reduction, and hydroxylation reactions. The CYP family of enzymes generally catalyzes the oxidative reactions. Phase II reactions are conjugation reactions involving glucuronic acid or sulfates in which conjugated product is made more polar, allowing it to be excreted into the urine or bile. Conjugation reactions can involve either the drug (primary conjugation) or the metabolite of a phase I reaction (132).

The CYP system consists of a family of closely related enzymes known as isoenzymes, each of which catalyzes the metabolism of a unique set of substrates. Table 4-2 lists the major isoenzymes that catalyze the metabolism of numerous neurologic drugs. Available evidence indicates that CYP metabolizing activity declines approximately 1% a year beginning at age 40, although substantial intrapatient variability is seen (115). Antipyrine metabolism is associated with CYP metabolism, and clearance of antipyrine declines with age, as shown in Figure 4-2.

Many CNS drugs that undergo either primary or secondary metabolism via conjugation reactions with glucuronic acid are mediated by uridine glucuronyl transferases (UGT) (4,125). As with the CYP system, UGTs are composed of isoenzymes with specific drug substrates (99). The effect of age on glucuronidation is less well understood than the CYP system. Greenblatt et al. (45,46) and Divoll et al. (21) studied the pharmacokinetics of several benzodiazepines (oxazepam, temazepam, and lorazepam) that undergo extensive glucuronidation in elderly patients, most of whom ranged in age from 65 to 75 years. Drug clearance was similar in elderly and younger subjects. The studies gave rise to the view that glucuronidation activity is spared in the elderly.

EXCRETION

Many drugs and their metabolites are eliminated completely or partly by the kidney. Age-related changes in renal function are well established (71,82,93,109). Anatomic changes result in decreased kidney size, decreased renal blood flow, a loss of glomeruli, and renal tubular changes (82,93). Functional changes include a decrease in glomerular filtration, decreased creatinine clearance, and increased serum creatinine concentrations (108). Renal function decreases begin at age 40, resulting in

a 40% decline in renal function by age 70 as compared with age 30 (72).

Reductions in renal function will result in a decrease in the clearance of drugs eliminated by the kidney. Serum creatinine is not a reliable marker of renal function in the elderly because creatinine is a byproduct of muscle and, as individuals age, lean body mass and serum creatinine decline (86). For example, a serum creatinine level (SCr) of 1.0 mg/dL, which is within the normal range, does not accurately estimate the creatinine clearance in a 41-kg woman who is 80 years of age. An estimated creatinine clearance (ClCr) adjusted for age, gender, and weight (when a patient is within 30% of his or her ideal body weight) provides a better indicator of renal function in the elderly (17). In most patients, an estimate of creatinine clearance can be used to adjust dosage. One such method is the Cockcroft-Gault equation:

$$ClCr = \frac{(140 - age)(wt\ in\ kg) * (0.85\ if\ patient\ is\ female)}{72 * Scr}$$

Using this equation, a woman 80 years of age would have an estimated creatinine clearance of 25 mL/min, necessitating a substantial change in dose for drugs such as gabapentin, which is virtually 100% renally eliminated. In contrast a 65-kg woman who is 30 years of age with a serum creatinine of 1.0 mg/dL would have an estimated creatinine clearance of 84 mL/min. Although an improvement over the use of an unadjusted SCr, the Cockcroft-Gault equation has its own limitations. In a healthy elderly patient, it may underpredict renal function, resulting in subtherapeutic dosing, and if the patient is frail, it may overpredict renal function, resulting in unexpected toxicity (30). The available evidence supports the conclusion that drug elimination via renal excretion or metabolism by either phase I or phase II declines with advancing age, although there is considerable variability. As a general rule, elderly patients should initiate therapy at a dose 30% to 50% less than younger adults, and dosing intervals can be extended as the elimination half-life is prolonged.

PHARMACODYNAMICS

Pharmacodynamics is the major source of variation in drug response (67). Age-related changes in pharmacodynamics are drug specific and can result in greater or diminished responses (16). Studies indicate that the elderly are more sensitive to CNS depressants than younger adults. Following administration of the same dose of diazepam, elderly patients experienced more pronounced sedative effects, although unbound serum concentrations were comparable to those observed in

Table 4-2. *CYP Enzymes Responsible for Neurologic Drug Metabolism and Their Induction and Inhibition*

1A2	2C9	2C19	2D6	3A4
Substrates				
Caffeine	Fluoxetine	Citalopram	Amitriptyline	Alprazolam
Carbamazepine	Phenytoin	Clomipramine	Desipramine	Carbamazepine
Clozapine	Valproic Acid	Diazepam	Donepezil	Citalopram
Fluvoxamine		Felbamate	Duloxetine	Clonazepam
Mirtazapine (minor)		Imipramine	Fluoxetine (minor)	Clozapine
Olanzapine		Phenytoin (minor)	Fluvoxamine	Donepezil
Ropinirole		Sertraline (minor)	Galantamine	Eszopiclone
Tacrine			Haloperidol	Galantamine
			Imipramine	Haloperidol
			Mirtazapine (minor)	Midazolam
			Nortriptyline	Mirtazapine
			Paroxetine	Nefazodone
			Perphenazine	Ropinirole (minor)
			Risperidone	Sertraline (major)
			Sertraline	Tiagabine
			Thioridazine	Triazolam
			Venlafaxine	Zaleplon
				Ziprasidone
				Zolipidem
				Zonisamide
Inducers				
Omeprazole	Carbamazepine	Carbamazepine		Carbamazepine
Tobacco	Phenobarbital	Phenytoin		Oxcarbazepine
	Rifampin	Rifampin		Phenobarbital
				Phenytoin
				Rifampin
				St. John's Wort
Inhibitors				
Cimetidine	Fluconazole	Cimetidine	Bupropion	Clarithromycin
Ciprofloxacin	Fluoxetine	Felbamate	Cimetidine	Diltiazem
Fluvoxamine	Fluvoxamine (moderate)	Fluconazole	Clomipramine	Erythromycin
		Fluoxetine	Duloxetine (moderate)	Fluconazole
		Fluvoxamine	Fluoxetine	Fluoxetine (moderate)
		Omeprazole	Paroxetine	Fluvoxamine (moderate)
		Oxcarbazepine		Grapefruit juice substances
		Sertraline (moderate)		Itraconazole
		Topiramate		Ketoconazole
				Nefazodone

Note: This table is not all inclusive. The authors recommend that all practitioners use drug interaction references or databases to check for potential interactions when prescribing medications.

younger adults (18). Older adults also exhibited exaggerated sedative effects after administration of midazolam, although the dose was reduced for the elderly study group and both groups had similar plasma concentrations (98). Little information is found about altered pharmacodynamics of other CNS drugs with age. It is reasonable to conclude that CNS depressants are likely to produce a greater effect in the elderly than in younger adults, even when doses are adjusted.

DRUG INTERACTIONS

The probability of a drug interaction increases significantly with the number of medications a person takes (92). The elderly have an increased risk of an unintended drug interactions because of the larger number of medications they take, age-related reductions in clearance, and greater sensitivity to drug effects. Drug interactions fall into two categories: pharmacokinetic and pharmacodynamic. In the former, one or both drugs affect the concentration of the other. In the latter, a drug combination can produce an additive (or supra-additive) effect, in which the desired or toxic response is exaggerated, or an antagonistic effect, in which one drug diminishes the desired effect of another. Advances in clinical pharmacology now provide clinicians with a better understanding of the underlying mechanisms and probability of drug interactions.

Knowledge of a drug's metabolic pathway and its activity as an inhibitor or inducer of metabolizing enzymes permits the prediction of drug combinations that are likely to interact. This allows the clinician to either select drugs without interaction potential or implement a plan to manage an interaction through patient education, monitoring, and dosage adjustment.

PHARMACOKINETIC DRUG INTERACTIONS

Absorption

Most medications are prescribed as oral dosage forms, which makes them susceptible to absorption interactions. Interactions can affect both the rate and extent of absorption. Changes in the rate of absorption will either increase or decrease the maximal plasma concentration (C_{max}) depending on the effect of the interacting drug. Such interactions are important for medications, such as analgesics or sedatives, in which C_{max} is an important contributor to response. Interactions resulting in either an increase or decrease in the extent of absorption (bioavailability) affects the total drug exposure. Changes in bioavailability are known to alter the response to antiepileptic drugs. Several different mechanisms reduce the absorption of drug from the gastrointestinal tract. Absorption will be hindered if the active medication binds to a cation to form an insoluble chelate. This interaction occurs when phenytoin is taken in combination with calcium-containing antacids (63). This can be a particularly relevant drug interaction because the older adult is more likely to use antacids to treat dyspepsia. Medications, disease, or aging can induce alterations in gastrointestinal tract motility. Anticholinergic medications (amitriptyline) and opioids decrease gastrointestinal motility, whereas prokinetic medications (metoclopramide) have the opposite effect (29). The bioavailability of drugs that are slowly absorbed (e.g., phenytoin and carbamazepine) or are given as controlled-release formulations can decrease with prokinetic medications. The bioavailability of drugs that are incompletely and slowly absorbed can increase in the presence of reduced gastrointestinal motility.

Inhibition or induction of P-gp can affect drug response. The best characterized interaction is P-gp inhibition by quinidine, which results in digoxin toxicity (35). Conversely, induction of P-gp will result in decreased bioavailability of susceptible drugs, although little is known about the importance of this transporter enzyme in the absorption of neurologic drugs. Rifampin is an inducer of P-gp as well as CYP isoenzymes (48,126). Serum concentrations of neurologic drugs that are substrates for both P-gp and CYP enzymes can be significantly reduced in the presence of rifampin or other inducers affecting both systems. Additional research is necessary to determine which neurologic drugs are transported by P-gp and how P-gp inhibition and induction affect the absorption of these drugs.

Protein Binding

Certain drugs can displace others from protein-binding sites. As discussed earlier in this chapter, the net result of such an interaction is a decrease in total but not unbound steady-state drug concentration. This interaction is only apparent for drugs in which plasma concentrations are measured. In most cases, protein-binding interactions do not require any adjustment in dosage.

Metabolism

The most clinically important drug interactions involve inhibition or induction of metabolism. Drug–drug interactions can be unilateral (i.e., one drug affects the other) or bilateral (each drug affects the other). Interactions can produce significant increases or decreases in the concentration of the affected drugs. Drugs that are metabolized by the same isoenzyme are more likely to interact; however, an inhibitor can bind to isoenzymes other than the one that mediates its metabolism. For example, fluoxetine is primarily metabolized by CYP2D6 but is an intermediate inhibitor of 3A4 in vitro (102). The extent of an inhibition interaction is determined by the fraction of the affected drug metabolized by the inhibited pathway and the concentration of the inhibitor relative to its inhibitory constant (Ki).

Inhibition of a CYP enzyme occurs via three mechanisms: reversible inhibition, quasi-irreversible inhibition, and irreversible inhibition (68). The most common mechanism is reversible inhibition that results from competition at the enzyme site. The time course for inhibition is dependent on the half-lives and the time to steady-state of the interacting drugs (83). As the inhibitor concentration approaches its Ki, the clearance of the affected drug decreases, and the plasma level rises. This can occur with the first dose of the inhibitor. The full effect of an inhibition reaction can take several days or longer because it is dependent on the new, prolonged half-life of the affected drug.

The most complex drug interactions are those that alter protein binding and metabolism simultaneously. As shown in Figure 4-3, valproate displaces phenytoin

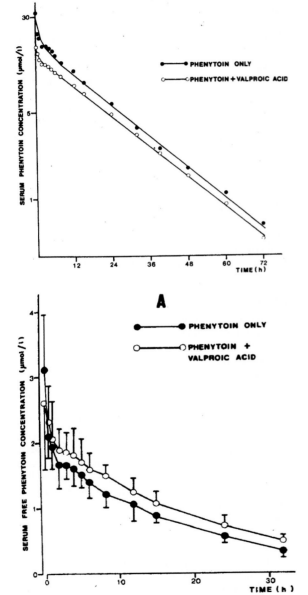

Figure 4-3. Effect of valproic acid on phenytoin total and unbound drug. (From Perucca E, Hebdige S, Frigo GM, et al. Interaction between phenytoin and valproic acid: plasma protein binding and metabolic effects. *Clin Pharmacol Ther.* 1980;28:779–789.)

from protein-binding sites, thus lowering total plasma PHT levels. At clinically relevant concentrations, valproate modestly inhibits phenytoin metabolism, resulting in an increase in unbound PHT levels. Depending on the extent of each interaction, a patient may present with symptoms of blurred vision and ataxia with total PHT concentrations that are unchanged or decreased.

Deinhibition of the enzyme is dependent on the elimination half-life of the inhibiting drug (83). The time for the affected drug to adjust to deinhibition is determined by its half-life to reach a new steady-state. As the concentration of the inhibitor falls below its Ki, the affected drug concentration will begin to decrease.

Induction of metabolic enzymes occurs when a stimulus causes more enzyme to be synthesized. The time course for induction is dependent on the rate of degradation of enzyme and the formation of new enzyme (94). It also appears that the half-life of a drug that triggers induction may partially account for the rate of induction. Rifampin has a half-life of 3 to 4 hours and demonstrates induction at 2 to 3 days, whereas phenobarbital has a half-life of up to 140 hours and takes several weeks to exert its effect (83).

The implication of enzyme inhibition and induction interactions is that the drug interaction may not be immediately clinically evident. It can take days to several weeks for a patient to become dizzy and unsteady on a dose that was changed 2 weeks previously. If the medication that causes the enzyme induction or inhibition is discontinued, the patient might begin to experience toxicity, or the drug may lose efficacy (Table 4-2).

Renal Elimination

Drug interactions involving elimination can occur. A few medications can inhibit tubular secretion and cause the clearance of affected drugs to decrease. The most common example of this interaction is the concomitant administration of probenecid with penicillin. Probenecid inhibits the secretion of penicillin into the urine, thereby decreasing its clearance (37).

Many medications and their metabolites are eliminated via glomerular filtration. The elderly may have decreased renal function and may take medications that acutely alter their renal function. Nonsteroidal anti-inflammatory drugs (NSAIDs) can inhibit prostaglandins that are necessary to maintain blood flow to the kidney, thereby decreasing glomerular filtration and the clearance of the medication or active metabolite. Generally, renal function is restored when the drug is discontinued (8,130).

PHARMACODYNAMICS

Understanding pharmacology helps predict possible drug interactions caused by pharmacodynamics. Medications that exert their effect on similar receptors can create an interaction. For example, administering haloperidol to a patient on levodopa may result in blocking the effects of the levodopa on dopamine receptors (133). Another interaction is the additive effect that two medications may have on a patient (e.g., amitriptyline and diphenhydramine). Amitriptyline has a high incidence of anticholinergic side effects when administered alone. When a patient adds diphenhydramine (an over-the-counter antihistamine), the patient increases his or her chance of having additional anticholinergic side effects (9). Also, a risk exists of a medication with an unknown mechanism or multiple mechanisms of action creating a pharmacodynamic effect that was not intuitively predictable; hence, greater vigilance by the practitioner is required. Although consideration of the above factors improves the ability to prevent or manage drug interactions, they remain difficult to predict because of interpatient variability in pharmacokinetics and pharmacodynamics.

ADVERSE DRUG REACTIONS

Adverse drug reactions (ADRs) are defined by the World Health Organization to be "any response to a drug that is noxious or unintended, and which occurs at doses used in man for prophylaxis, diagnosis, or therapy" (127). ADRs have been estimated to account for 7.9% to 24% of all hospitalizations of elderly patients (50,74). In a study by Hanlon et al. (52), an examination of veteran outpatients taking at least five medications demonstrated that the second most common cause of adverse reactions were CNS drugs.

Minimizing the number of medications is the key to reducing the risk of ADRs in the elderly. Assessing all medications a patient takes, including over-the-counter products, prescription drugs, and dietary supplements, is essential to prevent or to manage predictable adverse reactions before they occur (19).

Drugs that are not benefiting the patient should be discontinued. In some situations, a less toxic drug can be substituted for one causing side effects without loss of therapeutic effect. ADRs associated with CNS drugs can also result from changes in health status such as the onset of dementia or the development of tremor. The clinician should ascertain whether the ADR is a symptom of a medical problem or is exacerbated by that problem. Dosage requirements for older adults are generally reduced. The initial maintenance dose should be lower than that used in younger adults, and dose titration should proceed more slowly. Ensuring medication compliance, implementing therapeutic drug monitoring strategies, and periodically checking laboratory tests are other important steps associated with reducing the risk of ADR.

Discontinuing medications also puts the patient at risk for ADRs (42). Benzodiazepines can cause withdrawal symptoms and need to be slowly tapered. Medications that inhibit or induce drug-metabolizing enzymes can cause ADRs when they are being discontinued due to alterations in the concentration of the affected drug as the liver returns to its baseline metabolic activity. See the earlier Drug Interactions section for further discussion.

ADRs can be divided into two classes: type A (dose related) and type B (non–dose related). Dose-related drug effects are adverse effects that tend to be an exaggeration of a medication's pharmacology; they are predictable and dose related. Examples of dose-related ADRs include drowsiness, headache, and nausea, which account for 70% to 80% of all side effects, most of which are preventable (25,88). Non–dose-related drug effects occur unpredictably and can be severe reactions that are occasionally associated with significant morbidity and mortality such as Stevens-Johnson rash, acute organ failure, and blood dyscrasias. Some of the more commonly prescribed neurologic drugs have adverse reactions that can be particularly troublesome for older adults.

ANTIEPILEPTIC DRUGS

All of the older antiepileptic drugs (AED)—phenobarbital, phenytoin, carbamazepine, and valproic acid—are associated with numerous ADRs, including concentration-dependent CNS effects resulting in dizziness, unsteadiness, nystagmus, and diplopia. Carbamazepine-induced hyponatremia is more prevalent in the elderly (22,84). A major disadvantage to phenobarbital therapy is sedation, particularly in a population that may already have decreased mentation. All of the older AED medications have been associated with an increased risk of syncope and falls in the elderly (26,32).

The newer AEDs (felbamate, gabapentin, topiramate, tiagabine, lamotrigine, oxcarbazepine, levetiracetam, zonisamide, and pregabalin) also cause CNS adverse reactions including dizziness, headache, and somnolence similar to the older AEDs. Felbamate is rarely used because of the risk of aplastic anemia and hepatic failure. Lamotrigine is associated with a 7% occurrence of nonserious rash and a 1% occurrence of serious rash (i.e., Stevens-Johnson syndrome) (131). It should be dosed and monitored carefully when given concomitantly with valproic acid, as the latter inhibits lamotrigine's metabolism and greatly increases the risk of rash (81). A recent study that compared carbamazepine, lamotrigine, and gabapentin use in an elderly veteran population observed rash most frequently in the carbamazepine group (107). Oxcarbazepine can cause hyponatremia, which requires medication discontinuation (22,95). Patients also taking diuretics are at particular risk for becoming hyponatremic, and monitoring sodium is recommended (110). Tiagabine may cause dizziness, nervousness, tremor, and depression. Topiramate can cause significant cognitive impairment in younger adults and should be titrated carefully in the older adult (1). It can also cause weight loss (100) and renal calculi (64), which can be problematic in the frail older adult. Zonisamide can also cause CNS side effects and renal calculi (66). Levetiracetam has been shown to have an increased incidence of dizziness and somnolence in a younger adult population, which may be magnified when it is administered to an older population (15). Pregabalin is associated with dizziness, peripheral edema, and weight gain in older adults (33).

ANTIDEPRESSANTS

Antidepressants are used in the geriatric population for various reasons, including pain, headache, and depression. ADRs commonly occur with both tricyclic antidepressants (TCAs) and selective serotonin reuptake inhibitors (SSRIs). TCAs are noted for their anticholinergic effects that result in dry mouth, blurred vision, tachycardia, constipation, urinary retention, and confusion, all of which can be problematic in an elderly patient. Tricyclics can also cause orthostatic hypotension, seizures, and cardiac arrhythmias that may be magnified in the elderly (87). SSRIs and the newer antidepressants lack the cardiac side effects of tricyclic antidepressants, making them the preferred medications for initial treatment of depression in the elderly (2). The most frequent adverse reactions associated with SSRIs are insomnia, nausea, loose stools, and sexual dysfunction (80). Weight changes can also occur (101). The most common adverse reactions to bupropion are insomnia and headache, although it can cause seizures if the dose is increased quickly or exceeds 450 mg/d (20). The risk of seizures is significantly less with the extended-release formulations (112). It is not clear whether elderly patients are more likely to have seizures than younger adults. Venlafaxine, in a small percentage of older adults, caused a dose-related increase in blood pressure, which should be recognized as a potential adverse reaction and, therefore, should reduce the addition of potentially unnecessary treatment for hypertension (117). Nefazodone causes dose-related sedation, somnolence, dizziness, lightheadedness, blurred vision, and asthenia (104). Its use is limited by acute hepatic toxicity (13). Mirtazapine has been associated with transient somnolence (28). Duloxetine is associated with dry mouth, constipation, decreased appetite, insomnia, and fatigue when compared with placebo (89).

Although adverse reactions to antidepressants can occur at any age, it is clear that the risk for cognitive impairment is greater when administering TCAs in elderly patients (85). Adverse reactions to which younger adults can adjust may have a greater impact on an older adult's ability to function.

BENZODIAZEPINES

Approximately 10% of the elderly take a benzodiazepine (40,43). Benzodiazepines, commonly cause adverse events in the older adult, can result in side effects and falls. Medications with an extremely long half-life can cause daytime somnolence, confusion, and increased risk of falls (114). Although the older adult may have a similar plasma concentration of drug as their younger counterparts, they have significantly more CNS depression (14,47,123).

PARKINSON'S MEDICATIONS

Patients with Parkinson's disease are a challenge to dose and monitor because the disease has many symptoms that mirror the common adverse reactions to medications, including lethargy, cognitive impairment, falls, and sedation (6). Medications are classified as presynaptic drugs (e.g., carbidopa or levodopa, tolcapone, selegiline, and amantadine) and postsynaptic drugs (e.g., pergolide, bromocriptine, pramipexole, and ropinirole). The most common adverse reactions associated with these medications are abdominal discomfort and nausea at the initiation of therapy (61). Increased peripheral dopamine levels are associated with hypotension, nausea, and vomiting. These effects are decreased by an adequate carbidopa dose (62).

ALZHEIMER DRUGS

Pharmacotherapy for Alzheimer's disease is limited. The use of tacrine is limited by a high incidence of nausea, vomiting, diarrhea, dyspepsia, myalgias, and elevations in liver enzymes (7,41). Donepezil, rivastigmine, and glantamine are all associated with gastrointestinal reactions that generally occur while the dose is being titrated upward (36,105,106). Patients may overcome the gastrointestinal adverse reactions if therapy is initiated at the lowest dose available and gradually titrated up to the desired level. Memantine is well tolerated compared with placebo, with agitation occasionally occurring (97).

ANTIPSYCHOTICS

Some conditions that occur in the elderly (e.g., Alzheimer's and Parkinson's diseases) have symptoms of dementia. Adverse reactions associated with all of the antipsychotic drugs can be serious and irreversible. Older antipsychotics (i.e., haloperidol) can cause drug-induced parkinsonism in the older adult (122). The risk of developing tardive dyskinesia is greater in the elderly, and the risk is increased after as few as 3 months of antipsychotic drug therapy (39,58,121). Atypical antipsychotics have equal efficacy compared with the older drugs but with fewer extrapyramidal side effects (79). All of the atypical antipsychotics are associated with somnolence in the elderly (59). Clozapine causes orthostatic hypotension and requires a slow titration to overcome this adverse effect (76). Blood counts should be monitored weekly for the first 6 months, or until stable, and then biweekly indefinitely during clozapine treatment because of the possible development of agranulocytosis, for which age is thought to be a risk factor (3). Risperidone can cause extrapyramidal symptoms at higher doses; therefore, therapy should begin with a low dose (75). Olanzapine appears to be well tolerated in the older adult, although abnormal gait and metabolic changes, including weight gain, fasting blood glucose increases, and elevations in lipid panels, can occur (56,120). Quetiapine also appears to be tolerated, with the most common adverse reactions being somnolence, dizziness, postural hypotension, and agitation. Extrapyramidal adverse effects can also occur (78).

CONCLUSION

Neurologic drug therapy in the elderly presents formidable challenges for the clinician. Alterations in pharmacokinetics and pharmacodynamics because of aging and disease affect response and increase the risk of adverse reactions. Although drug elimination declines with advancing age, there is substantial interpatient variability, which complicates dose estimation. The use of multiple prescription and over-the-counter drugs, vitamins, and natural products significantly increases the likelihood of drug interactions. Minimizing the number of drugs, maintaining up-to-date records on medication use, ensuring good compliance, starting with low doses, and slowly titrating a drug are important factors in providing safe and effective therapy. Patients need to be told to advise their physicians when they are starting or discontinuing a medication or natural product. Application of basic principles will result in improved outcomes, a lower risk of adverse reactions, and the ability to prevent or manage interactions.

REFERENCES

1. Aldenkamp AP, Baker G, Mulder OG, et al. A multicenter, randomized clinical study to evaluate the effect on cognitive function of topiramate compared with valproate as add-on therapy to carbamazepine in patients with partial-onset seizures. *Epilepsia.* 2000;41:1167–1178.
2. Alexopoulos GS. Depression in the elderly. *Lancet.* 2005;365:1961–1970.
3. Alvir JM, Lieberman JA, Safferman AZ, et al. Clozapine-induced agranulocytosis. Incidence and risk factors in the United States. *N Engl J Med.* 1993;329:162–167.
4. Anderson GD. A mechanistic approach to antiepileptic drug interactions. *Ann Pharmacother.* 1998;32:554–563.
5. Bender AD. Effect of age on intestinal absorption: implications for drug absorption in the elderly. *J Am Geriatr Soc.* 1968;16:1331–1339.
6. Berchou RC. Maximizing the benefit of pharmacotherapy in Parkinson's disease. *Pharmacotherapy.* 2000;20:33S–42S.
7. Blackard WG Jr, Sood GK, Crowe DR, et al. Tacrine. A cause of fatal hepatotoxicity? *J Clin Gastroenterol.* 1998;26:57–59.
8. Blackshear JL, Davidman M, Stillman MT. Identification of risk for renal insufficiency from nonsteroidal anti-inflammatory drugs. *Arch Intern Med.* 1983;143:1130–1134.
9. Blazer DG 2nd, Federspiel CF, Ray WA, et al. The risk of anticholinergic toxicity in the elderly: a study of prescribing practices in two populations. *J Gerontol.* 1983;38:31–35.
10. Budnitz DS, Pollock DA, Weidenbach KN, et al. National surveillance of emergency department visits for outpatient adverse drug events. *JAMA.* 2006;296:1858–1866.
11. Campion EW, deLabry LO, Glynn RJ. The effect of age on serum albumin in healthy males: report from the Normative Aging Study. *J Gerontol.* 1988;43:M18–M20.
12. Carbonin P, Pahor M, Bernabei R, et al. Is age an independent risk factor of adverse drug reactions in hospitalized medical patients? *J Am Geriatr Soc.* 1991;39:1093–1099.
13. Carvajal Garcia-Pando A, Garcia del Pozo J, Sanchez AS, et al. Hepatotoxicity associated with the new antidepressants. *J Clin Psychiatry.* 2002;63:135–137.
14. Castleden CM, George CF, Marcer D, et al. Increased sensitivity to nitrazepam in old age. *Br Med J.* 1977;1:10–12.
15. Cereghino JJ, Biton V, Abou-Khalil B, et al. Levetiracetam for partial seizures: results of a double-blind, randomized clinical trial. *Neurology.* 2000;55:236–242.
16. Chapron D. Drug disposition and response. In: Delafuente J, Stewart R, eds. *Therapeutics in the elderly.* Cincinnati: Harvey Whitney Books Company; 2001:257–288.
17. Cockcroft DW, Gault MH. Prediction of creatinine clearance from serum creatinine. *Nephron.* 1976;16:31–41.
18. Cook PJ, Flanagan R, James IM. Diazepam tolerance: effect of age, regular sedation, and alcohol. *Br Med J (Clin Res Ed).* 1984;289: 351–353.
19. Cunningham G. Adverse drug reactions in the elderly and their prevention. *Scott Med J.* 1997; 42:136–137.
20. Davidson J. Seizures and bupropion: a review. *J Clin Psychiatry.* 1989;50:256–261.

21. Divoll M, Greenblatt DJ, Harmatz JS, et al. Effect of age and gender on disposition of temazepam. *J Pharm Sci.* 1981;70:1104–1107.

22. Dong X, Leppik IE, White J, et al. Hyponatremia from oxcarbazepine and carbamazepine. *Neurology.* 2005;65:1976–1978.

23. Doshi JA, Shaffer T, Briesacher BA. National estimates of medication use in nursing homes: findings from the 1997 Medicare current beneficiary survey and the 1996 medical expenditure survey. *J Am Geriatr Soc.* 2005;53:438–443.

24. Edelman IS, Leibman J. Anatomy of body water and electrolytes. *Am J Med.* 1959;27:256–277.

25. Edwards IR, Aronson JK. Adverse drug reactions: definitions, diagnosis, and management. *Lancet.* 2000;356:1255–1259.

26. Ensrud KE, Blackwell TL, Mangione CM, et al. Central nervous system-active medications and risk for falls in older women. *J Am Geriatr Soc.* 2002;50:1629–1637.

27. Evans MA, Triggs EJ, Cheung M, et al. Gastric emptying rate in the elderly: implications for drug therapy. *J Am Geriatr Soc.* 1981;29:201–205.

28. Fawcett J, Barkin RL. Review of the results from clinical studies on the efficacy, safety and tolerability of mirtazapine for the treatment of patients with major depression. *J Affect Disord.* 1998;51:267–285.

29. Fleisher D, Li C, Zhou Y, et al. Drug, meal and formulation interactions influencing drug absorption after oral administration. Clinical implications. *Clin Pharmacokinet.* 1999;36:233–254.

30. Fliser D, Franek E, Joest M, et al. Renal function in the elderly: impact of hypertension and cardiac function. *Kidney Int.* 1997;51:1196–1204.

31. Forbes GB, Reina JC. Adult lean body mass declines with age: some longitudinal observations. *Metabolism.* 1970;19:653–663.

32. French DD, Campbell R, Spehar A, et al. Drugs and falls in community-dwelling older people: a national veterans study. *Clin Ther.* 2006;28:619–630.

33. Freynhagen R, Strojek K, Griesing T, et al. Efficacy of pregabalin in neuropathic pain evaluated in a 12-week, randomised, double-blind, multicentre, placebo-controlled trial of flexible- and fixed-dose regimens. *Pain.* 2005;115:254–263.

34. Fromm MF. P-glycoprotein: a defense mechanism limiting oral bioavailability and CNS accumulation of drugs. *Int J Clin Pharmacol Ther.* 2000;38:69–74.

35. Fromm MF, Kim RB, Stein CM, et al. Inhibition of P-glycoprotein-mediated drug transport: a unifying mechanism to explain the interaction between digoxin and quinidine. *Circulation.* 1999;99:552–557.

36. Fulton B, Benfield P. Galanthamine. *Drugs Aging.* 1996;9:60–65.

37. Gibaldi M, Schwartz MA. Apparent effect of probenecid on the distribution of penicillins in man. *Clin Pharmacol Ther.* 1968;9:345–349.

38. Gidal BE, Lensmeyer GL. Therapeutic monitoring of topiramate: evaluation of the saturable distribution between erythrocytes and plasma of whole blood using an optimized high-pressure liquid chromatography method. *Ther Drug Monit.* 1999;21:567–576.

39. Glazer WM, Morgenstern H, Doucette JT. Predicting the long-term risk of tardive dyskinesia in outpatients maintained on neuroleptic medications. *J Clin Psychiatry.* 1993;54:133–139.

40. Gleason PP, Schulz R, Smith NL, et al. Correlates and prevalence of benzodiazepine use in community-dwelling elderly. *J Gen Intern Med.* 1998;13:243–250.

41. Gracon SI, Knapp MJ, Berghoff WG, et al. Safety of tacrine: clinical trials, treatment IND, and postmarketing experience. *Alzheimer Dis Assoc Disord.* 1998;12:93–101.

42. Graves T, Hanlon JT, Schmader KE, et al. Adverse events after discontinuing medications in elderly outpatients. *Arch Intern Med.* 1997;157:2205–2210.

43. Gray SL, Eggen AE, Blough D, et al. Benzodiazepine use in older adults enrolled in a health maintenance organization. *Am J Geriatr Psychiatry.* 2003;11:568–576.

44. Greenblatt DJ. Reduced serum albumin concentration in the elderly: a report from the Boston Collaborative Drug Surveillance Program. *J Am Geriatr Soc.* 1979;27:20–22.

45. Greenblatt DJ, Divoll M, Harmatz JS, et al. Oxazepam kinetics: effects of age and sex. *J Pharmacol Exp Ther.* 1980;215:86–91.

46. Greenblatt DJ, Harmatz JS, Shader RI. Clinical pharmacokinetics of anxiolytics and hypnotics in the elderly. Therapeutic considerations (Part I). *Clin Pharmacokinet.* 1991;21:165–177.

47. Greenblatt DJ, Harmatz JS, von Moltke LL, et al. Age and gender effects on the pharmacokinetics and pharmacodynamics of triazolam, a cytochrome P450 3A substrate. *Clin Pharmacol Ther.* 2004;76:467–479.

48. Greiner B, Eichelbaum M, Fritz P, et al. The role of intestinal P-glycoprotein in the interaction of digoxin and rifampin. *J Clin Invest.* 1999;104:147–153.

49. Grymonpre RE, Mitenko PA, Sitar DS, et al. Drug-associated hospital admissions in older medical patients. *J Am Geriatr Soc.* 1988;36:1092–1098.

50. Hallas J, Gram LF, Grodum E, et al. Drug related admissions to medical wards: a population based survey. *Br J Clin Pharmacol*. 1992;33:61–68.

51. Hanlon JT, Gray SL, Schmader KE. Adverse drug reactions. In: Delafuente J, Stewart R, eds. *Therapeutics in the elderly*. Cincinnati: Harvey Whitney Books Company; 2001:289–314.

52. Hanlon JT, Schmader KE, Koronkowski MJ, et al. Adverse drug events in high risk older outpatients. *J Am Geriatr Soc*. 1997;45:945–948.

53. Hoffman C, Rice D, Sung HY. Persons with chronic conditions. Their prevalence and costs *JAMA*. 1996;276:1473–1479.

54. Hurwitz A, Brady DA, Schaal SE, et al. Gastric acidity in older adults. *JAMA*. 1997;278:659–662.

55. Hurwit A, Ruhl CE, Kimler BF, et al. Gastric function in the elderly: effects on absorption of ketoconazole. *J Clin Pharmacol*. 2003;43:996–1002.

56. Hwang JP, Yang CH, Lee TW, et al. The efficacy and safety of olanzapine for the treatment of geriatric psychosis. *J Clin Psychopharmacol*. 2003;23:113–118.

57. Iber FL, Murphy PA, Connor ES. Age-related changes in the gastrointestinal system. Effects on drug therapy. *Drugs Aging*. 1994;5:34–48.

58. Jeste DV, Caligiuri MP, Paulsen JS, et al. Risk of tardive dyskinesia in older patients. A prospective longitudinal study of 266 outpatients. *Arch Gen Psychiatry*. 1995;52:756–765.

59. Jeste DV, Dolder CR, Nayak GV, et al. Atypical antipsychotics in elderly patients with dementia or schizophrenia: review of recent literature. *Harv Rev Psychiatry*. 2005;13:340–351.

60. Jusko WJ, Gretch M. Plasma and tissue protein binding of drugs in pharmacokinetics. *Drug Metab Rev*. 1976;5:43–140.

61. Koller WC. Levodopa in the treatment of Parkinson's disease. *Neurology*. 2000;55(11 suppl 4):S2–S7.

62. Koller WC, Pahwa R. Treating motor fluctuations with controlled-release levodopa preparations. *Neurology*. 1994;44(7 suppl 6):S23–S28.

63. Kulshrestha VK, Thomas M, Wadsworth J, et al. Interaction between phenytoin and antacids. *Br J Clin Pharmacol*. 1978;6:177–179.

64. Lamb EJ, Stevens PE, Nashef L. Topiramate increases biochemical risk of nephrolithiasis. *Ann Clin Biochem*. 2004;41:166–169.

65. Larson EB, Kukull WA, Buchner D, et al. Adverse drug reactions associated with global cognitive impairment in elderly persons. *Ann Intern Med*. 1987;107:169–173.

66. Leppik IE. Practical prescribing and long-term efficacy and safety of zonisamide. *Epilepsy Res*. 2006;68(suppl 2):S17–S24.

67. Levy G. Predicting effective drug concentrations for individual patients. Determinants of pharmacodynamic variability. *Clin Pharmacokinet*. 1998;34:323–333.

68. Lin JH, Lu AY. Inhibition and induction of cytochrome P450 and the clinical implications. *Clin Pharmacokinet*. 1998;35:361–390.

69. Lin JH, Yamazaki M. Role of P-glycoprotein in pharmacokinetics: clinical implications. *Clin Pharmacokinet*. 2003;42:59–98.

70. Lindell M, Karlsson MO, Lennernas H, et al. Variable expression of CYP and Pgp genes in the human small intestine. *Eur J Clin Invest*. 2003;33:493–499.

71. Lindeman RD. Overview: renal physiology and pathophysiology of aging. *Am J Kidney Dis*. 1990;16:275–282.

72. Lindeman RD, Tobin J, Shock NW. Longitudinal studies on the rate of decline in renal function with age. *J Am Geriatr Soc*. 1985;33:278–285.

73. Lovat LB. Age related changes in gut physiology and nutritional status. *Gut*. 1996;38:306–309.

74. Mannesse CK, Derkx FH, de Ridder MA, et al. Adverse drug reactions in elderly patients as contributing factor for hospital admission: cross sectional study. *BMJ*. 1997;315:1057–1058.

75. Marder SR, Meibach RC. Risperidone in the treatment of schizophrenia. *Am J Psychiatry*. 1994;151:825–835.

76. Masand PS. Side effects of antipsychotics in the elderly. *J Clin Psychiatry*. 2000;61(suppl 8):43–49.

77. Mayer U, Wagenaar E, Beijnen JH, et al. Substantial excretion of digoxin via the intestinal mucosa and prevention of long-term digoxin accumulation in the brain by the mdr 1a P-glycoprotein. *Br J Pharmacol*. 1996;119:1038–1044.

78. McManus DQ, Arvanitis LA, Kowalcyk BB. Quetiapine, a novel antipsychotic: experience in elderly patients with psychotic disorders. Seroquel Trial 48 Study Group. *J Clin Psychiatry*. 1999;60:292–298.

79. Meltzer HY. Serotonin receptors and antipsychotic drug action. *Psychopharmacol. Ser*. 1993;10:70–81.

80. Menting JE, Honig A, Verhey FR, et al. Selective serotonin reuptake inhibitors (SSRIs) in the treatment of elderly depressed patients: a qualitative analysis of the literature on their efficacy and side-effects. *Int Clin Psychopharmacol*. 1996;11:165–175.

81. Messenheimer J, Mullens EL, Giorgi L, et al. Safety review of adult clinical trial experience with lamotrigine. *Drug Saf*. 1998;18:281–296.

82. Meyer BR. Renal function in aging. *J Am Geriatr Soc*. 1989;37:791–800.

83. Michalets EL. Update: clinically significant cytochrome P-450 drug interactions. *Pharmacotherapy.* 1998;18:84–112.

84. Miller M. Renal and hormonal changes affecting fluid and electrolyte balance in the elderly. In: Rowan AJ, Ramsay RE, eds. *Seizures and epilepsy in the elderly.* Boston: Butterworth-Heinemann; 1997:29–43.

85. Moore AR, O'Keeffe ST. Drug-induced cognitive impairment in the elderly. *Drugs Aging.* 1999;15:15–28.

86. Muhlberg W, Platt D. Age-dependent changes of the kidneys: pharmacological implications. *Gerontology.* 1999;45:243–253.

87. Naranjo CA, Herrmann N, Mittmann N, et al. Recent advances in geriatric psychopharmacology. *Drugs Aging.* 1995;7:184–202.

88. Nebeker JR, Barach P, Samore MH. Clarifying adverse drug events: a clinician's guide to terminology, documentation, and reporting. *Ann Intern Med.* 2004;140:795–801.

89. Nelson JC, Wohlreich MM, Mallinckrodt CH, et al. Duloxetine for the treatment of major depressive disorder in older patients. *Am J Geriatr Psychiatry.* 2005;13:227–235.

90. Nielsen OA, Johannessen AC, Bardrum B. Oxcarbazepine-induced hyponatremia, a cross-sectional study. *Epilepsy Res.* 1988;2:269–271.

91. Nishiguchi K, Ohnishi N, Iwakawa S, et al. Pharmacokinetics of zonisamide; saturable distribution into human and rat erythrocytes and into rat brain. *J Pharmacobiodyn.* 1992;15:409–415.

92. Nolan L, O'Malley K. Adverse drug reactions in the elderly. *Br J Hosp Med.* 1989;41:446, 448, 452–457.

93. Nyengaard JR, Bendtsen TF. Glomerular number and size in relation to age, kidney weight, and body surface in normal man. *Anat Rec.* 1992;232:194–201.

94. Okey AB. Enzyme induction in the cytochrome P-450 system. *Pharmacol Ther.* 1990;45:241–298.

95. Pendlebury SC, Moses DK, Eadie MJ. Hyponatraemia during oxcarbazepine therapy. *Hum Toxicol.* 1989;8:337–344.

96. Pentikainen PJ, Valisalmi L, Himberg JJ, et al. Pharmacokinetics of midazolam following intravenous and oral administration in patients with chronic liver disease and in healthy subjects. *J Clin Pharmacol.*1989;29:272–277.

97. Peskind ER, Potkin SG, Pomara N, et al. Memantine treatment in mild to moderate Alzheimer's disease: a 24-week randomized, controlled trial. *Am J Geriatr Psychiatry.* 2006; 14(8):704–715.

98. Platten HP, Schweizer E, Dilger K, et al. Pharmacokinetics and the pharmacodynamic action of midazolam in young and elderly patients undergoing tooth extraction. *Clin Pharmacol Ther.* 1998;63:552–560.

99. Radominska-Pandya A, Czernik PJ, Little JM, et al. Structural and functional studies of UDP-glucuronosyltransferases. *Drug Metab Rev.* 1999;31:817–899.

100. Raskin P, Donofrio PD, Rosenthal NR, et al. Topiramate vs placebo in painful diabetic neuropathy: analgesic and metabolic effects. *Neurology.* 2004;63:865–873.

101. Rigler SK, Webb MJ, Redford L, et al. Weight outcomes among antidepressant users in nursing facilities. *J Am Geriatr Soc.* 2001;49:49–55.

102. Ring BJ, Binkley SN, Roskos L, et al. Effect of fluoxetine, norfluoxetine, sertraline and desmethyl sertraline on human CYP3A catalyzed 1′-hydroxy midazolam formation in vitro. *J Pharmacol Exp Ther.* 1995;275:1131–1135.

103. Roberts J, Tumer N. Pharmacodynamic basis for altered drug action in the elderly. *Clin Geriatr Med.* 1988;4:127–149.

104. Robinson DS, Roberts DL, Smith JM, et al. The safety profile of nefazodone. *J Clin Psychiatry.* 1996;57(suppl 2):31–38.

105. Rogers SL, Friedhoff LT. The efficacy and safety of donepezil in patients with Alzheimer's disease: results of a US multicenter, randomized, double-blind, placebo-controlled trial. The Donepezil Study Group. *Dementia.* 1996;7:293–303.

106. Rosler M, Anand R, Cicin-Sain A, et al. Efficacy and safety of rivastigmine in patients with Alzheimer's disease: international randomised controlled trial. *BMJ.* 1999;318:633–638.

107. Rowan AJ, Ramsay RE, Collins JF, et al. New onset geriatric epilepsy: a randomized study of gabapentin, lamotrigine, and carbamazepine. *Neurology.* 2005;64:1868–1873.

108. Rowe JW, Andres R, Tobin JD, et al. The effect of age on creatinine clearance in men: a cross-sectional and longitudinal study. *J Gerontol.* 1976;31:155–163.

109. Roxe DM. Aging and renal function. *Compr Ther.* 1991;17:13–19.

110. Schmidt D, Arroyo S, Baulac M, et al. Recommendations on the clinical use of oxcarbazepine in the treatment of epilepsy: a consensus view. *Acta Neurol Scand.* 2001;104:167–170.

111. Schor JD, Levkoff SE, Lipsitz LA, et al. Risk factors for delirium in hospitalized elderly. *JAMA.* 1992;267:827–831.

112. Settle EC Jr. Bupropion sustained release: side effect profile. *J Clin Psychiatry.* 1998;59(suppl 4):32–36.

113. Shock NW, Watkin DM, Yiengst MJ, et al. Age differences in the water content of the body as

related to basal oxygen consumption in males. *J Gerontol.* 1963;18:1–8.

114. Sorock GS, Shimkin EE. Benzodiazepine sedatives and the risk of falling in a community-dwelling elderly cohort. *Arch Intern Med.* 1988;148:2441–2444.

115. Sotaniemi EA, Arranto AJ, Pelkonen O, et al. Age and cytochrome P450-linked drug metabolism in humans: an analysis of 226 subjects with equal histopathologic conditions. *Clin Pharmacol Ther.* 1997;61:331–339.

116. Soumerai SB, Ross-Degnan D. Inadequate prescription-drug coverage for Medicare enrollees: a call to action. *N Engl J Med.* 1999;340:722–728.

117. Staab JP, Evans DL. Efficacy of venlafaxine in geriatric depression. *Depress Anxiety.* 2000; 12(suppl 1):63–68.

118. Stewart BH, Kugler AR, Thompson PR, et al. A saturable transport mechanism in the intestinal absorption of gabapentin is the underlying cause of the lack of proportionality between increasing dose and drug levels in plasma. *Pharm Res.* 1993;10:276–281.

119. Stewart RB. Drug use in the elderly. In: Delafuente J, Stewart R, eds. *Therapeutics in the elderly.* Cincinnati: Harvey Whitney; 2001:235–256.

120. Street JS, Clark WS, Gannon KS, et al. Olanzapine treatment of psychotic and behavioral symptoms in patients with Alzheimer's disease in nursing care facilities: a double-blind, randomized, placebo-controlled trial. The HGEU Study Group. *Arch Gen Psychiatry.* 2000;57:968–976.

121. Sweet RA, Mulsant BH, Gupta B, et al. Duration of neuroleptic treatment and prevalence of tardive dyskinesia in late life. *Arch Gen Psychiatry.* 1995;52:478–486.

122. Sweet RA, Pollock BG. Neuroleptics in the elderly: guidelines for monitoring. *Harv Rev Psychiatry.* 1995;2:327–335.

123. Swift CG, Swift MR, Ankier SI, et al. Single dose pharmacokinetics and pharmacodynamics of oral loprazolam in the elderly. *Br J Clin Pharmacol.* 1985;20:119–128.

124. Taeuber CM. Numerical growth. Current population reports sixty-five plus in America. 1992.

125. Tephly T, Green M, Puig J, et al. Endogenous substrates for UDP-glucuronosyltransferases. *Xenobiotica.* 1988;18:1201–1210.

126. Teunissen MW, Bakker W, Meerburg-Van der Torren JE, et al. Influence of rifampicin treatment on antipyrine clearance and metabolite formation in patients with tuberculosis. *Br J Clin Pharmacol.* 1984;18:701–706.

127. Venulet J, ten Ham M. Methods for monitoring and documenting adverse drug reactions. *Int J Clin Pharmacol Ther.* 1996;34:112–129.

128. Wallace SM, Verbeeck RK. Plasma protein binding of drugs in the elderly. *Clin Pharmacokinet.* 1987;12:41–72.

129. Watkins PB. The barrier function of CYP3A4 and P-glycoprotein in the small bowel. *Adv Drug Deliv Rev.* 1997;27:161–170.

130. Whelton A, Schulman G, Wallemark C, et al. Effects of celecoxib and naproxen on renal function in the elderly. *Arch Intern Med.* 2000; 160:1465–1470.

131. Wong IC, Mawer GE, Sander JW. Factors influencing the incidence of lamotrigine-related skin rash. *Ann Pharmacother.* 1999;33:1037–1042.

132. Woodhouse K, Wynne HA. Age-related changes in hepatic function. Implications for drug therapy. *Drugs Aging.* 1992;2:243–255.

133. Wright J. Drug interactions. In: Carruthers S, Hoffman B, Melmon L, eds. *Melmon and Morrelli's clinical pharmacology.* New York: McGraw-Hill; 2000:1257–1266.

134. Wynne HA, Cope LH, Mutch E, et al. The effect of age upon liver volume and apparent liver blood flow in healthy man. *Hepatology.* 1989;9:297–301.

135. Zhang QY, Dunbar D, Ostrowska A, et al. Characterization of human small intestinal cytochromes P-450. *Drug Metab Dispos.* 1999; 27:804–809.

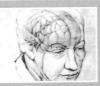

CHAPTER 5

Neurologic Considerations in the Postmenopausal Woman

Joyce Liporace, Kathryn Willcox, and David A. Thomas

Menopause is often ascribed with a whole host of physical and mental symptoms in mature women. Although it is not the root of all ills, it is true that hormones play a critical role in the regulation and maintenance of normal health and in the expression of disease. We live in a society where women can expect to live another three or four decades after menopause, representing a major portion of a woman's life. Therefore, practicing neurologists need to be aware of the complex issues that surround neurologic health and hormones.

At age 50, a woman's average life expectancy in the United States is 81.6 years (34). Her lifetime risk of developing stroke is 20%, and her risk of dying from it is 8%. For Alzheimer dementia, her risk of disease increases rapidly after age 65, with a 50% risk after age 85. For epilepsy, she faces a second peak in incidence after age 60.

Endogenous and supplemental steroid hormones alter the expression of these and other neurologic disorders. It is important that physicians understand the implications that hormonal changes have on both acute and chronic disease. Efforts to improve the quality of health care for individuals with dementia, stroke, epilepsy, and other chronic illnesses will have an important value to society.

Results from the Women's Health Initiative clinical trials have dramatically altered our thinking about the use of supplemental hormone replacement therapy (HRT) for perimenopausal and postmenopausal women (2,44). These randomized trials were designed to assess major disease outcomes among healthy women and raised concerns about adverse outcomes linked with estrogen replacement (Table 5-1). Both estrogen and progesterone supplements and estrogen alone increased the risk of ischemic stroke by 40%. Furthermore, hormonal replacement did not preserve cognitive function, prevent dementia, or treat the memory decline of Alzheimer's disease.

This chapter addresses special neurologic concerns for postmenopausal women and provides a rationale for strategies to improve health care for the mature woman. An overview of menopause and the interactions of steroid hormones and the brain are discussed, followed by a presentation of specific diseases.

MENOPAUSE

Menopause is the permanent cessation of menstruation after the loss of ovarian function. The median age at menopause in the United States is 52.6 years, with 1% of women experiencing menopause before age 40 (43). Menopause is a process (derived from the Greek words *meno* or month and *pausis* or cessation) that can only be defined retrospectively after 12 months of amenorrhea. The phase from the onset of

Table 5-1. *Relative Risks of Disease Outcomes from the Women's Health Initiative Trials*

Outcome	Estrogen Plus Progestin[a]	Risk[b]	Estrogen Alone[c]	Risk[b]
	Relative Risk (95% CI)		*Relative Risk (95% CI)*	
Stroke	1.41 (1.07–1.85)	0.20	1.39 (1.10–1.77)	0.20
Heart disease	1.29 (1.02–1.63)	0.26	0.91 (0.75–1.12)	—
Pulmonary embolus	2.13 (1.39–3.25)	0.45	1.34 (0.87–2.06)	—
Invasive breast cancer	1.26 (1.00–1.59)	0.93	0.77 (0.59–1.01)	—

[a]Postmenopausal women with a uterus (n = 16,608) were randomly assigned to 0.625 mg of conjugated estrogen and 2.5 mg of medroxyprogesterone or an identical placebo for an average of 5.2 years.
[b]The absolute difference in risk equals the rate per 1,000 women per year from age 50 to 54 years who were treated with hormones minus the rate in untreated women the same age.
[c]Postmenopausal women with a hysterectomy (n = 10,739) were randomly assigned to 0.625 mg of conjugated estrogen daily or an identical placebo for an average of 6.8 years.

irregular menses to menopause is called "perimenopause," which has an average duration of 5 years. It includes the year after cessation of menses. This time is also referred to as the "climacteric," which is the transition from reproductive to nonreproductive life. A woman is perimenopausal if serial follicle-stimulating hormone (FSH) levels are elevated (>20 IU/L) and estradiol is low (<60 pg/mL). During perimenopause, ovarian function is variable, with a shortened follicular phase and an increase in defective ovulation and anovulation. Other symptoms (e.g., hot flashes and night sweats) also occur. It is not a time of steady estrogen decline; instead, it is marked by peaks and valleys. This feature can be clinically frustrating because it can lead to fluctuating symptoms (e.g., changes in seizure and headache frequency).

The hypothalamic-pituitary axis changes dramatically during and before menopause. The most marked change is the increased secretion of FSH by the pituitary gland. Luteinizing hormone (LH) levels remain in the normal range despite a rise in FSH before menopause. With menopause, LH levels rise and plateau. The increased levels of FSH and LH are secondary to loss of negative feedback from lower circulating estrogen levels. Additionally, ovarian follicles no longer release inhibin, which normally suppresses FSH.

With cessation of menstruation, a decline occurs in estradiol concentration that is dramatic for the first 12 months; the decline then becomes gradual. The concentration of estrone, a weaker estrogen, also falls after menopause. Peripheral aromatization of adrenal androgens in adipose tissue, muscle, and skin becomes the major source of estrogens after menopause. Obese postmenopausal women have higher levels of circulating estrogen because of increased aromatization in adipose tissues.

Progesterone levels in perimenopausal women can be normal, but luteal-phase progesterone typically declines. Women can go through long phases of amenorrhea with absent progesterone secretion. With menopause, levels decline to approximately 30% of the concentration present in young women during the follicular phase of the menstrual cycle. The main source of progesterone becomes the adrenal gland. Peripheral conversion of steroids to progesterone is not seen in nonpregnant women.

With aging, ovarian androgen secretion declines. A shift in the pattern of androgen secretion occurs with the maintenance of testosterone at the expense of androstenedione. With the fall in androstenedione, a major source of testosterone, circulating levels of testosterone cannot be maintained, and serum levels decline. Typically, the decline in circulating androgens begins before menopause.

STEROID HORMONES AND THE BRAIN

Steroid hormones exert powerful effects on the brain, beginning shortly after conception and continuing throughout life. Sex steroids are highly lipophilic and readily cross the blood–brain barrier. The brain is well known as a target site of peripheral steroid hormones; however, it is also the site of de novo synthesis of steroid hormones from cholesterol (55). Steroid hormones influence function by immediate membrane effects and by genomic effects. Genomic effects are delayed, taking days to occur, and their effects are sustained for days to weeks after hormone exposure. Steroid hormones bind intranuclear receptors and act as transcription factors that regulate gene expression. Their diversity and magnitude suggest that hormonal therapy may be helpful to treat or prevent neurologic conditions that are sensitive to hormones.

ESTROGEN

The ovary converts acetate to cholesterol and subsequently to other steroids. FSH regulates the formation of estrogen by the ovarian follicle. Additionally, peripheral tissues including liver, fat, skeletal muscle, and hair follicles can convert adrenal androstenedione and testosterone to estrogen. This is the major source of estrogen in men and in postmenopausal women.

During reproductive years, the dominant follicle and its corpus luteum are the main sources of estrogen production. Natural estrogens include estradiol, estrone, estriol, and their conjugates. Of the three main human estrogens, estradiol-17β is the most potent. Estradiol is the principal estrogen produced in menstruating women. Estrone, the second major estrogen and the main estrogen in postmenopausal women, is metabolized from estradiol and from peripheral aromatization.

All estrogens circulate in blood, either free or bound to sex hormone–binding globulin (SHBG) or nonspecifically to albumin. Changes in SHBG occur secondary to some medications, for example, enzyme-inducing antiepileptic drugs. Alterations in SHBG alter the concentration of free estradiol and affect bioavailability.

Estrogen has both direct and inductive effects on neurons, glia, and microglia. Neurons contain nuclear receptors for estrogen, predominantly in the pituitary gland, hypothalamus, amygdala, hippocampus, raphe nuclei, and cerebral cortex. As transcriptional regulators, activated estrogen receptors direct or modulate synthesis of many neurotransmitters and neuropeptides. Estrogen increases acetylcholine (Ach) by inducing choline acetyltransferase, the rate-limiting step of production. In the hippocampus, estrogen upregulates

N-methyl-D-aspartic acid (NMDA) glutamate receptor subtype. It downregulates gamma-aminobutyric acid (GABA)-A receptor subunits and the synthesis of GABA. Neuronal excitability is further increased by induction of synaptic sprouting. Morphologic studies have shown that estrogen and progesterone induce anatomic changes in neurons of the CA1 region of the hippocampus, a structure critical in memory processing and learning, which has implications for aging, Alzheimer's disease (AD), and epilepsy. Within 12 to 24 hours after estrogen exposure in animals, hippocampal neurons form new dendritic spines and increase synaptic connections (61). The increase in dendritic spine density is reversed with progesterone.

PROGESTERONE

A progestin is a substance that binds to the progesterone receptor and has progestational activity. The most widely recognized progestational activity is transformation of proliferative to secretory endometrium in an estrogen-primed uterus. Progestins can be divided into two groups: natural (the only one is progesterone) and synthetic. All synthetic progesterones are not equal; some are derived from progesterone, whereas others are an alteration of testosterone with greater androgenic properties. Natural progesterone is secreted by the ovary mainly from the corpus luteum during the second half of the menstrual cycle. LH controls progesterone secretion. Progesterone circulates primarily bound to albumin and is extensively metabolized. Its half-life in blood is just a few minutes, although its actions on tissues continue after it has disappeared from serum.

Progesterone receptors are found in the hypothalamus and hippocampus and diffusely throughout the cerebral cortex, a distribution similar to estrogen, although progesterone receptors are more widespread throughout the neocortex. Progesterone and several of its metabolites induce sedation and decrease neuronal excitability. Its anxiolytic and hypnotic effects are partly mediated by enhancement of the inhibitory action of the neurotransmitter GABA. Additionally, progesterone reduces glutamate excitation. Genomic effects include upregulation of GABA and GABA-A receptor subunits.

ANDROGENS

Traditionally, androgens are thought of as male hormones. However, they clearly are important in women, playing a role in sexual drive, enhancement of insulin effect, cognition, bone health, sexual hair development, muscle mass, stature, and development of the immune system.

Women have androgen receptors in the brain, as do men. As with estrogen and progesterone, androgens can modify nervous system structures, cognition, and mood. The major sources for circulating androgens during the reproductive period are the ovary, the adrenal cortex,

and peripheral conversion of dehydroepiandrosterone and androstenedione. After menopause, the main source of circulating testosterone is peripheral conversion of adrenal androstenedione. Decreased adrenal androgen production is noted with age but is independent of menopause. Adrenal and ovarian production of androgens declines beginning at age 20, and serum androgen levels are decreased by half at age 40. Smaller changes are seen after age 60 (18).

STROKE

Stroke, one of the leading causes of death in the United States, is a primary cause of adult disability. Although stroke is more common in men, the overall mortality rate is higher in postmenopausal women (14% vs. 20%) (10). Aspirin may be less effective in platelet aggregation inhibition in women compared to men with a prior history of ischemic cerebrovascular disease (13). Gender also plays a role in response to carotid endarterectomy. Restenosis rates are significantly higher in women (14%) versus men (3.9%), with a mean follow-up period of 25 months (28).

Stroke risk factors are identical in men and women, although women carry the added burden of risks associated with pregnancy, hormonal contraception, and the effects of hormonal decline after ovarian failure. Basic science research suggests favorable neuroprotection and reduced neuronal injury after ischemic stroke with estrogen, but clinical trials do not support the basic research predictions (Table 5-2). Vascular endothelium and smooth muscle bind estrogen with high affinity. Estrogen promotes vasodilatation

Table 5-2. *Sex Steroid Effects on the Brain Related to Stroke*

Sex Steroid	Effects
Estrogen	Increased vasodilatation Decreased total and LDL cholesterol Increased HDL cholesterol Decreased fibrinogen and antithrombin III Increased nitric oxide Antioxidant effects
Progesterone	Increased LDL cholesterol Decreased HDL cholesterol Decreased vasodilatation
Testosterone	Decreased plasminogen activator inhibitor Decreased lipoprotein Enhanced fibrinolysis

HDL, high-density lipoprotein; LDL, low-density lipoprotein.

and alters both short-term and long-term vasomotor tone. Its actions depend on changes in renin, angiotensin-converting enzyme, nitric oxide, and prostaglandins (38). Estrogen favorably alters serum lipid concentrations through mediation of hepatic apoprotein genes. It decreases serum cholesterol, lowers low-density lipoprotein (LDL) cholesterol, and increases serum high-density lipoprotein (HDL) cholesterol. Coadministration of progesterone blunts these lipid effects because progesterone alone tends to raise LDL and lower HDL cholesterol.

There are four large clinical trials that have evaluated the effects of HRT on stroke risk and do not support a role in prevention. The Framingham Heart Study showed that postmenopausal use of HRT resulted in an increased risk of stroke (30). The Women's Estrogen for Stroke Trial did not find a significant effect on stroke prevention for oral estradiol versus placebo in women with a recent stroke or transient ischemic attack (57). The same results were found for women with coronary heart disease who were treated with oral conjugated equine estrogen and progesterone in the Heart and Estrogen-Progestin Replacement Study (50). The Women's Health Initiative study examined healthy women taking conjugated equine estrogen alone if they had a prior hysterectomy or in combination with medroxyprogesterone if they had an intact uterus (2,60). Women were between the ages of 50 and 79 years at baseline and were generally healthy. Women taking estrogen and progesterone had an elevated overall stroke risk of 30% compared with women taking placebo, and ischemic stroke was increased by 40%. For women without an intact uterus on estrogen alone, the risk of ischemic stroke was increased by 40% compared with women on placebo. Neurologists now inform patients that HRT cannot be recommended for stroke prevention.

MEMORY AND DEMENTIA

Neuropsychological reviews indicate that, although healthy women and men demonstrate similar performance on many cognitive tasks, men score better on constructional, visuospatial, and objective manipulation tasks, whereas women excel in verbal memory, word discrimination, and verbal fluency measures. Such differences may be mediated by both long-term and short-term exposure to steroid hormones.

Evidence indicates that specific aspects of memory covary with sex steroids in men and women. Alterations in performance are noted across the menstrual cycle in normal women, with higher estradiol levels linked to better verbal memory (41). In postmenopausal women, estrogen users attained higher scores on specific cognitive tasks of immediate and delayed paragraph recall. No changes were found in other cognitive

tasks or in tests of spatial memory (29). This suggests a specific—not global—effect in some women. In contrast, progesterone can reduce cognitive performance. In one study, oral progesterone given to healthy young women resulted in impaired symbol copying, fatigue, and confusion, along with reduced immediate verbal recall scores (21).

Alzheimer's disease (AD), the most common of the dementias, is a degenerative disease characterized by the gradual onset of progressive symptoms, including memory loss and other cognitive deficits, personality change, and executive dysfunction, ultimately requiring monitored assistance with activities of daily living. Currently, 4.5 million Americans are affected, and by 2050, 14 million will suffer from this disease (15). Incidence increases with age; one in 10 people are affected by age 65, and nearly one in two people are affected by age 85. Women have a higher predilection for Alzheimer's disease, independent of age.

Studies regarding the use of sex hormones to thwart the progression or appearance of Alzheimer's disease are conflicting. A number of estrogen effects may be relevant to AD (Table 5-3). Estrogen modulates growth factors, reduces oxidative stress, and promotes the formation of synaptic connections. It influences several neurotransmitters, including acetylcholine, which plays a critical role in AD. Additionally, estrogen increases the expression of apolipoprotein E and may reduce the formation of β-amyloid protein.

A meta-analysis of 10 studies (including eight case-control studies) suggested that neurologically normal estrogen users had a 29% lower rate of developing AD (62). Two large, prospective, community-based studies investigated the association of estrogen replacement therapy (ERT) and the risk of developing AD (31,53). They provided additional clinical support for a protective role of estrogen. In these studies, oral estrogen used during the postmenopausal period delayed the development of AD and lowered the risk of the disease by 60%. This risk reduction remained significant after adjusting for age, education,

Table 5-3. *Sex Steroid Effects on the Brain Related to Alzheimer's Disease*

Sex Steroid	Effects
Estrogen	Increased cholinergic transmission
	Antioxidant effect
	Increased apolipoprotein E
	Decreased β-amyloid protein
	Stimulation of synaptic density in hippocampal neurons
	Modulation of growth factors
Progesterone	Reduction of synaptic density in hippocampal neurons

ethnicity, and apolipoprotein E genotype. A magnetic resonance imaging (MRI) voxel-based morphometry study of postmenopausal women suggests that estrogen use may be linked to preserved gray matter volume, even when estrogen use is remote (8).

In contrast to these positive studies, others have found no effect of conjugated estrogen on the treatment of women with mild to moderate AD (27,39,58). Low-dose estrogen had no effect on mood, behavior, cognitive performance, or cerebral perfusion in a 12-week study of 50 women (58).

The most influential trial to date is the randomized, multicenter Women's Health Initiative Memory Study (WHIMS), which revealed negative results, with an increased risk of dementia and mild cognitive impairment for older women taking estrogen replacement (48). The timing of the replacement may have been an important factor, and a critical period of intervention may have been lost. In this study, women over the age of 65 clearly did not experience any cognitive benefit from estrogen use. Questions remain regarding the potential benefit of estrogen exposure in younger women for dementia risk modification.

Estrogen replacement is currently not recommended for women with dementia as we await future investigations to clarify its selective influence on each of the multiple pathways leading to neurodegeneration and cognitive decline.

EPILEPSY

Sex hormones influence the electrical activity of the brain through immediate membrane effects and genomic mechanisms (Table 5-4). Both estrogen and progesterone exert membrane effects, in part, at the GABA-A receptor complex. Animal models of epilepsy demonstrate that estrogen lowers the threshold for seizures. Topical application of estradiol to the brains of rabbits produces paroxysmal epileptiform discharges (35). Estradiol acts as an agonist at the NMDA receptor, which increases excitation. It also binds the GABA-A receptor, alters chloride conductance, and reduces GABA-mediated inhibition. Genomic effects of estrogen include reduction of GABA concentration and a reduction in GABA-A receptor subunits. Exposure to estrogen affects neuronal morphology, which promotes synaptogenesis (see Steroid Hormones and the Brain). Progesterone has the opposite effect and protects against seizures. It enhances GABA-mediated neuronal inhibition and reduces glutamate excitation. In humans, intravenous progesterone diminishes epileptic discharges (6). Little is known about the association of testosterone with neuronal excitability, and the effect appears to vary with age and gender.

Interestingly, age of menopause is affected by epilepsy and linked to seizure frequency (25). Earlier menopause is present with epilepsy, and greater seizure frequency is associated with up to a 3-year decline in the age of menopause (Table 5-5).

Seizures linked to the menstrual cycle are termed "catamenial epilepsy." With ovulatory cycles, the relatively high estrogen-to-progesterone ratio at ovulation and the rapid progesterone withdrawal just before menses are linked with seizure exacerbation. With anovulatory cycles, seizures are noted throughout the entire luteal phase because of the unopposed action of estrogen. These hormonal influences would also be expected to alter the expression of seizures after menopause. Many women with catamenial seizure patterns hope for improved seizure control following menopause.

Limited information is available concerning the effects of menopause on epilepsy. Because menopause is a complex process, it is difficult to study, and thus, good prospective studies are lacking. Early in menopause, an increase occurs in anovulatory cycles and in the estrogen-to-progesterone ratio. This would be expected to promote seizures. At the end of menopause, estrogen declines, which may reduce seizures. It can also be predicted that ERT might worsen seizure control.

In a retrospective study based on self-report, most women with epilepsy noted a change in their seizure pattern with menopause: 41% noted worsening, whereas 29% experienced improved seizure control.

Table 5-4. *Sex Steroid Effects on the Brain Related to Epilepsy*

	Estrogen	Progesterone
GABA-A chloride conductance	Decreased	Increased
GABA synthesis	Increased	Decreased
Excitatory response to glutamate	Increased	Decreased
Hippocampal dendritic synapses	Increased	Decreased
GABA-A receptor subunit mRNA	Decreased	Increased

GABA, gamma-aminobutyric acid.

Table 5-5. *Age of Menopause for Women with Epilepsy*

Group	Age of Menopause (years)
Controls	51.3
Frequent seizures (1/month)	46.7
Occasional seizure	47.7
Rare seizures (<20/life)	49.9

Additionally, it was suggested that menopause may be a risk factor for seizures; 20% of women in that study had new-onset seizures coincident with menopause (1). In another self-reported study, 68% of women with catamenial epilepsy reported increased seizures during perimenopause and a subsequent decline in seizures after menopause. This study also found that menopausal women given HRT were at increased risk for seizure exacerbation (63% vs. 12% not receiving HRT) (26). There was a single, randomized, placebo-controlled, double-blind trial of the effect of HRT on seizure control in postmenopausal women. Women were randomized to placebo, a single dose of 6.25 mg of conjugated estrogen with 2.5 mg of medroxypro-gesterone, or a double-dose hormonal therapy for 3 months (24). Seizure worsening was noted in 17% of patients on placebo, 50% of patients on single-dose HRT, and 71% of patients on double HRT, showing a dose-related increase in seizure frequency in this small study population (n = 21). Additionally, HRT was found to have a drug interaction with mainte-nance antiepileptic therapy, with a reduction in lam-otrigine blood levels. The safety of HRT in women with epilepsy needs to be further evaluated. Women with epilepsy who are prescribed hormones should be monitored carefully for change in seizure patterns, and medication levels need to be followed closely.

HEADACHE

No gender differences are seen in migraine prevalence before puberty. However, after puberty, more women (17.6%) than men (6%) have migraine (33). Peak incidence in women occurs at menarche. Migraines commonly occur in association with menses, with 60% of women experiencing catamenial headaches. The primary trigger appears to be estrogen withdrawal; however, fluctuations in estrogen play a key role. Although prevalence decreases with age, migraine can either improve or worsen with menopause. Typically, migraine without aura increases in frequency and severity with perimenopause; however, after natural menopause, two-thirds of women note substantial improvement in their headaches (5). For migraine with aura, postmenopausal women often note the aura with-out the headache. Surgical menopause can exacerbate migraine, probably because of the abrupt decline in estradiol. The favorable response of migraine in the postmenopausal period is attributed to the lack of vari-ation in sex hormones. Cluster headache in women is less likely to be influenced by menopause (56).

Women with hormonal responsive migraines may experience headache exacerbation with initiation of cyclic HRT. Reducing the estrogen dose or using continuous administration instead of interrupted estrogen replacement may be effective in treating headaches. Androgens may also be useful for treatment of headache (49). No evidence supports hysterectomy or oophorectomy to treat refractory migraine at any age.

PARKINSON'S DISEASE

Dopamine depletion in the nigrostriatal system gives rise to the bradykinesia, resting tremor, rigidity, postural instability, and gait disturbance that we clas-sify as Parkinson's disease. Women have a lower inci-dence of Parkinson's disease, and sex steroids have been implicated in this gender difference (16). Estrogen modulates dopaminergic activity in the nigrostriatal system and may influence disease (Table 5-6). It has a direct stimulatory effect on the synthesis of dopamine by activation of tyrosine hydroxylase, the rate-limiting enzyme. Additionally, physiologic levels of estrogen can increase dopamine by reducing catechol-O-methyltransferase (COMT) transcription by as much as 50%, resulting in reduced dopamine degradation (54).

Conflicting studies exist regarding the effects of estrogen on clinical signs. Dyskinesias are increased mid-cycle when estrogen levels are high, and bradyki-nesia is increased just before menses when estrogen levels decline (52). Additionally, pregnancy can induce chorea in susceptible women that resolves postpartum once hormone levels fall. In one study, low-dose estrogen replacement alone in 40 postmenopausal women with Parkinson's disease significantly reduced motor fluctuation compared with placebo, improving both "on" time and "off" time, based on patients' diaries (54). However, other reports suggest that estrogen has the opposite effect. During the luteal phase of the menstrual cycle when both estrogen and progesterone levels are high, some women need an increased dose of levodopa therapy. This indirect sign has been interpreted as an antidopaminergic effect of estrogen (22); however, it may represent a proges-terone effect. A double-blind, placebo-controlled study in postmenopausal women with Parkinson's dis-ease found no effect on symptoms when estradiol was given but did note that progesterone worsened both objective motor scores and subjective reports (52).

Table 5-6. *Sex Steroid Effects on the Brain Important in Parkinson's Disease*

Sex Steroid	Effects
Estrogen	Increased dopamine synthesis
	Increased dopamine release
	Increased D1 and D2 receptors
	Decreased catechol-O-methyltransferase
	Protection from apoptosis

Symptomatic Parkinson's disease in women may be delayed by higher physiologic striatal dopamine levels. This benefit is related to estrogen status, since parity, age at menopause, and duration of fertile lifespan are all associated with a later age at onset of clinical disease (23).

Supplemental estrogen does not seem to reduce disease risk. ERT did not affect the development of Parkinson's disease in 989 healthy postmenopausal women, but it was found to protect against dementia in women with established disease, after adjusting for age, education, and ethnicity (37). In the Nurses' Health Study, HRT was linked with a reduced incidence of Parkinson's disease but only among women who did not consume caffeinated beverages; the risk was elevated in women who did consume them (4). Needless to say, the literature regarding HRT and Parkinson's disease is murky.

SLEEP

Hypothalamic nuclei and periaqueductal gray are brain areas involved in the regulation of sleep. Because these regions have a high content of estrogen and progesterone receptors, sex steroids can influence sleep architecture. The loss of these hormones during menopause often interrupts sleep. Loss of sleep is associated with psychological and somatic distress, decreased cognitive function, and daytime fatigue (42). Insomnia and obstructive sleep apnea are the two most common sleep problems that affect menopausal women.

Although sleep apnea is usually more common in men, the severity and prevalence of sleep-disordered breathing increases in postmenopausal women, when compared to premenopausal women, which indicates a hormonal link (3). This may be due to progesterone stimulating breathing. Another possible explanation for the increase may be related to decreased respiratory drive and upper airway muscular tone (59).

Severe hot flashes are correlated with chronic insomnia (40). However, objective testing suggests that hot flashes have been overdiagnosed as the cause of insomnia (20). Sleep complaints in midlife should not routinely be attributed to hot flashes; instead, primary sleep disorders and medications need to be ruled out. Additionally, REM sleep has been found to suppress hot flashes in the second half of the night (19).

Hormonal therapy has been shown to be beneficial in cases of sleep apnea. The incidence of sleep-disordered breathing in hormone replacement users was half that of non–hormone replacement users, with the occurrence of sleep-disordered breathing similar to that of premenopausal women (46). Estrogen appears to have a significant beneficial effect on sleep-disordered breathing, whereas the addition of progesterone does not provide additional benefits (36).

If hot flashes have been isolated as the cause of insomnia, estrogen use has been found to reduce their occurrence by 80% to 90%. If estrogen is not a viable option, newer antidepressant agents have also been shown to decrease the incidence of hot flashes (47). There are many successful treatments that may be used to alleviate insomnia that is not caused by hot flashes. These include diet and lifestyle changes, cognitive behavioral therapy, and pharmacologic treatment (32).

MULTIPLE SCLEROSIS

Multiple sclerosis, a progressively disabling disease, has a strong gender preference that affects twice as many women as men. The exception to this preference is primary progressive disease, which occurs equally in men and women. Onset of symptoms typically begins between 15 and 40 years of age, with a steep decline in frequency after age 45 to 50. Disease onset is often within a few years of puberty. Because of the strong gender link, there is speculation that a relationship exists between sex hormones and disease prevalence.

The cause of multiple sclerosis remains unknown, but autoimmune processes are critical in development of the disease. Research supports the concept that gender and sex hormones influence autoimmune reactions. Much of the data come from in vitro studies, which may not necessarily apply to in vivo functioning. Nevertheless, the following observations can be made. Estrogens have both immunosuppressive and immunostimulatory properties. Progesterone and androgens tend to suppress the immune system. In vitro studies show that progesterone and androgens downregulate T-cell proliferative response to mitogens. Estrogen modulates cytokine expression. Cytokines are responsible for neuronal apoptosis, changes in the blood–brain permeability, and induction of myelin damage. Animal models of experimental allergic encephalitis (EAE) show gender-specific changes in cytokines (17).

Clinical data concerning the hormonal effects of multiple sclerosis during pregnancy suggest that menopause may also modulate multiple sclerosis. High estrogen levels found in the third trimester of pregnancy bring about a reduction in the rate of multiple sclerosis relapse, whereas the sudden withdrawal of estrogen characterizing the postpartum period is associated with a two- to threefold increase in relapse rate (51). In a self-report study of 149 women with multiple sclerosis, many (60%) noted increased symptoms 1 week before the onset of menses (30). These reports, along with the observation that young women with multiple sclerosis seemed less disabled when taking oral contraception, suggest that estrogen exerts a stabilizing or protective effect on the clinical manifestations of multiple sclerosis (7). A pilot study involving HRT for pre- and postmenopausal women with multiple sclerosis showed a beneficial effect. Of the postmenopausal women, 54% reported a worsening of symptoms with menopause, and 75% of those who had tried HRT reported an improvement (51).

The protective role of estrogens in the general health of women with multiple sclerosis is further supported by improvement in bone health with supplementation. Although osteoporosis is linked to menopause and age, patients with multiple sclerosis compound their risk for even greater bone loss as a result of common steroid treatments and immobility. The majority of women with multiple sclerosis do not obtain needed preventive health care (45). Further studies to clarify the role of combined hormonal replacement in multiple sclerosis are needed.

NEURO-ONCOLOGIC DISEASES

The scope of neuro-oncologic disease in mature women includes primary as well as metastatic tumors of the central nervous system (CNS). Although the incidence of primary brain tumors is greater in men than in women (9.2/100,000 vs. 8.7/100,000, respectively), meningiomas occur most commonly in women (14).

Meningiomas contain hormonal receptors; consequently, they can become more aggressive during pregnancy or during the luteal phase of the menstrual cycle. High proportions of progesterone and androgen receptors are found in meningiomas. Interestingly, normal adult meninges express very low levels of progesterone receptors. Progesterone may be responsible for meningioma growth (11), although additional studies to clarify the effects of estrogen are needed with the discovery of a second estrogen receptor (12). Interruption of hormone therapy in postmenopausal women with small or asymptomatic meningiomas does not seem warranted; instead, serial imaging is needed (9).

For women, breast tumors account for 27% of all cancers and are the leading cause of brain metastases. Prevalence increases with age. Notably, postmenopausal obesity, which is associated with higher estrogen levels, is associated with a higher risk of breast cancer. Transition to menopause does not affect survival for those diagnosed with cancer early in life; however, HRT increases the risk of developing breast cancer.

SUMMARY

Gender-based differences in health and disease need to be considered by health care providers. We still face the challenge of fully understanding the complex interaction of sex hormones and the brain, along with their relationship to expression of disease. Menopause is a time in a woman's life when hormonal changes cause clinical symptoms and can alter the expression of neurologic disease. It represents an ideal time for assessment of risk for chronic disease and initiation of health maintenance (Table 5-7) to improve quality of life.

Table 5-7. *Screening Tests for Chronic Disease in Menopausal Women*

12-hour fasting lipid panel
Thyroid function tests
Electrocardiogram
Mini-mental status examination
Papanicolaou smear
Mammogram
Bone density scan

REFERENCES

1. Abbasi F, Krumholz A, Kittner S, et al. Effects of menopause on seizures in women with epilepsy. *Epilepsia.* 1999;40:205–210.
2. Anderson GL, Limacher M, Assaf AR, et al. Effects of conjugated equine estrogen in postmenopausal women with hysterectomy: the Women's Health Initiative randomized controlled trial. *JAMA.* 2004;291:1701–1712.
3. Anttaalainen U, Saaresranta T, Aittokallio J, et al. Impact of menopause on the manifestation and severity of sleep-disordered breathing. *Acta Obstet Gynecol Scand.* 2006;85:1381–1388.
4. Ascherio A, Chen H, Schwarzschild MA, et al. Caffeine, postmenopausal estrogen, and the risk of Parkinson's disease. *Neurology.* 2003;60:790–795.
5. Ashkenazi A, Silberstein S. Hormone-related headache: pathophysiology and treatment. *CNS Drugs.* 2006;20:125–141.
6. Backstrom T, Zetterlund B, Blom S, et al. Effects of intravenous progesterone infusions on the epileptic discharge frequency in women with partial epilepsy. *Acta Neurol Scand.* 1984;69:240–248.
7. Bauer H, Hanefeld F. *Multiple Sclerosis: Its Impact from Childhood to Old Age.* London: WB Saunders Company, Ltd.; 1993.
8. Boccardi M, Ghidoni R, Govoni S, et al. Effects of hormone therapy on brain morphology of healthy postmenopausal women: a voxel-based morphometry study. *Menopause.* 2006;13:584–591.
9. Boullot P, Pellissier JF, Devictor B. Quantitative imaging of estrogen and progesterone receptors, estrogen-related protein, and growth fraction: Immunocytochemical assays in 52 meningiomas. correlation with clinical and morphological data. *J Neurosurg.* 1994;81:765.

10. Caradung R, Seshadri S, Beiser A, et al. Trends in incidence, lifetime risk, severity, and 30-day mortality of stroke over the past 50 years. *JAMA.* 2006;296:2939–2946.

11. Carroll RS, Glowacka D, Dashner K. Progesterone receptor expression in meningiomas. *Cancer Res* 1993;53:1312–1316.

12. Carroll RS, Zhang J, Black PM. Expression of estrogen receptors alpha and beta in human meningiomas. *J Neurooncol.* 1999;42:109–116.

13. Cavallari LH, Helgason CM, Brace LD, et al. Sex difference in antiplatelet effect of aspirin in patients with stroke. *Ann Pharmacother.* 2006;40: 812–817.

14. Cudlowicz M, Irizarry M, eds. *Neurologic disorders in women.* Boston: Butterworth-Heinemann; 1997.

15. Cummings JL. Alzheimer's disease. *N Engl J Med.* 2004;35:56–67.

16. Currie LJ, Harrison MB, Trugman JM, et al. Postmenopausal estrogen use affects risk for Parkinson's disease. *Arch Neurol.* 2004;61:886–888.

17. Czlonkowska A, Ciesielska A, Gromadzka G, et al. Gender differences in neurological disease: role of estrogens and cytokines. *Endocrine.* 2006;29: 243–256.

18. Davidson SL, Bell R. Androgen physiology. *Semin Reprod Med.* 2006;24:71–77.

19. Freedman RR, Roehrs TA. Effects of REM sleep and ambient temperature on hot flash induced sleep disturbance. *Menopause.* 2006;13:549–552.

20. Freedman RR, Roehrs TA. Lack of sleep disturbance from menopausal hot flashes. *Fertil Steril.* 2004;82:138–144.

21. Freeman E, Purdy R, Coutifaris C, et al. Anxiolytic metabolites of progesterone: correlation with mood and performance measures following oral progesterone administration to healthy female volunteers. *Clin Neuroendocrinol.* 1993;58:478–484.

22. Giladi N, Honigman S. Hormones and Parkinson's disease. *Neurology.* 1995;45:1028.

23. Haaxma CA, Bloem BR, Borm GF, et al. Gender differences in Parkinson's disease. *J Neurol Neurosurg Psychiatry.* 2007;78:819–824.

24. Harden CL, Herzog AG, Nikolov BG, et al. Hormone replacement therapy in women with epilepsy: a randomized, double-blind, placebo-controlled study. *Epilepsia.* 2006;47:1447–1451.

25. Harden CL, Koppel BS, Herzog A, et al. Seizure frequency is associated with age at menopause in women with epilepsy. *Neurology.* 2003;61:451–455.

26. Harden CL, Pulver M, Ravdin L, et al. The effect of menopause and perimenopause on the course of epilepsy. *Epilepsia.* 1999;40:1402–1407.

27. Henderson VW, Paganini-Hill A, Miller BL, et al. Estrogen for Alzheimer's disease in women: randomized, double-blind, placebo-controlled trial. *Neurology.* 2000;54:295–301.

28. Hugl B, Oldenburg WA, Neuhauser B, et al. Effect of age and gender on restenosis after carotid endarterectomy. *Ann Vasc Surg.* 2006;20:602–608.

29. Kampen D, Sherwin B. Estrogen use and verbal memory in healthy postmenopausal women. *Obstet Gynecol.* 1994;83:979–983.

30. Kaplan P. *Neurologic Disease in Women.* 1st ed. New York: Demos Medical Publishing; 1998.

31. Kawas C, Resnick S, Morrison A, et al. A prospective study of estrogen replacement therapy and the risk of developing Alzheimer's disease: the Baltimore Longitudinal Study of Aging. *Neurology.* 1997;48:1517–1521.

32. Lee K. Sleep dysfunction in women and its management. *Curr Treat Options Neurol.* 2006;8: 376–386.

33. Lipton R, Stewart W. Migraine in the United States: a review of epidemiology and health care use. *Neurology.* 1993;43(suppl 3):S6–S10.

34. Lobo RA. *Treatment of the Postmenopausal Woman: Basic and Clinical Aspects.* 2nd ed. Philadelphia: Lippincott Williams & Wilkins; 1999.

35. Logothesis J, Harner R. Electrocortical activation by estrogens. *Arch Neurol.* 1960;9:352–360.

36. Manber R, Kuo TF, Cataldo N, et al. The effects of hormone replacement therapy on sleep disordered breathing in postmenopausal women: a pilot study. *Sleep.* 2003;26:163–168.

37. Marder K, Tang M-X, Alfaro B, et al. Postmenopausal estrogen use and Parkinson's disease with and without dementia. *Neurology.* 1998;50: 1141–1143.

38. Mendelsohn M, Karas R. The protective effects of estrogen on the cardiovascular system. *N Engl J Med.* 1998;340:1801–1811.

39. Mulnard R, Cotman CW, Kawas C, et al. Estrogen replacement therapy for treatment of mild to moderate Alzheimer's disease: a 1-year randomized controlled trial. *JAMA.* 2000;283:1007–1015.

40. Ohayon MM. Severe hot flashes are associated with chronic insomnia. *Arch Intern Med.* 2006; 166:1262–1268.

41. Phillips S, Sherwin B. Variations in memory function and sex steroid hormones across the menstrual cycle. *Psychoneuroendocrinology.* 1992;17:497–506.

42. Regestein QR, Friebely J, Shifren JL, et al. Self-reported sleep in postmenopausal women. *Menopause.* 2004;11:198–207.

43. Reynolds RF, Obermeyer CM. Age at natural menopause in Spain and the United States: results from the DAMES project. *Am J Hum Biol.* 2005;17:331–340.

44. Rossouw JE, Anderson GL, Prentice RL, et al. Risks and benefits of estrogen plus progestin in

healthy postmenopausal women: principal results from the Women's Health Initiative randomized controlled trial. *JAMA*. 2002;288:321–333.

45. Shabas D, Weinreb H. Preventive healthcare in women with multiple sclerosis. *J Womens Health Gend Based Med*. 2000;9:389–395.

46. Shahar E, Redline S, Young T, et al. Hormone replacement therapy and sleep-disordered breathing. *Am J Respir Crit Care Med*. 2003;167:1186–1192.

47. Shanafelt TD, Barton DL, Adjei AA, et al. Pathophysiology and treatment of hot flashes. *Mayo Clinic Proc*. 2002;77:1207–1218.

48. Shumaker SA, Legault C, Kuller LH, et al. Conjugated equine estrogens and incidence of probable dementia and mild cognitive impairment in postmenopausal women: Women's Health Initiative Memory Study. *JAMA*. 2004;291:2947–2958.

49. Silberstein S, Merriam G. Estrogens, progestins, and headache. *Neurology*. 1991;41:786–793.

50. Simon JA, Hsia J, Cauley JA, et al. Postmenopausal hormonal therapy and risk of stroke: the Heart and Estrogen-progestin Replacement Therapy Study (HERS). *Circulation*. 2001;103:638–642.

51. Smith R, Studd J. A pilot study of the effect upon multiple sclerosis of the menopause, hormone replacement therapy, and the cycle. *J R Soc Med*. 1992;85:612–613.

52. Strijks E, Kremer J, Horstink M. Effects of female sex steroids on Parkinson's disease in postmenopausal women. *Clin Neuropharmacol*. 1999:22:93–97.

53. Tang M-X, Jacobs D, Stern Y, et al. Effect of oestrogen during menopause on the risk and age at onset of Alzheimer's disease: a population-based study in Rochester, Minnesota. *Lancet*. 1996;348:429–432.

54. Tsang K, Ho S, Lo S. Estrogen improves motor disability in parkinsonian postmenopausal women with motor fluctuations. *Neurology*. 2000;54:2292–2298.

55. Tsutsui K, Ukena K, Usui M, et al. Novel brain function: biosynthesis and actions of neurosteroids in neurons. *Neurosci Res*. 2000;36:261–273.

56. vanVliet JA, Favier I, Helmerhorst FM, et al. Cluster headache in women: relation with menstruation, use of oral contraceptives, pregnancy, and menopause. *J Neurol Neurosurg Psychiatry*. 2006;77:690–692.

57. Viscoli CM, Brass LM, Kernan WN. A clinical trial of estrogen replacement therapy after ischemic stroke. *N Engl J Med*. 2001;345:1243–1249.

58. Wang PN, Liao SQ, Liu R, et al. Effects of estrogen on cognition, mood, and cerebral blood flow in AD. *Neurology*. 2000;54:2062–2066.

59. Ware JC, McBrayer R, Scott JA. Influence of sex and age on duration and frequency of sleep apnea events. *Sleep*. 2000;23:165–170.

60. Wassertheil-Smoller S, Hendrix S, Limacher M, et al. Effect of estrogen plus progestin on stroke in postmenopausal women: the Women's Health Initiative—A randomized trial. *JAMA*. 2003;289:2673–2684.

61. Wooley C, McEwen B. Roles of estradiol and progesterone in regulation of hippocampal dendritic spine density during the estrus cycle in the rat. *J Comp Neurol*. 1993;336:293–306.

62. Yaffe K, Sawaya G, Lieberburg I, et al. Estrogen therapy in postmenopausal women: effects on cognitive function and dementia. *JAMA*. 1998;279:688–695.

WEBSITES OF NATIONAL SUPPORT GROUPS

American College of Obstetricians and Gynecologists: http://www.acog.org

American Epilepsy Society: http://www.aesnet.org

American Medical Women's Association: http://amwa-doc.org

Association of Reproductive Health Professionals: http://www.arhp.org

National Institutes of Health, Women's Health Initiative: http://www.healthtouch.com

National Osteoporosis Foundation: http://www.nof.org

Chat rooms: www.DrKoop.com; www.ivillage.com; www.webMD.com

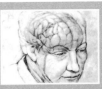

CHAPTER 6

Cognitive Changes Associated with Normal Aging

Julie L. Pickholtz and Barbara L. Malamut

With advances in health care in the United States and other industrialized countries, adults have been increasingly able to sustain their health status well into their 70s, 80s, and beyond. Associated with the improvement in health in older adults is a decrease in disease-related cognitive impairment. Thus, the significant mental decline that was once thought to be an inevitable part of the aging process is not considered characteristic of normal healthy aging. Adult offspring have been found to exhibit significantly less cognitive decline from their 60s to early 70s than their parents, providing evidence that cognitive aging has slowed (117). However, even though cognitive stability is greater than was once expected, specific age-related cognitive changes occur, even in healthy individuals. It is estimated that two of three intact elderly individuals exhibit some degree of performance decrement on neuropsychological testing (63). Research findings concerning the age at which decline begins and the trajectory of decline vary depending on the abilities studied and the study design (107). Some studies demonstrate that age-related cognitive changes decrease in a continuous fashion across the life span from as early as the 20s (87), while others indicate an acceleration of cognitive decline in later years (121).

There is an abundance of evidence in the aging literature that decline occurs in a number of areas of cognitive functioning in healthy, nondemented older adults. Although the focus of this chapter is on the neuropsychological, rather than biologic, aspects of aging, a short discussion of normal age-related changes in the brain is included because these neuropathologic events play a role in the cognitive changes.

NEUROPATHOLOGY

With aging, it is generally accepted that a number of changes in the brain occur universally, which are considered normal and are independent of disease processes (105). For example, there is evidence for age-related decreases in dopamine markers throughout the cortex and in the hippocampus, amygdala, and thalamus (7). Layer II of entorhinal cortex, an area necessary for forming new memories, shows pathology in virtually all humans over the age of 55 (78). Research also suggests that, as the nervous system ages, there are changes in the microvasculature in some regions of the brain (103).

Computed tomography (CT) and magnetic resonance imaging (MRI) studies have shown that aging is associated with enlargement of the cerebral ventricles and sulci and a decline in gray and white matter volumes (14,94,95). Gray matter loss is more pronounced than white matter loss in the overall brain. The age at which brain changes occur has been found to differ between men and women. A precipitous increase in ventricular volume begins in the fifth decade in men and the sixth decade in women, with an approximate 20% increase in ventricular volume per decade for both sexes (62).

Longitudinal MRI studies looking at regional differences indicate that age-specific volume changes do not appear to be uniform across brain areas. For both men and women, age differences are greatest in the parietal region compared with the frontal, temporal, and occipital areas. However, men show a greater loss of brain volume in all cortical regions (26,81,99). Loss of hippocampal volume has also been found to be greater for men than for women (26,99). In fact, volume decline in the hippocampus was found to begin as early as the third decade in men (92). With regard to gender-specific differences among brain regions, the greatest difference between the sexes appears to be in the volumes of the frontal and temporal regions.

The relationship between these age-related structural changes and functional decrements is less clear. Because normal aging affects some brain areas more than others, a decline would be expected in the cognitive functions supported by those regions. However, increase in ventricle volume independent of age did not explain normal age-related declines seen in intelligence scores (62). Similarly, when the effects of age were controlled in a different study, variations in total and limbic brain volumes were not predictive of memory test performance (129). In a cross-sectional MRI study of memory across the adult life span, changes in right-sided hippocampal volume with age were not related to steeper rates of forgetting for visual spatial material. However, cortical volumes were also measured and found to be a better predictor of recognition memory than hippocampal volume (42). No age-related differences were found between the two structures in their predictive power of recall abilities.

Functional imaging studies have raised the issue that aging may involve a functional plasticity or reallocation of brain network operations when performing a cognitive task. For example, when old and young subjects were compared using positron emission tomography (PET) during a verbal memory task, hypometabolism in the frontal region and greater activation in the occipital region were associated with age-related decline (50). Similarly, results from another PET study comparing young and old subjects who were matched for level of performance suggested that a different hippocampal network was activated during a visual memory test in the older subjects (36). A general trend has emerged from many functional neuroimaging studies of aging that suggests that activation is more lateralized in younger individuals and bilateral and more diffuse in older adults when performing the same task (19). Overall, these studies provide evidence that, when older subjects perform the same task as younger individuals, they use different brain pathways, but it is not yet known whether older individuals go about the task using different strategies.

AREAS OF COGNITIVE DECLINE IN NORMAL AGING

INTELLECTUAL ABILITIES

Intelligence can be conceptualized as consisting of two broad factors: fluid abilities, which reflect neurobiologic processes, and crystallized abilities, which depend more on experience and sociocultural influences (21,55). The basic trend in general intellectual abilities over time is for slight improvement in these abilities in early adulthood, stability in the middle years, and decline in later years (69). However, the decline is not uniform.

In general, fluid intelligence is vulnerable to the effects of aging, whereas crystallized intelligence is relatively spared. Fluid abilities such as processing speed, memory, and fluid reasoning are particularly vulnerable to the effects of aging, whereas crystallized abilities such as vocabulary and general knowledge remain stable (29,121). Many of these age-related changes are reflected on standardized intellectual testing. On the Wechsler Adult Intelligence Scale (WAIS), decline on Performance scales occurs at about the age of 60, whereas decline on the Verbal scales occurs at around age 80 (1,137). Research investigating differential life-span trajectories indicates that fluid intelligence reaches

a peak in the mid-20s, with decline starting by the mid-30s and continuing into old age (70). In contrast, crystallized intelligence does not peak until the 40s and remains stable for several decades, with some studies suggesting decline as early as the early 70s (70) and others not until the 90s (121).

PERFORMANCE SPEED

Aging is associated with slowing of many motor, perceptual, and cognitive behaviors and is most readily seen on timed tests. Age-related changes in motor and cognitive speed play a role in lower scores on the performance subtests of the WAIS because many of the subtests are timed (63). It has been found that performance on simple reaction time tests starts to decline at approximately age 50 (37). Speed of motor performance is inversely related to age on measures of walking speed and finger-tapping (109). However, performance decrements noted on many timed measures are not caused simply by motor slowing, but involve slowing of higher level cognitive processes as well (37,45). Thus, any reaction-time task that involves initiation, redirection, or decision making may be slowed because of slowed mental processing. An even more direct measure of cognitive slowing that assesses central processing time (i.e., event-related P300 and other evoked potentials) demonstrates a positive relationship between increasing age and longer latency intervals. It has been suggested that slowing of information processing is ubiquitous among people over 60 years old (9,117), whereas Salthouse (112) has found that processing speed declines from the 20s through old age. In adults over the age of 70, perceptual speed declines at increasingly rapid rates as times goes on (121). Processing of emotional stimuli, such as identification of facial expression, is also slower in older adults (64).

MEMORY

The most common cognitive complaint among elderly people is a change in memory. However, complaints about declining memory do not always correlate with poor performance on tests of memory (96,141,144). As seen in Table 6-1 and discussed in the following sections, memory can be divided into several components (i.e., immediate, declarative, nondeclarative, and remote), and studies have shown that different aspects of memory are sensitive to aging in various degrees.

Immediate Memory Span

Immediate memory is the ability to retain small amounts of information that remain untransformed for a very short period of time. Immediate memory span is usually measured with the number of digits one can repeat in correct sequential order immediately after presentation (i.e., digit span). Older adults perform

Table 6-1. *Changes in Memory Functioning with Normal Aging*

Memory Type	Change
Immediate memory	Unchanged
Short-term memory	Reduced
Long-term memory	Variable
Declarative	
Semantic	Unchanged up to age 70 years
Episodic	Reduced
Free recall	Reduced
Cued recall	Large benefit
Recognition	Unchanged
Acquisition	Reduced
Retrieval	Reduced
Percent retention	Unchanged
Source memory	Reduced
Nondeclarative	Mild decline
Remote memory	Unchanged

more poorly on tests of immediate memory than younger adults (147), although recent studies have suggested that the reduction of performance on traditional immediate memory tests may be related to factors other than memory. For example, some evidence indicates that the slower articulation rate of older adults contributes to their reduced span measures, and, when the rate of presentation is slowed, older adults perform equivalent to younger adults (80). Furthermore, items from early trials involving digit span have been found to interfere with performance on later trials. Because older adults are more susceptible to interference, they are at a disadvantage on later trials, which are used to measure higher levels of memory span (73).

Short-Term Memory

Short-term memory refers to the ability to recall larger amounts of new information very shortly after it is presented. Studies have shown significant age-related declines in the immediate recall of stories, word lists, and designs. This is due to difficulties in accessing stored information (31). As with immediate memory, age-related effects can be attenuated when information is presented at a slower pace, cuing is provided, and rehearsal is allowed (80).

Long-Term Memory

Long-term memory refers to the ability to learn and retain large amounts of newly learned information over a relatively long period of time. It involves encoding, consolidating, and retrieving the material. Long-term memory can be subdivided into declarative and nondeclarative memory.

Declarative Memory Declarative memory, which is also known as "explicit memory," refers to conscious

learning and remembering of events and facts and is tested by measures of recall and recognition. Many studies have shown that declarative or explicit memory declines with age, but the degree of change depends on the testing method. In general, older people perform significantly worse on free recall than recognition tests. Furthermore, age-related decline is not uniform across all of its components (63). Declarative memory can be further subdivided into semantic and episodic memory.

Semantic memory, which refers to memory for factual information or general word knowledge, is relatively resilient to the effects of aging. Research demonstrates an increase in general knowledge until early to middle old age and thereafter a modest decrease (83,87,107).

Episodic memory, which involves memories for personally experienced events that occur at a specific place and time (130), has been shown to be more age sensitive than semantic memory (83) and declines more rapidly (107). Such decline has been reported in both the verbal and visuospatial modalities (87). The ability to acquire episodic memory appears to decline progressively after the age of 70 years (22,122). The age-related changes are not limited to performance on standard memory tests, but also occur on batteries of tasks that are designed to emulate memory in everyday life such as prospective remembering of tasks (41,93). Aging is also associated with a decline in source memory (i.e., remembering specific information about the circumstances under which an event is encountered) (139). It has been found that older adults have more difficulty than younger adults in remembering the time, place, and other contextual features of events (39).

Although a reduction in the acquisition of new information can occur, healthy aging individuals do not tend to lose stores of information that have been learned. However, difficulty in retrieving that information has been observed. There is considerable evidence that the ability for strategic and effortful retrieval of newly learned information appears to be at least partially responsible for the decline in episodic memory. First, older adults have a lowered tendency for spontaneously using an organizational strategy when learning new information (126). Second, recall performance of older adults improves when retrieval cues are provided (89). Third, older adults perform more favorably on tests of recognition than on tests of free recall (32,83), which require more strategic and effortful functions. Hedden et al. (53) found evidence that working memory, which plays a role in strategic processing, has stronger relationships to free recall tasks and weaker relationships to cued recall and recognition tasks. Since working memory declines significantly with age, performance decline is less notable on tasks that provide an increasing level of environmental support (i.e., cued recall and recognition tasks).

In clinical settings, it is often difficult to detect declines in memory because elderly individuals are sometimes able to provide elaborate autobiographic information about their remote history. Evidence suggests that, in old age, personal experiences from early in life are remembered more easily than experiences from later in life. In contrast, younger adults show the reverse pattern, remembering recent events more easily than more remote events (93).

Nondeclarative Memory Nondeclarative memory, also known as "implicit memory," refers to learning as a result of prior experience without conscious reference to that experience. It has been noted that implicit memory declines less dramatically with age than explicit memory (63,93). One measure of nondeclarative memory is skill learning, in which improvement in speed or accuracy on a challenging task is measured. Some of the limited studies that have been performed with respect to aging have generally suggested that, relative to younger adults, the rate of skill learning in older adults is slower (145).

To summarize, aging is associated with a decline in declarative short-term and long-term memory, particularly for new episodic information. This memory decline is most pronounced when strategies are required for new learning. Aged individuals perform most favorably when asked to recognize rather than recall information. Furthermore, semantic information is remembered more easily than episodic information. Some evidence also suggests that certain types of nondeclarative memory decline with aging, although to a lesser extent than declarative memory.

ATTENTION

Attention is composed of a complex set of functions responsible for maintaining focus and selecting and processing certain aspects of experience. As is the case with memory, different aspects of attention are affected in aging to varying degrees.

Selective Attention

The ability to attend selectively to specific aspects of the environment is important for everyday behaviors that require an individual to ignore irrelevant information. Selective attention is important for such tasks as driving an automobile and conversing in noisy environments. Studies have demonstrated that older adults are more negatively affected by the presence of distracting information when engaged in a task (20,40). Relative to younger adults, they tend to have greater difficulty ignoring irrelevant information (73) and are more distracted by both visual (136) and auditory information (4).

Divided Attention

It has been noted that older subjects are more penalized than younger subjects when they must divide their attention between two sources (30). Although experimental findings have varied, task difficulty and task novelty have been found to mediate the degree to which age differences in divided attention are demonstrated (114,131). Thus, declines in divided attention are most apparent in aging adults when the task is novel or at a high level of difficulty.

Sustained Attention

Sustained attention, also known as "vigilance," refers to the ability to maintain concentration or focus over time. The studies that have investigated age differences in vigilance task performance have generally demonstrated little evidence for age-related declines (73). However, some evidence indicates that, under conditions when task difficulty is increased, sustained attention performance declines with age (79).

EXECUTIVE

Executive functions encompass a broad range of cognitive skills that rely on the functions of the prefrontal cortex, including monitoring of behavior, generating goals, memory of temporal sequences, inhibiting overlearned responses, and alternating behavioral responses in response to feedback. The prefrontal cortex is among the first parts of the aging brain to be affected (94). Therefore, it is not surprising that literature implicates change in executive functions as underlying many of the age-related decrements in cognition (48, 140). Executive functions are comprised of a number of heterogeneous skills, with some measures declining with age and others remaining relatively stable.

A classic example of an executive task is the Wisconsin Card Sorting Test (WCST), which involves problem solving and the ability to shift mental set when provided feedback (52). Aged individuals have been shown to make more perseverative errors on this task (i.e., persist in using a failed strategy) than their younger counterparts (94). These age-related increases in perseverative errors in healthy adults are associated with reduced volume of the prefrontal cortex and greater frontal subcortical white matter intensities on magnetic resonance imaging (47). Older individuals also make more perseverative errors on a variety of other cognitive tasks (34), suggesting a decline in mental flexibility. It has been suggested that these perseverative errors occur because older adults have more difficulty switching rapidly between sets of rules (148).

Abstract reasoning ability is another skill that relies on executive functions (e.g., flexible thinking) that has been found to decline with old age. Older people often approach reasoning tasks in a rigid way and are more likely than young adults to give concrete responses to proverb interpretation (69). Associations have also been found with age and tests of everyday problem solving and reasoning in community-dwelling nondemented older adults (18).

Aging has been associated with a decline in the ability to judge the order in which new information is presented. Studies have shown a decreased ability in the elderly to judge the relative recency of presentation for both pictures and words (76). This temporal tagging of information is considered to be a frontally mediated executive task. Older adults are also slower than young adults to think of an item they just saw, and this decrement is associated with reduced activation of the dorsolateral prefrontal cortex using functional magnetic resonance imaging (fMRI) (59).

The ability to inhibit automatic responses is an aspect of executive function that has shown varying results in the aging literature. One measure of inhibition that tends to remain relatively stable is the stop-signal task, which requires subjects to refrain from responding in response to a stimulus. Older subjects do not show decline in performance when the stimulus remains the same throughout the task; however, age-related decline is demonstrated if subjects must refrain from responding with one stimulus but not with another (12). Aging has also been found to have a negative effect on a person's ability to inhibit a usual response in a situation in favor of producing a novel response (138).

WORKING MEMORY

Working memory refers to an individual's ability to momentarily hold information in mind and simultaneously manipulate that information. For example,

digit span backward requires working memory because a person must hold all the numbers in abeyance to recall them in reverse. Age-related changes have been demonstrated in working memory and are thought to be related to disruption in executive functions as well as encoding and retrieval systems in the brain (63). Many studies have demonstrated that older people show moderate deficits on a variety of working memory tasks (111). For example, older subjects have more difficulty with a task that requires them to read a sentence while concurrently maintaining target words (85). Likewise, the ability to hold auditory instructions in a theoretical "phonologic loop" while delaying the execution of a task declines with age (65). Event-related potential studies suggest that age-associated disturbances in frontal lobe function contribute to the decline in working memory in normal aging (23). Decreased activation of the anterior cingulate cortex has also been associated with age-related decline in working memory (85). PET studies comparing young and old subjects have reported increased metabolism in several frontal lobe regions during working memory tasks in older subjects, which is thought to be caused by their need for compensatory strategies (43). Whereas better performance on working memory tests in younger adults is associated with decreased dorsolateral prefrontal cortical activity on functional MRI, older adults show increased activity in this area with better performance (110), supporting the idea that, as individuals age, an increased physiologic recruitment of frontal cortical areas is required to compensate.

LANGUAGE

Normal aging is associated with a decline in specific language skills. Reading abilities (108), fund of vocabulary (121), and functional knowledge of syntax and grammar (69) are essentially preserved. This relatively spared verbal knowledge can support performance on some memory tasks where knowledge can play a role. Furthermore, older adults are more likely than younger adults to take advantage of the application of verbal knowledge in such tasks (53). Other aspects of language change significantly with age. The most frequent language complaint of older individuals involves difficulty in retrieving names of people, places, and objects. Indeed, studies have shown that problems in accessing words (also known as lexical retrieval or the "tip-of-the-tongue" phenomenon) are greater for older than younger adults (16).

Performance on confrontational naming tests tends to remain stable between the ages of 30 and 50 years, decline slightly in the 60s, and clearly decrease among people aged 70 years or older (15,68). Qualitative changes in errors made on naming tests are also seen. These errors include: (a) circumlocutions, or using more words than necessary to provide accurate information; (b) nominalizations, or words describing the function of the pictured object (e.g., "mouth organ" for harmonica); (c) visual-perceptual errors, or misidentifications of the stimulus (e.g., "motel" for harmonica); and (d) semantic association errors, or responses that name an associate of the pictured object (e.g., "dice" for dominoes). These errors indicate that older people are familiar with information about the objects that they are asked to name but that they may have difficulty retrieving specific words. Thus, they "know" an item but cannot think of its name (69). More recent research suggests that aging negatively affects the retrieval of proper names more than other types of words (58,97).

Lowered performance in rate of verbal output (i.e., fluency) has been found to be affected from the age of 70 onward (83,84,106). Comprehension of spoken language has been found to be affected at an older age than naming and fluency and does not begin to decline until around the age of 80 years (106).

OTHER FACTORS AFFECTING COGNITION IN THE ELDERLY

Growing evidence indicates that many environmental and individual factors can influence cognitive function in aging. The next section includes a discussion of some of the variables shown to affect cognition in older individuals.

HEALTH STATUS

Even in the absence of medical illness, subtle changes in health status among intact older adults can be associated with cognitive changes. The presence of mild age-related health problems such as hypertension, diabetes, and mild cardiopathy, even when controlled by medications, has a negative impact on both cognition and waking cerebral electrical activity in the elderly (35).

Biologic age (as measured by biologic markers sensitive to aging, such as pulmonary capacity, sensory status, and muscle strength) accounts for a significant amount of age-related variance in cognitive performance, after controlling for health status and chronologic age (135). Likewise, baseline measures of cardiorespiratory fitness in healthy older adults were associated with preservation of cognitive function 6 years later (10).

Diminished gastrointestinal absorption associated with aging can compromise nutritional status (63) and, therefore, affect cognitive functioning. Because low vitamin levels are more prevalent in old age (8), vitamin status should be considered when an older individual complains of cognitive changes. Some studies show that an inverse relationship exists between levels of vitamin B_{12} and folic acid and performance on various tests of visuospatial functioning, attention, and memory (104). It has recently been found that high serum folate is associated with lower cognitive performance in seniors with low vitamin B_{12} status. When vitamin B_{12} status is normal, however, high serum folate has been associated with protection against cognitive impairment (77).

LIFESTYLE

Evidence is mounting for the importance of good cardiovascular conditioning and healthful diet in maintaining brain function. Research suggests that aerobic fitness can improve certain aspects of attention and memory performance (17,49,66) and reaction time (24). For example, fitness level has been shown to affect performance on sustained attention tasks in the elderly (17), whereas fitness is unrelated to sustained attention in young adults. Furthermore, there is evidence that improvement in cognition can occur in response to cardiovascular training (27,28,74).

Smoking also affects cognition in the elderly. Chronic smokers have been found to show lower scores than nonsmokers on tests of fluid intelligence (147). Older adult smokers also demonstrate a greater decline relative to nonsmokers on measures of information processing speed when tested 2 years after baseline (123). Furthermore, higher cigarette pack per year exposure is correlated with a significantly higher rate of decline in nondemented elderly adults (86).

Longitudinal data from the Nurses' Health Study indicated that total vegetable intake was significantly associated with less cognitive decline among older women, whereas fruits were not associated with cognition. The strongest associations occurred with greater intake of green leafy and cruciferous vegetables (60).

There is an increasing amount of evidence that older adults who lead a more active lifestyle can preserve their cognitive functioning (56,82,115). A cognitively and socially enriched lifestyle may slow the rate of cognitive decline in healthy older adults. Involvement in nonphysical leisure activities (e.g., chess, church, theatre, music) in middle adulthood is associated with slower decline in verbal memory in later life (102).

SENSORY FUNCTIONS

Hearing and vision commonly decline in old age. There is a growing body of research that supports a strong connection between sensory and cognitive functioning in aging individuals, even when accounting for compromised test performance as a result of sensory deficits. Longitudinal research has found that changes in sensory acuity are associated with changes in many cognitive abilities, even in the absence of overt sensory impairments. Some studies have found a relationship between both visual and auditory functioning and cognitive performance (71,132). Others suggest that decline in visual, but not auditory, modalities predicts decline in mental status test performance (101) and memory (5). Age-related reduction in vision is associated with reduced performance on mental status exam and verbal fluency (25). Some research has found improvements in mental status after cataract surgery that is not accounted for by restoration of visual acuity (127), whereas other studies show no evidence of long-term beneficial effect of improvement of sensory function on cognitive variables (132).

MEDICATIONS

Given increasing health complaints in the elderly, it is not surprising that aging adults take medication more frequently than younger adults. Diminished medication metabolism in older people can result in lowered tolerance, which often has negative effects on cognitive function (63). In particular, several studies have found that benzodiazepines can cause decline in cognitive performance among elderly individuals (128). For example, use of benzodiazepines is associated with decreases in episodic memory performance (67,91). Longitudinal data reveal that polypharmacy has a detrimental effect on cognitive ability in nondemented elderly subjects, whereas statins have a beneficial effect (124). In Chapter 4, the actions of specific medications are discussed in detail. When a change in cognition is presented, it is important to consider the possibility of medication change. Over-the-counter medications including vitamins also need to be considered because they can also cause significant cognitive problems on their own or through interactions with other medications.

HORMONE REPLACEMENT THERAPY

Results from studies linking estrogen levels and cognitive performance in women have yielded conflicting results. Several studies have demonstrated that hormone replacement therapy (HRT) in postmenopausal women may have a protective effect on cognitive performance compared with women not using HRT (61,98). Verbal fluency has been shown to benefit from HRT (46,146). It has also been suggested that HRT enhances verbal and visual memory in women and may forestall deterioration in short- and long-term memory that occurs with normal aging (100,119). Because of these cognitive benefits, it was hypothesized that HRT could potentially delay the onset of dementia. However, other studies have not found any cognitive benefit from HRT in postmenopausal women (11,72). Results of the large Women's Health Initiative Memory Study suggest that estrogen alone and combined estrogen and progesterone therapy may actually have an adverse effect on cognition

(120). Complicating this issue further are the findings of newer studies showing an increased risk of stroke in postmenopausal women on HRT (3). At this time, because the risks appear to outweigh the possible cognitive benefits, neurologists no longer recommend HRT in postmenopausal women. For more information about the medical effects of HRT, the reader is referred to Chapter 5.

DEPRESSION

Depression is common in elderly populations, with a prevalence ranging between 7.2% and 49% (38). Because depression is associated with declines in overall cognitive performance, particularly attention and memory (44), elderly individuals can often appear as if they have a dementia when they are actually depressed. This misdiagnosis is common because it is more difficult to detect depression in the elderly because depression in old age is more chronic in nature than that which occurs in younger adults. The lengthy development of depression in elderly adults, in contrast with the short clinical onset of depression in younger adults, can lead to undiagnosed depressive symptoms in the earlier stages of the disorder in older individuals (2). Some studies have found reduced levels of memory performance in depressed older adults on tasks with high demands on effortful encoding of information. Additionally, depressed older adults tend to benefit less from being provided with an inherent organizational structure when learning new material (6). Subjective memory complaints are more common among depressed than nondepressed older adults, even in the absence of memory deficits (141,144). Complicating the clinical picture of depressed older adults, depressive symptoms such as fatigue, apathy, and social withdrawal may be indicative of prodromal dementia (44,88).

EDUCATION

In general, level of education has been found to have significant associations with performance on neuropsychological measures (90). Studies among healthy elderly individuals suggest that those with higher levels of education tend to have better cognitive functioning and that this functioning is less likely to decline over time (57,116). In particular, highly educated individuals appear to have an advantage on tests that depend on the use of previously learned materials (e.g., tests of language and conceptualization). Education appears to be strongly related to abstraction and naming and less related to recognition and some recall memory measures (57). Lower education is also associated with larger age-related differences in memory for word lists (134). Exposure to languages also appears to protect against cognitive decline later in life. Compared with monolinguals, bilingual adults demonstrate better cognitive control, with older groups of adults showing the largest advantage (13).

Many plausible explanations are seen for the relationship between education and cognitive performance. For example, education is positively related to nutritional habits and health behaviors and, thus, may serve as a marker for better health, resulting in superior cognitive performance. Moreover, education increases exposure to general experiences and knowledge, which provides a larger context for problem solving and reasoning. These experiences may enable elderly educated individuals to develop compensatory strategies and adapt to cognitive losses more effectively (29). The "cognitive reserve" hypothesis provides some explanation for the protective effects of education and states that education may provide a buffer or reserve for the detrimental effects of aging on the brain (125).

LIVING ENVIRONMENT

In old age, a significant interaction occurs between psychosocial and neuropsychological factors. The living environment of older people has been shown to relate to their level of cognitive functioning. For example, in comparing older individuals living in a community with their counterparts living in institutions (e.g., senior citizen residents), those in the former group significantly out-performed the institutional group on tests of cognitive functioning, despite being matched for age, education, IQ, and health status (143). Although marked variability existed within both elderly groups, people living in institutions demonstrated greater cognitive variability, particularly in memory and functions associated with the frontal lobes, than people living in the community. No clear explanation is found for this difference between groups, but longitudinal studies of aging adults have shown that the level of cognitive functioning within an individual is not necessarily stable and will vary in parallel with variations in some psychosocial variables. In particular, two psychosocial variables—optimism and locus of control (i.e., belief in whether a person controls his or her own life or whether it is controlled by external forces)—best predicted level of cognitive functioning for both community- and institution-dwelling individuals over time (142). Likewise, higher control or self-efficacy beliefs are associated with better future performance or maintenance of ability over time (54). Therefore, it is possible that older people living in institutions may experience greater difficulties in relation to their environments that affect their optimism and feelings of control.

Marital status and living situation can also influence cognitive status. Van Gelder et al. (133) found that older men who lost a partner, who were unmarried, who started to live alone, or who lived alone in a 5-year period had significantly more cognitive decline compared with older men who were married or who lived with someone in those years. Possible explanations for these findings are that living alone or the loss of a partner can result in decreased social and leisure activities, higher risk of depression, and changes in diet and exercise patterns.

EMPLOYMENT

The number of older workers is projected to increase significantly over the next decade. It is estimated that individuals over age 55 will comprise as much as 20% of the workforce by 2015 (51). Given the age-related cognitive declines discussed in this chapter, an important question is whether job performance is compromised in older workers. Reviews of research on this issue have generally concluded that there is little evidence for a relationship between age and job performance (75). With a greater amount of work experience, older workers are likely to have acquired more job-related knowledge than younger workers, which is a very important predictor of job performance (118). According to Salthouse (113), older workers may compensate for cognitive decline by using their accumulated experience and knowledge because many job-related tasks rely more on crystallized abilities rather than fluid abilities.

Older workers' performance may be compromised in work situations where a high level of fluid abilities, such as response speed and working memory, are required. Czaja and Sharit (33) found that older subjects were significantly slower than younger subjects on computer-based tasks designed to simulate real-life jobs, controlling for prior computer experience. Although slower, they were as accurate in their responses as younger subjects. More specifically, the age-related differences were explained by slower psychomotor speed on a data entry task and poorer working memory on an account balancing task. In these situations, environmental accommodations and/or reallocation of job responsibilities may be warranted for older workers, particularly in occupations with high safety risk (e.g., vehicle operators, air traffic controllers, and police officers). In general, healthy aging workers can not only expect to remain a valuable part of the workforce, but the mental and social stimulation that employment provides may help protect older adults against age-related cognitive decline.

SUMMARY

Cognition in healthy aging people is a complex process that involves an interaction between psychosocial adjustment, premorbid cognitive functioning, level of education, nutritional and health status, environmental factors, and changes in the brain itself. Although many cognitive changes are associated with aging, the decline is not a universal process and, depending on the situation, may be slowed or even reversed. Finally, most healthy elderly people have the cognitive resources to function well in their own environments and to make appropriate accommodations when necessary.

REFERENCES

1. Albert MS, Moss MB. *Geriatric Neuropsychology.* New York: Guilford Press; 1988.
2. American Psychiatric Association. *Diagnostic and Statistical Manual of Mental Disorders.* 4th ed. Washington, DC: American Psychiatric Association; 1994.
3. Anderson GL, Limacher M, Assaf AR, et al. Effects of conjugated equine estrogen in post-menopausal women with hysterectomy: the Women's Health Initiative randomized controlled trial. *JAMA.* 2004;291:1701–1712.
4. Andres P, Parmentier FBR, Escera C. The effect of age on involuntary capture of attention by irrelevant sounds: a test of the frontal hypothesis of aging. *Neuropsychologia.* 2006;44:2564–2568.
5. Anstey KJ, Luszcz MA, Sanchez L. Two-year decline in vision but not hearing is associated with memory decline in very old adults in a population-based sample. *Gerontology.* 2001; 47:289–293.
6. Backman L, Forsell Y. Episodic memory functioning in a community-based sample of old adults with major depression: utilization of cognitive support. *J Abnorm Psychol.* 1994;103:361–370.
7. Backman L, Nyberg L, Lindenberger U, et al. The correlative triad among aging, dopamine, and cognition: current status and future prospects. *Neurosci ΩBiobehav Rev.* 2006;30:791–807.
8. Backman L, Small BJ, Wahling A. Cognitive functioning in very old age. In: Craik FI, Salthouse TA, eds. *The handbook of aging and cognition.* 2nd ed. Mahwah, NJ: Lawrence Erlbaum Associates; 2000.
9. Band GPH, Ridderinkhof KR, Segalowitz S. Explaining neurocognitive aging: is one factor enough? *Brain Cogn.* 2002;49:259–267.
10. Barnes DE, Yaffe K, Satariano WA, et al. A longitudinal study of cardiorespiratory fitness and cognitive function in healthy older adults. *J Am Geriatr Soc.* 2003;51:459–465.
11. Barret-Connor E. Hormone replacement. *Am J Geriatr Cardiol.* 1993;2:36–37.
12. Bedard AC, Nichols S, Barbosa JA, et al. The development of selective inhibitory control across the life span. *Dev Neuropsychol.* 2002;21:93–111.
13. Bialystok E, Craik FIM, Klein R, et al. Bilingualism, aging, and cognitive control: evidence from the Simon task. *Psychol Aging.* 2004;19:290–303.
14. Blatter DD, Bigler ED, Gade SD, et al. Quantitative volumetric analysis of brain MR: normative database spanning 5 decades of life. *Am J Neuroradiol.* 1995;16:241–251.
15. Borod JD, Goodglass H, Kaplan E. Normative data on the Boston Diagnostic Aphasia Examinations. *J Clin Neuropsychol.* 1980;2:209–215.
16. Bowles NL, Poon LW. Aging and retrieval of words in semantic memory. *J Gerontol.* 1985; 40:71–77.
17. Bunce DJ, Warr PB, Cochrane T. Blocks in choice responding as a function of age and physical fitness. *Psychol Aging.* 1993;8:26–33.
18. Burton CL, Strauss E, Hultsch DF, et al. Cognitive functioning and everyday problem solving in older adults. *Clin Neuropsychol.* 2006; 20:432–452.
19. Cabeza R. Hemispheric asymmetry reduction in older adults: the HAROLD model. *Psychol Aging.* 2002;17:85–100.
20. Carlson MC, Hasher L, Connelly SL, et al. Aging, distraction, and the benefits of predictable location. *Psychol Aging.* 1995;10:427–436.
21. Cattell RB. *Abilities: Their Structure, Growth and Action.* Boston: Houghton Mifflin; 1971.
22. Celsis P. Age-related cognitive decline, mild cognitive impairment or preclinical Alzheimer's disease. *Ann Med.* 2000;32:6–14.
23. Chao LL, Knight RT. Age-related prefrontal alterations during auditory memory. *Neurobiol Aging.* 1997;18:87–95.
24. Clarkson-Smith L, Hartley AA. Relationships between physical exercise and cognitive abilities in older adults. *Psychol Aging.* 1989;4:183–189.
25. Clemons TE, Rankin MW, McBee WL. Cognitive impairment in the age-related eye disease study. *Arch Ophthalmol.* 2006;124:537–543.
26. Coffey CE, Lucke JF, Saxton JA, et al. Sex differences in brain aging: a quantitative magnetic resonance imaging study. *Arch Neurol.* 1998; 55:169–179.
27. Colcombe SJ, Kramer AF. Fitness effects on the cognitive function of older adults: a meta-analytic study. *Psychol Sci* 2003;14:125–130.
28. Colcombe SJ, Kramer AF, Erickson KI, et al. Cardiovascular fitness, cortical plasticity, and aging. *Proc Natl Acad Sci USA.* 2004;101: 3316–3321.
29. Compton DM, Bachman LD, Brand D, et al. Age-associated changes in cognitive function in highly educated adults: emerging myths and realities. *Int J Geriatr Psychiatry.* 2000;15:75–85.
30. Craik FIM. Age differences in human memory. In: Birren JE, Schaie KW, eds. *Handbook of the psychology of aging.* New York: Van Nostrand Reinhold; 1977.
31. Craik FIM, Bialystok E. Cognition through the lifespan: mechanisms of change. *Trends Cogn Sci.* 2006;10:131–138.
32. Craik FIM, McDowd JM. Age differences in recall and recognition. *J Exp Psychol Learn Mem Cogn.* 1987;13:474–479.
33. Czaja S, Sharit J. Ability-performance relationships as a function of age and task experience for a data entry task. *J Exp Psychol Appl.* 1998;4:332–351.

34. Daignealt S, Braun CMJ, Whitaker HA. Early effects of normal aging on perseverative and non-perseverative prefrontal measures. *Dev Neuropsychol.* 1999;8:99–114.

35. Decary S, Vedette M, Massicotte-Marquez J, et al. A preliminary study of the impact of age-related pathologies on cognitive functioning and waking EEG. *North Am J Psychol.* 2005; 7:469–480.

36. Della-Maggiore V, Sekuler AB, Grady CL, et al. Corticolimbic interactions associated with performance on a short-term memory task are modified by age. *J Neurosci.* 2000; 20:8410–8416.

37. Der G, Deary IJ. Age and sex differences in reaction time in adulthood: results from the United Kingdom health and lifestyle survey. *Psychol Aging.* 2006;21:62–73.

38. Djernes JK. Prevalence and predictors of depression in populations of elderly: a review. *Acta Psychiatr Scand.* 2006;113:372–387.

39. Dodson CS, Bawa CS, Slotnick SD. Aging, source memory, and misrecollections. *J Exp Psychol.* 2007;33:169–181.

40. Earles JL, Connor LT, Frieske D, et al. Age differences in inhibition: possible causes and consequences. *Aging Neuropsychol Cogn.* 1997;4: 45–57.

41. Farrimond S, Knight RG, Titov N. The effects of aging on remembering intentions: performance on a simulated shopping task. *Appl Cogn Psychol.* 2006;20:533–555.

42. Fjell AM, Walhovd KB, Reinvang I, et al. Age does not increase rate of forgetting over weeks: neuroanatomical volumes and visual memory across the adult life-span. *J Int Neuropsychol Soc.* 2005;11:2–15.

43. Furey ML, Pietrini P, Haxby JV. Cholinergic stimulation alters performance and task-specific regional cerebral blood flow during working memory. *Proc Natl Acad Sci USA.* 1997; 94:6512–6516.

44. Ganguli M, Du Y, Dodge H, et al. Depressive symptoms and cognitive decline in late life. *Arch Gen Psychiatry.* 2006;63:153–160.

45. Gilmore R. Evoked potentials in the elderly. *J Clin Neurophysiol.* 1995;12:132–138.

46. Grodstein F, Chen J, Pollen DA, et al. Postmenopausal hormone therapy and cognitive function in healthy older women. *J Am Geriatr Soc.* 2000;48:746–752.

47. Gunning-Dixon FM, Raz N. Neuroanatomical correlates of selected executive functions in middle-aged and older adults: a prospective MRI study. *Neuropsychologia.* 2003;41:1929–1941.

48. Gunstead J, Paul RH, Brickman AM, et al. Patterns of cognitive performance in middle-aged and older adults: a cluster analytic examination. *J Geriatr Psychiatry Neurol.* 2006;19:59–64.

49. Hawkins HL, Kramer AF, Capaldi D. Aging, exercise and attention. *Psychol Aging.* 1992; 7:643–653.

50. Hazlett EA, Buchsbaum MS, Mohs RC, et al. Age-related shift in brain region activity during successful memory performance. *Neurobiol Aging.* 1998;19:437–445.

51. Head L, Baker PM, Bagwell B, et al. Barriers to evidence based practice in accommodations for an aging workforce. *Work.* 2006;27:391–396.

52. Heaton RK, Chelune GJ, Talley JL, et al. *Wisconsin Card Sorting Test manual: revised and expanded.* Odessa, FL: Psychological Assessment Resources; 1993.

53. Hedden T, Lautenschlager G, Park DC. Contributions of processing ability and knowledge to verbal memory tasks across the adult life-span. *Q J Exp Psychol.* 2005;58A:169–190.

54. Hess TM. Memory and aging in context. *Psychol Bull.* 2005;131:383–406.

55. Horn JL. Organization of abilities and the development of intelligence. *Psychol Rev.* 1968;75:242–259.

56. Hultsch DF, Hertzog C, Small BJ, et al. Use it or lose it: engaged lifestyle as a buffer of cognitive decline in aging? *Psychol Aging.* 1999; 14:245–263.

57. Inouye SK, Albert MS, Mohs R, et al. Cognitive performance in a high-functioning community-dwelling elderly population. *J Gerontol.* 1993;48: M146–M151.

58. James LE. Specific effects of aging on proper name retrieval: now you see them, now you don't. *J Gerontol.* 2006;61B:P180–P183.

59. Johnson MK, Mitchell KJ, Raye CL, et al. An age-related deficit in prefrontal cortical function associated with refreshing information. *Psychol Sci.* 2004;15:127–132.

60. Kang JH, Ascherio A, Grodstein F. Fruit and vegetable consumption and cognitive decline in aging women. *Ann Neurol.* 2005;57:713–720.

61. Kampen D, Sherwin BB. Estrogen use and verbal memory in healthy postmenopausal women. *Obstet Gynecol.* 1994;83:979–983.

62. Kaye JA, DeCarli C, Luxenberg JS, et al. The significance of age-related enlargement of the cerebral ventricles in healthy men and women measured by quantitative computed x-ray tomography. *J Am Geriatric Soc.* 1992;40:225–231.

63. Keefover RW. Aging and cognition. *Neurol Clin.* 1998;16:635–648.

64. Keightley ML, Winocur G, Burianova H, et al. Age effects on social cognition: faces tell a different story. *Psychol Aging.* 2006;21:558–572.

65. Kliegel M, Jager T. Delayed-execute prospective memory performance: the effects of age and working memory. *Dev Neuropsychol* 2006; 30:819–843.

66. Kramer A, Hahn S, Banich M, et al. Influence of aerobic fitness on the neurocognitive function of sedentary older adults. Poster session presented at the Cognitive Aging Conference, Atlanta, GA, 1998.

67. Kruse WH. Problems and pitfalls in the use of benzodiazepines in the elderly. *Drug Saf.* 1990; 7:328–344.

68. LaBarge E, Edwards D, Knesevich JW. Performance of normal elderly on the Boston Naming Test. *Brain Lang.* 1986;27:380–384.

69. La Rue A. *Aging and Neuropsychological Assessment.* New York: Plenum Press; 1992.

70. Li S, Lindenberger U, Hommel B, et al. Transformations in the couplings among intellectual abilities and constituent cognitive processes across the life span. *Psychol Sci.* 2004;15:155–163.

71. Lin MY, Gutierrez MS, Stone KL, et al. Vision impairment and combined vision and hearing impairment predict cognitive and functional decline in older women. *J Am Geriatr Soc.* 2004; 52:1996–2002.

72. Low L, Anstey KJ, Jorm AF, et al. Hormone replacement therapy and cognition in an Australian representative sample aged 60-64 years. *Maturitas.* 2006;54:86–94.

73. McDowd JM, Shaw RJ. Attention and aging: a functional perspective. In: Craik FI, Salthouse TA, eds. *The handbook of aging and cognition.* 2nd ed. Mahwah, NJ: Lawrence Erlbaum; 2000.

74. McDowell K, Kerick SE, Santa Maria DL, et al. Aging, physical activity, and cognitive processing: an examination of P300. *Neurobiol Aging.* 2003; 24:597–606.

75. McEvoy GM, Cascio WF. Cumulative evidence of the relationship between employee age and job performance. *J Appl Psychol.* 1989;74:11–17.

76. Mittenberg W, Seidenberg M, O'Learly DS, et al. Changes in cerebral functioning associated with normal aging. *J Clin Exp Neuropsychol.* 1989; 11:918–932.

77. Morris MS, Jacques PF, Rosenberg IH, et al. Folate and vitamin B-12 status in relation to anemia, macrocytosis, and cognitive impairment in older Americans in the age of folic acid fortification. *Am J Clin Nutr.* 2007;85:193–200.

78. Morrison HJ, Hof PR. Changes in cortical circuits during aging. *Clin Neurosci Res.* 2003; 2:294–304.

79. Mouloua M, Parasuraman R. Aging and cognitive vigilance: effects of spatial uncertainty and event rate. *Exp Aging Res.* 1995;21:17–32.

80. Multhaup KS, Balota DA, Cowan N. Implications of aging lexicality, and item length for the mechanisms underlying memory span. *Psychon Bull Rev.* 1996;3:112–120.

81. Murphy DG, DeCarli C, McIntosh AR, et al. Sex differences in human brain morphometry and metabolism: an in vivo quantitative magnetic resonance imaging and positron emission tomography study on the effect of aging. *Arch Gen Psychiatry.* 1996;53:585–594.

82. Newson RS, Kemps EB. General lifestyle activities as a predictor of current cognition and cognitive change in older adults: a cross-sectional and longitudinal examination. *J Gerontol.* 2005;60B:P113–P120.

83. Nyberg L, Ronnlund M, Dixon R, et al. Selective adult age differences in an age-invariant multifactor model of declarative memory. *Psychol Aging.* 2003;18:149–160.

84. Obler LK, Albert ML. Language skills across adulthood. In: Birren JE, Schaie KW, eds. *Handbook of the psychology of aging.* 2nd ed. New York: Van Nostrand Reinhold; 1985:463–473.

85. Otsuka Y, Osaka N, Morishita M, et al. Decreased activation of anterior cingulate cortex in the working memory of the elderly. *Neuroreport.* 2006;17:1479–1482.

86. Ott A, Andersen K, Dewey ME, et al. Effect of smoking on global cognitive function in nondemented elderly. *Neurology.* 2004;62:920–924.

87. Park DC, Hedden T, Davidson NS, et al. Models of visuospatial and verbal memory across the adult life span. *Psychol Aging.* 2002;17:299–320.

88. Paterniti S, Verdier-Taillefer M, Dufouil C, et al. Depressive symptoms and cognitive decline in elderly people. *Br J Psychiatry.* 2002;181:406–410.

89. Petersen R, Smith G, Kokmen E, et al. Memory function in normal aging. *Neurology.* 1992;42: 396–401.

90. Plassman BL, Welsh KA, Helms BS, et al. Intelligence and education as predictors of cognitive state in life. *Neurology.* 1995; 45:1446–1450.

91. Pomara N, Deptula D, Singh R, et al. Cognitive toxicity of benzodiazepines in the elderly. In: Salzman CL, Liebowitz B, eds. *Anxiety disorders and the elderly.* New York: Springer; 1991:175–196.

92. Pruessner JC, Collins DL, Pruessner M, et al. Age and gender predict volume decline in the anterior and posterior hippocampus in early adulthood. *J Neurosci.* 2001;21:194–200.

93. Prull MW, Gabrieli JD, Bunge SA. Age-related changes in memory: a cognitive neuroscience perspective. In: Craik FI, Salthouse TA, eds. *The handbook of aging and cognition.* 2nd ed. Mahwah, NJ: Lawrence Erlbaum Associates; 1999.

94. Raz N. Aging of the brain and its impact on cognitive performance: integration of structural and functional findings. In: Craik FI, Salthouse TA, eds. *The handbook of aging and cognition.* 2nd ed.

Mahwah, NJ: Lawrence Erlbaum Associates; 1999.

95. Raz N, Gunning-Dixon FM, Head D, et al. Neuroanatomical correlates of cognitive aging: evidence from structural magnetic resonance imaging. *Neuropsychology.* 1998;12:95–114.

96. Reese CM, Cherry KE. Effects of age and ability on self-reported memory functioning and knowledge of memory aging. *J Genet Psychol.* 2006;167:221–240.

97. Rendell PG, Castel AD, Craig FIM. Memory for proper names in old age: a disproportionate impairment? *Q J Exp Psychol.* 2005; 58A:54–71.

98. Resnick SM. Estrogen replacement therapy and cognitive aging. In: Keenan PA, Chairman. Neuroendocrinological influences on cognition. Symposium conducted at the American Psychological Association Convention, New York, NY, 1995. *Clin Neuropsychol.* 1995;9:3.

99. Resnick SM, Goldszal AF, Davatzikos C, et al. One-year age changes in MRI brain volumes in older adults. *Cereb Cortex.* 2000;10:464–472.

100. Resnick SM, Metter J, Zonderman AB. Estrogen replacement therapy and longitudinal decline in visual memory: a possible protective effect? *Neurology.* 1997;49:1491–1497.

101. Reyes-Ortiz CA, Kuo Y, DiNuzzo AR, et al. Near vision impairment predicts cognitive decline: data from the Hispanic established populations for epidemiologic studies of the elderly. *J Am Geriatr Soc.* 2005;53:681–686.

102. Richards M, Hardy R, Wadsworth MEG. Does active leisure protect cognition? Evidence from a national birth cohort. *Soc Sci Med.* 2003; 56:785–792.

103. Riddle DR, Sonntag WE, Lichtenwalter RJ. Microvascular plasticity in aging. *Ageing Res Rev.* 2003;2:149–168.

104. Riggs KM, Spiro A, Tucker K, et al. Relations of vitamin B-12, vitamin B-6, folate, and homocysteine to cognitive performance in the Normative Aging Study. *Am J Clin Nutr.* 1996; 63:306–314.

105. Ritchie K, Ledesert B, Touchon J. Subclinical cognitive impairment: epidemiology and clinical characteristics. *Compr Psychiatry* 2000;41:61–65.

106. Ritchie K, Touchon J, Ledesert B, et al. Establishing the limits and characteristics of normal age-related cognitive decline. *Rev Epidemiol Sante Publique.* 1997;45:373–381.

107. Ronnlund M, Nyberg L, Backman L, et al. Stability, growth, and decline in adult life span development of declarative memory: cross-sectional and longitudinal data from a population-based study. *Psychol Aging.* 2005;20:3–18.

108. Rubin E, Storandt M, Miller J, et al. A prospective study of cognitive function and onset of dementia in cognitively healthy elders. *Arch Neurol.* 1998;55:395–401.

109. Ruff RM, Parker SB. Gender and age-specific changes in motor speed and eye-hand coordination in adults: normative values for the Finger Tapping and Grooved Pegboard tests. *Percept Mot Skills.* 1993;76:1219–1230.

110. Rypma B, D'Esposito M. Isolating the neural mechanisms of age-related changes in human working memory. *Nat Neurosci.* 2000;3:509–515.

111. Salthouse TA. Age-related differences in basic cognitive processes: implications for work. *Exp Aging Res.* 1994;29:249–255.

112. Salthouse TA. Interrelations of aging, knowledge, and cognitive performance. In: Staudinger U, Lindenberger U, eds. *Understanding human development: dialogues with lifespan psychology.* Dordrecht, Netherlands: Kluwer Academic Publishers; 2003:265–287.

113. Salthouse TA. The aging of working memory. *Neuropsychology.* 1994;8:535–543.

114. Salthouse TA, Fristoe NM, Lineweaver TT, et al. Aging of attention: does the ability to divide decline? *Mem Cognit.* 1995;23:59–71.

115. Scarmeas N, Stern Y. Cognitive reserve and lifestyle. *J Clin Exp Neuropsychol.* 2003;25:625–633.

116. Schaie KW. The optimization of cognitive functioning in old age; predictions based on cohort-sequential and longitudinal data. In: Baltes PB, Baltes MM, eds. *Successful aging: perspectives from the behavioral sciences.* Cambridge, UK: Cambridge University Press; 1990:94–117.

117. Schaie KW. What can we learn from longitudinal studies of adult development? *Res Hum Dev.* 2005;2:133–158.

118. Schmidt FL, Hunter JE, Outerbridge AN. Impact of job experience and ability on job knowledge, work sample performance, and supervisory ratings of job performance. *J Appl Psychol.* 1986;7:432–439.

119. Sherwin BB. Can estrogen keep you smart? Evidence from clinical studies. *J Psychiatry Neurosci.* 1999;24:315–321.

120. Shumaker SA, Legault C, Kuller L, et al. Conjugated equine estrogens and incidence of probably dementia and mild cognitive impairment in postmenopausal women: Women's Health Initiative Memory Study. *JAMA.* 2004;291: 2947–2958.

121. Singer T, Verhaeghen P, Ghisletta P, et al. The fate of cognition in very old age: Six-year longitudinal findings in the Berlin Aging Study (BASE). *Psychol Aging.* 2003;18:318–331.

122. Small S, Stern Y, Tang M, et al. Selective decline in memory function among healthy elderly. *Neurology.* 1999;52:1392–1396.

123. Starr JM, Deary IJ, Fox HC, et al. Smoking and cognitive change from age 11 to 66 years: a confirmatory investigation. *Addict Behav.* 2007;32: 63–68.

124. Starr JM, McGurn B, Whiteman M, et al. Life long changes in cognitive ability are associated with prescribed medications in old age. *Int J Geriatr Psychiatry.* 2004;19:327–332.

125. Stern Y. What is cognitive reserve? theory and research application of the reserve concept. *J Int Neuropsychol Soc.* 2002;8:448–460.

126. Stuss DT, Craik FIM, Sayer L, et al. Comparison of older people and patients with frontal lesions: evidence of wordlist learning. *Psychol Aging.* 1996;11:387–395.

127. Tamura H, Tsukamoto H, Mukai S, et al. Improvement in cognitive impairment after cataract surgery in elderly patients. *J Cataract Refract Surg.* 2004;30:598–602.

128. Taylor JL, Tinklenberg JR. Cognitive impairment and benzodiazepines. In: Melzer HY, ed. *Psychopharmacology: the third generation of progress.* New York: Raven Press; 1987: 1449–1454.

129. Tisserand DJ, Visser PJ, van Boxtel MP, et al. The relation between global and limbic brain volumes on MRI and cognitive performance in healthy individuals across the age range. *Neurobiol Aging.* 2000;21:569–576.

130. Tulving E. *Elements of Episodic Memory.* New York: Oxford University Press; 1983.

131. Tun PA, Wingfield A. Does dividing attention become harder with age? Findings from the Divided Attention questionnaire. *Aging Cogn.* 1995;2:39–66.

132. Valentijn S, van Boxtel M, van Hooren S. Change in sensory functioning predicts change in cognitive functioning: results from a 6-year follow-up in the Maastricht aging study. *J Am Geriatr Soc.* 2005;53:374–380.

133. Van Gelder MB, Tijhuis M, Kalmijn S, et al. Marital status and living situation during a 5-year period are associated with subsequent 10-year cognitive decline in older men: the FINE Study. *J Gerontol.* 2006;61B: P213–P219.

134. Verhaeghen P, Marcoen A, Goossens L. Facts and fiction about memory aging: a quantitative integration of research findings. *J Gerontol.* 1993;48:157–171.

135. Wahlin A, deFrias C, MacDonald SWS, et al. How do health and biological age influence chronological age and sex differences in cognitive aging: moderating, mediating, or both? *Psychol Aging.* 2006;21:318–332.

136. Watson DG, Maylor EA. Aging and visual marking: selective deficits for moving stimuli. *Psychol Aging.* 2000;17:321–339.

137. Wechsler D. *WAIS-R Manual.* New York: The Psychological Corporation; 1981.

138. Wecker NA, Kramer JH, Wisniewski A, et al. Age effects on executive ability. *Neuropsychology.* 2000;14:409–414.

139. Wegesin DJ, Jacobs DM, Zubin NR, et al. Source memory and encoding strategy in normal aging. *J Clin Exp Neuropsychol.* 2000;22:455–464.

140. West R, Schwarb H. The influence of aging and frontal function on the neural correlates of regulative and evaluative aspects of cognitive control. *Neuropsychology.* 2006;20:468–481.

141. Williams JMG, Little MM, Scates S, et al. Memory complaints and abilities among depressed older adults. *J Consult Clin Psychol.* 1987;55:595–598.

142. Winocur G, Moscovitch M. A comparison of cognitive function in institutionalized and community-dwelling old people of normal intelligence. *Can J Psychol.* 1990;44:435–444.

143. Winocur G, Moscovitch M, Freedman J. An investigation of cognitive function in relation to psychosocial variables in institutionalized old people. *Can J Psychol.* 1987;41:257–269.

144. Wong C, Lam, L, Lui V, et al. Subjective complaints and self-evaluation of memory test performance in questionable dementia. *Int J Geriatr Psychiatry.* 2006;21:937–944.

145. Wright BM, Payne RB. Effects of aging on sex differences in psychomotor reminiscence and tracking proficiency. *J Gerontol.* 1985;40: 179–184.

146. Yonker JE, Adolfsson R, Eriksson E, et al. Verified hormone therapy improves episodic memory performance in healthy postmenopausal women. *Neuropsychol Dev Cogn B Aging Neuropsychol Cogn.* 2006;13:291–307.

147. Zacks RT, Hasher L, Li KZH. Human memory. In: Craik FI, Salthouse TA, eds. *The handbook of aging and cognition.* 2nd ed. Mahwah, NJ: Lawrence Erlbaum Associates; 2000.

148. Zelazo PD, Craik FIM, Booth L. Executive function across the life span. *Acta Psychol.* 2004; 115:167–183.

SUGGESTED WEBSITES

National Institute on Aging: http://www.nih.gov/nia/health

Health and Age: http://www.healthandage.com

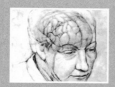

SECTION II

COMMON SIGNS AND SYMPTOMS IN THE OLDER ADULT

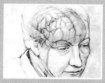

CHAPTER 7

Transient Loss of Consciousness: Seizures and Syncope

Maromi Nei and Reginald T. Ho

Transient loss of consciousness in the elderly often presents one of the most difficult diagnostic challenges, particularly because of the high incidence of chronic medical conditions and associated medication usage and the fact that so many conditions may lead to loss of consciousness.

The major differential diagnoses include neurologic and cardiovascular causes, with seizures and syncope leading the list. Seizures, which often present in the elderly, frequently are related to vascular and neurodegenerative conditions. Syncope refers to transient loss of consciousness often accompanied by loss of postural tone and generally results from inadequate global cerebral nutrient perfusion (34). Sudden cessation of cerebral perfusion for only 6 to 8 seconds can cause syncope and diffuse slowing on an electroencephalogram (EEG) (Fig. 7-1) (48). Its incidence increases with age due in part to greater medication

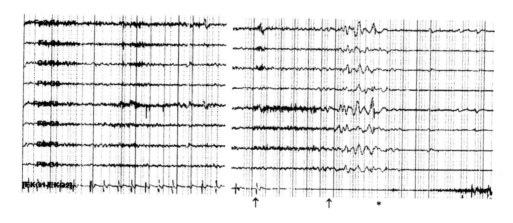

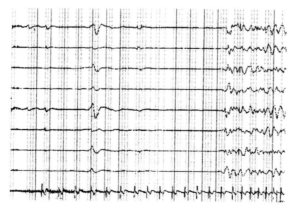

Figure 7-1. The electrocardiogram (ECG) reveals asystole for approximately 15.5 seconds, beginning at the *bold arrow*. Diffuse slowing of the electroencephalogram (EEG) follows 6 seconds later, and suppression of cerebral activity follows 10 seconds later. The suppression continues for approximately 18 seconds, including 12 seconds after return of the cardiac rhythm. This is again followed by diffuse slowing of the EEG, which is later followed by return of the EEG to a normal waking pattern (not shown).

usage and cardiovascular disease in elderly individuals (37,50,52).

PRESENTATION AND DIFFERENTIAL DIAGNOSIS

Details regarding the symptoms preceding and following the event are critical to determining the cause for loss of consciousness (8,32,35). A history regarding specific symptoms preceding loss of consciousness, particularly the duration and quality, should be elicited, and any triggering events should be identified (Tables 7-1 and 7-2).

SEIZURES

Seizures generally present as stereotyped spells that follow a specific and consistent progression of symptoms during each event. In partial-onset seizures, a specific aura can occur before the onset of alteration in level of consciousness. A clue may be a specific aura occurring in isolation as well as at the onset of a complex partial

Table 7-1. *Spells in the Elderly: Differential Diagnosis*

Neurologic
 Seizure
  Complex partial
  Secondarily generalized tonic-clonic
  Absence
  Nonconvulsive status epilepticus
 Transient ischemic attack
  Basilar artery ischemia
 Transient global amnesia
 Migraine
 Sleep disorder
 Nonepileptic psychogenic seizure
Cardiac
 Obstruction to outflow (aortic stenosis, idiopathic
  hypertrophic subaortic stenosis, pulmonary
  embolus)
 Loss of effective pump function (myocardial
  infarction, tamponade)
 Arrhythmias (bradyarrhythmias, tachyarrhythmias)
Reflexogenic
 Vasovagal syncope
 Situational syncope (cough, micturition, swallowing)
 Carotid sinus hypersensitivity
Orthostatic hypotension
 Medication effect
 Hypovolemic
 Neurogenic
Metabolic
 Hypoglycemia
 Hyperventilation

seizure (those associated with alteration in level of consciousness but without generalization) or secondarily as a generalized tonic-clonic seizure. The duration of seizures is brief, generally less than 2 minutes. However, in seizures associated with an alteration in level of consciousness, patients often experience amnesia of the seizure itself and may not recall events immediately preceding or following the seizure. Postictal confusion can last for several minutes to hours.

FOCAL CEREBRAL ISCHEMIA

Focal cerebral ischemia resulting in transient alteration in level of consciousness is not common. Normal consciousness depends on the functioning of both cerebral hemispheres, the reticular formation, other upper brainstem structures, the thalamus, and the hypothalamus (44). Thus, focal cerebral ischemia, as during a transient ischemic attack or stroke, must involve either both cerebral hemispheres or the brainstem and other deeper structures to result in alteration in level of consciousness. Posterior circulation ischemia or massive hemisphere infarction with shift can present with alteration in level of consciousness. Posterior circulation ischemia generally results in focal signs and symptoms (e.g., diplopia, eye movement abnormalities, other cranial nerve abnormalities, cerebellar dysfunction, motor and sensory dysfunction), which aid in the diagnosis. Massive infarction, of course, results in a sustained alteration in level of consciousness.

TRANSIENT GLOBAL AMNESIA

Transient global amnesia (TGA) presents with marked anterograde amnesia that generally persists for hours, as well as retrograde amnesia. Although patients may be disoriented to time and place, they retain knowledge of their identity. The patient often repeatedly asks the same questions and has difficulty encoding new memories during this event. No focal neurologic deficits are seen, and the patient is fully conscious throughout the episode, unlike during a complex partial seizure. The pathophysiology is debated but may be related to either cerebral ischemia or seizure. The finding of reversible changes in the CA-1 sector of the hippocampus on high-resolution magnetic resonance imaging (MRI) suggests that this area may be involved in the pathophysiology of TGA (6). The incidence of TGA has been estimated to be approximately five in 100,000 persons. Less than 25% of patients experience recurrent episodes (2,41).

SLEEP DISORDERS

Sleep disorders (e.g., sleep apnea or narcolepsy) present with other symptoms that suggest a sleep

Table 7-2. *Variables That Distinguish Common Spells in the Elderly*

Variable	Seizure	Syncope	TIA	TGA
Premonitory symptoms	None vs. aura	None vs. N/V, lightheadedness Diaphoresis	None	None
Posture effect	None	Often erect	None	None
Onset	Acute	Variable	Acute	Acute
Bystander observations				
Duration	1–2 minutes	Seconds to minutes	Minutes to hours	Hours
Movements	Variable tonic-clonic movements	Loss of tone Clonic jerks	Deficits along vascular pattern	None
Incontinence	Variable	None	None	None
Heart rate	Increased or decreased	Variable	Normal	Normal
Electroencephalogram during ictus	Epileptiform pattern	Diffuse Slowing	Focal Slowing or normal	Rare Slowing
Trauma	Tongue laceration or ecchymoses	Ecchymoses or fracture	None	None
Offset	Confusion Sleep	Alert or mild confusion	Alert	Alert

N/V, nausea and vomiting; TGA, transient global amnesia; TIA, transient ischemic attack.

disorder, particularly excessive daytime sleepiness, which results in lapses in consciousness. However, a history of sedation and concomitant symptoms (e.g., snoring or apnea) clearly differentiates the diagnosis of sleep disorders from other disorders.

NONEPILEPTIC PSYCHOGENIC SEIZURES

Nonepileptic psychogenic seizures are more common in younger individuals; however, they also occur in the elderly. A variety of different types of presentations are seen. Although slumping and sudden apparent loss of consciousness can occur, shaking and other movements can occur as well. Common features include (a) nonstereotyped spells; (b) irregular, nonrhythmic movements; (c) eye closure during the event; (d) waxing and waning of symptoms; (e) prolonged symptoms over several minutes to hours; (f) no history of spells arising directly from sleep; and (g) no history of severe injury (e.g., fracture, burn) during the spells. The patient may have a history of sexual or physical abuse, lack of response to anticonvulsant medication, and history of a psychiatric disorder. Recent data suggest that, in the elderly, a history of severe physical health problems or health-related traumatic experiences may be a prominent risk factor in this age group (20). Video-electroencephalographic (VEEG) monitoring (1) or EEG and observation of the episode are helpful in establishing the diagnosis.

SYNCOPE

Because syncope has a myriad of etiologies, it is useful to classify its causes into (a) cardiovascular, (b) neurally mediated (reflexogenic), (c) orthostatic (postural), and (d) metabolic because the diagnostic evaluation and prognosis in each category differ. Cardiovascular causes of syncope include arrhythmias and structural cardiopulmonary disease, and they should be considered in any elderly patient with significant heart disease (e.g., myocardial infarction, congestive heart failure). Arrhythmic syncope is often abrupt, and such an episode in a patient with left ventricular dysfunction or conduction abnormalities (e.g., bundle branch block) should raise suspicion for ventricular tachyarrhythmias and bradyarrhythmias, respectively. Structural cardiopulmonary disease causing syncope reduces cerebral perfusion by obstructing blood flow (e.g., aortic stenosis, hypertrophic obstructive cardiomyopathy) or decreasing cardiac output (e.g., myocardial infarction, tamponade).

Neurally mediated syncope includes vasovagal, viscerovagal (situational), and carotid sinus hypersensitivity and is due to an exaggerated reflex that increases vagal tone (causing bradycardia) while reducing sympathetic outflow (causing hypotension). Such forms of syncope often have a triggering event (e.g., prolonged standing, defecation, coughing). The classical prodromal symptoms of vasovagal syncope (warmth, nausea, lightheadedness, and diaphoresis) might be absent in an elderly patient. Abrupt syncope without prodrome can even occur (malignant vasovagal syncope). Orthostatic syncope is due to an abrupt drop in blood pressure while assuming an erect posture and is common in the elderly (54). Autonomic dysfunction, loss of baroreceptor responses, and frequent use of multiple medications predispose elderly individuals to orthostatic syncope. Primary autonomic failure can be caused by multiple system atrophy, which is generally associated with brainstem dysfunction or parkinsonism. The Shy-Drager and Bradbury-Eggleston types of autonomic failure are associated with other evidence of autonomic dysfunction, including sexual and bladder dysfunction and anhidrosis. Secondary autonomic dysfunction can result from an autonomic neuropathy, often associated with a peripheral neuropathy, which may be seen in diabetes mellitus, chronic inflammatory demyelinating neuropathy, amyloidosis, and other types of neuropathy. Metabolic abnormalities causing syncope are rare. These include high-altitude sickness [causing low partial pressure of oxygen (PO_2)], acute hyperventilation [causing low partial pressure of carbon dioxide (PCO_2) and cerebral vasoconstriction], and hypoglycemia. Insulinomas can cause repetitive seizurelike spells due to recurrent hypoglycemia (7). Hypoglycemia is also often associated with neuro-adrenergic symptoms (e.g., diaphoresis and tremors).

SEIZURES

Seizures are among the most common causes of transient loss of consciousness in the elderly. The incidence of both acute symptomatic and unprovoked seizures increases with age. The incidence of acute symptomatic seizures is approximately 100 in 100,000 persons older than 60 years of age (5,39). These seizures may be caused by acute cerebrovascular ischemia (40% to 50%), metabolic derangements (10% to 15%), drug withdrawal, central nervous system (CNS) infection, acute trauma, or toxic insults (5,39). The incidence of unprovoked seizures exceeds 100 in 100,000 persons in this same age group (25). Unprovoked seizures can occur as the result of a prior stroke or head trauma or in association with degenerative diseases such as Alzheimer's disease. However, a definitive cause for epilepsy (having two or more unprovoked seizures) is identified only in the minority of patients (30% to 50%) (5,39).

Risk factors for the development of epilepsy include a history of stroke, which is associated with a more than 20-fold increase in the risk of epilepsy; brain neoplasm; neurodegenerative disease; drug or alcohol withdrawal; CNS infection, which is associated with a threefold increase in risk; and head trauma, which is associated with a threefold increase in risk

(33,49). Alzheimer's disease is associated with a five- to 10-fold increase in risk for epilepsy (18,27,29,40,46). Major depression may also be a risk factor for seizures in the elderly (30).

Multiple seizure types may be seen. Partial-onset seizures, often related to degenerative, vascular, or neoplastic causes, are most common. However, generalized seizures related to toxic-metabolic encephalopathies and, perhaps, to genetic predisposition also occur.

TEMPORAL LOBE SEIZURES

Temporal lobe seizures are the most common type of seizure in the adult population, although extratemporal seizures may be more common in the elderly than in other age groups. Temporal lobe seizures can begin with an aura, such as a feeling of epigastric discomfort, an indescribable sensation, déjà vu, fear, or tinnitus. Although seizures are typically associated with positive phenomena, rather than the absence of normal function, both types of symptoms can be seen. During the seizure, speech arrest can occur, particularly in seizures originating in the left hemisphere. Complex partial seizures (those associated with an alteration in level of consciousness) arising from the temporal lobe may be manifested by automatisms, lip smacking, teeth grinding, chewing, and the utterance of phrases or sentences that can be unintelligible or repetitive. Staring without automatisms is a common presentation in this age group, and head or eye deviation or dystonic posturing can occur. Postictally, confusion can last for several minutes to hours, and the patient may experience amnesia of the seizure. Because the temporal lobes are important for memory, patients with seizures arising from this area often complain of memory difficulty interictally as well.

Because of connections to the hypothalamus, temporal lobe seizures can be associated with autonomic changes. These include pupillary dilatation, apnea, hyperventilation, flushing, diaphoresis, urinary urgency or incontinence, and heart rate and rhythm changes. Both ictal tachycardia and bradycardia can occur during seizures arising from the temporal lobes. Most temporal lobe seizures are associated with an increase in heart rate, but supraventricular tachycardia, sinus arrest, atrial fibrillation, and frequent premature atrial and ventricular depolarizations can occur (11,43). This association is particularly important to keep in mind when interpreting electrocardiographic (ECG) telemetry data during a typical spell. The ECG data alone without concomitant EEG during the spell may suggest that the event is primarily arrhythmic in origin, when in reality, the seizure is the primary event. Thus, simultaneous EEG-ECG monitoring is important in these cases.

EXTRATEMPORAL SEIZURES

Partial seizures arising from other areas of the brain can also produce characteristic symptoms. Frontal lobe seizures are typically brief; they often occur in clusters (particularly nocturnally) and are often mistaken for nonepileptic events because of the irregular limb movements that are sometimes seen. Violent movements of the extremities, at times accompanied by vocalizations, are seen, as are focal clonic movements, forced eye and head deviation, and rapid secondary generalization. Other seizures, such as those arising from the supplementary motor cortex unilaterally, can result in complex movements of the limbs bilaterally or in asymmetric posturing. The diagnosis can be difficult, particularly because the EEG may be normal both interictally and during the seizure. An EEG revealing frontal spikes or neuroimaging demonstrating a frontal lobe lesion may suggest the diagnosis. Additionally, a history of symptoms arising directly from sleep is helpful. Although the individual can be confused postictally, he or she may regain full consciousness quickly after the seizure.

Seizures can also arise from the parietal or occipital lobes, and seizures arising from these areas may be more common in the elderly than in younger populations. Parietal lobe seizures can present with numbness, tingling, or other sensations on the side contralateral to the seizure focus. Both occipital and parietal lobe seizures can present with visual symptoms as well. Nystagmus or eye deviation can occur during occipital lobe seizures.

Alteration of level of consciousness can also occur in the setting of nonconvulsive status epilepticus. Patients may present with waxing and waning confusion, which is oftentimes accompanied by subtle facial twitching, nystagmus, or other focal twitching. The diffuse encephalopathy that can accompany this entity can be erroneously attributed solely to a toxic-metabolic derangement or medication effect, rather than to seizures. An EEG is invaluable in the diagnosis of this entity.

SYNCOPE

Syncope accounts for 1% of hospital admissions and 3% of emergency room visits, and its incidence increases with age, particularly after age 70 (35). In the Framingham Heart Study, syncope occurred in 5.4 to 5.7 of 1,000 person-years, 11.1 of 1,000 person-years, and 16.9 to 19.5 of 1,000 person-years in age categories of 60 to 69 years, 70 to 79 years, and ≥80 years, respectively (52). Cardiovascular syncope carries a 1-year mortality rate of 30%; whereas neurally mediated syncope has a benign prognosis (36,52). Therefore, it is crucial that a cardiovascular cause of syncope be identified or excluded.

The most important part of the initial evaluation is a meticulous history and physical examination (12,34,53). The history provides the patient's underlying medical conditions (e.g., prior myocardial infarction), medication regimen (e.g., antihypertensive drugs), context of prior syncopal episodes, pertinent family history, alcohol use, and specific details of the event. These details should include: (a) triggering mechanisms; (b) prodromal symptoms; (c) body posture during syncope; (d) onset, duration, and offset of syncope; and (e) bystander observations. Syncope triggered by exertion suggests a cardiovascular cause (e.g., aortic stenosis, exercise-induced ventricular tachycardia) (17). Emotional distress or pain (e.g., blood draws) can provoke a vasovagal episode. Viscerovagal reflexes have specific, identifiable triggers (e.g., defecation, micturition), whereas neck manipulation (e.g., massaging, shaving) can precipitate a hypersensitive carotid sinus response. Chest pain and shortness of breath should raise suspicion for myocardial infarction or pulmonary embolus. Palpitations can be seen with both tachyarrhythmias and vasovagal syncope. Additional symptoms of a vasovagal episode include warmth, nausea, lightheadedness, and diaphoresis. It is important to remember, however, that elderly patients can present atypically (17). Syncope after prolonged standing or upright posture is characteristic of vasovagal or orthostatic syncope, respectively, whereas syncope during supine position suggests a cardiovascular etiology (17). By impeding mitral inflow, atrial myxomas cause syncope when bending over. Syncope is typically brief (12). Abrupt-onset syncope without prodrome suggests acute, complete cessation of cerebral perfusion as occurs with arrhythmic syncope, but it can also be seen with malignant vasovagal and orthostatic episodes.

Delayed and diminished reflexes in elderly patients make them particularly prone to trauma. Syncope preceded by prodromal symptoms is more characteristic of vasovagal syncope. Orientation after syncope (offset) is also important. Postevent confusion can occur with hypoglycemia or seizures, whereas preserved orientation is typical of cardiovascular syncope. Fatigue is common after a vasovagal episode. Because retrograde amnesia after syncope is common in elderly patients, particularly after head trauma, patient-derived medical histories are of limited value (17). Bystander observations, therefore, become very important. Medically trained bystanders might provide critical information on the patient's blood pressure and pulse. Observing flaccid collapse suggests syncope, whereas stiffness (tonic phase) and tongue biting suggest seizure. Prolonged cerebral hypoperfusion can cause myoclonic movements (convulsive syncope) that might be mistaken for a seizure (4,55).

The physical examination should focus on the (a) medical stability of the patient (vital signs), (b) clues that may provide a cause for syncope, and (c) areas of trauma that require medical attention. Therefore, a complete neurologic and cardiovascular examination including orthostatic blood pressure measurements is essential. Postural changes in blood pressure suggest orthostatic syncope. A carotid bruit might suggest the possibility of carotid sinus hypersensitivity. Congestive heart failure (elevated neck veins, peripheral edema) points toward cardiovascular syncope. A late-peaking, harsh systolic murmur in the left second intercostal space, soft second heart sound, and low-amplitude, delayed carotid pulses are findings of calcific aortic stenosis in the elderly.

CARDIOVASCULAR SYNCOPE

Cardiovascular syncope can be divided into arrhythmias and structural cardiopulmonary disease. Arrhythmias include both bradyarrhythmias and tachyarrhythmias. Bradyarrhythmias [sick sinus syndrome, atrioventricular (AV) block] increase in the elderly not only because of age-related sclerodegenerative changes of the sinus node and conduction system, but also because of medication side effects (e.g., beta-blockers). Supraventricular tachycardias (e.g., atrial fibrillation) are infrequent causes of syncope in the elderly and are due to rapid ventricular rates in stiff, noncompliant ventricles. Ventricular tachyarrhythmias should be considered in any elderly patient with prior myocardial infarction, bundle branch block, or left ventricular dysfunction. Structural cardiopulmonary diseases cause syncope by (a) obstructing right or left ventricular outflow (pulmonary embolus or aortic stenosis) or (b) causing ineffective pump function (myocardial infarction, tamponade). Aortic stenosis causing syncope is associated with a poor long-term prognosis, with an average survival of 3 years if untreated (47).

NEURALLY MEDIATED (REFLEXOGENIC) SYNCOPE

In vasovagal syncope, reduced venous return (e.g., prolonged standing) increases cardiac contractility and activates ventricular mechanoreceptors (C fibers). These fibers transmit afferent signals to the nucleus tractus solitarius (vasodepressor region) of the medulla. Efferent outputs from this center increase parasympathetic and decrease sympathetic outflow, leading to bradycardia and hypotension, respectively. Vasovagal syncope tends to have a benign prognosis (52). Carotid sinus hypersensitivity is generally a disease of older patients and is associated with atherosclerotic carotid artery disease and prior neck surgery. Syncope classically occurs during neck manipulation

(e.g., shaving). Diagnosis can be confirmed by gentle carotid massage (in the absence of a bruit) during continuous electrocardiographic monitoring. Three types of carotid sinus hypersensitivity responses are cardioinhibitory (asystole >3 seconds), vasodepressor (>50 mmHg drop in blood pressure), and mixed (combination of both types).

ORTHOSTATIC SYNCOPE

Orthostatic syncope is common in the elderly (54). Elderly patients are particularly prone to postural changes in blood pressure because of inadequate vasoconstrictor mechanisms, volume depletion (reduced thirst, diuretics), and medication use.

DIAGNOSTIC EVALUATION

SEIZURE LIKELY
Initial Evaluation

Based on the clinical presentation, the diagnosis of either seizure or syncope may be more likely. When the most likely diagnosis is seizure (Fig. 7-2), the initial workup should include an evaluation for possible metabolic derangements that may account for an acute seizure. Measurements of blood chemistry, including glucose, sodium, urea nitrogen, calcium, and magnesium, as well as an assessment of oxygenation status, are vital in the acute setting. If a CNS infection is suspected, a lumbar puncture should be performed. Medications should be carefully evaluated, and the evaluation of the past medical history should include any alcohol or illicit drug use. Toxicologic tests should be performed as clinically indicated.

Seek a history of head trauma, which may not necessarily immediately precede the seizure. The elderly are at increased risk for subdural hematomas, which can develop even after relatively mild head trauma. Oftentimes, subtle or no obvious neurologic deficits are seen in such cases. If the history includes recent head trauma, focal neurologic deficits, or a postictal Todd paralysis, computed tomography (CT) scan or MRI of the head should be done in the acute setting to exclude a contusion, mass lesion, stroke, or hemorrhage. An EEG may be helpful in the acute setting to rule out possible nonconvulsive status epilepticus, if clinically indicated.

Neuroimaging

All adults who present with a probable epileptic seizure should have an MRI of the brain performed, barring no contraindications. In the acute setting, a CT of the head may be adequate; however, a head CT does not adequately assess for the possibility of a neoplastic lesion.

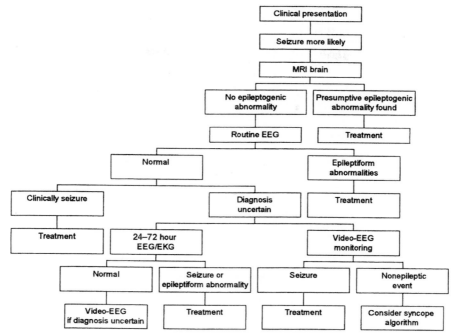

Figure 7-2. Transient loss of consciousness: seizure more likely.

Electroencephalography and Long-Term Monitoring

If uncertain whether a spell may have represented a seizure, additional tests may be helpful in making the diagnosis. A routine EEG, particularly if sleep is captured (the frequency of epileptiform abnormalities generally increases during sleep), may reveal epileptiform abnormalities. Nonspecific epileptiform abnormalities (sharp waves or spikes) in the EEG support the diagnosis of epilepsy. However, a normal EEG or one that reveals focal or generalized nonepileptogenic abnormalities does not exclude the diagnosis of epilepsy. In the elderly, it has been estimated that the frequency of interictal epileptiform activity is 26% to 35% on an initial EEG and is lower than in the general population of patients with epilepsy, in whom 51% to 56% have interictal epileptiform abnormalities on an initial EEG (3,19).

If a routine EEG does not reveal interictal epileptiform abnormalities and the diagnosis is still uncertain, prolonged EEG monitoring is helpful, particularly if the spells are recurrent and frequent. Ambulatory EEG-ECG monitoring over a 24- to 72-hour period has three major advantages over the routine EEG: (a) increased likelihood of detecting interictal epileptiform abnormalities because of the lengthy recording duration, particularly during sleep; (b) increased likelihood of recording the EEG during a typical spell; and (c) an evaluation for possible subclinical or nocturnal seizures. EEG-ECG monitoring is particularly helpful when the spells are frequent and it is unclear whether the spell is related to a seizure or an arrhythmia.

Another option in uncertain cases is video-EEG monitoring performed in the inpatient setting over several days. Advantages over ambulatory EEG monitoring include (a) decreased likelihood of artifact, which often arises during long-term outpatient EEG-ECG recording, and (b) visual characterization of the spells in question and the ability to correlate EEG changes with clinical observation. This type of monitoring is particularly useful in the diagnosis of nonepileptic psychogenic seizures, during which seizurelike activity may be observed without accompanying ictal changes on the EEG. However, some caution should be used in making this diagnosis because simple partial seizures and some types of complex partial seizures, particularly those of frontal origin, can have a normal EEG during the event in question.

SYNCOPE LIKELY

Initial Evaluation

The initial evaluation (history, physical examination, 12-lead electrocardiogram) provides a presumptive diagnosis in 50% to 60% of cases of syncope (Fig. 7-3). Particular attention should be paid to identifying or

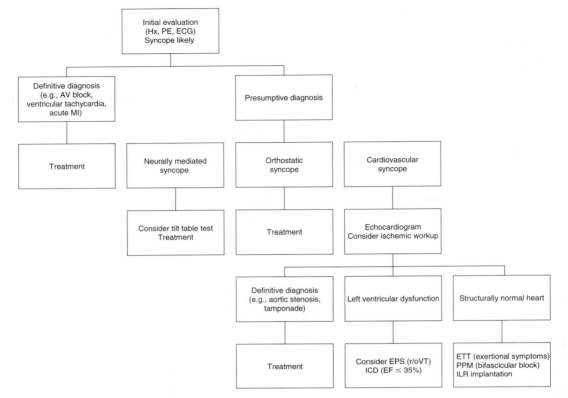

Figure 7-3. Transient loss of consciousness: syncope more likely. Hx, history; PE, physical examination; AV, atrioventricular; MI, myocardial infarction; EPS, electrophysiologic study; ETT, exercise treadmill test; PPM, permanent pacemaker; ICD, implantable cardioverter-defibrillator; ILR, implantable loop recorder.

excluding cardiovascular syncope because of its overall poor prognosis. For patients presenting to the emergency department, specifically designated syncope units can improve the diagnostic yield of syncope while reducing hospital admissions and length of stay (51).

Electrocardiogram

The 12-lead electrocardiogram is a simple, inexpensive test that is essential to the evaluation of syncope. Specific clues suggesting a bradyarrhythmia include impairments of impulse formation (sinus bradycardia or pauses) and conduction (atrioventricular block and bundle branch block). Infarct patterns, left ventricular hypertrophy, bundle branch block, and QT interval prolongation also raise the possibility of ventricular tachycardia.

Echocardiography

The transthoracic echocardiogram is the best noninvasive tool to provide information on heart chamber size and function, valvular disease, and pericardial anatomy. Although it might diagnose a structural

cardiopulmonary cause for syncope (e.g., aortic stenosis, hypertrophic obstructive cardiomyopathy, tamponade, pulmonary embolus-in-transit), it also has value in identifying a patient at high risk for arrhythmic syncope (left ventricular dysfunction).

Electrophysiologic Testing

The electrophysiologic study is an invasive test that attempts to identify an arrhythmic etiology for syncope. Electrocardiographic correlation between arrhythmia and syncope is often difficult because of the intermittent and sporadic nature of syncope. Induction of an arrhythmia in the electrophysiology laboratory provides a probable cause for syncope when other etiologies have been excluded. The test is indicated in elderly patients with undiagnosed syncope and structural heart disease (56).

Tilt Table Testing

Head-up tilt table testing identifies patients susceptible to vasovagal syncope with a specificity of approximately 90% (9,23). It can also identify elderly patients with orthostatic intolerance. However, given the high incidence of cardiovascular disease in the elderly, it is important that more malignant cardiovascular causes of syncope be excluded first in these patients.

Exercise Testing

Exercise testing is not routinely helpful in the diagnosis of syncope. Structural cardiopulmonary disease causing effort syncope (e.g., aortic stenosis, hypertrophic obstructive cardiomyopathy) is best diagnosed by echocardiography. Cardiac catheterization is preferable to exercise testing when chemically triggered ventricular tachyarrhythmia is a possibility. However, exercise testing can be helpful when syncope occurs with exertion (e.g., exercise-induced atrioventricular block) but remains undiagnosed despite a thorough cardiac evaluation.

Outpatient Monitoring

Outpatient monitoring can provide symptom-arrhythmia correlation, which is often absent on single "snapshot" ECGs. Outpatient monitoring should not be performed on patients at high risk for malignant arrhythmias (e.g., left ventricular dysfunction, bundle branch block) because attempts to record such episodes can be fatal. Such patients should be admitted to a hospital for diagnosis with telemetry monitoring. However, when arrhythmic syncope is suspected but remains undiagnosed despite an otherwise thorough cardiac evaluation, outpatient recording devices can be rewarding (21). Short-term monitors (e.g., 24-hour Holter) are generally not helpful because of the low likelihood of syncope during the recording period. Thirty-day event monitors are limited by the requirement for patient activation, which can be difficult after a syncopal episode. In contrast, long-term implantable loop recorders (REVEAL, Medtronic Inc., Minneapolis, MN) have been shown to be useful in the diagnostic evaluation of syncope in the elderly (13,38). In addition, generalized tonic-clonic seizures can also be detected on the implantable loop recorder by producing specific myopotential artifact patterns (31).

TREATMENT

SEIZURE AND EPILEPSY

When the diagnosis, based on the clinical evaluation, is of seizure, the decision must be made whether the patient should be treated with prophylactic medication. If the seizure is an acute symptomatic seizure related to a specific precipitating factor not associated with recurrent seizures, then treatment should be directed at eliminating the offending agent. When a specific precipitant cannot be found, other factors must be considered. Overall, approximately 33% to 50% of patients who experience one seizure will have

a second seizure (10,26). Specific factors can increase the likelihood that someone will experience recurrent seizures. MRI of the brain revealing a focal cortical abnormality, a history of a previous neurologic insult, a history of Todd paresis, status epilepticus, and an abnormal EEG increase the likelihood of recurrent seizures. In these cases, treatment with prophylactic medication may be considered. In cases of brain neoplasms, the likelihood of recurrent seizures is particularly high; thus, anticonvulsant medication is generally begun after an initial seizure. If a second seizure occurs, approximately three fourths of patients will experience recurrent seizures, and most would opt to treat at this point (28). Many personal factors can also affect the decision to treat a single seizure, including the need to drive again and employment concerns. Before beginning an anticonvulsant medication, discuss the pros and cons of medication, including the patient's individual likelihood of having recurrent seizures based on the clinical data, efficacy of the drugs, and potential side effects.

Medication Selection

When the decision is made to treat with an anticonvulsant medication, any concomitant medical conditions and current medications (including over-the-counter and nontraditional medications and supplements) should be evaluated carefully. Additional factors that can affect the medication choice include cost, dosing schedule, need for blood monitoring, potential side effects of the medications, history of drug allergies, and preferred route and form of drug administration.

Most patients' seizures can be controlled with the use of antiepileptic drugs (AEDs). The likelihood of control with medication should be discussed with the patient. It should be clear that the first medication may not result in complete control. In the general population, approximately 35% of patients will be refractory to medications. However, the longer a patient is seizure-free on medication, the less likely recurrent seizures will occur.

Certain side effects are possible with most of the currently available AEDs, including sedation, diplopia, nausea, and ataxia, particularly at higher levels (14,16,42,45,49). Slow medication titration and careful monitoring of serum drug levels can help prevent many of these side effects. Monitoring of drug levels is also helpful in the assessment of medication compliance, which can be difficult in the elderly because of the greater likelihood of memory difficulties and concomitant use of multiple other medications.

Among the older AEDs, carbamazepine (Tegretol), phenytoin (Dilantin), and valproic acid (Depakote, Depakene) appear to be equally efficacious in the treatment of partial seizures. Because carbamazepine, phenytoin, and valproic acid are highly protein bound, measurement of free levels is more helpful than total AED levels in this population. Carbamazepine is generally well tolerated but can cause ataxia or adverse cognitive effects at higher levels, as can phenytoin. Valproic acid often causes a tremor at therapeutic levels and can result in a tremor resembling that seen in Parkinson's disease. Phenobarbital and primidone (Mysoline), although effective, are more likely to result in significant cognitive side effects and are generally considered to be second-line medications.

As seen in Table 7-3, many of the newer anticonvulsant medications have favorable side effect profiles

and pharmacokinetics, making them attractive for use in this age group (15,24,42).

SYNCOPE

Treatment of syncope depends on its underlying etiology. Structural cardiopulmonary disease with correctable lesions can be treated by surgery (i.e., aortic valve replacement for aortic stenosis) or catheter-based interventions (i.e., pericardial drainage of tamponade). Permanent pacemaker implantation is indicated in patients (a) with syncope resulting from bradyarrhythmias (Class I) or (b) at high risk (e.g., bifascicular block) for bradyarrhythmias (Class II) (22). (Class I indicates evidence and/or general agreement

Table 7-3. *Medication Chart: Epilepsy, Syncope, and Orthostatic Hypotension*

Drug	Typical Dose	Side Effects/Risks	Cost/Month ($)
Phenytoin (Dilantin)	300–500 mg/d	Sedation, ataxia, gingival-hyperplasia, diplopia, hirsutism	<50
Carbamazepine (Tegretol)	400–800 mg/d	Sedation, nausea, ataxia, rash, diplopia, hyponatremia	<50
Valproic acid (Depakote)	750–3,000 mg/d	Sedation, pancreatitis, hepatitis, weight gain, tremor	>50
Tiagabine (Gabitril)	32–52 mg/d	Sedation, cognitive side effects	>50
Gabapentin (Neurontin)	900–3,600 mg/d	Sedation, weight gain, edema	>50
Lamotrigine (Lamictal)	300–800 mg/d	Rash, sedation, ataxia	>50
Topiramate (Topamax)	100–500 mg/d	Sedation, cognitive problems, nephrolithiasis	>50
Zonisamide (Zonegran)	200–600 mg/d	Sedation, nephrolithiasis, rash	>50
Oxcarbazepine (Trileptal)	600–2,400 mg/d	Sedation, rash, hyponatremia	>50
Levetiracetam (Keppra)	1,000–3,000 mg/d	Sedation, depression, psychosis	>50
Pregabalin (Lyrica)	150–600 mg/day	Sedation, weight gain, edema	>50
Fludrocortisone (Florinef)	0.3–1 mg/d	CHF, edema, headache, HTN hypokalemia, weight gain	<50
Indomethacin (Indocin)	25–50 mg t.i.d.	Interstitial nephritis, gastrointestinal upset, liver toxicity	<50
Ephedrine	12.5–25 mg t.i.d.	Anxiety, tachycardia, tremor	<50
Methylphenidate (Ritalin)	5–10 mg t.i.d.	Anxiety, tachycardia, tremor	>50
Midodrine (ProAmitine)	2.5–5 mg t.i.d. NTE 30 mg/d	Hypertension, piloerection, pruritis	>50
Phenylpropanolamine	25–75 mg b.i.d.	Hypertension	<50
Atenolol (Tenormin)	25–100 mg q.d.	CHF, hypotension, bradycardia, fatigue, exercise intolerance	<50
Metoprolol (Lopressor)	25–50 mg b.i.d.	CHF, hypotension, bradycardia, fatigue, exercise intolerance	<50
Theophylline (Theo-Dur)	200–300 mg q.d.	Nausea, vomiting, tremors Overdose: arrhythmia, seizure	<50
Scopolamine	1 patch q3d	Anticholinergic side effects: dry mouth, blurry vision, urinary retention	>50
Disopyramide (Norpace)	600 mg/d (dosing b.i.d. or q.i.d.)	CHF, anticholinergic side effects: dry mouth, blurry vision, urinary retention	>50

b.i.d., two times per day; CHF, congestive heart failure; HTN, hypertension; NTE, not to exceed; q, every; q.d., every day; q.i.d., four times per day; t.i.d., three times per day.

that the treatment is beneficial, useful, and effective; Class II indicates conflicting evidence and/or divergence of opinion about the usefulness/efficacy of the treatment.) Similarly, implantable cardioverter-defibrillator implantation is indicated in patients (a) with syncope resulting from ventricular tachyarrhythmias (Class I) or (b) at high risk (e.g., left ventricular dysfunction) for ventricular tachyarrhythmias (Class II) (22). Supraventricular tachyarrhythmias can be treated by either pharmacologic or ablative therapies. Nonpharmacologic therapy for neurally mediated syncope should include behavior modification to avoid triggering mechanisms (e.g., prolonged standing, neck manipulation). Pharmacologic therapies for vasovagal syncope include beta-blockers, volume expanders (salt tablets, mineralocorticoids), vasoconstrictors (midodrine), anticholinergic agents (scopolamine, disopyramide), selective serotonin reuptake inhibitors (paroxetine, sertraline), and theophylline. Selected individuals with recurrent vasovagal symptoms refractory to medical therapy might benefit from permanent pacemaker implantation, as can patients with the cardioinhibitory form of carotid sinus hypersensitivity (22).

Recurrent orthostatic syncope can be difficult to treat. Patients should avoid abrupt changes in posture. Offending medications should be reduced or eliminated. Tight-fitting leg stockings might help to increase venous return. Pharmacologic treatments include volume expanders (salt tablets, mineralocorticoids) and vasoconstrictors (midodrine), but the high incidence of hypertension in the elderly limits the usefulness of these therapies.

SUMMARY AND ADVICE

A careful clinical evaluation with appropriately guided tests will reveal a likely cause for transient loss of consciousness in most patients. However, the diagnosis can remain elusive despite a thorough evaluation, particularly with sporadic episodes. In these patients, re-evaluation may be necessary. Therapeutic trials can be useful in selected patients. Lack of response to therapy may also indicate that the true cause remains undiagnosed. Fortunately, the cause for transient loss of consciousness can be determined for most individuals.

REFERENCES

1. Abubakr A, Wambacq I. Seizures in the elderly: video/EEG analysis. *Epilepsy Behav.* 2005;7:447–450.
2. Adams RD, Victor M, Ropper AH. *Principles of Neurology.* 6th ed. New York: McGraw-Hill; 1997.
3. Ajmone-Marsan C, Zivin LS. Factors related to the occurrence of typical paroxysmal abnormalities in the EEG records of epileptic patients. *Epilepsia.* 1970;11:361–381.
4. Aminoff MJ, Scheinman MM, Griffin JC, et al. Electrocerebral accompaniments of syncope associated with malignant ventricular arrhythmias. *Ann Intern Med.* 1988;108:791–796.
5. Annegers JF, Hauser WA, Lee JR-J, et al. Acute symptomatic seizures in Rochester, Minnesota, 1935–1984. *Epilepsia.* 1995;36:327–333.
6. Bartsch T, Alfke T, Stingele R, et al. Selective affection of hippocampal CA-1 neurons in patients with transient global amnesia without long-term sequelae. *Brain.* 2006;129:2874–28 .
7. Bazil CW, Pack A. Insulinoma presenting a a seizure disorder. *Neurology.* 2001;56:817–818.
8. Benbadis SR, Wolfamuth BR, Goren H, et al. Value of tongue biting in the diagnosis of seizures. *Arch Intern Med.* 1995;155:2346–2349.
9. Benditt DG, Ferguson DW, Grubb BP, et al. Tilt-table testing for assessing syncope. An American College of Cardiology expert consensus document. *J Am Coll Cardiol.* 1996;28:263–275.
10. Berg AT, Shinnar S. The risk of seizure recurrence following a first unprovoked seizure: a quantitative review. *Neurology.* 1991;41:965–972.
11. Blumhardt LD, Smith PE, Owen L. Electrocardiographic accompaniments of temporal lobe epileptic seizures. *Lancet.* 1986;1:1051–1056.
12. Brignole M, Alboni P, Benditt D, et al. Guidelines on management (diagnosis and treatment) of syncope: update 2004. *Europace.* 2004;6:467–537.
13. Brignole M, Menozzi C, Maggi R, et al. The usage and diagnostic yield of the implantable loop-recorder in detection of the mechanism of syncope and in guiding effective antiarrhythmic therapy in older people. *Europace.* 2005;7:273–279.
14. Brodie MJ, Overstall PW, Giorgi L. Multicentre, double-blind, randomised comparison between lamotrigine and carbamazepine in elderly patients with newly diagnosed epilepsy. *Epilepsy Res.* 1999; 37:81–87.
15. Brodie MJ, Richens A, Yuen AWC. Double-blind comparison of lamotrigine and carbamazepine in newly diagnosed epilepsy. *Lancet.* 1996; 346: 476–479.
16. Craig I, Tallis R. Impact of valproate and phenytoin on cognitive function in elderly patients: results of a single-blind randomized comparative study. *Epilepsia.* 1994;35:381–390.
17. Del Rosso A, Alboni P, Brignole M, et al. Relation of clinical presentation of syncope to the age of patients. *Am J Cardiol.* 2005;96:1431–1435.
18. Dichter M, Weinberger LM. Epileptogenesis and the aging brain. In: Rowan AJ, Ramsay RE,

eds. *Seizures and epilepsy in the elderly*. Boston: Butterworth-Heinemann; 1997.

19. Drury I, Beydoun A. Interictal epileptiform activity in elderly patients with epilepsy. *Electroencephalogr Clin Neurophysiol*. 1998;106:369–373.

20. Duncan R, Oto M, Martin E, et al. Late onset psychogenic nonepileptic attacks. *Neurology*. 2006; 66:1644–1647.

21. Fogel RI, Evans JJ, Prystowsky EN. Utility and cost of event recorders in the diagnosis of palpitations, presyncope, and syncope. *Am J Cardiol*. 1997;79:207–208.

22. Gregoratos G, Abrams J, Epstein AE, et al. ACC/AHA/NASPE 2002 guideline update for implantation of cardiac pacemakers and antiarrhythmia devices: summary article: a report of the ACC/AHA Task Force on Practice Guidelines. *Circulation*. 2002;106:2145–2161.

23. Grubb BP, Wolfe D, Samiol D, et al. Recurrent unexplained syncope in the elderly: the use of head-upright tilt table testing in evaluation and management. *J Am Geriatr Soc*. 1992;40:1123–1128.

24. Haria M, Balfour JA. Levetiracetam. *Drugs*. 1997;7:159–164.

25. Hauser WA, Anneger JF, Kurland LT. Incidence of epilepsy and unprovoked seizures in Rochester, Minnesota: 1935–1984. *Epilepsia*. 1993;34:453–468.

26. Hauser WA, Hesdorffer DC. Incidence and prevalence. In: Hauser WA, Hesdorffer DC, eds. *Epilepsy: frequency, causes and consequences*. New York: Demos; 1990:1–51.

27. Hauser WA, Morris ML, Hewton LL, et al. Seizures and myoclonus in patients with Alzheimer's disease. *Neurology*. 1986;36:1226–1230.

28. Hauser WA, Rich SS, Lee JRJ, et al. Risk of recurrent seizures after two unprovoked seizures. *N Engl J Med*. 1998;338:429–434.

29. Hesdorffer DC, Hauser WA, Annegers JF, et al. Dementia and adult onset unprovoked seizures. *Neurology*. 1996;46:727–730.

30. Hesdorffer DC, Hauser WA, Annegers JF, et al. Major depression in a risk factor for seizures in older adults. *Ann Neurol*. 2000;47:246–249.

31. Ho RT, Wicks T, Wyeth D, et al. Generalized tonic-clonic seizures detected by REVEAL devices: diagnosing more than cardiac arrhythmias. *Heart Rhythm*. 2006;3:857–861.

32. Hoefnagels WAJ, Padberg GW, Overweg J, et al. Transient loss of consciousness: the value of the history for distinguishing seizure from syncope. *J Neurol*. 1991;238:39–43.

33. Holt-Seitz A, Wirrell EC, Sundaram MB. Seizures in the elderly: etiology and prognosis. *Can J Neurol Sci*. 1999;26:110–114.

34. Jhanjee R, Gert Van Dijk J, Sakaguchi S, et al. Syncope in adults: terminology, classification, and diagnostic strategy. *Pacing Clin Electrophysiol*. 2006;29:1160–1169.

35. Kapoor WN. Evaluation and outcome of patients with syncope. *Medicine*. 1990;69:160–175.

36. Kapoor WN, Karpf M, Wieand S, et al. A prospective evaluation and follow-up of patients with syncope. *N Engl J Med*. 1983;309:197–204.

37. Kapoor WN, Snustad D, Peterson J, et al. Syncope in the elderly. *Am J Med*. 1986;80:419–428.

38. Krahn AD, Klein GJ, Yee R, et al. Use of an extended monitoring strategy in patients with problematic syncope. *Circulation*. 1999;99:406–410.

39. Loiseau J, Loiseau P, Duche B, et al. A survey of epileptic disorders in southwest France: seizures in elderly patients. *Ann Neurol*. 1990;27:232–237.

40. McAreavey MJ, Ballinger BR, Fenton GW. Epileptic seizures in elderly patients with dementia. *Epilepsia*. 1992;33:657–660.

41. Miller JW, Petersen RD, Metter EJ, et al. Transient global amnesia: clinical characteristics and prognosis. *Neurology*. 1987;37:733–737.

42. Moshe SL. Mechanisms of action of anticonvulsant agents. *Neurology*. 2000;55[suppl 1]:32–40.

43. Nei M, Ho RT, Sperling MR. EKG abnormalities during partial seizures in refractory epilepsy. *Epilepsia*. 2000;41:542–548.

44. Plum F, Posner JB. The pathologic physiology of signs and symptoms of coma. In: *The diagnosis of stupor and coma*. 3rd ed. Philadelphia: FA Davis; 1980.

45. Ramsay RE, Pryor F. Epilepsy in the elderly. *Neurology*. 2000;55[suppl 1]:9–14.

46. Romanelli MF, Morris JC, Ashkin K, et al. Advanced Alzheimer's disease is a risk factor for late onset seizures. *Arch Neurol*. 1990;47:847–850.

47. Ross J Jr, Braunwald E. Aortic stenosis. *Circulation*. 1968;38[suppl 5]:61–67.

48. Rossen R, Kabat H, Anderson JP. Acute arrest of cerebral circulation in man. *Arch Neurol Psychiatry*. 1943;50:510–528.

49. Rowan AJ, Ramsay RE, eds. *Seizures and Epilepsy in the Elderly*. Boston: Butterworth-Heinemann; 1997.

50. Savage DD, Corwin L, Mcgee DL, et al. Epidemiologic features of isolated syncope: the Framingham study. *Stroke*. 1985;16:626–629.

51. Shen WK, Decker WW, Smars PA, et al. Syncope evaluation in the emergency departments study (SEEDS). A multidisciplinary approach to syncope management. *Circulation*. 2004;110:3636-3645.

52. Soteriades ES, Evans JC, Martin GL, et al. Incidence and prognosis of syncope. *N Engl J Med*. 2002;347:878–885.

53. Strickberger SA, Benson DW, Biaggioni I, et al. AHA/ACCF scientific statement on the evaluation of syncope. *Circulation*. 2006;113:316–327.

54. Ungar A, Mussi C, Del Rosso A, et al. Diagnosis and characteristics of syncope in older patients referred to geriatric departments. *J Am Geriatr Soc*. 2006;54:1531–1536.

55. Zaidi A, Clough P, Cooper P, et al. Misdiagnosis of epilepsy: many seizure-like attacks have a cardiovascular cause. *J Am Coll Cardiol*. 2000;36:181–184.

56. Zipes DP, DiMarco JP, Gillette PC, et al. Guidelines for clinical intracardiac electrophysiological and catheter ablation procedures. *J Am Coll Cardiol*. 1995;26:555–573.

SUGGESTED READINGS

Calkins H. Syncope. In: Zipes DP, Jalife J, eds. *Cardiac electrophysiology from cell to bedside*. 3rd ed. Philadelphia: WB Saunders; 2000:873–881.

Martin JB, Ruskin J. Faintness, syncope, and seizures. In: Wilson JD, Braunwald E, Isselbacher KJ, et al., eds. *Harrison's principles of internal medicine*. 12th ed. New York: McGraw-Hill; 1991:134–142.

Stein B, Roberts R. Syncope, presyncope, palpitations, and sudden death. In: Schlant RC, Alexander RW, eds. *Hurst's the heart*. 8th ed. New York: McGraw-Hill; 1994:475–479.

CHAPTER **8**

Dizziness and Vertigo in Older Adults

David Solomon, David E. Newman-Toker, and Jeffrey S. Durmer

This chapter reviews the epidemiology, causes, pathogenesis, diagnosis, and treatment strategies for the most frequently encountered causes of dizziness in the elderly patient. Although a complaint of dizziness might seem enigmatic at first, rational ways exist to evaluate this sensation and establish a cause based on a number of well-recognized health problems that affect many elderly patients (i.e., cardiovascular disease, depression, cervical spondylosis, polypharmacy, deconditioning). The vestibular system encompasses sensory structures in the labyrinth of the inner ear but also integrates visual and somatosensory information in service of three essential roles of the nervous system: maintenance of upright posture during standing and locomotion, stabilizing vision during head motion, and regulation of autonomic tone in response to orthostatic changes. Because of the multitude of underlying health conditions and situations that can cause dizziness, many different physicians and health care professionals encounter patient complaints of dizziness. Internists, geriatricians, family care physicians, neurologists, otorhinolaryngologists, psychiatrists, physiatrists, emergency physicians, and physical therapists all have the opportunity to diagnose and treat many patients with dizziness. This chapter is intended to help organize the approach to the elderly dizzy patient given the latest clinical and basic research on the causes and treatments of dizziness.

EPIDEMIOLOGY OF DIZZINESS

Dizziness is reported in approximately 30% of all people over the age of 65 (19,97). In the United States, it is the most common presenting complaint to office practices among patients over the age of 75 (50). The physician consultation rate in 1981 for the symptom of dizziness in the United Kingdom was approximately 54 in 1,000 for people aged 65 to 74 years and 76 in 1,000 for people aged 75 years or older (87). One of the most serious consequences of dizziness is falls. The National Health Interview Survey Supplement on Aging in 1986 determined that more than 18% of all persons 65 to 74 years of age and

more than 25% of all those 75 years of age or older had fallen in the previous year. In these groups, 15% to 23% fell because of dizziness alone (40). The same survey reported that a staggering 34% of persons 65 to 74 years old and 37% of persons older than 75 years had limited their activity because of dizziness. Smaller studies using more select populations of older people find that between 20% and 30% of falls are caused by dizziness (3,117). Some of these studies also suggest that patients who are older than 60 years have an increased incidence of potentially treatable diseases as a cause for their dizziness (3,54).

Another consequence of falling is the subsequent deterioration of function after the fall. Many elderly people who fall develop a fear of falling that limits their daily activity. This has a significant impact on mobility and can be quantified easily and reliably (78). Restriction of activities due to lack of confidence leads to more deconditioning, further increasing the risk of falling. Dynamic posturography studies of elderly people with dizziness and without dizziness show that a fear of falling is associated with an increased sway velocity and risk for fall, regardless of dizziness status (4). Clearly, with advancing age, dizziness is more common, and it represents an increasing risk for falls, as well as for syncope, functional disability, nursing home placement, stroke, and death (12,33,51,97,110).

The characteristics of dizziness in older people are different than the characteristics in younger people. In 1992, Kroenke et al. (51) studied 185 consecutive outpatients with a chief complaint of dizziness. Within a subgroup of 85 younger patients (average age, 49 years), they found that the symptoms of dizziness differed from the 100 older remaining patients (average age, 61 years). The older group was significantly more likely to have daily dizziness, limitation of function because of dizziness, fear of underlying illness, and increased use of medications for dizziness (51). These findings may mean that older individuals who experience dizziness are less able to compensate for the dizziness, have more severe dizziness, or report dizziness more often.

The presence of dizziness has a negative impact on quality of life in patients over 60 years of age and is associated with role limitations in physical and emotional spheres. When dizziness is episodic, the frequency of attacks correlates with perceived disability, resulting in additional psychological distress (43).

The differential diagnosis of dizziness in elderly patients is extensive. Studies designed to determine the cause of dizziness in geriatric patients have returned highly variable results, partly because of the different populations, criteria, and study designs used. Alternatively, dizziness is a highly variable symptom with a number of conditions that predispose to it. Tinetti et al. (112), using Drachman's categorization of dizziness symptoms, determined the prevalence of dizziness subtypes and associated treatable factors in a population of 1,087 independent people 72 years of age and older. The study, conducted over an 11-year period, showed that 29% of individuals experienced dizziness. No single cause for dizziness was found in this study, although many factors were related to its development. The authors suggest that dizziness can occur with either severe impairment of a single system (vision, vestibular, sensory, motor, or cerebellar) or with mild to moderate impairment of several systems. They conclude that dizziness should be considered a geriatric syndrome so that physicians will regard the symptom as a complex of interrelated systems, which, when perturbed, results in the disorienting sensation (112).

In the German National Telephone Health Interview Survey of 2003, participants were asked about the type of dizziness, duration, provoking factors, impact of dizziness, health care utilization, and previous diagnoses. The prevalence of vestibular vertigo was 16% for individuals 60 years of age and older (20% of women and 11% of men) (70). The prevalence of vertigo, dizziness, and disequilibrium was determined in a longitudinal and cross-sectional study from Sweden in cohorts between 70 and 90 years old. The prevalence of balance problems at age 70 was 36% for women and 29% for men and increased to 51% of women and 45% of men in the oldest age group (44).

DESCRIPTIONS OF DIZZINESS

When a patient complains of being dizzy, the subjective experience can be described with a perplexing number of seemingly equally nebulous terms: swimming, floating, lightheadedness, whirling, fainting, disorientation, unsteadiness, rocking, giddiness, dissociation, imbalance, or spinning.

Traditionally, the patient's description and history have guided subsequent questioning, examination, and testing. Some studies suggest that a careful history can predict the eventual diagnosis in 70% of chronically dizzy geriatric patients (97,98). However,

this does not necessarily imply that what the term "dizziness" means to any given patient must be defined unequivocally in order to achieve diagnostic accuracy. Nevertheless, much of the literature assumes this premise, attempting to divide patients' dizziness into one of four proposed subcategories (23). These dizziness subtypes include:

- Vertigo: a sensation of rotational, spinning movement
- Presyncope: a sensation of fainting or "passing out"
- Disequilibrium: a sensation of imbalance while standing or walking with no abnormal sensation in the head
- Other sensations: loosely defined as nonspecific dizziness, floating, giddiness, or other descriptions that fall outside of the previous categories

One difficulty with this type of scheme is that up to 60% of individuals fall into more than one symptom category (18,51,97,112). Alternative algorithms for anamnestic diagnosis focus not only on the type of dizziness, but also rely heavily on the timing of symptoms and the presence or absence of auditory complaints (47).

Risk factors associated with developing dizziness in old age include angina, hypertension, myocardial infarction (MI), stroke, Parkinson's disease, arthritis, diabetes, syncope, neurosensory impairment, alcohol use, smoking, nervousness, and medication use. In terms of medication use, antihypertensive agents, anticonvulsants, anxiolytics, antidepressants, and antipsychotics carry the highest risk for causing dizziness. A population-based cross-sectional study of 1,087 independent healthy people older than 72 years of age sought predisposing characteristics and situational factors associated with dizziness (112). Seven associated characteristics were identified with significant relative risk for dizziness (Table 8-1).

When they compared the 29% of the study population who reported dizziness with those who were not

Table 8-1. *Adjusted Relative Risks for Characteristics Associated with Dizziness*

Associated Characteristic	Relative Risk
Anxiety	1.69
Depression	1.36
Impaired balance	1.34
Past MI	1.31
Postural hypotension	1.31
Five or more medications	1.30
Impaired hearing	1.27

MI, myocardial infarction

dizzy, each of the four types of dizziness was associated with a significantly higher number of these characteristics (2.0 to 2.5 on average) than the nondizzy group (1.5 on average). Therefore, when assessing a geriatric patient even without a primary complaint of dizziness, recognition of one or more of these characteristics may help in uncovering an unreported problem. Also, recognition of the "syndrome" should not preclude a search for a specific cause (22).

Vertigo, defined as the perception of motion, has a prevalence of 25% to 54% in elderly persons complaining of dizziness (18,51,97,112). A careful history of dizziness has been shown to be 87% sensitive for vestibular disorder (51). Other symptoms often associated with vertigo include nausea, vomiting, unsteadiness, and sometimes hearing loss. The underlying mechanisms implicated include disorders of the peripheral or vestibular system and the cerebellar system. Specific diseases are discussed in the text that follows.

In elderly patients complaining of dizziness, presyncope, defined as a feeling of fainting, has a prevalence of 11% to 42% (97,112). History alone carries a sensitivity of 74% for cardiovascular (51). Associated symptoms include pallor, perspiration, palpitations, and syncope. The underlying mechanisms of presyncope stem from decreased cerebral perfusion caused by cardiovascular disease, hypovolemia, overmedication, orthostatic intolerance, dysautonomia, and hypercapnia.

Disequilibrium, as a category of dizziness, includes people with a sensation of imbalance while on their feet. The symptom of dizziness is not directly referred to as a sensation in the head and is usually dependent on standing, movement, or both. Therefore, this type of dizziness can include people suffering from gait abnormalities (e.g., disequilibrium syndrome, presbyastasis, or senile gait). In clinical studies of geriatric patients who complain of dizziness, 28% to 78% are diagnosed with disequilibrium (18,51,97,112). Extreme variability in the prevalence of this problem primarily results from the different patient populations under consideration. For example, some investigations that study nursing home residents show significantly higher numbers of a disequilibrium type of dizziness than similar outpatient community-based studies. The higher rate of disequilibrium in the nursing home population is likely because of the fact that placement in a nursing home environment is often predicated on mobility problems. Also, independent elderly outpatients with a gait abnormality are less likely to remain in the general community. A retrospective study of 116 neuro-otology clinic patients with an average age of 75 years and with the presenting complaint of dizziness showed that disequilibrium was the dizziness type most frequently reported to occur in combination with other types (55% of cases). As the primary type, it was seen in 28% of cases (97).

Because studies show that up to 50% to 60% of people with dizziness above the age of 65 years experience more than one dizziness symptom (18,96,97, 112), disequilibrium is likely a part of many geriatric causes of dizziness. The underlying mechanisms for disequilibrium vary, but disorders of the visual, vestibulospinal, proprioceptive, somatosensory, cerebellar, pyramidal, and extrapyramidal motor systems can all cause this type of dizziness.

In most studies of older people, the category of nonspecific dizziness comprises 17% to 33% of the study samples (18,26,51,97,99,112). An important reason for this variability in prevalence is the difference in how each study accounts for various psychiatric problems (e.g., panic disorders, anxiety, and obsessive-compulsive and mood disorders). It is also likely that cognitive decline in some older people makes reporting of symptoms, especially in large epidemiologic surveys, inaccurate or vague.

ANATOMY AND PHYSIOLOGY OF DIZZINESS

Before a discussion of the multiple causes of dizziness can begin, it is important to appreciate some of the anatomic and physiologic changes that occur with age in the nervous system. Age-related degeneration of the vestibular, cerebellar, visual, somatosensory, and proprioceptive systems can all have important implications for the development of different types of dizziness. Disequilibrium can result from the accumulation of mild to moderate deficits in multiple systems or from more severe deficits in one sensory system. Presyncope usually results from vascular or cardiac causes, and nonspecific light-headedness can have many causes without a clear pathophysiology. In particular, vertigo is attributable to processes that affect the peripheral and central vestibular systems. To appreciate the effects of age-related degeneration on the systems that are known to result in symptoms of vertigo and imbalance requires a familiarity with the normal anatomy and physiology of the vestibular system. Furthermore, central nervous system, visual, and somatosensory signals are as important as labyrinthine input in processing vestibular information. The sense of motion, therefore, is truly multimodal.

PERIPHERAL VESTIBULAR SYSTEM

The human vestibular system is composed of peripheral and central components. Both components function to maintain visual and postural stability during movement and provide sensory input to a perceptual mechanism subserving spatial orientation and navigation. The peripheral system begins with the end organs that transform angular and linear accelerations of the head into neural signals. These transformations occur in two endolymph-filled, paired membranous labyrinths in the petrous portion of each temporal bone. Within each labyrinth is a specialized sensory neuroepithelium arranged in two types of unique sensory receptors: (a) the three semicircular canals (SCCs)—posterior, anterior, and lateral—and (b) the two otolith organs—utricle and saccule. The three SCCs are oriented orthogonally to transduce head rotation about any axis. These function in pairs with a contralateral canal that lies in the same plane (e.g., the lateral SCC pair, the left anterior and the right posterior SCC pair). The otolith organs sense linear acceleration caused by gravity or translation, with the utricular maculae roughly in the same horizontal plane and the saccular maculae close to the midsagittal plane.

Mechanical transduction occurs at specialized projections at the apices of the hair cells. Each SCC has a patch of neuroepithelium at a widening of the canal termed the "ampulla," where hair cells can be deflected by movement of the cupula, a structure that spans the inner diameter of each canal. When the head is at rest, primary vestibular afferents in the VIIIth nerve have a spontaneous discharge rate, so input from each side is balanced. When the head is accelerated about an axis that lies perpendicular to the plane containing an SCC pair, the cupula is pushed into the column of fluid (endolymph) contained within the canal. The cupula is deflected, exciting hair cells innervating the canal toward which the head is rotating and inhibiting the afferents from the contralateral canal in a push-pull manner. For example, rotation of the head to the right increases the firing rate of VIIIth nerve fibers on the right and decreases in the firing rate of primary vestibular afferents on the left. The brain receives more neural activity from the right compared to the left and correctly interprets this information as rightward head turning in space. This generates leftward slow-phase eye velocity and rightward quick phases of nystagmus. This is the basis for the vestibular ocular reflex (VOR), which provides stable gaze despite head movements during locomotion. The absence of the VOR leads to oscillopsia (i.e., movement of the visual image on the retina) during head movement.

The hair cell processes of the otolith organs are in contact with the otoconial membrane, a structure embedded with calcium carbonate crystals. These "ear stones" are subjected to linear accelerations when the head is tilted with respect to gravity or with changes in linear velocity, generating a shear force that deflects the hair cells. While a normal constituent of the labyrinth, otoconia may become dislodged from an otolith organ and migrate into an SCC, making the canal sensitive to gravity when it normally only responds to head rotation. This is the mechanism of benign paroxysmal positional vertigo (BPPV), discussed later.

Additional peripheral vestibular structures include the cell bodies of primary vestibular afferent neurons in the Scarpa ganglion, with their peripheral process innervating the hair cells and their central processes, which are the Schwann cell-myelinated axons of the vestibular nerve. The VIIIth nerve travels through the internal auditory canal along with the facial nerve, traverses the subarachnoid space, and enters the lateral brainstem at the pontomedullary level. Vestibular nerve axons terminate within the vestibular nuclei and the flocculonodular lobe of the cerebellum.

CENTRAL VESTIBULAR SYSTEM

The central vestibular system is composed of projections from the four vestibular nuclei (superior, inferior, medial, and lateral) and the vestibulocerebellum (flocculonodular lobe and posterior vermis). These nuclei project to brainstem, thalamic, and spinal cord targets involved in orienting and reflexive righting movements of the eyes (VOR), head and neck (vestibulocolic system), and body (vestibulospinal system). The cerebellum is crucial for adaptation through inhibition of the brainstem vestibular neurons via direct Purkinje cell projections, and it influences ocular motor function via fibers from the fastigial nucleus. The nodulus of the cerebellum and commissural brainstem connections play a role in the central velocity storage mechanism, which is responsible for the duration of nystagmus following labyrinthine stimulation. To summarize the activity of the central vestibular system is well beyond the scope of this chapter, and the reader is referred to texts devoted to this topic (56). However, central vestibular structures involved in the generation of horizontal and vertical VOR eye movements are important for clinicians caring for patients with dizziness to understand because nystagmus is a compelling and informative examination finding in many of these patients.

Movement of the head about the yaw axis of the body (horizontally, as if saying "no-no") stimulates the lateral SCC, as mentioned earlier. To maintain fixation on a salient visual target, such as an oncoming car, the eyes are moved in a lateral conjugate fashion away from the direction of head movement. The distance and speed that the eyes move are dictated by the neural activity initiated by the magnitude and velocity of the response from the lateral SCC. Many pathways are shared with the saccadic system, which organizes a coordinated burst of activity required to move the eyes and shift gaze onto a target. The paramedian pontine reticular formation (PPRF) is the burst generator for horizontal rapid eye movements (saccades and quick phases of nystagmus), whereas another pontine nucleus, the nucleus prepositus hypoglossi (NPH), integrates the burst signal to an eye position signal. This latter function maintains final eye position achieved by the burst and allows for stabilization of the eyes in an eccentric position in the orbit. A similar midbrain system initiates and maintains eye movements in response to head movements about the pitch axis (vertically, as if saying "yes-yes"). The PPRF counterpart in the vertical system is the rostral interstitial nucleus of the medial longitudinal fasciculus (riMLF), and the corresponding integrator is the interstitial nucleus of Cajal (INC). Deficits in gaze holding, caused by structural or toxic metabolic damage, compromise these neural integrators and result in direction-changing, gaze-evoked nystagmus with quick phases in the direction of attempted gaze. Cerebellar dysfunction also causes an ipsilateral deficit in gaze holding and a gaze-evoked nystagmus. This should be distinguished from nystagmus that occurs following a unilateral vestibular loss, which is a direction-fixed spontaneous nystagmus that may be observed with the eyes in the straight-ahead position (especially with fixation removed).

One important anatomic fact allows for the rapid excitation of the proper eye muscles via VOR pathways. Individual SCCs excite only the specific oculomotor nuclei necessary to move the eyes in the opposite direction of the head movement responsible for the activation of that SCC. In other words, the VOR acts to maintain stable gaze by activating the eye muscles needed to precisely counteract any three-dimensional head movement. Thus, pathologic nystagmus can reveal its vestibular origins when it occurs in a direction predicted by dysfunction of one or more SCCs. All of these reflexive movements of the eye are under the influence of the cerebellum, cortex, and sensory systems. A loss of vestibulocerebellar function alone can lead to inaccurate eye movements, nystagmus, and sensations of vertigo. A loss of cortical activity leads to a lack of saccadic eye movement necessary for rapid fixation of a visual target. A loss of visual sensation often leads to a spontaneous horizontal and vertical nystagmus and drift.

Two additional basic principles are worth mentioning. First, the central vestibular system has the ability to adapt to changes in peripheral sensitivity with time. After an acute unilateral loss of labyrinthine function, for instance, the initial response to the altered input is nausea, ataxia, and a sensation of vertigo, with nystagmus beating toward the intact side. Many days later, the vertigo and associated symptoms dissipate, and only careful examination may reveal the imbalance between the two ears. This adaptive response to an acute change requires an intact central vestibular system and cerebellum, and this capacity for plasticity is reduced with age (75). Second, the central vestibular system works with cortical structures to maintain posture and a sense of position in space. This can be important in conditions that mainly affect the cortex and deep white matter projections such as multi-infarct dementia and frontotemporal atrophy.

AGE-RELATED CHANGES IN THE ANATOMY AND PHYSIOLOGY OF DIZZINESS

Peripheral and central vestibular structures degenerate with age (Table 8-2). The functional implications that are suggested by the loss of these structures are multiple. Loss of peripheral vestibular components such as hair cells (up to 40% in crista ampullaris and 30% in the maculae), Scarpa ganglion cells (especially over 60 years of age), and saccular and utricular nerve degeneration can all lead to increased neural

Table 8-2. *Age-Dependent Changes in the Vestibular System*

Labyrinths	Deformation of walls, abnormal endolymphatic flow
Cupula	Deposition of debris, inaccurate response to movements
Otoconia	Fragmentation, formation of endolymphatic debris
Hair cells	Apices accumulate lipofuscin
	Cilial derangement, fusion, formation of giant cilia
	Loss in cristae (40%), loss in maculae (20% to 30%)
Scarpa ganglion	Large decrease in number of neurons over 60 years
Saccular nerve	Degeneration of small and large fibers
Utricular nerve	Degeneration of small and large fibers
Vestibular nerve	Decrease in number of myelinated fibers over 40 years
	Slower conduction times with age
Vestibular nucleus	Loss of neurons (3% per decade) between ages 40 and 90 years
Cerebellum	Dramatic decrease in Purkinje cell number over 60 years

response times (81,83,84). After the age of 40, a selective loss of large-fiber vestibular axons also results in increased conduction times (9,10). Within the labyrinths, otoconia fragmentation and deposition on the cupula have been demonstrated to occur with aging (85). The increased incidence of BPPV as a function of age may be related to this anatomic change (74). Others claim that changes, such as deformation of the labyrinthine walls, that occur with age can lead to altered endolymphatic flow and symptoms of vertigo (90).

Central vestibular structures also undergo changes with age. It is estimated that a 3% decrease occurs per decade in the number of neurons in the vestibular nuclear complex in humans (57). Age-induced loss of cerebellar Purkinje cells can decrease the coordination of movements and visual-vestibular adaptability (36,113). In a study of 90 healthy people of widely varying ages, a 2.5% per decade decrease in Purkinje cell number from ages 0 to 100 years was found. The relationship between age and cell loss was curvilinear and showed no profound difference until the fifth or sixth decade, when a precipitous drop in cell number was noted (36). It is thought that the age-dependent atrophy of the cerebellar vermis, especially lobes 6 and 7, may also play a role in disorders of the visual-vestibular system that result in sensations of dizziness (80).

Impairment of distal somatosensory function and proprioception also occurs with age and can lead to feelings of disequilibrium or "spindle vertigo" (26,58,95). As vestibular degeneration accumulates with age, reliance on somatosensory systems for balance is increased. In a study of 30 healthy people aged 20 to 81 years, the subjective sensation of straight-ahead was demonstrated using a subject-controlled laser pointer on a blank screen. The head-fixed measurement was made with and without unilateral neck vibratory stimulation. Both young and old subjects showed that subjective straight-ahead moved toward the side of vibratory stimulation (presumably because of compensation secondary to the illusion of movement away from the side being vibrated). However, older subjects showed significantly greater changes from true straight-ahead than the younger subjects (106). This implies that compensatory systems are part of a normal sensory substitution process in the course of aging. It is already known that an increase in the gain of the cervico-ocular reflex occurs after bilateral vestibular lesions in humans (89). Thus, even a mild to moderate deficiency in visual or somatosensory systems can be an important predisposing risk factor for the development of dizziness or unsteadiness.

Degenerative changes in the vestibular system attributable to age are well known; however, the func-

tional implications of these changes are less well understood. The VOR can be tested in humans using electronystagmography (ENG), in which eye movements are recorded using electro-oculography (EOG) or video-oculography during caloric irrigation of each ear and positional testing. Caloric testing is helpful mainly for determining the symmetry of labyrinthine responses, and results do not correlate with either age-related anatomic findings or functional imbalance (60). Rotational chair studies provide quantitative assessment of VOR gain and phase. The clinical applications of these tests are discussed later in this chapter. Vestibulospinal and vestibulocolic reflexes are also testable in humans with posturography. Normative data for elderly subjects in VOR testing demonstrate a clear decline in function with age. In a 5-year longitudinal study of 110 healthy people aged 75 or older, a decrease in central VOR responses was demonstrated as a function of age. Rotary chair data demonstrated that gain (or the size of response) of the VOR was decreased and the phase lead of the VOR was increased with age (24). Additionally, a significant drop was noted in the average gain of visual-vestibular reflexes and optokinetic nystagmus (OKN). The basis for this may be related to the rapid drop-off in Purkinje cell number after the sixth decade, as previously discussed (36). However, the neural systems responsible for OKN and visual-vestibular responses include many different structures such as the primary visual cortex, frontal and parietal visual motor centers, thalamic and brainstem nuclei, and cerebellum. The authors of this study pointed out that the abnormal visual-vestibular responses they observed could lead to deficits in VOR function with normal head movements, resulting in sensations of dizziness. Plasticity in these pathways is required with changes in spectacle correction or while using bifocals, as many elderly do, which challenges the system even more. Other studies of the VOR and visual-vestibular responses in healthy elderly volunteers show age-related functional changes such as an amplitude-dependent decrease in VOR gain and a shorter dominant VOR time constant (increased phase lead) (5,26,75,77). Thus, as evidence supporting the natural aging process as a predisposing factor for dizziness develops, it is important to remember to use age-adjusted normative reference values for comparison.

Colledge et al. (18) reported such a high prevalence of asymptomatic abnormalities in healthy control subjects over the age of 65 years with routine ENG, electrocardiogram (ECG), and magnetic resonance imaging (MRI) testing that these tests had no value in screening for causes of dizziness in the elderly. They did find that posturography was sensitive for symptomatic dizziness, but it lacked specificity. In a separate study, a significant difference in dynamic posturography testing was seen between younger and older healthy people (4). A significant increase was seen in sway velocity for older people with dizziness and imbalance than for older people who were healthy. Increased sway velocity also correlated with an increased chance of falling (4). Other studies find similar results with increased sway velocity and disequilibrium (26). Thus, even if they lack specificity, abnormal sway velocities and dynamic posturography studies may help determine the elderly at risk for falling.

The caloric test, which has also been shown to be of little value in discerning age-dependent changes in healthy individuals (24,77,106), is generally useful in indicating an asymmetry between the two lateral SCC but not in quantifying the overall level of vestibular function. The exception would be in a patient with a significant bilateral peripheral weakness, which is seen following aminoglycoside (usually gentamicin) ototoxicity or with neurofibromatosis Type II. Normal caloric responses have been reported in persons with up to 25% reduction in crista ampullaris hair cells (15,67).

SPECIFIC CAUSES OF DIZZINESS IN THE ELDERLY

Dizziness has many causes in older people. Chronic medical problems, medications, deconditioning, depression, and degenerative diseases are just a few of the factors that play a role in producing dizziness. In elderly patients, the fact that they may be taking multiple medications and have multiple medical, neurologic, or psychiatric problems makes the task of organizing the possibilities more difficult. Since only about 50% of elderly individuals will endorse a single type of dizziness symptom (96,97) and patient reports of dizziness type are unreliable (72a), it is important to understand the temporal onset of symptoms and what environments, activities, or positions provoke the symptoms (timing and triggers) (72), rather than concentrating on eliciting a definitive description of the dizziness itself (71).

MULTISENSORY DIZZINESS

Although decreased vestibular sensitivity with aging is well established, it occurs slowly and, by itself, is unlikely to be the sole cause of dizziness. Simultaneous changes in compensatory sensory (vision and somatosensory) and motor (pyramidal and extrapyramidal) systems also contribute to age-associated dizziness, given the large number of medical conditions that affect these compensatory systems and that often present with dizziness as a primary symptom.

In addition to visual loss, which is common in the elderly due to macular degeneration and cataracts, there is an important iatrogenic cause that can be relatively easily addressed: multifocal spectacle correction. In a prospective cohort study of 156 community-dwelling

people aged 63 to 90 years, the 87 individuals (56%) who regularly wore spectacles with bifocal, trifocal, or progressive lenses performed significantly worse in visual tests (distant depth perception and distant edge-contrast sensitivity) when viewing stimuli at critical distances for detecting obstacles in the environment. Even when adjusting for age, poor vision, reduced lower limb sensation and strength, slow reaction time, and increased postural sway, multifocal glass wearers were more than twice as likely to fall over a 1-year period (59). Falls tended to be due to tripping on stairs or when the participants were outside their homes. Therefore, clinicians are justified in suggesting that older patients have a pair of single-correction spectacles for use when negotiating stairs and in unfamiliar settings.

Patients have been seen who complain of vague dizziness following unilateral cataract extraction with intraocular lens implantation. This frequently results in spectacle correction being used only for the nonoperated eye. This presents a problem to the vestibular system; although both the spectacle and intraocular lenses magnify or shrink the visual surround, one moves with the eyes and one is fixed to the head, necessitating nonconjugate eye movements for perfect gaze stability.

VERTIGO

Vertigo is often caused by peripheral vestibular and central vestibular disease (Table 8-3). Acute diseases that affect the peripheral vestibular system unilaterally cause vertigo of exquisite intensity, termed "peripheral" (or "true" spinning) vertigo. The intense nature of this vertigo usually remits over days because of central vestibular compensation; however, this is not always the case with purely *episodic* peripheral vertigo. In some studies of chronic dizziness, the symptom of vertigo is found in up to 50% of persons over the age of 66 years (51).

Labyrinthitis (vestibular and auditory loss) and, vestibular neuritis (vestibular loss only) are also common causes for peripheral vertigo. The symptoms, which are acute in onset and last for days to weeks, usually are preceded by an upper respiratory tract infection. A predilection is seen for the spring and early summer months (3), and herpes simplex virus is thought to play a disproportionate role in the pathogenesis of these disorders (107). Ménière disease infrequently develops in the elderly. It is characterized by recurrent bouts of peripheral vertigo lasting hours; associated with unilateral, low-frequency fluctuating hearing loss; and preceded by a sensation of fullness in the ear and tinnitus. Some investigators suggest that, in older people, ischemia of the inner ear is a more common cause for vertigo than infection (96). Labyrinthine infarction caused by isolated occlusion of the internal auditory artery (IAA) is rare but can be associated with a severe peripheral vertigo and hearing loss from ischemia in the posterior intracranial circulation.

Table 8-3. *Typical symptoms of vestibular disorders, by symmetry and temporal onset*

	Acute/Rapid Onset	Chronic/Insidious Onset
Unilateral (asymmetric)	*Examples*: • vestibular neuritis • acute brainstem or cerebellar stroke *Typical symptoms*: • continuous, severe dizziness (often with the perception of spinning vertigo), exacerbated by head movement • severe, spontaneous oscillopsia without head movement • severe nausea *Typical signs*: • severe gait unsteadiness • spontaneous nystagmus • abnormal VOR (unilateral) • vomiting, blood pressure lability	*Examples*: • recovery after unilateral vestibular loss • vestibular schwannoma *Typical symptoms*: • mild dizziness brought on or exacerbated by head movement • mild oscillopsia mainly with horizontal head movement • presence or absence of mild nausea *Typical signs*: • mild gait unsteadiness • nystagmus induced by provocative maneuvers • abnormal VOR (unilateral) • no vomiting or autonomic instability
Bilateral (symmetric)	*Examples*: • vestibular ototoxicity (aminoglycoside therapy) *Typical symptoms*: • moderate dizziness (usually nonvertiginous) independent of head motion • severe oscillopsia with head movement, vertical image instability during walking • mild to no nausea *Typical signs*: • gait unsteadiness, abnormal Romberg on foam • absence of nystagmus • abnormal VOR (bilateral) • poor DVA	*Examples*: • hereditary bilateral vestibular loss (neurofibromatosis type II) • age-related vestibular loss *Typical symptoms*: • mild nonvertiginous dizziness independent of head motion • severe oscillopsia with head movement • immune to motion sickness *Typical signs*: • gait unsteadiness in darkness and on uneven surfaces • absence of nystagmus • abnormal VOR (bilateral) • poor DVA

VOR, vestibular ocular reflex; DVA, dynamic visual acuity.
Adapted from Newman-Toker DE. Diagnosing dizziness in the emergency department: why "What do you mean by 'dizzy'?" should not be the first question you ask. Doctoral Dissertation, Clinical Investigation, Bloomberg School of Public Health. Baltimore: Johns Hopkins University; 2007.

Recurrent symptoms consistent with a Ménière-like presentation but without the aural and auditory symptoms are often referred to as "recurrent vestibulopathy" or "vestibular Ménière." This may actually represent a variant of migraine, although the link is often overlooked. Patients with migrainous vertigo generally do not have vertigo temporally associated with their headaches (21), and onset of vertigo symptoms is frequently later than onset of headache, with vestibular complaints beginning in some patients as late as the seventh decade of life (69).

The most common presenting symptom of vertebrobasilar transient ischemic attacks (VBTIA) is episodic vertigo. In fact, rotatory dizziness is considered to be a risk factor for stroke, whereas nonrotatory dizziness is not (96). Although vertigo can be a symptom of VBTIA, it classically occurs with other posterior fossa symptoms such as visual loss, dysarthria, dysmetria, diplopia, or dysphagia (31). Although recurrent, isolated episodes of vertigo, with or without hearing loss, are not usually cerebrovascular in origin, exceptions are known to occur (31, 55a). Patients with arteriosclerosis, postural hypotension, cervical spondylosis, arteritis, thromboembolic disease, polycythemia, and hypercoagulable states may experience vertigo caused by VBTIA. Basilar migraine has similar symptoms to VBTIA but is less common. It usually occurs in young women but can also affect the elderly. Symptoms can include headache and marching paresthesias, but radiologic and serum examinations are routinely normal.

Stroke is associated with persistent central vertigo of acute onset. Central vertigo is more likely to persist for weeks after an acute event than peripheral vertigo because vestibular adaptation relies on intact brainstem and cerebellar systems. Nystagmus associated with peripheral lesions tends to be proportional to the intensity of vertigo; with acute central lesions, nystagmus may be severe, even with relatively mild vertigo. Vertebral artery occlusion or, less often, posterior inferior cerebellar artery (PICA) occlusion causes the lateral medullary, or Wallenberg syndrome. Vertigo is associated with ipsilateral facial analgesia and Horner's syndrome, contralateral loss of pain and temperature sensation on the body, ipsipulsion of the eyes and body, dysarthria, dysphagia, nausea, hiccups, and oscillopsia. Anterior inferior cerebellar artery (AICA) infarct (73) causes hearing loss and continuous vertigo almost indistinguishable from benign causes of peripheral vertigo because it damages the labyrinths within the IAA territory (55). In addition, the inferolateral cerebellum and dorsolateral pons are often damaged, causing ataxia, dysmetria, and facial paralysis.

Isolated cerebellar infarcts caused by superior cerebellar artery (SCA), vertebral artery, PICA, or AICA occlusion initially can look similar to acute labyrinthitis with vertigo, nausea, vomiting, and ataxia. After swelling begins to compress the fourth ventricle, brainstem structures in the dorsal pons, such as the facial colliculi, can become involved. Thus, it is crucial to be able to distinguish between vertigo caused by cerebellar infarction, which sometimes causes a spontaneous purely vertical or direction-changing gaze-evoked nystagmus, and a more benign peripheral process that typically causes a unilateral vestibular loss and a direction-fixed nystagmus.

Other processes that cause central vertigo include tumors of the posterior fossa. Typically, because of the insidious onset of any associated vestibular imbalance, vertiginous symptoms are generally mild. Hemorrhage into such lesions, however, tends to produce acute vestibular presentations similar to those described above.

PRESYNCOPE

Sensations of near fainting, especially on standing, are associated with medical conditions that affect blood flow to the brain or decreased oxygen delivery to the brain.

Problems of the cardiovascular system are sometimes treated with medications that can increase dizziness symptoms. Some of these are discussed in the Medications section later in this chapter. Studies that delineate presyncope from other types of dizziness have generally evaluated orthostatic blood pressure changes in relationship to symptoms. Comparing recumbent to standing systolic or diastolic blood pressures and using the criteria of a drop in systolic blood pressure of 20 mm Hg or more or a 10-mm Hg drop in diastolic blood pressure after standing for 2 minutes are typical end points. Studies taking this approach in otherwise healthy elderly populations indicate that presyncope is associated with recurrent episodes of orthostatic blood pressure changes, higher mean supine blood pressures, and lower body mass indexes (79). In the Cardiovascular Health Study, 14.8% of those aged 65 to 69 years were diagnosed with orthostatic hypotension, and the percentage jumped to 26% in persons over the age of 85 years (88). Thus, presyncopal dizziness increases with age.

Many studies use systolic blood pressure changes within 2 minutes of standing to determine orthostatic hypotension; (97). However, the actual prevalence of presyncopal dizziness related to postural shifts in blood pressure may be higher than estimated in such studies. (54). Recently researchers have shown that mean arterial pressure (MAP) is a more sensitive measure for orthostatic hypotension because it is a better indicator of cerebral perfusion pressure (112). Some older individuals with *postural dizziness without postural hypotension* may be able to pool enough blood in their lower extremities to affect cerebral perfusion but not lower their systemic blood pressure enough (by the strict systolic and diastolic criteria) to be considered hypotensive (34,39). Also, a number of older people do not become immediately hypotensive on standing, but rather have delayed orthostatic hypotension (sometimes up to 30 minutes later) (104).

Conditions that predispose to presyncope include physical deconditioning, depression, autonomic dysfunction such as parasympathetic hyperactivity and vasovagal reactions to emotions, neurodegenerative diseases (e.g., Shy-Drager syndrome), progressive supranuclear palsy, Parkinson's disease, Alzheimer's disease, cardiovascular disease, and hyperventilation. Because the causes for presyncope are so common and varied, individuals often have multiple problems that contribute to their symptoms, and sometimes multiple professionals are required for successful treatment.

Other symptoms of episodic autonomic dysregulation such as flushing, diarrhea, or labile blood pressure should prompt consideration of neuroendocrine malignancies such as pheochromocytoma or medullary thyroid carcinoma (114). Niacin, prescribed for hyperlipidemia, can have similar effects.

DISEQUILIBRIUM

Of all the subcategories of dizziness, disequilibrium is the most pervasive in elderly people. As discussed, the multifactorial nature of this symptom leads to it being a component of dizziness in many older people. Degenerative changes that occur with age and disease in the visual, vestibular somatosensory, motor, and cerebellar systems can lead to disequilibrium. In terms of causes, visual loss and vestibular loss can often be the most incapacitating and result in the most severe disturbances of balance and gait. Visual disturbances caused by refractive errors, cataracts, glaucoma, and macular degeneration can all have a dramatic effect on equilibrium in older people. Vision is also extremely important as a compensatory sensory input for balance and orientation. This is why imbalance problems of primarily non-visual cause in the elderly are often worse when it is dark. For instance, bilateral vestibular loss caused by ototoxic medications results in symptoms of continuous unsteadiness and head-motion-associated oscillopsia because of loss of VOR and these symptoms are usually worse in darkness (3). Gentamicin-induced ototoxicity is not uncommon; as a rule, it occurs without vertigo or hearing loss and need not be associated with abnormal peak or trough levels or renal failure (38). Unilateral vestibular dysfunction usually results in vertigo, but slow-growing tumors (e.g., vestibular schwannomas) can cause imbalance that is less dramatic.

Though progressive decreases in vestibular function, visual acuity, hearing and vibration sensation are observed in normal elderly, decrements in gait and balance performance correlate best with the burden of white matter hyperintensity on MRI (7). Severe problems with balance and orientation can be caused by central nervous system disorders, such as frontal atrophy (e.g., frontotemporal dementia), diffuse white matter degeneration, Parkinson's disease, Binswanger's disease, cerebral autosomal dominant arteriopathy with subcortical infarct and leukoencephalopathy (CADASIL), hydrocephalus, and other neurodegenerative diseases (3,8,26,49,96,117,118). In studies designed to determine the neuropathology of disequilibrium, four common factors were found on postmortem analysis of patients with undiagnosed disequilibrium: (a) prominent frontal atrophy; (b) ventriculomegaly; (c) reactive astrocytes in the periventricular white matter; and (d) increased arteriolar wall thickness (118). These findings correspond well with MRI findings of ventriculomegaly and frontal atrophy in similar patients (6,8,61).

The presumed mechanism of disequilibrium in these patients is disruption of long-loop reflex fibers traversing the deep periventricular white matter (61). A slowing of righting reflexes in the lower extremities would result, and sensory-motor integration would be delayed. Evidence indicates slowed reaction times in older healthy individuals (92). In addition, central processing time, increases with age (30). Thus, systemic conditions and behavioral risk factors that might predispose to subcortical strokes (e.g., hypertension, diabetes, hyperlipidemia, hypercholesterolemia, hypercoagulable states, sleep apnea, smoking, and illicit drug use) should be considered by physicians caring for patients with disequilibrium.

Cerebellar and motor system dysfunction can also precipitate disequilibrium. As mentioned, Parkinson's disease and other neuromuscular diseases can lead to disequilibrium. Leg weakness is often seen with deconditioning in older people and can add to a feeling of imbalance and dizziness when standing. Primary cerebellar disorders can affect motor system coordination and modulation of vestibular-initiated righting reflexes. These disorders include Chiari malformations, spinocerebellar atrophy, paraneoplastic syndromes, vitamin E deficiency (Bassen-Kornzweig syndrome), medication or toxin exposure (alcohol, anticonvulsants, lithium, and organic solvents), and infections (101). Many of these disorders will have associated cerebellar findings such as ataxia, dysmetria, impaired smooth pursuit eye movements, OKN, and reduced ability to suppress VOR with fixation. Sensory abnormalities, often seen with toxin exposures and vitamin deficiencies, can also be associated with cerebellar disease.

Somatosensory deficits occur with age and disease and alter the perception of body position with regard to space. Often referred to as "multineurosensory impairment," the loss of proprioception in combination with any of the other sensory systems can lead to a pervasive disequilibrium. The symptoms of disequilibrium are often worse in the dark and are readily quantifiable by electrodiagnostic criteria and physical examination. Some conditions that predispose to sensory loss and disequilibrium include diabetes, renal disease, liver disease, cervical osteoarthritis, toxin exposures (e.g., acrylamide, thallium, arsenic), vitamin deficiencies (e.g., E, thiamine, pyridoxine, folate, and pantothenic acid), vitamin B_6 overdose, and medication exposures (e.g., neoplastic agents, amiodarone, almitrine, dapsone, disulfuram, isoniazid, metronidazole, phenytoin, and hydralazine).

Primary orthostatic tremor causes a disabling sense of unsteadiness that is worst when standing still and often improves with sitting or walking. The amount of subjective disability often appears disproportionate to any objective disequilibrium (28), leading to misdiagnosis of a psychogenic condition. This can be diagnosed from posturography (14) and was found in 0.7% of patients evaluated in a balance clinic (46). Treatment with clonazepam, pramipexole (27), and gabapentin (82) has been effective.

ADULT HYDROCEPHALUS

Patients may have subjective sensations of dizziness or instability early in the course of hydrocephalus.

At this stage, there may be no objective evidence of any gait disorder. With mild impairment, one might observe a cautious gait, and patients may have difficulty with tandem walking. Evidence of further progression includes obvious instability when walking, and decreased speed and stride length are observed. In general, walking speed is slowed, and steps are shorter. Step height is reduced, decreasing the clearance of the foot relative to the floor. Although the gait and posture control disturbance in normal pressure hydrocephalus (NPH) is nonspecific, some features have been stressed (32). There is both difficulty in standing from a seated position and imbalance while walking. Gait has a slowed speed and smaller step size, and difficulty in turning is noted early and is performed using multiple steps rather than a pivot. A wide-based gait is common, and patients often collapse into the chair when sitting. In the classic description, the feet may seem to stick to the ground with initiation (so-called "magnetic gait"). A diagnosis of NPH should be considered in patients with ventriculomegaly whose gait impairment is characterized by reduced walking speed, short stride length, decreased step height, and a widened base (100).

CHRONIC SUBJECTIVE DIZZINESS

Many patients describe a chronic nonvertiginous dizziness that is usually associated with decreased tolerance for motion stimuli and subjective unsteadiness. Often, this has been regarded as "psychogenic" dizziness. Most studies that attempt to divide dizziness into subtypes report that between 17% and 33% of dizzy patients fall into this designation. Many of these people may have psychiatric diagnoses in the realm of anxiety and panic disorders, mood disorders, or personality disorders. Studies indicate that psychiatric causes of dizziness in older individuals account for between 5% and 37% of cases (18,23,45,51,54,62,68, 94,97,98,99,112). People with anxiety and panic disorders present with complaints of dizziness in 18% of cases (45). In one study of patients attending a dizziness clinic, 20% met the criteria for the diagnosis of panic disorder (17).

Psychiatric causes for dizziness can create symptoms reminiscent of any of the other three categories; however, symptoms that occur in specific situations or environments or that occur continuously without evidence of systemic medical or neurologic disease suggest a psychiatric etiology. Some researchers have suggested that psychiatric causes of dizziness are not as prevalent in the elderly as in younger groups (54,97). Other studies illustrate a strong link between depression, anxiety, somatoform disorders, and dizziness in geriatric patients (4,51,52,99,112). In a study of 56 chronically dizzy elderly patients, 37% had psychiatric diagnoses contributing to their dizziness, including

anxiety disorders, depression, and adjustment disorders (99). Only 5% had primary psychiatric disorders, including panic disorder, obsessive-compulsive disorder, and conversion disorder, as the primary reason for their dizziness.

A common problem in all persons with dizziness is the subsequent increase in psychological stress (99). The presence of dizziness and the debilitating effect that it has on daily activities account for more than 25% of dizzy people reporting symptoms of agoraphobia and panic (119,121). Patients with mixed physical and psychiatric symptoms also tend to have the highest level of handicap from dizziness. In longitudinal studies of dizziness in both primary care and community-based populations, patients with the most severe, persistent, and numerous physical and psychiatric symptoms remained symptomatic and handicapped the longest (2,121). Thus, psychiatric disorders can cause (or more frequently be caused by) either an episode of dizziness or fear of future episodes of dizziness. In any case, it is clear that an increase in the chronicity of symptoms occurs by erosion of the physical and psychological state of the individual. This seems especially pertinent to elderly patients with dizziness who may be more likely to suffer from other physical ailments and degenerative diseases that increase the incidence of depression, anxiety, and panic disorder.

Progress is being made in the understanding of chronic subjective dizziness (CSD), with the development of working diagnostic criteria and reports of successful interventions. CSD has been defined as "a specific clinical syndrome with the cardinal feature of persistent nonspecific dizziness that cannot be explained by active medical conditions" (102). This is not a "wastebasket" diagnosis of exclusion, but rather, CSD is identified by the symptoms and physical examination findings listed in Table 8-4.

CSD has been diagnosed in patients ranging in age from 13 to 81 years. Three subtypes can be defined: otogenic CSD, psychogenic CSD, and interactive CSD. Otogenic CSD describes patients with no history of anxiety prior to the onset of their dizziness. CSD and anxiety begin after a transient (or prolonged) medical condition that affected balance function, such as vestibular neuronitis or BPPV. Patients with psychogenic CSD have no medical cause of dizziness, and symptoms develop during the course of their anxiety disorders. Interactive CSD is a term applied to patients with a predisposition to or preexisting anxiety disorders or who developed CSD and worsening anxiety after a transient medical condition that caused dizziness. Regardless of the subtype, treatment with selective serotonin reuptake inhibitor (SSRI) medications was effective in relieving dizziness in the majority of patients in an open-label prospective

Table 8-4. *Features Defining the Clinical Syndrome of Chronic Subjective Dizziness*

1. Persistent (duration of >3 months) sensations of nonvertiginous dizziness, light-headedness, heavy-headedness, or subjective imbalance present on most days.
2. Chronic (duration of >3 months) hypersensitivity to one's own motion, which is not direction specific, and to the movements of objects in the environment.
3. Exacerbation of symptoms in settings with complex visual stimuli such as grocery stores or shopping malls or when performing precision visual tasks such as reading or using a computer.
4. Absence of currently active physical neurotologic illnesses, definite medical conditions, use of medications that may cause dizziness, or inability of such conditions to account for the full extent of dizziness or disability. Medical history could include episodes of true vertigo or ataxia as long as the conditions causing those symptoms were resolved.
5. Absence of neurotologically significant anatomic lesions on brain imaging.
6. Normal or nondiagnostic findings on balance function tests, results consistent with fully compensated vestibular deficits, or isolated test abnormalities that could not explain their presenting symptoms.

Data from Staab JP, Ruckenstein MJ. Expanding the differential diagnosis of chronic dizziness. *Arch Otolaryngol Head Neck Surg.* 2007;133:170–176.

study (103). Interestingly, the response rates did not differ between patients with major psychiatric disorders and those with lesser psychiatric symptoms with coexisting peripheral vestibular conditions or migraine headaches. Prior to enrollment in the trial, two thirds of the patients failed treatment with meclizine hydrochloride and/or benzodiazepines.

MEDICATIONS

Approximately 13% of the US population is over the age of 65 years and accounts for more than 30% of all medications prescribed (65). Dizziness is listed as an adverse side effect for 90% of all oral medications in the *Physicians' Desk Reference*. National health expenditures for drugs in the United States have increased from $10 billion in 1965 to $20 billion in 1980 and to $60 billion in 1995 (1). The classes of medications most often associated with dizziness are antiarrhythmics, anticonvulsants, antidepressants, anxiolytics, antipsychotics, sedatives or hypnotics, muscle relaxants, and nonsteroidal anti-inflammatory drugs (NSAIDs) (64,96,112). A clear medication effect alone is difficult to ascertain, given that most of the conditions being treated with these types of medications are known to cause dizziness themselves. Depression, anxiety, panic disorders, dementia, arthritis, cardiovascular disease, and stroke are all conditions that can cause dizziness or are treated with medications that can cause dizziness.

The mechanisms by which medications cause symptoms differ, but a few factors make older people more vulnerable to medication effects than younger people. With age comes an increase in body fat percentage percentage (up to 35% between the ages of 20 and 70 years) and a small decrease in plasma volume (lower by 8%) (91). An age-dependent decrease has been demonstrated in cytochrome P450 system efficiency in the liver (115). Also, a decline in renal clearance by 30% to 50% between the ages of 30 and 80 years has been shown (86). Thus, elderly people are more likely to suffer the unwanted effects of any drug. Because falls are an easily measured outcome of interest in elderly populations, many studies focus on the relationship between medication use and falls, rather than dizziness, per se. In a study of 1,358 community-dwelling persons 65 years of age or older, benzodiazepines, digoxin, laxatives, diuretics, and diltiazem were shown to be associated with presyncope, syncope, and falls (20). A prospective study of older people on medications showed a substantially increased risk of falling while taking sedatives (odds ratio 28.3) (111). A prospective cohort study of people over age 65 living in nursing homes demonstrated that use of benzodiazepines, tricyclic antidepressants, or multiple psychotropic medications more than doubled their risk for recurrent falls (109). In the same study, 36% of all falls were directly attributed to medications. In a cross-sectional investigation of 1,087 people aged 72 years or older, antidepressant medication use, depression, and use of five or more medications were significantly associated with dizziness (112). In summary, studies concerned with the association of medication use with dizziness and risk of falls in older people support the following: (a) shorter-acting medications, especially sedatives and anxiolytics, are preferable; (b) care in the prescription of blood pressure lowering agents is advisable because of the risk of orthostatic hypotension; (c) antidepressants and depression itself can contribute to dizziness and falls; and (d) any medication, especially those that are psychoactive in nature, can have prolonged or enhanced effects because of the reduced ability to metabolize and clear drugs in older people.

INITIAL DIAGNOSIS AND MANAGEMENT OF THE DIZZY PATIENT

In the acute setting, emphasis should be on identifying potentially dangerous cardiovascular or cerebrovascular conditions, and differentiating them from non-emergent, more common causes (Table 8-5). Because dizziness is the primary reason for 4% of emergency department (ED) visits (16) and is a secondary complaint in another 24% of ED patients (71), there are many opportunities for misdiagnosis to have devastating consequences. Dizziness is the ED symptom most commonly associated with a missed diagnosis of stroke (66), and the population-based estimate of misdiagnosis rate for cerebrovascular events may be as high as 35% (48).

Position- or head- motion-provoked episodes of brief dizziness are more common than unprovoked episodes and are more likely to indicate a benign disorder (e.g., benign paroxysmal positioning vertigo, drug-induced orthostatic hypotension) (72). Syncope is rare in migraine, panic attack, and Ménière's disease, but near-syncope or drop attacks can occur with these disorders. Drop attacks are sudden falls without frank loss of consciousness, which are also seen with carotid sinus hypersensitivity or transient ischemic attacks, particularly in the vertebrobasilar circulation. Patients with brief, unprovoked, episodic vertigo (particularly with an

Table 8-5. *Causes of Unprovoked, Brief Episodic Dizziness (whether vertiginous or not)*

Nonurgent
  Migraine
  Neurocardiogenic presyncope
  Ménière's disease
  Panic attack
  Seizure*

Urgent
  Cardiac arrhythmia
  Transient ischemic attack
  Aortic dissection
  Colloid cyst of the third ventricle
  Myocardial ischemia
  Neurohumoral neoplasm
  Pulmonary embolus
  Subarachnoid hemorrhage

* Although much has been written on the subject of "epilepsia tornado," seizures represent a rare cause of isolated recurrent, episodic dizziness.
Adapted from Newman-Toker DE, Camargo CA Jr. 'Cardiogenic vertigo'-true vertigo as the presenting manifestation of primary cardiac disease. *Nat Clin Pract Neurol.* 2006; 2:167–172.

associated history of presyncope or syncope) should be evaluated for potentially serious arrhythmia; the presence of vertigo does not always indicate a disease of the peripheral labyrinth or central vestibular structures (72).

Patients with sudden onset of unilateral vestibular loss with no hearing changes or evidence of cerebrovascular cause are diagnosed with vestibular neuritis. Acute treatment of this condition with methylprednisolone (but not valacyclovir) was shown to improve the recovery of peripheral vestibular function (108).

Perhaps one of the most important questions to ask in the outpatient evaluation of chronic dizziness is whether or not symptoms are made worse by head movements. If head movements *do* exacerbate dizziness, then a simple program of vestibular exercises can provide significant relief of symptoms and improve postural stability and dizziness-related handicap in 67% of patients. This treatment requires only one 30- to 40-minute visit with a primary care nurse to initiate (120). This important study clearly demonstrated that effective, inexpensive, and convenient treatment can be delivered through a primary care practice, even when patients have longstanding symptoms of dizziness (mean duration of participants' dizziness was 8 years). Fewer than 3% of patients had previously been offered vestibular rehabilitation.

When taking the patient's history, attempt to distinguish the nature of the symptoms (e.g., vertigo vs. presyncope), the actual duration of any vertigo, whether any brainstem or cerebellar symptoms are also present (indicating a central or vascular cause), and whether unilateral hearing or aural symptoms indicate the side of peripheral involvement (Fig. 8-1). Determine whether symptoms are truly spontaneous and episodic (migraine, Ménière's disease, VBTIA), provoked by rolling over in bed (BPPV), or elicited by rich visual motion environments (migraine, chronic subjective dizziness). Ask whether patients are avoiding any activities, locations, or head movements and whether symptoms are chronically elicited by these activities; encourage a vestibular rehabilitation evaluation (41), habituation exercises, or tai chi (35).

An excellent description of the bedside vestibular and ocular motor examination is recommended for a more complete treatment of this topic (116). Spontaneous peripheral vestibular nystagmus is direction fixed, present in straight-ahead gaze, and suppressed with visual fixation, and is mixed horizontal torsional with quick phases beating toward the more active ear. It can be brought out by removing fixation with the use of Frenzel lenses or by performing occlusive ophthalmoscopy (look for systematic drift of the nerve head while covering the fellow eye). Nystagmus caused by brainstem or cerebellar disease is often direction-changing, gaze-evoked, and sometimes associated with vertical ocular misalignment (skew deviation)

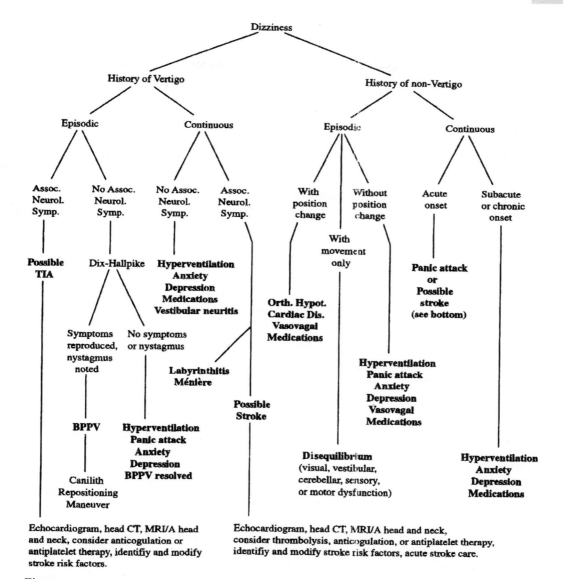

Figure 8-1. Algorithm for dizziness in elderly patients.

(17a); it is generally not suppressed with vision and can be disconjugate (as with an internuclear ophthalmoplegia). A *purely* vertical or torsional nystagmus should prompt evaluation for central disease, although mixed vertical-torsional nystagmus is prototypical of posterior semicircular canal BPPV.

DIAGNOSTIC TESTS

Basic laboratory tests in a neuro-otologic workup include an audiogram and ENG (ocular motor studies and caloric testing). An audiogram would be expected to show symmetric, high-frequency sensorineural hearing loss (SNHL) that is consistent with normal aging. Any asymmetry in pure-tone thresholds unexplained

by a conductive hearing loss or other known etiology should prompt an imaging study to rule out a schwannoma of the VIIIth nerve. The ideal study is a gadolinium-enhanced MRI, with attention to the internal auditory canals (IAC). A unilateral, low-frequency SNHL is consistent with Ménière's disease, especially if fluctuations can be documented.

Emergent imaging is recommended when transient vertigo is associated with unilateral or asymmetric hearing loss, brainstem or cerebellar symptoms other than vertigo (diplopia, dysarthria, appendicular dysmetria, dysphagia, downbeat or direction-changing nystagmus, Horner's syndrome, face or body sensory or motor changes), stroke risk factors (diabetes, hypertension, history of MI), acute-onset neck pain (magnetic resonance angiography to rule out dissection), new-onset severe headache, or the inability to stand or walk.

Ocular motor studies typically include tests of the smooth pursuit, fixation, and saccadic systems. Smooth pursuit deficits are normally seen in the aging population; responses that are asymmetric, however, should prompt concern about cerebellar pathology. An excess number of square wave jerks during visual fixation (0.5- to 5-degree saccades made away from and back to fixation at a frequency no greater than two per second) may be associated with progressive supranuclear palsy. Any spontaneous nystagmus recorded with the eyes straight ahead is abnormal; purely vertical nystagmus is indicative of brainstem or cerebellar pathology but can be seen with medication toxicity (lithium). Gaze-evoked (direction-changing) nystagmus recorded when upright similarly suggests cerebellar dysfunction or a toxic or metabolic derangement. A direction-fixed, mixed horizontal-torsional nystagmus seen in primary gaze (that increases when fixation is removed and with gaze in the quick-phase direction) is consistent with an acute unilateral vestibular loss. Caloric studies should confirm a peripheral weakness in the ear contralateral to the nystagmus quick-phase direction. This can also be confirmed at the bedside using the head impulse test (37). Screening for bilateral labyrinthine loss can be accomplished at the bedside by asking the patient to read an eye chart while the examiner oscillates the patient's head in the horizontal and vertical planes (so-called "dynamic visual acuity"). Loss of several lines of visual acuity suggests vestibular hypofunction (89a). Positional nystagmus is elicited both in static head orientations (supine with head turned left and right) and with the Dix-Hallpike maneuver, which is used to diagnose BPPV.

Patients with brief episodes of vertigo or imbalance associated with loud noises (Tullio phenomenon), nose blowing, or Valsalva maneuver may have dehiscence of superior semicircular canal (63). This can be further evaluated with vestibular-evoked myogenic potential testing (105) and with high-resolution computed tomography (CT) scanning of the temporal bone (42). Surgical repair through a middle cranial fossa approach can effectively alleviate symptoms in severe cases.

Benign Paroxysmal Positional Vertigo

BPPV is provoked by movement of the head with respect to gravity (rolling over or getting in and out of bed, looking up, or bending over). BPPV is by far the most common cause for peripheral vertigo in elderly patients (11). BPPV occurs in women twice as often as in men. A peak incidence for idiopathic BPPV occurs in the sixth decade. Post-viral cases peak in the fourth and fifth decades, and traumatic BPPV is seen with equal frequency across all ages (3). Studies of chronically dizzy

geriatric patients report that BPPV is the primary cause in 16% to 23% of cases (51,54,97). In a cross-sectional study of 100 healthy inner-city geriatric patients, 9% were diagnosed with unrecognized BPPV (74). These individuals were more likely to have lower activities of daily living scores, to have fallen in the previous 3 months, and to be depressed. This high incidence of unrecognized BPPV likely causes a significant amount of avoidable morbidity because more than 90% of BPPV cases can be treated successfully with a particle-repositioning maneuver [for review, see Furman and Cass (29) and Lanska and Remlar (53)].

The pathophysiology of BPPV is related to the effects of free-floating debris (usually degenerating or damaged otoconia) in the posterior semicircular canal (76). A sudden change in position of the head causes debris to slowly settle within the labyrinth by the force of gravity causing a sense of rotation. The symptoms have a latency of 2 to 10 seconds before onset and can last up to 45 seconds. Other medical conditions that can cause positional vertigo include alcohol intoxication and, rarely, macroglobulinemia (13).

Typically, vertigo emanates from a single posterior SCC, lasts less than 60 seconds, and may be worse in the morning (matutinal vertigo). It is diagnosed by performing the Dix-Hallpike maneuver to each side, with the patient returning to the upright position between each maneuver. The first two panels in Figure 8-2 demonstrate this maneuver for the right posterior SCC. When positive, a mixed vertical-torsional nystagmus (upbeat with torsion towards dependent ear) is observed, with slow phases downward (with respect to the head) and the top of the eyes rolling away from the dependent ear. The nystagmus can appear more vertical when looking toward the up ear and more torsional when looking toward the undermost ear. After being placed in the Dix-Hallpike position, nystagmus and vertigo should have a latency of several seconds (rarely up to 45 seconds) and are transient (usually less than 30 seconds). On returning to the upright position, the nystagmus may reverse direction and have a downbeating component.

The maneuver shown in Figure 8-2 is based on Epley's description (25). While seated, rotate the head 45 degrees toward the affected ear. Lay the patient back to the supine position, and maintain this position until the nystagmus decays completely. While supine, rotate the head 90 degrees toward the unaffected side, and hold this position for the same duration. Rotate the whole body 90 degrees with the patient in the lateral decubitus position, and again maintain this position. Sit the patient upright, keeping the head turned and chin down. The maneuver is best repeated to ensure that it was successful, and treatment can be repeated as often as necessary. Limitations on postural activities after treatment are not necessary (93).

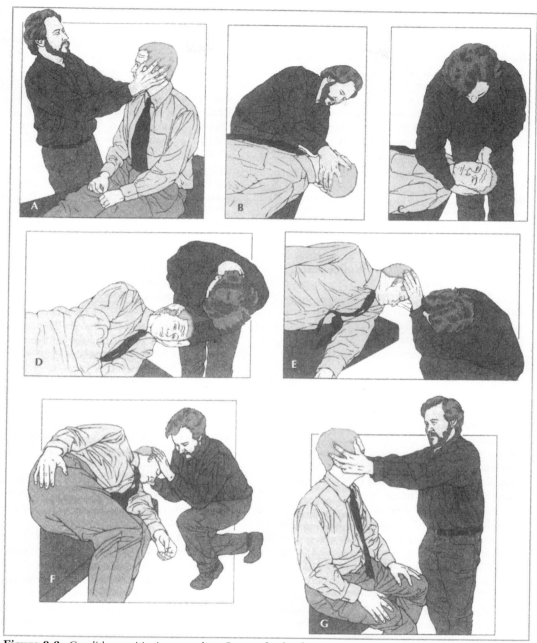

Figure 8-2. Canalith repositioning procedure. See text for details.

REFERENCES

1. Avron J. Medication use and the elderly: current status and opportunities. *Health Aff*. 1995;14: 276–286.
2. Bailey KE, Sloane PD, Mitchell M, et al. Which primary care patients with dizziness will develop persistent impairment? *Arch Fam Med*. 1993;2: 847–852.
3. Baloh RW. Dizziness in older people. *J Am Geriatr Soc*. 1992;40:713–721.
4. Baloh RW, Jacobson KM, Enrietto JA, et al. Balance disorders in older persons: quantification with posturography. *Otolaryngol Head Neck Surg*. 1998;119:89–92.

5. Baloh RW, Jacobson KM, Socotch TM. The effect of aging on visual-vestibuloocular responses. *Exp Brain Res*. 1993;95:509–516.

6. Baloh RW, Vinters HV. White matter lesions and disequilibrium in older people. II. Clinicopathologic correlation. *Arch Neurol*. 1995;52:975–981.

7. Baloh RW, Ying SH, Jacobson KM. A longitudinal study of gait and balance dysfunction in normal older people. *Arch Neurol*. 2003;60:835–839.

8. Baloh RW, Yue Q, Socotch TM, et al. White matter lesions and disequilibrium in older people. I. Case-controlled comparison. *Arch Neurol*. 1995;52:970–974.

9. Bergstrom B. Morphology of the vestibular nerve. II. The number of myelinated vestibular nerve fibers in man at various ages. *Acta Otolaryngol*. 1973;76:173–179.

10. Bergstrom B. Morphology of the vestibular nerve. III. Analysis of the calibers of the myelinated vestibular nerve fibers in man at various ages. *Acta Otolaryngol*. 1973;76:331–338.

11. Bloom J, Katsarkas A. Paroxysmal positional vertigo in the elderly. *J Otolaryngol*. 1989;18:96–98.

12. Boult C, Murphy J, Sloane P, et al. The relation of dizziness to functional decline. *J Am Geriatr Soc*. 1991;39:858–861.

13. Brandt T. Positional and positioning vertigo and nystagmus. *J Neurol Sci*. 1990;95:3–28.

14. Bronstein AM, Guerrez M. Visual-vestibular control of posture and gait: physiological mechanisms and disorders. *Curr Opin Neurol*. 1999;12:5–11.

15. Bruner A, Norris TW. Age-related changes in caloric nystagmus. *Acta Otolaryngol*. 1971;282:1–24.

16. Cappello M, di Blasi U, di Piazza L, et al. Dizziness and vertigo in a department of emergency medicine. *Eur J Emerg Med*. 1995;2:201–211.

17. Clark DB, Hirsch BE, Smith MG, et al. Panic in otolaryngology patients presenting with dizziness or hearing loss. *Am J Psychiatry*. 1994; 151:1223–1225.

17a. Cnyrim CD, Newman-Toker DE, Karch C, Brandt T, Strupp M. Bedside differentiation of vestibular neuritis from central "vestibular pseudoneuritis." Journal of Neurology, Neurosurgery, and Psychiatry 2008 (*in press*).

18. Colledge NR, Barr-Hamilton RM, Lewis SJ, et al. Evaluation of investigations to diagnose the cause of dizziness in elderly people: a community based controlled study. *BMJ*. 1996;313:788–792.

19. Colledge NR, Wilson JA, Macintyre CC, et al. The prevalence and characteristics of dizziness in an elderly community. *Age Ageing*. 1994; 23:117–120.

20. Cumming RG, Miller JP, Kelsey JL, et al. Medications and multiple falls in elderly people: the St. Louis OASIS Study. *Age Ageing*. 1991; 20:455–461.

21. Cutrer FM, Baloh RW. Migraine associated dizziness. *Headache*. 1992;32:300–304.

22. Drachman DA. Occam's razor, geriatric syndromes, and the dizzy patient. *Ann Intern Med*. 2000;132:403–404.

23. Drachman DA, Hart CW. An approach to the dizzy patient. *Neurology*. 1972;22:323–334.

24. Enrietto JA, Jacobson KM, Baloh RW. Aging effects on auditory and vestibular responses: a longitudinal study. *Am J Otolaryngol*. 1999; 20:371–378.

25. Epley JM. The canalith repositioning procedure for treatment of benign paroxysmal positional vertigo. *Otolaryngol Head Neck Surg*. 1992;107: 399–404.

26. Fife TD, Baloh RW. Disequilibrium of unknown cause in older people. *Ann Neurol*. 1993; 34:694–702.

27. Finkel MF. Pramipexole is a possible effective treatment for primary orthostatic tremor (shaky leg syndrome). *Arch Neurol*. 2000;57:1519–1520.

28. Fung VS, Sauner D, Day BL. A dissociation between subjective and objective unsteadiness in primary orthostatic tremor. *Brain*. 2001;124(2):322–330.

29. Furman JM, Cass S. Benign paroxysmal positional vertigo. *N Engl J Med*. 1999;341:1590–1596.

30. Grabiner MD, Jahnigen DW. Modeling recovery from stumbles: preliminary data on variable selection and classification efficiency. *J Am Geriatr Soc*. 1992;40:910–913.

31. Grad A, Baloh RW. Vertigo of vascular origin. Clinical and electronystagmographic features in 84 cases. *Arch Neurol*. 1989;46:281–284.

32. Graff-Radford NR, Godersky JC. Normal-pressure hydrocephalus. Onset of gait abnormality before dementia predicts good surgical outcome. *Arch Neurol*. 1986;43:940–942.

33. Grimby A, Rosenhall U. Health-related quality of life and dizziness in old age. *Gerontology*. 1995;41:286–298.

34. Hackel A, Linzer M, Anderson N. Cardiovascular and catecholamine responses to head-up tilt in the diagnosis of recurrent unexplained syncope in elderly patients. *J Am Geriatr Soc*. 1991; 39:663–668.

35. Hain TC, Fuller L, Weil L, et al. Effects of tai chi on balance. *Arch Otolaryngol Head Neck Surg*. 1999;125:1191–1195.

36. Hall TC, Miller KH, Corsallis JAN. Variations in the human Purkinje cell population according to age and sex. *Neuropathol Appl Neurobiol*. 1975; 1:267–292.

37. Halmagyi GM, Curthoys IS. A clinical sign of canal paresis. *Arch Neurol*. 1988;45:737–739.

38. Halmagyi GM, Fattore CM, Curthoys IS, et al. Gentamicin vestibulotoxicity. *Otolaryngol Head Neck Surg*. 1994;111:571–574.

39. Hargreaves A, Muir A. Lack of variation in venous tone potentiates vasovagal syncope. *Br Heart J.* 1992;67:486–490.

40. Havlik RJ. Aging in the eighties, impaired senses for sound and light in persons age 65 and over. Preliminary data from the Supplement on Aging to the National Health Interview Survey, United States January–June 1984. Hyattsville, MD: National Center for Health Care Statistics, Public Health Service; 1986.

41. Herdman SJ. Physical therapy management of vestibular disorders in older patients. *Phys Ther Pract.* 1992;1:77–87.

42. Hirvonen TP, Weg N, Zinreich SJ, et al. High-resolution CT findings suggest a developmental abnormality underlying superior canal dehiscence syndrome. *Acta Otolaryngol.* 2003;123:477–481.

43. Hsu LC, Hu HH, Wong WJ, et al. Quality of life in elderly patients with dizziness: analysis of the short-form health survey in 197 patients. *Acta Otolaryngol.* 2005;25:55–59.

44. Jonsson R, Sixt E, Landahl S, et al. Prevalence of dizziness and vertigo in an urban elderly population. *J Vestib Res.* 2004;14:47–52.

45. Kanton W. Panic disorder and somatization. *Am J Med.* 1984;77:101–106.

46. Karlberg M, Fransson PA, Magnusson M. Posturography can be used to screen for primary orthostatic tremor, a rare cause of dizziness. *Otol Neurotol.* 2005;26:1200–1203.

47. Kentala E, Rauch SD. A practical assessment algorithm for diagnosis of dizziness. *Otolaryngol Head Neck Surg.* 2003;128:54–59.

48. Kerber KA, Brown DL, Lisabeth LD, et al. Stroke among patients with dizziness, vertigo, and imbalance in the emergency department: a population-based study. *Stroke.* 2006;37:2484–2487.

49. Kerber KA, Enrietto JA, Jacobson KM, et al. Disequilibrium in older people; a prospective study. *Neurology.* 1998;51:574–580.

50. Koch H, Smith MC. Office-based ambulatory care for patients 75 years and over. National Ambulatory Medical Care Survey, 1980 and 1981. Hyattsville, MD: National Center for Health Statistics, Public Health Service; 1985.

51. Kroenke K, Lucas CA, Rosenberg ML, et al. Causes of persistent dizziness: a prospective study of 100 patients in ambulatory care. *Ann Intern Med.* 1992;117:898–904.

52. Kroenke K, Lucas CA, Rosenberg ML, et al. Psychiatric disorders and functional impairment in patients with persistent dizziness. *J Gen Intern Med.* 1993;8:530–535.

53. Lanska DJ, Remler B. Benign paroxysmal positioning vertigo: classic descriptions, origins of the provocative positioning technique, and conceptual developments. *Neurology.* 1997;48:1167–1177.

54. Lawson J, Fitzgerald J, Birchall J, et al. Diagnosis of geriatric patients with severe dizziness. *J Am Geriatr Soc.* 1999;47:12–17.

55. Lee H, Sohn SI, Jung DK, et al. Sudden deafness and anterior inferior cerebellar artery infarction. *Stroke.* 2002;33:2807–2812.

55a. Lee H, Yi HA, Baloh RW. Sudden bilateral simultaneous deafness with vertigo as a sole manifestation of vertebrobasilar insufficiency. *J Neurol Neurosurg Psychiatry.* 2003 April;74(4):539–41.

56. Leigh RJ, Zee DW, eds. *The neurology of eye movements.* 4th ed. Oxford: Oxford University Press; 2006.

57. Lopez I, Honrubia V, Baloh RW. Aging and the human vestibular nucleus. *J Vestib Res.* 1997;7:77–85.

58. Lord SR, Clark RD, Webster IW. Postural stability and associated physiological factors in a population of aged persons. *J Gerontol.* 1991;46:M69–M76.

59. Lord SR, Dayhew J, Howland A. Multifocal glasses impair edge-contrast sensitivity and depth perception and increase the risk of falls in older people. *J Am Geriatr Soc.* 2002;50:1760–1766.

60. Mallinson AI, Longridge NS. Caloric response does not decline with age. *J Vestib Res.* 2004;14:393–396.

61. Masdeu JC, Wolfson L, Lantos G, et al. Brain white-matter changes in the elderly prone to falling. *Arch Neurol.* 1989;46:1292–1296.

62. McRae D. The neurologic aspects of vertigo. *California Med.* 1960;92:255–259.

63. Minor LB, Solomon D, Zinreich JS, et al. Sound- and/or pressure-induced vertigo due to bone dehiscence of the superior semicircular canal. *Arch Otolaryngol Head Neck Surg.* 1998;124:249–258.

64. Monane M, Avorn J. Medications and falls: causation, correlation and prevention. *Clin Geriatr Med.* 1996;12:847–858.

65. Montamat SC, Cusack BJ, Vestal RE. Management of drug therapy in the elderly. *N Engl J Med.* 1989;321:303–309.

66. Moulin T, Sablot D, Vidry E, et al. Impact of emergency room neurologists on patient management and outcome. *Eur Neurol.* 2003;50:207–214.

67. Nadol JB, Schuknecht HF. The pathology of peripheral vestibular disorders in the elderly. *Ear Nose Throat J.* 1989;68:930–933.

68. Nedzelski JM, Barber HO, McIlmoyl L. Diagnoses in a dizziness unit. *J Otolaryngol.* 1986;15:101–104.

69. Neuhauser HK, Leopold M, von Brevern M, et al. The interrelations of migraine, vertigo, and migrainous vertigo. *Neurology*. 2001;56:436–441.

70. Neuhauser HK, von Brevern M, Radtke A, et al. Epidemiology of vestibular vertigo: a neurotologic survey of the general population. *Neurology*. 2005;65:898–904.

71. Newman-Toker DE. Diagnosing dizziness in the emergency department: Why "What do you mean by 'dizzy'?" should not be the first question you ask. Doctoral Dissertation, Clinical Investigation, Bloomberg School of Public Health. Baltimore: Johns Hopkins University; 2007.

72. Newman-Toker DE, Camargo CA Jr. 'Cardiogenic vertigo'—true vertigo as the presenting manifestation of primary cardiac disease. *Nat Clin Pract Neurol*. 2006;2:167–172.

72a. Newman-Toker DE, Cannon LM, Stofferahn ME, Rothman RE, Hsieh YH, Zee DS. Imprecision in patient reports of dizziness symptom quality: a cross-sectional study conducted in an acute-care setting. *Mayo Clin Proc*. 2007;82:1329–1340.

73. Oas JG, Baloh RW. Vertigo and the anterior inferior cerebellar artery syndrome. *Neurology*. 1992;42:2274–2279.

74. Oghalai JS, Manolidis S, Barth JL, et al. Unrecognized benign paroxysmal positional vertigo in elderly patients. *Otolaryngol Head Neck Surg*. 2000;122:630–634.

75. Paige GD. Senescence of human visual-vestibular interactions. 1. Vestibulo-ocular reflex and adaptive plasticity with aging. *Exp Brain Res*. 1992;2:133–151.

76. Parnes LS, McClure JA. Free-floating endolymph particles: a new operative finding during posterior semicircular canal occlusion. *Laryngoscope*. 1992;102:988–992.

77. Paterka RJ, Black FO, Schoenhoff MB. Age-related changes in human vestibulo-ocular reflexes: sinusoidal rotation and caloric tests. *J Vestib Res*. 1990;1:49–59.

78. Peretz C, Herman T, Hausdorff JM, et al. Assessing fear of falling: can a short version of the Activities-specific Balance Confidence scale be useful? *Mov Disord*. 2006;21:2101–2105.

79. Puisieux F, Boumbar Y, Bulckaen H, et al. Intraindividual variability in orthostatic blood pressure changes among older adults: the influence of meals. *J Am Geriatr Soc*. 1999;47:1332–1336.

80. Raz N, Torres IJ, Spencer WD. Age-related regional differences in cerebellar vermis observed in vivo. *Arch Neurol*. 1992;49:412–416.

81. Richter E. Quantitative study of human Scarpa's ganglion and vestibular sensory epithelium. *Acta Otolaryngol*. 1980;90:199–208.

82. Rodrigues JP, Edwards DJ, Walters SE, et al. Blinded placebo crossover study of gabapentin in primary orthostatic tremor. *Mov Disord*. 2006;21:900–905.

83. Rosenhall U. Mapping of the crista ampullares in man. *Ann Otol Rhinol Laryngol*. 1972;81:882–889.

84. Rosenhall U. Vestibular macular mapping in man. *Ann Otol Rhinol Laryngol*. 1972;81:339–351.

85. Ross MD, Peacor D, Johnson LG. Observations on normal and degenerating human otoconia. *Ann Otol Rhinol Laryngol*. 1976;85:310–326.

86. Rowe JW, Andres R, Tobin JD, et al. The effect of age on creatinine clearance in man: a cross-sectional and longitudinal study. *J Gerontol*. 1976;31:155–163.

87. Royal College of General Practitioners, Office of Population Censuses and Surveys, Department of Health and Social Security. Morbidity statistics from general practice. Third national study 1981–1982. London: Her Majesty's Stationary Office; 1986.

88. Rutan GH, Hermanson B, Bild DE. Orthostatic hypotension in older adults: the Cardiovascular Health Study. *Hypertension*. 1992;19:508–519.

89. Sawyer RN Jr, Thurston SE, Becker KR, et al. The cervico-ocular reflex of normal human subjects in response to transient and sinusoidal trunk rotations. *J Vestib Res*. 1994;4:245–249.

89a. Schubert MC, Herdman SJ, Tusa RJ. Vertical dynamic visual acuity in normal subjects and patients with vestibular hypofunction. *Otol and Neurotol*. 23:373–377, 2002.

90. Schuknecht HF, Merchant SN. Vestibular atelectasis. *Ann Otol Rhinol Laryngol*. 1988;97:565–576.

91. Shader RI, Greenblatt DJ, Harmatz JS, et al. Absorption and disposition of chlordiazepoxide in young and elderly male volunteers. *J Clin Pharmacol*. 1977;17:709–718.

92. Shaw NA. Age-dependent changes in central somatosensory conduction time. *Clin Electroencephalogr*. 1992;23:105–110.

93. Simoceli L, Bittar RS, Greters ME. Posture restrictions do not interfere in the results of canalith repositioning maneuver. *Rev Bras Otorrinolaringol*. 2005;71:55–59.

94. Simpson RB, Nedzelski JM, Barber HO, et al. Psychiatric diagnoses in patients with psychogenic dizziness or severe tinnitus. *J Otolaryngol*. 1988;17:325–330.

95. Skinner HB, Barrack RL, Cook SD, et al. Joint position sense in total knee arthroplasty. *J Orthop Res*. 1984;1:276–283.

96. Sloane D. Evaluation and management of dizziness in the older patient. *Clin Geriatr Med.* 1996;12:785–801.

97. Sloane D, Baloh RW. Persistent dizziness in geriatric patients. *J Am Geriatr Soc.* 1989; 37:1031–1038.

98. Sloane D, Blazer D, George LK. Dizziness in a community elderly population. *J Am Geriatr Soc.* 1989;37:101–108.

99. Sloane D, Hartman M, Mitchell M. Ppychological factors associated with chronic dizziness in patients aged 60 and older. *J Am Geriatr Soc.* 1994;42:847–852.

100. Snijders AH, van de Warrenburg BP, Giladi N, et al. Neurological gait disorders in elderly people: clinical approach and classification. *Lancet Neurol.* 2007;6:63–74.

101. Solomon D. Distinguishing and treating causes of central vertigo. *Otolaryngol Clin North Am.* 2000;33:579–601.

102. Staab JP, Ruckenstein MJ. Expanding the differential diagnosis of chronic dizziness. *Arch Otolaryngol Head Neck Surg.* 2007;133: 170–176.

103. Staab JP, Ruckenstein MJ, Solomon D, et al. Serotonin reuptake inhibitors for dizziness with psychiatric symptoms. *Arch Otolaryngol Head Neck Surg.* 2002;128:554–560.

104. Streeten D. Delayed orthostatic intolerance. *Arch Intern Med.* 1992;152:1066–1072.

105. Streubel SO, Cremer PD, Carey JP, et al. Vestibular-evoked myogenic potentials in the diagnosis of superior canal dehiscence syndrome. *Acta Otolaryngol Suppl.* 2001;545:41–49.

106. Strupp M, Arbusow V, Borges Pereira C, et al. Subjective straight-ahead during neck muscle vibration: effects of ageing. *Neuroreport.* 1999; 10:3191–3194.

107. Strupp M, Brandt T. Vestibular neuritis. *Adv Otorhinolaryngol.* 1999;55:111–136.

108. Strupp M, Zingler VC, Arbusow V, et al. Methylprednisolone, valacyclovir, or the combination for vestibular neuritis. *N Engl J Med.* 2004;351:354–361.

109. Thapa PB, Gideon P, Fought RL, et al. Psychotropic drugs and risk of recurrent falls in ambulatory nursing home residents. *Am J Epidemiol.* 1995;142:202–211.

110. Tilvis RS, Hakala SM, Valvanne J, et al. Postural hypotension and dizziness in a general aged population: a four-year follow-up of the Helsinki Aging Study. *J Am Geriatr Soc.* 1996;44:809–814.

111. Tinneti ME, Speechley M, Ginter SF. Risk factors for falls among elderly persons living in the community. *N Engl J Med.* 1988;319:1701–1707.

112. Tinetti ME, Williams CS, Gill TM. Dizziness among older adults: a possible geriatric syndrome. *Ann Intern Med.* 2000;132:337–344.

113. Torvik A, Torp S, Lindboe CF. Atrophy of the cerebellar vermis in ageing: a morphometric and histologic study. *J Neurol Sci.* 1986; 76:283–294.

114. Tritos NA, Clerkin EP, Dugan JM, et al. Dizzy and red-faced. *Am J Med.* 2007;120:412–414.

115. Vestal RE, Montamat SC, Nielson C. Drugs in special patient groups: the elderly. In: Melmon KL, et al., eds. *Clinical pharmacology.* New York: McGraw Hill; 1992:851–874.

116. Walker MF, Zee DS. Bedside vestibular examination. In: Shepard NT, Solomon D, eds. *Practical issues in the management of the dizzy and balance patient.* Philadelphia: WB Saunders; 2000:495–506.

117. Weindruch R, Korper S, Hadley E. The prevalence of dysequilibrium and related disorders in older persons. *Ear Nose Throat J.* 1989; 68:925–929.

118. Whitman GT, DiPatre PL, Lopez IA, et al. Neuropathology in older people with disequilibrium of unknown cause. *Neurology.* 1999; 53:375–382.

119. Yardley L. Overview of psychologic effects of chronic dizziness and balance disorders. *Otolaryngol Clin North Am.* 2000;33:603–616.

120. Yardley L, Donovan-Hall M, et al. Effectiveness of primary care-based vestibular rehabilitation for chronic dizziness. *Ann Intern Med.* 2004; 141:598–605.

121. Yardley L, Owen N, Nazareth I, et al. Prevalence and presentation of dizziness in a general practice community sample of working age people. *Br J Gen Pract.* 1998;48:1131–1135.

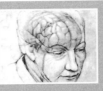

CHAPTER 9.1

Definition and Epidemiology of Falls and Gait Disorders

Neil B. Alexander

INTRODUCTION

FALLS

A fall is a sudden, unintentional change in position causing an individual to land at a lower level, on an object, or on the ground. Because most falls are not associated with syncope, most investigators exclude falls associated with loss of consciousness (e.g., as from a seizure), although loss of consciousness can occur after the fall. Other overwhelming events (e.g., sustaining a violent blow or sudden onset of paralysis) are also not as common as nonsyncopal falls. Annually, falls occur in approximately one third of community-dwelling older adults and one half of nursing home residents. The nursing home resident rate (1.5 falls per bed annually) is likely caused by the increased frailty of these residents and the increased reporting in this setting (30). Depending on the published series, although up to 2% of falls result in hip fractures, other fractures can occur in up to 5% of falls, and other serious injuries (e.g., head injury) can occur in up to 10%. Often, more than 50% of persons who fall sustain at least some minor injury (e.g., a laceration); more importantly, however, these and others who fall can develop fear of falling and restrict their activity. Those who fall, particularly repeat fallers, tend to have activities of daily living (ADL) and instrumental ADL disability and are at high risk for subsequent hospitalization, further disability, institutionalization, and death (19,40,41).

GAIT DISORDERS

Determining that a gait is "disordered" is difficult because no clearly accepted standards are generally seen for "normal" gait in older adults. Some believe that slowed gait speed suggests a disorder, whereas others believe that deviations in smoothness, symmetry, and synchrony of movement patterns suggest a disorder. However, a slowed and aesthetically abnormal gait, in fact, can provide the older adult with a safe, independent gait pattern. Self-reports of difficulty walking are common. At least 20% of noninstitutionalized older adults admit to having difficulty

walking or require the assistance of another person or special equipment to walk (23). Limitations in walking also increase with age. In some samples of noninstitutionalized older adults aged 85 years and older, the incidence of limitation in walking can be more than 54% (23). Although age-related gait changes (e.g., in speed) are most apparent past age 75 or 80, most gait disorders appear in connection with underlying diseases, particularly as disease severity increases. Attributing a gait disorder to one disease cause in older adults is particularly difficult because similar gait abnormalities are common to many diseases (2).

CAUSES, RISK FACTORS, AND CLINICAL MANIFESTATIONS

Multiple factors frequently contribute to falls, fall-related injury, and gait disorders. In falls, often a complex interaction occurs between individual impairments (intrinsic factors), situational factors (aspects related to the ADL task being performed), and extrinsic factors (environmental demands and hazards). In terms of intrinsic factors, the diseases and impairments that are implicated in gait disorders are similar to those that place an older adult at risk for falls and fall-related injury. At least seven major intrinsic factors or conditions can be implicated, and although age-related changes can be present (such as in reduction of leg strength), the major contributors to risk of fall and gait disorders are the diseases that influence each factor (Table 9-1). These functions include vestibular, proprioceptive, and visual function; cognition; and musculoskeletal factors. For example, patients with leg arthritis (with associated pain and limited range of motion and strength) and dementia (with associated lack of judgment, inattention, and confusion) are at risk for falls. Medications are also major risk factors and are categorized according to their major mechanism of effect (Table 9-2). Extrinsic and situational factors (Table 9-3) contribute to the risk of falls and fall-related injury when (a) environmental hazards are present; (b) the environment or tasks performed demand

This chapter is reprinted from the 2002 edition of *Clinical Neurology of the Older Adult*.

Table 9-1. *Intrinsic Factors Contributing to Risk of Falls, Fall-Related Injury, and Gait Disorders*

Factor	Typical Diseases Involved
Central processing	Dementia
Neuromotor	Parkinson's disease, stroke, myelopathy (such as from cervical or lumbar spondylosis), cerebellar degeneration, carotid sinus hypersensitivity, peripheral neuropathy, vertebrobasilar insufficiency
Vision	Cataracts, glaucoma, age-related macular degeneration
Vestibular	Acute labyrinthitis, Ménière's disease, paroxysmal positional vertigo
proprioception	Peripheral neuropathy (such as from diabetes mellitus), B_{12} deficiency
Musculoskeletal	Arthritis, foot disorders
Systemic	Postural hypotension, metabolic disease (e.g., thyroid), cardiopulmonary disease, other acute illness (e.g., sepsis)

greater postural control and mobility; and (c) situations require changing positions (such as transferring and turning). For example, a patient with Parkinson's disease (intrinsic factor) may trip over a rug (extrinsic factor) but only under certain situations, such as when walking to the bathroom at night (situational factor). Situational factors are particularly important when an injury results from a fall (37). For example, major injuries are more likely when falling from an upright position (with greater potential energy to be dissipated) and when falling laterally, with direct impact on the hip. Other environmental factors (e.g., hardness of impact surface) and other intrinsic factors (e.g., low femoral bone mineral density and body mass index) also contribute to increased risk of fall-related injury (9,15).

The relative contribution of intrinsic, extrinsic, and situational factors also depends on the person

falling and the environment in which that person is living. Community-dwelling fallers tend to be exposed to greater environmental demand and hazards and tend to be less physically impaired; thus, extrinsic factors make more contributions to fall and fall injury risk (19). Nursing home fallers are usually more physically impaired and are exposed to fewer environmental hazards and demand; thus, intrinsic factors such as weakness and balance disorders contribute more to falls and fall injury risk (30).

ASSESSMENT OF GAIT DISORDERS AND FALL RISK

DIAGNOSES CONTRIBUTING TO FALLS AND GAIT DISORDERS

Disordered gait may not be an inevitable consequence of aging, but rather a reflection of the increased prevalence and severity of age-associated diseases.

Table 9-2. *Medications Contributing to Risk of Falls, Fall-Related Injury, and Gait Disorders*

Medication Category	Typical Medications
Reduce alertness or retard central processing	Analgesics (especially narcotics) Psychotropics (especially tricyclics, long-acting benzodiazepines, phenothiazines)
Impair cerebral perfusion	Antihypertensives (especially vasodilators) Antiarrhythmics Diuretics (especially when dehydration occurs)
Direct vestibular toxicity	Aminoglycosides High-dose loop diuretics
Extrapyramidal syndromes	Phenothiazines

Table 9-3. *Extrinsic and Situational Factors Contributing to Risk of Falls and Fall-Related Injury*

Factor	Examples
Environmental hazard	Slippery or uneven walking surface, poor lighting
Increased environmental demand	Using stairs, rising from low chair
Situational	Changing position, risk-taking behavior, recent relocation to new nursing home

From author's own original work and adapted from King MB, Tinetti ME. Falls in community-dwelling older persons. *J Am Geriatr Soc.*1995;43:1146–1154.

These underlying diseases, both neurologic and non-neurologic, are the major contributors to disordered gait. In a primary care setting, patients consider pain, stiffness, dizziness, numbness, weakness, and sensations of abnormal movement to be the most common contributors to their walking difficulties (17). The most common diagnoses found in a primary care setting thought to contribute to gait disorders include degenerative joint disease, acquired musculoskeletal deformities, intermittent claudication, postorthopedic surgery and poststroke impairments, and postural hypotension (17). Usually, more than one contributing diagnosis is found. Factors such as dementia and fear of falling also contribute to gait disorders. The diagnoses found in a neurologic referral population are primarily neurologically oriented (12, 34): frontal gait disorders [usually related to normal pressure hydrocephalus (NPH) and cerebrovascular processes]; sensory disorders (also involving vestibular and visual function); myelopathy; previously undiagnosed Parkinson's disease or parkinsonian syndromes; and cerebellar disease. Known conditions causing severe impairment (e.g., hemiplegia and severe hip or knee disease) are frequently not referred to a neurologist. Thus, many gait disorders, particularly those that are classical and discrete (e.g., related to stroke and osteoarthritis) and those that are mild or may relate to irreversible disease (e.g., multi-infarct dementia), are presumably diagnosed in a primary care setting and treated without a referral to a neurologist. Other less common contributors to gait disorders include metabolic disorders (related to renal or hepatic disease), central nervous system (CNS) tumors or subdural hematoma, depression, and psychotropic medications. Case reports also document reversible gait disorders caused by clinically overt hypo- or hyperthyroidism and vitamin B_{12} and folate deficiency [for detailed review, see Alexander (2)].

A potentially useful classification system [based on Nutt et al. (22) and elaborated in Alexander (1)] (Table 9-4) categorizes these diseases according to the sensorimotor levels that are affected. Diseases considered part of the low sensorimotor level can be divided into peripheral sensory and peripheral motor dysfunction, including musculoskeletal (arthritic) and myopathic or neuropathic disorders that cause weakness. These disorders are generally distal to the CNS. With peripheral sensory impairment, vestibular disorders, peripheral neuropathy, posterior column (proprioceptive) deficits, and visual impairment commonly cause unsteady and tentative gait. With peripheral motor impairment, a number of classical gait patterns emerge, including obvious compensatory maneuvers. These conditions involve extremity (both body segment and joint) deformities, painful weight bearing, and focal myopathic and neuropathic weakness. Note

that, if the gait disorder is limited to this low sensorimotor level (i.e., the CNS is intact), the person adapts well to the gait disorder, compensating with an assistive device or learning to negotiate the environment safely. At the middle level, the execution of centrally selected postural and locomotor responses is faulty, and the sensory and motor modulation of gait is disrupted. Gait can be initiated normally, but stepping patterns are abnormal. Examples include diseases causing spasticity (e.g., related to myelopathy, vitamin B_{12} deficiency, and stroke), parkinsonism (idiopathic as well as drug induced), and cerebellar disease (e.g., alcohol induced). Classical gait patterns appear when the spasticity is sufficient to cause leg circumduction and fixed deformities (e.g., equinovarus), the parkinsonism produces shuffling steps and reduced arm swing, and the cerebellar ataxia increases trunk sway sufficiently to require a broad base of gait support. At the high level, the gait characteristics become more nonspecific, and cognitive dysfunction and slowed cognitive processing become more prominent. Behavioral aspects such as fear of falling are also important, particularly in cautious gait. Frontal-related gait disorders often have a cerebrovascular component and are not merely the result of frontal masses and NPH. The severity of the frontal-related disorders runs a spectrum from gait ignition failure (i.e., difficulty with initiation) to frontal disequilibrium, where unsupported stance is not possible. Cognitive, pyramidal, and urinary disturbances can also accompany a gait disorder. Gait disorders that might fall into this category have been given a number of overlapping descriptions, including gait apraxia, marche à petit pas, and arteriosclerotic parkinsonism.

Note that more than one disease or impairment is likely present that contributes to a gait disorder; one example could be the long-standing diabetic patient with peripheral neuropathy or a recent stroke who is now very fearful of falls. Certain disorders can actually involve multiple levels, such as Parkinson's disease affecting high (cortical) and middle (subcortical) structures. Drug-metabolic causes (e.g., from sedatives, tranquilizers, and anticonvulsants) can involve more than one level; phenothiazines, for example, can cause high (sedation) and middle (extrapyramidal) level effects.

Other factors that contribute to gait disorders that are frequently disease associated (e.g., related to cardiopulmonary disease) but are often assessed separately include marked reductions in activity and aerobic fitness, reductions in joint strength and range of motion, and previous falls.

Although older adults may maintain a relatively normal gait pattern well into their 80s, some slowing occurs, and decreased stride length becomes a common feature described in older adult gait disorders

Table 9-4. *Gait Disorders Classified by Sensorimotor Level, with a Description of the Specific Pathologic Condition and Associated Gait Findings**

Sensorimotor Level	Within Level Classification	Condition (pathology, symptoms, signs)	Typical Gait Findings
Low	Peripheral sensory	Sensory ataxia (posterior column, peripheral nerves)	Unsteady, uncoordinated
		Vestibular ataxia	Unsteady, weaving (*drunken*)
		Visual ataxia	Tentative, uncertain
	Peripheral motor	Arthritic (antalgic; joint deformity)	Avoids weight bearing on affected side, shorten stance phase.
			Painful hip may produce *Trendelenberg* (trunk shift over affected side).
			Painful knee is flexed.
			Painful spine produces short, slow steps and decreased lumbar lordosis.
			Other nonantalgic features: contractures, deformity-limited motion, buckling with weight bearing.
			Kyphosis and ankylosing spondylosis produce stooped posture.
			Unequal leg length can produce trunk and pelvic motion abnormalities (including *Trendelenberg*).
		Myopathic and neuropathic (weakness)	Pelvic girdle weakness produces exaggerated lumbar lordosis and lateral trunk flexion (*Trendelenberg* and *waddling* gait).
			Proximal motor neuropathy produces *waddling* and *foot slap*.
			Distal motor neuropathy produces distal weakness (especially ankle dorsiflexion, foot *drop*), which may lead to exaggerated hip flexion/foot lifting (*steppage gait* and *foot slap*).
Middle	Spasticity	Hemiplegia/paresis	Leg swings outward in semicircle from hip (circumduction). Knee may hyperextend (*genu recurvatum*), and ankle may excessively plantar flex and invert (*equinovarus*).
		Paraplegia/paresis	With less paresis, some may only lose arms swing and only drag or scrape the foot. Both legs circumduct, steps are short shuffling and scraping, and when severe, hip adducts so that knees cross in front of each other (*scissoring*).
	Parkinsonism		Small shuffling steps, hesitation, acceleration (*festination*), falling forward (*propulsion*), falling backward (*retropulsion*), moving the whole body while turning (*turning en bloc*), absent arm swing.
	Cerebellar ataxia		Wide-based with increased trunk sway, irregular stepping, especially on turns.
	Cautious gait		Fear of falling with appropriate postural responses, normal to widened base, shortened stride, decreased velocity, and *en bloc* turns.
High	Frontal-related gait disorders, other white matter lesions	Cerebrovascular, normal pressure hydrocephalus	Proposed spectrum ranges from gait ignition failure, to frontal gait disorder, to frontal disequilibrium. May also have cognitive, pyramidal, and urinary disturbances.
			Gait ignition failure: difficulty initiating gait, short shuffling gait, may freeze with diversion of attention or turning.
			Frontal gait disorder: similar to Parkinson's but wider base, upright posture, preservation of arm swing.
			Frontal disequilibrium: cannot stand unsupported.

*See text for additional details.

Adapted from Alexander NB. Differential diagnosis of gait disorders in older adults. *Clin Geriatr Med.* 1996;12:697–698.

[reviewed by Alexander (2)]. Some authors have proposed the emergence of an age-related gait disorder without accompanying clinical abnormalities (i.e., essential "senile" gait disorder) (20). This gait pattern is described as broad based with small steps, diminished arm swing, stooped posture, flexion of the hips and knees, uncertainty and stiffness in turning, occasional difficulty initiating steps, and a tendency toward falling. These and other nonspecific findings (e.g., inability to perform tandem gait) are similar to gait patterns found in a number of other diseases, and yet the clinical abnormalities are insufficient to make a specific diagnosis. This "disorder" may be a precursor to an as-yet-asymptomatic disease (e.g., related to subtle extrapyramidal signs) and is likely to be a manifestation of concurrent, progressive cognitive impairment (e.g., Alzheimer's disease or vascular dementia) (10). Thus, "senile" gait disorder potentially reflects a number of potential disease causes and is generally not useful in labeling gait disorders in older adults.

HISTORY AND PHYSICAL EXAMINATION

Emphasis should be placed on assessing the cardiovascular, visual, vestibular, musculoskeletal, and neurologic systems, as well as assessing medication use. A history of the fall and the circumstances surrounding it, including associated symptoms and associated movements or activities that may have elicited the fall, are useful. Subject reports of premonitory or associated symptoms (e.g., palpitations, shortness of breath, chest pain, vertigo, light-headedness, and associated activities) help determine contributing medical conditions. Of particular importance is the determination of syncope or near-syncope, which leads to a different differential diagnosis and workup, including Holter monitor, tilt table, and carotid massage. Recent data from selected populations suggest underrecognition of near-syncope as caused by carotid sinus hypersensitivity (CSH) (3,45), but the contribution of CSH to an actual fall is not completely clear. Symptoms that are postprandial or postmicturition can help better define accompanying risk. The vestibular or cardiovascular origin of dizziness or light-headedness, particularly when positional, is sometimes difficult to differentiate (see examination discussed below). A careful medical history and a review of the factors given in Table 9-1 will help elucidate the multiple factors contributing to the fall. A brief systemic evaluation for evidence of subacute metabolic disease (e.g., thyroid disorders), acute cardiopulmonary disorders (e.g., myocardial infarction), or other acute illness (e.g., sepsis) is warranted because falling may be the presenting feature of acute and subacute systemic decompensation in an older adult. An assessment of mobility is also indicated to include ADL function and ambulation (i.e., wheelchair use, distance ambulated, and the extent of human or device assistance required; see below).

Using the factors given in Table 9-1, the physical examination should include an attempt to identify motion-related factors, such as by provoking both objective and subjective responses to the Dix-Hallpike maneuver and to supine and standing blood pressure and pulse measurements. In the Dix-Hallpike maneuver, while the patient is seated on an examination table, the examiner holds the patient's head, turns the head to one side, and lowers the head to the level of the table, classically 30 degrees below the table level. The patient then sits up, and the maneuver is repeated again to the other side. Blood pressure should be measured with the patient both supine and standing to rule out orthostatic hypotension. Vision screening, at least for acuity, is essential. Examining the cardiovascular system helps exclude arrhythmia, valvular heart disease, and heart failure. The neck, spine, extremities, and feet should be evaluated for deformities and pain or limitations in range of motion. A formal neurologic assessment is critical and should include assessment of strength and tone, sensation (including proprioception), coordination (including cerebellar function), and station and gait. In regard to the latter, the Romberg test screens for simple postural control and whether the proprioceptive and vestibular systems are functional. Some investigators have proposed one-legged stance time less than 5 seconds as a risk factor for injurious falls (43), although even relatively healthy older adults aged 70 can have difficulty with one-legged stance (29). Given the importance of cognition as a risk factor, screening for mental status is also indicated.

PERFORMANCE-BASED FUNCTIONAL ASSESSMENT

Technologically oriented assessments involving formal kinematic and kinetic analyses have not been applied widely in clinical assessments of older adult balance and gait disorders. Using a functional gait and balance battery, which includes aspects such as turning while standing, has been proposed as a means to detect and quantify abnormalities and direct interventions. Fall risk, for example, can be increased with more abnormal gait and balance scale scores (39). Clinical gait assessments use a battery of items, either timed or scored semiquantitatively, usually based on whether a subject is able to perform the task and, if able, how normal or abnormal the performance was. Batteries that focus primarily on gait include the following:

- Functional Ambulation Classification Scale (16) rates the use of assistive devices, the degree of human assistance (either manual or verbal), the distance the patient can walk, and the types of surfaces the patient can negotiate.

- Performance-Oriented Balance and Mobility Assessment (POMA) gait subsection (35) is a rating of gait initiation, turning, step length and height, step symmetry and continuity, path deviation, and trunk sway.
- Get Up and Go Test (24) is a timed sequence of rising from a chair, walking 3 m, turning, and returning to the chair.
- Dynamic Gait Index (33) is a rating of a series of tasks, including turning, walking while turning the head, clearing obstacles, and using stairs.
- Functional Obstacle Course (21) is a timed test of negotiating different floor textures, graded surfaces, stairs, and simultaneous functional activities while walking (e.g., opening and closing doors).
- Gait Abnormality Rating Scale (42) is modified to score gait variability, guardedness, staggering, foot contact, hip range of motion, shoulder extension, and arm-heel synchrony.
- Emory Functional Ambulation Profile (47) is a battery of timed tasks, including walking on a hard floor, walking on a carpeted surface, stepping over an obstacle, and walking up and down four stairs.

These scales were used reliably in smaller, selected published samples, although perhaps less reliably in larger epidemiologic settings [e.g., see Rockwood et al. (28) for critique of Get Up and Go Test].

Comfortable gait speed has become a powerful assessment and outcome measure. Measured as part of a timed short-distance (e.g., 8 feet) walk or as measured in terms of distance walked over time (such as 6 minutes), gait speed predicts disease activity (e.g., arthritis), cardiac and pulmonary function (particularly in congestive heart failure), and ultimately mobility and ADL disability, institutionalization, and mortality [for review, see Alexander (2)].

LABORATORY AND DIAGNOSTIC TESTS

Depending on the history and physical examination, further laboratory and diagnostic evaluation may be warranted. Tests such as electrocardiograms, Holter monitors, cardiac enzymes, and echocardiograms are not routinely recommended unless a cardiac source is suspected. Similarly, complete blood count, chemistries, and stool for occult blood are useful only when acute systemic disease is suspected. Head or spine imaging, including X-ray study, computed tomography (CT), or magnetic resonance imaging (MRI), are of unclear use unless the history and physical examination suggest neurologic abnormalities, either preceding or of recent onset, related to the gait disorder. A possible exception relates to cerebral white matter changes on CT scan considered to be ischemic in nature (termed

"leukoaraiosis"), which can cause nonspecific gait disorders. Recently, periventricular high-signal measurements on MRI as well as increased ventricular volume, even in apparently healthy older adults [see discussion in Camicoli et al. (4) for review of previous studies], have been associated with gait slowing. Age-specific guidelines, sensitivity, specificity, and cost effectiveness of these workups remain to be determined.

INTERVENTIONS TO REDUCE FALLS, FALL-RELATED INJURY, AND GAIT DISORDERS

FALLS

Interventions to reduce falls, fall-related injury, and gait disorders attempt to improve functional capacity, decrease falls, and decrease injuries, but sometimes patterns of independence are altered as well (i.e., for safety reasons, ambulating in inclement weather conditions is discouraged). Interventions can be divided into at least four categories (Table 9-5). Interventions that deal directly with intrinsic factors focus on decreasing disease-related impairment and providing therapy. Extrinsic factor interventions have thus far focused primarily on decreasing hazards and environmental demand. Examples of these extrinsic interventions include improving lighting, adding grab bars, raising the toilet seat, finding an appropriate bed height, and providing an appropriately structured environment for those who are cognitively impaired. Because restraint use may be associated with more falls and injuries (6), reducing active mechanical restraints (e.g., vests) may not necessarily increase falls or fall-related injury. More passive alternatives, such as wheelchair adaptations, removable belts, and wedge seating, can apparently provide adequate fall protection with less mobility limitation. Few controlled studies have addressed situational factors, although caregiver or nurse surveillance, particularly with those who are considered for restraint, may be useful. Use of motion detectors has a mixed benefit because a staff person still needs to be present to respond to the triggered alarm. Finally, protective padding worn over the hip can be a useful alternative for fallers at risk for hip injury. A recent randomized, community-based study found a reduction in hip fractures (relative hazard = 0.4) in those wearing hip protector pads (18). In this study, most hip fractures in the hip pad group occurred in those who were not wearing the pad at the time of the fall. Note, however, as in previous hip pad studies, that compliance was still a problem; 31% of those randomized to the hip pad group refused to wear the pad. Alternatively, flooring materials exist that will help dissipate the impact force, although a floor that is too compliant may be destabilizing by itself.

Table 9-5. *Interventions to Reduce Falls, Fall-Related Injury, and Gait Disorders*

Intrinsic
    Treat the underlying disease
    Eliminate drugs or reduce dosages
    Initiate physical therapy program
        Balance and gait training (including training
            with an assistive device)
        Vestibular rehabilitation and habituation training
    Initiate exercise program
        Tai chi
        Resistive (strength) training
        Other balance training
Extrinsic
    Reduce environmental hazards
    Reduce active restraints
    Improve fall surveillance
        Identify those at risk
        Increase staff proximity and ratio
        Improve motion detection
    Decrease or dissipate impact force
        Protective pads and flooring

A multifactorial approach seems most appropriate, individualizing a combination of medical, rehabilitative, environmental, and intervention strategies for each faller or potential faller (11). In a multifactorial approach (36) for nonsyncopal falls, in-home interventions were performed in community-dwelling older adults with at least one of the following risk factors: postural hypotension, use of benzodiazepines or hypnotic sedatives, use of four or more prescription medications, inability to transfer safely to a bathtub or toilet, environmental hazards for falls or tripping, gait impairment, balance impairment, and arm and leg strength or range-of-motion impairment. Although 47% of the controls fell during the 1-year follow-up, only 35% of the intervention group fell (36). Reductions in postural blood pressure changes (and medication use) and in balance, gait, and transfer problems contributed the most to reducing falls (38). The intervention group had a lower incidence of injurious falls and hospitalizations, but the difference did not reach statistical significance. However, given the financial costs of the injuries and medical care required, average costs for the controls exceeded that of those in the intervention group (27). A bidisciplinary intervention (medical and single occupational therapy home visit) also showed a reduction in falls (odds ratio = 0.39 vs. controls) in community-dwelling emergency room patients seen for nonsyncopal and syncopal falls (7). A randomized trial of a fall reduction consultation service used in 14 nursing homes showed a decline in the proportion of recurrent fallers

(44% in intervention homes vs. 54% in control homes) and a trend toward a lower incidence of injurious falls (26). The consultation service made a series of recommendations according to domains (in order of most to least commonly recommended) related to wheelchairs, the environment, transferring and ambulation, and psychotropic medication use.

Other controlled studies provide more caveats about the effect of interventions on fall reduction. No fall prevention study has had sufficient power to show a reduction in serious fall injuries, such as hip fracture (13), although a reduction in hip fracture was recently noted with the use of hip pads (see above). Some studies demonstrate no change in falls, but because of the multidisciplinary evaluation, other comorbid conditions are identified that might lead to improved overall health and decreased hospitalizations (31). Some studies suggest that environmental hazards relate poorly to fall occurrence (32), and even home modification interventions may reduce falls by mechanisms unrelated to the modifications themselves (8,14). Also of note is the success of fall reduction with the withdrawal of psychotropic medications (66% reduction in falls); however, by 1 month following study completion, 47% of patients had restarted their psychotropic medications (5). Studies that focus on low-intensity exercise or behavioral interventions find small and transient, if any, effects on fall reduction, with the greatest effects in targeted high-risk groups who are given individually tailored exercise programs (11). A recent meta-analysis of seven independent, randomized clinical studies suggests that intervention programs that include exercise and balance training, in particular, can reduce falls by 10% (25). Moreover, one recent controlled study found that a 15-week program of tai chi reduced the risk of falls by 48% (46).

GAIT DISORDERS

Even if a diagnosable condition is found on evaluation, many conditions causing a gait disorder, at best, are only partially treatable [for a more extensive review of the following studies, see Alexander (2)]. The patient is often left with at least some residual disability. However, other functional outcomes (e.g., reduction in weight-bearing pain) can be equally important in justifying treatment. Achievement of premorbid gait patterns may be unrealistic, and improvement in measures such as gait speed is reasonable as long as gait remains safe. Comorbidity, disease severity, and overall health status tend to strongly influence treatment outcome.

Many of the reports dealing with treatment and rehabilitation of gait disorders in older adults are retrospective chart reviews and case studies. Gait disorders, presumably secondary to vitamin B_{12} deficiency, folate deficiency, hypothyroidism, hyperthyroidism, knee osteoarthritis, Parkinson's disease, and inflammatory polyneuropathy show improvement in ambulation as a result of medical therapy. A variety of modes of physical therapy for diseases such as Parkinson's disease, knee osteoarthritis, and stroke also result in modest improvements but continued residual disability. Recent studies suggest that the use of a special apparatus and techniques for gait rehabilitation of patients with specific diseases and impairments (e.g., body weight support and a treadmill) enhances post-stroke gait retraining (44).

Modest improvement and residual disability are also the result of surgical treatment for compressive cervical myelopathy, lumbar stenosis, and NPH. Few controlled prospective studies and randomized studies address the outcome of surgical treatment for compressive cervical myelopathy, lumbar stenosis, and NPH. A number of problems plague the available series: outcomes (e.g., pain and walking disability) are not reported separately; the source of the outcome rating is not clearly identified or blinded; the criteria for classifying outcomes differ; the follow-up intervals are variable; the selection factors for conservative versus surgical treatment between studies differ or are unspecified; and publication bias exists (only positive results are published). Most of the surgical series include all ages, although the mean age is usually above 60 years. Many older adults have reduced pain and increased maximal walking distance following laminectomies and lumbar fusion surgery, although they have continued residual disability. A few studies document equivalent surgical outcomes with conservative, nonsurgical treatment. Finally, it is unclear how many of the initial postoperative gains are maintained long term, particularly in NPH.

Outcomes for hip and knee replacement surgery for osteoarthritis are better, although some of the same methodologic problems exist with these studies. Other than pain relief, sizable gains in gait speed and joint motion occur, although residual walking disability continues for a number of reasons, including residual pathology on the operated side and symptoms on the nonoperated side.

REFERENCES

1. Alexander NB. Differential diagnosis of gait disorders in older adults. *Clin Geriatr Med.* 1996;12:697–698.
2. Alexander NB. Gait disorders in older adults. *J Am Geriatr Soc.* 1996;44:434–451.
3. Allcock LM, O'Shea D. Diagnostic yield and development of a neurocardiovascular investigation unit for older adults in a district hospital. *J Gerontol.* 2000;55A:M458–M462.
4. Camicoli R, Moore MM, Sexton G, et al. Age-related changes associated with motor function in healthy older people. *J Am Geriatr Soc.* 1999;47:330–334.
5. Campbell AJ, Robertson MC, Gardner MM, et al. Psychotropic medication withdrawal and a home-based exercise program to prevent falls: a randomized controlled trial. *J Am Geriatr Soc.* 1999;47:850–853.
6. Capezuti E, Strumpf NE, Evans LK, et al. The relationship between physical restraint removal and falls and injuries among nursing home residents. *J Gerontol.* 1998;3A:M47–M52.
7. Close J, Ellis M, Hooper R, et al. Prevention of falls in the elderly (PROFET): a randomized controlled trial. *Lancet.* 1999;353:93–97.
8. Cumming RG, Thomas M, Szonyi G, et al. Home visits by occupational therapists for assessment and modification of environmental hazards: a randomized trial of falls prevention. *J Am Geriatr Soc.* 1999;47:1397–1402.
9. Cummings SR, Nevitt MC. A hypothesis: the causes of hip fractures. *J Gerontol.* 1989;44:M107–M111.
10. Elble RJ, Hughes L, Higgins C. The syndrome of senile gait. *J Neurol.* 1992;239:71–75.
11. Feder G, Cryer C, Donovan S, et al. Guidelines for the prevention of falls in people over 65. *BMJ.* 2000;321:1007–1011.
12. Fuh JL, Lin KN, Wang SJ, et al. Neurologic diseases presenting with gait impairment in the elderly. *J Geriatr Psychiatry Neurol.* 1994;7:89–92.
13. Gardner MM, Robertson MC, Campbell AJ. Exercise in preventing falls and fall related injuries in older people: a review of randomized controlled trials. *Br J Sports Med.* 2000;34:7–17.
14. Gill TM. Preventing falls: to modify the environment or the individual? *J Am Geriatr Soc.* 1999;47:1471–1472.
15. Greenspan SL, Myers ER, Maitland LA, et al. Fall severity and bone mineral density as risk factors for hip fracture in ambulatory elderly. *JAMA.* 1994;271:128–133.
16. Holden MK, Gill KM, Magliozzi MR. Gait assessment for neurologically impaired patients: standards for outcome assessment. *Phys Ther.* 1986;66:1530–1539.
17. Hough JC, McHenry MP, Kammer LM. Gait disorders in the elderly. *Am Fam Pract.* 1987;30:191–196.
18. Kannus P, Parkkari J, Niemi S, et al. Prevention of hip fracture in elderly people with use of a hip protector. *N Engl J Med.* 2000;343:1506–1513.
19. King MB, Tinetti ME. Falls in community-dwelling older persons. *J Am Geriatr Soc.* 1995;43:1146–1154.

20. Koller WC, Wilson RS, Glatt SL, et al. Senile gait: correlation with computed tomographic scans. *Ann Neurol*. 1983;13:343–344.

21. Means KM, Rodell DE, O'Sullivan PS, et al. Comparison of a functional obstacle course with an index of clinical gait and balance and postural sway. *J Gerontol*. 1998;53A:M331–M335.

22. Nutt JG, Marsden CD, Thompson PD. Human walking and higher-level gait disorders, particularly in the elderly. *Neurology*. 1993;43:268–279.

23. Oschiega Y, Harris TB, Hirsch R, et al. The prevalence of functional limitations and disability in older persons in the US: data from the National Health and Nutrition Examination survey III. *J Am Geriatr Soc*. 2000;48:1132–1135.

24. Posiadlo D, Richardson S. The timed "Up & Go": a test of basic functional mobility for frail elderly persons. *J Am Geriatr Soc*. 1991;39:142–148.

25. Province MA, Hadley EC, Hornbrook MC, et al. The effects of exercise on falls in elderly persons: a population-based randomized trial. *JAMA*. 1995;273:1341–1347.

26. Ray WA, Taylor JA, Meador KG, et al. A randomized trial of a consultation service to reduce falls in nursing homes. *JAMA*. 1997;278:557–562.

27. Rizzo JA, Baker DI, McAvay G, et al. The cost-effectiveness of a multifactorial targeted prevention program for falls among community elderly persons. *Med Care*. 1996;34:954–969.

28. Rockwood K, Awalt E, Carver D, et al. Feasibility and measurement properties of the functional reach and timed up and go tests in the Canadian Study of Health and Aging. *J Gerontol*. 2000;55A:M70–M73.

29. Rossiter-Fornoff JE, Wolf SL, Wolfson LI, et al. A cross-validation study of the FICSIT common data base static balance measures. *J Gerontol*. 1995;50A:M291–M297.

30. Rubinstein LZ, Josephson KR, Robins AS. Falls in the nursing home. *Ann Intern Med*. 1994;121:442–451.

31. Rubinstein LZ, Ribbins A, Josephson K, et al. The value of assessing falls in the elderly population: a randomized clinical trial. *Ann Intern Med*. 1990;113:308–316.

32. Sattin RW, Rodriguez JG, DeVito CA, et al. Home environmental hazards and the risk of falling injury events among community-dwelling older persons. *J Am Geriatr Soc*. 1998;46:669–676.

33. Shumway-Cook A, Woollacott MH. Assessment and treatment of the patient with mobility disorders. In: *Motor control: theory and practical applications*. 1st ed. Baltimore: Williams & Wilkins; 1995.

34. Sudarsky L, Rontal M. Gait disorders among elderly patients: a survey study of 50 patients. *Arch Neurol*. 1983;40:740–743.

35. Tinetti ME. Performance-oriented assessment of mobility problems in elderly patients. *J Am Geriatr Soc*. 1986;34:119–126.

36. Tinetti ME, Baker DI, McAvay G, et al. A multifactorial intervention to reduce the risk of falling among elderly people living in the community. *N Engl J Med*. 1994;331:821–827.

37. Tinetti ME, Douchette JT, Claus EB. The contribution of predisposing and situational risk factors to serious fall injuries. *J Am Geriatr Soc*. 1995;43:1207–1213.

38. Tinetti ME, McAvay G, Claus E. Does multiple risk factor reduction explain the reduction in fall rate in the Yale FICSIT trial? *Am J Epidemiol*. 1996;144:389–399.

39. Tinetti ME, Speechley M, Ginter SF. Risk factors for falls among elderly persons living in the community. *N Engl J Med*. 1988;319:1701–1707.

40. Tinetti ME, Williams CS. Falls, injuries due to falls, and the risk of admission to a nursing home. *N Engl J Med*. 1997;337:1279–1284.

41. Tinetti ME, Williams CS. The effect of falls and fall injuries on functioning in community-dwelling older persons. *J Gerontol*. 1998;53A:M112–M119.

42. Van Swearingen JM, Paschall KA, Bonino P, et al. Assessing recurrent fall risk of community-dwelling frail older veterans using specific tests of mobility and the physical performance test of function. *J Gerontol*. 1998;53A:M457–M464.

43. Vellas BJ, Wayne SJ, Romero L, et al. One-leg balance is an important predictor of injurious falls in older persons. *J Am Geriatr Soc*. 1997;45:735–738.

44. Visintin M, Barbeau H, Korner-Bitensky N, et al. A new approach to retrain gait in stroke patients through body weight support and treadmill stimulation. *Stroke*. 1998;29:1122–1128.

45. Ward CR, McIntosh S, Kenny RA. Carotid sinus hypersensitivity—a modifiable risk factor for fractured neck of the femur. *Age Ageing*. 1999;28:127–133.

46. Wolf SL, Barnhart HX, Kutner NG, et al. Reducing frailty and falls in older persons: an investigation of tai chi and computerized balance training. *J Am Geriatr Soc*. 1996;44:489–497.

47. Wolf SL, Catlin PA, Gage K, et al. Establishing the reliability and validity of measurements of walking time using the Emory Functional Ambulation Profile. *Phys Ther*. 1999;79:1122–1133.

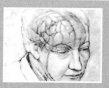

CHAPTER 9.2

Interventions for Preventing and Treating Falls

Stacie Segebart

Falls are the leading cause of injury death among persons aged 65 years and older. Between 30% and 40% of community-dwelling adults fall each year (4). Fall-related death rates and hip fracture hospitalizations have been increasing over the years (13).

This chapter covers a generalized approach of physical therapy evaluation and intervention for prevention and management of falls. Therapeutic intervention is based on various components of a comprehensive evaluation. A systems model will be discussed in a broad spectrum that will help to drive treatment focus and intervention with each individual's presentation. Common clinical tests of impairments and function will be overviewed along with computerized dynamic posturography.

EVALUATION

Effective patient management requires a multidisciplinary approach that focuses on pathology, impairments, and resultant functional limitations. The therapy evaluation is pertinent in driving the choice of therapy intervention.

As seen in Figure 9-1, there are multiple variables that have an effect on a person's balance. Problems within any of these components can result in a loss of balance and falls. Therefore, a comprehensive evaluation that considers all of these systems is critical when setting up a treatment regimen to establish optimal balance rehabilitation and fall prevention (6).

The muscular contractile component, along with joint mobility, refers to sequencing, scaling, and timing of muscular contractions and plays a role in body position and movement, as well as posture and alignment during standing and sitting.

Balance involves the interaction between three sensory systems: visual, vestibular, and somatosensory. Visual input relays information about our environment and our body location. It measures head and eye position relative to the surroundings. Information relating to movement of our body and joints is provided by the somatosensory system. It associates our body location in relationship with our support surface and gravity. The vestibular system measures the head position relative to our self and gravity.

Age-related changes affect the sensory systems and motor components, which coincide with issues involving balance (2). In order to maintain postural stability, the sensory system needs to effectively detect movement, while the motor systems strategize to move the center of mass. Attention to the organization and processing of these senses is also compromised by age-associated changes. Our environment constantly challenges us as individuals. Although hearing plays a minor role in fall prevention, it should also be considered during treatment intervention because an individual may react to a loud noise by turning their head and causing them to react to a weight shift and vestibulo-ocular response requirements.

Various movement strategies, such as the ankle strategy, hip strategy, and stepping response, are used for postural control during an external perturbation. These strategies are based on the size of the perturbation and the size of the support surface. For example, the ankle strategy is used in situations of small perturbation, whereas the hip strategy is used during larger perturbations. The stepping response occurs when the movement of the center of mass moves outside the base of support. Due to the importance of each response in preventing falls, therapy intervention should focus on developing the ability to use the appropriate strategy at the right time in both static and dynamic situations.

The cognitive status of a patient will also determine the success of balance management for several reasons. First, one must determine whether the patient is able to learn and adapt to various environmental situations. Second, the patient will also need to be capable of integrating the various strategies in an environmental challenge. Therefore, greater understanding of the cognitive capacity and attention span of the patient will help to strategize your therapy intervention.

The patient's overall health status will make a difference in treatment approach as well. Cardiovascular changes as a result of aging or pathology could result in lowered aerobic capacity, decreased exercise tolerance, or orthostatic hypotension. Questioning the individual about their activity levels can help to drive the treatment and length of intervention. The 6-minute walk test, which measures the distance an

Figure 9-1. Systems Model. Adapted from Shumway-Cook A, Woollacott MH. *Motor Control: Theory and Practical Applications*. Baltimore: Williams & Wilkins, 1995:121; and Neurocom International, Inc. *Clinical Integration Seminar*. Clackamas, OR: Neurocom International; 2005–2006:5.

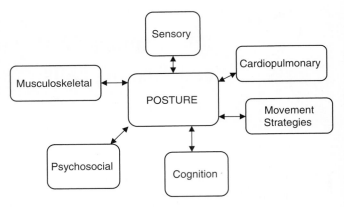

individual walks in 6 minutes, is a tool used in therapy to help document a patient's overall functional endurance during ambulation.

The psychological status of a patient is another critical variable in determining outcome of therapy. Depression can have a direct and indirect impact. It can affect postural control. Abnormal extensor muscle tone may limit the patient's ability for good postural control and alignment. The patient's motivation can also limit the treatment avenues and functional outcomes.

Patients are not always ready to accept certain safety measures, or they can become resistant to using an assistive device. If a patient has a positively skewed sense of self-efficacy, he or she may feel that a device is not necessary. In contrast, a patient's fear of falling can be great enough to result in avoidance of situations considered to be risky.

The treatment of these challenging patients is approached in numerous ways depending upon the individual. At times, the objectivity of a functional test may be proof enough to the patient that they are at risk of falling. To help objectively measure a person's fear of falling, several scales have been developed. The Falls Efficacy Scale (FES) has been developed for measuring fear of falling (14). Also correlated with the FES test is the Activities-Specific Balance Confidence (ABC) scale, which is administered to the patient addressing any fears of falling that impact life's activities. The ABC test has a wider continuum of activity difficulty in regard to activities of daily living (8). The Dizziness Handicap Inventory (DHI) is a multidimensional self-assessment tool that addresses the emotional, functional, and physical aspects that quantify the level of disability and handicap of a patient. The test measures the self-perceived impact that imbalance or dizziness has on the quality of life and psychosocial well-being of the patient (3). In the evaluation process, detection of individuals at risk for falls is an important concept that should be used in any health care setting.

Having a simplified systematic tool for detection of fall prevention should be integrated into the therapy evaluation process. At the beginning of therapy, the patient should be asked to complete a generalized form, and then the questions can be discussed in the subjective format of the therapy evaluation. Questions should be concise and include the various risk factors of falling so that treatment intervention can be targeted specifically for home safety and modifications can be made to prevent falls (9).

FUNCTIONAL TESTS

Functional testing helps to summarize the nature of a balance problem and provides objectivity in an evaluation. The results help physical therapists to direct treatment and focus on objective goal setting. Table 9-6 lists the most commonly used functional balance tests.

The Balance Evaluation Systems Test (BESTest) is a comprehensive tool that is divided into six sections: Biomechanical Constraints, Stability Limits/Verticality, Transitions/Anticipatory, Reactive, Sensory Orientation, and Stability in Gait. The test was designed by Fay Horak to identify principal issues of a patient's balance problem.

The Timed Up and Go (TUG) is a quick testing tool to implement in the clinic. For this measure, the subject stands up from a standard chair and walks 3 m, turns around, and then returns to sitting while being timed. This test has been shown to be a sensitive and specific measure for identifying community-dwelling

Table 9-6. *Common Functional Balance Tests*

Balance Evaluation Systems Test (BESTest)
Timed Up and Go (TUG)
Functional Reach Test (FRT)
Berg Balance Scale (BBS)
Dynamic Gait Index (DGI)
Functional Gait Assessment (FGA)

Table 9-7. *Predictive Results of Timed Up and Go Test*

Seconds	Rating
<10	Freely mobile
<20	Mostly independent
20–29	Variable mobility
>30	Impaired mobility

Adapted from Podsiadlo D, Richardson S. The timed "Up & Go": a test of basic functional mobility for frail elderly persons. *J Am Geriatr Soc.* 1991;39:142–148.

adults who are at risk for falls (11). Scoring is represented in Table 9-7.

The Functional Reach Test (FRT) is another simple and inexpensive task to administer and demonstrates correlation with postural control (5). This test was first administered for anterior and posterior dynamic stability; however, it may be adapted to perform a lateral reaching task. The test is administered by having the patient reach forward with feet shoulder distance apart and arms raised at 90 degrees of flexion. The individual then reaches as far forward as possible while maintaining balance, and the length of reach is measured. The functional reach norms are presented in Table 9-8.

The Berg Balance Scale (BBS) is predominantly a static balance test used in the older adult population. The test tends to be more beneficial when administered to lower to mid-functioning adults secondary to its artificial ceiling effect. It is based on 14 tasks that the patient performs. The items include ability to sit, stand, lean, and turn and upright posture on one leg (1,2). The score is then calculated, and patients are categorized into one of three levels for risk of falls. See Table 9-9 for a calculation of percent probability of falling based on the BBS (10).

The Dynamic Gait Index (DGI) is a test that measures eight components of functional balance. The test evaluates the patient's ability to modify gait in response to changing task demands (12). It is used to determine the likelihood of falling in the older adult and has been validated for use in the vestibular-impaired individual (15). Another test that is based on

Table 9-8. *Functional Reach Norms*

Norms	Men (inches)	Women (inches)
20–40 yrs	16.7	14.6
41–69 yrs	14.9	13.8
70–87 yrs	13.2	10.5

Adapted from Duncan PW, Weiner DK, Chandler J, et al. Functional reach: a new clinical measure of balance. *J Gerontol.* 1990;45:M192–M197.

the DGI is known as Functional Gait Assessment (FGA). This is comprised of 10 tasks of variations of gait speed, surface, visual variance, and steps (15).

The choice of which assessment tool to use will be based on your clinical assessment and functional independence of the patient. A combination of assessment tools may be the best choice for your patient because each test has a certain aspect of focus.

COMPUTERIZED DYNAMIC POSTUROGRAPHY

Computerized dynamic posturography (CDP) was developed by Neurocom and uses a computerized force plate system to objectively quantify and assess the possible sensory, motor, and central adaptive impairments that may affect balance control (7). Table 9-10 lists the various impairment and functional tests. The objective measures obtained through the use of CDP, sway, and postural reactions help to quantify the effectiveness of therapeutic interventions.

The dynamic control of the center of gravity can be regulated by reflexes, automatic or anticipatory postural responses, or voluntary movements. The motor impairment tests help to differentiate between these balance lines of defense, as signified in Table 9-10.

The generation of a motor response is reflective of the environmental situation along with the patient's experience of the condition. The motor control test (MCT) consists of a platform translating forward and backward at three different amplitudes while measuring the timing, direction, and strength of the patient's motor response. This activity relates information about the patient's automatic motor system and the efficiency, latency, and symmetry of muscular response to the external stimuli.

Adaptive motor responses are measured using the adaptation test (ADT). This test measures the patient's ability to minimize sway during five sequenced inclinations of toes up and down. The interpretation of the ADT can indicate musculoskeletal limitations (e.g., ankle mobility) or inadequate muscle strength or timing. Fear of falling can also be demonstrated on this test.

Limits of stability (LOS) represent voluntary motor control as a patient performs timed weight shifting in a targeted conelike fashion. This test provides information pertaining to movement timing and control, limits of perceived and actual stability, and reaction times. This information can help to guide focus on appropriate treatment management.

Rhythmic weight shifting (RWS) tests the patient's ability to weight shift in the sagittal and frontal plane at three different paces using a visual target. RWS correlates information in the nature of speed, timing,

Table 9-9. *Percent Probability of Falling Based on Berg Balance Score (BBS) and Fall History*

Berg Score	No Falls in the Last 6 Months (%)	One Fall in the Last 6 Months (%)
56	3	23
55	4	28
54	5	33
53	6	39
52	7	45
51	9	51
50	12	60
49	14	63
48	18	69
47	22	74
46	26	78
45	31	82
44	37	86
43	43	88
42	49	91
41	55	93
40	61	94
39	67	95
38	72	96
37	77	97
36	80	98
35	85	99
34	88	99
33	90	99

BBS: 0 to 20 = high risk for falling; 21 to 40 = medium risk for falling; and 41 to 56 = low risk for falling.
Calculated by Diane Wrisley, PhD, PT, NCS from equation in Shumway-Cook A, Baldwin M, Polissar NL, et al. Predicting the probability for falls in community dwelling older adults. *Phys Ther.* 1997;77:812–819. As outlined in Herdman 2003.

amplitude, and directional control including the patient's ability to reverse direction.

Weight-bearing squat (WBS) measures the lower extremity symmetry while performing a squat at 0, 30, 60, and 90 degrees. These findings can drive treatment intervention for strength, pain management, postural alignment, or further sensory testing.

The unilateral stance (US) test indicates whether there is a biomechanical dysfunction or somatosensory involvement. During US, three trials of single-leg stance are performed with eyes open and eyes closed.

Sensory and motor impairments lead to a level of functional limitation. The functional tests from the Neurocom system, as listed in Table 9-10, are other options to use to quantify patient dysfunction and for treatment intervention.

INTERVENTION

Specific therapeutic interventions for fall prevention are dependent on an individual patient's needs and presentation. Assessment of the overall patient's dysfunction gathered from the evaluation and functional measures is the key component in driving a successful intervention. A thorough evaluation can help to focus therapy on the underlying causes of a balance dysfunction.

Some patients do return to therapy for further intervention for the same diagnosis. Diagnosis can be looked at as stages beginning to end. Intervention and treatment choice should be based on the patient's best interest in regard to safety and promoting functional independence.

Conventional methods are not always the answer, and creativity does play into the art of therapy as we strive for positive outcomes for our patients. Some patients have limitations that do not coincide with their expectations. Listen to the patient's goals, but remain realistic; consider those impairments that are permanent, and focus on those that are more adaptable. Compensatory strategies for balance may be employed in certain patient cases.

Table 9-10. *Computerized Dynamic Posturography*

Sensory Impairment Tests
  Modified Clinical Test of Sensory
    Interaction on Balance (mCTSIB)
  Sensory Organization Test (SOT)
Motor Impairment Tests
  Voluntary Motor
    Limits of Stability (LOS)
    Rhythmic Weight Shift (RWS)
    Weight-Bearing Squat (WBS)
    Unilateral Stance (US)
  Adaptive and Automatic Motor
    Adaptation Test (ADT)
    Motor Control Test (MCT)
Functional Limitation Tests
  Sit to Stand (STS)
  Walk Across (WA)
  Tandem Walk (TW)
  Step Quick Turn (SQT)
  Step Up and Over (SUO)
  Forward Lunge (FL)

Each balance program will be specific to the individual because the impairments and functional limitations can vary in presentation from patient to patient. The uniqueness of the therapy program will be based on the various factors touched on from the systems model and from a multifactorial medical history and environmental screening. A multifactorial intervention will include therapy intervention addressing exercise programs, balance and gait training, modification and education on environmental hazards (e.g., flooring, footwear, and lighting) and home safety, medical management and modification of medications, and treatment and management of systemic processes such as hypotension (9).

SUMMARY

Therapy intervention needs to be a multidisciplinary and integrated approach for the optimal management of balance in elderly patients. There is no set program. Each case needs to be individually evaluated, and treatment plans need to be formulated according to the medical, psychological, cognitive, and environmental needs of each patient. Creative approaches to patient care are more successful than the most basic of balance programs when appropriate. A complex and interactive treatment intervention can help to challenge and strengthen the multifaceted balance system.

REFERENCES

1. Berg K. Balance and its measure in the elderly: a review. *Physiother Can.* 1989;41:240–246.
2. Berg K, Wood-Dauphinee SL, Williams JI, et al. Measuring balance in the elderly: preliminary development of an instrument. *Physiother Can.* 1989;41:304–311.
3. Cattaneo D, Regola A, Meotti M. Validity of six balance disorders scales in persons with multiple sclerosis. *Disabil Rehabil.* 2006;28:789–795.
4. Centers for Disease Control and Prevention. Web-Based Injury Statistics Query and Reporting System (WISQARS). National Center for Injury Prevention and Control, Centers for Disease Control and Prevention. 2001. Available at http://www.cdc.gov/ncipc/wisqars/.
5. Duncan PW, Weiner DK, Chandler J, et al. Functional reach: a new clinical measure of balance. *J Gerontol.* 1990;45:M192–M197.
6. Horak FB. Postural orientation and equilibrium: what do we need to know about neural control of balance to prevent falls? *Age Ageing.* 2006;35: ii7–ii11.
7. Neurocom International, Inc. Computerized Dynamic Posturography. 2007. Available at http://onbalance.com/program/role/cdp/index.aspx.
8. Powell LE, Myers AM. The activities-specific balance confidence (ABC) scale. *J Gerontol A Biol Sci Med Sci.* 1995;50A:M28–M34.
9. Rao SS. Prevention of falls in older patients. *Am Fam Physician.* 2005;72:81–88.
10. Shumway-Cook A, Baldwin M, Polissar NL, et al. Predicting the probability for falls in community dwelling older adults. *Phys Ther.* 1997;77:812–819.
11. Shumway-Cook A, Brauer S, Woollacott M. Predicting the probability for falls in community-dwelling older adults using the timed Up & Go Test. *Phys Ther.* 2000;80:896–903.
12. Shumway-Cook A, Woollacott MH. *Motor Control: Theory and Practical Applications.* Baltimore: Williams & Wilkins; 1995.
13. Stevens JA, Hasbrouck L, Durant TM, et al. Surveillance for injuries and violence among older adults. *MMWR CDC Surveill Summ.* 1999;48:27–50.
14. Tinetti ME, Powell L. Fear of falling and low self-efficacy: a cause of dependence in elderly persons. *J Gerontol.* 1993;48:35–38.
15. Wrisley DM, Marchetti GF, Kuharsky DK, et al. Reliability, internal consistency, and validity of data obtained with the functional gait assessment. *Phys Ther.* 2004;84:906–918.

CHAPTER 10

Acquired Disorders of Swallowing, Cognition, Speech, and Language in the Older Adult

Karen T. McNett and Alice P. Armbruster

It is the coalescence of remediation and compensation along with providing counseling, education, and information that comprises treatment for acquired dysphagia, cognitive-linguistic, speech, and/or language impairment. The effectiveness of treatment is dependent upon accurate diagnosis. Therefore, this chapter will discuss and provide an overview of various diagnostic and treatment approaches used by the medical speech-language pathologist for acquired disorders of swallowing, cognition, speech, and language in the older adult.

Accurate diagnosis is dependent upon the education, knowledge, and experience of the clinician, use of appropriate diagnostic tools that are valid and reliable, an understanding of normal versus abnormal, and knowledge of the differences between "normal limits" and "functional limits." Furthermore, delineating strengths and weaknesses in a hierarchical fashion is helpful in developing a plan of action that takes into consideration the patient's desires and those of his or her family and caregivers. The ultimate objective of therapy is to return a patient to the highest level of function with the least amount of support possible.

Obtaining objective and standardized data will help delineate specific deficits relative to an individual's peer group by determining any deviance from the mean and ranking the severity of that deviance. Consideration must be given to the patient's baseline normal and whether that deviated from peers. Evaluation of how deficits impact function to determine whether the deficits lead to impairment for the individual is also essential. Finally, it is a healthy fear, or respect, for the impact of labels that should provide a cautionary guide in the analysis and interpretation stages of diagnosis, particularly as it relates to cognitive-linguistic deficits and disorders.

There has been increasing interest in and focus on evidence-based practice (EBP) in the field of Speech-Language Pathology (SLP) over recent years. EBP is a diagnostic and treatment process in which the clinician uses the best evidence available in conjunction with clinical expertise and the patient's values to decide on the options that suit the patient best (2). EBP guidelines have been developed by the Academy of Neurologic Communication Disorders and Sciences (ANCDS) in collaboration with the American Speech Language Hearing Association and the US Department of Veterans Affairs. There has been criticism within the scientific process that few, if any, high-powered, randomized, controlled trials support the efficacy of speech therapy. Some argue that a randomized controlled trial does not lend itself well to the unique and individual variances that comprise each patient's deficits within the clinical environment, particularly a heterogeneous population such as those with acquired brain injury. While the research and debate continue, there are fundamental methods, approaches, and techniques supported in the literature.

The process of evaluation and diagnosis begins with obtaining a thorough review of the patient's history and physical information and a consult with the patient's family and/or caregivers. If the client is an inpatient in the hospital, the SLP will communicate with the patient's nurse to determine whether the patient is able to proceed with an evaluation.

Most often in the medical setting, the first and foremost reason to consult a SLP is to determine a patient's ability to engage in safe oral intake; the risk for aspiration with oral intake; the ability to maintain nutrition and hydration via safe oral intake; the need for an alternate source to provide nutrition, hydration, and medication; and a prognosis of whether that required alternate source will be temporary or long term.

THE ORAL MOTOR EXAMINATION

The oral motor examination (OME) is an assessment of structure and function. The SLP will assess oral structure, mucosa, and cranial nerve function because they impact speech and swallowing and because they may signal neuropathology. Respiration, resonance, and articulation will be assessed at rest, during structured tasks, and dynamically in open context conversation. First, the SLP will assess facial symmetry both at rest and upon movement. Next, labial closure, rounding, and retraction will be tested. The tongue will be examined for lingual extension, and any deviation or

Table 10-1. *Sustained Phonation Maximum in Seconds for the Vowel /ah/*

	Median	Minimum	Maximum
Young males	28.5 (8.4)	22.6 (5.5)	34.6 (11.4)
Young females	22.7 (5.7)	15.2 (4.1)	26.5 (11.3)
Elderly males	13.8 (6.3)	13.0 (5.9)	18.1 (6.6)
Elderly females	14.4 (5.7)	10.0 (5.6)	15.4 (5.8)
AMRs and SMRs for Normal Adults			
/puh/	6.3 (0.7)	5.0 (0.4)	7.1 (1.2)
/tuh/	6.2 (0.8)	4.8 (0.4)	7.1 (1.1)
/kuh/	5.8 (0.8)	4.4 (0.6)	6.4 (1.1)
/puh-tuh-kuh/	5.0 (0.7)	3.6 (0.3)	7.5 (1.3)

Derived from Duffy J. *Motor Speech Disorders: Substrates, Differential Diagnosis, and Management.* St. Louis: Mosby; 1995.

fasciculations are noted; the tongue will also be examined for lateralization, atrophy, and strength against applied pressure. Speech alternating motion rates (AMRs) and sequential motion rates (SMRs) will also be evaluated. The hard and soft palates will be examined, noting any deformity and any deviation from complete, full, and strong retraction upon phonation. Vocal quality will be perceptually rated for vocal frequency, intensity, quality, and resonance (Table 10-1). Particular attention will be paid to the coordination of the articulatory, resonatory, and respiratory systems as they relate to speech, swallowing, and communicative ability.

It is a complete and thorough OME that belies evaluation of dysarthria, oral or verbal apraxia, dysphagia, cognitive-communicative disorder, and aphasia. Any deviation from that which is considered within functional limits will be noted. Any deviation from that which is considered within normal limits will trigger further evaluation. For example, the OME of an individual who is edentulous and has no dentures is certainly not within "normal" limits; however, it may well be within "functional" limits. This individual may have been edentulous and eating a regular-consistency diet for many years with no difficulty. Another example may be an individual who underwent partial glossectomy secondary to cancer several years earlier, who has been eating a regular-consistency diet without difficulty. The key piece of information is whether the deviance from "normal" impacts safe and efficient oral intake and efficient and effective speech or communication.

ACQUIRED NEUROMUSCULAR SPEECH DISORDERS

Neuromuscular speech disorders include dysarthria and apraxia, two distinctly different disorders. Dysarthria refers to a speech disorder that results from a disturbance in muscular control over the speech mechanism due to damage of the central or peripheral nervous system, resulting in paralysis, weakness, or incoordination of the speech mechanism and leading to difficulty with oral communication (7). Dysarthria, in its most severe form, is characterized by anarthria (failure of structures to articulate).

The terms oral apraxia and verbal apraxia refer to a disorder of motor sequencing that is present in the absence of neuromuscular weakness. Severe oral and verbal apraxia is characterized by effortful articulatory groping to produce speech sounds; however, in its mild form, it may merely present as phonemic substitutions during open context conversation.

DYSARTHRIA ASSESSMENT

The diagnosis of dysarthria is based upon complete assessment of five characteristics: respiration, phonation, resonance, articulation, and prosody (Table 10-2). Standardized articulation protocols are more commonly used with children to determine whether the child is exhibiting a disorder of articulation or phonologic processes. This is not the case in the adult population. The Frenchay Dysarthria Assessment (11) is one commonly used protocol in the adult population. The Assessment of Intelligibility of Dysarthric Speech (AIDS) (29) is another.

While there are a few standardized articulation protocols that may be used with adults, they are infrequently used in deference to a "speech sample" that is both tape recorded and transcribed and possibly videotaped in order to provide the patient with visual feedback of his or her own communication skills. As mentioned earlier, the combination of speech AMRs and SMRs and speech intelligibility for verbal production of basic needs/wants words, phrases, sentences, and paragraph levels are assessed. The most commonly used paragraphs are presented

Table 10-2. *Differentiating the Dysarthrias*

	Lower Motor Neuron (LMN)	Upper Motor Neuron (UMN)	Unilateral Upper Motor Neuron (UUMN)	Hypokinetic	Hyperkinetic	Ataxic
Articulation	Imprecise; weak and floppy	Imprecise consonants	Imprecise; weakness on one side only—contralateral to lesion	Reduced lingual phoneme strength; increased rate	Involuntary movement; inconsistent overshooting for target consonant articulation	Inconsistent; imprecise consonants; excess and unequal stress; distorted vowels
Respiration	Breathy	Grunts at end of phrase	May be reduced capacity; may see clavicular breathing	Reduced capacity; increased rate; latency to begin exhalation	Myoclonic displacement of abdominal wall	Inconsistent
Phonation	Hypernasal	Strain-strangle; bulbar cry (sounds like a motor winding down)	Harsh	Hypophonic; monopitch; monoloud	Abnormal vowel prolongation	Pitch variation; intensity or loudness variation
Prosody	Short phrases	Slow; excess and equal stress	Slow	Rushes of short, blurred phrases	Variable rate; inappropriate silences	Staccato; inconsistent excess stress
Overall	Weakness; labial or lingual fasciculations are hallmark	Spasticity; strain-strangle vocal quality; bulbar cry is hallmark	Unilateral weakness; most amenable to voluntary control; thick-tongued sounding	Masked facies; festinating gait; rigidity; hypophonic, monopitch, monoloud vocal quality with rushes of blurred, short phrases	Involuntary movements	Discoordination; (to the untrained ear, sounds as if drunk)

This is not intended to be a comprehensive list and does not include the various mixed dysarthrias.

in Figure 10-1. Both paragraphs contain a fair sampling of all phonemes and phoneme combinations in the English language. In addition to having the patient read these passages, speech intelligibility is perceptually rated in open context conversation. Some individuals may not be able to see or read; therefore, accommodating the individual's abilities and needs is essential in order to determine the patient's baseline level and current status and assess for confirmatory signs.

DYSARTHRIA TYPES AND HALLMARK SIGNS

There are seven types of dysarthria that are dependent upon the location of the lesion (8). These are as follows:

Flaccid dysarthria is caused by a lesion in the lower motor neuron or final common pathway, resulting in weakness, paresis, paralysis, hypotonia, and atrophy. The presence of fasciculations is a confirmatory sign.

Rainbow Passage

When the sunlight strikes raindrops in the air, they act like a prism and form a rainbow. The rainbow is a division of white light into many beautiful colors. These take the shape of a long round arch, with its path high above and its two ends apparently beyond the horizon. There is, according to legend, a boiling pot of gold at one end. People look, but no one ever finds it. When a man looks for something beyond his reach, his friends say he is looking for the pot of gold at the end of the rainbow.

(Fairbanks, 1960)

Zoo Passage

Look at this book with us. It's a story about a zoo. That is where bears go. Today it's very cold out of doors, but we see a cloud overhead that's a pretty, white, fluffy shape. We hear that straw covers the floor of cages to keep the chill away; yet a deer walks through the trees with her head high. They feed seeds to birds so they're able to fly.

(Fletcher, 1972)

Figure 10-1. Phonemically balanced passages commonly used for speech sampling. © 2000 Douglas N. Honorof, Jill McCullough & Barbara Somerville. All rights reserved.

Unilateral upper motor neuron dysarthria is caused by a unilateral lesion located in the upper motor neuron. Speech intelligibility is impacted by location of weakness and compounded by discoordination. Speech will sound slurred, slow, and thick. Oral dysphagia is frequently a concomitant problem.

In *spastic dysarthria*, the lesion occurs in the upper motor neuron bilaterally and results in spastic, tight muscles. All five speech characteristics are affected. Often, short phrases are produced in a low monopitch. Resonance is hypernasal. A strain-strangled vocal cry or pseudobulbar cry is frequently seen. Hallmark signs include spasticity; weak, slow, reduced range of motion; degenerative conditions; slow and effortful articulation; appear to be speaking against resistance; fatigue; hypernasality; dysphagia; drooling; and emotional lability.

Ataxic dysarthria is typically noted when there is a cerebellar or brainstem lesion. Coordination and integration are affected. To the untrained ear, this speech disorder sounds much like "drunken speech." Excessive loudness and unequal stress are features.

Hypokinetic dysarthria typically results from a lesion in the basal ganglia. Reduced range and amplitude of movement are exhibited. Speech articulation sounds are blurred, and voice is quiet. Patients typically benefit from use of prosodic cues such as a metronome and compensatory strategies that enable improved vocal intensity.

Hyperkinetic dysarthria also occurs in a basal ganglia lesion. Excessive, uncontrollable movement, involuntary hyperkinesias, and chorea are exhibited. Vocal quality is typically hypernasal, harsh, and loud in intensity. Speech articulation is characterized by inconsistent articulatory breakdown; there is no pattern. Dyskinesias are further broken down into nine types: hyperkinesia, myoclonus, tic, chorea, ballism, athetosis, dystonia, spasm, and tremor. Hyperkinetic dysarthria is not amenable to a specific dysarthria treatment unless the underlying movement disorder is medicated. Speech therapy services are beneficial to individuals and their family or caregivers initially and for a brief duration to provide education and counseling.

Mixed dysarthria lesions are, as the name implies, mixed or diffuse. This can be seen in traumatic brain injury (TBI), closed head injury (CHI), multiple sclerosis (MS), and amyotrophic lateral sclerosis (ALS). Therapy techniques are highly individualized and based upon which component contributes most to unintelligibility.

In *anarthria*, the lesions are typically in the cortex and cerebellum. If a patient's mutism is related to a single lesion, it is likely brainstem. Patients are often speechless due to loss of neuromuscular control over the speech mechanism.

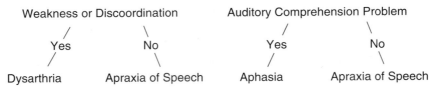

Figure 10-2. Flowchart for differentiating dysarthria from apraxia.

APRAXIA ASSESSMENT

Apraxia is an impairment in motor programming and is not due to weakness or paralysis of structures. Traditional characteristics include phonemic errors, perseverative and anticipatory misarticulations, and inconsistent articulatory approximations. Errors vary with increased complexity. For example, an individual may have little difficulty producing automatic speech phrases or overlearned passages or songs but increased difficulty for novel verbal productions. The patient will usually exhibit awareness of misarticulations and a great deal of frustration. Because of this frustration, the focus of therapy is initially generally placed on getting the message out and later on fine tuning the use of compensatory strategies such as slow rate, even stress, and even spacing between words.

APRAXIA VERSUS DYSARTHRIA

When determining whether a person has apraxia or dysarthria, the first characteristic to which attention must be paid is the patient's struggle or "articulatory groping" as speech is attempted. The SLP will have previously noted on the OME whether the patient demonstrated "articulatory groping" when attempting various oral postures upon command (e.g., grimacing when asked to open the mouth, lingual extension when asked to puff up the cheeks, squinting when asked to demonstrate pursing the lips and blowing). If no asymmetry or weakness is demonstrated on OME and no effortful struggle is apparent when performing volitional oral postures, verbal apraxia may be present. Phonemic substitutions are quite commonly exhibited in verbal apraxia, even if no effortful articulatory groping is demonstrated when volitionally producing various oral postures for the OME. For example, an individual may say "The <u>c</u>log jumped off the cliff" or "The dog jumped off the <u>d</u>iff" when asked to read "The dog jumped off the cliff." Individuals with verbal apraxia will likely exhibit difficulty repeating words of increasing length (e.g., back, backhand, backhanded; increase, increasing, increasingly). Difficulty will be exhibited for multisyllabic words. They will often report, "I know the word, I just can't say it." They may well exhibit no difficulty when reading a printed paragraph aloud and then an inordinate amount of difficulty during conversation.

Differentiating between apraxia and dysarthria is fundamental in order to initiate the correct treatment approach. Excessive repetition and practice are essential treatment techniques for verbal apraxia; whereas, they would be ineffective and inappropriate for some types of dysarthria (e.g., mixed flaccid-spastic dysarthria seen in ALS or flaccid dysarthria seen with myasthenia gravis). Figure 10-2 illustrates basic considerations for diagnostic differentiation of dysarthria and apraxia.

DYSARTHRIA TREATMENT

A very broad and basic tenet applies in the treatment of dysarthria: if it's tight, relax it; if it's weak, tighten it up. The rule in the treatment of apraxia is *repetition, repetition, repetition*. First, however, before the appropriate treatment can be identified and initiated, a thorough evaluation of the speech mechanism and its subsystems must be performed to delineate the nature and extent of any impairment. As mentioned previously, the subsystems of: respiration, phonation, articulation, resonation, and prosody must be profiled (10). Speech therapy aims to maximize effectiveness, efficiency, and naturalness of communication through restoration, compensation, and adjustment (1). Dependent upon the patient's underlying cognitive status, awareness, insight and stimulability for use of compensatory strategies awareness, and insight and ability to be stimulated for use of compensatory strategies, dysarthria treatment may be brief, while apraxia treatment may be long term. Some individuals with severe apraxia may require evaluation for and fitting with a speech-generating device.

Approaches to management of neuromuscular speech disorders include medical, pharmacologic, behavioral, and prosthetic. Again, looking at the substrates, the underlying characteristics of the dysarthria, is essential. If the patient exhibits poor respiratory support, then restoring or compensating for it will facilitate phonation for speech. If velopharyngeal insufficiency is resulting in hypernasal speech, a palatal lift may be required. If incomplete vocal fold adduction is resulting in reduced vocal intensity, perhaps pushing/pulling techniques may be beneficial to facilitate the patient's ability to achieve a Valsalva and improved vocal fold adduction for phonation and cough. Frequently, teaching the patient to control or manage phonation and articulation while coordinating these with respiration and prosody results in improved speech intelligibility. Techniques vary widely and are highly individualized.

Physiologic support for speech includes posture, strength, and coordination. Facilitating the patient's awareness of his or her speech intelligibility through feedback is essential. Providing education and information to the patient and his or her family and caregivers is essential so that they understand the underlying theory and can carry it over during activities of daily life. Enabling the patient to become responsible for self-monitoring of speech through tallying and daily record sheets is beneficial. Always providing therapeutic activities at a level just above the most advanced skill demonstrated during assessment is ideal to challenge the patient.

Efficacy of treatment, as mentioned earlier, is not well supported in the literature, primarily due to the lack of large randomized controlled studies to provide data with significant weight to demonstrate one technique over another in certain populations. However, smaller studies and case studies report success of various techniques and approaches. Most patients measure the efficacy of a given treatment technique by their improved functional skills and abilities in their daily life. Most family members and caregivers measure the efficacy of a given treatment technique by their ability to carry over or implement it in daily life. All patients, families, and caregivers measure the efficacy of given treatments by their ease of communication during activities of daily life and ability to remain engaged in social interaction.

Approaches to treatment include *speaker oriented*, where the focus is on structural support and behavioral modification, and *communication oriented*, where the focus is placed on the communication environment and involves family members and caregivers. Individualized assessment and goal setting are key to successful outcomes.

Melodic intonation therapy is a technique frequently used during treatment for apraxia and aphasia (21). The rhythm and music facilitate verbal production during an overlearned motor sequence, enabling the patient to achieve success. As skills improve, the musical and prosodic supports are faded, and the patient transitions to verbal production of novel concepts in natural settings.

Listener skills, attitudes, and experience contribute in important ways to the "range of intelligibility potentials" for speakers with severe dysarthria. Listeners must be viewed as active participants in the message construction process. Therefore, information and

training are critical. Clinical information might come in the form of comparisons of their performance with less familiar partners. Because familiar listeners may underestimate the problems that less experienced listeners encounter, such information should be provided as part of the clinical decision-making process that leads to the selection of speech supplementation strategies (17).

According to ANCDS EBP Guidelines for Dysarthria and a systematic review of speech strategies by Hanson et al. (16), compensatory speech strategies may be useful for speakers with severe or profound dysarthria, and the best candidates are those whose communication functions in natural settings have been impaired, have adequate pragmatic and cognitive skills, and have sufficient motor function to generate the cues. Selection among the various strategies must be made on an individual basis because each strategy has unique advantages and disadvantages. Additionally, communication partners play a critical role in ensuring the successful use of strategies; therefore, family and caregiver education and training should be included as an important element of intervention.

Acquired voice disorders are frequently treated by both the otorhinolaryngologist and SLP. The use of instrumentation for visualization of the vocal cords can provide objective data to guide diagnosis and treatment.

Psychogenic speech and voice disorders can be successfully managed with SLP involvement. The SLP does not attempt to treat the disorder; rather, the SLP attempts to treat the speech symptoms and facilitate the patient's ability to relearn proper techniques or behaviors. Medication and SLP therapy are a powerful therapeutic combination to aid communication.

DYSPHAGIA

The definition of dysphagia is impairment that occurs during any one of the four phases of swallowing or, quite simply, difficulty in propelling liquid or solid food from the oropharynx to the upper esophagus (9). Unlike speech, which is relatively impervious to the effects of age, swallowing, even in healthy adults, shows some decrements with time. Many of these changes are subclinical and do not constitute a disorder. It is widely acknowledged that dysphagia in the elderly can be mainly attributed to various neurologic or systemic conditions and is not a part of normal aging (27).

The four stages of swallowing are as follows: oral preparatory stage, oral stage, pharyngeal stage, and esophageal stage (23). The oral cavity, pharynx, and esophagus are three distinct anatomic regions that can function separately but, in swallowing, effectively integrate their functions through a neuronal network (24). It is important to understand normal function during each of the stages to fully understand disordered deglutition.

The act of swallowing is elicited by a combination of conscious and subconscious cues. A typical individual swallows approximately 600 times a day (350 times while awake, 200 times while eating, and about 50 times while sleeping) without giving any significant thought or effort to this activity (22).

We would be unable to state when our last saliva swallow occurred because it is reflexive. We do know, however, that drooling is not present, so we rightfully deduce that swallowing occurred.

A total of 30 paired striated muscles are used in oropharyngeal swallowing. The synchronous movement of the muscles of swallowing may be likened to the precise movement of a finely tuned instrument. It does not require much deviance to disrupt the symphony of preciseness that is critical to protection of the upper airway (26).

Neural control of swallowing consists of three major parts: (a) sensory afferent fibers contained in the cranial nerves, (b) central organizing centers, and (c) efferent motor fibers contained in the cranial nerves and ansa cervicalis (26).

The oral preparatory stage involves sensation, taste, and recognition of the constitution of the bolus of food or liquid being placed in the mouth. The oral region encompasses the anterior portal of the gastrointestinal tract and possesses the hardest articulating surfaces of the body, the dentition of the two arches (24). Food, liquid, and medications must be maintained in the oral cavity with adequate seal of the lips. An estimate of range of lip seal to cup, straw, fork, or spoon is learned by trial and error. Being fed, such as with patients with cognitive impairment, or feeding oneself affects acceptance of food and liquid. The pacing of the eating/feeding process is governed by many factors including appetite, taste preference, mood, and mentation.

The gastrointestinal system is a fairly smart system. Referred sensation of fullness or impaired motility from the distal esophagus may have an effect on the oral acceptance of food. Intact dentition that includes one's own teeth or dentures is extremely important for preparing food for eventual transit. Rotary mastication is achieved by adequate range, direction, and velocity of movement of the mandible and maxilla. Saliva moistens the oral cavity and is mixed with food to facilitate the formation of a cohesive, transportable, manageable bolus. Saliva is also important for keeping food parts from sticking to the gums, teeth, and palate. The tongue must achieve an appropriate shape to accommodate, maintain, and control the bolus, whether liquid, solid, or pill. There is

certainly a cognitive component that is required for effective pill swallowing. Adequate buccal strength is required for maintaining the bolus on the tongue. The velopharyngeal port must seal to prevent food and liquid from entering the nasal passages.

The oral stage of swallowing is initiated when the tongue begins posterior movement of the bolus and takes less than 1 to 1.5 seconds to complete (23). The convexity of the tongue maintains the bolus without premature spillage over the base of the tongue. Symmetric, sequential, peristaltic movement of the anterior two thirds of the tongue transports boluses posteriorly. The tip of the tongue makes contact with the hard palate and is achieved with results in negative pressure. The tongue base retracts and bulks, acting like a piston to propel the food, liquid, or pill bolus into the hypopharynx.

The pharyngeal stage of swallowing occurs when the bolus is sucked into the laryngopharynx by production of a zone of negative pressure (15). Closure of the velopharyngeal complex is achieved. The pharynx, although anatomically joined to the oral region, really serves as a conduit for two completely different functions: moving boluses of air to and from the lungs and transferring boluses of food and liquids from the oral cavity toward the stomach via the esophagus (24). The swallow is triggered within 1 second or less. The vocal folds adduct, and a period of apnea occurs. The larynx elevates and moves anteriorly and places itself under the base of the tongue to protect it from passing food and liquid. The epiglottis, which is attached by ligaments to the hyoid bone, inverts and covers the airway. Food, liquids, and pills move through the pharynx by peristaltic movement of the pharyngeal muscles. Aspiration is defined as the entry of food or liquid into the airway below the true cords. Penetration is defined as the entry of food or liquid into the laryngeal vestibule at some level down to but not below the true vocal cords (23). Good examples of disrupting the normal period of apnea during swallowing are laughing and talking mid-swallow with subsequent vestibular penetration or tracheal aspiration. Finally, the cricopharyngeus muscle relaxes, and the bolus enters the upper esophageal sphincter (UES).

The esophageal stage, compared to the complexity of the oral and pharyngeal stages of swallowing, consists of the simple task of transporting the bolus from the pharynx to the stomach (6). Esophageal peristalsis is initiated shortly after the bolus traverses the UES. The peristaltic contraction moves from the striated muscle of the upper portion of the esophageal body to the smooth muscle of the distal portion of the esophagus at a speed between 2 and 4 cm per sec (18).

There are five cranial nerves that contribute to swallowing and are involved in the regulation of deglutition (6):

Table 10-3. *Conditions in Which Dysphagia Is Frequently Noted*

Alzheimer/dementia	Hiatal hernia
C-P hypertrophy	Large osteophytes/DISH
Head/neck CA	Loss of appetite
Chronic aspiration	Loss of taste
Confusion (post surg/post anesthesia)	Postsurgical debilitation
COPD	Presbyesophagus
CVA	Mastication problems (ill-fitting dentures)
Debilitation, nonsurgical	Progressive neurologic diseases (Parkinson/ALS/PSP)
Effects of medication	Malnutrition (begets more malnutrition)
Disproportionate decompensation	Radiation (including latent effects)
Esophageal stricture	Surgical changes
GERD	TBI

ALS, amyotrophic lateral sclerosis; CA, cancer; COPD, chronic obstructive pulmonary disease; C-P, cricopharyngeal; CVA, cerebrovascular accident; DISH, diffuse ideopathic skeletal hyperostosis; GERD, gastroesophageal reflux disease; PSP, progressive supranuclear palsy; TBI, traumatic brain injury.

Trigeminal nerve (CN V): The major sensory nerve for the head and face and the motor nerve for the muscles of mastication.

Facial nerve (CN VII): Supplies the motor innervation to the muscles of expression and the platysma and buccinator muscles.

Glossopharyngeal nerve (CN IX): Provides sensory innervation to the pharynx and taste to the posterior third of the tongue.

Vagus nerve (CN X): Is both sensory and motor. It supplies innervation to the pharynx, larynx, and esophagus. Pharyngeal branches provide motor innervation to the levator veli palatini, the stylopharyngeus, and the constrictor muscles of the pharynx.

Hypoglossal nerve (CN XII): Supplies motor innervation to the tongue.

Dysphagia may result from a variety of etiologies and is frequently multifactorial. Some disorders in which dysphagia is commonly seen are listed in Table 10-3.

There are many signs and symptoms of dysphagia, and it is not uncommon for a patient to present with the following symptoms:

Poor appetite, anorexia, avoidance of social dining, and complaint that eating is undesirable
Anterior labial leakage of liquids, solids, or pills due to poor lip closure
Impaired mastication (dentures are improperly fitting)
Impaired lingual transit of solids, liquids, or pills
Buccal stasis
Nasal regurgitation
Excessive aerophagia
Audible swallow
Globus sensation
Repetitive swallows needed to clear bolus

Coughing or choking when eating or drinking
Food, liquid, or pills that stick in the throat area or are regurgitated
Necessity for liquid wash when eating solids
Complaint that food or liquids "go into the wrong pipe"
Unintentional weight loss
Congestion that is chronic/recurrent pneumonia
Elevated temperature
Wet/gurgly vocal quality
Chronic throat clearing related to eating/drinking

DYSPHAGIA EVALUATION

A complete clinical swallowing examination (CSE) is always performed prior to utilization of other diagnostic tests. The patient should be sufficiently alert and participative in the exam, and this is a good example of the common sense component of swallowing. It is also necessary to be able to sustain alertness to minimally meet the body's need for adequate nutrition and hydration. After the current state of mentation is established, the patient is positioned upright at 90 degrees. The CSE begins with a thorough examination of the oral mechanism. This includes testing of the cranial nerves that are involved in swallowing. Modeling may be needed for patients with cognitive impairment, aphasia, or apraxia. Assessment of ability to handle oral secretions is performed. Pooling of oral secretions and wet-sounding vocal quality are indications that the patient's swallowing may be impaired. Symmetry, strength, range, direction, and velocity of movement of the oral structures are assessed. Lingual and speech AMRs and SMRs are performed to determine whether rapid and precise movement is present. Dysarthria or oral apraxia (motor planning impairment) may be revealed. Status of cognitive/communicative skills is at the very least perfunctorily assessed.

Videofluoroscopic swallow study (VFSS) is considered to be the "gold standard" among diagnostic tools for identifying and defining disorders of the swallowing mechanism. The videofluoroscopic procedure is "your friend, your ally" for the many reasons that will be outlined. If there is debate regarding the need to perform this test on a particular patient, we should err on the side of proactivity. Recovery from elaborate surgery or cerebrovascular accident (CVA) should never be jeopardized by acquisition of preventable aspiration pneumonia. VFSS is a noninvasive test. It is relatively inexpensive and provides an excellent view of the entire deglutitive process. It takes only about 3 to 5 minutes to complete from start to finish. The radiation that the patient is subjected to is less than from a chest X-ray. It involves only eating, drinking, and pill swallowing. There are no tubes or probes introduced. You are able to view the entire swallowing mechanism and the integration of each of the four phases, including the esophageal stage.

Lip seal for maintenance of liquid and solid boluses, mastication, lingual collection, and transport of food and liquids are assessed. The most pertinent concern is presence of risk to the upper airway. Risk to the airway may be present at any one of the four levels. This is the platform to try any and all strategies that will afford a patient the opportunity to eat and drink safely. Although prescribed aspiration precautions may be analogous to the writings of Tolstoy, compensatory strategies are evidence based. A chin tuck is at times recommended to the dysphagic patient by other health professionals due to the mentality of "one size fits all." In fact, a chin tuck maneuver facilitates aspiration in some patients. The only professional who should make recommendations regarding positional changes is a speech pathologist. Frequently, the patient and family members are shown the VFSS tape so that the etiology of the dysphagia is better understood. This is particularly beneficial with "silent" aspiration, that is, aspiration that does not trigger a cough or throat clear. Videoendoscopy [fiberoptic endoscopic examination of swallowing (FEES) is another method of diagnosing dysphagia using a flexible scope. Velopharyngeal competence and pharyngeal status before and after may be assessed depending on placement of the endoscope. With FEES, unlike VFSS, there is a period of "white out" or blocking of the image when the swallow occurs due to the closure of the pharynx around the scope. It is not possible to evaluate the oral stage of the swallow using FEES. Because treatment for oropharyngeal swallowing disorders is directed largely at the motor activity during the swallow, FEES makes it difficult to define the exact nature of the patient's physiologic disorder and the effectiveness of treatment strategies (23). Additionally, activity or, in some cases, inactivity during the esophageal stage is not visualized at all.

DYSPHAGIA TREATMENT

Dysphagia treatment may include all of the following: education, strategies, exercises, surgery, and intervention from colleagues. One of the most important elements of successful swallowing rehabilitation is education. This is reiterated in this section because patients and their primary caregivers respond to treatment more effectively and enthusiastically as a result. It has been our practice to provide evidence-based research coupled with the expectation that compliance with recommendations will be forthcoming.

Compensatory strategies may include any combination of the following. These should not be confused with dysphagia exercises.

- Communication aids: facilitate a patient's ability to express nutritional wants/needs
- Liquid/solid consistency modification
- Liquid wash for residual that may be present in the oral cavity or hypopharynx
- Increasing accessibility to food or drink: snacks/containers of fluids that are within reach; utensils that ease access to food items
- Decreasing accessibility to food or drink; controlled portions
- Increasing meal frequency
- Removing distractions
- Increasing caloric intake
- Dietician's role: calorie count, ways to increase caloric intake, counseling for patient/family
- Signs/symptoms of dysphagia or aspiration (pulmonary, pneumonias, coughing, choking, loss of appetite, malnutrition, dehydration)
- Supervision or companionship during meals

In sum, eating and drinking are an integral part of our existence on many levels including sustaining life and psychosocial attachment to eating and drinking. Many of our interactions with family, friends, and colleagues involve the taking of meals. This transcends cultures and may be likened to a universal language. Globally aphasic patients can connect to their environment on a simple level when determined to be safe for beginning oral intake. As clinicians, our most difficult message is that food and liquid must be modified or even withheld in some cases. The diagnosis and treatment of dysphagia are based upon discrete, scientific, and evidence-based processes.

ALEXIA AND AGRAPHIA

Acquired agraphia (dysgraphia) is a disorder of one's ability to use graphemic symbols. The dysgraphias can be divided into two subcategories: amnemonic (central, linguistic) and atactic (peripheral, motor). The central agraphias can be further subdivided: phonologic, lexical, semantic, and deep. The peripheral agraphias can be further subdivided: apraxic, allographic, spatial, and other as in the micrographia seen in Parkinson's disease.

Acquired alexia (dyslexia) is a disorder of one's ability to comprehend written symbols. There are two main categories: alexia (or dyslexia) without agraphia and alexia (or dyslexia) with agraphia.

Alexia without agraphia (pure alexia) is associated with lesions of the left medial occipital lobe and splenium. Visual input from both occipital areas to the left angular gyrus, where written information is decoded, is lost. Perisylvian language areas are intact; therefore, writing and oral spelling are preserved (4). An individual with pure alexia or alexia without agraphia demonstrates compromised reading comprehension but normal or near-normal auditory comprehension and verbal expression. The ability to copy is usually impaired and may tend to worsen over time. Written acalculia and color anomia are often present. A right homonymous hemianopsia is almost always present, but a right hemiparesis is rare. A visual agnosia for objects and/or colors occasionally accompanies the syndrome. The patient with alexia without agraphia often is noted to read in a "letter-by-letter" fashion. Each letter of the word is named, often aloud, before the word is identified. Comprehension of words spelled aloud is usually good (21).

Acalculia refers to lost numeric calculation ability. Gerstmann syndrome is comprised of four features: finger agnosia, right-left discrimination, acalculia, and dysgraphia. It is typically seen with a left parietal lesion (21). Alexia, agraphia, and acalculia relate to one's communication skills within their environment; therefore, these deficits are typically assessed and treatment initiated by the SLP.

Regardless of the therapy activity or the treatment program, the SLP who practices EBP will use any technique or strategy supported in the literature that facilitates the patient's improved language skills and compensates for their deficits to achieve the patient's goals for improved functional communication.

COGNITIVE-COMMUNICATION DISORDERS

Aphasia can be simply defined as a loss of language skills and can be identified and profiled with a variety of approaches, including: *systems classification* which

identifies aphasia as anterior v. posterior, fluent v. nonfluent; a *unidimensional approach* which views aphasia as a general language breakdown that crosses all modalities: speaking, listening, reading, and writing (25); a *multidimensional definition* which associates function with cerebral localization of lesion. The Bostonian Classification System is such an approach and is commonly used today. A variety of aphasia treatment models exist, including: stimulation-facilitation, modality, linguistic, processing, minor hemisphere mediation, and functional communication model. Regardless, the majority of practicing speech-language pathologists use a hybrid approach referred to as "multitheoretical" (6).

In terms of actual treatment, this means that receptive and expressive language deficits will be remediated by excessive stimulation and elicited responses via a structured therapy task, using application of a hierarchical set of cues to provide effortless learning to the patient in order that the patient may realize positive feedback. For those skills that do not show remediation within a reasonable period of time, compensatory strategies will be developed unique to the patient's deficits, skills, and home environment. Counseling, education and information will be provided to the patient, the patient's family and caregivers. When improvement plateaus, a home program is typically developed and taught to the patient, patient's family and caregivers. If an augmentative communication device or speech generating device is indicated, the SLP will evaluate to determine the type of device most appropriate for the patient, "fit" the patient with the device and provide training regarding its use.

Understanding the hierarchy of cognitive-linguistic skills is required to assess their impact upon communication. Sustained attention is the foundation and is followed by the ability to divide attention and then to multitask. Working and immediate memory underlie short-term memory. As cognitive processing occurs, information is either dumped or stored, ultimately being placed in long-term memory. Organization and reasoning skills build upon attention and memory to support abstract reasoning and problem solving. The executive function skills of goal setting, planning, judgment, and self-monitoring complete the higher level cognitive skills. All of these skills underlie effective communication and independent functioning within one's environment. If there are deficits in these underlying cognitive-linguistic skills, communication will be impaired, and safety may be at risk.

The American Speech-Language-Hearing Association (ASHA) defines cognitive-communication disorder as difficulty with any aspect of communication that is affected by disruption of cognition. Communication includes listening, speaking, gesturing, reading, and writing in all domains of language (phonologic, morphologic, syntactic, semantic, and pragmatic). Cognition includes cognitive processes and systems (e.g., attention, memory, organization, executive functions). Areas of function affected by cognitive impairments include behavioral self-regulation, social interaction, activities of daily living, learning and academic performance, and vocational performance (3). Kennedy (20) defines cognitive-communicative rehabilitation after TBI as including the assessment and treatment of underlying cognitive processes as they interact and are manifest in communication behavior, broadly understood (listening, reading, writing, speaking, and gesturing), and at all levels of language (phonologic, morphologic, syntactic, semantic, and pragmatic).

RIGHT CVA (RIGHT HEMISPHERE DYSFUNCTION)

The left hemisphere of the brain is typically dominant for language; however, frequently individuals with right hemisphere lesions or diffuse neuropathology seen in CHI or TBI, encephalopathy, and/or dementia exhibit communication impairment. The SLP will administer standardized cognitive-linguistic and aphasia testing to determine what impact the underlying cognitive-linguistic deficits have on communication ability.

Individuals with right hemisphere dysfunction may exhibit communication impairment for linguistic, extralinguistic, and nonlinguistic skills. Naming and verbal fluency may be impaired. Language skills are usually intact; however, functional communication is impaired. Extralinguistic deficits appear for failing to interpret cues and organize information efficiently; there is difficulty with differentiating significant from irrelevant information. The big picture is lost to the details. Difficulty is often exhibited for integration and interpretation, inhibition of impulsive responses, and understanding figurative and implied meanings. There may also be difficulty with ability to maintain topic and a tendency to overpersonalize information, which can lead to digression and tangentiality. Problems also surface for presupposition and failing to recognize and appreciate the communication situation and the communicative partner's knowledge. Difficulty for recognizing and producing emotional responses can be present. Nonlinguistic deficits appear as attentional disorders (auditory, visual, and spatial) and perceptual disorders. The individual may focus on minute details of their environment rather than the whole, neglect items in the left hemispace, or exhibit anosagnosia (an unawareness of their deficits) or prosopagnosia (an inability to recognize faces).

Outcomes for treatment of individuals with right hemisphere dysfunction are generally poor because lack of awareness, insight, integration, ability to stay on task, and ability to understand the need to stay on task and participate in treatment all contribute to poor motivation and participation. Treatment focuses excessively on awareness of deficits and facilitating the patient's ability to appreciate their need for therapy.

ACQUIRED BRAIN INJURY

Head injury can be traumatic (penetrating) or closed (nonpenetrating), focal or diffuse, mild or severe. Early intense therapy results in the best outcome. Family and/or caregiver involvement is essential. Provision of education and information to the patient, family, and caregivers is key. Direct training of isolated cognitive-linguistic skills through various structured tasks in the therapy treatment room, in addition to metacognitive work with the patient and their caregivers, and then functional activities within the patient's home and/or community environment to exercise the skills at a level just above the patient's capability to challenge the individual, along with provision of positive feedback or errorless learning is a most successful treatment approach (19). Evaluation, assessment, and standardized testing in the head-injured population requires an experienced SLP and administration of a battery of tests because no one test can accurately tease out all deficits (28).

SUMMARY

Practitioners must look at diagnostic opinions and treatments with scientific skepticism. A valid diagnostic opinion will be clear, concise, and based in longstanding theoretical classifications; it will not be obtuse and general. A valid treatment approach will be supported in the literature, not just touted by anecdotal reports and testimonials. We all must take care to not only trust our own clinical experience, but also to consult with others who have different or perhaps more clinical experience. Ultimately, we must make our patient's best interests most important and meet our ethical and professional responsibilities to them (13).

REFERENCES

1. Adamovich B, Henderson JA, Auerbach S. *Cognitive Rehabilitation of Closed Head Injured Patients*. Austin: Pro-Ed, Inc; 1985.
2. American Speech-Language-Hearing Association. *Perspectives on Neurophysiology and Neurogenic Speech and Language Disorders*. Vol. 16, No. 3. Rockville, MD: American Speech-Language-Hearing Association; 2006.

3. American Speech-Language-Hearing Association. Roles of speech language pathologists in the identification, diagnosis, and treatment of individuals with cognitive-communication disorders. Practice guidelines and policies. Rockville, MD: American Speech-Language-Hearing Association; 2004:24 (Suppl).

4. Armbruster A, Wijdicks E. Pure alexia: past and present. *Mayo Clin Proc.* 2006;81:3975.

5. Chapey R. *Language intervention strategies in adult aphasia.* Baltimore: Williams & Wilkins, 1994.

6. Cunningham ET, Donner MW, Jones B, et al. Anatomical and physiological overview. In: Jones B, Donner M, eds. *Normal and abnormal swallowing imaging in diagnosis and therapy.* New York: Springer-Verlag; 1991:7–32.

7. Darley F, Aronson A, Brown J. *Motor Speech Disorders.* Philadelphia: W.B. Saunders; 1975.

8. Duffy J. *Motor Speech Disorders; Substrates, Differential Diagnosis, and Management.* Boston: Mosby; 1995.

9. Duranceau A, Lafontaine ER, Taillefer R, et al. Oropharyngeal dysphagia and operations on the upper esophageal sphincter. *Surg Annu.* 1987;19: 317–362.

10. Dworkin J. *Motor Speech Disorders: A Treatment Guide.* Baltimore: Mosby; 1991.

11. Enderby P. *The Frenchay Dysarthria Assessment.* San Diego: College Hill Press; 1983.

12. Fairbanks G. *Voice and Articulation Drillbook.* 2nd ed. New York: Harper & Row; 1960.

13. Finn P, Bothe AK, Bramlett RE. Science and pseudoscience in communication disorders: criteria and applications. *Am J Speech Lang Pathol.* 2005;14:172–186.

14. Fletcher S. Contingencies for bioelectronic modification of nasality. *J Speech Hear Disord.* 1972;37:329–346.

15. Groher M. *Dysphagia, Diagnosis and Management.* 2nd ed. Newton: Butterworth-Heinemann; 1992.

16. Hanson EK, Yorkston KM, Beukelman DR. Speech supplementation techniques for dysarthria: a systematic review. *J Med Speech Lang Pathol.* 2004;12:ix–xxix.

17. Hustad KC, Beukelman DR. Integrating AAC strategies with natural speech. In: Beukelman DR, Yorkston KM, Reichle J, eds. *Augmentative and alternative communication for adults with acquired neurologic disabilities.* Baltimore: Paul H. Brookes Publishing; 2000:89–113.

18. Kahrilas PJ. The anatomy and physiology of dysphagia. In: Gelfand DW, Richter JE, eds. *Dysphagia: diagnosis and management.* New York: Igaku-Shoin; 1989:11–28.

19. Kennedy M. Making clinical decisions for managing cognitive-communication disorders after traumatic brain injury. Chicago: Rehabilitation Institute of Chicago, August 8-9, 2006.

20. Kennedy MRT. Cognitive-communication treatment after traumatic brain injury. *Neurophys Neurogenic Speech Lang Disord.* 2002;12:1–32.

21. LaPointe L. *Aphasia and Related Neurogenic Language Disorders.* 2nd ed. New York: Thieme; 1997.

22. Lear CSC, Flanagan JB, Moorrees CFS. The frequency of deglutition in man. *Arch Oral Biol.* 1965;10:83–89.

23. Logemann JA. *Evaluation and Treatment of Swallowing Disorders.* Austin: Pro-Ed, Inc.; 1998.

24. Miller AJ. Overview of oral, pharyngeal and esophageal swallowing. In: Rosenbeck J, ed. *Neuroscientific principles of swallowing and dysphagia.* San Diego: Singular Publishing Group, Inc.; 1999:1–1125.

25. Schuell H. *Differential diagnosis of aphasia with the Minnesota test.* Minneapolis: University of Minnesota Press, 1973.

26. Shaker R. Oropharyngeal dysphagia: practical approach to diagnosis and management. *Semin Gastroint Disord.* 1992;3:115–119.

27. Sonies B. The aging oropharyngeal system. In: Ripich D, ed. *Handbook of geriatric communication disorders.* Texas: Pro-Ed, Inc.; 1991.

28. Turkstra L, Ylvisaker M, Coelho C, et al. Practice guidelines for standardized assessment for persons with traumatic brain injury. *J Med Speech Lang Pathol.* 2005;13:ix–xxviii.

29. Yorkston KM, Beukelman DR. *Assessment of Intelligibility of Dysarthric Speech.* Austin: Pro-Ed, Inc.; 1981.

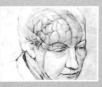

CHAPTER 11

Tremor

Tanya Simuni

INTRODUCTION AND DEFINITIONS

Tremor is defined as a rhythmic involuntary oscillatory movement of a body part (6). The visibility and unique characteristics of tremor make it easy to recognize; however, defining the type of tremor can be more challenging. Classification of tremor is based on its clinical characteristics. Agreement between the observers on the terms is essential for correct classification, which ultimately will lead to accurate diagnosis and treatment. As explained below, tremor is described according to the behavioral circumstances in which it occurs.

I. Rest tremor occurs in a body part that is not voluntarily activated and is completely supported against gravity (e.g., as when resting on a couch or arm rest).
II. Action tremor occurs during any voluntary contraction of skeletal muscle and can be a combination of postural, kinetic, and isometric tremor.
   A. Postural tremor occurs in an attempt to hold a body part motionless against gravity (e.g., outstretched arms).
   B. Kinetic tremor occurs during a voluntary movement and can be of three types:
      1. Isometric tremor occurs during a muscle contraction against a stationary rigid object (pushing against a wall).
      2. With intention tremor, tremor amplitude increases as the limb approaches the target during a visually guided movement (finger-to-nose testing).
      3. Task-specific tremor appears or becomes exacerbated during specific tasks (e.g., primary writing tremor or occupational tremors).

TREMOR EPIDEMIOLOGY

Tremor is the most common type of all movement disorders, and the incidence of tremor increases with age, independent of the cause. Considering that tremor can be a manifestation of a variety of neurologic conditions, prevalence data are available only

with respect to the most common diagnostic entities, specifically essential tremor (ET), which is a monosymptomatic disorder with no neurologic signs other than postural or action tremor, and parkinsonian tremor. Even in those settings, the numbers are inconsistent. Reported ET prevalence varies from 0.0005% to 5.5% (1,27), depending on the study methodology and the population age. Despite such a wide range, unanimous agreement exists between investigators of the increasing prevalence of ET with age. Larson and Sjogren (18) reported a twofold increase of tremor prevalence rate in the population over the age of 40 years compared with the general population. Another study reported a 10-fold increase in prevalence of ET in persons 70 to 79 years of age compared with those 40 to 69 years of age (11). It is estimated that about 5 million individuals over the age of 40 are affected by ET in the United States, making it undoubtedly the most common movement disorder (8,15).

Similar to ET, a clear age-dependent increase is seen in the prevalence of parkinsonian tremors. It is estimated that Parkinson's disease affects 1% of the population over the age of 65 (31). Generally, tremor is present in 75% of patients with Parkinson's disease, making Parkinson's disease tremor (PDT) the second most common cause of tremor. Prevalence of tremor in the setting of various metabolic derangements (e.g., renal, hepatic encephalopathy, hypoglycemia, hyperthyroidism) is unknown; however, the incidence of these conditions is clearly age dependent. The same is true for drug-induced tremor, considering the exponential increase of medication intake with age.

TREMOR PATHOPHYSIOLOGY

Despite the high prevalence of tremor, knowledge of its pathophysiology and anatomic generators is limited. Central versus peripheral nervous system origin of tremor is still debated. It remains unclear whether tremor generators are disease specific or a common final pathway exists that is independent of tremor cause. Four mechanisms have been postulated (12,30):

1. Mechanical oscillation of the extremity is based on simple mechanical properties of any mass-spring system. An extremity attached to a stiff joint oscillates after a mechanical perturbation. The resonance frequency is inversely related to the mass of the body part, and it can be measured by a sensitive accelerometer attached to the outstretched limb. This mechanism can potentially explain physiologic tremor but doubtfully represents a solo mechanism of pathologic tremors.
2. Reflex activation of tremor is based on the muscle stretch reflex. The oscillation of a limb activates muscle spindle receptors, which, via the Ia afferents, monosynaptically connect to the motor neuron and through the motor axon back to the extrafusal muscle fibers. This creates a reflex loop. These reflex loops, if appropriately timed, can produce rhythmic bursts of muscle activity, consistent with tremor.
3. Central oscillator likely plays the major role in tremor generation. Specific cell populations within the central nervous system have the capacity to fire repetitively because of the unique properties of their membrane potential. Single-cell oscillation is insufficient to produce a visible tremor in the periphery. However, if cell activity is synchronized, the synchronized volley can cause sufficient motor neuron pool activation to produce a visible tremor. Two regions within the central motor pathways demonstrate oscillatory behavior under certain conditions: the inferior olive and the relay nuclei of the thalamus. It is believed that the pattern of tremor produced is oscillator dependent. Essential type tremor has been linked to the inferior olive, whereas parkinsonian tremor has been linked to the basal ganglia region, with the thalamus being the potential cortical projection relay nuclei for both. This hypothesis would explain the effectiveness of thalamic target for surgical treatment of both types of tremor.
4. Cerebellar lesions can be associated with tremor. It is unlikely that the cerebellum has an independent tremor oscillator region, but it can participate in tremor generation by altering feedforward and feedback loops. Based on positron emission tomography (PET) data, cerebellar blood flow is increased in almost all types of tremor (3). Such nonselective activation supports the hypothesis that the cerebellum is likely a relay site for tremor rather than the primary generator, although the data are inconclusive.

It is still unclear whether one mechanism plays a leading role in a particular tremor generation versus occurring in parallel or whether the mechanisms might be additive. It seems, at least in the setting of ET and Parkinson's disease, that a central tremor generator exists, the activity of which can be augmented or modified by the peripheral input.

TREMOR CAUSE

Table 11-1 summarizes multiple potential causes of tremor. It is beyond the scope of this chapter to discuss each of them. From a clinical standpoint, it is useful to define the tremor syndrome, which will narrow the causative differential diagnosis and guide in the choice of therapeutic intervention (6).

PHYSIOLOGIC TREMOR

In every healthy subject, physiologic tremor is present in the joint or muscle that is free to oscillate. It has low amplitude and high frequency. Usually, it is not visible, except for intermittent finger tremors.

ENHANCED PHYSIOLOGIC TREMOR

Enhanced physiologic tremor (EPT) has the same frequency characteristics as physiologic tremor but is easily visible. It is mainly postural. The diagnosis should not be made in the presence of an underlying neurologic pathology. This form of tremor overlaps the category of drug- or toxin-induced tremor. Screening for potential metabolic derangements associated with tremor should be performed (Table 11-2). Distinction between EPT and mild forms of ET is arbitrary and usually is based on the presence of functional disability with the latter.

ESSENTIAL TREMOR

The diagnosis of ET is based on the presence of bilateral, largely symmetric, postural or kinetic tremor that involves hands and forearms and that is visible and persistent (6,8). Tremor can involve head and voice; however, chin or leg involvement is atypical. In cases of severe ET, resting tremor can be present; however, the possibility of coexisting Parkinson's disease (PD) has to be ruled out. Tremor frequency is 4 to 12 Hz. Some patients, especially women, can present with head tremor as an isolated manifestation of ET. Caution should be taken to rule out an underlying cervical dystonia with a prominent tremor component. The possibility of an underlying symptomatic cause, such as drugs, toxins, or metabolic abnormalities, should be excluded before making the diagnosis of ET. A distinction should be made between ET as the causative entity, also referred to as benign familial essential tremor, versus ET as a clinical syndrome, which defines tremor of a particular type that potentially can be associated with other neurologic findings. The former is labeled as definite ET in the Tremor Investigation Group (TRIG) nomenclature, whereas the latter is labeled as probable versus possible,

Table 11-1. *Tremor: Etiologic Classification*

Physiologic tremor
    Enhanced physiologic tremor
Pathologic tremors
    Hereditary, degenerative, and idiopathic disease
        Essential tremor
            Definite essential tremor (ET) (monosymptomatic ET)
            Probable ET (ET with atypical distribution of tremor)
            Possible ET (ET + other neurologic findings)
        Parkinsonian tremor
            Parkinson's disease
            Other parkinsonian syndromes (e.g., multiple system atrophy, progressive supranuclear palsy, Wilson's disease)
        Task-specific tremor (e.g., writers tremor, voice tremor)
        Dystonic tremor syndromes (generalized or focal dystonia + tremor in the affected body part)
        Cerebellar tremor syndromes (e.g., spinocerebellar degenerations, olivopontocerebellar atrophy)
    Cerebral diseases of various etiologies
        Central nervous system infections (e.g., neurosyphilis, neuroborreliosis, HIV, smallpox)
        Inflammatory conditions (multiple sclerosis)
        Space occupying lesions (e.g., tumors, cerebrovascular insults, atrioventricular malformation)
        Posttraumatic tremor
    Metabolic diseases
        Hyper/hypothyroidism
        Hyperparathyroidism
        Hypocalcemia
        Hypomagnesimia
        Hypoglycemia
        Hepatic encephalopathy
        Renal encephalopathy
    Drug-induced
        Centrally acting substances (e.g., neuroleptics, antidepressants—especially tricyclics, lithium, cocaine, alcohol, caffeine)
        Sympathornimetics (bronchodilators)
        Steroids
        Miscellaneous (valproate, perhexiline, amiodarone, mexilitine, vincristine, cyclosporine A)
    Toxin-induced (mercury, lead, manganese, cyanide, carbon monoxide, nicotine, arsenic, alcohol)
    Peripheral neuropathies
        Roussy—Lévy syndrome
        Other hereditary neuropathies
        Polyneuropathy of various origin (diabetes, uremia, porphyria)
    Other disorders with tremor symptoms
        Emotions, fatigue, cooling
        Drug withdrawal
        Psychogenic tremor

Modified from Deuschl G, Bain P, Brin M. Consensus statement of the Movement Disorder Society on Termor. Ad Hoc Scientific Committee. *Mov Disord.* 1998;13[Suppl 3]:2–23, with permission.

depending on the type of associated neurologic findings (2). Definite ET is a monosymptomatic disease, meaning that no other abnormal neurologic findings should be present. It has strong familial predisposition, with about 50% of patients having a positive family history for tremor, pointing to likely autosomal dominant inheritance, although the gene has yet to be identified (9). Conversely, lack of family history does not preclude the diagnosis of ET. Symptoms have an insidious onset with a variable rate of progression. The most disabling feature of ET is action or kinetic tremor of the arms, which interferes with the patient's ability to perform the simplest daily activities (e.g., eating, drinking, writing). Patients with severe ET

Table 11-2. *Screening for Potential Symptomatic Causes of Tremor*

1. Thyroid function (thyroid-stimulating hormone, T3, T4)
2. Metabolic screen (Na, K, Cl, Ca, Mg, creatinin, blood urea nitrogen, glucose)
3. Liver function tests (alanine aminotransferase, aspartate aminotransferase)
4. Ceruloplasmin, serum and urine copper[a]
5. Cortisol, parathyroid hormones[a]
6. Toxicology test[a]

[a]To be performed only when clinically indicated.

can be completely disabled, so the label of benign is a misnomer. A number of patients have a combination of ET and other movement disorders (e.g., dystonia, parkinsonism, myoclonus, restless legs syndrome). Those patients are classified as possible ET according to TRIG criteria (2).

PRIMARY ORTHOSTATIC TREMOR

Primary orthostatic tremor is a unique syndrome characterized by the presence of high-frequency (13 to 18 Hz) tremor of the trunk and legs that occurs only with stance (4). The patients are asymptomatic when lying down or sitting. Rarely, symptoms persist with walking. Subjectively, patients report a feeling of unsteadiness when standing up. Constant change of the position of the feet relieves the symptoms; thus, patients quickly learn to march in one spot. The clinical examination finding is benign, except for minimally visible and sometimes only palpable fine-amplitude rippling of the leg muscles. The diagnosis can be confirmed by an electromyographic (EMG) study of the quadriceps muscles, which records a typical tremor pattern of 13 to 18 Hz. Symptoms respond to low-dose clonazepam. A recent study also demonstrated the benefit of gabapentin, although the number of study subjects was small (29).

TASK- AND POSITION-SPECIFIC TREMOR

Task- and position-specific tremors comprise a group of tremor syndromes that share a common feature of tremor activation when engaged in a specific task. The most common type is primary writing tremor, when symptoms appear only or predominantly with that particular activity. Use of the limb with other activities (e.g., eating, weight lifting) is not associated with tremor. Other examples include task-specific tremors of musicians and athletes, as well as isolated voice tremor. Some of these patients have dystonic posturing of the limb in conjunction with tremor. These cases should be classified as focal dystonia with dystonic tremor.

DYSTONIC TREMOR SYNDROMES

Tremor in a body part affected by dystonia is a well-known phenomenon, although its mechanism is unknown. The pattern of tremor differs from ET; it is localized to the dystonic body part, has an irregular pattern with variable frequency, and usually resolves with complete rest. Gestes antagonistes, a sensory trick used by a lot of patients to overcome dystonic movement by touching the involved body part, such as placing the hand on the cheek in cases of cervical dystonia, frequently reduces tremor. This type of tremor responds to botulinum toxin injections. Sometimes patients with dystonia (e.g., patients with cervical dystonia and upper limb postural tremor) may have an ET type of tremor in the body part not affected by dystonia. These patients should not be classified as having dystonic tremor. They likely have an ET–dystonia overlap syndrome.

PARKINSONIAN TREMOR SYNDROMES

Parkinsonism is a clinical syndrome, not a disease entity. However, parkinsonian tremor has unique characteristics believed to be stigmata of striatonigral dysfunction. Classic parkinsonian tremor occurs in a resting limb, has a pill-rolling pattern, and is low frequency (4 to 6 Hz). It characteristically diminishes with activity of the affected limb. Tremor can be accelerated with mental activity, with stress, or when movement of another body part is performed. As noted earlier, parkinsonian tremor is not an obligatory sign of PD; however, it is present in 75% of patients with PD. Alternatively, rest tremor is unusual in patients with atypical parkinsonian syndromes (e.g., multiple system atrophy, progressive supranuclear palsy). Tremor in PD typically involves distal arms but also legs and chin; head or voice tremor is atypical in these patients. PD tremor is asymmetric or at least initially starts on one side of the body. Tremor usually is not the major cause of disability because it abates when the limb is involved in action. Aside from classic resting tremor, patients with PD can have various degrees of postural and action tremor. That tremor component can be either at the same frequency as a resting tremor or it can be faster and nonharmonically related to the resting tremor. The former type is believed to be the continuation of rest tremor under postural or kinetic conditions, whereas the mechanism of the latter is unknown. Few patients with PD have pure postural or kinetic tremor with no rest tremor component. However, some patients will have postural or kinetic tremor at the onset of the disease and develop the classical rest tremor pattern later on.

Generally, distinction between classic ET and a parkinsonian-type tremor is straightforward based on the distinct tremor characteristics. In some cases, however, distinction can be difficult, especially at the early stages of the disease. It is estimated that about 20% of patients with ET are misdiagnosed for PD and vice versa (10). The differential diagnosis criteria are summarized in Table 11-3.

MONOSYMPTOMATIC REST TREMOR

Some patients exhibit isolated rest tremor without evidence of associated parkinsonian signs (e.g., bradykinesia, rigidity). According to the Brain Bank Parkinson's disease diagnostic criteria, the diagnosis of PD should not be made in the absence of bradykinesia, although PET data in some of these patients provide evidence of dopaminergic dysfunction to the degree similar to otherwise typical PD (5). However, for clinical purposes, these patients should be labeled as having "monosymptomatic rest tremor," unless they develop other clinical signs of PD.

CEREBELLAR TREMOR SYNDROMES

Various types of tremor have been described in cerebellar disorders; however, the most common type, considered to be the stigmata of cerebellar dysfunction, is intentional tremor. As discussed, it is a kinetic tremor, the amplitude of which increases during a visually guided movement toward a target. It frequently is irregular and unilateral, having a frequency below 5 Hz and no rest tremor component. It typically involves the limbs and is elicited on the finger-to-nose or heel-to-chin tests. The pathophysiologic basis of cerebellar tremor is unknown, although anatomically, it is associated with the damage of either superior cerebellar peduncles or dentate nuclei. Another pattern of tremor associated with cerebellar pathology is slow-frequency oscillation of the body trunk or head, the amplitude of which increases with movement. That pattern is known as titubation.

HOLMES TREMOR

Holmes tremor, also known as midbrain tremor, rubral tremor, or myorhythmia, is a unique tremor syndrome usually of symptomatic origin caused by a lesion of the central nervous system. Originally, it was believed to be associated with lesions in red nuclei or midbrain, hence the name (24). Recently, however, more and more cases have been reported in which the lesion was located outside the midbrain. The pattern of tremor is a combination of resting and intention. It frequently is irregular and has slow frequency (<4.5 Hz). The proximal muscles can be involved more than distal muscles, unlike other tremor types. Tremor frequently is unilateral. In cases of cerebrovascular events as the cause of the structural lesion, a delay is seen to the time of tremor onset, which can be up to 2 years (16). Pathophysiology of this type of tremor is unknown, but PET data suggest that it is caused by a combined lesion of cerebellothalamic and nigrostriatal pathways (28).

PALATAL TREMOR SYNDROMES

Palatal tremor was formally classified as palatal myoclonus; however, rhythmicity of movement is consistent with the tremor pattern. Palatal tremor can

Table 11-3. *Differential Diagnosis of Essential Tremor and Parkinsonian Tremor*

	Essential tremor[a]	Parkinson's disease
Resting tremor	+	+++
Postural or action tremor	+++	+
Tremor asymmetry	+	+++
Rigidity	±	+++
Bradykinesia	−	+++
Chin tremor	−	++
Leg tremor	±	+++
Voice tremor	+++	−
Head tremor	+++	−
Hereditary tremor	+++	−
Response to alcohol	+++	−
Response to dopaminergic (+/−)	−	+++

[a]± indicate presence versus absence and the severity of the symptoms on a scale from one to three, with three being most severe.
Adapted from Deuschl G, Krack P. Tremors: differential diagnosis, neurophysiology, and pharmacology. In: Jankovic J, Tolosa E, eds. *Parkinson's disease and movement disorders.* Baltimore: Williams & Wilkins; 1998:419–452.

be either symptomatic or essential (7,34). Symptomatic causes of tremor include preceding brainstem or cerebellum lesion with subsequent inferior olivary hypertrophy, which can be demonstrated on a magnetic resonance imaging (MRI) scan. Rhythmic movement may not be limited to the soft palate and can also involve other brainstem innervated muscles (frequently, extraocular musculature). In essential cases, by definition, no identifiable underlying structural lesion exists, and the MRI scan is normal. Clinically, signs are limited to the soft palate, and the patients usually have an ear click, which is a rhythmic sound in the ears.

DRUG-INDUCED AND TOXIC TREMOR SYNDROMES

The incidence of toxin- or drug-induced tremor is unknown; however, potentially it can be the most common cause of tremor, exceeding ET and tremors of Parkinson's disease, especially in the elderly. The pattern of tremor can be variable, depending on the agent and individual predisposition. The most common pattern is enhanced physiologic tremor that occurs when using tremorogenic drugs. The list of the potential offending agents is extensive; however, the most frequently cited ones are sympathomimetics, stimulants, steroids, and antidepressants (6). For patients with an acute onset of tremor, medication lists must be carefully reviewed for a potential causative relationship to the symptoms. Tremorogenic effects might not be limited to the pharmaceutic agent but can be associated with certain foods and beverages (caffeinated drinks). Another common pattern of drug-induced tremor is parkinsonian tremor with the use of dopamine-blocking agents (19). The best recognized offending agents are neuroleptics because of their ability to block postsynaptic dopamine receptors. However, less well-known and less used presynaptic dopamine-depleting agents (e.g., reserpine and tetrabenazine) can cause the same syndrome (20). The effect of dopamine-blocking agents is not limited to tremor; they cause the full triad of parkinsonian symptoms. Withdrawal of the offending agent should lead to resolution of tremor and other symptoms within 3 weeks to 6 months. Rare cases of persistent symptoms have been reported, despite withdrawal of the offending agents (13). Such cases raise the possibility of underlying Parkinson's disease in those individuals that was clinically unveiled by neuroleptic exposure.

The association of tremor with toxin exposure has been known for some time, and the list of potential offending agents is long (21). A detailed history, especially in the setting of acute onset of tremor, will help to isolate the potential toxin or drug and proceed with the appropriate investigation.

TREMOR SYNDROMES IN PERIPHERAL NEUROPATHY

Tremor has been described with various kinds of peripheral neuropathies; however, they have been most commonly linked with demyelinating neuropathies (32). The pattern of tremor is usually postural or kinetic. Roussy-Lévy is the syndrome characterized by the presence of demyelinating hereditary motor sensory neuropathy (HSMN type I) and essential type tremor (26). In some patients, tremor responds to alcohol and propranolol. The pathophysiology of tremor in neuropathies is unclear, but it is believed to involve both peripheral and central mechanisms.

PSYCHOGENIC TREMOR

Generally, the diagnosis of psychogenic movement disorder is the most challenging, even for an experienced movement disorder neurologist. Clues to the diagnosis have been established and include (6,14,17) the following:

- Acute onset of the symptoms or spontaneous remissions
- Pattern of tremor inconsistent with any known syndrome
- Distractibility of symptoms
- Ability to provoke symptoms with suggestion
- History of somatization in the past
- Additional nonphysiologic signs found on neurologic examination
- Presence of secondary gain

These are only clues to the diagnosis. Careful examination by an experienced professional allows the correct diagnosis to be made in most cases, while avoiding unnecessary testing and pharmacologic exposure. Nonconfrontational counseling and referral to a psychologist are essential; however, they do not always guarantee a good recovery.

DIFFERENTIAL DIAGNOSIS OF TREMOR

In most cases, tremor is easy to recognize and distinguish from other types of movement disorders based on its clinical characteristics. Rhythmicity of the movement differentiates it from chorea and hemiballism. Oscillatory pattern of movement distinguishes tremor from dystonia or myoclonus, even in cases when the latter carry pseudoperiodic patterns. Tics can be rhythmic, but their rapid speed and stereotypy allow separating them from tremor. Rhythmicity and oscillating pattern of movement differentiate tremor from asterixis, which is a negative myoclonus usually seen in the setting of metabolic encephalopathy.

Epilepsia partialis continua is rarely misinterpreted as tremor because of the presence of rhythmic jerks. However, acute onset of symptoms, lack of prior history of tremor, localization of symptoms to one limb, and electroencephalogram data allow differentiation of these syndromes. Clonus can be rhythmic; however, localization of the symptoms around the joint and presence of other pyramidal findings make it unlikely to be confused with tremor. Despite unique characteristics of tremor that distinguish it from other movements, differentiating the type of tremor can be more challenging. Differential diagnosis of tremor syndromes, discussed earlier, is summarized in Table 11-4. The major source of confusion is distinguishing ET and Parkinson's disease tremor (PDT), especially at the early stages. Table 11-3 summarizes criteria for differentiating tremor in these two common entities.

APPROACH TO THE DIAGNOSIS AND MANAGEMENT OF TREMOR

When a clinician evaluates a patient with any kind of involuntary movement, the first step is to define the type of movement disorder. The following is the suggested stepwise approach to evaluation of patients with tremor (Fig. 11-1):

Step 1. Does the patient have a tremor?
Step 2. What is the pattern of tremor (resting, postural, kinetic, goal directed)?

Step 3. What is the distribution of tremor (head, chin, voice, upper or lower limbs, trunk)?
Step 4. What is the tremor frequency (fast, >7 Hz; medium, 4 to 7 Hz; low, <4 Hz)?
Step 5. Are there any other positive findings on the neurologic examination (bradykinesia, rigidity, gait abnormality, pyramidal findings, cerebellar signs, dystonia, neuropathic signs)?
Step 6. Based on the data from the previous steps, define the tremor syndrome:
  1. Physiologic
  2. Parkinsonian
  3. Essential
  4. Other
Step 7. Review medical history for:
  1. Mode of tremor onset (acute vs. insidious)
  2. Family history of neurologic disease (specifically tremor)
  3. Alcohol sensitivity
  4. History of medication exposure
  5. History of toxin exposure
Step 8. Determine the cause of the tremor syndrome based on the data from Step 2-7 (not always possible).
Step 9. Decide if additional testing is necessary.
Step 10. Evaluate treatment options based on the type of tremor syndrome (essential vs. parkinsonian).
Step 11. Treat only if symptoms produce functional compromise and no reversible cause is identified.
Step 12. Re-evaluate the diagnosis, if necessary, based on the treatment response and the cause of the disease (appearance of new neurologic findings).

Table 11-4. *Tremor Syndromes: Differential Diagnosis*

Tremor diagnosis	Distribution	Activation by[a]			Frequency (Hz)
		Rest	Posture	Action[a]	
Physiologic	Arms	−	+	+	8–12
Enhanced physiologic	Arms	−	+	+	8–12
Essential	Arms, head, voice	−	++	++	4–12
Dystonic	Part of body with dystonia	−	+	++	<7
Primary writing	Arm	−	+	+++	5–10
Orthostatic	Legs, trunk	−	+++	+	13–18
Parkinson's	Arms, legs, chin	+++	+	+	4–6
Cerebellar	Arms, head, trunk	−	+	+++ Intention	<5
Holmes (rubral)	Arm, leg; usually unilateral	+++	+	+++	<4.5
Neuropathic	Limbs	−	++	+	3–10
Drug-induced	Limbs[a]	+++	++	++	[b]
Psychogenic	Any body part	Any combination, inconsistent pattern			

[a]± indicate presence versus absence and the severity of the symptoms on a scale from one to three, with three being most severe.
[b]Depending on the type of medication, can be predominantly essential or parkinsonian type.

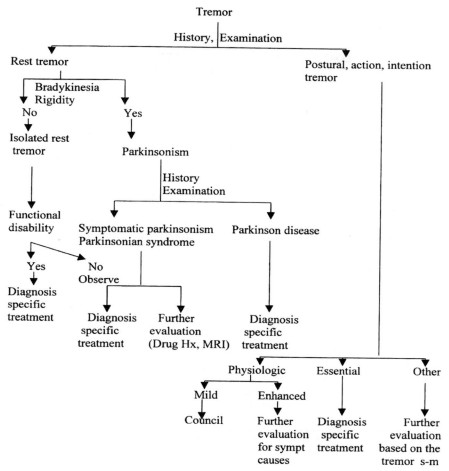

Figure 11-1. Tremor evaluation algorithm.

DIAGNOSTIC STUDIES

The diagnosis of tremor is a clinical one based on the history and examination. Diagnostic studies to confirm tremor as the type of movement disorder are rarely necessary. Surface electromyography can be performed to clarify tremor frequency and is most useful to confirm the diagnosis of orthostatic tremor (high-frequency tremor) (23). EMG can also be a useful tool when psychogenic tremor is suspected because it will reveal an inconsistent muscle-firing pattern (22,25). Nerve conduction study in conjunction with EMG should be performed if a neurogenic cause (peripheral neuropathy) of tremor is suspected.

Screening for potential symptomatic causes of tremor should be performed in all cases of acute onset of symptoms. The suggested evaluation panel is presented in Table 11-2. The extent of testing should be geared to each particular case. Thyroid studies should be performed in all patients with the syndrome of enhanced physiologic tremor.

Patients with tremor and an otherwise normal neurologic examination do not require neuroimaging. Neuroimaging, preferably MRI, should be performed in the presence of other positive focal findings on examination (e.g., pyramidal or cerebellar signs) to rule out an underlying structural lesion.

TREATMENT OPTIONS

Choice of tremor therapy is based on the tremor syndrome (33). The major distinction is between essential and parkinsonian type tremor. Physiologic tremor does not require pharmacologic therapy. In the setting of enhanced physiologic tremor, the primary objective is to find and correct the potential underlying symptomatic cause. Treatment should be attempted only if the investigation is not revealing and symptoms produce a functional compromise. The choice of therapy is the same as for ET; however, the treatment should be started with a long-acting benzodiazepine (clonazepam). Some patients benefit from use of

Table 11-5. *Medication Chart: Tremor*

Medication	Dose	Risks	Cost/month ($)
Parkinson's tremor Levodopa/carbidopa Dopamine agonists	25/100 mg 3–6/d	Orthostasis, confusion, nausea, hallucinations	>50.00 Much more expensive than 50.00
Pramipexole Ropinirole Pergolide Bromocriptine	0.75-3.0 mg/d 3–16 mg/d 0.75–3 mg/d 7.5–30 mg/d	Orthostasis, confusion, nausea, hallucinations, somnolence	
Amantadine	100–300 mg/d	Confusion, LE edema	>50.00
Trihexyphenidyl	1–2 mg three times daily	Confusion, dry mouth, urinary retention; should not be used in patients with glaucoma	<50.00
Clozapine	25–50 mg/d	Neutropenia, sedation	Much more expensive than 50.00
Essential tremor Propranolol	60–320 mg/d	Orthostasis, sleep disturbance, depression; contraindicated in asthma, diabetes, heart block	<50.00
Primidone	50–250 mg/d	Sedation, confusion	<50.00
Clonazepam	0.5–3.0 mg/d	Sedation	<50.00
Enhanced physiologic tremor Propranolol	10 mg as needed		<50.00
Clonazepam	0.5 mg at bedtime		<50.00
Cerebellar tremor	No effective therapy, essential tremor (ET) medications can be tried		
Holmes tremor	No effective therapy, parkinsonian and ET medications can be tried		

LE, Lower extremities.

propranolol (10 mg) on an as-needed basis. A recently published practice parameter summarized data on the treatment choices for ET (35). The major groups of medications used for treatment of parkinsonian and ET tremor are presented in Table 11-5.

SUMMARY

Tremor is a common neurologic sign, especially in the elderly. It can be a symptom of a variety of underlying medical and neurologic conditions. A complete history, careful examination, and stepwise approach to defining the type of tremor are essential for correct diagnosis and appropriate management.

REFERENCES

1. Aiyesimoju AB, Osuntokun BO, Bademosi O, et al. Hereditary neurodegenerative disorders in Nigerian Africans. *Neurology.* 1984;34:361–362.
2. Bain P, Brin M, Deuschl G, et al. Criteria for the diagnosis of essential tremor. *Neurology.* 2000; 54[Suppl 4]:S7–S7.
3. Boecker H, Brooks DJ. Functional imaging of tremor. *Mov Disord.* 1998;13[Suppl 3]:64–72.
4. Britton TC, Thompson PD. Primary orthostatic tremor. *BMJ.* 1995;310:143–144.
5. Brooks DJ, Playford ED, Ibanez V, et al. Isolated tremor and disruption of the nigrostriatal dopaminergic system: an 18F-dopa PET study. *Neurology.* 1992;42:1554–1560.
6. Deuschl G, Bain P, Brin M. Consensus statement of the Movement Disorder Society on Tremor. Ad Hoc Scientific Committee. *Mov Disord.* 1998;13[Suppl 3]:2–23.
7. Deuschl G, Toro C, Hallett M. Symptomatic and essential palatal tremor. 2. Differences of palatal movements. *Mov Disord.* 1994;9:676–678.
8. Elble RJ. Report from a U.S. conference on essential tremor. *Mov Disord.* 2006;21:2052–2061.
9. Findley LJ. Epidemiology and genetics of essential tremor. *Neurology.* 2000;54[Suppl 4]:S8–S13.
10. Findley LJ, Koller WC. Essential tremor: a review. *Neurology.* 1987;37:1194–1197.
11. Haerer AF, Anderson DW, Schoenberg BS. Prevalence of essential tremor. Results from

the Copiah County study. *Arch Neurol.* 1982; 39:750–751.

12. Hallett M. Overview of human tremor physiology. *Mov Disord.* 1998;[Suppl 3]:43–48.
13. Klawans HLJ, Bergen D, Bruyn GW. Prolonged drug-induced Parkinsonism. *Confin Neurol.* 1973; 35:368–377.
14. Koller W, Lang A, Vetere-Overfield B, et al. Psychogenic tremors. *Neurology.* 1989;39:1094–1099.
15. Koller WC. Essential tremor: the beginning of a new era. *Mov Disord* 1997;12:841.
16. Krack P, Deuschl G, Kaps M, et al. Delayed onset of "rubral tremor" 23 years after brainstem trauma. *Mov Disord.* 1994;9:240–242.
17. Lang AE, Koller WC, Fahn S. Psychogenic parkinsonism. *Arch Neurol.* 1995;52:802–810.
18. Larson T, Sjogren T. Essential tremor: a clinical and genetic population study. *Acta Psychiatr Neurol Scand.* 1960;44:36.
19. Llau ME, Nguyen L, Senard JM, et al. Drug-induced parkinsonian syndromes: a 10-year experience at a regional center of pharmaco-vigilance. *Rev Neurol (Paris).* 1994;150:757–762.
20. Lorenc-Koci E, Ossowska K, Wardas J, et al. Does reserpine induce parkinsonian rigidity? *J Neural Transm Park Dis Dement Sect.* 1995; 9:211–223.
21. Manyam BV. Uncommon forms of tremor. In: Jankovic J, Tolosa E, eds. *Parkinson's disease and movement disorders.* Baltimore: Williams & Wilkins; 1998:387–403.
22. McAuley JH, Rothwell JC, Marsden CD, et al. Electrophysiological aids in distinguishing organic from psychogenic tremor. *Neurology.* 1998; 50:1882–1884.
23. McManis PG, Sharbrough FW. Orthostatic tremor: clinical and electrophysiologic characteristics. *Muscle Nerve.* 1993;16:1254–1260.
24. Paviour DC, Jager HR, Wilkinson L, et al. Holmes tremor: application of modern neuroimaging techniques. *Mov Disord.* 2006;21:2260–2262.
25. Piboolnurak P, Rothey N, Ahmed A, et al. Psychogenic tremor disorders identified using tree-based statistical algorithms and quantitative tremor analysis. *Mov Disord.* 2005; 20:1543–1549.
26. Plante-Bordeneuve V, Guiochon-Mantel A, Lacroix C, et al. The Roussy-Levy family: from the original description to the gene. *Ann Neurol.* 1999;46:770–773.
27. Rautakorpi I, Takala J, Marttila RJ, et al. Essential tremor in a Finnish population. *Acta Neurol Scand.* 1982;66:58–67.
28. Remy P, de Recondo A, Defer G, et al. Peduncular "rubral" tremor and dopaminergic denervation: a PET study. *Neurology.* 1995;45:472–477.
29. Rodrigues JP, Edwards DJ, Walters SE, et al. Blinded placebo crossover study of gabapentin in primary orthostatic tremor. *Mov Disord.* 2006; 21:900–905.
30. Rothwell JC. Physiology and anatomy of possible oscillators in the central nervous system. *Mov Disord.* 1998;13:24–28.
31. Tanner CM, Aston DA. Epidemiology of Parkinson's disease and akinetic syndromes. *Curr Opin Neurol.* 2000;13:427–430.
32. Thomas PK. Overview of Charcot-Marie-Tooth disease type 1A. *Ann NY Acad Sci.* 1999;883:1–5.
33. Wasielewski PG, Burns JM, Koller WC. Pharmacologic treatment of tremor. *Mov Disord.* 1998;13:90–100.
34. Zadikoff CA, Lang E, Klein C. The 'essentials' of essential palatal tremor: a reappraisal of the nosology. *Brain.* 2006;129:832–840.
35. Zesiewicz TA, Elble R, Louis ED, et al. Practice parameter: therapies for essential tremor: report of the Quality Standards Subcommittee of the American Academy of Neurology. *Neurology.* 2005;64:2008–2020.

SUGGESTED READING

Deuschl G, ed. Tremor: basic mechanisms and clinical aspects. *Mov Disord.* 1998;13[Suppl 3].

Deuschl G, Krack P. Tremors: differential diagnosis, neurophysiology, and pharmacology. In: Jankovic J, Tolosa E, eds. *Parkinson's disease and movement disorders.* Baltimore: Williams & Wilkins; 1998: 419–452.

Koller WC, ed. Essential tremor. *Neurology.* 2000; 54[Suppl 4].

Zesiewicz TA, Elble R, Louis ED, et al. Practice parameter: therapies for essential tremor: Report of the Quality Standards Subcommittee of the American Academy of Neurology. *Neurology.* 2005; 64:2008–2020.

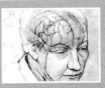

CHAPTER 12

Neuro-Ophthalmology

Benjamin J. Osborne, Rod Foroozan, and Mark L. Moster

In this chapter, we discuss the common neuro-ophthalmic disorders that occur in the elderly, including causes of visual loss from vascular occlusive disease [including giant cell arteritis (GCA)], optic disc swelling, orbital disease (including thyroid eye disease), disorders of ocular motility [including myasthenia gravis (MG)], and disorders of the face and eyelid.

Many neuro-ophthalmic disorders can be diagnosed solely by a complete ocular history. A thorough ocular history should include the onset and severity of visual dysfunction, the timing and progression of the visual disturbance, the presence of pain, and exacerbating and relieving factors. Specific attention should be paid to establishing whether the ocular complaint is unilateral or bilateral. A prior ocular history, including a history of strabismus, surgery, and trauma, should be sought, and any family history of ocular disease should be noted. The use of medications, both systemic and topical preparations, should be recorded in a general review of the medical history. During the examination, both eyes must be assessed, even if the patient believes that the problem is unilateral.

An important assessment of central visual function can be made by testing the best-corrected visual acuity, and each eye should be tested separately. Although most measures of visual acuity depend on subjective responses, electrophysiologic testing can be used to gain some objective measure of visual function.

Pupillary reactivity should be assessed in the dark by instructing the patient to view a distant target, eliminating the miosis that occurs with accommodation and the near response. The response depends on the intensity of light projected and the efficiency of transmission through the afferent visual pathway (Fig. 12-1). This response is dependent on a difference between the conduction of the two afferent pupillary pathways, hence the designation relative afferent pupillary defect (RAPD), also known as a Marcus Gunn pupil (77). Patients with symmetric deficits in the afferent pupillary pathway may not have a RAPD. Instead, they show a pattern similar to that seen with a less intense light source because the conduction of the afferent pathway is less efficient.

Assessment of the afferent visual system must include confrontation visual field testing. Each eye is tested separately by fully occluding the opposite eye (Fig. 12-2). The superior visual field is tested by asking the patient to count the number of fingers seen on each hand of the examiner. An impairment of either the nasal or temporal portion of the superior visual field can be confirmed by retesting each quadrant individually. Similarly, testing of the inferior visual field is performed by presenting fingers just below the level of the patient's chin; then test the fellow eye in a similar fashion.

Electrophysiologic testing is generally not required in the evaluation of the afferent visual system but can be helpful in cases of unexplained visual loss (13). The electroretinogram (ERG) represents the sum of the response of retinal photoreceptors, and specific testing conditions can aid in differentiating the cone and rod responses. Multifocal electroretinography is a relatively new technology that measures retinal function in the central 40 to 50 degrees of the retina. It is helpful in accessing retinal disease in cases of medication toxicities (such as amiodarone, hydroxychloroquine, and ethambutol), paraneoplastic retinopathies, and retinal vascular occlusions (46). The visual evoked potential (VEP) can assess the latency and amplitude of the afferent visual response, including the visual cortex, but typically is not specific enough to determine the site of visual dysfunction.

RETINAL DISORDERS

RETINAL ARTERIAL OCCLUSIONS

Acute visual loss from retinal disease is most commonly from vascular disease. Retinal arterial occlusion, both central retinal artery occlusion (CRAO) and branch retinal artery occlusion (BRAO), causes painless loss of vision that is acute and often catastrophic. Patients with retinal artery obstruction will have visual field loss consistent with the area of occlusion, and those with CRAO will have a small RAPD. Seventy-five to 80% of patients with a CRAO will have visual acuity of counting fingers or worse (32),

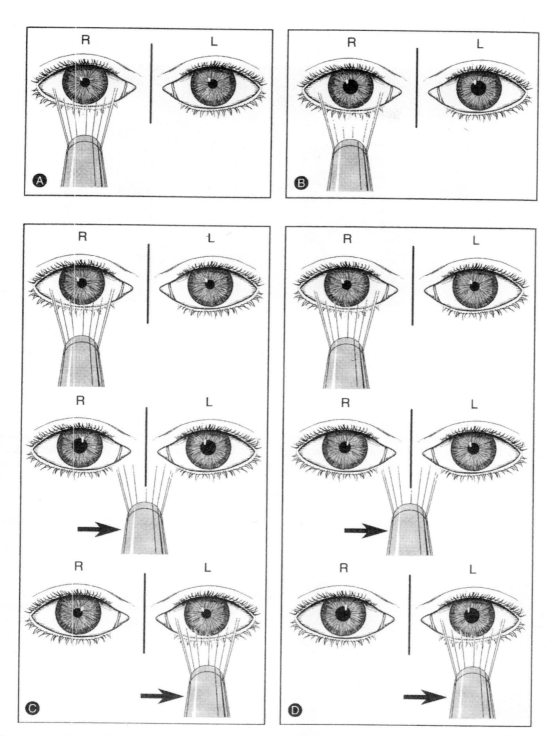

Figure 12-1. The pupillary response. **A:** Light projected into the right eye causes constriction of both pupils. **B:** Light of lesser intensity than that in **(A)** causes pupillary constriction that is less brisk. **C:** Light first projected into the right eye is then moved to the other eye. As the light moves between the eyes, pupillary dilation occurs. This is followed by constriction when light is shown into the left eye (a normal pupillary response). **D:** Light first projected into the right eye causes constriction of both pupils. On swinging the light to the left eye, the pupils continue to dilate rather than constrict (a relative afferent pupillary defect of the left eye, also known as a Marcus Gunn pupil). (From Foroozan R, Bailey RS. Essentials of the ophthalmologic examination. In: Maus M, Jeffers JB, Holleran DK, eds. *The clinics atlas of office procedures: essentials of ophthalmology.* Philadelphia: WB Saunders; 2000, with permission.)

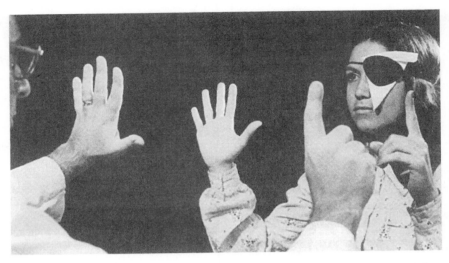

Figure 12-2. Testing visual fields. The examiner holds each hand at one arm's length from the patient. The patient's left eye is occluded, and the patient is then asked to count the number of fingers presented in the superior portion of the visual field. This should then be repeated in the inferior portion of the visual field. Alternatively, each quadrant of the visual field can be tested separately. (From Skarf B, Glaser JS, Trick GL, et al. Neuro-ophthalmologic examination: the visual sensory system. In: Glaser JS, ed. *Neuro-Ophthalmology*. 3rd ed. Philadelphia: Lippincott Williams & Wilkins; 1999.)

and those with BRAOs tend to have better final visual acuities (86). Funduscopy reveals retinal whitening (a marker of ischemia) in the area of obstruction (Fig. 12-3), which may enhance the darker appearance of the fovea ("cherry red spot"), as well as attenuation of the retinal arterioles and, occasionally, stagnant arterial blood flow ("box-carring") (11). Patients with a cilioretinal artery, which has a separate blood supply than the central retinal artery, may have sparing of the macula with preserved visual acuity. The most common type of ocular arterial obstruction, CRAO, is thought to be caused by emboli, thrombosis, vasculitis, arterial spasm, and trauma. The most common visual field defect is a central scotoma followed by generalized peripheral constriction (33).

Patients with retinal vascular arterial occlusions most commonly have vasculopathic risk factors (e.g., hypertension and diabetes), and an increase in mortality from cardiac disease and stroke has been documented in patients with visible retinal arterial emboli (43,71). The evaluation of patients with retinal arterial occlusions remains controversial, but many authors suggest carotid ultrasonography and echocardiography as screening tests (73). It is important to assess elderly patients with retinal vascular occlusions for signs and symptoms of GCA because this inflammatory disorder has been estimated to account for 1% of central retinal arterial occlusions. Hence, a careful funduscopic examination should document the presence of arterial emboli (Fig. 12-4), which would largely exclude GCA as a cause of arterial occlusion.

An improvement in visual outcome has been noted in anecdotal reports of CRAO with intra-arterial thrombolytic therapy, hyperbaric oxygen, ocular massage, and anterior chamber paracentesis but only early in the course (within the first 1 to 2 hours of symptoms) (68). Despite the many treatments that have been proposed for patients presenting acutely with retinal arterial occlusions, no therapy has shown a

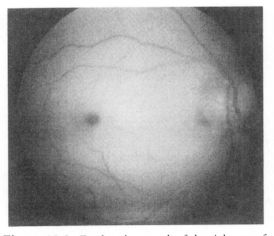

Figure 12-3. Fundus photograph of the right eye of a patient with a central retinal arterial occlusion shows pallor within the macula and a cherry red spot. (Courtesy of the Resident Slide Collection of the Wills Eye Hospital.)

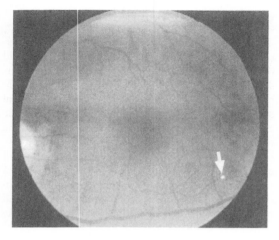

Figure 12-4. Fundus photograph of the left eye of a patient with a retinal embolus (*arrow*). (Courtesy of the Resident Slide Collection of the Wills Eye Hospital.)

definitive benefit when compared with observation. The European Assessment Group for Lysis in the Eye (EAGLE) study is an ongoing prospective, randomized, multicenter study started in 2002 that is currently evaluating visual acuity 1 month after CRAO. Patients are being randomized to either a conservative treatment arm [including ocular massage and lowering intraocular pressure (IOP) with eye drops] or intra-arterial tissue-type plasminogen activator (tPA) within 20 hours of vision loss (21).

AMAUROSIS FUGAX

Amaurosis fugax, or a temporary loss of vision, is thought to occur from a transient occlusion of the ophthalmic circulation and is a known risk factor for acute stroke. Patients often report a dimming of the vision that lasts 10 to 20 minutes before resolution. Funduscopic findings are most commonly normal but can reveal evidence of prior retinal arterial emboli or arterial attenuation, which is an associated finding of hypertension. Elderly patients with amaurosis fugax should have carotid ultrasonography and cardiac echography in an attempt to find a source for the embolic phenomena (6).

Amaurosis fugax was one of the three symptoms evaluated in the North American Symptomatic Carotid Endarterectomy Trial (NASCET). Patients with carotid stenosis of 70% to 99% by ultrasonography who had endarterectomy had a reduced risk of subsequent stroke (9%) compared with those treated medically (26%) 2 years after treatment (58). A retrospective analysis of the NASCET trial found that patients with amaurosis fugax who had at least three of the following characteristics had a significant

benefit from carotid endarterectomy: age >75 years old, history of hemispheric transient ischemic attack (TIA) or stroke, history of intermittent calf claudication, male sex, ipsilateral internal carotid artery stenosis of 80% to 94%, and no collaterals see on cerebral angiography (5). In the absence of visible emboli, patients with amaurosis fugax should be evaluated for GCA with an erythrocyte sedimentation rate (ESR) and C-reactive protein (CRP) because elderly patients with this disorder can present with transient episodes of visual loss.

RETINAL VENOUS OBSTRUCTIONS

Acute painless loss of vision occurs with central retinal vein occlusion (CRVO). Risk factors for CRVO include hypertension, diabetes mellitus, and glaucoma (14). Funduscopy reveals hemorrhagic optic disc swelling, with diffuse surrounding retinal hemorrhages and dilated and tortuous retinal veins (Fig. 12-5). Exudate and subretinal fluid within the macula—the most important prognostic factors in patients presenting with vein occlusions—are chiefly responsible for the decrease in vision at presentation. Bilateral vein occlusions are atypical and should prompt a hematologic assessment for severe anemia, hypertension, thrombocytopenia, and other blood dyscrasias.

Patients with CRVO typically have visual acuities of 20/40 or worse. Ophthalmologic follow-up is essential because as many as 30% of patients with CRVO can develop neovascularization of the iris,

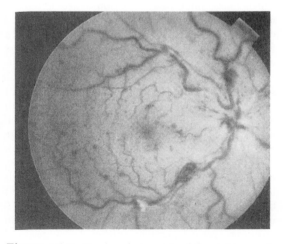

Figure 12-5. Fundus photograph of the right eye of a patient with a central retinal vein occlusion shows hemorrhagic optic disc swelling, dilated and tortuous retinal veins, and scattered intraretinal hemorrhages. (Courtesy of the Resident Slide Collection of the Wills Eye Hospital.)

leading to an aggressive form of glaucoma, which requires retinal laser photocoagulation (15).

OCULAR ISCHEMIC SYNDROME

Similar fundus findings as seen in patients with CRVO can occur in patients with carotid occlusive disease. A 90% or greater occlusion of the carotid artery can lead to chronic ipsilateral diffuse retinal hemorrhages, mostly in the midperipheral retina, and dilated retinal veins in the ocular ischemic syndrome (OIS) (10). Patients often complain of photophobia, ocular pain, and decreased visual acuity with bright light because the hypoxia caused by carotid insufficiency is believed to cause impairment in photoreceptor metabolism, which is accentuated in bright light. Patients can have mild corneal edema and inflammation within the anterior chamber that can cause the eye to appear red from conjunctival injection. OIS is distinguished from CRVO by its chronic course, absence of optic nerve swelling, and absence of tortuous retinal veins. Patients with OIS should have close ophthalmologic follow-up because chronic hypoxia of the retina predisposes to neovascularization of the iris and can cause neovascular glaucoma (51).

ACQUIRED RETINAL DEGENERATION

Retinal dysfunction can occur in cases of cancer-associated retinopathy (CAR, or MAR for melanoma-associated retinopathy). This is a paraneoplastic syndrome caused by antibodies to retinal elements, which causes photopsia (sensation of seeing lights), nyctalopia (difficulty seeing at night), and constricted visual fields associated with retinal degeneration (42). Patients may present with sudden or subacute painless vision loss. Serum autoantibodies against retinal proteins (such as recoverin and alpha-enolase) may be seen in patients with CAR, and autoantibodies against rod bipolar cells may be seen in MAR. Patients with MAR typically already have a history of melanoma, whereas CAR usually precedes the diagnosis of the causative malignancy (usually small-cell lung cancer). No abnormality may be seen during funduscopy, especially early on in the disorder, and electrophysiologic studies with ERG may be required to document the reduced photoreceptor amplitudes. Several months later, patients may develop attenuated retinal arterioles, retinal pigment epithelial changes, and mild optic disc pallor. Intravenous methylprednisolone and plasmapheresis have been shown in some case reports to be associated with variable improvements in visual acuity, color vision, and visual fields (16).

OPTIC NEUROPATHY

The causes of optic neuropathy are extensive; however, optic nerve dysfunction, including RAPD, visual field defect, acquired color vision deficit (dyschromatopsia), and impaired contrast sensitivity, is invariably present. The onset, duration, and progression of visual symptoms will help differentiate acute from chronic causes of optic nerve dysfunction. Funduscopy in optic neuropathy often shows optic disc swelling acutely; over time, however, all causes of optic neuropathy will cause the optic nerve to appear pale. In many cases (e.g., traumatic optic neuropathy and neuropathy from compressive lesions), disc swelling may not be noted because the site of pathology lies posterior to the optic nerve head.

OPTIC DISC SWELLING (DISC EDEMA)

The presence of bilateral disc edema requires immediate attention. Associated retinal hemorrhages and cotton wool spots, including cotton wool spots of the optic nerve, are suggestive of hypertensive retinopathy. Central nervous system tumors can cause bilateral disc swelling secondary to increased intracranial pressure. Thus, patients with bilateral disc edema should have their blood pressure taken, and neuroimaging should be performed emergently to exclude a compressive lesion (see Fig. 12-6 for assessment of the elderly patient with optic disc swelling).

Unilateral disc swelling in elderly patients most commonly results from anterior ischemic optic neuropathy (AION). Nonarteritic ischemic optic neuropathy (NAION) occurs most commonly in vasculopathic patients in the fifth and sixth decades. Patients with NAION have an abrupt onset of painless visual loss (with visual acuities typically in the 20/60 to 20/200 range), often in the early morning hours, and an altitudinal visual field defect (36). Disc swelling, thought to be secondary to vascular insufficiency of the short posterior ciliary circulation that supplies the optic nerve head, is most often hyperemic and may be sectoral with splinter nerve fiber layer (NFL) hemorrhages. Examination of the uninvolved eye often reveals a small optic cup, suggesting a "disc at risk" for ischemia and crowding of the retinal blood vessels (19). Because NAION has only rarely been associated with embolic phenomena, carotid and cardiac ultrasonography are not indicated in the evaluation of patients with typical NAION. Some risk factors for NAION have been identified, including diabetes mellitus, hypertension, smoking, and nocturnal hypotension. In patients with NAION, the risk of infarction of the fellow optic nerve over 5 years is approximately 15% (57). The risk for ipsilat-

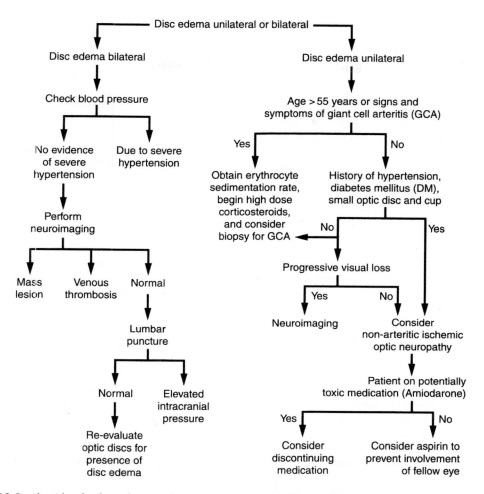

Figure 12-6. Algorithm for the evaluation of common causes of optic disc swelling in the elderly.

eral recurrence is quite small, at approximately 6% (30). Although some patients with NAION may have an improvement in visual acuity over the ensuing months, most will be left with a significant visual deficit. Inferior altitudinal and inferior nasal defects are the most common field cuts associated with NAION (33). No medical or surgical therapy has shown consistent benefit for patients with NAION. Some authors have suggested that aspirin may prevent infarction of the fellow eye (4), but long-term benefit has not been proven.

A number of patients using the antiarrhythmic amiodarone have been noted to have disc swelling that is virtually indistinguishable from that caused by NAION (49,56,61). However, patients in some of these cases have shown a more progressive visual deficit and bilateral involvement, which are uncommon in NAION. Amiodarone also causes crystalline deposits within the superficial cornea, in a whorl-like

fashion, that are not visually disabling. Because the progression of visual loss has been halted in some patients after discontinuing this agent, patients on amiodarone with what appears to be NAION should be carefully observed for progression and fellow eye involvement (8). Patients should not discontinue amiodarone without first consulting their cardiologist (55).

Recently, there have been reports in the medical literature of an association between NAION and the use of erectile dysfunction medications, such as sildenafil, tadalafil, and vardenafil (81). It is unclear whether there is a causal relationship because some of the patients using erectile dysfunction medications have some vascular risk factors that are also associated with NAION, such as diabetes, hypertension, and hypercholesterolemia.

Patients with diabetes mellitus, often with poorly controlled blood sugar levels, may present with hyperemic disc swelling and mild visual dysfunction (sometimes without visual complaints), which are consistent with diabetic papillopathy (65). The disc swelling and visual deficit will typically resolve weeks to months after the onset of symptoms.

AION from GCA occurs most commonly in patients in their sixth through eighth decades (mean age, 75 years), and women are affected more commonly than men. GCA is more common in whites and people from Northern Europe and is quite rare in African-Americans and Asians (63). Acute visual loss may occur after a history of brief episodes of transient visual loss. Visual acuities and visual field defects in AION caused by GCA are more commonly worse than those in patients with NAION. The disc edema of GCA is often noted to be "chalky white" in appearance because of the diffuse pallid swelling (Fig. 12-7). A history of headache, scalp tenderness, jaw claudication, fever, malaise, decreased appetite, weight loss, and symptoms of polymyalgia rheumatica should be sought (23). Other causes of vision loss from GCA include branch and CRAO and posterior ischemic optic neuropathy (PION). In addition to optic neuropathy from AION, other cranial nerves can be affected in GCA, and diplopia, facial nerve palsy, and facial pain have been noted.

Patients suspected of having GCA should have ESR and CRP drawn and be placed on corticosteroids without delay to prevent visual loss in the fellow eye; visual loss in the affected eye is typically irreversible. Although most patients with GCA will have an elevated ESR (estimates of up to 24% of biopsy-proved cases may not), those patients suspected of having GCA should have biopsy of the superficial temporal artery to confirm the diagnosis. An elevated CRP level may be helpful in suspicious cases with a normal ESR, and bilateral biopsy should be considered in cases with a high clinical suspicion because skip lesions can lead to a false-negative biopsy result. The variables with the highest positive predictive value for a positive temporal artery biopsy are jaw claudication, scalp tenderness, new headache, and vision loss (85). Most patients require high doses of corticosteroids (prednisone, 60 to 100 mg) for at least 6 months to 1 year. Attempts to taper steroid therapy should be very gradual, with close monitoring of visual function, ESR, and CRP.

Despite the differences outlined above, the disc swelling from NAION can be difficult to distinguish from that caused by GCA, and ESR and CRP studies are warranted in all patients >55 years with optic disc edema thought to be caused by ischemic optic neuropathy.

Optic nerve tumors (e.g., malignant optic gliomas and meningiomas) can cause optic disc swelling; however, more commonly, optic atrophy is present with these lesions. Patients may present with findings suggestive of an acute optic neuropathy without evidence of optic disc swelling, the so-called "posterior ischemic optic neuropathy" (PION) thought to be caused by ischemia of the retrobulbar circulation of the optic nerve (35). The average age of patients with PION is 52 years old (12). Optic neuropathy from PION has been noted after acute ischemic states, such as after cardiac bypass or spine surgery, and in patients with GCA. PION is a rare complication of spinal surgery and has been associated with spinal surgeries with blood loss of more than 1 L and anesthesia duration over 6 hours. Usually the vision loss is bilateral and severe (47). Patients suspected of having PION, without a history of an acute ischemic event, should have an ESR and CRP drawn to rule out GCA (31). Electrophysiologic testing showing a normal ERG and absent VEP is suggestive of PION and can help confirm the diagnosis.

A rare cause of vision loss in patients with cancer is paraneoplastic optic neuropathy. The vision loss is typically acute to subacute and painless. Patients may have associated neurologic signs such as chorea, ataxia, peripheral neuropathy, and dementia. Funduscopy shows bilateral optic disk swelling. Autoantibodies against collapsing response-mediating protein-5 (CRMP-5) are commonly found and are predominantly associated with small cell lung cancer (16).

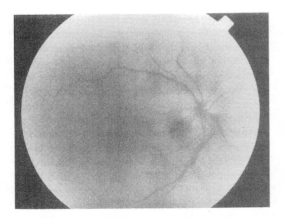

Figure 12-7. Fundus photograph of the right eye of a patient with arteritic AION from GCA shows pale swelling of the optic nerve head. (Courtesy of the Resident Slide Collection of the Wills Eye Hospital.) AION, anterior ischemic optic neuropathy; GCA, giant cell arteritis.

OPTIC ATROPHY

GLAUCOMA

Glaucomatous optic atrophy is characterized by optic nerve cupping and elevated intraocular pressure (IOP) in the presence of visual field defects. It is estimated that 1% to 2% of the population has glaucoma, and 50% are thought to be unaware of the diagnosis (62). Hence, a screening fundus examination is paramount to the diagnosis. Elevated IOP, the only known modifiable risk factor, is not present in all cases of glaucomatous optic neuropathy. Typically, involvement is bilateral, but it can be asymmetric. Older age is an important risk factor for glaucomatous optic atrophy, and a family history of glaucoma is frequently present in first-degree relatives. Optic atrophy in glaucoma is typically associated with disc pallor within the area of cupping (Fig. 12-8), but pallor that appears to be out of proportion to the degree of cupping should prompt further investigation (2). Visual loss in glaucoma is most often progressive, with loss of the peripheral visual field occurring before loss of central fixation. It is often difficult to make a diagnosis solely on one encounter because IOP can fluctuate, and close follow-up with quantitative visual field testing is important.

Although open angle glaucoma accounts for more than 90% of all patients with glaucoma in the United States, angle closure glaucoma can result in diffuse conjunctival injection, ocular pain, nausea, and vomiting from an extreme rise in IOP (2). However, some cases of chronic angle closure may not manifest these more acute findings and will require ophthalmologic examination to reveal the cause of visual dysfunction.

OPTIC NERVE MENINGIOMAS

Meningiomas of the sphenoid wing and, less commonly, the optic nerve cause progressive visual loss, optic disc pallor, and sometimes optic disc venous collaterals or "shunt vessels" (20). Meningiomas are most commonly found in middle-aged and elderly women, and an external examination may reveal a mass within the temporal fossa. Although surgery is often recom-

mended for external compression, radiation is very helpful, particularly for optic nerve sheath meningiomas. More than half of patients treated with stereotactic fractionated radiotherapy will show some improvement in their vision within 3 months (50,53).

OTHER CAUSES OF OPTIC ATROPHY

The finding of unexplained optic atrophy requires investigation. A family history of visual loss may suggest a hereditary optic neuropathy, and a remote history of trauma may suggest traumatic optic neuropathy. Patients with a history of alcohol abuse and smokers are at risk for developing a form of toxic optic neuropathy characterized by visual field defects that involve fixation and the blind spot (cecocentral scotomas) (66). In addition, a dietary history should be obtained because many of these patients are deficient in the essential B vitamins. A long list of medications is associated with optic neuropathy, which can first present acutely with disc swelling and show progressive disc pallor.

It is important to assess potentially treatable conditions that can cause unexplained optic atrophy; hence, neuroimaging with attention to the optic nerves is recommended. In addition, testing for syphilis, sarcoidosis, Lyme disease, and nutritional deficiency (vitamin B_{12} and folate) should be considered.

OPTIC CHIASM AND OPTIC TRACTS

Vascular insufficiency and mass lesions most frequently cause disorders of the optic chiasm and optic tracts. Involvement of the optic chiasm or tracts causes similar signs and symptoms, as found in patients with optic neuropathy, but because of decussation of the nasal retinal ganglion cells, these more posterior lesions cause binocular visual field defects.

Pituitary adenomas are the most common cause of chiasmal dysfunction and, as these tumors enlarge

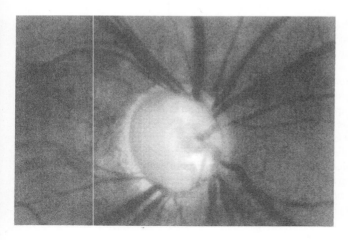

Figure 12-8. Fundus photograph of a patient with advanced glaucomatous optic disc cupping, with loss of the neuroretinal rim. (Courtesy of the Resident Slide Collection of the Wills Eye Hospital.)

superiorly, involvement of the chiasm progresses. Visual acuity may be normal, and the only finding may be a bitemporal visual field defect because of the involvement of the crossing nasal fibers of each optic nerve. However, progression of the lesion will cause optic neuropathy and decreased vision, which can occur acutely if the tumor hemorrhages, as in pituitary apoplexy. Chronic compression of the optic chiasm will result in optic neuropathy, which can be bilateral. Hemorrhage of enlarging pituitary adenomas can cause compression within the cavernous sinus and multiple cranial nerve palsies. Pituitary apoplexy is an ophthalmic, endocrinologic, and neurosurgical emergency because infarction can lead to both acute cortisol insufficiency, requiring intravenous corticosteroids, and blindness from chiasmal compression (25). Other lesions that can cause chiasmal dysfunction include craniopharyngiomas (a second peak of incidence occurs in the elderly), meningiomas, and arterial aneurysms.

Lesions of the optic tract result in homonymous hemianopsia because they contain ipsilateral temporal retinal fibers and contralateral nasal retinal fibers. In addition, there can be a contralateral RAPD with optic tract lesions. The cause of optic tract lesions is similar to that of chiasmal lesions, and long-standing lesions result in optic atrophy.

POSTERIOR AFFERENT PATHWAY

Unilateral involvement of the lateral geniculate nucleus (LGN), optic radiations, and occipital cortex, most commonly from cerebrovascular disease, results in binocular visual field defects without affecting visual acuity. In general, the more posterior the lesion, the more congruous the visual field defect, although this point is controversial (67).

Patients with homonymous hemianopsias from parietal lobe disease may have an associated disturbance of higher cortical function (e.g., agnosia, alexia, and dyscalculia). Visual loss from bilateral occipital disease results in a visual deficit with normal pupillary responses (67). Patients with cortical visual loss may not be aware of their deficit (Anton's syndrome) and claim that they can see, in the absence of dementia or delirium.

Bilateral involvement of the mesial anterior and mesial occipital lobes will result in cerebral dyschromatopsia, most commonly with an associated superior visual field defect. Loss of facial recognition, prosopagnosia, is also thought to be caused by disorders of the medial occipitotemporal cortex. Cortical disconnection syndromes (e.g., alexia without agraphia), in which the patient can write but cannot read because of involvement of the splenium of the corpus callosum and the dominant occipital cortex, demonstrate the complexity of higher cortical function.

Visual hallucinations associated with visual deficits (Charles Bonnet syndrome) have been well described, especially in the elderly. These hallucinations are commonly formed and occur in a lucid state, with patients commonly aware that what they are "seeing" is really not there. Most hallucinations are well tolerated, especially with reassurance (76). The most common cause of Charles Bonnet syndrome is macular degeneration.

Patients with neurodegenerative disorders may present with visual complaints, despite normal visual acuity and a normal ocular examination. Disturbances can include visual blurring, difficulty reaching for objects, and impaired depth perception. However, these rarely occur in isolation and are often associated with other disorders of higher cortical function. Late in the course, these patients may develop visual hallucinations (67).

EFFERENT VISUAL SYSTEM

ASSESSMENT OF OCULAR ALIGNMENT AND EXTRAOCULAR MOTILITY

To assess ocular alignment and extraocular motility, the patient should fixate at a distant object, while the examiner occludes one eye. If the uncovered eye turns to achieve fixation, this implies that the eye was not previously in alignment. If the refixation movement is in the nasal direction, then the eye was initially temporal and the deviation is known as an "exodeviation." If the refixation movement is in the temporal direction, an esodeviation is present. Prisms can be used to quantitate the angle of deviation.

The actions of the six extraocular muscles (Table 12-1) should be tested by instructing the patient to look in the direction of the muscle's greatest action. Each muscle and its yoke-pair act to move the eyes in the same direction of gaze. In right gaze, for example, the right lateral rectus muscle abducts the right eye, while the left medial rectus muscle adducts the left eye.

DIPLOPIA

Patients with diplopia often report perceiving two images of a single object, with the image of the more dominant eye being clearer than that of the fellow eye. However, diplopia from a small ocular misalignment can produce blurred images as the brain attempts to fuse the two images. Hence, the evaluation of unexplained visual blurring should also assess the ocular motor system.

In evaluating a patient with diplopia, establish whether the symptoms occur under monocular or binocular conditions. Diplopia that persists despite occlusion of the fellow eye is, with rare exception,

Table 12-1. *Primary Functions of the Extraocular Muscles*

Muscle	Function	Innervation
Lateral rectus	Abduction	VI cranial nerve
Medial rectus	Adduction	III cranial nerve
Superior rectus	Elevation	III cranial nerve
Inferior rectus	Depression	III cranial nerve
Superior oblique	Intorsion	IV cranial nerve
Inferior oblique	Extorsion	III cranial nerve

secondary to an ocular media disturbance (e.g., corneal irregularity, cataract, subluxed lens). Patients with monocular diplopia often report that they see blurred, multiple, or "ghost" images rather than two distinct images, and a pinhole (2 to 3 mm in diameter) placed in front of the eye will often eliminate the blurred images.

Diplopia that is relieved with occlusion of one eye is suggestive of an ocular misalignment. By quantifying the deviation in primary gaze (straight gaze), in left, right, up, and down gaze, and on head tilt to the right and left, the examiner can determine whether the deviation is comitant (the same or similar in each position of gaze) or incomitant (different, depending on gaze direction) (54).

THIRD NERVE PALSY

The oculomotor nerve is composed of parasympathetic fibers from the Edinger-Westphal nucleus and fibers of the subnuclei of motor neurons to each of the extraocular muscles. The nuclear centers for the third cranial nerve are in the midbrain, at the level of the red nuclei. The oculomotor nerves run anteriorly in the midbrain, adjacent to the cerebral peduncles, and into the subarachnoid space to lie between the superior cerebellar and the posterior cerebral arteries (26). The third nerve then courses into the wall of the cavernous sinus and enters the superior orbital fissure, branching into superior (supplying the levator palpebrae superioris and superior rectus muscles) and inferior (supplying the inferior oblique, inferior rectus, and medial rectus muscles, and the parasympathetic fibers to the ciliary ganglion, which innervate the iris sphincter) divisions. In addition to the iris sphincter, the ciliary ganglion also innervates the ciliary muscle, which stimulates accommodation of the lens. Only isolated third nerve palsy (TNP) will be discussed here, and any patient with evidence of dysfunction of more than a single cranial nerve requires further investigation. Patients with TNP may complain of pain, horizontal diplopia (in cases of incomplete ptosis), or ptosis (26).

Nuclear and fascicular lesions, which frequently have accompanying neurologic signs [contralateral tremor from involvement of the red nuclei (Benedikt syndrome), contralateral hemiparesis from involvement of the cerebral peduncles (Weber syndrome), and contralateral ataxia from involvement of the superior cerebellar peduncle (Nothnagel syndrome)], are most commonly caused by ischemic injury. Because of the anatomy of the third nerve nucleus, an isolated unilateral complete TNP is unlikely to be from a nuclear lesion.

In the subarachnoid space, the third nerve is vulnerable to mass lesions, the most common being cerebral arterial aneurysms. Because the parasympathetic fibers course in the periphery of the nerve, compressive lesions causing complete TNP involve the pupil in addition to the extraocular muscles. However, in incomplete TNP, the pupil may not be affected initially; hence, these patients should be followed daily for at least 1 week to confirm that the pupil does not dilate.

Vascular insufficiency is the most common cause of TNP in the elderly, with most patients having a history of diabetes mellitus or hypertension. GCA rarely causes TNP, and elderly patients with diplopia should be questioned for symptoms of GCA. Because the pupillary fibers course in the periphery of the nerve, collateral blood flow is thought to spare the parasympathetic fibers in cases of vascular TNP. Despite this, pupillary dysfunction indistinguishable from that caused by mass lesions can still occur in vascular TNP; thus, any patient with TNP who has pupillary involvement should have a neuroimaging study with magnetic resonance imaging (MRI) and magnetic resonance angiography (MRA), computed tomography angiography (CTA), or routine angiography. The role of MRA or CTA versus routine angiography is controversial; however, angiography is currently the standard because smaller aneurysms capable of causing a TNP may rarely be missed with MRA or CTA.

Vascular TNP typically improves within 2 to 4 months after the onset of symptoms; thus, patients suspected of having a vascular TNP should have a neuroimaging study if progression of the TNP is noted or the symptoms fail to improve.

Lesions within the cavernous sinus, superior orbital fissure, and orbit rarely cause isolated TNP because of involvement of the surrounding structures. However, both isolated superior and inferior division TNPs do occur. Because it is rare for the muscles innervated by the oculomotor nerve to be involved singly and in isolation, other conditions such as thyroid eye disease and MG should be considered in these cases.

Aberrant regeneration, an anomalous rewiring of damaged neurons, can occur months after the onset of TNP from compressive lesions. Neuronal misdirection can result in abnormal movements such as eyelid elevation on downgaze and pupillary constriction with adduction. Because this neuronal miswiring occurs almost exclusively with compressive lesions, patients followed for presumed vascular TNP should have a neuroimaging study if aberrant regeneration is noted.

FOURTH NERVE PALSY

The fourth nerve nuclei, which lie caudal to the third nerve nuclei within the midbrain, send crossed fibers that exit dorsally from the brainstem (26). These fibers run anteriorly to enter the wall of the cavernous sinus and then through the superior orbital fissure to innervate the superior oblique muscle. Trauma, in which patients often have bilateral involvement, and ischemic injury are the most common causes of fourth nerve paresis.

Patients with fourth nerve palsies typically complain of vertical diplopia because the superior oblique muscle acts to infraduct the eye, and they may adopt a compensatory head tilt, which can diminish the vertical deviation. The superior rectus and superior oblique muscles act to intort the eye (rotate the 12 o'clock meridian inward, toward the patient's nose), whereas the inferior rectus and oblique muscles act to extort the eye. Thus, fourth nerve palsies will result in extorsion as well as supraduction of the affected eye. The diagnosis should be made using the three-step test for vertical diplopia described elsewhere (26). Bilateral fourth nerve palsies characteristically will have a right hypertropia on right gaze, left hypertropia on left gaze, V pattern esotropia, and excyclotorsion of the eyes greater than 10 degrees.

Vasculopathic patients with isolated acquired fourth nerve palsies may be observed (see earlier discussion of TNP). If the fourth nerve palsy is progressive or if symptoms do not improve after several months, neuroimaging should be performed.

SIXTH NERVE PALSY

The sixth cranial nerves arise in the pons and exit the brainstem anteriorly to rise up the clivus (where the two nerves are closest together) and pierce the dura at the Dorello canal, which bridges the petrous portion of the temporal bone (26). The sixth nerve travels in the cavernous sinus under the internal carotid artery (where it can be compressed by an aneurysm of the carotid artery) and anteriorly to enter the superior orbital fissure and innervate the lateral rectus muscle. Patients with sixth nerve palsies will present with esotropia, which increases with gaze toward the affected side. Patients may adopt a head turn toward the involved side to put the affected eye in an adducted position and minimize the diplopia.

Within the brainstem, the sixth nerve nucleus lies adjacent to the horizontal gaze center and has neurons destined for the contralateral medial rectus subnucleus, so that a nuclear sixth lesion, most commonly from ischemia, will produce an ipsilateral gaze palsy. Fascicular lesions involving the pyramidal tract can cause an ipsilateral abduction deficit, ipsilateral facial weakness, and contralateral hemiplegia (Millard-Gubler syndrome).

At the Dorello canal, the sixth nerve is vulnerable to compressive forces that are generated with increased intracranial pressure. Thus, any cause of increased intracranial pressure, including central nervous system masses and venous sinus thrombosis, can cause unilateral or bilateral sixth nerve palsies. Inflammation of the petrous portion of the temporal bone can affect the sixth nerve (Gradenigo syndrome), and inflammation of the adjacent fifth nerve ganglion can cause a painful sixth nerve palsy. Within the cavernous sinus, superior orbital fissure, and orbit, the sixth nerve is rarely affected in isolation.

As with isolated third and fourth nerve palsy, vasculopathic patients with sixth nerve palsy initially may be observed. All elderly patients should be questioned regarding signs and symptoms of GCA because sixth nerve palsy has rarely been a presenting manifestation of this disorder. Ischemic sixth nerve palsies usually completely resolve, but up to one third of patients may later have a recurrent ocular motor nerve palsy (70).

THYROID EYE DISEASE

Thyroid eye disease is the most frequent cause of acquired diplopia that is not secondary to extraocular muscle palsy (72). It occurs more frequently in women than men, and although thyroid function testing is abnormal in most cases, patients with thyroid eye disease can be hyperthyroid, hypothyroid, or euthyroid. Furthermore, systemic treatment of thyroid dysfunction may have little or no change on the signs and symptoms of thyroid eye disease. The pathogenesis for this disorder remains unknown, but the clinical manifestations are well recognized.

Patients present with painless proptosis (thyroid eye disease is the most common cause of unilateral or bilateral proptosis in adults), eyelid retraction (in part because of sympathetic stimulation of the Müller's muscle in the upper and lower eyelids) causing the thyroid

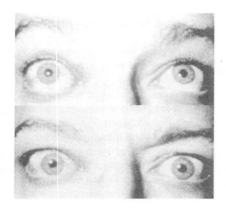

Figure 12-9. Composite external photographs of a patient with thyroid eye disease show restriction in upgaze (*top*), proptosis with bilateral eyelid retraction (*bottom*), and conjunctival injection over the insertion of the right lateral rectus muscle (*both*). (Courtesy of the Resident Slide Collection of the Wills Eye Hospital.)

Enlargement of the extraocular muscles can result in compression of the optic nerve at the orbital apex and subsequent visual loss with associated visual field defects. Lid and periorbital swelling may be noted, and examination of the conjunctiva may reveal chemosis (edema of the conjunctiva) and engorged vessels over the insertions of the extraocular muscles. The proptosis can lead to vision-threatening corneal exposure from inadequate eyelid closure. Corneal exposure should be managed with lubricant ointments and can rarely require surgical therapy.

Smoking has been associated with an increased risk of thyroid eye disease in patients with thyroid dysfunction and in a worsening of ocular symptoms in patients with pre-existing thyroid eye disease (9). Some studies suggest that treatment with radioactive iodine, without concurrent steroid treatment, has an adverse effect on thyroid eye disease (64). Systemic corticosteroids can be used for patients who have acute exacerbations of thyroid eye disease. Patients who respond will typically do so within the first several weeks of therapy, and thus, prolonged courses with steroids should be avoided. Low-dose orbital radiation (20 Gy) is controversial (27) but may cause involution of active inflammation; however, acute congestion with optic neuropathy sometimes requires surgical orbital decompression to relieve crowding of the orbital apex.

"stare," eyelid lag in downgaze, and disturbances in ocular motility (Fig. 12-9). Involvement of the inferior rectus muscle is most common, followed by the medial rectus, superior rectus, and lateral rectus muscles. Thus, limitation in upgaze is the most common abnormality of ocular motility, although nearly any pattern of abnormal extraocular motility can be seen. Orbital imaging with computed tomography (CT) scan or MRI shows enlargement of the extraocular muscles with sparing of the muscle tendons, including in asymptomatic patients with thyroid eye disease (78).

The differential diagnosis of thyroid eye disease (Table 12-2) should include idiopathic orbital pseudotumor, which is an orbital inflammatory disorder of unknown cause that can present with proptosis, ocular pain, and injection that mimics orbital cellulitis

Table 12-2. *Differential Diagnosis of Common Orbital Diseases of the Elderly*

	Thyroid Eye Disease	Orbital Pseudotumor	Orbital Infection	Arteriovenous Fistula
Ocular signs and symptoms	Proptosis, corneal exposure, eyelid lag, eyelid retraction, rarely visual loss, diplopia	Proptosis, pain, conjunctival injection, rarely visual loss, eyelid swelling, and erythema	Ophthalmoplegia, visual loss, eyelid swelling, and erythema	Proptosis, injection, elevated intraocular pressure, pulsatile tinnitus
Orbital imaging	Enlargement of extraocular muscles sparing tendons	Enlargement of extraocular muscles, including tendons, enlargement of lacrimal gland, inflammation of orbital fat	Contiguous sinus disease, involvement of cavernous sinus	Enlargement of extraocular muscles, dilated superior ophthalmic vein
Systemic findings	History of thyroid disease, may be euthyroid	Occasional association with collagen vascular disease	Fever, immunosuppression (especially diabetes mellitus)	Hypertension

(17). Orbital imaging shows inflammatory signs of the involved tissue (lacrimal gland, orbital fat, or extraocular muscles) and, in the case of extraocular muscle involvement, involvement of the tendinous insertion. Findings that help differentiate this inflammatory disorder from infection typically include the lack of fever, neutrophilia, and other systemic symptoms. Patients with orbital pseudotumor show dramatic improvement with corticosteroid therapy.

Immunosuppressed patients with ophthalmoplegia, especially diabetics, should be evaluated for fungal infections. Invasive fungal infections, such as those caused by mucormycosis, can cause progressive ophthalmoplegia with invasion of the cavernous sinus that is life threatening, even in the absence of obvious ocular inflammatory signs (22). An otolaryngologic consultation to assess the nasal and sinus mucosa may reveal the characteristic black mucosal eschar.

Elderly patients, especially women, are at risk for developing spontaneous, low-flow, dural-venous fistulas that result in proptosis, mild ocular discomfort, and conjunctival injection (80). These low-flow fistulae, which most commonly occur from the communication between small meningeal arteries and the cavernous sinus, can cause pulsatile tinnitus. Impaired venous return from orbital congestion can cause elevated IOP. Angiography with embolization can close these fistulas, although many will close spontaneously.

MYASTHENIA GRAVIS

MG is a disorder of the voluntary muscles that commonly involves the face, limb girdle, extraocular muscles, and eyelids. Antibodies to the acetylcholine receptors found on striated muscle endplates are responsible for impaired synaptic transmission, which worsens with prolonged stimulation. Although many patients will have systemic involvement, up to 75% of them will present with only ocular involvement (84).

The earliest signs of MG may be ptosis and ophthalmoplegia. The ptosis is often worse at the end of the day and improves with rest. The ice test (a surgical glove filled with ice and placed over the eyelids for 2 minutes) frequently improves the ptosis caused by MG (45). The ophthalmoplegia of MG can involve any of the extraocular muscles and produce any pattern of strabismus; however, MG does not cause clinical pupillary dysfunction. Sustained upgaze can be tested to fatigue the extraocular muscles and eyelids and elicit an ocular deviation or ptosis that may not be apparent during the initial assessment. Testing orbicularis oculi strength may reveal impairment of voluntary eyelid closure.

Although the diagnosis of MG is primarily a clinical one, several tests can aid the clinician, especially in atypical cases. Intravenous injection of edrophonium (Tensilon), a short-acting antiacetylcholinesterase agent, can improve the signs of MG within minutes after infusion (Fig. 12-10). Side effects of Tensilon include bradycardia and bronchospasm, which are potentially lethal in the elderly; hence, some are reluctant to perform Tensilon testing in an office setting. Antiacetylcholine receptor antibodies, which are found in 80% to 90% of patients with generalized MG, are seen in 50% to 60% of patients with isolated ocular myasthenia (82). Nerve conduction studies with repetitive stimulation show an abnormal decrement in approximately 70% of patients with ocular MG. Single-fiber electromyography of the orbicularis oculi muscle demonstrates impaired impulses, which are seen in at least 90% of ocular MG (59). Because thymomas occur in 10% of patients with MG, a CT scan of the mediastinum should be performed.

Although anticholinesterase agents have been the mainstay for treatment of MG, ocular myasthenia often does not respond adequately to the typical doses used for systemic MG. Corticosteroids can ease the diplopia in some patients and may reduce the risk of progression to generalized MG but not without the risk of steroid-induced side effects (40). Immunosuppressive agents (e.g., azathioprine and cyclosporine) can be considered in patients who do not respond to pyridostigmine or prednisone.

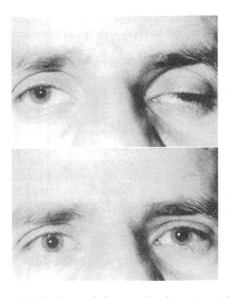

Figure 12-10. External photographs of a patient with left upper eyelid ptosis from myasthenia gravis before edrophonium (Tensilon) (*top*) injection and improvement of ptosis after injection of Tensilon (*bottom*). (Courtesy of the Resident Slide Collection of the Wills Eye Hospital.)

DISORDERS OF GAZE

DORSAL MIDBRAIN SYNDROME
The dorsal midbrain syndrome consists of deficiency of upgaze, poorly reactive pupils that show light-near dissociation, and convergence-retraction movements with attempted upgaze. Most commonly, this occurs with mass lesions in the area of the dorsal midbrain (48).

PROGRESSIVE SUPRANUCLEAR PALSY
Progressive supranuclear palsy is a progressive disorder of vertical gaze that typically begins with impaired downgaze greater than upgaze, prompting many patients to note an inability to see food at mealtime and difficulty walking down steps (48). The supranuclear origin of this disorder implies that the brainstem-mediated reflexes (e.g., the oculovestibular reflex) are intact. Saccadic eye movements are affected more commonly than smooth pursuit, and patients may have a parkinsonian gait and rigidity, especially of the neck.

VERTICAL OCULAR DEVIATIONS
Rapid downward movements of the eyes followed by a slower return are seen in ocular bobbing, most commonly from pontine lesions (18). Damage within the brainstem, most commonly from ischemic insults, results in slow, pendular vertical eye movements that appear to be rhythmic with movements of the palate in oculopalatal myoclonus. A skew deviation is an acquired vertical deviation (often comitant) due to a deficit within the vestibulocerebellar pathways and cannot be ascribed to dysfunction of a single cranial nerve or extraocular muscle (48). Skew deviation causes vertical diplopia, which often results from ischemic insults within the posterior fossa.

INTERNUCLEAR OPHTHALMOPLEGIA
Internuclear ophthalmoplegia (INO) results from disruption of the medial longitudinal fasciculus (MLF), which ascends from the sixth nerve nucleus to the contralateral medial rectus subnucleus within the brainstem (29). Ischemic stroke is the most common cause of INO in the elderly. Interruption of the MLF results in an ipsilateral adduction deficit, and the fellow eye will often show a jerk nystagmus that increases with abduction.

CONVERGENCE INSUFFICIENCY
The area responsible for convergence lies within the midbrain. Patients with convergence insufficiency may have diplopia or blurring of near vision, with the ability to fuse at distance (74). Examination will reveal fusion at distance but an exodeviation near, despite the presence of normal extraocular motility. Patients with this finding should have a neuroimaging study to exclude a midbrain lesion.

DIVERGENCE INSUFFICIENCY
Divergence insufficiency results in a symptomatic comitant esodeviation at distance with fusion at near vision. The patients have a full and normal extraocular motility exam. It is a nonlocalizing cause of diplopia that, in the elderly, often results from pontine ischemia, although the center for divergence in the brain is unknown (48). If the patient has no other neurologic abnormalities, the likelihood of finding a lesion on brain MRI or head CT is quite low, and the diplopia may resolve spontaneously after several months (37).

NYSTAGMUS

Nystagmus is an oscillatory movement of the globes characterized by a rhythmic to-and-fro movement caused by a breakdown in fusional or gaze mechanisms (18). It is categorized as "pendular" if the movements are of equal velocity in each direction and "jerk" if the movements are slow in one direction and fast in another. The direction of nystagmus is defined as the direction of the fast phase. Other descriptive features (e.g., amplitude, frequency, velocity, and axis of rotation) are used clinically to characterize the different forms of nystagmus.

Patients with acquired nystagmus often complain of oscillopsia, a visual shaking, and blurred vision; to minimize their symptoms, patients may hold their head in a position (the null point) that minimizes the nystagmus. Either pendular or jerk nystagmus can be seen in patients with poor visual acuity of long-standing duration.

GAZE-EVOKED NYSTAGMUS
Gaze-evoked nystagmus is a jerk nystagmus that occurs in the affected direction but not in primary gaze. This type of nystagmus is nonlocalizing but often occurs from medications (e.g., ethanol, sedatives, illicit drugs) or lesions within the posterior fossa (18). Poor cerebellar control is thought to contribute to impairment of the ability to hold the eyes in eccentric gaze.

PERIODIC ALTERNATING NYSTAGMUS
Periodic alternating nystagmus (PAN) is a horizontal jerk nystagmus that is intermittent, lasting 1 to 2 minutes before spontaneously reversing (18). Lesions of the cervicomedullary junction or cerebellum often cause this type of nystagmus. Treatment with baclofen has been successful in some of these patients.

CONVERGENCE-RETRACTION NYSTAGMUS

Convergence-retraction nystagmus is characteristic of the dorsal midbrain syndrome that consists of light-near dissociation and impaired upgaze (18). This eye movement, although not true nystagmus, is best elicited by downward rotation of a vertical optokinetic stimulus, which produces fast upward reflexive saccades. Instead of the normal reflexive upward movement, the globes retract, and the palpebral fissures narrow.

SEE-SAW NYSTAGMUS

Parachiasmal and upper midbrain lesions rarely result in a dissociated nystagmus in which one eye rises and intorts, while the other eye falls and extorts, similar to a see-saw (18).

DOWNBEAT NYSTAGMUS

Downbeat nystagmus is a jerk nystagmus, with the fast phase downward, that increases in downgaze (18). Patients are particularly bothered when reading because of the increase in intensity on downgaze. Disorders of the cervicomedullary junction (especially the Arnold-Chiari malformation), drug intoxication, magnesium deficiency, vitamin deficiency, lithium toxicity, cerebellar degeneration, and ischemic stroke have all caused this form of nystagmus.

OPSOCLONUS

Opsoclonus is a random movement of the eyes that can be intermittent or constant. The rapid saccadic movements are in all directions and appear chaotic, without an identifiable pattern. Opsoclonus can be a marker of an underlying malignancy, most commonly a paraneoplastic syndrome, or can occur after viral encephalitis (34).

ANISOCORIA AND PUPILLARY DYSFUNCTION

Anisocoria is a difference in pupillary size (diameter), and a difference in pupillary diameters of 1 mm or greater is generally accepted as clinically significant (41). To establish which eye is abnormal, measure the pupil size in light and then in dark, and record the pupillary diameters. Disparity in pupil size that remains the same in light and dark is characteristic of physiologic anisocoria. To avoid the miosis that occurs with the near response, examine the pupils while the patient views a distant object.

Disparity in pupil size that increases in dark is characteristic of Horner's syndrome, with the miotic pupil failing to dilate appropriately. The presence of Horner's syndrome can be confirmed by looking for delayed dilation of the miotic pupil with darkness (dilation lag). Pharmacologic testing with 4% to 10% cocaine in each eye will fail to dilate the miotic pupil normally in a patient with Horner's syndrome. Cocaine availability may be limited to most clinicians, and there are some studies suggesting that apraclonidine 0.5% drops can be used as an alternative test. Apraclonidine is an alpha-adrenergic sympathomimetic that dilates the supersensitive denervated miotic pupil but does not dilate the normal pupil (44). Hydroxyamphetamine drops can localize (preganglionic vs. postganglionic; see below) the Horner's syndrome.

Disparity in pupil size that is greater in light is generally from one of four causes: iris trauma, Adie's pupil, TNP, or pharmacologic dilation. Pupils that are abnormally large in light may show irregularities along the pupillary border or evidence of prior surgery, which can impair constriction to light.

An Adie's pupil (tonic pupil) is an irregularly dilated pupil that shows minimal reaction to light and is slow to constrict with convergence (41). With slit lamp examination, sectoral constriction of the pupil may be seen, with one portion of the iris showing undulating movements. Most commonly, it occurs in women and is unilateral. Because the Adie's pupil is thought to occur from neuronal denervation, the iris demonstrates supersensitivity and constricts with 0.125% pilocarpine drops. Systemic findings can occur with decreased deep tendon reflexes (Adie's syndrome), and further evaluation rarely may be necessary because the tonic pupil has been seen in patients with syphilis and Lyme disease.

The pupillary dilation of TNP rarely occurs in the absence of other signs of third nerve dysfunction. However, in cases requiring confirmation of pupillary involvement, 1% pilocarpine instilled into the affected eye will constrict the pupil, whereas 0.125% pilocarpine generally will not (41), although supersensitivity has been described in some cases of TNP. Pharmacologic dilation, whether knowingly self-induced or accidental, will not typically respond to 1% pilocarpine, and the pupil will remain dilated.

LIGHT-NEAR DISSOCIATION

Light-near dissociation occurs when the pupils fail to react to light but constrict with convergence. Historically, this finding was associated with tertiary syphilis (Argyll Robertson pupils), but it can be seen in diabetics, TNP with aberrant regeneration, bilateral optic nerve disease, dorsal midbrain syndrome, central nervous system lesions, and Adie's pupils (75).

HORNER'S SYNDROME

Horner's syndrome results from a disturbance in the sympathetic pathway, which contains three neurons.

The first neuron begins in the hypothalamus and descends to synapse in the cervical and superior thoracic spinal cord. The second neuron, with its cell body within the spinal cord, ascends to synapse in the superior cervical ganglion in the region of the angle of the mandible. The third neuron, with its body in the superior cervical ganglion, ascends with the carotid artery, through the cavernous sinus and orbital fissures, to innervate the dilator muscle of the iris via the long ciliary nerves.

Patients with Horner's syndrome may present because of ptosis or miosis or may be diagnosed on screening examination (Fig. 12-11). Ptosis of the upper eyelid caused by Horner's syndrome is rarely greater than 2 mm and occurs because of interruption of the sympathetic pathway to the Müller's muscle. The miosis and resultant pupil disparity that occur in Horner's syndrome are more apparent in dark than in light.

The causes of Horner's syndrome vary depending on which neuron is involved (41). The most common cause of first-order Horner's syndrome in the elderly is vascular insufficiency in the brainstem, and often patients will have other neurologic signs and symptoms. Lung masses are the most common cause of second-order lesions because the apex of the lung rests adjacent to the pathway of the fibers headed to the superior cervical ganglion. Third-order Horner's syndrome is frequently associated with headache syndromes (e.g., cluster headaches and migraine), cavernous sinus lesions, and internal carotid dissection.

Determining the order of the lesion in Horner's syndrome can be achieved by pharmacologic testing. Hydroxyamphetamine (1%), which stimulates the sympathetic nerve terminals to release norepinephrine, causes pupillary dilation in first- and second-order

Horner's syndrome. Third-order lesions involve the adrenergic nerve endings, which are responsible for the release of norepinephrine; hence, the pupil in these lesions will not dilate with hydroxyamphetamine. It is important to note that testing with cocaine and hydroxyamphetamine should be separated by 24 hours.

An important cause of third-order Horner's syndrome is internal carotid dissection. Although a history of trauma is often elicited, spontaneous dissection or exertion from the Valsalva maneuver or repetitive coughing can lead to disruption of the sympathetic chain. Patients may complain of head and neck pain, dysgeusia, pulsatile tinnitus, and transient visual loss. These patients require immediate attention with MRI and MRA of the neck and brain to identify the intraluminal flap characteristic of carotid dissection because, within 6 days of symptom onset, 30% of patients with internal carotid dissection will have a stroke, which may be prevented by anticoagulation (7).

NEURO-OPHTHALMIC DISORDERS OF THE EYELID AND FACE

BLEPHAROPTOSIS (PTOSIS)

Blepharoptosis (ptosis) is the term used when the upper eyelid margin hangs lower than its normal position. The upper eyelid normally covers the superior sclera completely, with the margin of the eyelid lying between the limbus superiorly and the superior pupillary margin. The lower lid margin rests just at the inferior limbus.

Causes of acquired ptosis are divided into the following categories: mechanical, aponeurotic, neurogenic, and myogenic. Mechanical ptosis arises from a compression of the upper lid, most commonly from mass lesions, scarring, and redundant skin folds. Obvious mass lesions can often be palpated through the eyelid skin. Lifting redundant eyelid skin may reveal a normal upper lid margin and eyelid function. Aponeurotic ptosis results from a dehiscence of the tendon of the levator muscle from the superior tarsus.

The most important causes of neurogenic ptosis are from TNP and Horner's syndrome. Complete TNP results in complete ptosis from involvement of the nerve to the levator; hence, levator function is impaired, but the position of the lid crease is normal. Thus, patients with TNP may not complain of diplopia because of occlusion of the involved visual axis. Incomplete TNP often results in incomplete ptosis, which is typically greater than 1 to 2 mm. Ptosis in Horner's syndrome occurs because of dysfunction of the Müller's muscle, resulting in a mild neurogenic ptosis (1 to 2 mm). Myogenic ptosis most frequently occurs from MG. A less common cause of myogenic ptosis is chronic progressive external ophthalmoplegia

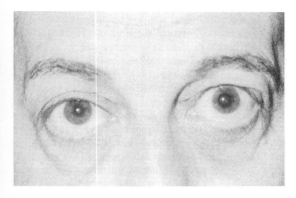

Figure 12-11. External photograph of a patient with Horner's syndrome on the right shows miosis of the right pupil and mild ptosis of the right upper eyelid. (Courtesy of the Resident Slide Collection of the Wills Eye Hospital.)

(CPEO), which results from a mitochondrial abnormality. Patients present with progressive ophthalmoplegia and ptosis, which are typically bilateral. Patients with CPEO can have an associated retinal pigmentary degeneration and cardiac conduction defects (Kearns-Sayre syndrome) (52).

TRIGEMINAL NEURALGIA

Rapid attacks of sharp, jabbing pain (lasting seconds) within the distribution of the trigeminal nerve are characteristic of trigeminal neuralgia (79). The onset is most common in the sixth and seventh decades, occurring more commonly in women than men. In some cases, an aberrant vessel is believed to compress the fifth nerve sensory root as it enters the pons, although multiple sclerosis (especially if bilateral) and tumors are other causes. Carbamazepine and baclofen have been used successfully in many patients, although some require surgical intervention, such as microvascular decompression, percutaneous rhizotomy, or stereotactic radiosurgery.

BELL'S PALSY

Bell's palsy is the most common cause of facial nerve dysfunction, with an increasing incidence with age. Although the pathophysiology of Bell's palsy is unknown, antecedent viral illnesses (including that from herpes zoster and simplex), diabetes mellitus, and thyroid dysfunction are predisposing factors.

Signs and symptoms develop over hours to days, with unilateral facial weakness, impaired eyelid closure, and tearing. Evaluation of patients with Bell's palsy should exclude central nervous system involvement or evidence of other cranial nerve palsies, which require neuroimaging. Other secondary causes of facial dysfunction include Lyme disease, sarcoidosis, HIV infection, Sjögren syndrome, and amyloidosis. Examination of the ear, tongue, and oral mucosa should exclude vesicular eruptions due to herpes zoster virus (Ramsay Hunt syndrome).

Ocular involvement should be assessed by testing orbicularis oculi strength, looking for lagophthalmos (inability to achieve full eyelid closure), and testing of the Bell's phenomenon (reflexive rotation of the globes superiorly with forced eyelid closure). Each of these tests will aid in determining the risk of corneal exposure.

Although 80% to 90% of patients with Bell's palsy will have spontaneous recovery, improvement of facial nerve function is most often incomplete, and elderly patients have a poorer prognosis (60). Aberrant regeneration of the facial nerve can lead to abnormal facial muscle activity with movement of the mouth or excessive tearing with mastication (crocodile tears).

Corticosteroids have had a beneficial effect on the recovery of some patients with Bell's palsy. Because cases of Bell's palsy have been associated with herpes virus infections, acyclovir may be considered in these patients as well (1,24,28). Patients at risk for corneal exposure can be treated with topical lubricants, eyelid taping, and moisture chambers. Some patients may require surgical intervention with tarsorrhaphy and implanted eyelid weights to achieve eyelid closure and preserve corneal integrity.

BENIGN ESSENTIAL BLEPHAROSPASM

Benign essential blepharospasm (BEB) is a repetitive, bilateral contraction of the facial musculature, most commonly affecting the orbicularis oculi and periocular muscles. BEB occurs more commonly in women and rarely under the age of 50. Frequently, the duration and frequency of contractions increase as the disorder progresses, and complete eyelid closure can lead to a functional impairment of vision in some patients.

Examination of the ocular surface for irritants, signs of dry eye syndrome (e.g., keratopathy or poor tear film), and ocular inflammation is necessary because each of these disorders can cause a repetitive eyelid closure that mimics essential blepharospasm.

Treatment with local intramuscular injections of botulinum toxin (BTX), which interrupts release of acetylcholine from the nerve terminals, has been shown to be effective in reducing the contractions in essential blepharospasm (39). In most patients, the effect lasts 3 to 6 months, with the need for further injections as the treatment effect wanes. Although local effects (e.g., ptosis, diplopia, and ecchymosis) can occur, reports of systemic toxicity from BTX are rare. Extensive myectomy (Anderson procedure) for patients unresponsive to BTX has been reported in some centers (39).

HEMIFACIAL SPASM

Repetitive, unilateral facial contractions are characteristic of hemifacial spasm. As with essential blepharospasm, the contractions, which can be localized, can progressively involve the entire side of the face (Fig. 12-12). Some patients with hemifacial spasm may have an aberrant course of a small artery that compresses the facial nerve, whereas other cases have been rarely associated with tumors of the parotid gland and cerebellopontine angle. Therefore, neuroimaging of the course of the facial nerve should be performed. Treatment with BTX (see previous section) has been effective; however, some patients have undergone surgical microvascular decompression of the facial nerve at the skull base (Jannetta procedure) (38). Eighty-four to 92% of patients are reported to be symptom free after microvascular decompression surgery for hemifacial spasm. The most common side effect of the procedure is ipsilateral deafness (2% to 8%) (3,69).

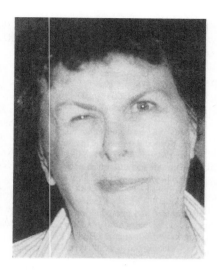

Figure 12-12. External photograph of a patient with hemifacial spasm shows involuntary contraction of the musculature of the right side of the face. (Courtesy of the Resident Slide Collection of the Wills Eye Hospital.)

EYELID MYOKYMIA

Eyelid myokymia, which is characterized by a fine, intermittent quivering movement of the eyelids, is generally a benign condition associated with stress, fatigue, and nicotine or caffeine use; however, some pontine lesions (gliomas) can cause progressive myokymia that typically involves the platysma and other facial muscles (83).

REFERENCES

1. Adour KK, Ruboyianes JM, Von Doersten PG, et al. Bell's palsy treatment with acyclovir and prednisone compared with prednisone alone: a double-blind randomized controlled trial. *Ann Otol Rhinol Laryngol.* 1996;105:371–378.
2. American Academy of Ophthalmology. *Basic and Clinical Science Course: Section 10. Glaucoma.* San Francisco: American Academy of Ophthalmology; 2007–2008.
3. Barker FG, Jannetta PG, Bissonette DJ, et al. Microvascular decompression for hemifacial spasm. *J Neurosurg.* 1995;82:201–210.
4. Beck RW, Hayreh SS, Podhajsky PA, et al. Aspirin in nonarteritic anterior ischemic optic neuropathy. *Am J Ophthalmol.* 1997;123:212–217.
5. Benavente O, Eliasziw M, Steifler JY, et al. Prognosis after transient monocular blindness associated with carotid artery stenosis. *N Engl J Med.* 2001;345:1084–1090.
6. Biousse V. Carotid disease and the eye. *Curr Opin Ophthalmol.* 1997;8:16–26.
7. Biousse V, Touboul PJ, D'Anglejan-Chatillon J, et al. Ophthalmologic manifestations of internal carotid artery dissection. *Am J Ophthalmol.* 1998; 126:565–577.
8. Brazis PW, Lee AG. Neuro-ophthalmic problems caused by medications. *Focal Points.* 1998; 16:1–14.
9. Brix TH, Hansen PS, Kyvik KO, et al. Cigarette smoking and risk of clinically overt thyroid disease. *Arch Intern Med.* 2000;160:661–666.
10. Brown GC, Green WR. The ocular ischemic syndrome. *Curr Opin Ophthalmol.* 1994;5:14–20.
11. Brown GC, Magargal LE. Central retinal artery obstruction and visual acuity. *Ophthalmology.* 1982;89:14–19.
12. Buono LM, Foroozan R. Perioperative posterior ischemic optic neuropathy: review of the literature. *Surv Ophthalmol.* 2005;50:15–26.
13. Carr RE, Siegel IM. *Visual Electrodiagnostic Testing: A Practical Guide for the Clinician.* 2nd ed. Baltimore: Williams & Wilkins; 1990.
14. Central Vein Occlusion Study Group. Baseline and early natural history report. The central vein occlusion study. *Arch Ophthalmol.* 1993; 111:1087–1095.
15. Central Vein Occlusion Study Group. Natural history and clinical management of central retinal vein occlusion. *Arch Ophthalmol.* 1997;115:486–491.
16. Chan, JW. Paraneoplastic retinopathies and optic neuropathies. *Surv Ophthalmol.* 2003;48:12–38.
17. Chavis RM, Garner A, Wright JE. Inflammatory orbital pseudotumor. A clinicopathologic study. *Arch Ophthalmol.* 1978;96:1817–1822.
18. Dell'Osso LF, Daroff RB. Nystagmus and saccadic intrusions and oscillations. In: Glaser JS, ed. *Neuro-Ophthalmology.* 3rd ed. Philadelphia: Lippincott Williams & Wilkins; 1999:369–401.
19. Doro S, Lessell S. Cup-disc ratio and ischemic optic neuropathy. *Arch Ophthalmol.* 1985;103: 1143–1144.
20. Dutton JJ. Optic nerve sheath meningiomas. *Surv Ophthalmol.* 1992;37:167–183.
21. Feltgen N, Neubauer A, Jurklies B, et al. Multicenter Study of the European Assessment Group for Lysis in the Eye (EAGLE) for the treatment of central retinal artery occlusion: design issues and implications. EAGLE Study report no. 1. *Graefes Arch Clin Exp Ophthalmol.* 2006;244:950–956.
22. Ferry AP, Abedi S. Diagnosis and management of rhino-orbitocerebral mucormycosis (phycomycosis). A report of 16 personally observed cases. *Ophthalmology.* 1983;90:1096–1104.
23. Ghanchi FD, Dutton GN. Current concepts in giant cell (temporal) arteritis. *Surv Ophthalmol.* 1997;42:99–123.

24. Gilden DH. Bell's palsy. *N Engl J Med*. 2004; 351:1323–1331.

25. Glaser JS. Topical diagnosis: the optic chiasm. In: Glaser JS, ed. *Neuro-Ophthalmology*. 3rd ed. Philadelphia: Lippincott Williams & Wilkins; 1999:199–238.

26. Glaser JS, Siatkowski M. Infranuclear disorders of eye movement. In: Glaser JS, ed. *Neuro-Ophthalmology*. 3rd ed. Philadelphia: Lippincott Williams & Wilkins; 1999:405–460.

27. Gorman CA, Garrity JA, Fatourechi V, et al. A prospective, randomized, double-blind, placebo-controlled study of orbital radiotherapy for Grave's ophthalmopathy. *Ophthalmology*. 2001; 108:1523–1534.

28. Grogan PM, Gronseth GS. Practice parameter: steroids, acyclovir, and surgery for Bell's palsy (an evidence-based review). *Neurology*. 2001;56: 830–836.

29. Hamilton SR. Neuro-ophthalmology of eye-movement disorders. *Curr Opin Ophthalmol*. 1999;10:405–410.

30. Hayreh SS, Podhajsky PA, Zimmerman B. Ipsilateral recurrence of nonarteritic anterior ischemic optic neuropathy. *Am J Ophthalmol*. 2001;132:734–742.

31. Hayreh SS, Podhajsky PA, Zimmerman B. Ocular manifestations of giant cell arteritis. *Am J Ophthalmol*. 1998;125:509–520.

32. Hayreh SS, Zimmerman MB. Central retinal artery occlusion: visual outcome. *Am J Ophthalmol*. 2005;140:376–391.

33. Hayreh SS, Zimmerman B. Visual field abnormalities in nonarteritic anterior ischemic optic neuropathy. *Arch Ophthalmol*. 2005;123:1554–1562.

34. Herishanu Y, Apte R, Kuperman O. Immunological abnormalities in opsoclonus cerebellopathy. *Neuro-Ophthalmol*. 1985;5:271–276.

35. Isayama Y, Takahashi T, Inoue M, et al. Posterior ischemic optic neuropathy. Clinical diagnosis. *Ophthalmologica*. 1983;187:141–147.

36. Ischemic Optic Neuropathy Decompression Trial Study Group. Characteristics of patients with nonarteritic anterior ischemic optic neuropathy eligible for the Ischemic Optic Neuropathy Decompression Trial. *Arch Ophthalmol*. 1996; 114:1366–1374.

37. Jacobson DM. Divergence insufficiency revisited: natural history of idiopathic cases and neurologic associations. *Arch Ophthalmol*. 2000;118:1237–1241.

38. Jannetta PT, Abbasy M, Marion JC. Etiology and definitive microsurgical treatment of hemifacial spasm: operative techniques and results in 47 patients. *J Neurosurg*. 1977;47:321–328.

39. Jordan DR, Patrinely JR, Anderson RL, et al. Essential blepharospasm and related dystonias. *Surv Ophthalmol*. 1989;34:123–132.

40. Kaminski HJ, Daroff RB. Treatment of ocular myasthenia. Steroids only when compelled. *Arch Neurol*. 2000;57:752–753.

41. Kawasaki A. Physiology, assessment, and disorders of the pupil. *Curr Opin Ophthalmol*. 1999; 10:394–400.

42. Keltner JL, Thirkill CE, Tyler NK, et al. Management and monitoring of cancer-associated retinopathy. *Arch Ophthalmol*. 1992;110:48–53.

43. Klein R, Klein BEK, Jensen SC, et al. Retinal emboli and stroke: the Beaver Dam eye study. *Arch Ophthalmol*. 1999;117:1063–1068.

44. Koc F, Kavuncu S, Kansu T, et al. The sensitivity and specificity of 0.5% apraclonidine in the diagnosis of oculosympathetic paresis. *Br J Ophthalmol*. 2005;89:1442–1444.

45. Kubis KC, Danesh-Meyer HV, Savino PJ, et al. The ice test versus the rest test in myasthenia gravis. *Ophthalmology*. 2000;107:1995–1998.

46. Lai TY, Chan WM, Lai RY, et al. The clinical applications of multifocal electroretinography: A systematic review. *Surv Ophthalmol*. 2007;52:61–96.

47. Lee LA, Roth S, Posner KL, et al. The American Society of Anesthesiologists Postoperative Visual Loss Registry. *Anesthesiology*. 2006;105:652–659.

48. Leigh JR, Daroff RB, Troost BT. Supranuclear disorders of eye movements. In: Glaser JS, ed. *Neuro-Ophthalmology*. 3rd ed. Philadelphia: Lippincott Williams & Wilkins; 1999:345–368.

49. Mantayjarvi M, Tuppurainen K, Ikaheimo K. Ocular side effects of amiodarone. *Surv Ophthalmol*. 1988;42:360–366.

50. Miller NR. New concepts in the diagnosis and management of optic nerve sheath meningioma. *J Neuroophthalmol*. 2006;26:200–208.

51. Mizener JB, Podhajsky P, Hayreh SS. Ocular ischemic syndrome. *Ophthalmology*. 1997;104: 859–864.

52. Moraes CT, DiMauro S, Zeviani M, et al. Mitochondrial DNA deletions in progressive external ophthalmoplegia and Kearns-Sayre syndrome. *N Engl J Med*. 1989;320:1293–1299.

53. Moster ML. Detection and treatment of optic nerve sheath meningioma. *Curr Neurol Neurosci Rep*. 2005;5:367–375.

54. Moster ML. Paresis of isolated and multiple cranial nerves and painful ophthalmoplegia. In: Yanoff M, Duker JS, eds. *Ophthalmology*. 3rd ed. St. Louis: Mosby; 2007.

55. Murphy MA, Murphy JF. Amiodarone and optic neuropathy: the heart of the matter. *J Neuroophthalmol*. 2005;25:232–236.

56. Nagra PK, Foroozan R, Savino PJ, et al. Amiodarone induced optic neuropathy. *Br J Ophthalmol*. 2003;87:420–422.

57. Newman NJ, Scherer R, Langenberg P, et al. The fellow eye in NAION: Report from the ischemic

optic neuropathy decompression trial follow-up study. *Am J Ophthalmol.* 2002;134:317–328.

58. North American Symptomatic Carotid Endarterectomy Trial Collaborators. Beneficial effect of carotid endarterectomy in symptomatic patients with high-grade carotid stenosis. *N Engl J Med.* 1991;325:445–453.

59. Padua L, Stalberg E, LoMonaco M, et al. SFEMG in ocular myasthenia gravis diagnosis. *Clin Neurophysiol.* 2000;111:1203–1207.

60. Peitersen E. The natural history of Bell's palsy. *Am J Otol.* 1982;4:107–111.

61. Purvin V, Kawasaki A, Borruat FX. Optic neuropathy in patients using amiodarone. *Arch Ophthalmol.* 2006;124:696–701.

62. Quality of Care Committee, Glaucoma Panel. *Primary Open-Angle Glaucoma. Preferred Practice Pattern.* San Francisco: American Academy of Ophthalmology; 1992.

63. Rahman W, Rahman FZ. Giant cell (temporal) arteritis: an overview and update. *Surv Ophthalmol.* 2005;50:415–428.

64. Rasmussen AK, Nygaard B, Feldt-Rasmussen U. (131)I and thyroid-associated ophthalmopathy. *Eur J Endocrinol.* 2000;143:155–160.

65. Regillo CD, Brown GC, Savino PJ, et al. Diabetic papillopathy: patient characteristics and fundus findings. *Arch Ophthalmol.* 1995;113:889–895.

66. Rizzo JF, Lessell S. Tobacco amblyopia. *Am J Ophthalmol.* 1993;116:84–87.

67. Rizzo M, Barton JJ. Retrochiasmal visual pathways and higher cortical function. In: Glaser JS, ed. *Neuro-Ophthalmology.* 3rd ed. Philadelphia: Lippincott Williams & Wilkins; 1999:239–291.

68. Rumelt S, Dorenboim Y, Rehany U. Aggressive systematic treatment for central retinal artery occlusion. *Am J Ophthalmol.* 1999;128:733–738.

69. Samii M, Günther T, Iaconetta G, et al. Microvascular decompression to treat hemifacial spasm: long-term results for a consecutive series of 143 patients. *Neurosurgery.* 2002;50:712–719.

70. Sanders SK, Kawasaki A, Purvin VA. Long-term prognosis in patients with vasculopathic sixth nerve palsy. *Am J Ophthalmol.* 2002;134:81–84.

71. Savino PJ, Glaser JS, Cassady J. Retinal stroke: is the patient at risk? *Arch Ophthalmol.* 1977;95:1185–1189.

72. Scott IU, Siatkowski MR. Thyroid eye disease. *Semin Ophthalmol.* 1999;14:52–61.

73. Sharma S. The systemic evaluation of acute retinal artery occlusion. *Curr Opin Ophthalmol.* 1998;9:1–5.

74. Siatkowski MR, Glaser JB. Pediatric neuro-ophthalmology. In: Glaser JS, ed. *Neuro-Ophthalmology.* 3rd ed. Philadelphia: Lippincott Williams & Wilkins; 1999:461–487.

75. Slamovits TL, Glaser JS. The pupils and accommodation. In: Glaser JS, ed. *Neuro-Ophthalmology.* 3rd ed. Philadelphia: Lippincott Williams & Wilkins; 1999:527–552.

76. Teunisse RJ, Cruysberg JRM, Verbeek A, et al. The Charles Bonnet syndrome: a large prospective study in the Netherlands. *Br J Psychiatry.* 1995;166:254–257.

77. Thompson HS, Corbett JJ, Cox TA. How to measure the relative afferent pupillary defect. *Surv Ophthalmol.* 1981;26:39–42.

78. Trokel SL, Hilal SK. Recognition and differential diagnosis of enlarged extraocular muscles in computed tomography. *Am J Ophthalmol.* 1979;87:503–512.

79. Troost BT. Migraine and other headaches. In: Glaser JS, ed. *Neuro-Ophthalmology.* 3rd ed. Philadelphia: Lippincott Williams & Wilkins; 1999:553–587.

80. Troost BT, Glaser JS, Morris PP. Aneurysms, arteriovenous communications, and related vascular malformations. In: Glaser JS, ed. *Neuro-Ophthalmology.* 3rd ed. Philadelphia: Lippincott Williams & Wilkins; 1999:589–628.

81. United States Food and Drug Administration. Alert for healthcare professionals: Sildenafil citrate. 2005. Available at: http://www.fda.gov/cder/drug/Infosheets/HCP/sildenafilHCP.htm.

82. Vincent A, Newsom-Davis J. Acetylcholine receptor antibody characteristics in myasthenia gravis. *Clin Exp Immunol.* 1982;49:266–272.

83. Waybright EA, Gutman L, Chou SM. Facial myokymia. Pathological features. *Arch Neurol.* 1979;36:244–245.

84. Weinberg DA, Lesser RL, Vollmer TL. Ocular myasthenia: a protean disorder. *Surv Ophthalmol.* 1994;39:169–210.

85. Younge BR, Cook BE, Bartley GB, et al. Initiation of glucocorticoid therapy: before or after temporal artery biopsy? *Mayo Clin Proc.* 2004;79:483–491.

86. Yuzurihara D, Iijima H. Visual outcome in central retinal and branch retinal artery occlusion. *Jpn J Ophthalmol.* 2004;48:490–492.

SUGGESTED READINGS

American Academy of Ophthalmology. *Basic and Clinical Science Course: Section 5. Neuro-Ophthalmology.* San Francisco: American Academy of Ophthalmology; 2007–2008.

Foroozan R, Bailey RS. Essentials of the ophthalmologic examination. In: Maus M, Jeffers JB, Holleran DK, eds. *The clinics atlas of office procedures: essentials of ophthalmology.* Philadelphia: WB Saunders; 2000.

Glaser JS. *Neuro-Ophthalmology*. 3rd ed. Philadelphia: Lippincott Williams & Wilkins; 1999.

Kunimoto DY, Kanitkar KD, Makar M, et al. *The Wills Eye Manual: Office and Emergency Room Diagnosis and Treatment of Eye Disease*. 4th ed. Philadelphia: Lippincott Williams & Wilkins; 2004.

Liu GT, Volpe NJ, Galetta SL. *Neuro-Ophthalmology: Diagnosis and Management*. New York: WB Saunders; 2000.

Miller NR, Newman NJ. *Walsh & Hoyt's Clinical Neuro-Ophthalmology*. 6th ed. Vol. 1–3. Baltimore: Lippincott Williams & Wilkins; 2005.

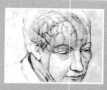

CHAPTER 13

Sleep in the Older Person

Alon Y. Avidan

By the year 2050, it is predicted that approximately one fifth of the population will be over 65 years of age. In 1900, only 4% of the population was over 65. This increase will have profound medical, economic, and psychosocial consequences. Because sleep complaints increase with age, the medical community needs to educate itself on changes in sleep with age. This chapter describes those changes as well as the most common diagnoses and treatments of sleep disorders seen in the elderly patient with neurodegenerative disease.

Although the normal sleep architecture changes with age, with less time spent in the deeper levels of sleep, sleep disturbances in the older population are often multifactorial. The sleep disturbance may be due to a primary sleep disorder, such as obstructive sleep apnea (OSA), periodic limb movements of sleep (PLMS), or restless leg syndrome (RLS), or it may be secondary to circadian rhythm changes, medical problems, psychiatric conditions, polypharmacy, or psychosocial factors. Conversely, when sleep disorders become chronic, they may exacerbate medical and psychiatric illnesses. Chronic sleep disorders or associated excessive daytime sleepiness (EDS) may result in disturbed intellect, impaired cognition, confusion, psychomotor retardation, or increased risk of injury, any of which can alter an individual's quality of life or create social and economic burdens for caregivers.

SLEEP TESTS

Sleep is evaluated by recording electrical potentials from the brain [electroencephalography (EEG)], eye movements [electro-oculography (EOG)], muscle activity [electromyography (EMG)], heart rhythm [electrocardiogram (EKG)], body position (supine, left, right), oximetry, and respiratory activity (airflow, thoracic and abdominal excursion). Traditionally, sleep is generally recorded in the laboratory setting for one full night. This full night sleep recording is called a polysomnograph (PSG). It is a method of continuous and simultaneous recording of physiologic variables during sleep (249). It is indicated for the evaluation of patients suspected of having a sleep-related breathing disorder, unusual nocturnal spells, or unusual movements. A second recording, the Multiple Sleep Latency Test (MSLT) may be useful in quantitating the degree of sleepiness. This test measures an individual's ability to fall asleep when given four or five nap opportunities throughout an average day. The MSLT is done during the day, following a nocturnal polysomnogram (249).

When patients are first recorded in the sleep laboratory, their anxiety about sleeping in a new and unfamiliar environment may lead to a recording that is not representative of their usual sleep. This is called the first night effect (3). Recently, technical advances allow for these types of recordings to be done in the home. Patients are set up with instrumentation in the laboratory, sent home, and asked to come back the following day after spending the night in their own bed. These home recordings or unattended monitoring reduce the first night effect, reduce costs, increase comfort, and reduce the waiting time for a study in some cases.

SLEEP STAGING

Sleep is divided into two states: nonrapid eye movement (NREM) sleep and REM sleep. NREM and REM sleep alternate throughout the night in a cyclical pattern. NREM sleep is further subdivided into stages 1, 2, 3, and 4. NREM sleep progresses from stage 1 (light sleep) to slow-wave sleep (SWS) (stages 3 and 4). With this progression from stage 1 to 4, there is a relative increase in the depth of sleep and the threshold for spontaneous arousals. Stage 1 sleep is a transition between wakefulness and sleep. Its characteristics include low-voltage, mixed-frequency EEG and slow rolling eye movements. The signatures of stage 2 sleep include sleep spindles and K-complexes. SWS refers to stages 3 and 4 sleep. It is characterized by high-amplitude (75 μV), slow-frequency (delta) waves (62). REM sleep is very distinct from light and SWS and is characterized by increased sympathetic activity, rapid eye movements, dreaming, and an increase in the depth and rate of breathing. REM sleep is accompanied by a low-voltage, mixed-frequency EEG and reduction of the EMG tone (muscle atonia). This is when the most elaborate dreams emerge. A physiologic sleep paralysis manifested by low EMG tone on the polysomnogram protects the patient from acting out dreams.

AGE-RELATED CHANGES IN SLEEP

With aging, the amount of time spent in SWS decreases; thus, the time spent in lighter levels of sleep increases. The proportion of REM sleep is generally preserved. However, the latency to the first REM period decreases, and the overall amount of REM sleep may decrease as a result of an overall reduction in nocturnal sleep time. Older adults also take longer to initiate sleep. They have a reduced total sleep time, frequent awakenings, and early morning awakenings and are more likely to have diurnal naps (83,167).

The prevalence of napping in older adults ranges from 25% to 80% (200,263). Studies that have used the MSLT to evaluate sleepiness in older persons have shown that, given the opportunity, they tend to fall asleep during the day faster than younger patients (61). This daytime sleepiness suggests that the older adults are not getting sufficient sleep at night. This is interpreted to mean that the need for sleep in older adults is not reduced, but rather that the ability to sleep is changed (10).

Studies that have looked at gender differences in the sleep of healthy elderly have found that women sleep better than men (38) and maintain sleep better than men (203). Recent studies evaluating the effects of menopause on sleep have found associated subjective complaints of insomnia. Objectively, menopause was found to prolong sleep latency, reduce REM sleep, and reduce total sleep time. Treatment with estrogen replacement therapy may alleviate these problems (268).

CLINICAL HISTORY

The clinical evaluation of an elderly patient with a sleep complaint involves a multidisciplinary approach. First, the clinical approach begins with a careful history taking of the present and past sleep history, as well as a detailed history of specific sleep complaints. Family history is always important as well as social history, in particular regarding alcohol and caffeine intake. Questions regarding polypharmacy and particular use of psychiatric medications may be a key in the initial evaluation.

Important questions that need to be asked when obtaining the sleep history are as follows. This information is supplemented by having the patient keep a careful sleep diary for several weeks.

- *Do you have difficulty falling asleep?*
- *Do you feel that you are excessively sleepy?*
- *What is your sleep-wake schedule during the weekdays/weekends?*
- *How many hours do you sleep per night?*
- *How long does it take you to fall asleep after deciding to go to sleep?*
- *How many times do you wake up during a typical night?*
- *How long does it take you to "get going" after you get out of bed?*
- *Do you snore loudly or stop breathing at night?*
- *Do you have crawling or aching feelings in your legs when trying to fall asleep?*
- *Do you kick or twitch your arms or legs during sleep?*
- *Do you walk in your sleep?*
- *Do you act out your dreams?*

Questions regarding daytime behavior are also important, such as the general quality of sleep upon awakening, frequency of daytime napping, and propensity to fall asleep in unacceptable situations such as driving, during conversations, or while watching a movie. It is often crucial to interview the bed partner in addition to the patient to obtain information regarding the patient's sleep habits; daytime functioning; alcohol, tobacco, and caffeine use; snoring; recent changes in snoring intensity; apnea-like spells; nocturnal spells; morning headaches; confusion; and leg jerks. However, many older adults have no bed partners.

ASSESSMENT OF SLEEP DISORDERS IN THE OLDER PERSON

The polysomnogram is important in the assessment of specific sleep stage abnormalities, leg movements, unusual behaviors, and the presence of underlying sleep-related breathing disorders. The MSLT serves several functions. It is useful in an objective evaluation of sleepiness. It may also reveal narcolepsy, a very rare condition in the older person. The use of video PSG is especially important in the evaluation of parasomnias such as REM sleep behavior disorder (RBD). When patients are suspected of having RBD, it is helpful to place EMG leads on all four limbs during polysomnography.

SLEEP-RELATED BREATHING DISORDER

OBSTRUCTIVE SLEEP APNEA

Sleep-related breathing disorders are probably among the most serious of the sleep disorders. OSA is due to cessation of airflow caused by a complete or partial upper airway collapse at the level of the pharyngeal airways. Central sleep apnea (CSA) is due to cessation of both airflow and respiratory effort. Respiratory events are classified as either complete (apnea) or partial (hypopnea). The respiratory disturbance index (RDI) has been defined as the number of apneas and hypopneas per hour of sleep. At my center, an observation of at least five apneas and hypopneas per hour of sleep is thought to be consistent with a significant level of OSA. However, many older persons without symptoms meet these criteria, and whether they deserve treatment has not yet been well defined.

OSA is due to multiple factors that together can predispose an individual to develop collapse of the airways. Advanced age, neurologic and endocrine impairment, abnormal oral anatomy, obesity, and abnormal nocturnal respiratory reflexes can all contribute to the development of OSA (46,222).

OSA is more common in the older person compared to the young. In individuals >65 years of age, 24% have five or more apneas per hour of sleep, and 81% have >10 respiratory events per hour of sleep (21). A follow-up study from the same group examining a population of community-dwelling geriatric men and women found that those with severe OSA had a significantly shorter survival time on follow-up when compared to those with mild/moderate OSA or minimal/no OSA (19). OSA, however, was not a predictor of death, whereas cardiovascular disease and pulmonary disease were predictors.

Obesity is a central factor contributing to OSA. Although older patients are not as overweight as clinic patients, body mass index (BMI) is still the best predictor of whether an older individual will or will not have OSA (15,21). Elderly patients with OSA have significantly higher BMI compared with patients with minimal or no OSA, supporting the claim that obesity is a risk factor for OSA (19).

Excessive Daytime Sleepiness

EDS is a major symptom in patients with OSA. It is unclear whether the sleepiness is due to disruption of the sleep architecture caused by respiratory-related arousals, repeated episodes of hypoxemia, or factors not yet identified. The EDS may manifest itself as sleepiness during what might be considered inappropriate times. Patients with OSA with EDS report falling asleep while in conversations and while reading, watching television, and even driving.

EDS can also contribute to significant cognitive impairment. OSA is associated with difficulties with attention, memory decline, and concentrating during the day (43). Patients with OSA who experience nocturnal hypoxemia have been shown to possess reduced cognitive functioning (13). Treatment of the underlying sleep-disordered breathing may improve some of the cognitive deficiencies (84). Elderly patients with OSA have also been reported to be at risk for disturbed vigilance, impaired ability to rapidly solve complex problems, and impaired attention/concentration on formal testing of cognition when compared to subjects without OSA (42,102). Nocturnal hypoxemia may also contribute to fatal arrhythmia, hypertension, myocardial infarction, and stroke (223). Other consequences of OSA may include anoxia, cardiorespiratory failure, and ultimately death during sleep (19,24).

SNORING

Snoring may be a hallmark of a sleep-related breathing disorder. Snoring is often disruptive to the sleep of the bed partner who often is first to suspect that there is a problem. Snoring is due to an incomplete upper airway obstruction and is often associated with cardiovascular disease and hypertension (98). Snoring has been linked with hypertension. Research has shown that about one third of patients with hypertension have a sleep-related breathing disorder (12). Repeated or chronic nocturnal hypoxemia may result in impaired cerebral function and hypersomnolence (84).

TREATMENT OF OBSTRUCTIVE SLEEP APNEA

Continuous Positive Airway Pressure and Oral Appliances

Continuous positive airway pressure (CPAP) and sometimes bilevel positive airway pressure (BiPAP) are currently the main methods of treatment. Both work as a splint at the level of the upper airways to prevent their collapse (238,239). Surgery is often an alternative for those who are unable to tolerate CPAP or BiPAP, although it is effective only about 50% of the time. In the elderly, surgery should be considered only if there are no other medical problems that preclude it. Various oral appliances have been recently introduced for the management of mild/moderate OSA. These act by repositioning the mandible and tongue anteriorly (mandibular advancing device and tongue retaining device). The net effect is an improvement in the oropharyngeal airway space (34,156). Oral appliances would not be appropriate for older patients with dentures or for those who are missing a significant number of teeth.

Positional Therapy

Positional therapy may be appropriate for patients with mild OSA confined to supine sleep. Teaching patients to sleep in other positions may be accomplished by sewing a pocket with a tennis ball in the back portion of the pajamas or nightgowns (11).

Management of OSA in the Elderly

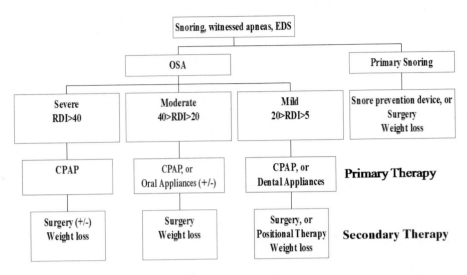

Figure 13-1. Algorithm: potential treatment of OSA in elderly patients. EDS, excessive daytime sleepiness; OSA, obstructive sleep apnea; RDI, respiratory disturbance index; CPAP, continuous positive airway pressure.

Medications

The role of medications such as tricyclic antidepressants, which may increase airway muscle tone and reduce apneas, is somewhat controversial in the elderly because of medication-related side effects and risks of polypharmacy. Previous findings report that medroxyprogesterone may be effective for patients with mild OSA (237).

Surgery

The treatment of OSA in the elderly poses a special problem. Since their sleep is lighter and more disrupted, many patients may not tolerate CPAP very well. Major surgical interventions for OSA, such as bimaxillary advancement, genioglossus advancement, and hyoid suspension, need to be considered with caution, especially if the patient has underlying cardiovascular disease.

Lifestyle

OSA may be potentiated or worsened by a variety of other factors. Many older patients who suffer from insomnia may "self-medicate" themselves with alcohol, which can exacerbate OSA (242). Sleeping in the supine position increases the respiratory disturbances (63). Medications such as benzodiazepines, barbiturates, and narcotics should be used with the utmost care as they may exacerbate respiratory disturbances and reduce a patient's ability to arouse when an apnea

occurs (12). Figure 13-1 outlines a possible algorithm for the management of OSA.

PERIODIC LIMB MOVEMENT DISORDER OF SLEEP

The hallmark of PLMS, also known as nocturnal myoclonus, is a repetitive and continuous leg jerk 0.5 to 5 seconds in duration typically occurring every 20 to 40 seconds during sleep and resulting in arousals (67). The polysomnographic diagnosis of PLMS is made when five or more of these movements are recorded per hour of sleep. Many patients with PLMS present to the clinician with nocturnal leg jerks associated with an uncomfortable sensation and urge to kick or move the involved limb (RLS). Moving the limb often dissipates the uncomfortable sensation. Patients may complain of a motor restlessness, difficulties initiating sleep, and multiple nocturnal awakenings, which result in hypersomnolence (68). Bed partners of patients with PLMS are often bothered by the leg jerks that may not bother the patients themselves. The polysomnogram is often the only reliable way to document the leg movements and thus to make the diagnosis.

RLS is often described as a "creeping" sensation in the lower extremities (41,260,261). This sensation is improved when patients move their legs but returns when the movement ceases. Patients with RLS often complain of difficulty falling asleep. The RLS may be

Table 13-1. *Medication Chart: Treatment of Restless Leg Syndrome (RLS) in the Older Adult*

Drug: Class (generic/brand)	Dose	Potential Side Effects
Iron:		
Ferrous Sulfate	325 mg bid/tid with vitamin C 100–200 mg; recommended for ferritin <45 µg/L	Gastrointestinal side effects: constipation
Dopamine Agonists:		
Pramipexole (Mirapex)[*]	0.125–1.5 mg, 1 hr before bedtime; start low and increase slowly	Sleep attacks, nausea, rare propensity for compulsive behavior (compulsive gambling)
Ropinirole (Requip)[*]	0.5–4 mg 1 hr before bedtime	
Dopaminergic Agents:		
Levodopa/Carbidopa (Sinemet)	25/200 mg; ½ tab–3 tabs 30 minutes before bedtime	Nausea, sleepiness, augmentation and rebound of daytime symptoms, insomnia, gastrointestinal disturbances
Anticonvulsants:		
Gabapentin (Neurontin)	300–2,700 mg/day divided tid	Daytime sleepiness, nausea
Clonidine:		
Catapres	0.1 mg bid; may be helpful in patients with hypertension	Dry mouth, drowsiness, constipation, sedation, weakness, depression (1%), hypotension
Opiates:		
Darvocet (Darvocet-N)	300 mg/day	Nausea, vomiting, restlessness, constipation; addiction, tolerance may be possible
Darvon (propoxyphene)	65–135 mg at bedtime	
Codeine	30 mg	

[*]Only FDA-indicated treatment for moderate-severe restless leg syndrome as of March, 2007.

exacerbated by rheumatoid arthritis, excessive caffeine intake, and iron deficiency. Most patients with RLS have PLMS. The converse, however, is not true. Polysomnography is not indicated for making the diagnosis of RLS.

It is estimated that between 5% and 6% of the population has PLMS. This disorder increases in frequency with older age. One study reported that 45% of older people may have this condition with no gender predilection (20). The diagnosis and treatment of this disorder is extremely important because it can lead to sleep initiation insomnia in the older person. It has been hypothesized that, since dopamine agonists and opiates improve the symptoms of RLS/PLMS, related transmitter systems may be involved in the pathogenesis of these conditions.

PLMS has traditionally been treated with benzodiazepines such as clonazepam or temazepam (171), levodopa/carbidopa (143), or opiates such as acetaminophen and codeine (144). More recently, dopamine agonists such as pramipexole and ropinirole have received approval from the Food and Drug Administration (FDA) for the specific treatment of RLS

(110,174,181,206). Table 13-1 outlines the current treatment approaches for patients with PLMS and RLS and possible side effects. Each pharmacologic modality has its advantages and disadvantages. As of today, the benefit-to-risk ratio is unresolved. Recently, iron has been implicated in playing a central role in the physiology of RLS. Iron deficiency can produce RLS symptoms, and iron replacement therapy results in improvement.

Many patients with OSA may also suffer from PLMS. It is prudent that careful analysis be made to determine whether OSA and PLMS coexist in the patient, since treatment of the underlying PLMS (with benzodiazepine) may worsen the OSA. Treatment of the sleep-related breathing disorder may improve or worsen the PLMS; further study of this possibility is needed.

INSOMNIA

Insomnia is the most common sleep complaint reported by older people. It is defined as the inability to either initiate or maintain sleep or as early morning awakening associated with disturbed daytime functioning (178). Older persons are likely to experience sleep maintenance insomnia (difficulty remaining asleep) and early morning awakening (waking early in the morning with the inability to reinitiate sleep). Epidemiologic data have shown a higher prevalence of insomnia in older persons when compared to younger individuals (107,147). In people over 60 years of age, up to 40% may experience insomnia, frequent awakening, and light and disrupted sleep (169).

Insomnia is a symptom, not a diagnosis. When the older person suffers from insomnia, the etiology can be multifactorial. Several factors that should be considered in the differential diagnosis include medical and psychiatric illnesses and polypharmacy. The duration of insomnia—transient (a few days), short term (a few weeks), or chronic (>1 month)— provides important diagnostic information.

In the evaluation of insomnia, a detailed medical and sleep history should be taken. Particular attention should be paid to the underlying medical conditions (heart disease, diabetes), medication use or misuse (polypharmacy), and substance use/misuse (alcohol, caffeine, and/or tobacco). Sleep history should be focused on the sleep hygiene (bedtime, sleep time, wake time). Sleep diaries (sleep logs) are crucial in the evaluation. These self-reported subjective measures allow for easy calculation of total time in bed, total sleep time, and sleep efficiency (116).

Polysomnograms are not necessary in the evaluation of most insomnia. A single PSG may not be representative of a patient's sleep at home and may not detect insomnia that is not present on a nightly basis (128). However, in the older patient with insomnia, a PSG may be indicated if the clinician suspects an underlying RLS, PLMS, or OSA (90). Others have advocated a formal PSG when traditional therapy of insomnia fails and the possibility of an underlying primary sleep disorder persists (154). Another objectively verifiable indicator of a sleep-wake schedule involves the use of an actigraph, a device worn on the wrist to record body movements (129,209).

There are many causes of insomnia in the older person. The most important group to consider in this age group is patients with insomnia due to medical factors. These factors include primary pulmonary disease [i.e., chronic obstructive pulmonary disease (COPD), asthma], neurologic and neurodegenerative disorders (e.g., parkinsonism, Alzheimer's disease, cerebrovascular accidents, headaches), nocturia, and pain syndromes. Underlying psychiatric conditions are important contributors to disruption of the sleep architecture. Up to 90% of patients with depression have an abnormal sleep architecture (205). The most striking polysomnographic features of depression include a decreased REM latency and early morning awakening (38).

In addition, older patients may have sleep disruption due to the use/abuse of alcohol, nicotine, and caffeine. In the sleep practice, it is not uncommon to see alcohol being used as a sleeping aid. Although initially it does decrease the sleep latency, it produces arousals, sleep fragmentation, REM deprivation, and REM rebound later during the night. Since the metabolism of alcohol is slower with advanced age, it has more powerful sedating effects (88). Stimulants (caffeine and medications containing stimulants) are notorious causes of insomnia (95). Caffeine is associated with increased sleep latency, reduced sleep efficiency, and spontaneous arousals. Caffeine withdrawal is associated with depression, irritability, and hypersomnolence. Nicotine induces insomnia and sleep fragmentation.

The role of polypharmacy is critical in assessing the older person with sleep disorders. Patients are often treated by multiple physicians who may prescribe several medications. Patients often use over-the-counter medications, vitamins, and herbal preparations.

INSOMNIA TREATMENT

Medications

Pharmacotherapy for insomnia in the older person is common but may be complicated by age-related changes in pharmacodynamics and pharmacokinetics (130). Some sleeping pills, particularly the longer acting ones, have multiple side effects in the older person. These range from hypersomnolence and being accident prone (207) to having disrupted sleep architecture (reduced REM and SWS). Tolerance is a major issue when long-acting sleeping pills are taken chronically, resulting in rebound insomnia and the need of higher dosage to achieve the same clinical efficacy.

Hypnotics

Hypnotics, when used in the older person, need to be given at the lowest possible dose for a short time. Shorter acting hypnotics are preferable, and patients need to be followed up closely. Potential side effects of hypnotics include anterograde amnesia and rebound insomnia. This is true for hypnotics with short or intermediate half-lives. All hypnotics will, if given in appropriate doses, improve insomnia. The goal is to use the medication with the fewest side effects at the lowest dose that will be clinically effective.

Hypnotics, when prescribed to patients with underlying OSA, may produce further nocturnal hypoxemia (115). Withdrawal from hypnotics may actually produce a worsening of insomnia and heightened anxiety. This is especially true with abrupt cessation from longer acting medications. The newer short-acting hypnotics do not have these same side effects and may be safer in the older patient. Examples

Table 13-2. *Medication Chart: Treatment of Insomnia—Newer Hypnotics Agents (as of March, 2007)*

Medication	Indication	Half-Life (hr)	Sleep Initiation	Sleep Maintenance	Approved Dose (mg)
Zaleplon	Short-term management of insomnia (improves sleep latency)	1	✔		5, 10
Zolpidem	Short-term management of insomnia (improves sleep latency and increases total sleep time)	2.5	✔		5, 10
Zolpidem CR	Insomnia characterized by difficulties with sleep onset and/or sleep maintenance	2.8	✔	✔	6.25, 12.5
Eszopiclone	Short- and long-term management of insomnia (improves sleep latency and increases total sleep time)	6–7	✔	✔	1, 2, 3
Ramelteon	Insomnia characterized by difficulty with sleep initiation (improves sleep latency and increases total sleep time)	1–2.6	✔		8

Source: *Physicians' Desk Reference.* 60th ed. Montvale, NJ: Thomson; 2005:1686–1691;2867–2871;3139–3143;3228–3231.

include zaleplon, which is a nonbenzodiazepine hypnotic from the pyrazolopyrimidine class selective for the benzodiazepine-1 receptor; zolpidem, which is a nonbenzodiazepine hypnotic of the imidazopyridine class selective for the type 1 $GABA_A$-benzodiazepine receptor; and eszopiclone, which is a nonbenzodiazepine agent that is a pyrrolopyrazine derivative of the cyclopyrrolone class (23,87,103,142,164,168). Zolpidem tartrate extended-release tablets have been introduced for the management of sleep maintenance insomnia. The drug consists of a coated two-layer tablet; one layer releases its drug content immediately, and another layer allows a slower release of additional drug content (173,179,185). In 2005, a new melatonin receptor agonist, ramelteon, was made available for the management of sleep initiation insomnia with the advantage of being a nonscheduled agent with zero evidence for abuse or tolerance. This agent selectively binds to the melatonin (MT1 and MT2) receptors in the suprachiasmatic nucleus (SCN), leading to the attenuation of the alerting signal generated by the SNC, which is thought to facilitate the onset of sleep (151,166,186,187). Table 13-2 lists currently available and approved hypnotic agents.

Sleep Hygiene

Drug therapy alone is not appropriate if one aims to eradicate chronic insomnia. Drug therapy, if used at all, must be combined with educational, behavioral, and cognitive interventions aimed at introducing adaptive behaviors. One of the most important educational approaches for insomnia includes modifying disadvantageous sleep hygiene habits that patients may have adopted over the years (124,127). Originally developed by Hauri (125,126), the basic elements of better sleep hygiene include limiting naps to less than 30 minutes a day, avoiding stimulants and sedatives, limiting liquids at bedtime, keeping a regular sleep schedule, and incorporating light exposure and exercise into the daily routines. Stimulus-control therapy, originally proposed by Bootzin and Nicassio (54), proposes that sleep disturbances are behaviorally conditioned and thus need to be reconditioned. The aim of this intervention is to recondition the bed/bedroom as cues for sleep. Patients are instructed to go to bed only when tired, to get out of bed after 20 minutes of being unable to fall asleep, and to return to bed when sleepy. They are also instructed to avoid looking at the clock, shorten daytime naps, use the bed only for sleep, and get up at a consistent time in the morning (94,95,220).

Sleep restriction therapy proposed by Spielman et al. (229) has in its merits the need to restrict time in bed to provide for better sleep efficiency. This technique involves curtailing time in bed and total sleep time, which may initially lead to a state of sleep deprivation. It works by preventing patients from becoming frustrated by restricting the time spent in bed. Other common therapeutic modalities for insomnia include cognitive intervention, which helps patients gain insight into maladaptive beliefs and attitudes toward sleep, and relaxation techniques and biofeedback, which help patients lower the degree of anxiety and arousal associated with insomnia (54).

CIRCADIAN RHYTHM ABNORMALITIES

The sleep-wake cycle is controlled by the circadian modulator located in the SCN of the anterior hypothalamus. Zeitgebers, external cues such as light, synchronize the circadian rhythms. Disturbances in circadian rhythms are due to a mismatch between the environmental cues and the endogenous circadian rhythms. The hypersomnolence seen in the older person may be due in part to a disintegration of the normal circadian rhythm (136).

Advanced sleep phase syndrome (ASPS) is very common among older patients. Patients with ASPS generally get sleepy early in the evening and wake up early in the morning being unable to reinitiate sleep. Although the older adult may get sleepier in the evening, he/she still tries to remain awake until a "more acceptable" time (e.g., 10:00 or 11:00 PM). Then when they wake up early unable to fall back to sleep, they have not even been in bed long enough to get the sleep they need, resulting in a state of sleep deprivation (10,12). ASPS can be treated with bright light therapy because light is one of the strongest cues for synchronizing circadian rhythms. Bright light therapy involves exposure of 2,500 lux of light at 1 meter eye level. Light exposure in the evening delays sleep initiation (58,59,76).

Melatonin, a neurohormone produced by the pineal gland, can reset sleep onset by synchronization of the internal circadian clock (80). With advanced age, less melatonin is produced (204). Melatonin replacement therapy may be a key for treating insomnia in the elderly. In 1995, Haimov et al. (122) showed a positive correlation between a lower peak level of melatonin and poor sleep efficiency in older patients with insomnia. Melatonin treatment early in the morning may also be used for ASPS. When melatonin is given a few hours prior to the onset of the endogenous production (which peaks around 3:00 to 5:00 AM), it will shift the circadian pacemaker to an earlier time and thus cause a phase advance (152,153,227). Currently, more data are needed to improve our understanding of the appropriate dosage, pharmacologic properties, and indications. More data are also needed regarding the appropriate safety and efficacy of this substance. Since the FDA does not regulate melatonin, care must be exercised when using it.

SLEEP DISORDERS IN NEUROLOGIC DISORDERS

Patients with a history of dementia may have a number of underlying sleep disturbances consisting of insomnia, hypersomnia, circadian rhythm disturbances, excessive motor activity at night, nocturnal agitation, and wandering and abnormal nocturnal behaviors (64). Dementia patients with sleep problems may be at increased risk for irritability, impaired motor and cognitive skills, depression, and fatigue (39). Patients with dementia are also at risk for additional sleep disturbances, such as OSA and PLMS, which occur at a higher incidence with aging. Many of these sleep disruptions can cause considerable caregiver burden and may put the patient at increased risk for institutionalization in nursing home facilities (155,197).

Sleep disturbances in dementia may be due to both underlying direct and indirect mechanisms (39,64). Direct mechanisms are related to specific lesions in the neuroanatomic pathways involved in sleep physiology and neurochemistry. Structural alteration of the sleep-wake–generating neurons located in the SCN is one example of the direct mechanism, whereas insufficient light exposure and excessive noise at the patient's living quarters are examples of the indirect or external mechanisms that disturb sleep (Fig. 13-2).

ALZHEIMER'S DISEASE

In Alzheimer's disease (AD), degeneration of the neurons of the SCN may be responsible for circadian rhythm abnormalities, sundowning syndrome, and other sleep-wake schedule disturbances (Fig. 13-3) (39,64). The severity of circadian rhythm disturbances is shown to be correlated with the severity of dementia (17,18). Sleep studies in patients with dementia demonstrate decreased sleep efficiency, increased diffuse slow-wave activity, and reversal of their circadian rhythmicity, which, after incontinence, is the second most common cause for institutionalization (196).

Degeneration of the cholinergic neurons in the nucleus basalis of Meynert, the pedunculopontine tegmental and laterodorsal tegmental nuclei, and noradrenergic neurons of the brainstem may be responsible for the predictable decreased REM sleep in AD patients (Fig. 13-3) (39,64). Degeneration of the brainstem respiratory neurons and the supramedullary respiratory pathways may cause sleep apnea and other respiratory dysrhythmias in sleep in AD (Fig. 13-3) (39,64).

Indirect mechanisms include pharmacologically related side effects, underlying psychiatric diagnosis such as mood disorders, increasing incidence of PLMS in elderly AD patients, and age-related alterations in sleep (Fig. 13-2). Other indirect mechanisms include general medical diseases affecting the

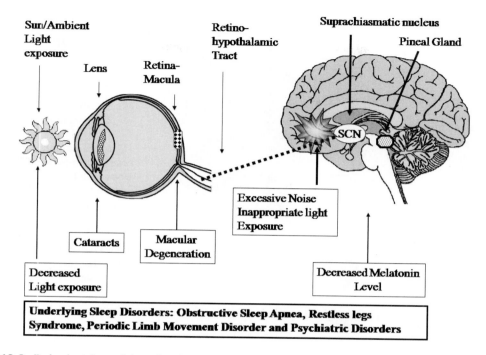

Figure 13-2. Pathophysiology of sleep disturbances in patients with dementia: potential external and intrinsic factors. (Modified from Avidan A. Sleep in dementia and other neurodegenerative disorders. In: Culebras A, ed. *Sleep disorders and neurologic diseases.* 2nd ed. New York: Taylor & Francis Group; 2007.)

cardiorespiratory system and environmental factors such as insufficient light and excessive environmental noise in nursing homes facilities or other long-term care institutions (Fig. 13-2).

Sleep Architecture in Alzheimer's Disease

Patients with AD have dramatic sleep architectural abnormalities. The signature findings include decrease in sleep efficiency, increase in NREM stage 1 sleep, increase in arousal and awakening frequency, and a reduction in total sleep time, sleep spindles, and K-complexes. A profound disruption in sleep-wake rhythmicity occurs primarily early in the onset of AD. Sleep fragmentation subsequently leads to hypersomnolence (increased daytime sleepiness), nocturnal insomnia, nocturnal wandering, increase in cognitive decline, increase in the number of daytime naps, increase in time in bed and time spent awake in bed, increase in the frequency of nocturnal wandering, disorientation, and confusion (47,64,255–259).

Later on, as AD progresses, patients may present with a more dramatic reduction of REM sleep, increased REM sleep latency, and a marked alteration of the circadian rhythm resulting in hypersomnolence (39). In fact, sleep and cognitive dysfunction are positively correlated in AD. Patients with AD are also susceptible to "sundowning," a term describing the nocturnal exacerbation of agitation or disruptive behavior in older patients (248). Sundowning is frequently encountered in dementia and remains a frequent cause of institutionalization in patients with AD. Inevitably, the medications often used to treat AD also affect sleep. Current pharmacotherapy for cognitive loss in AD involves the use of cholinesterase inhibitors, which may increase REM sleep and may also induce insomnia and vivid dreams (45).

Circadian Rhythm Disturbances in Alzheimer's Disease

The symptoms of insomnia and hypersomnia can reflect a primary circadian dysrhythmia. AD patients tend to sleep more during the day and be more active during the night. This increased motor activity at night is the major contributing factor to significant caregiver distress.

Direct mechanisms thought to contribute to circadian dysrhythmia in patients with AD and other dementing conditions are related to degenerative changes that take place in the SCN and to decreased melatonin production in the pineal gland (Figs. 13-1

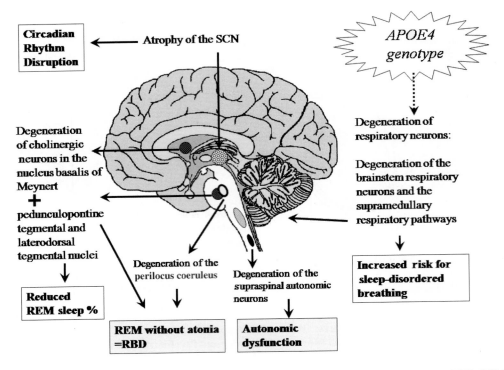

Figure 13-3. Pathophysiology of sleep disturbances in neurodegenerative disorders: direct mechanisms. RBD, REM sleep behavior disorder; SCN, suprachiasmatic nucleus; (*broken arrow*) demonstrates a hypothetical relationship (Modified from Avidan A. Sleep in dementia and other neurodegenerative disorders. In: Culebras A, ed. *Sleep disorders and neurologic diseases.* 2nd ed. New York: Taylor & Francis Group; 2007.)

and 13-2) (75,236,240,241). Indirect mechanisms include medications prescribed for these patients that cause nocturnal confusion, or sundowning. AD patients are commonly affected by the irregular sleep-wake rhythm (ISWR), which is characterized by a lack of discernable sleep-wake circadian rhythm. Instead of having a major sleep period, sleep is fragmented into three or more periods during the 24-hour day, with the longest sleep period occurring between 2:00 and 6:00 AM. Patients with ISWR may present with hypersomnia, insomnia, or the need for frequent naps throughout the day. The disorder also affects the sleep quality of the caregiver.

Important factors that may contribute to ISWR include weak external entraining stimuli such as reduced exposure to environmental light and diminished daytime activity. The diagnosis of ISWR is made by reviewing the patient's sleep log or actigraphy confirming the lack of periodic circadian rhythmicity. A history of isolation or reclusion may aid in diagnosis. The differential diagnosis of ISWR includes other sleep or psychiatric disorders that can cause fragmented sleep, poor sleep hygiene, and voluntary maintenance of irregular sleep schedules.

Sleep Disordered Breathing in Alzheimer's Disease

Sleep-related breathing disorders, such as OSA, are very common in AD patients compared to nondemented elderly and to younger adults (93,131). One study demonstrated that the severity of AD is proportional to the severity of the OSA (16,137). Furthermore, anecdotal reports of dementia-like symptoms associated with OSA have led to the speculation that there may be a causal relationship between sleep-disordered breathing and AD (219).

In AD, sleep apnea could be a consequence of cell loss in the brainstem respiratory center. Conversely, neuronal degradation in AD may be hastened by nightly insults of intermittent cerebral hypoxemia related to the underlying OSA. One of the key genotypic markers for AD is the apolipoprotein E epsilon 4 (APOE4) allele. A recent discovery that sleep-disordered breathing (SDB) is associated with the APOE4 allele in the general population has sparked an interest in this topic because OSA is characterized by multiple genetic vulnerabilities (44,141). In individuals under age 65, the APOE4 allele was more significantly associated with increased risk of OSA (201). However, other studies did not replicate the result in part because of different genetic populations and different age cohorts (106,208). In a recent study of 1,775 participants aged 40 to 100 years with an OSA prevalence rate of 19%, after adjustment for age, sex, and BMI, the presence of any APOE4 allele was associated with increased odds of having OSA (120).

Treatment of Sleep Disturbances in Alzheimer's Disease

SDB is related to agitation in AD, and treatment of the underlying SDB may improve the agitation, easing the burden of care giving and prolonging the time that patients are able to remain at home (112). Neuropsychological analyses have revealed that, in patients with OSA, cognitive flexibility, attention, processing speed, and memory all improve with CPAP therapy (9,30,31,66,163). Compliance with CPAP was also associated with greater improvements in attention, psychomotor speed, executive functioning, and nonverbal delayed recall (9).

Recent studies showed that melatonin, an indoleamine secreted by the pineal gland, may play an important role in aging and AD as an antioxidant and neuroprotector. Melatonin levels diminish with aging, and patients with AD have a more profound reduction in this hormone (269). Data from clinical trials indicate that melatonin replacement improves sleep and slows down the progression of cognitive impairment in AD (269). Other data show that melatonin may be protective of neuronal cells via antioxidant and antiamyloid-mediated activity properties, arrests the formation of amyloid fibrils, attenuates Alzheimer-like tau hyperphosphorylation, and protects cholinergic neurons but may not be an effective sleep agent (108,182,225,228,231,262). A misleading labeling of the hormone melatonin as a "food supplement" and the lack of quality control over melatonin preparations on the market (besides the fact that it is currently not regulated by the FDA in the United States) unfortunately continue to be serious concerns, and heath care providers should use caution when prescribing it to elderly patients with dementia (272). To date, there have been no randomized clinical trials of sedative-hypnotic medications specifically targeted at AD patients with sleep problems (45).

Treatment for Circadian Rhythm Disturbances in Alzheimer's Disease

Treatments for circadian rhythm sleep disorders including the irregular sleep-wake type are aimed at consolidating the sleep-wake cycle. Most of the studies have examined the effect of melatonin or the effect of increased bright light exposure in patients living in nursing homes. In one study, combination therapy of bright light, vitamin B_{12}, chronotherapy, and hypnotic agents produced a 45% success rate in one cohort of patients suffering from AD (28). However, a recent multicenter, randomized, double-blind, placebo-controlled clinical trial using actigraphically derived measures of sleep demonstrated no beneficial effects of melatonin 2.5 or 10.0 mg on sleep disturbance in a well-characterized, large AD population (n = 157) (45,225).

Light therapy has been shown to be effective in the management of circadian rhythm disturbances in patients with dementia; however, the optimal timing, duration, and intensity of light have not yet been determined (158,214). A more practical approach to the management of ISWR is to begin with behavioral and environmental strategies. In addition to increased bright light exposure, structured social and physical activities and avoidance of naps during the day have been shown to improve sleep (6–8,221). During the sleep period, the environment should be conducive to sleep and consist of minimal noise, a darkened room, and a comfortable room temperature. The use of hypnotic or sedating psychoactive medications should be used with caution in elderly patients with dementia. Time exposure to bright light in the morning may be helpful in some patients. Evening bright light pulses ameliorated sleep-wake cycle disturbances in some patients with AD (214). Ancoli-Israel et al. (14) examined the effect of light on sleep and circadian activity rhythms in nursing home patients with probable or possible AD. The results of her study showed that both morning and evening bright light resulted in more consolidated sleep at night, as measured with wrist actigraphy. The authors suggested that nursing homes increase ambient light in activity rooms where patients spend the majority of their days (14). The authors hypothesized that, although the SCN of patients with severe AD is more likely to be functioning abnormally or be degenerated and the circadian activity rhythms deteriorate as AD progresses, it is still possible that patients with more intact SCNs (i.e., patients with mild to moderate AD) might benefit from light treatment even more than patients with severe AD (22).

Data evaluating the use of antipsychotic agents and benzodiazepines have demonstrated improvements in sleep or nocturnal behavior but lacked real-time behavioral observations as relevant outcomes (165). Agents such as the antipsychotics often have adverse effects such as sedation, confusion, orthostatic hypotension, and parkinsonism, which are often clinically significant in elderly patients with dementia (165). The high-potency antipsychotics are associated with an increased risk of producing extrapyramidal side effects, whereas the low-potency agents have more sedating, anticholinergic, and orthostatic hypotensive properties (165).

PARKINSON'S DISEASE

Sleep disorders are encountered in the majority of Parkinson's disease (PD) patients, adversely affecting their quality of life (191). Pathologic hypersomnia and fatigue are common in patients with PD and are two of the most disabling features (96). Sleep problems in PD patients also correlate with increased severity of disease.

The frequency of sleep complaints in patients with PD is estimated to be between 60% and 90%. A variety of other mechanisms that are either disease-related or secondary mechanisms may come into play, including prescribed therapy for PD using dopaminergic treatment (233). PD patients may experience a number of sleep disorders including insomnia, parasomnia, and hypersomnia, including EDS and sleep attacks (39). Excessive nocturia can disturb sleep, particularly in those with severe PD, and may be related to the natural evolution of dysautonomia in PD (270).

Patients with PD often have difficulty or total inability to turn over during the night and get out of bed. This is most likely secondary to bradykinesia. Leg cramps, leg jerks, and dystonic spasms of the limbs, face, and back are also very common. One community-based survey evaluating 245 patients with PD demonstrated that nearly two thirds of patients reported sleep disorders, which is significantly more than among patients with diabetes (46%) and healthy control subjects (33%) (247). About one third of the patients with PD rated their overall nighttime problem as moderate to severe (247). The most commonly reported sleep disorders included frequent arousals leading to awakenings, which lead to sleep fragmentation, and early morning awakening, which ultimately results in a poor sleep efficiency (247). The study found a strong correlation between depression and sleep disorders in patients with PD, which underlines the importance of identifying and treating both conditions in these patients (247).

The underlying biologic basis of sleep disruption in PD is possibly related to the alteration of dopaminergic, noradrenergic, serotonergic, and cholinergic neurons in the brainstem (233). Typical sleep abnormalities include fragmented sleep with an increased number of arousals and awakenings and PD-specific motor phenomena such as nocturnal immobility, rest tremor, eye blinking, dyskinesias, and other phenomena such as PLMS, RLS, fragmentary myoclonus, and respiratory dysfunction in sleep (233). Sleep maintenance problems and difficulties with sleep initiation are the earliest and most frequent sleep disorders observed in these patients (233). Close to 90% of these patients often have sleep maintenance insomnia associated with frequent awakenings (64,109). Sleep fragmentation and spontaneous daytime dozing occurred much more frequently in PD patients than in controls (97). Sleep fragmentation in PD may be due to increased skeletal muscle activity, disturbed breathing, and REM–to–NREM variations of the dopaminergic receptor sensitivity (233).

These complaints manifest on polysomnographic recordings as reduction of sleep efficiency, increased wake after sleep onset (WASO), increased sleep fragmentation, reduction of SWS and REM sleep, disruption of NREM–to–REM cyclicity, loss of muscle atonia, and increased EMG activity, which is the basis for RBD (69,191,218).

Motor abnormalities in PD during sleep include the parkinsonism tremor and REM onset blepharospasm, which disappears during REM sleep. Patients have rapid blinking at sleep onset and REM intrusion into NREM sleep. RBD is very common in PD patients (64,69) and may also precede the onset of PD (246). Patients with PD who have posture reflex abnormalities and autonomic impairment are at an increased risk for sleep-related breathing disorder in the form of CSA, OSA, and alveolar hypoventilation syndrome (25). PD may lead to a restrictive pulmonary disease. Patients with PD are also found to have circadian rhythm abnormalities and depression (250). Circadian rhythm disturbances in PD may be related to mesocorticolimbic dopaminergic abnormalities and mesostriatal system abnormalities (233). Abnormalities of dopaminergic neurons in the ventral tegmentum area often lead to EEG desynchronization and abnormal sleep-wake schedule disorder (91). Additional attempts to explain the sleep-wake disruption in PD have been linked to reduction in serotonergic neurons of the dorsal raphe, noradrenergic neurons of the locus coeruleus, and cholinergic neurons of the pedunculopontine nucleus (233).

Patients with PD who are already on medications may have additional sleep difficulties. Low-dose dopaminergic agonists are often sedating. On the other hand, high-dose dopaminergic agonists may lead to increased hallucinations, nightmares, and increased arousals. Levodopa is often associated with increased sleep latency but an increased sleep continuity (29,188). In patients with PD who developed motor fluctuations (on-off phenomenon, wearing off) during the day, other common sleep-related motor complaints including nocturnal akinesia, dystonia, and painful cramps are observed (233). Chronic release formulation of levodopa/carbidopa (Sinemet CR) has been demonstrated to improve nocturnal akinesia and increase sleep efficiency of patients with PD with underlying sleep-related motor disturbances (233).

Treatment of sleep disorders in patients with PD deserves special consideration. Patients with PD who suffer from insomnia are often treated by improving sleep hygiene abnormalities. Pharmacologic treatment with small-dose dopaminergic preparations (e.g., levodopa/carbidopa 25/100) and small doses of sedating tricyclic antidepressants (TCAs) may be tried. Problems with bradykinesia and nocturia are often improved by providing patients with a portable bedside commode. For patients with RLS symptoms, evening and nocturnal doses of a dopaminergic agonist, such as carbidopa/levodopa, or a dopamine (D_3) agonist are useful (216). Patients with OSA are often improved with CPAP. Patients who are diagnosed with OSA in addition to autonomic dysfunction can be treated effectively with CPAP. However, a definitive treatment (with tracheostomy) is indicated and is often mandatory due to the increased risk of fatal cardiac arrhythmias.

REM SLEEP BEHAVIOR DISORDER

RBD is characterized by pathologic augmentation of skeletal muscle tone during REM sleep (Fig. 13-4). Patients present with unusual, complex, and intense motor activity during a dream sequence. The range of motor activities can vary from a simple limb movement to very complex quasi-purposeful movements suggestive of dream content enactment (64). The potential for self and bed partner injury is high, especially during severe episodes (4). Current speculations suggest that the pontine tegmentum is the locus of the muscle tone inhibitor system, which normally causes muscle atonia during REM sleep (Fig. 13-5) (216). The perilocus coeruleus of the rostral tegmentum of the pons produces activation of the medullary inhibitory zone via the tegmentoreticular tract. RBD is characterized by a loss of atonia

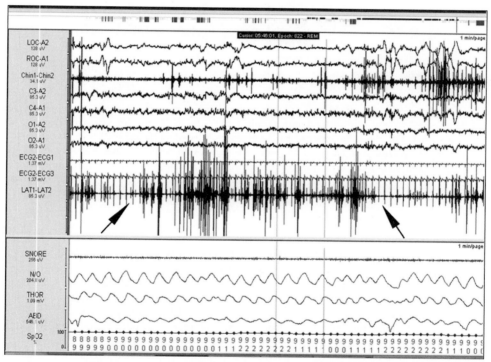

Figure 13-4. Polysomnographic example of REM sleep behavior disorder. A 60-second epoch from a diagnostic polysomnogram of an 80-year-old man with PD who was referred to the sleep disorders clinic for evaluation of recurrent violent nighttime awakenings. Illustrated in this figure is a typical spell that this patient was experiencing during the night. He was noted to yell, jump from bed, and have complex body movements. The figure shows abnormal augmentation REM muscle atonia in the left anterior tibialis muscle and chin EMG channel (note the *arrows* depicting a representative area). The patient was diagnosed with RBD and was treated successfully with clonazepam 0.25 mg. Channels are as follows: electro-oculogram (*left*: LOC-A2, *right*: ROC-A1), chin EMG, electroencephalogram (left central, right central, left occipital, right occipital), two ECG channels, limb EMG (LAT), snore channel, nasal-oral airflow, respiratory effort (thoracic, abdominal), and oxygen saturation (SaO2).
REM, rapid eye movement; PD, Parkinson's disease; RBD, REM sleep behavior disorder; EMG, electromyogram; ECG, electrocardiogram; EMG (LAT), EMG left anterior tibialis.

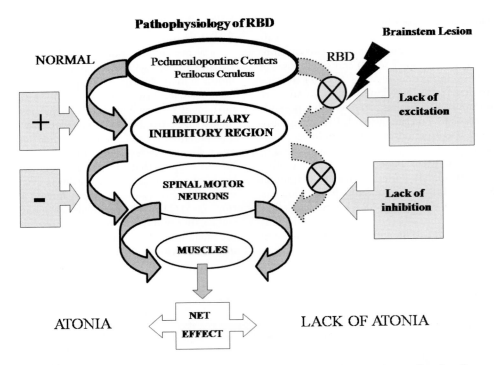

Figure 13-5. Pathophysiology of RBD. Muscle atonia during REM sleep results from pontine-mediated perilocus coeruleus inhibition of motor activity. This pontine activity exerts an excitatory influence on medullary inhibitory centers (magnocellularis neurons) via the lateral tegmentoreticular tract. These neuronal groups, in turn, hyperpolarize the spinal motor neuron postsynaptic membranes via the ventrolateral reticulospinal tract. In RBD, the brainstem mechanisms generating muscle become disrupted. The pathophysiology of RBD in humans is based on the cat model. In the cat model, bilateral pontine lesions result in a persistent absence of REM atonia associated with prominent motor activity during REM sleep, similar to that observed in RBD in humans. The pathophysiology of the idiopathic form of RBD in humans is still not very well understood but may be related to reduction of striatal presynaptic dopamine transporters. RBD, REM sleep disorder behavior; REM, rapid eye movement. (Modified from Avidan AY. Sleep disorders in the older person. *Prim Care.* 2005;32:563–586.)

during REM sleep, which facilitates the motor behaviors during dreaming (175,189,218). Figure 13-5 summarizes the possible neuroanatomic theory behind RBD.

REM-sleep behavior disorder is a common sleep disorder seen in PD (111,157). Recent findings from various studies suggest that a high percentage of patients with PD without sleep complaints may have subclinical or clinical RBD and that RBD can be the heralding manifestation of parkinsonism by many years in older male patients (1,49,51,111,150,198, 233,265). In addition to its high prevalence in patients with PD, RBD is a common sleep disturbance in other neurodegenerative disorders such as multiple system atrophy (MSA) and dementia with Lewy bodies [diffuse Lewy body disease (DLBD)] (1,134,195).

The majority of cases occur with advancing age; approximately 60% are idiopathic, whereas the remaining 40% may have an underlying neuropathology.

RBD typically manifests itself in the sixth or seventh decade of life. This disorder has a particular predilection to occur in a number of synucleinopathies and other neurodegenerative disorders in addition to PD, such as DLBD, olivopontocerebellar degeneration, Shy-Drager syndrome (SDS), and MSA (5,50,101, 160,195,215,218).

Secondary causes of RBD include diseases that disrupt brainstem centers involved in REM-generated muscle atonia such as multiple sclerosis (MS), cerebral vascular accidents, and brainstem neoplasm. Twenty-five percent of patients may have a prodrome of subclinical behavioral release during sleep. The acute onset of RBD is related to drugs such as tricyclic antidepressants (TCA), monoamine oxidase inhibitors (MAOI), and selective serotonin reuptake inhibitors (SSRI) and acute withdrawal of alcohol and barbiturates. In extreme cases, excessive caffeine intake has been implicated in RBD (101,160,218,235).

In many cases, the diagnosis is suspected clinically based on the patient's and the bed partner's reports of recurrent dream enacting and complex and potentially aggressive behaviors during the night. The diagnosis is confirmed by polysomnography using multiple-limb EMG leads (as in Fig. 13-4) along with simultaneous continuous video monitoring demonstrating evidence of increased electromyographic bursts of chin EMG or limb electrodes during REM sleep. Clinically, the diagnosis of RBD based on the International Classification of Sleep Disorders Revised (ICSD-R) has some intrinsic limitations based on the patient report and terminologic ambiguity, whereas diagnosis based on polysomnography has a better reliability (53,70). The sleep study may also capture the actual spells during which the abnormal activity is demonstrated (limb jerk or complex, vigorous, violent behaviors). If there is evidence of an abnormal neurologic examination, a full neurologic workup including a brain MRI may also be needed (160,216).

The differential diagnosis of RBD includes sleepwalking, nocturnal seizures, posttraumatic stress disorder (PTSD), sleep terrors, nocturnal panic disorders, delirium, sleep-related gastroesophageal reflux, PLMS, psychogenic dissociative state, and confusional arousals with sleep apnea (Table 13-3). Distinguishing RBD from nocturnal seizures may sometimes be difficult. However, unlike nocturnal seizures, the typical RBD spell is usually not stereotyped and is often variable (4,148,160,218). Additional laboratory studies may be needed, especially if the clinical history remains vague or ambiguous. When the possibility of nocturnal seizures cannot be reliably excluded, additional sleep testing may be warranted.

Treatment for Rapid Eye Movement Sleep Behavior Disorder

Environmental safety is crucial in every patient with likely RBD. This may include making the sleeping environment safe by removing sharp objects and padding the bed area. Suggested pharmacotherapy for RBD includes clonazepam (0.25 to 1 mg orally at bedtime), which is effective in 90% of cases (160). There is little evidence of tolerance or abuse with this form of treatment. Caution should be exercised when using it in patients with chronic respiratory diseases or impaired renal function, and it is contraindicated in patients with documented hypersensitivity, severe liver disease, or acute narrow angle glaucoma. Abrupt discontinuation of clonazepam can precipitate withdrawal symptoms (160). Other agents that can be helpful include imipramine (25 mg orally at bedtime), carbamazepine (100 mg orally three times a day), and levodopa in cases where RBD is associated with PD. Recent studies have also demonstrated improvement

with melatonin, which is believed to exert its therapeutic effect by restoring REM sleep atonia. One study reported that melatonin was effective in 87% of patients taking 3 to 9 mg at bedtime (245), whereas a later study reported resolution in those taking 6 to 12 mg of melatonin at bedtime (48). Tacrine, donepezil, and Serzone, which are drugs used in AD and other dementing disorders, may exacerbate RBD. Some antidepressants may potentially increase total REM sleep, which may worsen RBD.

DIFFUSE LEWY BODY DISEASE

Diffuse Lewy body disease (DLBD) is a neurodegenerative disorder characterized by parkinsonism, dementia, fluctuations in mental status, and hallucinations. RBD is now recognized as a feature of DLBD (50,251,271). Nightmares without atonia may be an early symptom of DLBD and is very often the initial manifestation of DLBD (50,81).

MULTIPLE-SYSTEM ATROPHY

Patients with MSA experience degeneration of the pontine tegmentum, nucleus tractus solitarius, nucleus ambiguous, hypoglossal nucleus, reticular formation of the brainstem, and at times, the cervical and thoracic spinal cord. Therefore, the diffuse neurodegenerative process that encompasses these key structures involved in the regulation of the sleep-wake transition and respiratory function in MSA may account for the most frequent sleep disturbances in MSA, SDB, and RBD (65,113).

Patients with MSA are commonly affected with RBD, which represents the most common clinical sleep manifestation and polysomnographic findings in patients with MSA. In a large study involving MSA patients, RBD was diagnosed by PSG monitoring in 90% of patients, dream-enacting behaviors were reported in 69% of patients, and RBD preceded the clinical presentation of MSA in 44% of patients (195). REM sleep behavior disorder can frequently herald the appearance of other MSA symptoms by years; therefore, expanded polysomnographic montage consisting of multiple limbs and video monitoring is recommended in patients MSA when these spells are suspected (195,216). Increasing evidence points to the role of basal ganglia dysfunction in the underlying pathophysiology of RBD in MSA. In fact, a recent study from our center has revealed that decreased nigrostriatal dopaminergic projections may contribute to RBD in MSA (117).

Patients with MSA frequently manifest a variety of sleep-related respiratory disturbances, some of which are life threatening. Above all, a common and serious complication is upper airway OSA associated with stridor, which is caused by vocal cord abductor paralysis (VCAP) and may lead to sudden death during

Table 13-3. *Differential Diagnosis of Nocturnal Spells in the Older Person*

Variable	Nocturnal Seizure	REM Sleep Behavior Disorder (RBD)	Somnambulism	Nocturnal Dissociative Disorder	Confusional Arousals	Sleep-Related Panic Attacks	Nightmares
Stage of Sleep	NREM > REM, ictal discharges facilitated by K-complexes	REM sleep	First 3rd of night, SWS		First 3rd of night, during SWS	Transition from NREM stage 2 to SWS	Second half of night during REM sleep, also NREM
Spell Symptoms	Generalized tonic-clonic activity: generalized epilepsy, partial epilepsy	Talking, arm movements, kicking, punching	Automatisms, getting out of bed, walking	Alteration of consciousness, identity, memory	Sudden arousal, confusion, disorientation, inappropriate behavior	Sudden awakening with subjective fear, impending doom	Sudden awakening with anxiety and dream recall
Duration	Seconds to minutes	Seconds to 20–30 minutes	1–5 minutes, 30–60 minutes rare		Seconds to 10 minutes	Several seconds to a few minutes	5–15 minutes
Postspell Symptoms	Unresponsiveness, confusion, weakness, incontinence (urine/stool), tongue biting	Detailed recall of an active dream with theme of violence	Confusion, amnesia to the event; recall is rare	Amnestic to event/dreamlike mentation	No recall of event	Excessive arousal, increased sympathetic activity	Vivid recall of a frightening dream
EEG Pattern During Spell	Ictal EEG pattern	REM Sleep	Transition from SWS to stage 1, diffuse and slow alpha, high-amplitude delta bursts		Slow-wave activity, microsleeps, poorly reactive alpha		Increased eye movements during REM
Pathophysiology	CNS vascular disease, neoplasm (in the older person)	Loss of muscle atonia, pontine/CNS lesions, stress, parkinsonian disorders	Predisposing psychopathology, sleep deprivation, alcohol, strong sleep pressure	Underlying serious psychopathology, abuse	Incomplete awakening from SWS	Predisposing anxiety disorder, depression, daytime panic attacks, alcohol abuse	Precipitated by daytime stress, drugs (beta-blockers), psychopathology
Potential Treatments	Appropriate antiepileptic drugs (i.e., valproate/phenyoin/carbamazepine)	Clonazepam (after management of potential OSA), levodopa-carbidopa, melatonin, dopamine agonists	Avoid injury, protect patient, avoid precipitating factors, hypnosis, psychotherapy, benzodiazepines, tricyclic antidepressants	Psychotherapy, psychopharmacology, resistant to treatment	Relaxation techniques, avoidance of stress	Treatment of the underlying anxiety disorder or panic disorder, psychotherapy, anxiolytics	Address underlying psychiatric illness, avoid stress, psychotherapy, improve sleep hygiene, rarely REM suppressants

sleep (177). For this reason, nocturnal stridor in MSA has been considered a poor prognostic feature (183). For the early diagnosis of VCAP, it is critical to perform laryngoscopy during sleep because VCAP does not appear during wakefulness in the early stage of MSA (210).

Polysomnography study should be obtained to assess the severity of respiratory disturbances, and tracheostomy is the most reliable treatment for respiratory disturbances due to VCAP. Although CPAP may be a useful treatment for some patients, absolute compliance is mandatory. Tracheostomy is probably the only effective measure for emergency treatment of severe respiratory dysfunction and hypoxia in patients with marked laryngeal stridor as can be seen in laryngeal abductor paralysis in patients with MSA (183,210).

OLIVOPONTOCEREBELLAR DEGENERATION

The sleep problems encountered in this condition include central, obstructive, and mixed sleep apnea probably caused by bulbar muscle weakness (39). Patients may also have nocturnal stridor as well as RBD (132,211). Patients, unaware of their nocturnal sleep disturbance, complain only of the resulting daytime tiredness and sleepiness (211). Patients may also have nocturnal stridor as well as RBD. Nocturnal polyuria has also been reported in olivopontocerebellar atrophy, possibly related to a disturbance in the circadian rhythm for arginine vasopressin secretion due to degeneration of SCN and marked increase in the secretion of atrial natriuretic peptide due to abnormal diurnal variation in blood pressure (172).

SHY-DRAGER SYNDROME

Patients with SDS most commonly present with sleep-related respiratory dysregulation with frequent arousals and hypoxemia (55). Apneas encountered in this syndrome include obstructive, mixed, and central apneas. Cheyne-Stokes respiratory dysfunction, apneustic breathing, and inspiratory gasping are commonly seen. The hypersomnia seen in these patients is probably secondary to the dramatic sleep disruption. Patients may be at risk of dying from sudden cardiac death related to the underlying sleep-related breathing disorder. RBD disorder and insomnia are also common in this disease.

The mechanism of sleep disruption in this condition is probably due to pathology in the brainstem structures regulating sleep-wake transition. Patients with SDS are at increased risk for developing brainstem ischemia secondary to nocturnal hypotensive episodes, which may subsequently potentiate the tendency to develop RBD (192). Sleep studies in patients with SDS demonstrate reduced SWS, reduced REM

sleep, reduced total sleep time, increased sleep latency, increased frequency of awakenings, absence of atonia in REM sleep, and increased respiratory dysrhythmias (39,64).

PROGRESSIVE SUPRANUCLEAR PALSY

Sleep disturbances are universal in progressive supranuclear palsy (PSP) (39,121). Insomnia is probably the most severe sleep problem noted by decreased total sleep time and significant sleep disruption without a specific clinical complaint (39). Insomnia in PSP is worse than insomnia in PD or AD and may be due to degenerative changes in brain structures responsible for sleep maintenance and marked nigrostriatal dopamine deficiency (5,146). Other sleep disturbances may be related to the well-documented immobility in bed and difficulty with transfers, depression, dysphagia, and frequent nocturia seen in PSP. REM sleep behavior disorder and SDB are not common features in PSP (39,121).

The polysomnographic features of PSP are unique. When one evaluates the eye leads of the recording, it is interesting to note the absence of vertical eye movement during REM sleep. Horizontal eye movements are present but are slower and reduced in amplitude. During REM sleep, polysomnography may show increased phasic twitching and increased fast activity with alpha intrusion. The minority of patients with PSP may have periodic leg movements of sleep and OSA. The sleep architecture profile consists of increased sleep latency, increased arousal and awakening frequency, decreased stage 2 NREM sleep, reduced REM sleep, and reduced REM latency (39,64).

EPILEPSY

Consideration of epilepsy and epileptic-like spells in the elderly is important because these are frequent problems in elderly patients referred to epilepsy centers. A recent study from the Cleveland Clinic Foundation looked at the frequency of nonepileptic seizures in elderly patients referred for epilepsy monitoring and found that 43% had a diagnosis other than epilepsy, including transient ischemic attacks, syncope, movement disorders, and sleep disorders (145). Although most of the patients did not have any evidence for epilepsy, more than two thirds of these patients had been placed on anticonvulsive drugs (145).

Sleep and epilepsy have a reciprocal relationship. Sleep can affect the frequency and distribution of epileptiform discharges, while epileptic discharges can change sleep regulation and induce sleep disruption. Patients with epilepsy complain of symptoms such as hypersomnia, insomnia, and even greater breakthrough seizures attributed to sleep disruptions.

Sleep disturbances in epilepsy patients probably indicate the presence of an underlying sleep disorder rather than the effect of epilepsy or medication on sleep. Physicians must be able to identify and differentiate between potential underlying sleep disorders and sleep dysfunction related to epilepsy and direct therapy to improve the patient's symptoms (252).

Sleep deprivation was noted to increase interictal discharges in patients with generalized epilepsy (82). The sleep state can promote interictal activity in as many as one third of patients with epilepsy and up to 90% of patients with sleep state–dependent epilepsy (86,252). Up to one third of patients with medically refractory epilepsy had evidence of OSA; treatment of the underlying sleep apnea with CPAP can improve seizure frequency (85,161,253).

Nocturnal seizures and certain types of parasomnias can have similar clinical semiologies and can become a diagnostic dilemma. Common sleep disorders and manifestations such as cataplexy, sleep attacks in the setting of narcolepsy, night terrors, and RBD may be confused with epilepsy (37). Some epilepsy syndromes such as benign rolandic and nocturnal frontal lobe epilepsies, occur predominantly or exclusively during sleep.

Antiepileptic drugs (AEDs) also affect sleep architecture (212). Phenytoin increases the amount of NREM sleep, decreases sleep efficiency, and reduces sleep latency (267). Carbamazepine increases the number of sleep-stage shifts and decreases REM sleep (114). Benzodiazepines decrease sleep latency and reduce SWS (71,212). Gabapentin has been shown to improve sleep efficiency and SWS and increase REM sleep (105,194). In clinical practice, understanding the unique effects of these AEDs may offer the clinician an opportunity to improve sleep and wakefulness; medications that improve sleep disorders may require tailored dosing schedules to maximize their benefit (252).

MULTIPLE SCLEROSIS

MS is the most common nontraumatic cause of neurologic disability in young adults (138). With improved therapy, many patients survive to older age. Sleep disturbances in MS are common but poorly recognized, and almost half of all patients demonstrate sleep disturbances due to leg spasms, pain, immobility, nocturia, or medication (243). Common sleep disorders in patients with MS include insomnia, RLS, narcolepsy, and RBD. Sleep disruption in MS may result in hypersomnolence, increased fatigue, and a lowered pain threshold. Therefore, an increased clinical awareness of sleep-related problems is warranted in this patient population because they are extremely common and have the potential to negatively impact overall health and quality of life (104).

SLEEP AND STROKE

The number of patients affected by stroke will increase as a function of aging (60). Sleep and stroke interact in a number of complex ways. Probably the most important of these interactions is the fact that patients with sleep apnea or nocturnal hypoxemia often present with cardiac arrhythmias, intellectual decline, and increased risk of stroke. Habitual snoring affects 4% to 24% of the adult population with a maximum prevalence around the age of 50 to 60 years and is strongly associated with OSA. Habitual snoring may have adverse effects on long-term stroke outcome. Snoring was found to adversely affect prognosis in stroke survivors (230). Hypersomnolence and prolonged sleep, which can be symptoms of SDB, may also represent independent risk factors for stroke (79,202). Sleep-disordered breathing is common among stroke patients as defined by an apnea-hypopnea index (AHI) ≥10 per hour (35,89,119).

Treatment of SDB has been recently shown to improve subjective well-being and mood in stroke patients with SDB (213,264). Based on the blood pressure lowering effects of CPAP, treatment of SDB may lead to a stroke risk reduction of about 20% (193). Currently, it remains to be established whether SDB represents an independent risk factor for stroke. The relationship may be a genetically determined one due to the increased vascular risk associated with SDB.

CSA and sometimes Cheyne-Stokes breathing may be latent phenomena after the stroke and may occur in as many as 30% to 40% of patients (135,190). Subsequent to the stroke, patients may present with the coexistence of both OSA during REM sleep and Cheyne-Stokes breathing during light NREM sleep (36,190,199). Central hypoventilation syndrome and failure of automatic breathing (Ondine curse) are more typically associated with brainstem strokes and are less common presentations (36).

Bilateral lacunar ischemic infarcts in the tegmentum of the pons and periventricular white matter damage can present as REM sleep without atonia, which leads to RBD (33,217). Patients with Binswanger's disease or subcortical leukoencephalopathy are at an increased risk for developing RBD primarily because white matter ischemia in the vicinity of the supratentorial system is often involved in modulating REM-related atonia. Brain MRI studies in patients with RBD with underlying strokes show ischemic lesions in the pontine tegmentum, which is the locus of the muscle tone inhibitor system. Stroke can impair the regulation of sleep-wake and breathing control mechanisms. Secondary consequences from the stroke, such as immobilization, pain, hypoxia, and depression, can also impact sleep.

AMYOTROPHIC LATERAL SCLEROSIS

Amyotrophic lateral sclerosis (ALS) is a neurodegenerative disease in middle-aged and elderly patients. ALS has a relentless progression with no impairment of the mental function, or sensorium. Respiratory failure in this disorder occurs late in the course of the disease and may also be the presenting feature of this disease. It is not uncommon for physicians to encounter patients with breathing difficulties, bulbar weakness, and stridor in the emergency room only to later diagnose ALS. The major sleep complaint of these patients is EDS, likely caused by sleep-related respiratory disturbances and insomnia (26,27,99,100).

The mechanism of respiratory disturbance in this disorder may be due to the weakness of the upper airways caused by bulbar weakness, diaphragmatic weakness (due to a phrenic nerve lesion), and intercostal muscle weakness (due to the degeneration of intercostal nerve nuclei). Degeneration of the central respiratory neurons accounts for both central and OSA. Polysomnographic findings include apneas in the form of central, obstructive, and mixed events, increased awakenings, sleep fragmentation, and reduced nocturnal oxygen saturation (2,72,99,100,170).

Noninvasive positive pressure upper airway ventilation provides a long-lasting benefit in symptoms and quality of life indicators for ALS patients and should be offered to all patients with symptoms of SDB or inspiratory muscle dysfunction (73). Positive pressure therapy can also prolong tracheostomy-free survival (57).

SPINAL CORD DISEASES

Patients with spinal cord injury (SCI) often present with sleep disturbances related to respiratory dysfunction, particularly when the lesion occurs in the upper cervical spinal cord within the vicinity of the phrenic nerve nuclei (74). Patients with SCI have a greater difficulty in falling asleep, describe more frequent awakenings, are more likely to be prescribed sleeping pills, sleep more hours, take more frequent and longer naps, and are more likely to snore compared to controls (40). In particular, spasms, pain, paresthesia, and voiding difficulties have a higher association with sleep problems (40).

The incidence of SDB in SCI is high in patients with tetraplegia, especially when the patient is elderly, has an increased large neck circumference, has a long duration of the disease, and is on cardiac medications (234). The increased use of cardiac medication in tetraplegics with SDB may implicate a link between SDB and cardiovascular morbidity, one of the leading causes of death in tetraplegia. OSA appears to be more common in older patients with spinal cord injury than in the general population and is related to ventilatory dysfunction secondary to spinal cord injury (224).

Neurologic conditions likely to damage and disrupt the phrenic and intercostal motor neurons in the spinal cord include poliomyelitis, ALS, spinal cord tumors, spinal trauma, spinal surgery (e.g., cervical cordotomy or anterior spinal surgery), and nonspecific or demyelinating myelitis (74). Patients with syringobulbia present with severe abnormalities in respiratory rhythm generation during sleep (180). The respiratory disturbances are not due to muscle weakness, and they are not correlated with the size of the cavity (180). Phrenic nerve damage may cause diaphragmatic paralysis, and although unilateral paralysis is asymptomatic, bilateral paralysis presents with orthopnea manifesting as difficulty on inspiration out of proportion to the cardiopulmonary status, which may be life threatening (74).

POST-POLIO SYNDROME

Post-polio syndrome (PPS) describes the new, late manifestations that occur in patients three to four decades after the occurrence of acute poliomyelitis (139). PPS is more common at the present time due to the large epidemics of poliomyelitis in the 1940s and 1950s. Neurologic manifestations of PPS consist of neurologic, musculoskeletal, and systemic symptoms and signs. The most prominent neurologic manifestation is a new progressive weakness at times accompanied by atrophy referred to as post-polio progressive muscular atrophy (PPMA) when affecting the extremities. However, a new weakness can also affect respiratory and bulbar muscles, which can be more serious and cause dysphagia, dysphonia, and respiratory failure (77,140). Respiratory failure in PPS may be treated with CPAP, BiPAP, or tracheotomy and permanent ventilation if necessary (32). Other sleep disturbances include random myoclonus, periodic movements in sleep with muscle contractions, ballistic movements of the legs, and restless legs syndrome (56). Poliovirus-induced damage to the spinal cord and brain may be implicated as a possible cause of these abnormal movements in sleep (56). It is suggested that polysomnography be performed on PPS patients with EDS and respiratory complaints (232).

HUNTINGTON'S DISEASE

Huntington's disease (HD) is a hereditary, progressive, neurodegenerative condition characterized by significant motor dysfunction that typically appears as involuntary and spasmodic movements, cognitive impairment, and psychiatric difficulties. It is caused by an expanded CAG repeat in the gene encoding huntingtin, a protein of unknown function. Sleep disturbances are common in HD and consist of disturbed sleep patterns with increased sleep onset latency, reduced sleep efficiency, increased arousals and sleep fragmentation, decreased SWS, frequent nocturnal awakenings, increased density of sleep spindles, increased time spent awake, and reduced sleep efficiency (92,123,266). Patients who have HD have also shown higher density sleep spindles, in contrast with findings in other neurodegenerative dementia populations (92). These abnormalities correlated in part with duration of illness, severity of clinical symptoms, and degree of atrophy of the caudate nucleus (266).

Based on actigraphy data, patients with HD demonstrate significant activity and spend more time making high-acceleration movements compared with age-matched controls (133). In contrast with findings in other neurodegenerative dementias, no increase in sleep-related breathing disorders has been demonstrated in HD (52). Circadian rhythm sleep disturbances, however, are an important pathologic feature of HD and may arise from a disruption of the expression of the circadian clock genes *mPer2* and *mBmal1* in the SCN, the principal circadian pacemaker in the brain (176).

MYOTONIC DYSTROPHY

Sleep abnormalities in patients with myotonic dystrophy include hypersomnia, sharing with narcolepsy a short sleep latency and the presence of sleep-onset REM periods during the MSLT (162). Hypersomnia is found in almost one third of patients with myotonic dystrophy, and the severity of daytime sleepiness correlates with the severity of muscular impairment (149). Corpus callosum atrophy might occur in myotonic dystrophy patients, and the size of the atrophy, especially in the anterior portion, might be associated with the hypersomnia (118). Patients with myotonic dystrophy report a longer sleep period, a less restorative sleep, difficulties with sleep initiation, and hypersomnia comparable with those found in idiopathic hypersomnia (149). In myotonic dystrophy, hypersomnia may be aggravated by alveolar hypoventilation and SDB but is not entirely reversed by satisfactory application of positive pressure airway ventilation, suggesting that hypersomnia is partially related to an intrinsic hypersomnia caused by central nervous system alteration (73).

A dysfunction of the hypothalamic hypocretin system has recently been found in patients with myotonic dystrophy and may mediate the underlying hypersomnia (162). Modafinil, a wake-promoting agent, was recently found to reduce hypersomnolence and improves mood, quality of life measures of energy, and health change in patients with myotonic dystrophy (78,159).

Patients with myotonic dystrophy have increased risk of OSA, CSA, and EDS (72,73,226). These patients are also thought to have a centrally mediated impairment in breathing probably related to a brainstem respiratory center disorder rather than respiratory muscle weakness (244,254). Nonobstructive sleep apneas and alveolar hypoventilation may be related to an underlying central neurologic pathology in myotonic dystrophy; muscle weakness and myotonia may underlie development of obstructive sleep disordered breathing (73).

Neuropathologic findings in patients with myotonic dystrophy consist of severe neuronal loss and gliosis in the midbrain and pontine raphe, particularly in the dorsal raphe nucleus and superior central nucleus and pontine and medullary reticular formation (184). Alveolar hypoventilation and the hypersomnia in myotonic dystrophy may be attributed to these morphologic abnormalities and would appear to be central in nature (184).

CONCLUSION

Sleep changes dramatically with old age. Both subjective and objective measures show increases in sleep-wake disturbances with age. What remains a controversial issue is whether it is a decreased need for sleep or a decreased ability to sleep that decreases with aging. The older person has a more fragmented sleep, sleeps less deeply, and tends to have early morning awakening. The aging process itself does not cause sleep problems. Sleep changes even more dramatically with dementia. When encountering daytime sleepiness in an older patient with neurologic and neurodegenerative disorders, it is crucial to first review the patient's medical history, psychiatric history, medications, underlying medical illnesses, and sleep-wake schedule pattern. The prevalence of SDB, PLMS, RLS, and RBD, many of which are comorbid with dementia, increases with age and may lead to EDS or insomnia. Many sleep disorders are potentially reversible. A carefully thought out clinical decision-making process can greatly benefit the patient and family. Sleep problems of the elderly contribute heavily to the decision to institutionalize an elder, largely by interfering with the sleep of caregivers. Thus, sleep problems greatly contribute to the social and economic cost of institutional care. As the population ages, the nature, prevalence, and treatability of the sleeping problems of both elders and their caregivers need further study.

REFERENCES

1. Abad VC, Guilleminault C. Review of rapid eye movement behavior sleep disorders. *Curr Neurol Neurosci Rep*. 2004;4:157–163.
2. Aboussouan LS, Lewis RA. Sleep, respiration and ALS. *J Neurol Sci*. 1999;164:1–2.
3. Agnew HW, Webb WB, Williams RL, et al. The first night effect: an EEG study of sleep. *Psychophysiology*. 1966;2:263–266.

4. Aldrich MS. *Sleep Medicine.* Oxford: Oxford University Press, Inc; 1999.

5. Aldrich MS, Foster NL, White RF, et al. Sleep abnormalities in progressive supranuclear palsy. *Ann Neurol.* 1989;25:577–581.

6. Alessi CA, Martin JL, Webber AP, et al. Randomized, controlled trial of a nonpharmacological intervention to improve abnormal sleep/wake patterns in nursing home residents. *J Am Geriatr Soc.* 2005;53:803–810.

7. Alessi CA, Schnelle JF, MacRae PG, et al. Does physical activity improve sleep in impaired nursing home residents? *J Am Geriatr Soc.* 1995; 43:1098–1102.

8. Alessi CA, Yoon EJ, Schnelle JF, et al. A randomized trial of a combined physical activity and environmental intervention in nursing home residents: do sleep and agitation improve? *J Am Geriatr Soc.* 1999;47:784–791.

9. Aloia MS, Di Dio P, Perlis ML, et al. Neuropsychological changes and treatment compliance in older adults with sleep apnea. *J Psychosom Res.* 2003;54:71–76.

10. Ancoli-Israel S. Sleep problems in older adults: putting myths to bed. *Geriatrics.* 1997;52:20–30.

11. Ancoli-Israel S, Alessi C. Sleep and aging. *Am J Geriatr Psychiatry.* 2005;13:341–343.

12. Ancoli-Israel S, Bliwise DL, Mant A. *Sleep and Breathing in the Elderly.* New York: Mercel Dekker, Inc.; 1993.

13. Ancoli-Israel S, Coy T. Are breathing disturbances in elderly equivalent to sleep apnea syndrome? *Sleep.* 1994;17:77–83.

14. Ancoli-Israel S, Gehrman P, Martin JL, et al. Increased light exposure consolidates sleep and strengthens circadian rhythms in severe Alzheimer's disease patients. *Behav Sleep Med.* 2003;1:22–36.

15. Ancoli-Israel S, Jones DW, Hanger MA, et al. *Sleep in the Nursing Home.* New York: Elsevier Press; 1991.

16. Ancoli-Israel S, Klaubner MR, Butters N, et al. Dementia in institutionalized elderly: relation to sleep apnea. *J Am Geriatr Soc.* 1991; 39:258–263.

17. Ancoli-Israel S, Klauber MR, Gillin JC, et al. Sleep in non-institutionalized Alzheimer's disease patients. *Aging (Milano).* 1994;6:451–458.

18. Ancoli-Israel S, Klauber MR, Jones DW, et al. Variations in circadian rhythms of activity, sleep, and light exposure related to dementia in nursing-home patients. *Sleep.* 1997;20:18–23.

19. Ancoli-Israel S, Kripke DF, Klauber MR, et al. Morbidity, mortality and sleep-disordered breathing in community dwelling elderly. *Sleep.* 1996;19:277–282.

20. Ancoli-Israel S, Kripke DF, Klauber MR, et al. Periodic limb movements in sleep in community-dwelling elderly. *Sleep.* 1991;14:496–500.

21. Ancoli-Israel S, Kripke DF, Klauber MR, et al. Sleep-disordered breathing in community-dwelling elderly. *Sleep.* 1991;14:486–495.

22. Ancoli-Israel S, Martin JL, Gehrman P, et al. Effect of light on agitation in institutionalized patients with severe Alzheimer's disease. *Am J Geriatr Psychiatry.* 2003;11:194–203.

23. Ancoli-Israel S, Richardson GS, Mangano RM, et al. Long-term use of sedative hypnotics in older patients with insomnia. *Sleep Med.* 2005; 6:107–113.

24. Ancoli-Israel S, Stepnowsky C, Engler R, et al. The relationship between congestive heart failure, sleep apnea, and mortality in older men. *Chest.* 2003;124:1400–1405.

25. Apps MC, Sheaff PC, Ingram DA, et al. Respiration and sleep in Parkinson's disease. *J Neurol Neurosurg Psychiatry.* 1985;48:1240–1245.

26. Arnulf I, Derenne JP. Respiratory disorders during sleep in degenerative diseases of the brain stem. *Rev Neurol (Paris).* 2001;157:S148–S151.

27. Arnulf I, Similowski T, Salachas F, et al. Sleep disorders and diaphragmatic function in patients with amyotrophic lateral sclerosis. *Am J Respir Crit Care Med.* 2000;161:849–856.

28. Asayama K, Yamadera H, Ito T, et al. Double blind study of melatonin effects on the sleep-wake rhythm, cognitive and non-cognitive functions in Alzheimer type dementia. *J Nippon Med Sch.* 2003;70:334–341.

29. Askenasy JJ, Yahr MD. Reversal of sleep disturbance in Parkinson's disease by antiparkinsonian therapy: a preliminary study. *Neurology.* 1985; 35:527–532.

30. Avidan AY. Sleep disorders in the older patient. *Prim Care.* 2005;32:563–586.

31. Avidan AY. Sleep in the geriatric patient population. *Semin Neurol.* 2005;25:52–63.

32. Bach JR. Management of post-polio respiratory sequelae. *Ann N Y Acad Sci.* 1995;753:96–102.

33. Bahro M, Katzmann KJ, Guckel F, et al. REM sleep parasomnia. *Nervenarzt.* 1994;65:568–571.

34. Bailey DR, Attanasio R. Dentistry's role in the management of sleep disorders. Recognition and management. *Dent Clin North Am.* 2001; 45:619–630.

35. Bassetti C, Aldrich M, Chervin R, et al. Sleep apnea in the acute phase of TIA and stroke. *Neurology.* 1996;47:1167–1173.

36. Bassetti C, Aldrich MS, Quint D, et al. Sleep-disordered breathing in patients with acute supra- and infratentorial stroke. *Stroke.* 1997; 28:1765–1772.

37. Bazil CW. Nocturnal seizures. *Semin Neurol.* 2004;24:293–300.

38. Benca RM, Obermeyer WH, Thisted RA, et al. Sleep and psychiatric disorders: a meta–analysis. *Arch Gen Psychiatry.* 1992;49:651–668.

39. Bhatt MH, Podder N, Chokroverty S, et al. Sleep and neurodegenerative diseases. *Semin Neurol.* 2005;25:39–51.

40. Biering-Sorensen F, Biering-Sorensen M. Sleep disturbances in the spinal cord injured: an epidemiological questionnaire investigation, including a normal population. *Spinal Cord.* 2001;39:505–513.

41. Bixler EO, Kales A, Vela-Bueno A, et al. Nocturnal myoclonus and nocturnal myoclonic activity in the normal population. *Res Commun Chem Pathol Pharmacol.* 1982;36:129–140.

42. Bliwise DL. *Cognitive Function and Sleep Disordered Breathing in Aging Adults.* New York: Elseiver; 1991.

43. Bliwise DL. Review: sleep in normal aging and dementia. *Sleep.* 1993;16:40–81.

44. Bliwise DL. Sleep apnea, APOE4 and Alzheimer's disease 20 years and counting? *J Psychosom Res.* 2002;53:539–546.

45. Bliwise DL. Sleep disorders in Alzheimer's disease and other dementias. *Clin Cornerstone.* 2004; 6[Suppl 1A]:S16–S28.

46. Bliwise DL, Feldman DE, Bliwise NG, et al. Risk factors for sleep disordered breathing in heterogeneous geriatric populations. *J Am Geriatr Soc.* 1987;35:132–141.

47. Bliwise DL, Tinklenberg J, Yesavage JA, et al. REM latency in Alzheimer's disease. *Biol Psychiatry.* 1989;25:320–328.

48. Boeve B. Melatonin for treatment of REM sleep behavior disorder: response in 8 patients. *Sleep.* 2001;24[Suppl]:A35.

49. Boeve BF, Silber MH, Ferman TJ, et al. Association of REM sleep behavior disorder and neurodegenerative disease may reflect an underlying synucleinopathy. *Mov Disord.* 2001;16:622–630.

50. Boeve BF, Silber MH, Ferman T, et al. REM sleep behavior disorder and degenerative dementia: an association likely reflecting Lewy body disease. *Neurology.* 1998;51:363–370.

51. Boeve BF, Silber MH, Ferman TJ, et al. REM sleep behavior disorder in Parkinson's disease and dementia with Lewy bodies. *J Geriatr Psychiatry Neurol.* 2004;17:146–157.

52. Bollen EL, Den Heijer JC, Ponsioen C, et al. Respiration during sleep in Huntington's chorea. *J Neurol Sci.* 1988;84:63–68.

53. Bologna, Geneva, Parma, and Pisa Universities Group for the Study of REM Sleep Behaviour Disorders in Parkinson's Disease. Interobserver reliability of ICSD–R criteria for REM sleep behaviour disorder. *J Sleep Res.* 2003;12:255–257.

54. Bootzin R, Nicassio P. *Behavioral Treatments for Insomnia.* New York: Academic Press, Inc.; 1978.

55. Briskin JG, Lehrman KL, et al. *Shy-Drager Syndrome and Sleep Apnea.* New York: Liss; 1978.

56. Bruno RL. Abnormal movements in sleep as a post-polio sequelae. *Am J Phys Med Rehabil.* 1998;77:339–343.

57. Butz M, Wollinsky KH, Wiedemuth-Catrinescu U, et al. Longitudinal effects of noninvasive positive-pressure ventilation in patients with amyotrophic lateral sclerosis. *Am J Phys Med Rehabil.* 2003; 82:597–604.

58. Campbell SS, Kripke DF, Gillin JC, et al. Exposure to light in healthy elderly subjects and Alzheimer's patients. *Physiol Behav.* 1988;42:141–144.

59. Campbell SS, Terman M, et al. Light treatment for sleep disorders: consensus report. V. Age-related disturbances. *J Biol Rhythms.* 1995; 10:151–154.

60. Carolei A, Sacco S, DeSantis F, et al. Epidemiology of stroke. *Clin Exp Hypertens.* 2002;24:479–483.

61. Carskadon MA, Brown ED, Dement WC. Sleep fragmentation in the elderly: relationship to daytime sleep tendency. *Neurobiol Aging.* 1982; 3:321–327.

62. Carskadon MA, Dement WC. *Normal Human Sleep: An Overview.* Philadelphia: W.B. Saunders Company; 2001.

63. Cartwright RD, Diaz F, Lloyd S. The effects of sleep posture and sleep stage on apnea frequency. *Sleep.* 1991;14:351–353.

64. Chokroverty S. Sleep and degenerative neurologic disorders. *Neurol Clin.* 1996;14:807–826.

65. Chokroverty S, Sharp JT, Barron KD. Periodic respiration in erect posture in Shy-Drager syndrome. *J Neurol Neurosurg Psychiatry.* 1978;41:980–986.

66. Cohen-Zion M, Stepnowsky C, Marler C, et al. Changes in cognitive function associated with sleep disordered breathing in older people. *J Am Geriatr Soc.* 2001;49:1622–1627.

67. Coleman RM. *Periodic Movements in Sleep (Nocturnal Myoclonus) and Restless Legs Syndrome.* Menlo Park, CA: Addison-Wesley Publishing Co; 1982.

68. Coleman RM, Bliwise DL, Sajben N. Daytime sleepiness in patients with periodic movements in sleep. *Sleep.* 1982;5:S191–S202.

69. Comella CL. Sleep disturbances in Parkinson's disease. *Curr Neurol Neurosci Rep.* 2003;3:173–180.

70. Consens FB, Chervin RD, Koeppe RA, et al. Validation of a polysomnographic score for REM sleep behavior disorder. *Sleep.* 2005;28:993–997.

71. Copinschi G, Van Onderbergen A, L'hermite-Baleriaux M, et al. Effects of the short-acting benzodiazepine triazolam, taken at bedtime, on

circadian and sleep-related hormonal profiles in normal men. *Sleep*. 1990; 13:232–244.

72. Culebras A. Sleep and neuromuscular disorders. *Neurol Clin*. 1996;14:791–805.

73. Culebras A. Sleep disorders and neuromuscular disease. *Semin Neurol*. 2005;25:33–38.

74. Culebras A. Sleep disorders associated with neuromuscular and spinal cord disorders. Neurology Medlink, 2006. Available at: http://www.medlink.com/medlinkcontent.asp.

75. Czeisler C, Dumont M, Duffy JF. Association of sleep-wake habits in older people with changes in output of circadian pacemaker. *Lancet*. 1992; 340:933–936.

76. Czeisler CA, Kronauer RE, Allan JS, et al. Bright light induction of strong (type 0) resetting of the human circadian pacemaker. *Science*. 1989;244:1328–1333.

77. Dalakas MC, Sever JL, Madden DL, et al. Late postpoliomyelitis muscular atrophy: clinical, virologic, and immunologic studies. *Rev Infect Dis*. 1984; 6:S562–S567.

78. Damian MS, Gerlach A, Schmidt F, et al. Modafinil for excessive daytime sleepiness in myotonic dystrophy. *Neurology*. 2001;56:794–796.

79. Davies DP, Rodgers H, Walshaw D, et al. Snoring, daytime sleepiness and stroke: a case-control study of first-ever stroke. *J Sleep Res*. 2003;12:313–318.

80. Dawson D, Encel N. Melatonin and sleep in humans. *J Pineal Res*. 1993;15:1–12.

81. de Brito-Marques PR, de Mello RV, Montenegro L. Nightmares without atonia as an early symptom of diffuse Lewy bodies disease. *Arq Neuropsiquiatr*. 2003;61:936–941.

82. Degen R, Degen HE. Sleep and sleep deprivation in epileptology. *Epilepsy Res Suppl*. 1991; 2:235–260.

83. Dement W, Richardson G, Prinz P, et al. *Changes of Sleep and Wakefulness with Age*. New York: Van Nostrand Reinhold; 1996.

84. Derderian SS, Rajagopal KR. Neuropsychologic symptoms in obstructive sleep apnea improve after treatment with nasal continuous positive airway pressure. *Chest*. 1988;94:1023–1027.

85. Devinsky O, Ehrenberg B, Barthlen GM, et al. Epilepsy and sleep apnea syndrome. *Neurology*. 1994;44:2060–2064.

86. Dinner DS. Effect of sleep on epilepsy. *J Clin Neurophysiol*. 2002;19:504–513.

87. Doghramji PP. Treatment of insomnia with zaleplon, a novel sleep medication. *Int J Clin Pract*. 2001;55:329–334.

88. Dufour MC, Archer L, Gordis E. Alcohol and the elderly. *Clin Geriatr Med*. 1992;8:127–141.

89. Dyken ME, Somers VK, Yamada T, et al. Investigating the relationship between stroke and obstructive sleep apnea. *Stroke*. 1996;27:401–407.

90. Edinger JD, Hoelscher TJ, Webb MD, et al. Polysomnographic assessment of DIMS: empirical evaluation of its diagnostic value. *Sleep*. 1989;12:315–322.

91. Eisensehr I, Linke R, Noachtar S, et al. Reduced striatal dopamine transporters in idiopathic rapid eye movement sleep behavior disorder. Comparison with Parkinson's disease and controls. *Brain*. 2000;123:1155–1160.

92. Emser W, Brenner M, Stober T, et al. Changes in nocturnal sleep in Huntington's and Parkinson's disease. *J Neurol*. 1988;235:177–179.

93. Erkinjuntti T, Sulkava PM, et al. Sleep apnea in multiinfarct dementia and Alzheimer's disease. *Sleep*. 1987;10:419–425.

94. Espie CA. Insomnia: conceptual issues in the development, persistence, and treatment of sleep disorder in adults. *Annu Rev Psychol*. 2002; 53:215–243.

95. Espie CA. *The Psychological Treatment of Insomnia*. Chichester, United Kingdom: John Wiley; 1991.

96. Fabbrini G, Barbanti P, Aurilia C, et al. Excessive daytime sleepiness in de novo and treated Parkinson's disease. *Mov Disord*. 2002;17: 1026–1030.

97. Factor SA, McAlarney T, Sanchez-Ramos JR, et al. Sleep disorders and sleep effect in Parkinson's disease. *Mov Disord*. 1990;5:280–285.

98. Fairbanks DNF, Fujita S, Ikematsu T, et al. *Snoring and Obstructive Sleep Apnea*. New York: Raven Press; 1987.

99. Ferguson KA, Strong MJ, Ahmad D, et al. Sleep and breathing in amyotrophic lateral sclerosis. *Sleep*. 1995;18:514.

100. Ferguson KA, Strong MJ, Ahmad D, et al. Sleep-disordered breathing in amyotrophic lateral sclerosis. *Chest*. 1996;110:664–669.

101. Ferini-Strambi L, Zucconi M. REM sleep behavior disorder. *Clin Neurophysiol*. 2000; 111(suppl 2): S136–S140.

102. Findley LJ, Presty SK, Barth J, et al. *Impaired Cognition and Vigilance in Elderly Subjects with Sleep Apnea*. New York: Elsevier; 1991.

103. Finucane TE. Treatment for insomnia. *Lancet*. 2002;359:1434.

104. Fleming WE, Pollak CP. Sleep disorders in multiple sclerosis. *Semin Neurol*. 2005;25:64–68.

105. Foldvary-Schaefer N, De Leon Sanchez I, et al. Gabapentin increases slow-wave sleep in normal adults. *Epilepsia*. 2002;43:1493–1497.

106. Foley DJ, Masaki K, White L, et al. Relationship between apolipoprotein E epsilon 4 and sleep-disordered breathing at different ages. *JAMA*. 2001;286: 1447–1448.

107. Ford DE, Kamerow DB. Epidemiologic study of sleep disturbances and psychiatric disorders. An opportunity for prevention. *JAMA*. 1989;262:1479–1484.

108. Frank B, Gupta S. A review of antioxidants and Alzheimer's disease. *Ann Clin Psychiatry*. 2005; 17:269–286.

109. Frucht S, Greene P, Fahn S. Sleep episodes in Parkinson's disease: a wake-up call. *Mov Disord*. 2002;15:601–603.

110. Fulda S, Wetter TC. Dopamine agonists for the treatment of restless legs syndrome. *Expert Opin Pharmacother*. 2005;6:2655–2666.

111. Gagnon JF, Bedard MA, Fantini ML, et al. REM sleep behavior disorder and REM sleep without atonia in Parkinson's disease. *Neurology*. 2002;59:585–589.

112. Gehrman PR, Martin JL, Shochat T, et al. Sleep-disordered breathing and agitation in institutionalized adults with Alzheimer's disease. *Am J Geriatr Psychiatry*. 2003;11:426–433.

113. Ghorayeb I, Bioulac B, Tison F. Sleep disorders in multiple system atrophy. *J Neural Transm*. 2005;112:1669–1675.

114. Gigli GL, Placidi F, Diomedi M, et al. Nocturnal sleep and daytime somnolence in untreated patients with temporal lobe epilepsy: changes after treatment with controlled-release carbamazepine. *Epilepsia*. 1997;38:696–701.

115. Gillin JC, Ancoli-Israel S. *The Impact of Age on Sleep and Sleep Disorders*. Baltimore: Williams & Wilkins; 1992.

116. Gillin JC, Byerley WF. The diagnosis and management of insomnia. *N Engl J Med*. 1990;322: 239–248.

117. Gilman S, Koeppe RA, Chervin RD, et al. REM sleep behavior disorder is related to striatal monoaminergic deficit in MSA. *Neurology*. 2003; 61:29–34.

118. Giubilei F, Iannilli M, Vitale A, et al. Sleep patterns in acute ischemic stroke. *Acta Neurol Scand*. 1992; 86:567–571.

119. Good DC, Henkle JQ, Gelber D, et al. Sleep-disordered breathing and poor functional outcome after stroke. *Stroke*. 1996;27:252–259.

120. Gottlieb DJ, DeStefano AL, Foley DJ, et al. APOE epsilon 4 is associated with obstructive sleep apnea/hypopnea: the Sleep Heart Health Study. *Neurology*. 2004;63:664–668.

121. Gross RA, Spehlmann R, Daniels JC. Sleep disturbances in progressive supranuclear palsy. *Electroencephalogr Clin Neurophysiol*. 1978; 45: 16–25.

122. Haimov I, Lavie P, Laudon M, et al. Melatonin replace-ment therapy of elderly insomniacs. *Sleep*. 1995;18:598–603.

123. Hansotia P, Wall R, Berendes J. Sleep disturbances and severity of Huntington's disease. *Neurology*. 1985;35:1672–1674.

124. Hauri PJ. Advances in the behavioral treatment of insomnia. *Sleep Med Rev*. 2003;7:201–202.

125. Hauri PJ. Behavioral treatment of insomnia. *Med Times*. 1979;107:36–47.

126. Hauri PJ. Insomnia. *Clin Chest Med*. 1998; 19:157–168.

127. Hauri PJ. *Primary Insomnia: Principles and Practice of Sleep Medicine*. Philadelphia: W.B. Saunders Company; 2003.

128. Hauri PJ, Olmstead E. What is the moment of sleep onset for insomniacs? *Sleep*. 1983;6:10–15.

129. Hauri PJ, Wisbey J. Wrist actigraphy in insomnia. *Sleep*. 1992;15:293–301.

130. Hicks R, Dysken MW, Davis JM, et al. The pharmacokinetics of psychotropic medication in the elderly: a review. *J Clin Psychiatry*. 1981;42:374–385.

131. Hoch CC, Kupfer DJ, et al. Sleep disordered breathing in normal and pathological aging. *J Clin Psychiatry*. 1986;47:499–503.

132. Hughes RJ, Sack RL, Lewy AJ. The role of melatonin and circadian phase in age-related sleep-maintenance insomnia: assessment in a clinical trial of melatonin replacement. *Sleep*. 1998;21:52–68.

133. Hurelbrink CB, Lewis SJ, Barker RA. The use of the Actiwatch-Neurologica system to objectively assess the involuntary movements and sleep-wake activity in patients with mild-moderate Huntington's disease. *J Neurol*. 2005;252:642–647.

134. Iranzo A, Santamaria J, Rye, et al. Characteristics of idiopathic REM sleep behavior disorder and that associated with MSA and PD. *Neurology*. 2005;65:247–252.

135. Iranzo A, Santamaria J, Berenguer J, et al. Prevalence and clinical importance of sleep apnea in the first night after cerebral infarction. *Neurology*. 2002;58:911–916.

136. Jacobs D, Ancoli-Israel S, Parker L, et al. Twenty-four-hour sleep-wake patterns in a nursing home population. *Psychol Aging*. 1989;4:352–356.

137. Janssens JP, Pautex S, Hilleret H, et al. Sleep disordered breathing in the elderly. *Aging (Milano)*. 2000;12:417–429.

138. Johnson RT. *Current Therapy in Neurologic Disease*. Philadelphia: Mosby; 1985.

139. Jubelt B. Post-polio syndrome. *Curr Treat Options Neurol*. 2004;6:87–93.

140. Jubelt B, Cashman NR. Neurological manifestations of the post-polio syndrome. *Crit Rev Neurobiol*. 1987;3:199–220.

141. Kadotani H, Kadotani T, Young T, et al. Association between apolipoprotein E epsilon 4 and sleep-disordered breathing in adults. *JAMA*. 2001;285:2888–2890.

142. Kamel NS, Gammack JK. Insomnia in the elderly: cause, approach, and treatment. *Am J Med*. 2006;119:463–469.

143. Kaplan B, Mason NA. Levodopa in restless legs syndrome. *Ann Pharmacother*. 1992;26:214–216.

144. Kavey N, Walters AS, Hening W, et al. Opioid treatment of periodic movements in sleep in patients without restless legs. *Neuropeptides.* 1988;11:181–184.

145. Kellinghaus C, Loddenkemper T, Dinner DS, et al. Non-epileptic seizures of the elderly. *J Neurol.* 2004;251:704–709.

146. Kish SJ, Chang LJ, Mirchandani L, et al. Progressive supranuclear palsy: relationship between extrapyramidal disturbances, dementia, and brain neurotransmitter markers. *Ann Neurol.* 1985;18: 530–536.

147. Klink ME, Quan SF, Kaltenborn WT, et al. Risk factors associated with complaints of insomnia in a general adult population. Influence of previous complaints of insomnia. *Arch Intern Med.* 1992;152:1634–1637.

148. Kowey PR, Mainchak RA, et al. Things that go bang in the night. *N Engl J Med.* 1992;327:1884.

149. Laberge L, Begin P, Montplaisir J, et al. Sleep complaints in patients with myotonic dystrophy. *J Sleep Res.* 2004;13:95–100.

150. Larsen JP, Tandberg E. Sleep disorders in patients with Parkinson's disease: epidemiology and management. *CNS Drugs.* 2001;15:267–275.

151. Laustsen G, Andersen M. Ramelteon (rozerem): a novel approach for insomnia treatment. *Nurse Pract.* 2006;31:52–55.

152. Lewy AJ, Ahmed S, Sack RL. Phase shifting the human circadian clock using melatonin. *Behav Brain Res.* 1996;73:131–134.

153. Lewy AJ, Emens J, Jackman A, et al. Circadian uses of melatonin in humans. *Chronobiol Int.* 2006; 23:403–412.

154. Lichstein KL, Reidel BW. Behavioral assessment and treatment of insomnia: a review with an emphasis on clinical application. *Behav Ther.* 1994;15:659–688.

155. Little JT, Satlin A, Sunderland T, et al. Sundown syndrome in severely demented patients with probable Alzheimer's disease. *J Geriatr Psychiatry Neurol.* 1995;8:103–106.

156. Lowe AA. *Dental Appliances for the Treatment of Snoring and Obstructive Sleep Apnea.* Philadelphia: W.B. Saunders; 1994.

157. Lowe AD. Sleep in Parkinson's disease. *J Psychosom Res.* 1998;44:613–617.

158. Lyketsos CG, Lindell Veiel L, Baker A, et al. A randomized, controlled trial of bright light therapy for agitated behaviors in dementia patients residing in long-term care. *Int J Geriatr Psychiatry.* 1990;14:520–525.

159. MacDonald JR, Hill JD, Tarnopolsky MA. Modafinil reduces excessive somnolence and enhances mood in patients with myotonic dystrophy. *Neurology.* 2002;59:1876–1880.

160. Mahowald MW, Schenck CH. *REM Sleep Behavior Disorder.* Philadelphia: WB Saunders; 1994.

161. Malow BA, Bowes RJ, Lin X. Predictors of sleepiness in epilepsy patients. *Sleep.* 1997;20:1105–1110.

162. Martinez-Rodriguez JE, Lin L, Iranzo A, et al. Decreased hypocretin-1 (orexin-A) levels in the cerebrospinal fluid of patients with myotonic dystrophy and excessive daytime sleepiness. *Sleep.* 2003;26:287–290.

163. Mazza M, Della Marca G, De Risio S, et al. Sleep disorders in the elderly. *Clin Ther.* 2004;155: 391–394.

164. McCall WV. Sleep in the elderly: burden, diagnosis, and treatment. *Prim Care.* 2004;6:9–20.

165. McGaffigan S, Bliwise DL. The treatment of sundowning. A selective review of pharmacological and nonpharmacological studies. *Drugs Aging.* 1997;10:10–17.

166. McGechan A, Wellington K. Ramelteon. *CNS Drugs.* 2005;19:1057–1065.

167. McGheie A, Russel S. The subjective assessment of normal sleep patterns. *J Mental Sci.* 1962; 108:642–654.

168. Melton ST, Wood JM, Kirkwood CK. Eszopiclone for insomnia. *Ann Pharmacother.* 2005;39: 1659–1665.

169. Miles L, Dement WC. Sleep and aging. *Sleep.* 1980;3:119–220.

170. Minz M, Autret A, Laffont F, et al. A study on sleep in amyotrophic lateral sclerosis. *Biomedicine.* 1979;30:40–46.

171. Mitler MM, Browman CP, Menn SJ, et al. Nocturnal myoclonus: treatment efficacy of clonazepam and temazepam. *Sleep.* 1986;9: 385–392.

172. Miyamoto T, Miyamoto M, Yokota N, et al. A case of nocturnal polyuria in olivopontocerebellar atrophy. *Psychiatry Clin Neurosci.* 1999;53:279–281.

173. Moen MD, Plosker GL. Zolpidem extended release in insomnia: profile report. *Drugs Aging.* 2006;23:843–846.

174. Montagna P. The treatment of restless legs syndrome. *Neurol Sci.* 2007;28:S61–S66.

175. Morrison AR. The pathophysiology of REM-sleep behavior disorder. *Sleep.* 1998;21:446–449.

176. Morton AJ, Wood NI, Hastings MH, et al. Disintegration of the sleep-wake cycle and circadian timing in Huntington's disease. *J Neurosci.* 2005; 25:157–163.

177. Munschauer FE, Mador J, Ahuja A, et al. Selective paralysis of voluntary but not limbically influenced automatic respiration. *Arch Neurol.* 1991; 48:1190–1192.

178. National Institutes of Health. NIH State-of-the-Science Conference Statement on manifestations and management of chronic insomnia in

adults. *NIH Consens State Sci Statements*. 2005; 22:1–30.

179. Neubauer DN. New approaches in managing chronic insomnia. *CNS Spectr*. 2006;11[Suppl 8]: 1–13.

180. Nogues M, Gene R, Benarroch E, et al. Respiratory disturbances during sleep in syringomyelia and syringobulbia. *Neurology*. 1999;52:1777–1783.

181. Oertel WH, Stiasny-Kolster K, Bergtholdt B, et al. Efficacy of pramipexole in restless legs syndrome: a six-week, multicenter, randomized, double-blind study (effect-RLS study). *Mov Disord*. 2007; 22:213–219.

182. Olakowska E, Marcol W, Kotulska K, et al. The role of melatonin in the neurodegenerative diseases. *Bratisl Lek Listy*. 2005;106:171–174.

183. Olson EJ, Boeve BF, Silber MH. Rapid eye movement sleep behaviour disorder: demographic, clinical and laboratory findings in 93 cases. *Brain*. 2000;123:331–339.

184. Ono S, Kurisaki H, Sakuma A, et al. Myotonic dystrophy with alveolar hypoventilation and hypersomnia: a clinicopathological study. *J Neurol Sci*. 1995;128:225–231.

185. Owen RT. Extended-release zolpidem: efficacy and tolerability profile. *Drugs Today (Barc)*. 2006;42:721–727.

186. Owen RT. Ramelteon: profile of a new sleep-promoting medication. *Drugs Today (Barc)*. 2006; 42:255–263.

187. Pandi-Perumal SR, Zisapel N, Srinivasan V, et al. Melatonin and sleep in aging population. *Exp Gerontol*. 2005;40:911–925.

188. Pappert EJ, Goetz CG, Niederman FG, et al. Hallucinations, sleep fragmentation, and altered dream phenomena in Parkinson's disease. *Mov Disord*. 1999;14:117–121.

189. Parkes JD. The parasomnias. *Lancet*. 1987; 2:1021–1025.

190. Parra O, Arboix A, Bechich S, et al. Time course of sleep-related breathing disorders in first-ever stroke or transient ischemic attack. *Am J Resp Crit Care Med*. 2000;161:375–380.

191. Partinen M. Sleep disorder related to Parkinson's disease. *J Neurol*. 1997;244:S3–S6.

192. Pauletto G, Belgrado E, Marinig R, et al. Sleep disorders and extrapyramidal diseases: an historical review. *Sleep Med*. 2004;5:163–167.

193. Pepperell JCT, Ramdassingh-Dow S, Crosthwaite N, et al. Ambulatory blood pressure after therapeutic and subtherapeutic nasal continuous positive airway pressure for obstructive sleep apnoea: a randomized parallel trial. *Lancet*. 2001;359: 204–210.

194. Placidi F, Diomedi M, Scalise A, et al. Effect of anticonvulsants on nocturnal sleep in epilepsy. *Neurology*. 2000;54:S25–S32.

195. Plazzi G, Corsinin R, et al. REM sleep behavior disorders in multiple system atrophy. *Neurology*. 1997;48:1094–1097.

196. Pollak CP, Perlick D. Sleep problems and institutionalization of the elderly. *J Geriatr Psychiatry Neurol*. 1991;4:204–210.

197. Pollak CP, Perlick D, Linsner JP, et al. Sleep problems in the community elderly as predictors of death and nursing home placement. *J Community Health*. 1990;15:123–135.

198. Poryazova RG, Zachariev ZI. REM sleep behavior disorder in patients with Parkinson's disease. *Folia Med (Plovdiv)*. 2005;47:5–10.

199. Power WR, Mosko SS, Sassin JF. Sleep-stage dependent Cheyne-Stokes respiration after cerebral infarct: a case study. *Neurology*. 1982;32: 763–766.

200. Prinz PN. Sleep patterns in the healthy aged: relationship with intellectual function. *J Gerontol*. 1977;32:179–185.

201. Punjabi NM, Shahar E, Redline S, et al. Sleep-disordered breathing, glucose intolerance, and insulin resistance: the Sleep Heart Health Study. *Am J Epidemiol*. 2004;160:521–530.

202. Qreshi AI, Giles WH, Croft JB, et al. Habitual sleep patterns and risk for stroke and coronary disease: a 10-year follow-up from NHANES I. *Neurology*. 1997;48:904–910.

203. Rediehs MH, Reis JS, Creason NS. Sleep in old age: focus on gender differences. *Sleep*. 1990;13: 410–424.

204. Reiter RJ. The pineal gland and melatonin in relation to aging: a summary of the theories and of the data. *Exp Gerontol*. 1995;30:199–212.

205. Reynolds CFI. *Sleep in Affective Disorders*. Philadelphia: Saunders Company; 1989.

206. Ropinirole (Requip) for restless legs syndrome. *Med Lett Drugs Ther*. 2005;47:62–64.

207. Roth T, Roehrs T, et al. *Pharmacological Treatment of Sleep Disorders*. New York: John Wiley & Sons; 1988.

208. Saarelainen S, Lehtimaki R, Kallonen E, et al. No relation between apolipoprotein E alleles and obstructive sleep apnea. *Clin Genet*. 1998;53: 147–148.

209. Sadeh A, Acebo C. The role of actigraphy in sleep medicine. *Sleep Med Rev*. 2002;6:113–124.

210. Sakakibara R, Odaka T, Uchiyama T, et al. Colonic transit time and rectoanal videomanometry in Parkinson's disease. *J Neurol Neurosurg Psychiatry*. 2003;74:268–272.

211. Salva MA, Guilleminault C. Olivopontocerebellar degeneration, abnormal sleep, and REM sleep without atonia. *Neurology*. 1986;36:576–577.

212. Sammaritano M, Sherwin A. Effect of anticonvulsants on sleep. *Neurology*. 2000;54:S16–S24.

213. Sandberg O, Franklin LA, Bucht G, et al. Nasal continuous positive airway pressure in stroke patients with sleep apnea: a randomized treatment study. *Eur Respir J*. 2001;18:619–622.
214. Satlin A, Volicer L, Ross V, et al. Bright light treatment of behavioral and sleep disturbances in patients with Alzheimer's disease. *Am J Psychiatry*. 1992;149:1028–1032.
215. Schenck CH, Bundlie SR, Mahowald MW. Delayed emergence of a parkinsonian disorder in 38% of 29 older men initially diagnosed with idiopathic rapid eye movement sleep behavior disorder. *Neurology*. 1996;46:388–393.
216. Schenck CH, Bundlie SR, Patterson AL, et al. Rapid eye movement sleep behavior disorder: a treatable parasomnia affecting older adults. *JAMA*. 1987;257:1786–1789.
217. Schenck CH, Mahowald MW. Injurious sleep behavior disorders (parasomnias) affecting patients on intensive care units. *Intensive Care Med*. 1991;17:219–224.
218. Schenck CH, Mahowald MW. REM sleep parasomnias. *Neurol Clin*. 1996;14:697–720.
219. Schletens PVF, Van Keimpema A, Lindebloom J, et al. Sleep apnea syndrome presenting with cognitive impairment. *Neurology*. 1991;41:155–156.
220. Schneider DL. Insomnia. Safe and effective therapy for sleep problems in the older patient. *Geriatrics*. 2002;57:24–26, 29, 32.
221. Schnelle JF, Cruise PA, Alessi CA, et al. Sleep hygiene in physically dependent nursing home residents: behavioral and environmental intervention implications. *Sleep*. 1998;21:515–523.
222. Shepard JW. *Cardiorespiratory Changes in Obstructive Sleep Apnea*. Philadelphia: W.B. Saunders Company; 1989.
223. Shepard JW. Hypertension, cardiac arrhythmias, myocardial infarction, and stroke in relation to obstructive sleep apnea. *Clin Chest Med*. 1992;13:437–458.
224. Short DJ, Stradling JR, Williams SJ. Prevalence of sleep apnoea in patients over 40 years of age with spinal cord lesions. *J Neurol Neurosurg Psychiatry*. 1992;55:1032–1036.
225. Singer C, Tractenberg ER, Kaye J, et al. A multicenter, placebo-controlled trial of melatonin for sleep disturbance in Alzheimer's disease. *Sleep*. 2003;26:893–901.
226. Sivak ED, Shefner JM, Sexton J. Neuromuscular disease and hypoventilation. *Curr Opin Pulm Med*. 1999;5:355–362.
227. Skene DJ, Deacon S, Arendt J. Use of melatonin in circadian rhythm disorders and following phase shifts. *Acta Neurobiol Exp (Wars)*. 1996;56:359–362.
228. Skene DJ, Swaab DF. Melatonin rhythmicity: effect of age and Alzheimer's disease. *Exp Gerontol*. 2003;38:199–206.
229. Spielman AJ, Saskin P, Thorpy MJ. Treatment of chronic insomnia by restriction of time in bed. *Sleep*. 1987;10:45–56.
230. Spriggs DA, French JM, Murdy JM, et al. Snoring increases the risk of stroke and adversely affects prognosis. *Q J Med*. 1992;303:555–562.
231. Srinivasan V, Pandi-Perumal SR, Maestroni GJ, et al. Role of melatonin in neurodegenerative diseases. *Neurotox Res*. 2005;7:293–318.
232. Steljes DG, Kryger MH, Kirk BW, et al. Sleep in postpolio syndrome. *Chest*. 1990;98:133–140.
233. Stocchi F, Barbato L, Nordera G, et al. Sleep disorders in Parkinson's disease. *J Neurol*. 1998;245:S15–S18.
234. Stockhammer E, Tobon A, Michel F, et al. Characteristics of sleep apnea syndrome in tetraplegic patients. *Spinal Cord*. 2002;40:286–294.
235. Stolz SE, Aldrich MS. REM sleep behavior disorder associated with caffeine abuse. *Sleep Res*. 1991;20:341.
236. Stopa EG, Volicer L, Kuo-Leblanc V, et al. Pathologic evaluation of the human suprachiasmatic nucleus in severe dementia. *J Neuropathol Exp Neurol*. 1999;58:29–39.
237. Strohl KP, Hensley MJ, Saunders NA, et al. Progesterone administration and progressive sleep apneas. *JAMA*. 1981;245:1230–1232.
238. Strollo PJ Jr, Atwood SM. Positive pressure therapy. *Clin Chest Med*. 1998;19:55–68.
239. Sullivan CE, Grunstein RR. *Continuous Positive Airway Pressure in Sleep-Disordered Breathing*. Philadelphia: WB Saunders Company; 1989.
240. Swaab DF, Fisser B, Kamphorst W, et al. The human suprachiasmatic nucleus; neuropeptide changes in senium and Alzheimer's disease. *Basic Appl Histochem*. 1988;32:43–54.
241. Swaab DF, Fliers E, Partiman TS. The suprachiasmatic nucleus of the human brain in relation to sex, age and senile dementia. *Brain Res*. 1985;342:37–44.
242. Taasan VC, Block AJ, Boysen PG, et al. Alcohol increases sleep apnea and oxygen desaturation in asymptomatic men. *Am J Med*. 1981;71:240–245.
243. Tachibana N, Howard RS, Hirsch NP, et al. Sleep problems in multiple sclerosis. *Eur Neurol*. 1994;34:320–323.
244. Takasugi T, Ishihara T, Kawamura J, et al. Respiratory failure: respiratory disorder during sleep in patients with myotonic dystrophy. *Rinsho Shinkeigaku*. 1995;35:1486–1488.
245. Takeuchi N, Uchimura N, Hashizume Y, et al. Melatonin therapy for REM sleep behavior disorder. *Psychiatry Clin Neurosci*. 2001;55:267–269.

246. Tan A, Salgado M, Fahn S. Rapid eye movement sleep behavior disorder preceding Parkinson's disease with therapeutic response to levodopa. *Mov Disord*. 1996;11:214–216.

247. Tandberg EJ, Larsen P, Karlsen K. A community-based study of sleep disorders in patients with Parkinson's disease. *Mov Disord*. 1998;13:895–899.

248. Taylor JL, Friedman L, Sheikh J, et al. Assessment and management of "sundowning" phenomena. *Semin Clin Neuropsychiatry*. 1997;2:113–122.

249. Thory MJ, Yager J. *The Encyclopedia of Sleep and Sleep Disorders*. New York: Facts on File, Inc.; 1991.

250. Trenkwalder C. Sleep dysfunction in Parkinson's disease. *Clin Neurosci*. 1998;5:107–114.

251. Turner RS, Chervin RD, Frey KA, et al. Probable diffuse Lewy body disease presenting as REM sleep behavior disorder. *Neurology*. 1997;49:523.

252. Vaughn BV, D'Cruz OF. Sleep and epilepsy. *Semin Neurol*. 2004;24:301–313.

253. Vaughn BV, D'Cruz OF, Beach R, et al. Improvement of epileptic seizure control with treatment of obstructive sleep apnoea. *Seizure*. 1996;5:73–78.

254. Ververs CC, Van der Meche FG, Verbraak AF, et al. Breathing pattern awake and asleep in myotonic dystrophy. *Respiration*. 1996;63:1–7.

255. Vitiello MV, Bliwise DL, Prinz PN. Sleep in Alzheimer's disease and the sundown syndrome. *Neurology*. 1992;42:83–93.

256. Vitiello MV, Borson S. Sleep disturbances in patients with Alzheimer's disease: epidemiology, pathophysiology and treatment. *CNS Drugs*. 2001;15:777–796.

257. Vitiello MV, Poceta JS, Prinz PN. Sleep in Alzheimer's disease and other dementing disorders. *Can J Psychol*. 1991;45:221–239.

258. Vitiello MV, Prinz PN. Alzheimer's disease. Sleep and sleep/wake patterns. *Clin Geriatr Med*. 1989;5:289–299.

259. Vitiello MV, Prinz PN, Williams DE, et al. Sleep disturbances in patients with mild-stage Alzheimer's disease. *J Gerontol*. 1990;45:M131–M138.

260. Walters AS. Toward a better definition of the restless legs syndrome. The International Restless Legs Syndrome Study Group. *Mov Disord*. 1995; 10:634–642.

261. Walters AS, Hickey K, Maltzman J, et al. A questionnaire study of 138 patients with restless legs syndrome: the "Night-Walkers" survey. *Neurology*. 1996;46:92–95.

262. Wang JZ, Wang ZF. Role of melatonin in Alzheimer-like neurodegeneration. *Acta Pharmacol Sin*. 2006;27:41–49.

263. Wauquier A, Van Sweden B, Lagaay AM, et al. Ambulatory monitoring of sleep-wakefulness patterns in healthy elderly males and females (> 88 years): the "Senieur" protocol. *J Am Ger Soc*. 1992;40:109–114.

264. Wessendorf TE, Wang YM, Thilmann AF, et al. Treatment of obstructive sleep apnoea with nasal continuous positive airway pressure. *Eur Respir J*. 2001;18:623–629.

265. Wetter TC, Trenkwalder C, Gershanik O, et al. Polysomno-graphic measures in Parkinson's disease: a comparison between patients with and without REM sleep disturbances. *Wien Klin Wochenschr*. 2001;113:249–253.

266. Wiegand M, Moller AA, Lauer CJ, et al. Nocturnal sleep in Huntington's disease. *J Neurol*. 1991;238:203–208.

267. Wolf PU, Roder-Wanner U, Brede M. Influence of therapeutic phenobarbital and phenytoin medication on the polygraphic sleep of patients with epilepsy. *Epilepsia*. 1984;25:467–475.

268. Wooten V. Medical causes of insomnia. In: Kryger MH, Dement WC, eds. *Principles and practice of sleep medicine*. Philadelphia: W.B. Saunders Company; 1994:456–475.

269. Wu YH, Swaab DF. The human pineal gland and melatonin in aging and Alzheimer's disease. *J Pineal Res*. 2005;38:145–152.

270. Young AM, Home M, Churchward T, et al. Comparison of sleep disturbance in mild versus severe Parkinson's disease. *Sleep*. 2002;25:573–577.

271. Zesiewicz TA, Baker MJ, Dunne PB, et al. Diffuse Lewy body disease. *Curr Treat Options Neurol*. 2001;3:507–518.

272. Zhdanova IV, Tucci V. Melatonin, circadian rhythms, and sleep. *Curr Treat Options Neurol*. 2003;5:225–229.

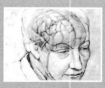

CHAPTER 14

Headaches

David W. Dodick and David J. Capobianco

Before considering the topic of headaches in the elderly, it is prudent to define the term "elderly." One definition is: "rather old; being past middle age" (32). Another equally nebulous definition requires one add "50 years to your own age" (anonymous). Nonetheless, age 65, the standard age for retirement, is often regarded as the beginning of old age.

The elderly are the fastest growing segment of the population. In the United States, over 34 million people are aged 65 years or older (17). If population trends continue, by 2030, it is estimated that 20% of the population (80 million persons) will be over the age of 65 (17).

Headache in the elderly, although less prevalent than in younger adults, is a common complaint that presents a special challenge to the physician. The clinician faces not only a broad differential diagnosis, but also must contend with the difficulty of managing headache when comorbid illnesses can contraindicate or complicate effective treatments. Headache in the elderly can conveniently be divided into primary and secondary headaches. Primary headache disorders, such as migraine, cluster headache, and tension-type headache (TTH), are diseases unto themselves (morbus suis generis). Secondary headache represents a symptom of an underlying disease such as an intracranial mass lesion or a metabolic disorder. Although the overall incidence of headache declines with advancing age, the relative proportion of secondary headaches increases, thus highlighting the importance of a careful evaluation and a high level of suspicion when evaluating an elderly patient with a complaint of headache.

EPIDEMIOLOGY

Headache prevalence declines with age. Although it is one of the most common symptoms in the young, headache declines in old age to become the tenth most common symptom of elderly women and the fourteenth most common symptom of elderly men (21). The prevalence of headache in women and men aged 55 to 74 years is approximately 66% and 53%, respectively, compared with 92% and 74%, respectively,

in their younger counterparts between the ages of 21 to 34 years (50). The prevalence declines even further in those over the age of 75 to 55% and 22% for women and men, respectively. Despite this age-related decline, the prevalence of headache in the elderly is still high. In a community survey, the prevalence of frequent headache in the elderly was 20% for women and 10% for men, a significant public health problem by any standard (9). A recent survey in the United Kingdom demonstrated a decline in the 3-month prevalence of headache for those over the age of 66 (40.6% in men and 49.7% in women) compared with younger individuals (4).

CAUSES

As in the younger age groups, "benign" primary headache disorders, such as migraine and TTH, account for most headaches that affect the elderly (Fig. 14-1). However, an important distinguishing feature is that secondary ("symptomatic") headaches are much more common in the aged, constituting up to 30% of all headache complaints (42). The underlying causes also differ qualitatively compared with the young, in that diseases such as giant cell arteritis (GCA) and subdural hematomas are mainly disorders of the elderly. Table 14-1 outlines the various primary and secondary headaches seen in the elderly population.

PRIMARY HEADACHES

MIGRAINE

Although migraine attenuates and often disappears with advancing age, approximately one third of individuals with migraine continue to suffer from recurrent attacks into older age. Although rare, some people (2% to 3%) may experience their first migraine attack after the age of 50 years. The prevalence of migraine in the elderly has been estimated to be between 2.9% (42) and 10.5% (41). Women continue to be affected more often than men.

The clinical features of the migraine attack may change over time. The pain may more commonly be

197

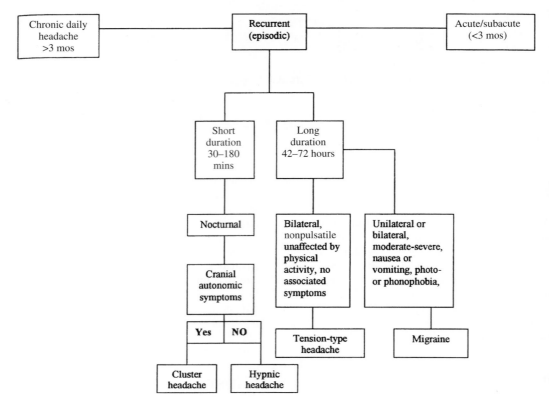

Figure 14-1. Headache in the elderly. *(Continued on next page)*

holocephalic rather than unilateral (29). The associated symptoms, mainly photophobia, phonophobia, and nausea and vomiting, occur less commonly in the elderly than in their younger counterparts (29). The headache may be accompanied by aura, or as frequently recognized in clinical practice, elderly patients may have recurrent attacks of painless aura (50). Aura without headache, referred to as "late-life migraine accompaniments," represents reversible focal cortical dysfunction and may take the form of a recurrent hemisensory disturbance (paresthesia) or a scintillating visual scotoma. These episodic focal neurologic disturbances can be easily confused with transient ischemic attacks (TIA). A careful evaluation is important in this setting, including a detailed history of prior migraine attacks, because the incidence and prevalence of cerebrovascular disease increase in the elderly. The key diagnostic features that differentiate late-life migraine accompaniments from TIA are listed in Table 14-2.

Although the effective therapeutic options for migraine are the same in the elderly, the therapeutic approach to these patients is sometimes a challenge because of coexisting medical illnesses. Managing the older patient with migraine requires a thorough

familiarity with the individual's health status and a practical knowledge of pharmacology (34). Vascular disease, for example, precludes the use of migraine-specific medications such as ergotamine derivatives and triptans. Beta-blockers and calcium channel blockers are best avoided in patients with depression or congestive heart failure, whereas prostatism, glaucoma, heart failure, or arrhythmias may preclude the use of tricyclic antidepressants. Moreover, even when these contraindications do not exist, the elderly are more likely to experience more side effects from certain medications, such as sedation and confusion with tricyclics or impaired renal function with nonsteroidal anti-inflammatory drugs (NSAIDs) because of diminished renal function and creatinine clearance (34).

In addition, medications used for certain medical disorders can exacerbate migraine in this population. For example, the use of vasodilating antihypertensive medications (e.g., nifedipine or methyldopa) can worsen migraine or lead to an increase in the frequency of attacks. Similarly, when used for ischemic heart disease, nitrates can precipitate an attack of migraine or cluster headache in those who are predisposed.

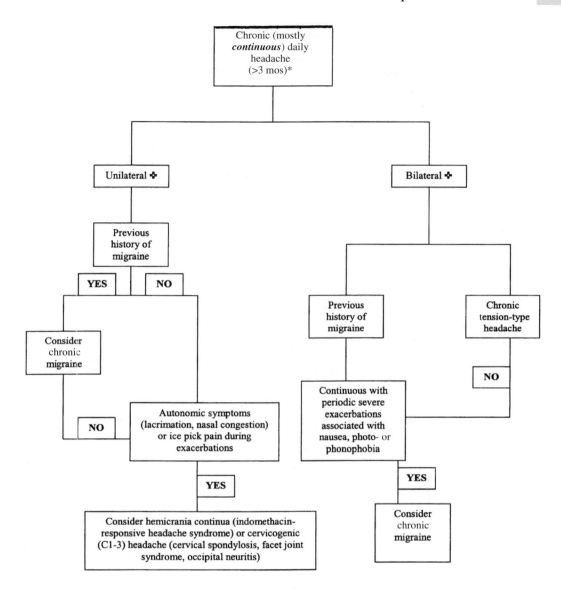

Figure 14-1. *Continued.*

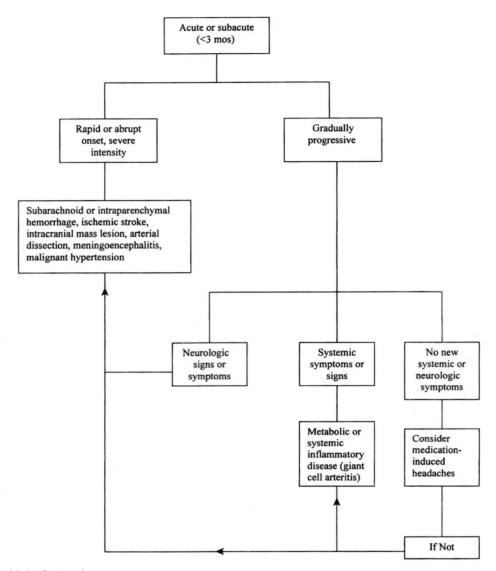

Figure 14-1. *Continued.*

TENSION-TYPE HEADACHE

TTH is a "featureless headache." It is a dull, bilateral, or diffuse headache, often described as a pressure or squeezing sensation of mild to moderate intensity. It has no accompanying migraine features (e.g., nausea, emesis, photophobia, phonophobia), and the pain is not worsened with movement and does not prohibit activity. No cranial autonomic symptoms are noted. When presenting as a new headache, especially in patients over the age of 40 years, it should be considered a diagnosis of exclusion because it is the headache phenotype most frequently mimicked by brain tumors and other organic causes of headache. The exact prevalence of TTH in the elderly is difficult to assess because of various definitions used across studies and the propensity for organic disease to masquerade as TTH in this age group. However, estimates range from 18% (45) to 52% (41). Although most elderly people have had TTH since youth or middle age, about 10% develop TTH after the age of 50 years. Again, a careful search for organic disease is imperative in this particular group because many underlying metabolic, systemic, and psychiatric (depression) disorders and structural intracranial disease present with

Table 14-1. *Primary and Secondary Headaches in the Elderly*

Primary headaches
    Migraine
    Tension-type
    Cluster
    Hypnic
Secondary headaches
    Inflammatory/infectious/structural
        Giant cell arteritis
        Cerebrovascular disease (ischemic and
            hemorrhagic stroke)
        Malignant hypertension
        Intracranial mass lesion (tumor, subdural
            hematoma)
        Intracranial injection (meningitis and
            encephalitis)
        Cervical spondylosis
        Fever or infection
Metabolic/systemic
    Medications (including rebound syndromes)
    Hypoxia or hypercapnia (chronic respiratory
        diseases, sleep apnea)
    Anemia, polycythemia
    Electrolyte disturbances (hypocalcemia,
        hyponatremia)
    Depression
    Chronic renal failure

ill-defined, nonpulsatile, bilateral headaches that could easily be mistaken for TTH.

The approach to treatment should involve nonpharmacologic treatment strategies as well as the judicious use of NSAIDs, analgesics, and tricyclic antidepressants for prophylaxis.

CLUSTER HEADACHE

Cluster headache is one of the most distinctive of the primary headaches, with an unmistakable attack profile. The pain is so excruciatingly intense that it has been termed the "suicide headache." It is often maximal in the orbital region and peaks in intensity within 5 minutes. It can occur during the day or, characteristically, awaken a patient out of a sound sleep. The pain lasts between 15 minutes and 2 hours, but the average duration is 60 minutes if untreated. One or more cranial autonomic features, such as lacrimation, nasal congestion, rhinorrhea, ptosis, meiosis, and conjunctival injection, are seen in more than 97% of patients. Rarely, cluster headache can begin as late as the eighth decade, although this type of headache in elderly individuals invariably will have started at a younger age. The average age of onset is approximately 28 years, and men are affected four times more often than women (13). Although cluster headache is uncommon in random surveys of the healthy elderly, it accounts for up to 4% of elderly patients presenting to headache clinics (42). New-onset cluster headache has been reported in the elderly (47), with the oldest age of onset being a 91-year-old woman (40).

As with migraine and TTH, the treatment of cluster headache in the elderly is frequently complicated by the presence of coexisting medical disorders. Subcutaneous sumatriptan, the most effective medication for the acute treatment of cluster headache, must be used with caution in those with cardiovascular risk factors, especially because cluster headache occurs more commonly in men, the majority of whom are chronic smokers. For patients with coexistent cardiovascular disease or significant risk factors, oxygen inhalation is the safest and most effective acute agent. Verapamil, usually combined with a short course of corticosteroids, is often highly effective in terminating a cluster period or reducing the frequency and intensity of attacks during this period (13).

HYPNIC HEADACHE

Hypnic headache, a primary headache disorder that primarily affects elderly individuals, occurs exclusively during sleep (12,37). The mean age of onset is approximately 60 years, and women are more often

Table 14-2. *Distinguishing Features of Late-Life Migraine Accompaniments versus TIA*

Migraine Aura	TIA
Positive visual phenomena (scintillating scotoma)	Negative symptoms (loss of vision)
Gradual buildup	Abrupt onset
Sequential progression from one modality to another (visual-sensory-speech)	Simultaneous appearance
Repetitive attacks of identical nature	Variable symptomatology
Average duration 20–30 minutes	Average duration <15 minutes
Flurry of attacks in mid-life common	Flurry of attacks not common
Mild headache following attack in 50%	Headache less likely with TIA

TIA, transient ischemic attack.

affected than men. The headache typically awakens the individual from sleep often at or near the same time each night, prompting the term "alarm-clock" headache. The headache is moderate to severe in intensity and often bilateral and squeezing, although the pain can be unilateral in up to one third of patients. Generally, no associated "migrainous" symptoms (e.g., nausea, emesis, photophobia, phonophobia) or cranial autonomic symptoms (e.g., lacrimation, rhinorrhea), as seen with cluster headache, occur. The pain usually lasts 30 to 60 minutes, although attacks can last several hours. Remaining in a supine position often exacerbates the pain; therefore, most individuals will report needing to rise from bed for relief. Nocturnal attacks often occur more than four nights per week, and some individuals may have several attacks through the night. In some patients, an attack can occur during a daytime nap.

Recently, a case of symptomatic hypnic headache has been reported (36). This underscores the need to proceed with appropriate neuroimaging to exclude a secondary headache disorder.

Lithium carbonate is an effective treatment, but the side effects in this age group sometimes preclude its long-term use (12,37). Caffeine, either by tablet or as a cup of coffee before bedtime, can be effective for some patients (12). Other medications reported to be effective for prophylaxis include flunarizine (33), indomethacin (11), melatonin (15), topiramate (20), and pregabalin (48).

SECONDARY HEADACHES

GIANT CELL ARTERITIS

GCA is a necrotizing granulomatous systemic arteritis that affects medium and large arteries, especially those branching from the proximal aorta. It occurs primarily in middle-aged and elderly persons. Although it is manifest by a wide range of clinical symptoms, headache is both the most common symptom and the reason why patients with GCA are seen by neurologists. The average age of onset is approximately 70 years, and the disease is rare before the age of 50. More than 90% of cases occur in those over 60 years of age. Women are affected about twice as commonly as men.

In a population-based study in Olmstead County, Minnesota, the incidence and prevalence of the disease over a 42-year period was found to be 17.8 and 200/100,000/year, respectively, in persons aged 50 years and older (38). The age-specific incidence rate increases from 2.1 per 100,000 in those 50 to 59 years of age to 49 per 100,000 in those above the age of 80, highlighting the dramatic increase in incidence with age. An autopsy series revealed arteritis in 1.6% of 899 postmortem cases, indicating that the disease may be more common than is clinically apparent (35).

Headache is the most frequent and most common initial symptom in patients with GCA. The location, quality, and severity of the headache vary from patient to patient. Although the headache is often moderate to severe, it can begin as an insidious and mild ache. The headache can be throbbing, boring, or lancinating in quality, and the pain can radiate to the neck, face, gums, jaw, or tongue. Although temporal headaches have become synonymous with this disease, the headache may be diffuse or localized to any head region, including the occiput. In one study of 24 biopsy-proven cases, headache was localized to the temporal region in only six patients, whereas seven patients had headache that did not even involve the temporal area (43). Scalp tenderness is usually localized to the temporal or, less commonly, the occipital arteries. It can be diffuse or even absent in up to one third of patients with headache. Headaches can be severe, even when the cranial arteries are normal to palpation, and may subside, even when the disease activity continues; therefore, in isolation, headaches cannot be used as a surrogate clinical marker for disease activity.

Polymyalgia rheumatica (PMR), malaise, and fatigue occur in over 50% of patients at some time during the illness. In several reports of GCA, PMR has been noted in 40% to 60% of patients and has been the initial symptom complex in 20% to 40% of patients (22).

Ocular involvement is a well-known and perhaps the most notorious complication of GCA. Visual symptoms, including amaurosis, diplopia, and permanent visual loss, are the most important early manifestations of the disease. Visual loss can be unilateral or bilateral, and sequential loss of vision in one eye and then the other is not unusual. If unilateral visual loss occurs and is left untreated, involvement of the contralateral eye can occur within 1 to 2 weeks. Onset of visual loss is often sudden and irreversible, but well-documented cases of gradually progressive visual loss with recovery of vision after treatment have been described (28). The incidence of blindness is between 8% and 20% but can approach 40% in those patients who are not treated. Blindness is preceded by amaurosis in only about 15% of patients, which underscores the need for early diagnosis and treatment. The most common cause of visual loss is ischemic anterior optic neuropathy, although ischemic posterior optic neuropathies without disc edema can occur. Reversible ischemia can also account for other visual phenomena in this illness, including orthostatic fluctuations in vision, transient monocular visual loss, and ocular motor disturbances.

GCA should be considered in the diagnosis of any patient older than 50 years of age who has a new form of headache, change in a previously stable pattern of headache, jaw claudication, weight loss, abrupt loss of vision, PMR, unexplained prolonged fever or anemia, or high erythrocyte sedimentation rate (ESR). Temporal artery biopsy is recommended for diagnosis in all patients, and when feasible and safe, the biopsy should be done before initiating treatment with steroids. The temporal artery is biopsied most frequently, but if the facial or occipital arteries are clearly involved, they can be sampled as well. If a focal abnormality can be palpated, a small biopsy of the affected segment can be performed. Skip lesions can occur pathologically, resulting in a false-positive rate of 4% to 5% (24). As such, when the arteries are normal on examination, a generous arterial specimen (3 to 5 cm) should be harvested, and multiple histologic sections at 1-mm levels should be analyzed. In patients with a negative biopsy finding, a contralateral biopsy should be performed. Sorenson and Lorenzen (44) found GCA-positive results in specimens from the contralateral temporal artery in seven of 13 patients who initially had negative biopsy results.

Elevated sedimentation rates are characteristic of both GCA and PMR. Sedimentation rates greater than 100 mm in 1 hour (Westergren method) are common, but biopsy-proven cases with normal (0 to 40 mm) sedimentation rates have been described (51). The prevalence of a normal ESR in patients with GCA is estimated to be between 2% and 8.7%. Other serum markers that are commonly elevated in patients with GCA include C-reactive protein, fibrinogen, alpha$_2$-globulin, gamma-globulin, complements, factor VIII or von Willebrand factor, and interleukin-6. A mild to moderate normochromic anemia, thrombocytosis, decreased albumin, and elevated liver function tests, particularly alkaline phosphatase, are usually seen as well.

Corticosteroid therapy is the treatment of choice in all cases of GCA and is the only therapy proved to be efficacious. In general, once the diagnosis is suggested, prednisone is initiated, irrespective of the type or number of clinical manifestations. After obtaining a complete blood count and sedimentation rate, prednisone is started immediately in patients with recent or impending vascular complications (e.g., visual loss or stroke). Steroid treatment does alter the histopathologic picture, and therefore, it is preferable to obtain an arterial biopsy before or shortly after initiating treatment. However, inflammatory changes in the temporal arteries can persist for 2 to 4 weeks after steroids are begun.

Although the ideal initial prednisone dose, tapering scheme, and duration of treatment are debated, an initial starting dose of 40 to 60 mg of prednisone in single or divided daily dosages is adequate for most patients. Progression to complete bilateral blindness can occur in patients with the use of lower dosages. Alternate-day steroid regimens are less effective than daily administration and cannot be relied on to control acute symptoms or disease activity. The dosage should be increased up to 120 mg per day in those who do not demonstrate a prompt clinical or laboratory response to lower dosages.

Patients with acute or impending visual loss or vascular complications should be hospitalized and administered intravenous methylprednisolone (1,000 mg/day over 3 to 5 days). Oral corticosteroids are then started at a dose of 1.5 to 2.0 mg/kg/day. The initial starting dosage is maintained until all reversible symptoms resolve and all aberrant laboratory parameters have normalized, which usually occurs within 2 to 4 weeks. Once resolution is maintained for 2 weeks, the dosage can be reduced by 10 mg every 2 weeks until a dose of 40 mg per day is attained. Thereafter, the dosage should not be decreased by more than 10% of the total daily dosage every 1 to 2 weeks. Once the total dosage is less than 10 mg, monthly tapering by 1 mg can be instituted. The alteration in steroid dosage should be based predominantly on clinical signs and symptoms. Most relapses appear to be related to inadequate suppression of a continuous inflammatory process rather than from spontaneous exacerbations. Although sedimentation rate and C-reactive protein studies now are generally considered to be the most sensitive and widely available surrogate laboratory markers of disease activity, an increase in either or both does not always predict relapse; relapse can occur despite these markers remaining within normal limits (26). This emphasizes the importance of close clinical monitoring to determine the rate and extent to which steroids are tapered.

Treatment of GCA with long-term daily corticosteroids at high dosages can lead to frequent and potentially serious consequences. Patients must be periodically monitored for a number of potential adverse events that are commonly associated with long-standing corticosteroid administration, including osteoporosis, hypertension, peptic ulcer disease, diabetes, and subcapsular cataracts. All patients on long-term corticosteroids should receive 1 to 2 g of supplemental calcium (calcium carbonate or citrate) and 400 to 800 U of vitamin D on a daily basis to prevent steroid-induced osteoporosis.

MASS LESIONS

In the elderly, the incidence of intracranial disease increases, including both metastatic and primary brain tumors (8,10). However, headache as the sole manifestation of brain tumor is uncommon in patients with a normal neurologic examination and no history of systemic cancer and occurs in only 1% of patients with brain tumors. The headache associated with intracranial mass lesions is usually intermittent and tends to develop and resolve over several hours. The most common type of brain tumor headache is a relatively bland "tension-type" headache, which is seen in more than two thirds of patients. Most patients describe the headache as a "dull ache" or "pressure" or "like a sinus headache." Migraine-like headaches are seen in about 10% of patients with brain tumors.

The classic brain tumor headache—severe headache that is worse in the morning and associated with vomiting—occurs in a minority (17%) of patients (16). In individuals with a past history of headache, the headache associated with intracranial lesions is similar to the patient's previous headaches. This highlights the importance of carefully evaluating an elderly individual complaining of a headache that is even slightly different, more severe, more frequent, or associated with neurologic signs or symptoms, including slowed mentation. A neuroimaging study should be obtained in such a circumstance.

Headache in patients with brain tumor is more likely to be a prominent symptom when the tumor involves the leptomeninges or infratentorial compartment, which increases the likelihood of obstruction of cerebrospinal fluid pathways. Headaches are also common in individuals with a prior history of headache, as well as in patients with raised intracranial pressure and in patients with tumors that are associated with edema or shift of midline structures.

Some unusual headache syndromes, although uncommon, should raise the suspicion of an underlying mass lesion. These include paroxysmal headaches that are sudden in onset and peak within seconds but last only minutes to hours. This type of headache may signify a colloid cyst of the third ventricle. In addition, when this type of headache is precipitated by a Valsalva maneuver (exertion, cough, strain), it may indicate an underlying structural lesion, sometimes seen at the cervicomedullary junction. Finally, atypical facial pain in an elderly patient has been described in patients with nonmetastatic lung cancer (1,6,14). A high index of suspicion is required in patients with facial pain, especially in those with a history of tobacco use or a recent history of weight loss.

Magnetic resonance imaging (MRI) with gadolinium is the imaging procedure of choice when evaluating an elderly patient with headache for an intracranial neoplasm. MRI is preferable to computed tomography (CT) because it detects smaller lesions, particularly in the brainstem or cerebellum, and leptomeningeal disease and will demonstrate involvement and enhancement of cranial nerves as well as thrombosis of venous sinuses, which is sometimes seen in these patients. It can

also assist with therapy if resection or focal radiation is contemplated.

The management of headache in a patient with a brain tumor is usually relatively straightforward. Before definitive therapy, if the headache is severe and requires analgesia, simple analgesics (e.g., acetaminophen) can be used first. In cases in which there is a significant amount of edema but central nervous system lymphoma is not in the differential diagnosis, dexamethasone (4 mg) two to four times daily is usually effective. Aspirin and other NSAIDs should generally be avoided if surgical intervention is likely because of the increased risk of bleeding. In refractory cases, opioids are effective. Codeine is usually effective but may not be converted to morphine and lack analgesic efficacy in the presence of medications such as cimetidine and fluoxetine, which compete for enzymatic binding sites. Hydromorphone, morphine, methadone, and fentanyl can be useful, whereas meperidine and mixed opioid agonist-antagonists (e.g., pentazocine, butorphanol) should be avoided because of toxic metabolites and the potential for reverse analgesia.

CEREBROVASCULAR DISEASE

ISCHEMIC STROKE

Headache can be an important but often neglected symptom of stroke because it is often overshadowed by other dramatic symptoms such as aphasia or hemiplegia. It is not widely recognized that ischemic strokes are associated with headache in about 25% of cases (23). Headache occurs more often with cortical rather than subcortical infarctions, and when infarctions are large, the headaches tend to be unilateral and ipsilateral to the side of the ischemia. Headache is important to recognize because it not only accompanies or follows the stroke, but it may also herald the ischemic event by days or even weeks and thus provide an opportunity for intervention and prevention. These "premonitory" headaches occur in up to 10% of patients with ischemic stroke (18). Headache is generally less common with TIA but can be more common when the TIA involves the vertebrobasilar rather than the carotid circulation.

Headache associated with cerebral ischemia is sometimes unilateral and focal but can be diffuse, nonlocalizing, and dull or throbbing in nature. The headache can last for more than 24 hours. The intensity ranges from being barely noticeable to moderately severe. Headaches associated with posterior circulation ischemia are usually more severe. When the headaches are classified according to the International Headache Society criteria, about 50% resemble TTH, and approximately 30% resemble migraine.

The pathophysiology is unclear, but it may be caused by vasodilation of pain-sensitive vessels by the release of vasoactive substances such as substance P, calcitonin gene-related polypeptide, and other peptides, which, with the cytokines, nitrous oxide, and bradykinins that are released from the vessel itself, contribute to increased nociceptive stimulation.

HEMORRHAGIC STROKE

Although headache is not universal in patients with hemorrhagic stroke, the frequency of headache is higher than in ischemic stroke and highest in patients with cerebellar and occipital hematomas. Overall, headache frequency appears to be in the range of 40% to 60%. When the intraparenchymal hematoma is small, headache may not be present.

SUBDURAL HEMATOMA

Headache is also a frequent accompaniment of subdural hematomas in the elderly. The incidence of headache increases with the duration of the hematoma, occurring in up to 80% of those with chronic subdural hematomas (30). Although a prominent complaint, few distinguishing features of the headache are reported in patients with subdural hematomas. They can be mild to moderate but are often reported as persistent and troublesome. The headache can be paroxysmal and irregular and occur intermittently throughout the day, sometimes with each episode lasting only minutes.

ISCHEMIC HEART DISEASE (CARDIAC CEPHALGIA)

Headache may occur as part of a constellation of symptoms in patients with symptomatic ischemic heart disease or, more rarely, as the sole manifestation of myocardial ischemia. In a study of 150 consecutive patients presenting with angina, 6% had head pain during at least some episodes of angina (39). As an isolated symptom, cardiac cephalgia typically occurs in the context of exertion or other activities that provoke angina. Accordingly it is an uncommon cause of exertional headache (27,49). The diagnosis is confirmed by a positive cardiac stress test, which demonstrates that the onset and resolution of headache coincide with the onset and resolution of cardiac ischemia. The mechanism of cardiac cephalgia is likely secondary to convergence of sympathetic or vagal afferent input with second-order neurons within the trigeminocervical complex (19).

HYPERTENSION

Although hypertension can exacerbate headache, because the two are highly prevalent conditions, the association between the two is often coincidental. Most large-scale epidemiologic studies have shown that headache in hypertensive individuals is not more prevalent than in normotensive controls. However, headache can be caused by severe hypertension, which is defined as a diastolic blood pressure greater than 130 mm Hg (2,5). Headache occurs in up to 80% of patients with paroxysmal hypertension secondary to pheochromocytoma.

The type of headache described in patients with diastolic pressure above 130 mm Hg is frequently diffuse, is present on awakening, and subsides over several hours. In contrast, the headache from paroxysmal hypertension is abrupt and throbbing and subsides within several minutes.

The pathophysiology of hypertension-related headache is uncertain but may result from hypertensive dilation and stretching of resistance vessels. In patients with malignant hypertension or paroxysmal hypertension, headache may, in part, be related to failure of autoregulation and the formation of brain edema with raised intracranial pressure.

Treatment of hypertensive headache involves aggressively treating the elevated blood pressure. Some drugs that dilate resistance vessels (e.g., calcium channel blockers and hydralazine) can exacerbate headache and are best avoided in this patient population.

MEDICATION-RELATED HEADACHE

The illnesses that attend older age often require medications, some of which can cause headache. Table 14-3 lists some of the medications more commonly associated with headache. Alcohol and caffeine, which are often not listed on a medication list, can cause headache from either their consumption or withdrawal. Their use should be carefully determined in elderly patients complaining of headache. In addition, the elderly suffer the same analgesic, ergot, and triptan rebound headaches that afflict younger age groups. Medication-induced headaches are entirely nonspecific but tend to be diffuse, sometimes throbbing, of mild to moderate intensity, and variable in duration. They can be persistent or episodic and temporally related to the administration of the medications (e.g., nitrates).

Treatment first and foremost involves tapering and withdrawal of the potentially offending agent(s). Withdrawal symptoms can be severe, depending on the medication being withdrawn, and therefore, it is prudent, particularly in the elderly, to taper medications slowly to avoid a withdrawal syndrome. If medication is necessary, it is prudent to start low and titrate slowly to the lowest effective dose.

CERVICAL SPONDYLOSIS

Cervical spondylosis, which is more common with aging, is said to represent a common cause of headache in the elderly. However, because radiographic evidence

Table 14-3. *Medications Causing Headaches in the Elderly*

Cardiovascular
　　Vasodilators (nitrates, nicotinic acid,
　　　　dipyridamole)
　　Antihypertensives (nifedipine, methyldopa,
　　　　reserpine, hydralazine)
　　Antiarrythmics (quinidine, digoxin)
Nonsteroidal anti-inflammatory drugs
　　Indomethacin, diclofenac, piroxicam
Antibiotics
　　Tetracyclines, trimethoprim-sulfamethoxazole,
　　　　isotretinoic
Gastrointestinal
　　Ranitidine, cimetidine, omeprazole
Reproductive
　　Estrogens
　　Sildafenil
Hematologic/oncologic
　　Erythropoietin
　　Chemotherapeutics (tamoxifen, cyclophos
　　　　phamide)
Bronchodilators
　　Aminophylline, theophylline, pseudoephedrine
Central nervous system
　　Sedatives (alcohol, barbiturates, benzodiazepines)
　　Stimulants (caffeine, methylphenidate)
　　Antiparkinsonian (amantadine, levodopa)
Antidepressant (trazodone and other selective
　　serotonin reuptake inhibitors)

of cervical spondylosis is ubiquitous in the elderly and because most headache syndromes are diffuse and involve the occipitonuchal region, cervical spondylosis as a cause for headache in the elderly is likely overdiagnosed. Nevertheless, when present, the features of cervicogenic headache include occipital pain and limitation of range of motion of the neck and spasm of cervical muscles. Associated abnormalities may be detected by physical examination of structures in the cervical root distribution, including sensory deficits, reflex changes, or muscle wasting in the arms. A local diagnostic block (short-acting local anesthetic and a corticosteroid) of the greater occipital nerve or the medial branch of C2 or a radiographically affected facet joint may provide a diagnostic clue to the inciting structure and provide temporary pain relief. Treatment with medication may be limited, although simple analgesics or NSAIDs can be tried in conjunction with a mild muscle relaxant. Other approaches (e.g., physiotherapy and massage treatments) should be considered.

METABOLIC HEADACHES

A number of metabolic and systemic disorders can cause headache in the elderly. According to the International Headache Society, metabolic headaches are those that occur during a metabolic disturbance and disappear within 7 days after corrective treatment.

Hypoxia-related headaches can occur in a variety of settings, including headache associated with chronic obstructive pulmonary disease, cardiac failure, and anemia. Hypoxia and hypercarbia can also occur in those with obstructive or central sleep apnea and lead to throbbing nocturnal or morning headaches that may clear after the patient rises from bed. Chronic renal failure, with or without associated anemia, can be associated with dull, diffuse, and chronic daily headaches. Dialysis can also lead to headaches, likely through an osmotic mechanism.

THE EYE AND HEADACHE

Many causes are found for eye pain. Ocular causes of eye pain or headache are invariably associated with a red eye, cloudy cornea (acute angle closure glaucoma), visual loss, diplopia, or an enlarged pupil. In general, "the white eye is not the cause of a painful eye." The only exceptions to this are posterior scleritis, which is best diagnosed by ultrasonography; optic neuritis, where the visual loss is sometimes preceded by mild pain; and subacute angle closure glaucoma, which can only be diagnosed by gonioscopy, a procedure not routinely performed during an ophthalmologic examination. Because the incidence of glaucoma increases with advancing age, an ophthalmologic evaluation should be considered in the elderly patient with new-onset ocular, frontal, or brow pain when no other cause is evident.

TRIGEMINAL NEURALGIA

Trigeminal neuralgia is the most common neuralgic syndrome in the elderly, with an average age of onset of 50 years. A female preponderance for trigeminal neuralgia is found, with an annual incidence rate of 4.7 and 7.2 and prevalence of 108 and 200 per 1 million population in men and women, respectively.

Trigeminal neuralgia is an exquisitely severe, unilateral facial pain syndrome characterized by lancinating electric shocklike jolts of pain that are confined to the distribution of one or more divisions of the trigeminal nerve. The ophthalmic division is affected in isolation in only 4% of patients. The maxillary or mandibular divisions are more commonly affected, and in more than two thirds of patients, two or more divisions of the trigeminal nerve are affected. The cardinal features of this disorder are listed in Table 14-4.

The cause of trigeminal neuralgia varies with age. Secondary trigeminal neuralgia caused by compressive mass lesions, demyelinating disease, or other structural lesions is more likely when the disorder presents before the fifth decade of life. In the elderly population, most patients have idiopathic trigeminal neuralgia, of whom approximately 80% have compression of the trigeminal root by an artery (superior cerebellar or anterior inferior cerebellar), vein, or both.

In one series of 2,972 patients with trigeminal neuralgia, 296 (10%) were found to have underlying intracranial tumors (7). Meningiomas and posterior fossa tumors were the tumors most commonly found, and although neurologic deficits developed on follow-up evaluation in 47% of the patients, most had no neurologic deficits, and the delay in eventual tumor diagnosis was 6.3 years. These patients were younger than those with idiopathic pain, and although carbamazepine was the most effective medication used in this group, the relief was usually temporary.

The results of these studies in patients with trigeminal neuralgia underscore the need for a careful clinical evaluation of every patient, and most authorities advocate a brain MRI during the initial evaluation, even in the absence of neurologic signs or symptoms. Special attention should be given to the cerebellopontine angle and the course of the trigeminal nerve.

A diagnosis of idiopathic (primary) trigeminal neuralgia is established by its typical clinical features: a normal neurologic examination, except for the presence of trigger points, and a normal cranial imaging procedure. Impaired sensation in the distribution of any branch of the trigeminal nerve or a diminished or absent corneal reflex should raise suspicion of a structural, demyelinating, or compressive trigeminal nerve lesion.

Other diagnostic possibilities to be considered in patients with atypical clinical features include dental pathology, tumor (intracranial, sinuses, nasopharynx, mouth, jaw, skull, chest), vascular (GCA, aneurysm or arteriovenous malformation, carotid dissection, carotidynia), ocular (iritis, uveitis, optic neuritis, glaucoma, Tolosa-Hunt syndrome, orbital pseudotumor), and idiopathic headache syndromes [cluster headache, migraine, chronic paroxysmal hemicrania, short-lasting unilateral neuralgiform pain with conjunctival injection and tearing (SUNCT)].

Medical Treatment

Medical therapy for trigeminal neuralgia is usually effective within 2 to 3 days. The most commonly used agents, dosages, efficacy, and classes of evidence are outlined in Table 14-5. Carbamazepine has been the drug of first choice, but a related drug, oxcarbazepine, may be as effective as carbamazepine with a better tolerability profile, fewer drug interactions, and no need for hematologic and hepatic enzyme monitoring. Baclofen is also a useful agent, particularly when used in combination with carbamazepine, wherein there may be a synergistic effect at lower dosages of each. More recently, some of the newer anticonvulsants (e.g., gabapentin and lamotrigine) have shown promise. Again, the effective medications for trigeminal neuralgia, the level of evidence supporting their use, and the main side effects and dosages are listed in Table 14-5.

A number of general caveats apply to the treatment of trigeminal neuralgia, irrespective of the agent used:

- Start low and titrate slowly to the lowest effective dosage.
- Because remissions are common, withdraw medication slowly after an effective course and complete remission for 1 to 2 months.
- Combinations of medications can have additive or synergistic effects and may allow a lower dose of each with fewer side effects.
- Pain response does not exclude underlying pathology; nonresponse to a medication does not exclude diagnosis.
- In general, monitoring blood levels in patient with trigeminal neuralgia is not helpful, except to monitor compliance.
- In general, medications become less effective over time.

Table 14-4. *Cardinal Features of the Pain of Trigeminal Neuralgia*

Paroxysmal jabs of pain
Brief: 2–120 seconds
Sudden, intense, stabbing, superficial
Precipitated by certain activities such as brushing, chewing, talking
Associated with trigger zones: medial face (nose, lips, gums)
Paroxysms of pain separated by pain-free intervals*
Refractory phase following a paroxysm of pain, which is proportional to the length and intensity of the paroxysm, and during which pain cannot even be elicited
Spontaneous remission periods are common (50% of patients), usually last 6 months or more, and occur more commonly early in the course of the illness
No cranial nerve deficit

Table 14-5. *Medical Treatment for Trigeminal Neuralgia*

Drug	Class of Evidence	Standard Dose (mg)	Main Side Effects	Special Points	Efficacy: % Response
Carbamazepine	Class I	Initial: 200–300 Final: 600–800	CNS (dose-dependent), rash (3%), neutropenia or pancytopenia, hyponatremia	Slow dose titration, divided dosages	60–80
L-baclofen	Class III	Initial: 15 Final: 60–80	CNS (dose-dependent)	Synergistic effect with carbamazepine	65–75
Phenytoin	Class III	Initial: 200 Final: 300–400	CNS (dose-dependent), rash, gingival hypertrophy, acne, hirsutism, folate and vitamin D deficiency	Multiple drug influence level of serum protein binding, less effective than carbamazepine, useful as intravenous fosphenytoin (250 mg) in acute setting	50
Gabapentin	Class III	Initial: 300 Final: 600–2400	CNS (dose-dependent)	May be especially useful in TN seconday to MS	60–80**
Oxcarbazepine	Class III	Initial: 600 Final: 600–2400	Same as carbamazepine, but better tolerated	May be as if not more effective than carbamazepine, no black box warning, no monitoring of hepatic enzymes or liver function tests, fewer drug interaction; however, 2% risk of hyponatremia	75–90
Lamotrigine	Class I	Initial: 25–50 Final: 200–400	CNS (dose-dependent), rare life-threatening rash (0.3%)	Caution with coadminstration with valproic acid, slow titration, slow titration	60–75
Clonazepam	Class III	Initial: 1 Final: 6–8	CNS (dose-dependent), habituation	Slow titration, gradual withdrawal	65
Valproic acid	Class III	Initial: 250–500 Final: 500–1500	CNS, tremor, alopecia, weight gain, anusea, pancreatitis, and hepatotoxicity (rare)	Teratogenicity (neural tube defects), enteric-coated form, SR form for one-daily dosing	50

CNS, central nervous system; MS, multiple sclerosis; SR, sustained release; TN, trigeminal neuralgia.

Table 14-6. *Surgical Therapies for Trigeminal Neuralgia*

Procedure	Efficacy	Recurrence	Complications	Special Points
Microvascular decompression	1 yr: 75% 10 yr: 64%	1 yr: 16% 10 yr: 33%	Persistent facial sensory loss (17%), hearing loss (2%), facial weakness (1% to 2%), cerebrospinal fluid leak (2%), major stroke/death (1%)	Recommended for patients with V1 pain, or pain involving all three divisions, who desire no sensory deficit
Stereotactic radiosurgery	2 yr: 58% to 75% initial response for tumor-related TN	2 yr: 6%	Transient facial paresthesias (<10%), sensory loss (3%)	Noninvasive, local anasthesia, no convelescent interval, mean delay to efficacy 1 month (but up to 3–6 months)
Radiofrequency thermal rhizotomy	Initial: 96% to 100%	10–18 yr: 25% to 31%	Dysesthesias up to 50% (severe in 2%), corneal anasthesia (2% to 10%; 15% in first division procedures), keratitis (0.5% to 3%)	Stroke, diplopia, abscess, seizures (rare); death (1 patient in series of 10,000)
Glycerol rhizotomy	Initial: 80% to 95%	1.5–4 yr: 30% to 50%	Similar to RF lesions, plus oral herpes lesions, chemical aseptic meningitis	Useful for those who wish to minimize facial sensory loss, first division pain, bilateral TN
Balloon compression	Initial: 90%	5–10 yr: 20% to 30%	Dysesthesisas (4%)	Nonselective, motor division invariably transiently (<1 yr) affected
Peripheral avulsion or chemical neurolysis (phenol or absolute alcohol)	Initital: 90%	3 yr: 70%	Sensory loss (majority)—returns by 6 months	Very low-risk procedure, 30% still have complete pain relief at 3 yr, may be considerred in elderly or those with high operative risk

RF, radiofrequency; TN, trigeminal neuralgia.

Surgical Treatment

Ultimately, approximately 30% of patients become resistant to or intolerant of drug therapy, and for these patients, interventional or surgical procedures are necessary. Numerous invasive approaches have been tried over the years, ranging from alcohol injection into peripheral trigeminal nerve branches to trigeminal root section. The most commonly used procedures are outlined in Table 14-6.

Opinions differ regarding the best surgical treatment for patients with trigeminal neuralgia. When comparing different surgical approaches, consider technical success and initial relief, long-term recurrence rate, facial numbness, facial dysesthesias, corneal anesthesia, trigeminal motor dysfunction, permanent cranial nerve deficits, intracranial hemorrhage and infarction, postoperative morbidity, and perioperative mortality.

In general, for healthy patients with idiopathic trigeminal neuralgia, a microvascular decompression is usually recommended if the first division or all three divisions are involved or the patient desires no sensory deficit (3,31). However, in some centers, stereotactic radiosurgery is becoming the treatment of first choice because it is noninvasive and associated with very low morbidity and risk for facial paresthesias (<10%) (25).

In many centers, a percutaneous technique, especially radiofrequency rhizotomy, is the procedure of choice for most patients having a first invasive surgical procedure (46). Compared with microvascular decompression, the results are comparable with radiofrequency rhizotomy, the side effects are less morbid, and it is more cost effective. The initial success rate is higher and recurrence rates are lower compared with glycerol rhizotomy and balloon compression, but the incidence of facial dysesthesias and corneal anesthesia may be higher. Of the percutaneous procedures directed at the gasserian ganglion, balloon compression has the lowest incidence of corneal anesthesia and keratitis.

The final decision on treatment is one that weighs the patient's preference and medical risk, the rate of initial and long-term relief versus the risk of facial sensory loss and perioperative morbidity, and the comfort and expertise of the treating neurosurgeon.

REFERENCES

1. Abraham PJ, Capobianco DJ, Cheshire WP. Facial pain as the presenting symptom of lung carcinoma with normal chest radiograph. *Headache*. 2003;43:499–504.
2. Badran RH, Weir RJ, McGuiness JB. Hypertension and headache. *Scand Med J*. 1970;15:48–51.
3. Barker FG 2nd, Janetta PJ, Bissonette DJ, et al. The long-term outcome of microvascular decompression for trigeminal neuralgia. *N Engl J Med*. 1996;334:1077–1083.
4. Boardman HF, Thomas E, Croft PR, et al. Epidemiology of headache in an English district. *Cephalalgia*. 2003;23:129–137.
5. Bulpitt CJ, Dollery CT, Carne S. Change in symptoms of hypertension after referral to hospital clinic. *Br Heart J*. 1976;38:121–128.
6. Capobianco DJ. Facial pain as a symptom of non-metastatic lung cancer. *Headache*. 1995;33:581–585.
7. Cheng TM, Cascino TL, Onofrio BM. Comprehensive study of diagnosis and treatment of trigeminal neuralgia secondary to tumors. *Neurology*. 1993;43;2298–2302.
8. Claus EB, Bondy ML, Schildkraut JM, et al. Epidemiology of intracranial meningioma. *Neurosurgery*. 2005;57:1088–1095.
9. Cook NR, Evans DA, Funkelstein HH, et al. Correlates of headache in a population-based cohort of elderly. *Arch Neurol*. 1989;46:1228–1244.
10. Deorah S, Lynch CF, Sibenaller ZA, et al. Trends in brain cancer incidence and survival in the United States: surveillance, epidemiology, and end results program, 1973 to 2001. *Neurosurg Focus*. 2006;20:E1.
11. Dodick DW, Jones JM, Capobianco DJ. The hypnic headache syndrome: another indomethacin responsive headache syndrome? *Headache*. 2000;40:830–835.
12. Dodick DW, Mosek A, Campbell JK. The hypnic (alarm-clock) headache syndrome. *Cephalalgia*. 1998;18:152–156.
13. Dodick DW, Rozen T, Silberstein SD, et al. Cluster headache. *Cephalalgia*. 2000;20:787–803.
14. Eross EJ, Dodick DW, Swanson JW, et al. A review of intractable facial pain secondary to underlying lung neoplasms. *Cephalalgia*. 2003;23:2–5.
15. Evers S, Goadsby PJ. Hypnic headache: clinical features, pathophysiology and treatment. *Neurology*. 2003;60:905–909.
16. Forsythe PA, Posner JB. Headaches in patients with brain tumors: a study of 111 patients. *Neurology*. 1993;43:1678–1683.
17. Giddens AN, Duneier M, Applebaum RP. *Introduction to Sociology*. New York: WW Norton Company; 2003.
18. Gorelick PB, Hier DB, Caplan LR, et al. Headache in acute cerebrovascular disease. *Neurology*. 1986;36:1445–1450.

19. Grace AJ, Horgan K, Breathnach K, et al. Anginal headache and its basis. *Cephalalgia*.1997;17: 195–196.

20. Guido N, Specchio LM. Successful treatment of hypnic headache with topiramate: a case report. *Headache*. 2006;46:1205–1206.

21. Hale WE, Perkins LL, May FE, et al. Symptom prevalence in the elderly. *J Am Geriatr Soc*. 1986;34:333–340.

22. Hunder GG. Giant cell arteritis and polymyalgia rheumatica. *Med Clin North Am*. 1997;81: 195–219.

23. Jensen TS, Gorelick PB. Headache associated with ischemic stroke and intracranial hematoma. In: Olesen J, Welch KMA, eds. *The headaches*. 2nd ed. Philadelphia: Lippincott Williams & Wilkins; 2000:781–787.

24. Klein, RG, Campbell RJ, Hunder GG. Skip lesions in temporal arteritis. *Mayo Clin Proc*. 1976;51:504–510.

25. Konzdiolka D, Perez B, Flickinger JC, et al. Gamma knife radiosurgery for trigeminal neuralgia. Results and expectations. *Arch Neurol*. 1998; 55:1524–1529.

26. Kyle V, Hazelman BL. Treatment of polymyalgia rheumatica and giant cell arteritis. I. Steroid regimens for the first two months. *Ann Rheum Dis*. 1998;48:658–661.

27. Lipton RB, Lowenkopf T, Bajwa ZH, et al. Cardiac cephalgia: a treatable form of exertional headache. *Neurology*. 1997;49:813–816.

28. Lipton RB, Soloman S, Wertenbaker C. Gradual loss and recovery of vision in temporal arteritis. *Arch Intern Med*. 1985;145:2252–2253.

29. Martins KM, Bordini CA, Bigal ME, et al. Migraine in the elderly: a comparison with migraine in young adults. *Headache*. 2006;46:312–316.

30. McKissock W. Subdural hematoma: a review of 389 cases. *Lancet*. 1960;1:1365–1370.

31. McLaughlin MR, Janetta PJ, Clyde BL, et al. Microvascular decompression of cranial nerves: lessons learned after 4400 operations. *J Neurosurg*. 1999;90:1–8.

32. Merriam-Webster Online. Accessed December 28, 2006. Available at http://www.m-w.com/.

33. Morales-Asin F, Mauri JA, Iniguez C, et al. The hypnic headache syndrome: report of three new cases. *Cephalalgia*. 1998;18:157–158.

34. Oates JA. The science of drug therapy. In: Brunton LL, Parker KL, Buxton ILO, et al., eds. *Goodman and Gilman's the pharmacological basis of therapeutics*. 11th ed. New York: McGraw Hill; 2005.

35. Ostberg G. Temporal arteritis in a large necropsy series. *Ann Rheum Dis*. 1971;30:224–235.

36. Peatfield RC, Mendoza ND. Posterior fossa meningioma presenting as hypnic headache. *Headache*. 2003;43:1007–1008.

37. Raskin NH. The hypnic headache syndrome. *Headache*. 1988;28:534–536.

38. Salvarani C, Gabriel SE, O'Fallon WM, et al. The incidence of giant cell arteritis in Olmstead County, Minnesota, apparent fluctuations in cyclic pattern. *Ann Intern Med*. 1995;123:192–194.

39. Sampson JJ, Cheitlin MD. Pathophysiology and differential diagnosis of cardiac pain. *Prog Cardiovacular Dis*. 1971;13:507–531.

40. Seidler S, Marthol H, Pawlowski M, et al. Cluster headache in a ninety one year old woman. *Headache*. 2006;46:179–180.

41. Serratrice G, Serbanesco S, Sanbuc R. Epidemiology of headache in elderly. Correlations with life conditions and socio-professional environment. *Headache*. 1985;25:85–89.

42. Solomon GD, Kunkel RS, Frame J. Demographics of headache in elderly patients. *Headache*. 1990; 30:273–276.

43. Solomon S, Cappa K-G. The headache of temporal arteritis. *J Am Geriatr Soc*. 1987;35:163–165.

44. Sorenson S, Lorenzen I. Giant-cell arteritis, temporal arteries and polymyalgia rheumatica: a retrospective study of 63 patients. *Acta Med Scand*. 1977;201:207–213.

45. Strikiathachorn A. Epidemiology of headache in Thai elderly: a study in the Bangkae Home for the Aged. *Headache*. 1991;31:677–681.

46. Taha JM, Tew JM. Comparison of surgical treatments for trigeminal neuralgia: reevaluation of radiofrequency rhizotomy. *Neurosurgery*. 1996;38: 865–871.

47. Torelli P, Beghi E, Manzoni GC. Cluster headache prevalence in the Italian general population. *Neurology*. 2005;64:469–474.

48. Ulrich K, Gunreben B, Lang E, et al. Pregabalin in the therapy of hypnic headache. *Cephalalgia*. 2006;26:1031–1032.

49. Vernay DD, Deffond P, Fraysse P et al. Walk headache: an unusual manifestation of ischemic heart disease. *Headache*. 1989;29:350–351.

50. Waters WE. The Pontypridd headache survey. *Headache*. 1974;14:81–90.

51. Wong RL, Kron JH. Temporal arteritis without an elevated erythrocyte sedimentation rate. *Am J Med*. 1986;80:959–964.

SUGGESTED READING

Forsythe PA, Posner JB. Headaches in patients with brain tumors: a study of 111 patients. *Neurology*. 1993;43:1678–1683.

Hunder GG. Giant cell arteritis and polymyalgia rheumatica. *Med Clin North Am*. 1997;81:195–219.

Kyle V, Hazelman BL. Treatment of polymyalgia rheumatica and giant cell arteritis. I. Steroid regimens for the first two months. *Ann Rheum Dis*. 1998;48:658–661.

Solomon GD, Kunkel RS, Frame J. Demographics of headache in elderly patients. *Headache*. 1990;30:273–276.

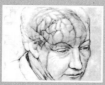

CHAPTER 15

Back and Neck Pain

H. Gordon Deen, Jr.

Acute pain in the back or neck is one of the most common symptoms experienced by older adults. Virtually every adult has experienced at least one episode of acute spinal pain. For most of these patients, extensive laboratory investigation and imaging tests are unnecessary; rapid improvement can be expected with only simple treatment measures. It should be emphasized, however, that a few patients have significant neurologic impairment or evidence of cancer or other serious underlying systemic illness. For these patients, an extensive differential diagnosis must be considered, and prompt workup and specialty consultation may be necessary.

DIFFERENTIAL DIAGNOSIS AND INITIAL ASSESSMENT

Primary care practitioners often do the initial evaluation and management of patients with acute back-related symptoms. The initial patient examination may be performed at the physician's office or in the hospital emergency department. A thorough clinical assessment is crucial to make the best decisions about diagnosis, laboratory testing, diagnostic imaging, and specialist referral. Usually, acute low back or neck pain resolves quickly, and a precise anatomic basis for the pain is never determined. These cases can be referred to as "uncomplicated" low back or neck pain. A nonspecific diagnosis such as lumbar or cervical strain is appropriate.

The clinical approach is quite different for patients with severe or persistent pain (5). In these cases, an extensive differential diagnosis must be considered (Tables 15-1 and 15-2). There are several "red flags" that may indicate the presence of a serious underlying disease. These include severe trauma (for example, motor vehicle accident or sports injury), severe or progressive neurologic deficit, unrelenting nocturnal pain, unexplained weight loss, history of cancer, and fever (Table 15-3). These can be considered to be indicators of "complicated" low back or neck pain.

Table 15-1. *Differential Diagnosis of Low Back Pain with or without Radiculopathy*

1. Discogenic or degenerative disease
   A. Herniated intervertebral disk
   B. Degenerative lumbar spondylosis
      –Central lumbar canal stenosis
      –Lateral recess stenosis
   C. Synovial cyst of facet joint
2. Tumor
   A. Primary intradural tumor of spinal cord, conus, or cauda equina
   B. Tumor of vertebral column or epidural space (or both)
      –Metastatic tumor
      –Plasmacytoma or multiple myeloma
      –Primary bone tumor (e.g., chordoma)
   C. Extraspinal retroperitoneal malignancy
3. Vascular lesion
   A. Arteriovenous malformation of the spinal cord
   B. Spinal dural arteriovenous fistula
4. Infection
   A. Intervertebral diskitis or osteomyelitis
   B. Epidural abscess
   C. Urinary tract infection
   D. Herpes zoster or other viral radiculopathy
5. Intra-abdominal or intrapelvic disease
   A. Abdominal aortic aneurysm
   B. Nephrolithiasis
   C. Posterior perforating duodenal ulcer
   D. Pancreatic disease
   E. Endometriosis
6. Degenerative hip disease
7. Neurologic complications of diabetes
   A. Peripheral neuropathy
   B. Radiculopathy
8. Congenital
   A. Tethered cord
   B. Intraspinal lipoma
9. Metabolic bone disease
   A. Osteoporotic compression fracture
10. Trauma

Table 15-2. *Differential Diagnosis of Neck Pain with or without Neurologic Involvement*

1. Discogenic or degenerative disease
   A. Herniated intervertebral disk
   B. Degenerative cervical spondylosis with canal stenosis
   C. Synovial cyst of facet joint
2. Tumor
   A. Primary intradural tumor of spinal cord or adjacent nerve roots
   B. Tumor of vertebral column or epidural space (or both)
      –Metastatic tumor
      –Plasmacytoma or multiple myeloma
      –Primary bone tumor (e.g., chordoma)
3. Vascular lesion
   A. Arteriovenous malformation of the spinal cord
   B. Spinal dural arteriovenous fistula
4. Infection
   A. Intervertebral diskitis or osteomyelitis
   B. Epidural abscess
   C. Herpes zoster or other viral radiculopathy
5. Degenerative shoulder disease
6. Neurologic complications of diabetes
7. Metabolic bone disease
   A. Osteoporotic compression fracture
8. Trauma

The presence of severe, unremitting pain, especially at night, may indicate the presence of a spinal tumor. This is especially true in the older adult. Any patient over age 65 with acute, severe pain at any level of the spinal column should be considered to have a spinal metastatic tumor until proven otherwise. This suspicion is heightened if the patient has a history of malignant disease or unexplained weight loss. The clinician should also be aware that low back pain may be a referred symptom and may indicate the presence of a serious disease of the abdomen or pelvis, such as abdominal aortic aneurysm, renal colic, pancreatitis, or retroperitoneal tumor. Low back pain may also be a manifestation of urinary tract infection, especially in

Table 15-3. *Indicators of Complicated Spinal Pain*

1. Severe trauma—for example, motor vehicle accident or serious sports injury
2. Severe or progressive neurologic deficit
   A. Loss of motor strength
   B. Numbness or loss of sensation
   C. Impaired bladder or bowel control
3. Unrelenting nocturnal pain
4. Unexplained weight loss (>4.5 kg in 6 months)
5. History of cancer
6. Fever

women. This relatively common problem must be excluded, or treated if present, before embarking on an extensive spinal evaluation.

Patients with low back pain may also have leg pain, often referred to as sciatica or radiculopathy. These terms refer to pain and paresthesias extending down the leg in a dermatomal pattern. The onset may be gradual or abrupt, and patients generally do not recall any trauma or unaccustomed physical activity. The most common cause of sciatica is a herniated lumbar intervertebral disk. In the general population, 95% of lumbar disk herniations occur at the L4-5 and L5-S1 levels. In older individuals, upper lumbar disk herniations at or above the L3-4 level are somewhat more common. Other compressive lesions that can cause sciatica include degenerative lumbar spinal stenosis, tumor, and epidural abscess. The clinician must also be aware of noncompressive causes of leg pain, including radiculopathy due to diabetes and herpes zoster (shingles). Pain in the hip and groin may occasionally indicate the presence of an upper lumbar radiculopathy, but more often it indicates the presence of degenerative hip disease, especially in the older adult.

Patients with disorders of the cervical spine can also have neurologic involvement, including cervical radiculopathy, myelopathy, or a combination of the two. Cervical radiculopathy refers to pain and paresthesias radiating to the arm in a specific dermatomal pattern. Cervical myelopathy refers to symptoms caused by spinal cord compression. These symptoms are more ominous and may include weakness and clumsiness of the arms and legs and bowel and bladder dysfunction.

CLINICAL ASSESSMENT

The importance of a detailed medical history cannot be overemphasized. The patient should be asked to describe the site, duration, and intensity of pain; extension of pain; body positions that relieve or exacerbate the pain; extremity weakness or sensory disturbance; and any bladder or bowel dysfunction. Any history of trauma, weight loss, malignant disease, or other systemic disease should be noted. The physician should carefully review the medication history and any other treatments that have been used. It is important to take the time to obtain an accurate and thorough medication history because some patients may obtain prescription and over-the-counter medications from multiple sources. Diet supplements and other "alternative medicine" remedies have become increasingly popular, and the clinician should ask about these as well. The physician should inquire about previous episodes of spinal pain and what treatments have been used.

An accurate history of tobacco use is essential. Smoking is a risk factor for osteoporosis and chronic back pain. Smoking may increase intradiskal pressure because of chronic coughing, jeopardize disk metabolism because of vascular effects of nicotine, and serve as a marker for psychosocial traits associated with frequent and prolonged pain.

Secondary gain phenomena such as litigation, workers compensation issues, job dissatisfaction, psychiatric problems, and narcotic abuse should be completely explored. These psychosocial issues appear to have an important influence in magnifying symptoms of back and neck pain. Waddell et al. (9) have described a group of nonorganic physical signs that are highly suggestive of psychosocial distress, rather than a structural lesion in the spine. These include tenderness that is superficial and nonanatomic, reproduction of low back pain by application of pressure to the top of the head, inconsistent responses to straight-leg raising with distraction, "give way" weakness, nonanatomic sensory findings, and an overreaction to routine examination maneuvers. These signs have withstood the test of time and continue to be very useful in the evaluation of spine patients with psychological overlay.

It is important to review the impact that the back pain is having on normal activities of daily living and employment. The physician should ask whether the patient requires a cane or other ambulation aid, whether the patient has fallen, and whether the patient can function independently. It is often helpful to note how the patient arrived for the examination. One can ask whether the patient had to rest between the parking lot and the examination room and whether a walker or wheelchair was needed. It is important to note whether the patient has missed work or stopped his/her usual recreational activities.

Most, but by no means all, elderly patients are retired, so employment status is a nonissue for many. The physician should ask these patients whether they have had to curtail shopping, travel, yard work, golfing, and other leisure activities.

Older adults may have pre-existing medical illnesses, such as congestive heart failure; neurologic disorders, such as Parkinson's disease; and musculoskeletal conditions, such as degenerative arthritis of the hip, that magnify the impact of acute spinal symptoms. For example, the patient with an acute lumbar disk herniation who also has Parkinson's disease may find that his/her functional status is much more severely compromised than a similar patient without Parkinson's disease.

The general physical examination should include an assessment of gait, straight-leg raising (Lasègue sign), spinal range of motion, and spinal tenderness or spasm. Straight-leg raising is the most sensitive indicator of nerve root compression. If straight-leg raising pain is absent, then another diagnosis (other than nerve root compression) should be considered. The presence of crossed straight-leg raising (exacerbation of leg pain when the contralateral leg, or the well leg, is raised) is strongly suggestive of lumbar disk herniation. Signs of malignant disease or infection should be noted. If hip and groin pain is present, the Fabere maneuvers (flexion, abduction, external rotation, and extension of the hip—also known as the Patrick test) should be performed. The trochanter should be palpated for evidence of tenderness or inflammation. Positive findings point to degenerative arthritis of the hip joint or trochanteric bursitis (or both). An inguinal hernia should be excluded.

In patients presenting with neck pain, the head and neck should be observed from all directions, looking for abnormal head posture such as seen in torticollis. Cervical range of motion should be assessed. The physician should check for a Spurling sign, radiating arm pain precipitated by head tilt or rotation to the symptomatic side. The patient should be asked whether cervical flexion produces an electric shock sensation in the torso or extremities (Lhermitte phenomenon). This finding suggests the presence of a cervical cord lesion, which could be compressive (tumor) or noncompressive (demyelinating disease). The shoulder is examined for evidence of a rotator cuff injury or degenerative joint disease.

A neurologic examination should include an assessment of strength, sensation, and deep tendon reflexes. If there is evidence of an acute myelopathy or cauda equina syndrome, perianal sensation and rectal tone should be assessed. A sensory level usually correlates with the anatomic level of the lesion. For example, a patient with a T10 cord lesion will usually have a T10 sensory level. In some cases, however, the sensory level may be several levels below the actual site of the lesion. For example, a patient harboring an intradural tumor at the T2 vertebral level might have a T8 dermatomal sensory level on initial evaluation.

On the basis of the initial assessment, a few patients will have a significant neurologic deficit (severe myelopathy, radiculopathy, or cauda equina syndrome) or evidence of a serious underlying disease such as cancer (Table 15-3). Patients with these findings have "complicated spinal pain" and warrant immediate radiographic investigation, usually with magnetic resonance imaging (MRI), and prompt surgical referral. Most patients, however, can be managed with simple measures, as described later.

It should be emphasized that incomplete clinical evaluation leads to an overreliance on diagnostic tests, notably MRI, which in turn leads to errors in diagnosis and treatment. Patients may be given the diagnosis of lumbar disk disease or lumbar spinal stenosis on the basis of an MRI, yet ultimately prove to have a completely different diagnosis. The author has seen patients referred for neurosurgical consultation for "lumbar disk disease" who are subsequently found to have completely different diagnoses, including spinal cord tumor, spinal arteriovenous malformation, metastatic carcinoma, abdominal aortic aneurysm, spinal infection, degenerative arthritis of the hip, inguinal hernia, peripheral neuropathy, and viral radiculitis due to herpes zoster. Thus, the physician must be aware of the broad differential diagnosis of spinal column pain and perform a thorough clinical assessment to establish the correct diagnosis and institute appropriate therapy.

INITIAL APPROACH TO DIAGNOSIS AND MANAGEMENT

The natural history of acute pain in the lower back or neck, in the absence of a tumor or other serious underlying disease process, is characterized by rapid improvement (Fig. 15-1). A substantial majority of patients will experience resolution of symptoms within 4 to 6 weeks. A nonspecific diagnosis such as lumbar or cervical strain is appropriate. Laboratory investigation and spinal imaging are usually not required (6).

The typical patient with "uncomplicated" acute spinal pain can be managed with short-term bed rest (1 to 2 days) and aspirin or nonsteroidal anti-inflammatory medications (NSAIDs), such as ibuprofen. Acetaminophen is a reasonable alternative if the patient cannot tolerate NSAIDs because of gastrointestinal distress or other side effects.

A new class of NSAIDs, the cyclo-oxygenase-2 (COX-2) inhibitors, initially showed great promise in the treatment of back and musculoskeletal pain because these medications were effective pain relievers and had fewer gastrointestinal side effects than older NSAIDs. More recently, use of this class of medications has declined dramatically as a result of data showing an increased risk of cardiovascular complications. For this reason, two popular COX-2 inhibitors, rofecoxib (Vioxx) and valdecoxib (Bextra), have been withdrawn from the market. The only COX-2 inhibitor currently available is celecoxib (Celebrex).

Muscle relaxants, such as cyclobenzaprine (Flexeril), may be useful on a short-term basis in selected patients if there is a pronounced degree of paraspinal muscle spasm. Narcotic analgesics are usually unnecessary.

Figure 15-1. Management of low back pain.

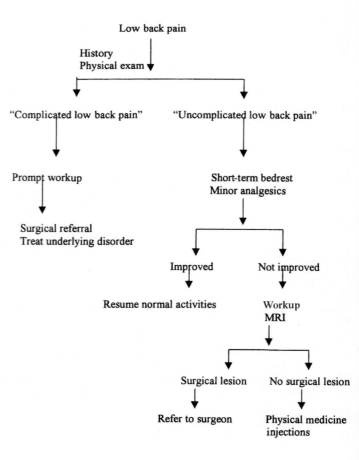

Table 15-4. *Medication Chart: Back and Neck Pain*

Drug	Dose	Risks	Cost/Month
Aspirin	325–650 mg qid prn pain; maximum: 2,600 mg/day	Gastrointestinal symptoms, tinnitus, asthma	$10
Ibuprofen	600–3,200 mg/day	Gastrointestinal symptoms	$20
Acetaminophen	1,000–4,000 mg/day	Hepatic toxicity	$10
Meloxicam (Mobic)	7.5–15 mg/day	Gastrointestinal symptoms	$180
Celecoxib (Celebrex)	100–200 mg/day	Gastrointestinal symptoms	$120
Cyclobenzaprine (Flexeril)	20–30 mg/day	Drowsiness, nausea	$100
Methylprednisolone dose pack	1-week tapering course	Gastrointestinal symptoms	$6 (1-week course)
Propoxyphene napsylate and acetaminophen	1–2 tablets qid prn pain; maximum: 6 tablets per day	Hepatic toxicity, nausea, constipation	$115

qid, four times a day; prn, as needed.

If narcotics are used, they should be prescribed in small quantities on a time-limited basis. A short course of oral steroids may be helpful in patients with acute radicular pain. These medications are outlined in Table 15-4.

Patients should be cautioned about side effects and maximum recommended doses of each medication. They should be informed when a medication has more than one active ingredient. An example of this is Darvocet-N 100, which contains propoxyphene napsylate (100 mg) and acetaminophen (650 mg). A patient who is taking Tylenol on a regular schedule and Darvocet-N 100 for breakthrough pain must avoid exceeding the maximum recommended daily dose of acetaminophen (4000 mg) to avoid potentially serious hepatic toxicity. In older patients, the adverse effects of pharmacologic therapy must be balanced against the positive effects of pain relief and functional improvement.

Diagnostic tests, physical therapy, back braces, imaging tests, and surgical referral are usually unnecessary for patients with acute spinal pain. Hospitalization is needed only in exceptional circumstances. It is very important to reassure the patient that he/she most likely has a benign, self-limited condition and that symptoms should rapidly resolve without active treatment. Terms like "ruptured disk" are alarming to patients and should be avoided. Patients may resume work and normal activities of daily living as symptoms allow. Aerobic exercise, weight control, and avoidance of tobacco use should be emphasized. Patients are instructed to avoid heavy lifting, to avoid repetitive bending and twisting of the lower back, to change positions frequently, and to use a chair with adequate lower back support. More than 90% of patients with nonspecific acute low back and neck pain will experience complete relief of symptoms by using these simple measures.

For the few patients who have not experienced improvement within 4 to 6 weeks, further assessment is warranted, and the physician should attempt to establish a more precise diagnosis. The following tests may be done: plain radiography of the painful spinal segment, complete blood cell count, erythrocyte sedimentation rate, chemistry profile, and urinalysis. The prostate-specific antigen level should be assessed in men older than age 50 years. The main reason for these tests is to screen for nondiscogenic causes of spinal pain.

SPINAL IMAGING

Plain radiographs may be very helpful in establishing the diagnosis of spinal compression fractures in the elderly. When seen in the lower thoracic and lumbar regions, these fractures are usually the result of osteoporosis. A compression fracture at or above the T6 level is usually not due to osteoporosis and should raise suspicion for a tumor.

MRI should be considered for patients with 4 to 6 weeks of persistent spinal pain, especially for those patients with neurologic symptoms or signs. This imaging test provides a wealth of anatomic information; however, the physician must be aware that the MRI is extremely sensitive and that many "abnormalities" demonstrated by this procedure simply represent normal aging changes in the spine. Many completely asymptomatic people will have abnormal findings on lumbar and cervical MRI; thus, test results must be interpreted cautiously (8). The phrase "gray hair of the spine" is an apt description that can be used to convey the significance of many of the positive findings seen on spinal MRI in the elderly in terms that can be understood by the lay person.

The so-called "open magnet" MRI is generally not helpful in the evaluation of spinal disorders. Although this type of MRI examination is better tolerated by claustrophobic patients, image quality is suboptimal. The image quality is generally not adequate for surgical planning or even for establishing a diagnosis. As a result, patients who undergo open magnet MRI frequently need to have additional spinal imaging, either standard MRI with sedation or computed tomography (CT)/myelography. This adds to the time, effort, and expense of the diagnostic workup.

MRI plays a major role in spinal imaging; however, situations exist in which this examination cannot be done. Absolute contraindications include the presence of pacemakers and ferromagnetic implants such as cochlear implants and certain intracranial aneurysm clips. Relative contraindications include claustrophobia, obesity, and the need for advanced life support in the critically ill patient. Another problem is the prolonged examination time, which can preclude technically satisfactory imaging in the patient with severe pain. These patients often are unable to hold still long enough to obtain a satisfactory MRI.

In situations where MRI would be contraindicated or technically difficult, myelography with water-soluble contrast medium followed by CT, the so-called myelogram-CT, remains an excellent diagnostic tool that is very useful in selected patients. This examination allows superb visualization of the spinal canal, subarachnoid space, spinal column, and extraspinal soft tissues. Bony detail is particularly well seen. The myelogram-CT, a minimally invasive procedure, involves a spinal tap, usually in the lumbar region, for injection of contrast material and should usually be ordered only after consultation with a neurologist or neurosurgeon. The myelogram-CT should generally be reserved for those patients who are being seriously considered for surgical treatment. Similar to MRI, the myelogram-CT has a significant incidence of positive findings in asymptomatic or minimally symptomatic patients. Therefore, the examination must be interpreted cautiously and in the context of the patient's clinical findings. Unlike MRI, the myelogram-CT gives the clinician the opportunity to examine the patient's cerebrospinal fluid (CSF), a small sample of which can be removed before the contrast material is injected. Routine CSF studies include protein, glucose, and cell count. A variety of cultures and stains can be obtained if infection is a consideration. Similarly, cytologic analysis looking for malignant cells can be very helpful in selected cases.

The most common complication of myelography is a spinal headache due to the lumbar puncture. This occurs in about 10% of cases. A much less common but more serious complication is neurologic deterioration in cases where there is a complete block of the spinal canal due to tumor or other compressive lesion. It is thought that withdrawing small amounts of CSF below a complete block can cause further compression of the spinal cord, like the effect of a cork being pushed further into a bottle. Another uncommon but potentially serious complication is anaphylactic reaction to the iodine-based contrast material. For this reason, any patient with a history of significant allergic reaction to iodine or shellfish should be pretreated with steroids and diphenhydramine prior to myelography. Oral anticoagulants, such as warfarin, must be discontinued for a few days prior to myelography to allow the international normalized ratio (INR) and prothrombin time to normalize. Fortunately, serious complications of myelography are very uncommon, and the myelogram-CT examination continues to play a major role in the evaluation of spinal disorders.

When used in patients with lower back and leg pain, both MRI and myelogram-CT should include the entire lumbar spine and the lower thoracic spine up to the T10 level to rule out intradural tumors and other lesions at the thoracolumbar junction. Stated another way, a lumbar MRI or myelogram-CT, which stops at L3 or even at L1, is inadequate. These examinations must image the entire spinal column from the sacrum up to T10. Close communication between the clinician and the radiologist is necessary to avoid imaging the wrong segment of the spinal column.

The use of CT without intrathecally administered contrast enhancement (noncontrast CT) should be discouraged. This examination does not visualize the subarachnoid space and, therefore, cannot diagnose cauda equina tumors and other intradural lesions that can mimic lumbar disk herniations. A "negative" noncontrast CT does not eliminate the need for MRI or myelogram-CT in the patient with unexplained acute back or neck pain. Similarly, the patient with a "positive" noncontrast CT will frequently still require MRI or myelogram-CT for surgical decision making.

Bone mineral density (BMD) should be measured in individuals at increased risk for osteoporosis, in patients under 50 years of age with atraumatic fractures, and in patients with osteopenia or spinal deformities noted on plain radiographs, MRI, or CT. Bone density testing can be used to establish a diagnosis of osteoporosis, to estimate future fracture risk, and to follow the response to treatment.

Dual-energy X-ray absorptiometry (DEXA) is the most widely used test for measuring BMD. DEXA can measure bone density in the lumbar spine and hip, two sites that are subject to the most clinically significant fractures. The DEXA test report includes a measure of BMD in grams per centimeter squared, a calculated T-score, and a calculated Z-score. The T-score represents the number of standard deviations (SD) a bone density is above or below the mean peak bone mass of the general population. T-scores are used to define the presence of osteoporosis. For example, a T-score between $+1.0$ and -1.0 is normal; a T-score between -1.0 and -2.5 indicates osteopenia (low bone mass); and a T-score below -2.5 indicates osteoporosis.

Radionuclide bone scanning is an important technique for evaluating the age of vertebral compression fractures. An acute or subacute fracture will show intense uptake at the fracture site, whereas a chronic fracture does not show uptake. This is a critically important piece of information because acute and subacute fractures may benefit from vertebral augmentation with polymethylmethacrylate, whereas a chronic fracture generally does not.

In patients who have sustained neck injury, plain film radiography has been replaced by helical CT scanning as the diagnostic procedure of choice. CT scanning is more sensitive than plain films in the diagnosis of cervical spine fracture, especially in older patients with advanced cervical spondylosis (4). CT scanning also has the advantage of being a faster examination and requiring less patient manipulation than traditional plain films. As a result, CT scanning is now the imaging procedure of choice for patients with acute cervical spine trauma.

If neck pain persists, the physician should consider reimaging the cervical spine after 3 to 6 weeks. Flexion-extension radiographs or MRI may be needed to evaluate for ligamentous instability, which may not be apparent on the initial imaging studies.

NEUROPHYSIOLOGIC TESTING

Electromyography (EMG) and nerve conduction velocity (NCV) studies can be helpful in patients with arm or leg pain. These studies can confirm a clinical impression of cervical or lumbar monoradiculopathy or may indicate the presence of an unsuspected polyradiculopathy or peripheral neuropathy. In patients with upper extremity symptoms, EMG and NCV studies may indicate the presence of carpal tunnel syndrome, ulnar neuropathy, or brachial plexus lesion, which can mimic a cervical radiculopathy. In patients with atypical limb pain, normal findings on EMG can also be helpful to exclude the presence of radiculopathy as a cause for their symptoms. Somatosensory evoked potentials (SSEPs) can be very useful in patients in whom cervical myelopathy is suspected. Generally, neurophysiologic testing is not useful in patients without evidence of radiculopathy or myelopathy (for example,

the patient with midline axial spinal column pain without neurologic involvement).

CONSERVATIVE TREATMENT

If the results of laboratory testing and imaging are unremarkable, a physical therapy program should be initiated after consultation with a physiatrist or physical therapist. Typically, a rehabilitation regimen begins with an exercise and stretching program. Physical therapy modalities such as traction, diathermy, application of heat or cold, ultrasound therapy, and transcutaneous electrical stimulation (TENS) may be added. If physical medicine is successful, a response is generally seen within 4 to 6 weeks. Epidural steroid injections may be of benefit in selected patients (7). These injections are frequently done in patients with lumbar symptoms. Cervical epidural steroid injections are less commonly done but can safely be performed by physicians experienced in the technique. Caudal blocks, selective nerve root injections, facet blocks, and trigger point injections may also be of benefit in selected patients. A substantial majority of patients with acute and subacute spinal pain will experience relief of symptoms with these simple, minimally invasive procedures.

For most patients with back and neck pain, aerobic exercise is the best long-term conservative treatment. Aerobic exercise helps improve overall conditioning and endurance, aids with weight loss, and increases endogenous endorphins, which decreases pain and improves the sense of well-being. Most patients, even the elderly, can usually find some form of aerobic activity that they can comfortably perform.

SURGICAL CONSULTATION

Surgical referral should be considered for patients with significant or progressing neurologic signs and symptoms and for patients who have failed conservative treatment and whose imaging studies show a lesion that seems to explain their symptoms. Patients with pain but no structural lesion are probably best served by referral to a pain management specialist or a neurologist, rather than to a surgeon. Surgical referral of these latter cases often adds nothing but time and expense to the patient's management.

Although older patients may take longer to recover from surgery and require more rehabilitation, the physician should be aware that advanced age does not preclude consideration of elective spinal surgery in the elderly. Overall health and "physiologic age" are more important than chronologic age. Healthy individuals older than 90 years of age can be expected to have good outcomes after spinal operations, provided they meet the same criteria for operation as younger patients.

To give one example, advanced age is not a predictor of poor outcome in patients undergoing lumbar decompressive laminectomy for spinal stenosis.

SURGICAL MANAGEMENT

The most common indication for surgical referral of the older patient is degenerative lumbar spinal stenosis with neurogenic claudication. The optimal candidate for surgery has leg symptoms, rather than low back pain, as the primary complaint. The MRI or myelogram-CT should show significant lumbar spinal canal or lateral recess stenosis that correlates with the clinical findings. The surgical treatment is lumbar decompressive laminectomy of the stenotic spinal segments. A fusion may be needed in some cases, especially those with spondylolisthesis and/or scoliosis. Lumbar decompressive laminectomy is the most common spinal operation performed on Medicare beneficiaries. Good or excellent results can be expected in 70% to 90% of cases. Although some patients may experience recurrent symptoms over time, recent data indicate that the benefits of surgery, in terms of relief of leg pain and functional status, are maintained at 10-year follow-up (3). Complication rates are higher in patients requiring spinal fusion.

Interspinous decompression with the X Stop device represents a new, minimally invasive option for selected patients with stenosis at one or two levels (1). This procedure involves placement of an oval spacer between the spinous processes at a stenotic segment, thereby opening up that segment through localized spine flexion. The device is Food and Drug Administration approved, and preliminary results are encouraging. The procedure can be done on an outpatient basis without a general anesthetic.

Lumbar disk herniation is seen more frequently in middle-aged adults but may also occur in the elderly. The optimal candidate for a lumbar disk operation has sciatica, rather than low-back pain, as the primary symptom; an objective neurologic deficit that involves one or more spinal nerve roots; and clear-cut evidence of a herniated disk on MRI or myelogram-CT that correlates precisely with the clinical findings. Operative intervention is almost never indicated if findings on imaging studies are normal.

Patients with mild to moderate neurologic deficit are considered for elective diskectomy if the conservative treatment measures outlined previously are unsuccessful. Urgent surgical treatment is usually indicated for patients with severe or rapidly progressive radiculopathy, and emergent surgical intervention should be considered for patients with an acute cauda equina syndrome. In properly selected patients, lumbar diskectomy can be expected to achieve excellent or good results in 80% to 90% of patients,

although some patients experience recurrent symptoms over long-term follow-up (2). A fusion is usually not required. Lumbar diskectomy is a relatively safe operation. Blood loss is usually minimal. Younger patients can sometimes undergo this surgery on an outpatient basis, but the older adult usually requires a short hospital stay of 1 to 2 days. Serious complications, such as death, paraplegia, and great vessel injury, can occur but are fortunately uncommon.

The indications for cervical diskectomy are similar to those of lumbar diskectomy. The optimal candidate for surgery has radicular symptoms (or myelopathy), rather than neck pain, as the primary symptom; an objective neurologic deficit; and clear-cut evidence of a herniated disk on MRI or myelogram-CT that correlates well with the clinical findings.

Patients with mild to moderate neurologic deficit are considered for elective surgery if they fail conservative treatment. Urgent surgery should be considered for those patients with severe or rapidly progressive neurologic deficit. In properly selected patients, cervical diskectomy can be expected to achieve results comparable to those seen with lumbar diskectomy, with excellent or good results in 80% to 90% of patients. The results are less favorable in patients with severe cervical myelopathy. Cervical diskectomy can be performed via anterior and posterior approaches, with or without fusion. The surgical approach will vary, depending on imaging results and surgeon preference. Serious complications, such as death and quadriplegia, can occur but fortunately are uncommon.

CONCLUSION

Acute pain in the low back or neck is one of the most common problems encountered in clinical practice. For the few patients who have complicated spinal pain, manifested by a severe neurologic deficit or evidence of cancer or other serious underlying illness, a broad differential diagnosis must be considered. Rapid workup and surgical referral may be needed in these cases. However, most patients with uncomplicated low back pain require no laboratory tests or imaging, and their symptoms improve with simple treatment measures. If symptoms do not improve within 4 to 6 weeks, further evaluation is required. These patients should undergo MRI or myelogram-CT of the symptomatic spinal segment. Physical therapy and various types of injections may be helpful in patients without clear-cut surgical lesions or in patients who wish to defer surgery. Surgical treatment of many common degenerative spinal disorders of the elderly can be accomplished safely and can be expected to achieve an excellent or good result in most cases. Advanced age is not a contraindication to elective spinal surgery provided that the patient is medically fit and meets the appropriate surgical indications.

REFERENCES

1. Anderson PA, Tribus CB, Kitchel SH. Treatment of neurogenic claudication by interspinous decompression: application of the X STOP device in patients with lumbar degenerative spondylolisthesis. *J Neurosurg Spine*. 2006;4:464–471.
2. Atlas SJ, Keller RB, Wu YA, et al. Long-term outcomes of surgical and nonsurgical management of sciatica secondary to a lumbar disc herniation: 10 year results from the Maine lumbar spine study. *Spine*. 2005;30:927–935.
3. Atlas SJ, Keller RB, Wu YA, et al. Long-term outcomes of surgical and nonsurgical management of lumbar spinal stenosis: 8 to 10 year results from the Maine lumbar spine study. *Spine*. 2005;30:936–943.
4. Berlin L. CT versus radiography for initial evaluation of cervical spine trauma: what is the standard of care? *Am J Roentgenol*. 2003;180:911–915.
5. Carragee EJ. Persistent low back pain. *New Engl J Med*. 2005;352:1891–1898.
6. Deyo RA, Weinstein JN. Low back pain. *N Engl J Med*. 2001;344:363–370.
7. Garfin SR. Clinical crossroads: a 50-year-old woman with disabling spinal stenosis. *JAMA*. 1995;274:1949–1954.
8. Jensen MC, Brant-Zawadzki MN, Obuchowski N, et al. Magnetic resonance imaging of the lumbar spine in people without back pain. *New Engl J Med*. 1994;331:69–73.
9. Waddell G, McCulloch JA, Kummel E, et al. Nonorganic physical signs in low-back pain. *Spine*. 1980;5:117–125.

SUGGESTED READING

Clark CR, ed. *The Cervical Spine*. 4th ed. Philadelphia: Lippincott Williams & Wilkins; 2005.

Fenton DS, Czervionke LF, eds. *Image-Guided Spine Intervention*. Philadelphia: Saunders; 2003.

Herkowitz HN, Dvorak J, Bell G, et al. *The Lumbar Spine*. 3rd ed. Philadelphia: Lippincott Williams & Wilkins; 2004.

Popp AJ, ed. *A Guide to the Primary Care of Neurological Disorders*. Park Ridge, IL: American Association of Neurological Surgeons; 1998:101–120.

Ropper AH, Brown RH, eds. *Adams and Victor's Principles of Neurology*. 8th ed. New York: McGraw-Hill; 2005.

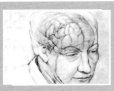

CHAPTER 16

Incontinence and Sexual Dysfunction in the Elderly

Edmund Y. Ko, Sneha S. Vaish, Donald E. Novicki, Dean M. Wingerchuk, and Elliot M. Frohman

Urinary incontinence (UI) is a very common complaint among the elderly and adversely affects the lives of millions of people. The prevalence of UI is 5% to 30% of people living in the community, 40% to 70% of elderly patients in an acute hospital setting, and up to 50% of people living in nursing homes (41). Currently, the health care cost of UI exceeds $20 billion annually in the United States (33). The total lifetime costs for treatment of UI in one older adult have been estimated at $60,000 (10).

Age-related changes of bladder function play a significant role in increasing UI. The aging bladder demonstrates increases in uninhibited detrusor contractions, impaired contractility, abnormal detrusor relaxation patterns, and reduced capacity. In addition, the aging population experiences a shift in nocturnal diuresis, and the frequency of nocturia increases (69). The aging male population can suffer from benign prostatic hyperplasia (BPH) with secondary bladder changes. BPH is evident in 50% of the male population by age 50 and 80% by age 80 (13). Beyond primary changes to the genitourinary tract, elderly adults can suffer from other risk factors that contribute to UI. These include decreased mobility and manual dexterity, difficulties accessing toilets, impaired mentation, and a variety of comorbid medical conditions and multiple medications outlined in Table 16-1.

Initial evaluation of elderly patients with UI should include a comprehensive history and physical exam including a thorough "brown bag review" of all medications used by the patient. The workup should include a comprehensive physical examination, a rapid screening for cognition using the Mini-Mental State Examination, neurologic exam, and evaluation of the patient's mobility and manual dexterity. Useful diagnostic tests include urinalysis, urine culture, urine cytology, free flow and postvoid residual by catheter or ultrasound, 72-hour voiding diary, cough stress test, and urodynamics if empirical treatment has failed. Combining information gleaned from these tests can allow identification of the cause and contributing factors leading to the UI and can help the health care team to formulate and initiate an appropriate treatment plan.

Table 16-1. *UI in the Older Adult: Risk and Predisposing Factors*

Comorbid Disease
Diabetes
Congestive heart failure
Degenerative joint disease
Sleep apnea
Severe constipation

Neurologic/Psychiatric
Stroke
Parkinson's disease
Dementia–all types
Depression
Normal pressure hydrocephalus

Medication
α-Adrenergic (blockers and agonists)
Cholinergics (blockers and agonist)
Angiotensin-converting enzyme inhibitors
Calcium blockers
Diuretics
Opiates
Anticholinergics
Antidepressants/antipsychotics

Functional
Impaired cognition
Impaired mobility
Inaccessibility of toilets
Lack of caregivers

Adapted from Dubeau CE. The aging lower urinary tract. *J Urol.* 2006;175:S11–S15.

BLADDER INNERVATION

An understanding of bladder innervation and physiology is required to diagnose and treat UI. The lower urinary tract is innervated by three sets of peripheral nerves involving the parasympathetic, sympathetic, and somatic nervous systems. Pelvic parasympathetic nerves arise from S2-4 of the spinal cord in a region termed the sacral parasympathetic nucleus (SPN); they send axons through the ventral roots to peripheral ganglia in the detrusor wall where they release acetylcholine. This action facilitates voiding by excitation of the detrusor muscle and relaxation of the urethra. Lumbar sympathetic fibers arising from the lumbar spinal cord follow a path through the sympathetic chain ganglion to the inferior mesenteric ganglia and then through the hypogastric nerve to pelvic ganglia. These fibers provide noradrenergic excitatory and inhibitory input, which relaxes the detrusor and contracts the sphincteric mechanism to facilitate urine storage. Finally, somatic influences are exerted via the pudendal nerve; motoneurons to the external urethral sphincter (EUS) arise from the lateral border of the ventral horn, known as the Onuf nucleus, and contract the EUS (16).

Afferent pathways through the pelvic, hypogastric, and pudendal nerves transmit information from the lower urinary tract to the lumbosacral spinal cord. Pelvic nerve afferents monitor the volume of the bladder and amplitude of bladder contractions via myelinated A-δ and unmyelinated C axons. A-δ fibers located in the bladder smooth muscle sense bladder fullness (i.e., wall tension) and serve as low-threshold mechanoreceptors. C fibers located in the mucosa respond to both stretch (i.e., bladder volume sensors) or nociception and overdistention. C fibers are largely insensitive to normal distention. They become mechanosensitive after activation by a chemical mediator during inflammation (16).

REFLEX CIRCUIT

The lower urinary tract has two major functions: (a) low-pressure bladder filling and storage of urine with continence and (b) low-pressure periodic voluntary emptying. The micturition cycle is organized via a simple on-off switching circuit (Fig. 16-1) that maintains a reciprocal relationship between the urinary bladder and the urethral outlet (16). During bladder filling and urine storage, three functions must occur: (a) the bladder must continue to maintain low pressure and accommodate an increasing volume of urine, (b) the bladder outlet must remain closed, and (c) there should be an absence of abnormal bladder contractions. In contrast, during bladder emptying/voiding three things must happen: (a) the bladder must contract for an adequate magnitude and duration, (b) a concomitant lowering of resistance at the level of the smooth and striated sphincter must occur, and (c) there must be an absence of anatomic obstruction (67).

Voiding dysfunction may occur from damage to the micturition reflex at the storage level or at the elimination level. Thus, voiding dysfunction may be categorized as the failure to store urine or the failure to empty urine secondary to the bladder or the outlet (Table 16-2). In addition, a mixture of both of these classifications can exist. By extrapolating from a basic switchlike framework, many different etiologic possibilities that affect storage, emptying, or both can be defined as illustrated in Table 16-3.

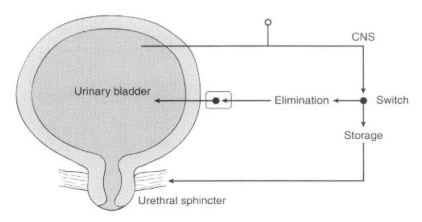

Figure 16-1. Diagram illustrating the anatomy of the lower urinary tract and the "switchlike" function of the micturition reflex pathway. During urine storage, a low level of afferent activity activates efferent input to the urethral sphincter. A high level of afferent activity induced by bladder distention activates the switching circuit in the CNS, producing firing in the efferent pathways to the bladder, inhibition of the efferent outflow to the sphincter, and urine elimination. CNS, central nervous system. (From Walsh PC, Retik AB, Vaughan ED, et al., eds. *Campbell's Urology.* 8th ed. Philadelphia: Saunders; 2002. Copyright © 2002 Saunders, An Imprint of Elsevier.)

Table 16-2. *Functional Classification of Voiding Dysfunction*

Failure to Store
  Bladder dysfunction
  Outlet dysfunction
Failure to Empty
  Bladder dysfunction
  Outlet dysfunction
Mixed Failure to Store and Empty

STORAGE AND ELIMINATION PHASES OF THE BLADDER

By viewing micturition as a simple on-off circuit, adding the complexity of the afferent and efferent neural control of the urinary tract yields a complex but understandable circuit, as described below (16). Intravesical pressure measurements during bladder

Table 16-3. *Types of Incontinence Based on Function*

Female
  Failure to Store
    Bladder dysfunction
      OAB–wet or dry
      Decreased bladder compliance
      Fistula
    Outlet dysfunction
      SI–anatomic urethral hypermobility
      Intrinsic sphincteric deficiency
  Failure to Empty
    Bladder dysfunction
      Detrusor decompensation
      Bladder denervation with hypocontractile bladder
    Outlet dysfunction
      Neurogenic sphincter dysfunction
      Iatrogenic urethral obstruction
  Combined
    Detrusor instability with hypocontractile bladder

Male
  Failure to Store
    Bladder dysfunction
      OAB–wet or dry
      OAB secondary to bladder outlet obstruction
      Decreased compliance
      Bladder decompensation with overflow incontinence
    Outlet dysfunction
      SI: iatrogenic after prostatectomy
      Neurogenic denervation
  Failure to Empty
    Bladder dysfunction
      Bladder decompensation
      Bladder denervation
    Outlet dysfunction
      Benign prostatic hyperplasia with obstruction
      Neurogenic sphincter dysfunction
  Combined
    OAB with hypocontractile bladder
    Parkinson's disease
    Cerebrovascular accident

OAB, overactive bladder; SI, stress incontinence.
Modified from Wein AJ. Pathophysiology and classification of voiding dysfunction. In: Walsh PC, Retik AB, Vaughan ED, et al., eds. *Campbell's urology*. 8th ed. Philadelphia: Saunders; 2002:887–899; and Kobashi KC, Leach GE. Bladder dysfunction and urinary incontinence. In: Noble J, Greene HL, Levinson W, et al., eds. *Noble: textbook of primary care medicine*. 3rd ed. St. Louis: Mosby; 2001:1409–1417.

filling should show constant low pressure and low levels of afferent pelvic nerve activity. The responding efferent pathways produce pudendal nerve outflow and contraction of the EUS, sympathetic nerve stimulation causing detrusor inhibition with activation of the continence mechanism, and finally, inactivation of the sacral parasympathetic outflow (Fig. 16-2A).

The initiation of micturition can be activated either voluntarily or involuntarily. The activation of micturition incites high levels of afferent pelvic nerve activity, which stimulates the brainstem micturition center. The pontine micturition center (PMC) then inhibits somatic nerve output (pudendal

nerve) to cause relaxation of the EUS and inhibits sympathetic outflow (hypogastric nerve) to cause a release of inhibition on the relaxation of bladder and contraction of the urethra. The PMC stimulates parasympathetic outflow, which excites the bladder and relaxes the internal sphincter smooth muscle of the urethra. Voiding occurs by initial relaxation of the urethral sphincter, and then a few seconds later, contraction of the bladder, increase in bladder pressure, and flow of urine.

Maintenance of the voiding reflex is through ascending afferent input from the spinal cord, which may pass through the periaqueductal gray matter (PAG) before reaching the PMC (Fig. 16-2B).

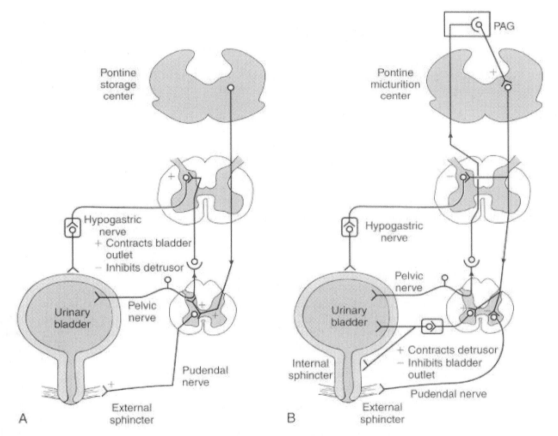

Figure 16-2. Mechanism of storage and voiding reflexes. **A:** Storage reflexes. During the storage of urine, distention of the bladder produces low-level bladder afferent firing. Afferent firing in turn stimulates (i) the sympathetic outflow to the bladder outlet (base and urethra) and (ii) pudendal outflow to the EUS. These responses occur by spinal reflex pathways and represent "guarding reflexes," which promote continence. Sympathetic firing also inhibits detrusor muscle and transmission in bladder ganglia. **B:** Voiding reflexes. At the initiation of micturition, intense vesical afferent activity activates the brainstem micturition center, which inhibits the spinal guarding reflexes (sympathetic and pudendal outflow to the urethra). The PMC also stimulates the parasympathetic outflow to the bladder and internal sphincter smooth muscle. Maintaining the voiding reflex is through ascending afferent input from the spinal cord, which may pass through the PAG before reaching the PMC. EUS, external urethral sphincter; PMC, pontine micturition center; PAG, periaqueductal gray matter. (From Walsh PC, Retik AB, Vaughan ED, et al., eds. *Campbell's Urology.* 8th ed. Philadelphia: Saunders; 2002. Copyright © 2002 Saunders, An Imprint of Elsevier.)

PATHOPHYSIOLOGY OF VOIDING DYSFUNCTION

Dysfunction at any level of the urinary mechanism outlined in the previous section can cause loss in the regulation of voiding and result in UI. Loss of detrusor inhibition and relaxation of the internal sphincter occur, which results in uninhibited bladder contractile activity, causing urgency and UI. Injuries to the PMC or to the descending spinal pathways cause a loss of coordination between the bladder and the urinary sphincter, which results in an uninhibited contraction and a nonrelaxing urinary sphincter (detrusor sphincteric dyssynergia). This causes a high-pressure, poor emptying bladder, which eventually can decompensate and cause upper urinary tract damage. This type of dysfunction is seen with dementia, stroke, multiple sclerosis (MS), tumors, or other brain injuries. Exceptions to this framework are lesions of the internal capsule (typically strokes), which result in uninhibited and poorly sustained detrusor contractions and inadequate voiding pressure with sphincteric dysfunction.

Injuries at the level of the spinal cord can be from trauma, disk herniation, vascular lesions, MS, tumors, syringomyelia, myelitis, or iatrogenic causes. In the acute phase, they lead to a hypocontractile bladder with low pressure and large bladder capacity. Over time, these injuries lead to a loss of innervation and sphincteric spasticity and voiding dyssynergia. Bladder wall fibrosis occurs and can result in detrusor hypertrophy, high voiding pressure, ureteral reflux or obstruction leading to renal damage, and UI. Cervical spinal cord injuries may cause autonomic dysreflexia. Injuries above the level of the sympathetic outflow from the cord result in hypertensive blood pressure fluctuations, bradycardia, and sweating with stimulation of the lower urinary tract.

Pathologic lesions that occur at or below the sacral micturition center (S2-4) may be caused by spinal cord injury, damage to the anterior horn cells from poliovirus or herpes zoster, or iatrogenic causes such as radiation or surgery. These lesions are often incomplete and cause a mixture of overactive bladder (OAB) activity with weakened muscle contractility. Sphincter tone is diminished, and bladder pressure is low, but capacity is high and can lead to UI. Voiding is accomplished through straining.

Hypocontractile bladders can result from other neurologic conditions including diabetes mellitus, tabes dorsalis, pernicious anemia, and posterior spinal cord lesions. The pathology is not damage to the detrusor muscle nucleus, but rather a loss of sensory input through the afferent feedback pathway. Eventually, this may lead to a loss of neurotransmission in the dorsal horn of the cord and loss of perception in bladder filling, resulting in overstretching of the detrusor. An atonic detrusor with a large volume capacity and high residual urine may eventually occur.

Pelvic trauma may injure the nerves to the sphincter, and selective denervation can lead to an incompetent sphincter mechanism and UI. Peripheral nerve injuries can also occur with radical pelvic surgeries or radiation therapy. During pelvic surgeries, damage to the peripheral nerves may result in a bladder that cannot accommodate with filling; the smooth muscle is intact, but no central reflex organizes muscle activity, and a hypertonic bladder wall with high-pressure filling and poor storage of urine can occur. Radiation can result in denervation of the detrusor or sphincter. At the detrusor level, it can cause fibrosis and loss of compliance of the detrusor, with failure to both store and empty urine adequately.

Incomplete neural lesions can cause variable lower urinary tract dysfunction that is often not predictable based on the level of the injury. In disease processes such as MS, the neural lesions can be present at multiple levels and can confuse clinical presentations in patients (16,39,63,67).

PERIPHERAL PHARMACOLOGY

Normal human detrusor muscle has been studied pharmacologically, yielding evidence for both prejunctional and postjunctional receptors as locations of action for potential drugs. At least five different cholinergic muscarinic receptor subtypes (M1 to M5) have been cloned. M1, M4, and M5 receptor subtypes are found in the human nervous system. M2 and M3 receptors are predominate as the cholinergic receptors in the bladder smooth muscle. M2 receptors play a role in inhibition of bladder relaxation and modulation of bladder contraction in denervation injuries or spinal cord disease, whereas M3 receptors mediate direct detrusor muscle contractions. In turn, multiple muscarinic receptor antagonists have been developed and are widely prescribed for the treatment of UI (3). Antimuscarinics depress both voluntary and involuntary bladder contractions and increase total bladder capacity. However, antimuscarinics lack receptor specificity, and side effects include dry mouth, tachycardia, constipation, and blurred vision from accommodation paralysis. Such adverse events may be unpleasant or annoying for younger individuals but dangerous for the elderly.

MECHANISTIC CLASSIFICATION OF UI

Defining the overarching causes of UI can be difficult due to nonstandard terminology. However, each clinician should choose one of the classifications and

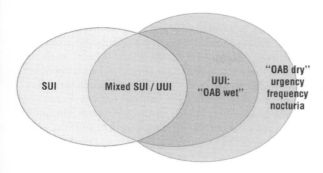

Figure 16-3. Urinary incontinence (UI) may be urge UI (UUI), stress UI (SUI), or mixed in any type. Overactive bladder (OAB) syndrome includes those who are wet and dry. (Adapted from Abrams P, Cardozo L, Fall M, et al. The standardisation of terminology in lower urinary tract function: report from the standardisation sub-committee of the International Continence Society. *Urology*. 2003;61:37–49.)

apply it to his or her practice. UI can be divided into five major categories: OAB, including both OAB wet and dry; stress incontinence (SI); overflow incontinence; functional incontinence; and mixed incontinence, which can have elements of all these categories (69). Figure 16-3 illustrates the extensive overlap between categories (2).

OVERACTIVE BLADDER

OAB is defined by the International Continence Society (ICS) as urgency with or without urge UI (UUI) usually associated with frequency and nocturia (2). The ICS defines urgency as "sudden compelling desire to void that is difficult to defer" (2). OAB overlaps with other subtypes of lower urinary tract symptoms (LUTS). Data from the National Overactive Bladder Evaluation study reveal that the prevalence of OAB is 16.5% of the general adult population, or approximately 33 million people in the United States. Of people meeting the criteria for OAB, only 37% of patients afflicted with OAB will experience UUI (OAB wet), whereas the remaining patients remain dry (OAB dry) (62). OAB has a significant impact on quality of life, affecting physical activity, psychological well-being, social activity, sexual activity, occupational productivity, and domestic logistics (38).

Many different causes of OAB have been described, including neurogenic and myogenic detrusor damage, bladder urothelium causes, and neurotransmitter abnormalities. In the neurogenic circumstance, the micturition reflex is disturbed; baseline bladder storage function occurs through relaxation of the bladder, activation of the sphincter, and deactivation of the parasympathetic neural stimulation. Suprapontine lesions can affect the reflex and cause increased lower urinary tract afferent nerve input, loss of peripheral inhibition, and enhancement of excitatory neurotransmission in the micturition reflex pathway (18). Common causes include stroke, Parkinson's disease, spinal cord injury, MS, and transverse myelitis.

The myogenic situation is applicable to individuals with bladder outlet obstruction. Over time, the increase in intravesical pressure causes partial neurologic denervation of the bladder smooth muscle. The smooth muscle denervation causes an increase in the number of spontaneous actions potentials, which in turn propagate from cell to cell causing "micromotions" in the detrusor. These micromotions increase vesicular pressure and activate the afferent receptors, and the feedback to the central nervous system (CNS) will cause the sensations associated with OAB (68).

Bladder urothelial–based causes occur when bladder distention increases the amount of acetylcholine released from the urothelium; this feedback to the CNS creates a sensation of urgency, which drives the OAB (19). A final hypothesis in patient with OAB is an abnormal leak of acetylcholine from efferent nerve fibers, which causes micromotions in the bladder smooth muscle that stimulate the CNS, recreating the sense of urgency in OAB (3).

The management of OAB includes a variety of treatments, ranging from noninvasive management with behavior modifications to pharmacologic therapy to treatment as invasive as surgery. Behavior modification is initially education for the patient about the micturition reflex and dysfunction and includes the use of a voiding diary to better elucidate the patient's voiding habits. Simple solutions include adjustment of fluid intake (time, quantity, or type) and a timed voiding regimen at predetermined intervals. Pelvic floor exercise and biofeedback can be introduced to abort unwanted sensation of urgency. Pharmacologic treatments include five antimuscarinics agents: darifenacin (Enablex), oxybutynin (Ditropan), solifenacin (VesiCare), tolterodine (Detrol), and chlordiazepoxide (Tropium); these drugs are currently approved for treatment of OAB in the United States. Studies of these drugs have shown similar efficacy (70% to 75%) in decreasing episodes of UUI (68).

Novel trends for treatment of OAB include injections of botulinum toxin (BTX) into the bladder or the urethra or sacral nerve stimulation (SNS) for those who are refractory to antimuscarinic therapy. BTX causes paralysis by inhibiting the release of acetylcholine from the motor nerve into the neuromuscular junction, leaving the bladder unable to contract. The temporary relaxation generally lasts between 3 and 6 months before full muscle strength returns (25). Neuromodulation through SNS involves percutaneous surgical placement of electrodes through the sacral foramen, typically S3, under local anesthesia. After a trial of 3 to 7 days, the temporary leads can be internalized with a permanent implant, currently produced under the name InterStim therapy. The electrical stimulation modulates neural reflexes to impact the bladder and pelvic floor to reduce the UUI. Brazzelli et al. (11) systematically reviewed the efficacy and safety of SNS for severe UUI, and results show that 67% of patients become dry or achieve a 50% improvement in symptoms after implantation.

STRESS INCONTINENCE

In women, stress UI is defined as anatomic incontinence secondary to the hypermobility of the vesicourethral segment due to pelvic floor weakness (63). Pregnancy and childbirth can affect the lower genitourinary tract through anatomic changes, denervation injury, or traumatic injury. Up to one third of premenopausal women and almost one half of postmenopausal women experience some type of pelvic floor disorder in their lifetime, including UI, anal incontinence, or pelvic organ prolapse. Pelvic organ prolapse is the herniation of the pelvic organs to or through the vaginal opening. One in nine women will have surgery for pelvic floor disorders by age 80, and 30% will require reoperation. Symptoms of pelvic organ prolapse include bulge sensation in the perineum, urinary or bowel symptoms, sexual symptoms, and pain (56). In neurologically healthy men, SI is very unusual and occurs only after lower urinary tract surgery, such as transurethral resection of the prostate (TURP) or radical prostatectomy (1). Symptoms generally present as involuntary loss of urine when a patient laughs, coughs, sneezes, changes position, or performs an activity that increases intraabdominal pressure.

Standard nonsurgical treatments include medications, biofeedback, pelvic floor exercises, behavioral therapy, periurethral injections, and corrective surgery. Pharmacologic agents include alpha-agonists, vaginal or oral estrogen, and tricyclic antidepressants. Pharmacologic intervention usually does not lead to a cure and is often combined with the behavioral therapy described earlier (55,58). Periurethral injections have been done with a variety of different substances, including collagen, fat, Teflon, and silicone polymers, and provide reasonably good short-term symptomatic improvement. The results are not long lasting in most individuals.

Surgical techniques to correct SI in female patients include pubovaginal slings, retropubic suspension, needle suspension, and anterior colporrhaphy. The history of bladder suspensions began with the Marshall-Marchetti-Krantz and Burch procedures (63). However, in the last 20 years, pubovaginal and needle suspension have become popular because of the ease and approach of the procedure. Slings are placed beneath the proximal urethra and bladder to provide a "hammock" for support and direct urethral compression. Pubovaginal slings have been created from a variety of materials, including synthetic, autologous, allogeneic, and xenogenic tissues (39).

The sling serves as a "backstop" to prevent urethral descent and opening when increased intraabdominal pressure occurs. Slings and retropubic suspensions maintain an 83% to 84% success rate beyond 48 months compared with a 67% success rate at approximately 48 months for needle suspensions. Overall, slings appear to be the most efficacious treatment at this time.

Male patients have the option of a male sling or the artificial genitourinary sphincter (AGUS), which remains a standard of treatment for incontinence. The male sling is a piece of synthetic mesh placed around the urethra similarly to the female sling; it applies pressure to the urethra and aids in continence. It is made from a single piece of mesh and has no parts that the patient needs to manipulate; however, it has higher failure rates. The AGUS is made of three parts: (a) a fluid-filled cuff placed around the bulbous urethra, which occludes the urinary channel; (b) a pressurized suprapubic reservoir; and (c) a pump located in the scrotum that is activated to move fluid from the cuff to the reservoir. When a patient wishes to void, he pumps the pump to cause temporary cuff deflation. This allows urine to pass, and the cuff will refill within 3 to 5 minutes, returning continence.

OVERFLOW INCONTINENCE

Overflow incontinence is defined by the chronic retention of urine. The patient voids small frequent amounts of urine. Overflow may be the result of detrusor hypocontractility from chronic medical conditions such as diabetes mellitus, vitamin B_{12} deficiency, or disorders with similar neurologic effects. In elderly male patients, the possibilities of bladder neck contractures, bladder neck dysfunction, and sphincter dyssynergia should all be entertained, but bladder decompensation is usually due to BPH. About 80% of men age 80 years will have evidence of BPH, and roughly 50% of men with documented bladder outlet obstruction suffer from detrusor overactivity with or without UI. Interestingly, with outlet correction, the overactivity often disappears (13).

Treatment of overflow incontinence involves treatment of the underlying medical condition, but effects on the bladder may be permanent. The goal of treatment is to empty the bladder and protect the upper tracts. This can be done with behavior modification via limitation of fluid intake, Valsalva and Credé voiding, and timed voiding. These maneuvers may not adequately empty the bladder, and clean intermittent catheterization or chronic indwelling catheter may be needed. For treatment of BPH, initial treatment involves the use of alpha-blockers (terazosin, doxazosin, tamsulosin, or alfuzosin) or the addition of a 5 α-reductase inhibitor (finasteride or dutasteride). Combination therapy with doxazosin and finasteride may be more effective in decreasing the risk of overall clinical progression of BPH than either drug alone (47). Additionally, in patients with BPH causing overflow, significant OAB may exist. For these patients, the addition of an antimuscarinic to alpha-blockers may improve quality of life (4). Surgical intervention is recommended in men when BPH is refractory to medical therapy or leads to renal insufficiency, urinary retention, recurrent urinary tract infections, bladder calculi, hydronephrosis, or high postvoid residual. Minimally invasive surgical approaches not requiring a general anesthetic can be accomplished through transurethral microwave (TUMT). More invasive surgical techniques include TURP, transurethral incision of the prostate (TUIP), transurethral laser prostatectomy, and open simple prostatectomy. The risks and benefits must be discussed extensively with the patients; the risk of an anesthetic must be weighed carefully with respect to the elderly patient's comorbidities.

FUNCTIONAL INCONTINENCE

Functional incontinence is defined as UI secondary to the inability to gain access to a toilet because of impaired mobility or manual dexterity, environment and access to toilets, impaired cognition, or limitation from medical conditions. Mobility affects the ability of many elderly patients to get to the bathroom in time to void. In addition, the manual dexterity required to undress may impact UI. If bathrooms are not easily accessible either inside or outside the homes, patients may be unable to prevent UI. Comorbid medical and neurologic conditions commonly result in UI. Medication side effects from narcotics, sedatives, or neuroleptic agents may also impair elderly patients and exacerbate UI (21,69). Other factors that influence functional incontinence specifically in the elderly are physical or chemical restraints, poor vision, depression, reduced exercise tolerance, gait abnormalities, or the fear of falling (69). Treatment of functional incontinence begins with primarily identifying the causes and taking actions to eliminate them.

SEXUAL DYSFUNCTION

Sexuality is the ability to experience or express sexual feelings. Human sexuality is determined by a combination of multiple influences. These include the emotional, psychological, spiritual, social, cultural, religious, and physiologic characteristics of sex and human sexual behavior, to name a few. Throughout life, human sexuality is molded by experiences and changes as one matures from adolescence into adulthood and inevitably to advanced age. Sexual dysfunction is an important issue in the elderly and is often multifactorial. Males and females are affected by sexual dysfunction as they age.

SEXUAL PHYSIOLOGY

Four stages comprise the sexual response cycle: (a) excitement, (b) plateau, (c) orgasm, and (d) resolution. Excitement is induced by multiple factors, including visual, tactile, olfactory, auditory, and mental stimuli. This leads to arousal. The plateau stage involves maintenance of the arousal. Orgasm is characterized by rhythmic muscular contractions associated with intense feelings and release of neurochemical transmitters through the CNS, leading to a sense of well-being. Resolution is the phase after orgasm when the body returns to the nonaroused state. During this time, the sexual organs become sensitive to touch and may be refractory to orgasm despite continued stimulation. Each of the stages is affected by the physiologic changes associated with aging.

Male Sexual Function

Normal male sexual function requires an intact libido, the ability to achieve and maintain an erection, orgasm/ejaculation, and detumescence. Libido refers to sexual desire and is affected by visual, olfactory, tactile, gustatory, auditory, mental, and hormonal stimuli. Libido can be increased with sex steroids (testosterone). Conversely, libido can be decreased by medications and hormonal, medical, physical, or psychiatric changes and disorders (48).

The penis is composed of three erectile bodies (two corpora cavernosa and one corpus spongiosum) filled with smooth muscle bundles. These bundles form endothelium-lined cavernous sinuses, which, when engorged with blood supplied by the pudendal artery, result in erection. These erectile bodies are surrounded by a sheath of elastic fibers known as the tunica albuginea. The tunica provides the penis with flexibility, rigidity, and tissue strength for an erection and exerts an active compressive force upon the venous system to prevent venous outflow to maintain an erection.

Two forms of innervation regulate penile activity: autonomic (sympathetic and parasympathetic) and somatic (sensory and motor). Sympathetic innervation originates at the T10 to L2 spinal segments and passes to the sympathetic chain ganglia. Nerve fibers from the ganglia travel through lumbar splanchnic nerves to the inferior mesenteric and superior hypogastric plexuses. Fibers reach the pelvic plexus traveling in the hypogastric nerves.

Parasympathetic innervation originates in the spinal erection center in the intermediolateral nuclei located at spinal cord levels S2-4. The parasympathetic nerves pass through the pelvic nerves to the pelvic plexus and join the sympathetic fibers originating from T10–L2. The autonomic nerves merge to form the cavernous nerves and dorsal nerve and regulate the neurovascular events that make up erection (parasympathetic) and detumescence (sympathetic) (44).

The somatosensory pathway begins at the sensory nerve endings and receptors in the genitalia. These receptors join, forming the dorsal nerve of the penis, which eventually becomes the pudendal nerve more proximally. The pudendal nerve joins the S2-4 nerve roots and concludes in the central gray region spinal neurons and interneurons of the lumbosacral segment. The spinothalamic and spinoreticular pathways in the spinal cord carry sensory messages of touch, temperature, and pain from the nerve endings of the genitalia to the thalamus and sensory cortex, resulting in sensory perception (44).

The integration center between the central and peripheral autonomic nervous system is located in the paraventricular nucleus (PVN) of the hypothalamus. Besides erectile function and sexual behavior, the PVN is also involved in feeding, metabolic balance, blood pressure, and heart rate (72).

Penile erection is a dynamic vascular event that is modulated by the nervous system. Cavernosal artery smooth muscle relaxation is an active process leading to an erection. Parasympathetic nerves in the S2-4 distribution release nitric oxide, which leads to increased cyclic guanosine monophosphate (cGMP). This decreases intracellular calcium, causing relaxation of smooth muscle. Smooth muscle relaxation leads to arterial and arteriolar dilation, resulting in increased penile blood flow. Blood is trapped within expanding sinusoids in the corpora, leading to compression of the subtunical venous sinuses, thereby decreasing venous outflow. The tunica albuginea also plays a role in erection by compressing the emissary veins between the inner circular and outer longitudinal layers, decreasing

venous outflow. All of these events lead to increased intracavernosal pressure, resulting in an erection (44). The active combination of the increased arterial blood inflow with the decreased venous outflow is required to maintain an erection. If either of these processes is disrupted, an erection may not occur.

Detumescence is a product of the sympathetic nervous system located in the thoracolumbar spinal segments (T12-L2). When these nerves are activated, contraction of corporal smooth muscle resumes, and arterial flow diminishes, leading to penile flaccidity (45).

Three types of erections can occur: reflexogenic, psychogenic, and nocturnal. Reflexogenic erections occur due to tactile stimulation of the genitals, which is mediated through a local neurologic loop. Genital stimulation is transmitted via somatic pathways through the pudendal nerve to S2-4 and then back to the genitals. Reflexogenic erections are conserved in upper spinal cord injury patients but are difficult to control by the individual and are usually short in duration.

Psychogenic erections are achieved by nontactile stimulation. These include visual, olfactory, auditory, or gustatory stimuli, memories, and/or fantasies. Internally generated imagery (i.e., sexual fantasies) often represents one of the most potent means to produce sexual arousal and erection. Nocturnal, or central, erections occur spontaneously without any tactile or psychogenic stimulation. They commonly occur during the sleep cycle during rapid eye movement (REM) sleep (43).

Orgasm is divided into two phases: emission and ejaculation. Both require stimulation of the external genitalia involving the parasympathetic pathways. Emission involves the active process of peristaltic contractions of the smooth muscles of the seminal tract resulting in secretion of fluids from the epididymis, seminal vesicles, and prostate into the posterior prostatic urethra. Subsequent bladder neck closure, relaxation of the EUS, and coordinated contractions of the bulbospongiosus and pelvic floor muscles propagate semen through the urethra and out the penile urethra, resulting in ejaculation. This involuntary process is mediated by the thoracolumbar (T10-L2) sympathetic and sacral (S2-4) parasympathetic pathways as well as somatosensory pathways. These pathways integrate peripheral and central signals into coordinated outputs to genitourinary structures, resulting in a normal emissary and ejaculatory process (29).

Female Sexual Function

Female sexual function is mediated through the neurovascular pathways similar to those described in men. Increased vaginal blood flow from arousal occurs with tactile stimulation of the genitals or from psychogenic measures, resulting in vaginal lubrication and swelling of the clitoris and labial tissues. Female orgasm involves synchronous contractions of the vaginal walls, lasting between 10 and 50 seconds. Unlike male orgasm, the female orgasm can be multiple, both in number and involved sites (26).

SEXUAL CHANGES WITH ADVANCING AGE

Multiple physiologic events associated with aging contribute to sexual dysfunction in men and women (Table 16-4). Men may notice a gradual decline in their libido and sexual ability. Changes include decline in excitement, plateau, orgasm, and resolution; increased time of stimulation to obtain an erection; difficulty in maintaining an adequate erection for intercourse; weaker orgasms; reduction in seminal volume; and prolongation of the refractory period after resolution between erections. These changes are mainly due to the gradual decrease in testosterone as men age (28).

Libido is strongly affected by testosterone levels. As men age, they experience a decrease in testicular function with a resultant decrease in testosterone production. Studies in the elderly have reported a reduc-

Table 16-4. *Sexual Physiologic Changes in Aging Men and Women*

Women

Decreased estrogen levels
Decreased vaginal lubrication
Atrophy of vulvar tissue
Thinning and increased friability of the
  vaginal mucosa
Reduced elasticity and muscle tone of vagina
Decreased vaginal length and width
Decrease in the size of the clitoris
Increased stimulation required to reach climax
Weaker orgasms and decreased duration

Men

Testosterone levels decline gradually
Decline/prolongation of sexual stages
Excitement, plateau, orgasm, and resolution
Increased genital stimulation required to obtain
  and maintain a sufficient erection
Orgasms weaker with shorter intervals
Reduction of semen volume
Rapid detumescence in resolution stage
Prolongation of refractory period between
  erections
Increased stimulation to achieve erection and
  reach climax

Adapted and modified with permission from Ginsberg TB. Aging and sexuality. *Med Clin North Am.* 2006;90:1025–1036.

tion in libido in 30% of male patients under the age of 65, a 31% decrease between the ages of 65 to 75, and a 47% decrease over the age of 75 (65). Although testosterone levels and erectile function diminish with aging, a consistent correlation between the two has not been established (40). Testosterone replacement can improve libido and may provide a subjective improvement in erectile function (59).

Genital sensation also declines in addition to the other sensory changes associated with aging (i.e., sight, smell, taste, hearing, balance, etc.). Studies have demonstrated that aging is associated with decreased genital electrical and vibrotactile thresholds as well as decreased pudendal somatosensory evoked potentials (36). As a result, increased tactile stimulation and manipulation may be required for arousal and orgasm to occur in older men (57).

Women may also notice a gradual decline in sexual function with aging. The most significant physiologic changes occur at or around the time of menopause, when the ovaries cease to produce estrogen (20). This signifies the end of menstruation and reproductive potential. Female sex steroids play an important role in maintaining anatomic and functional integrity of the sexual structures (52). Estrogen loss is a main factor affecting sexual function, leading to hot flashes, mood swings, irritability, diminished vaginal secretions and lubrication, pH changes in the vagina causing increased infections, changes in the vulvar tissue and thinning of vaginal mucosa, and loss of libido (22,28). Low estradiol levels are strongly correlated with the development of vaginal atrophy and dyspareunia and may also be associated with prolongation of time to achieve vaginal vasocongestion and lubrication. The number and intensity of vaginal and uterine contractions during orgasm may also decrease as a result of decreased estrogen levels. Such changes can be improved for many patients by local or systemic estrogen replacement therapy (30).

Sexual dysfunction is common in both sexes. It has been reported in the literature to affect 10% to 52% of men and 25% to 63% of women (42). The Massachusetts Male Aging Study (MMAS) reported that almost 35% of men between 40 and 70 years of age had moderate to complete erectile dysfunction (ED) that was strongly correlated to age, health status, and emotional function (24). The prevalence of sexual dysfunction in women was slightly higher at 43%, according to the National Health and Social Life Survey (42).

CONTRIBUTING FACTORS TO SEXUAL DYSFUNCTION

Medical problems and related treatments (i.e., surgery or medications) play a large role in sexual dysfunction in the aging population (Table 16-5). Most studies suggest that, although an organic cause

Table 16-5. *Potential Medical Causes of Sexual Dysfunction*

Surgery
Trauma
Pelvic pathology
Toxins (organic compounds, heavy metals, peptide neurotoxins, etc.)
Endocrine disorders (DM, hypothyroidism, hyperprolactinemia, uremia, etc.)
Infectious diseases (HIV, viral infections, leprosy, etc.)
Cardiovascular disorders (HTN, coronary artery disease, MI, etc.)
Rheumatologic disorders (lupus, etc.)
Hematologic disorders (hemochromatosis, sickle cell anemia, leukemia, etc.)
Neurologic disorders (MS, Parkinson, epilepsy, spinal cord injury, etc.)
Psychiatric disorders (depression, schizophrenia, anxiety, etc.)

DM, diabetes mellitus; HIV, human immunodeficiency virus; HTN, hypertension; MI, myocardial infarction; MS, multiple sclerosis.

is more often diagnosed as the factor leading to sexual dysfunction, psychosocial reasons should also be explored as causative factors (28). Many of the organic causes are intimately intertwined, and therefore, it may be difficult to define a single causative factor. Organic factors include cardiac and vascular disease, endocrine dysfunction, penile trauma and diseases, and neurogenic disorders. Other potential causes of sexual dysfunction include infectious diseases (human immunodeficiency virus), rheumatologic disorders (lupus), and hematologic disorders (sickle cell, leukemia).

ED is defined as the consistent inability to achieve or maintain an erection suitable for intercourse (53). Vascular disease, resulting in disturbance of blood flow to and from the penis, is the most common cause of ED (24). Hyperlipidemia, hypertension, and diabetes mellitus are some of the diseases that can lead to vascular disease and sexual dysfunction.

Arterial insufficiency and venous leakage are two vascular mechanisms that cause ED. Atherosclerosis of the pelvic arteries can lead to decreased perfusion pressure and arterial flow to the sinusoids of the corpora cavernosa. Cavernosal arteries can develop intimal and medial thickening and trabecular fibrosis, which prevents inflow of arterial blood into the sinusoids. Likewise, the loss in arterial compliance with aging also correlates with a loss in venous compliance. Structural changes to the fibroelastic structures of the corpora may result in a loss of compliance and an inability to compress the emissary veins against the tunica albuginea. Venous leakage through the subtunical venules, despite adequate inflow, prevents achievement of sufficient pressures within the corpora cavernosa to obtain and/or maintain an erection (50).

Diabetics are at increased risk of developing ED. According to the MMAS (24), the prevalence of ED is three times higher in diabetic men (28% compared with 9.6% in normal men) and ranges from 20% to 71% (23). It also occurs at an earlier age. Approximately 50% of diabetic men will experience ED at least once in their lifetime. The age-adjusted relative risk for developing ED for medically treated or untreated diabetic patients is 1.83 (95% confidence interval, 1.23 to 2.73) in the MMAS (35).

Diabetes may induce ED by altering peripheral nerve activity, vascular function, androgen secretion, endothelial cell function, and smooth muscle contractility. Diabetes medications, as well as concomitant diseases associated with diabetes seen in the metabolic syndrome (i.e., obesity, hypertension, lipid disorders, and coronary heart disease), also play a large role in diabetic ED. Glycemic control plays an important role in ED prevention (54). Although blood sugar management may prevent the development of ED in younger diabetics, it may only prevent further progression in a diabetic with ED (31).

The proposed mechanisms for diabetic-associated ED include central and autonomic neuropathy, endothelial cell dysfunction, and smooth muscle dysfunction. Nitric oxide and vasoactive intestinal peptide are two neurotransmitters that are adversely affected by diabetes. Peripheral neuropathy is also a consequence of diabetes and can result in decreased genital sensation, requiring increased stimulation to achieve an erection. Because of the coexistence of angiopathic and neuropathic changes in most diabetic patients, the precise pathophysiologic mechanisms in diabetic patients are usually not clear (72).

Other endocrine abnormalities such as hyperprolactinemia, Cushing's disease, thyroid dysfunction, and pituitary tumors may also result in decreased libido and impotence.

Peyronie's disease is an acquired benign condition that includes the presence of a plaque or induration of the tunica albuginea, penile curvature during erection, penile pain, and ED. It can occur after acute penile trauma or spontaneously. It has been associated with Dupuytren contractures of the hand. A fibrous plaque develops in the tunica albuginea of the penis. This plaque is often palpable on physical examination. This, in effect, tethers one side of the penis. When erection occurs, the side with the plaque will be shortened in comparison to the contralateral side, leading to penile curvature to the direction of the plaque. The curvature can be so severe that intercourse is not possible. This plaque can also be located circumferentially, forming a constricting band around the penis preventing tumescence distal to the plaque. Emissary veins may also be kept open, preventing venous constriction and thus preventing a full erection (27).

Neurogenic causes of ED can be associated with any disorder that affects the brain, spinal cord, or the autonomic fibers to the penis. This includes spinal cord injury, MS, tumors, syringomyelia, Parkinson's disease, cerebrovascular events, various dementias, epilepsy, peripheral neuropathy, disk disease, and transverse myelitis. This is by no means an exhaustive list, but it demonstrates the variety of etiologies of neurologic sexual dysfunction (64).

Spinal cord injury patients can retain a degree of erectile function depending on the level and completeness of their injury. Those with partial lesions or lesions to the upper parts of their cord are more likely to retain erections versus those with complete lesions or lower cord injuries. After a spinal cord injury, approximately 75% of patients will maintain some degree of erectile capability. Only 25% of the 75% will have an erection adequate enough for penetration (48).

Surgical procedures that disrupt the neural pathway can also be a cause of ED. Direct injury to the sacral plexus or pudendal or cavernosal nerves can occur during spinal, pelvic, rectal, or prostate surgeries.

Prostate cancer is one of the most common malignancies diagnosed in males according to the American Cancer Society. Radical prostatectomy is a common surgical procedure used to treat this disease. ED is a common phenomenon after surgery, even though in some cases the nerves responsible for erections can be spared. Potency preservation has been reported to be as high as 90% with nerve-sparing surgery (66), but in recent literature, erectile capacity with nerve-sparing techniques ranges from 35% to 68% (64).

The likelihood of the return of erectile activity is inversely correlated with the age of the patient and directly correlated with the quality of erections prior to surgery. The younger and the more potent the patient is prior to surgery, the more likely he will regain erections if the nerves are spared (51). Most erections after surgery will not be as good as before. Recovery of erections may take up to 12 to 18 months

postoperatively (64). Nonsurgical treatments for prostate cancer include radiation (external-beam or brachytherapy), cryotherapy, and androgen deprivation therapy. Each of these treatments is also likely to cause sexual dysfunction.

Although TURP for benign prostatic hypertrophy is unlikely to produce ED, some studies have documented a 3% to 37% incidence of sexual dysfunction postoperatively. This has been thought to be associated with perforation of the prostatic capsule or extensive electrocautery to the posterolateral capsule near the neurovascular bundles (32). Another study documented a subjective decrease in the quality of erections after TURP in up to 27.5% of patients, although 64% of this group equated retrograde ejaculation with decreased potency (60).

DRUG EFFECTS

Sexual dysfunction is a common side effect of many medications (Table 16-6), including antihypertensives, diuretics, cardiac medications, antihyperlipidemics, antidepressants, antipsychotics, anticholinergics, antiandrogens, many chemotherapeutic agents, tranquilizers, H_2 antagonists, and recreational drugs. Beta-blockers and thiazide diuretics are implicated most frequently among the antihypertensives. Medications used to treat BPH, including terazosin and finasteride, are also associated with ED. Antidepressants and antipsychotic medications, especially selective serotonin reuptake inhibitors, tricyclics, and neuroleptics, are associated with alterations in erectile, ejaculatory, and orgasmic function and sexual desire (64).

It is estimated that at least 25% of impotent men are affected by medication-induced ED. Although medications are associated with many sexual side effects, the patients taking them have multiple comorbidities that predispose them to sexual dysfunction. This may confound the clinical picture regarding the cause of the sexual disorder (i.e., is it the medication or the medical condition?) (48).

Abused drugs, including alcohol, amphetamines, cocaine, heroin, marijuana, and nicotine, can also impair sexual function. It is estimated that up to 95% of alcoholics suffer from sexual dysfunction, although the general effects of chronic alcoholism rather than alcohol itself may be the major cause. Current and former smokers also have an increased risk of developing ED and sexual dysfunction (6).

PSYCHOSOCIAL FACTORS

Although the mind can be a powerful source for sexual arousal and stimulation, it can also be a potent inhibitor of sexual function. Fear and anxiety are two themes that commonly lead to psychosocial sexual dysfunction. It may be something as simple as performance anxiety or

Table 16-6. *Medications Potentially Associated with Sexual Dysfunction*

Antihypertensives
  Alpha/Beta blockers
  Calcium channel blockers
  Clonidine
  Guanethidine
  Methyldopa
  Reserpine
Cardiac Medications
  Clofibrate
  Digoxin
Diuretics
  Spironolactone
  Thiazides
H₂ blockers
  Cimetidine
  Ranitidine
Chemotherapeutic agents

Antidepressants
  Monoamine oxidase inhibitors
  Selective serotonin reuptake inhibitors
  Tricyclic antidepressants
Anxiolytics
  Benzodiazepines
  Lithium
Antipsychotics
  Clozapine
  Haloperidol
  Risperidone
Alpha-antagonists (for benign prostatic hyperplasia)
  Tamsulosin
  Doxazosin
  Terazosin
Hormonal medications (for prostate cancer)
  Bicalutamide
  Finasteride
  Flutamide
  Leuprolide

can be as complex as a history of sexual abuse. Psychosocial factors include relationship conflict, loss of attraction and interest to a partner or sex in general, fear of sexually transmitted diseases, conflicts over sexual preference, work or family stress, anger or resentment with a partner, and depression (46).

EVALUATION OF SEXUAL DYSFUNCTION

The evaluation of sexual dysfunction begins with a thorough history and physical. Many patients may hesitate to discuss their sexual history candidly. A strong physician–patient relationship with an open, nonjudgmental, and nonthreatening atmosphere aids in obtaining often embarrassing yet vital information necessary to treating sexual dysfunction. Starting with open-ended questions will allow the patient to present any information that they are comfortable with and establish rapport. Essential components of a thorough sexual history address onset, duration, progression, and severity of ED; change in sexual desire; quality of ejaculation and orgasm; associated genital pain; lifestyle factors (i.e., sexual preference, spouse, or partner); and sexual function of the partner (12).

A thorough medical and sexual history should be obtained to elicit whether the cause is organic, psychogenic, or multifactorial. Information regarding medical comorbidities, prior surgical procedures, current and prior medications, abused substances and duration of use, psychiatric conditions, marital status, and current sexual status can aid in diagnosis. Prior treatments for sexual dysfunction, if any, can also aid in evaluation and diagnosis and guide the treatment course for the future.

Physical examination should include a basic evaluation of mental, neurologic, cardiovascular, pulmonary, and genitourinary status. Mental status changes, gait instability, visual field deficits, pulse deficits, cyanosis of fingers and toes, palpable penile plaques, penile curvature, testicular atrophy or asymmetry, vaginal tissue atrophy, gynecomastia, barrel chest, or pursed lip breathing may all give clues to the underlying etiology for sexual dysfunction. Mini-Mental State Examination, depression scales, and interviews with the patient's significant other may also reveal underlying psychological factors that are not initially apparent.

If hormone dysfunction is suspected, testosterone and luteinizing hormone levels in males and estradiol, follicle-stimulating hormone, and androgen levels in females should be obtained. Prolactin levels, thyroid function tests, renal function tests, fasting blood glucose, and glycosylated hemoglobin level can also be obtained selectively in both men and women with sexual dysfunction. Nocturnal penile tumescence testing (Rigi-Scan) to evaluate for nocturnal tumescence and rigidity of erectile episodes during REM sleep may be helpful in distinguishing functional from organic ED. Duplex Doppler ultrasound can also be performed to evaluate males with suspected arterial or venous disorders. Pelvic angiography is seldom used unless a vascular surgery is contemplated.

Ultimately, many patients with sexual dysfunction can benefit from referrals to a urologist, gynecologist, psychiatrist, or sex therapist for further evaluation and management.

TREATMENT OF SEXUAL DYSFUNCTION

The treatment of male sexual dysfunction depends on the patient's desire to pursue therapeutic options as well as the underlying etiology. If the cause is primarily psychogenic, counseling, sexual therapy, and psychiatric evaluation provide an adequate starting point. Organic or surgical causes of male sexual dysfunction can be treated medically or surgically (Table 16-7).

Medical therapies include oral medications, intraurethral suppositories, and intracavernosal injections. Oral medications available include sildenafil (Viagra), tadalafil (Cialis), and vardenafil (Levitra). These medications are phosphodiesterase (PDE) inhibitors that prevent the breakdown of cGMP, thus enhancing the effects of nitric oxide, leading to vasodilation (71). Efficacy ranges from 40% to 85% and depends on severity and cause of ED (61). When taken several hours prior to sexual activity, they can produce adequate erections for intercourse. Because of the noninvasive nature, ease of administration, effectiveness, and tolerance, PDE type 5 (PDE-5) inhibitors have been recommended by the World Health Organization (WHO) as first-line treatment for men with ED (34).

Common side effects of all three medications include headache, flushing, nasal congestion, abnor-mal vision, and dizziness. Serious side effects can include myocardial infarction, stroke, arrhythmias, severe hypotension, and priapism. Contraindications include the concurrent use of nitrates or antihypertensives, cardiovascular disease, and cardiac comorbidities. If there is any question of PDE-5 use in a patient, refer him to a specialist for evaluation before treatment.

Muse, or alprostadil (prostaglandin E1), is an intraurethral suppository that acts locally to relax arterial smooth muscle, producing vasodilation in the corpora cavernosa. Efficacy has been reported to be up to 70% (17). Patients are advised to empty their bladder prior to inserting the pellet into the urethral meatus. Onset of action usually is within 10 to 15 minutes after insertion. Side effects include penile pain, dysuria, urethral discharge, hematuria, and priapism. Although this medication has local effects, systemic side effects can include syncope, hypotension, dizziness, and headache.

Intracavernosal penile injection (PINJ) involves injecting medication directly into the corpora cavernosa with a small needle. Medications used in this method include alprostadil (prostaglandin E1), papaverine, which is a nonselective PDE inhibitor, and phentolamine, which is a competitive α_1- and α_2-adrenergic receptor antagonist. Papaverine has been used alone with efficacy up to 70%. Phentolamine is effective in up to 81% of men when used in a combination mixture along with papaverine and prostaglandin E1 (Tri-Mix) (61). The injection is started at a low dose and titrated to the desired effect by the patient. Injection should take place about 10 to 15 minutes prior to sexual activity. Intracavernosal agents require refrigeration and expire after several months. Side effects include pain, infection, bleeding, scar tissue leading to penile curvature, and priapism.

For patients with multiple medical comorbidities and taking multiple medications with possible interactions with ED medications, vacuum assist devices (i.e., penile pump) are available. Negative pressure is produced by placing a cylinder over the penis and activating the device with a hand pump or battery-driven pump. When the penis is erect, a constricting band is placed at the base of the penis to trap blood in the cavernosa. After sexual activity is complete, the band is removed, and detumescence ensues. Efficacy is reported to be between 67% and 92% (7,70). Although side effects are minimal, patients do complain about the unnatural nature of the device. It may be difficult for a patient or partner to manipulate the unit due to arthritis, movement disorders, or decreased dexterity.

Surgical implantation of a penile prosthesis may be considered as a secondary option. There are two basic types of prosthesis: inflatable or semi-rigid. In the

Table 16-7. *Treatment of Erectile Dysfunction*

Medical Therapy
Oral–phosphodiesterase (PDE-5) inhibitors
    Tadalafil (Cialis)
    Vardenafil (Levitra)
    Sildenafil (Viagra)
Intraurethral
    Alprostadil urethral (Muse)
Intracavernosal
    Alprostadil intracavernous, prostaglandin E1
      (Caverject, Edex)
    Phentolamine, papaverine, prostaglandin E1
      (Tri-Mix)

Surgical Therapy
Penile prosthesis
    Inflatable
    Semi-rigid/malleable

Mechanical Therapy
Vacuum assist device
Constrictor band

Counseling
Psychiatric counseling and therapy
Patient and partner education
Sexual therapy:
    Tactile stimulation

Section II • *Common Signs and Symptoms in the Older Adult*

United States, inflatable prostheses are implanted about 90% of the time, and semi-rigid rods are implanted about 10% of the time. Both prostheses involve placing mechanical devices in the corpora cavernosa on each side of the penis. Although a penile prosthesis is the most invasive technique used to treat ED, it has the highest satisfaction rate in patients (96% to 98% satisfaction rate) and their partners (91% to 96% satisfaction rate). The major source of dissatisfaction was shortening of the erect penis (49). Risks include bleeding, infection, pain, mechanical malfunction, erosion through the penis or urethra, decreased penile sensation, and penile shortening.

A surgical option that is not widely used includes vascular revascularization procedures for patients with arteriogenic ED. This procedure is not commonly performed in the United States and is recommended for younger patients (<50 years old with minimal comorbidities with ED). In a study group from Japan, the objective efficacy for penile revascularization in a select group of males was 85% at 3 years and 66% at 5 years of follow-up (37).

The treatment of sexual dysfunction in women is complicated and not as well defined as the treatment available for men (Table 16-8). In contrast to the male sexual response, the female response is more likely to be responsive rather than spontaneous. Because of the large psychological component of sexual arousal for women, pharmacotherapy for treatment of sexual dysfunction in women is not well defined. Counseling, including psychiatric evaluation, couples' therapy, and sex therapy, may play an important role in initial treatment for female sexual dysfunction.

If there is a hormonal deficiency, systemic estrogen may be used. If there is vaginal atrophy and/or dryness, local estrogen replacement with creams or suppositories and water-based lubricants have been found to be useful. Contraindications to estrogen replacement must be considered prior to initiating therapy. Androgen supplements, used in an off-label manner, may improve libido in women, although there are no Food and Drug Administration–approved formulations specifically for sexual dysfunction in women (5,30).

PDE inhibitors have been used off label to treat female sexual dysfunction. The results have been controversial. In an early study, sildenafil (Viagra) was shown to have no difference versus placebo in the treatment of estrogenized and estrogen-deficient women with sexual dysfunction (8,9). Conversely, in a study of healthy young females, Viagra was found to improve arousal, orgasm, and sexual enjoyment (14). Viagra has been demonstrated to improve subjective sexual function and clitoral blood flow in premenopausal diabetic women suffering from sexual dysfunction (15). At the time of this publication,

Table 16-8. *Treatment of Female Sexual Dysfunction*

Counseling and education of patient and partner
  Menopausal changes
    Hormonal changes
    Genitalia changes
  Basic female sexual health
  Body and mind relationships
Medical therapies
  Systemic estrogen therapy
    Oral tablets
    Vaginal suppository
    Vaginal rings
  Local estrogen therapy
    Estrogen creams
    Nonmedical therapies
Nonmedical therapies
  Physical
    Exercise
    Diet modification
    Weight control
    Lifestyle modification
  Psychosocial therapies
    Address psychiatric disorders
    Self-image modification
    Partner attention
    Sexual therapy

Viagra and other PDE-5 inhibitors are currently FDA approved only for treatment of male ED and pulmonary hypertension in adults. Any other use is considered off label.

SUMMARY

Urinary and sexual problems are common in the elderly population. Medical comorbidities may complicate these problems and create difficult treatment situations for the physician. An open-minded approach combined with multidisciplinary involvement can result in improved quality of life in this patient population.

REFERENCES

1. Abrams P. Describing bladder storage function: overactive bladder syndrome and detrusor overactivity. *Urology.* 2003;62:26–37.
2. Abrams P, Cardozo L, Fall M, et al. The standardisation of terminology in lower urinary tract function: report from the standardisation subcommittee of the International Continence Society. *Urology.* 2003;61:37–49.

3. Andersson KE. Antimuscarinics for treatment of overactive bladder. *Lancet Neurol.* 2004;3:46–53.

4. Athanasopoulos A, Gyftopoulos K, Giannitsas K, et al. Combination treatment with an α-blocker plus an anticholinergic for bladder outlet obstruction: a prospective, randomized, controlled study. *J Urol.* 2003;169:2253–2256.

5. Bachmann G, Oza D. Female androgen insufficiency. *Obstet Gynecol Clin North Am.* 2006;33: 589–598.

6. Bacon CG, Mittleman MA, Kawachi I, et al. A prospective study of risk factors for erectile dysfunction. *J Urol.* 2006;176:217–221.

7. Baltaci S, Aydos K, Kosar A, et al. Treating erectile dysfunction with a vacuum tumescence device: a retrospective analysis of acceptance and satisfaction. *Br J Urol.* 1995;76:757–760.

8. Basson R. Female sexual response: the role of drugs in the management of sexual dysfunction. *Obstet Gynecol.* 2001;98:350–353.

9. Basson R, McInnes R, Smith MD, et al. Efficacy and safety of sildenafil citrate in women with sexual dysfunction associated with female sexual arousal disorder. *J Womens Health Gend Based Med.* 2002;11:367–377.

10. Birnbaum H, Leong S, Kabra A. Lifetime medical costs for women: cardiovascular disease, diabetes, and stress urinary incontinence. *Womens Health Issues.* 2003;13:204–213.

11. Brazzelli M, Murray A, Fraser C. Efficacy and safety of sacral nerve stimulation for urinary urge incontinence: a systematic review. *J Urol.* 2006; 175:835–841.

12. Broderick GA. Oral pharmacotherapy and the contemporary evaluation and management of erectile dysfunction. *Rev Urol.* 2003;5[Suppl 7]: S9–S20.

13. Burnett AL, Wein AJ. Benign prostatic hyperplasia in primary care: what you need to know. *J Urol.* 2006;175:S19–S24.

14. Caruso S, Intelisano G, Farina M, et al. The function of sildenafil on female sexual pathways: a double-blind, cross-over, placebo-controlled study. *Eur J Obstet Gynecol Reprod Biol.* 2003;110: 201–206.

15. Caruso S, Rugolo S, Agnello C, et al. Sildenafil improves sexual functioning in premenopausal women with type 1 diabetes who are affected by sexual arousal disorder: a double-blind, crossover, placebo-controlled pilot study. *Fertil Steril.* 2006; 85:1496–1501.

16. Chancellor MB, Yoshimura N. Physiology and pharmacology of the bladder and urethra. In: Walsh PC, Retik AB, Vaughan ED, et al., eds. *Campbell's urology.* 8th ed. Philadelphia: WB Saunders; 2002:831–875.

17. Costabile RA. Alprostadil for the treatment of erectile dysfunction. *Expert Opin Investig Drugs.* 1999;8:844–884.

18. de Groat WC. A neurologic basis for the overactive bladder. *Urology.* 1997;50:36–52.

19. de Groat WC. The urothelium in overactive bladder: passive bystander or active participant? *Urology.* 2004;64:7–11.

20. Dennerstein L, Lehert P, Burger H, et al. Sexuality. *Am J Med.* 2005;118:59S–63S.

21. Dubeau CE. The aging lower urinary tract. *J Urol.* 2006;175:S11–S15.

22. Farage M, Maigach H. Lifetime changes in the vulva and vagina. *Arch Gynecol Obstet.* 2006;273: 195–202.

23. Fedele D, Bortolotti A, Coscelli C, et al. Erectile dysfunction in type 1 and type 2 diabetics in Italy. On behalf of Gruppo Italiano Studio Deficit Erettile nei Diabetici. *Int J Epidemiol.* 2000; 29:524–531.

24. Feldman HA, Goldstein I, Hatzichristou DG, et al. Impotence and its medical psychosocial correlates: results of the Massachusetts Male Aging Study. *J Urol.* 1994;151:54–61.

25. Frenkl TJ, Rackley RR. Injectable neuromodulatory agents: botulinum toxin therapy. *Urol Clin North Am.* 2005;32:89–99.

26. Fugl-Meyer KS, Oberg K, Lundberg PO, et al. On orgasm, sexual techniques, and erotic perceptions in 18- to 74-year-old Swedish women. *J Sex Med.* 2006;3:56–68.

27. Gelbard MK. Peyronie's disease. In: Ball TP, ed. *AUA update series.* Volume XXI. Houston: American Urological Association; 2002:226–231.

28. Ginsberg TB. Aging and sexuality. *Med Clin North Am.* 2006;90:1025–1036.

29. Giuliano F, Clement P. Serotonin and premature ejaculation: from physiology to patient management. *Eur Urol.* 2006;50:454–466.

30. Goldstein I, Alexander JL. Practical aspects in the management of vaginal atrophy and sexual dysfunction in perimenopausal and postmenopausal women. *J Sex Med.* 2005;2[Suppl 3]:154–165.

31. Goldstraw MA, Kirby MG, Bhardwa J, et al. Diabetes and the urologist: a growing problem. *BJU Int.* 2007;99:513–517.

32. Hansbury DC, Sethia KK. Erectile function following transurethral prostatectomy. *Br J Urol.* 1995;75:12–13.

33. Hu TK, Wagner TH, Bentkover JD, et al. Costs of urinary incontinence and overactive bladder in the United States: a comparative study. *Urology.* 2004;63:461–465.

34. Jardin A, Wagner G, Khoury S, et al. Recommendations of the 1st International Consultation on

Erectile Dysfunction. In: Jardin A, Wagner G, Khoury S, et al., eds. *Erectile dysfunction*. Plymouth, United Kingdom: Health Publications Ltd; 2000: 711–726.

35. Johannes CB, Araujo AB, Feldman HA, et al. Incidence of erectile dysfunction in men ages 40 to 69 years old: longitudinal results from the Massachusetts Male Aging Study. *J Urol*. 2000;163:460–463.

36. Johnson RD, Murray FT. Reduced sensitivity of penile mechanoreceptors in aging rats with sexual dysfunction. *Brain Res Bull*. 1992;28:61–64.

37. Kawanishi Y, Kimura K, Nakanishi R, et al. Penile revascularization surgery for arteriogenic erectile dysfunction: the long-term efficacy rate calculated by survival analysis. *BJU Int*. 2004;94:361–368.

38. Kelleher CJ, Reese PR, Pleil AM, et al. Health health-related quality of life of patients receiving extended-release tolterodine for overactive bladder. *Am J Manag Care*. 2002;8:S608–S615.

39. Kobashi KC, Leach GE. Bladder dysfunction and urinary incontinence. In: Noble J, Greene HL, Levinson W, et al., eds. *Noble: textbook of primary care medicine*. 3rd ed. St. Louis: Mosby; 2001: 1409–1417.

40. Kupelian V, Shabsigh R, Travison TG, et al. Is there a relationship between sex hormones and erectile dysfunction? Results from the Massachusetts Male Aging Study. *J Urol*. 2006; 176:2584–2588.

41. Landi F, Cesari M, Russo A, et al. Potentially reversible risk factors and urinary incontinence in frail older people living in community. *Age Aging*. 2003;32:194–199.

42. Laumann EO, Paik A, Rosen RC. Sexual dysfunction in the United States: prevalence and predictors. *JAMA*. 1999;281:537–544.

43. Lue TF. Male sexual dysfunction. In: Tanagho EA, McAninch JW, eds. *Smith's general urology*. 16th ed. New York: McGraw-Hill; 2004:592–611.

44. Lue TF. Physiology of penile erection and pathophysiology of erectile dysfunction. In: Kavoussi LR, Novick AC, Partin AW, et al., eds. *Campbell-Walsh urology*. 9th ed. Philadelphia: Saunders Elsevier; 2007:718–749.

45. Lue TF. Physiology of penile erection and pathophysiology of erectile dysfunction and priapism. In: Walsh PC, Retik AB, Vaughan ED Jr, et al., eds. *Campbell's urology*. 8th ed. Philadelphia: Saunders; 2002:1591–1618.

46. Mallis D, Moysidis K, Nakopoulou E, et al. Psychiatric morbidity is frequently undetected in patients with erectile dysfunction. *J Urol*. 2005;174:1913–1916.

47. McConnell JD, Roehrborn CG, Bautista OM, et al. The long-term effect of doxazosin, finasteride, and combination therapy on the clinical progression of benign prostatic hyperplasia. *N Engl J Med*. 2003;349:2387–2398.

48. McVary KT. Sexual dysfunction. In: Kasper DL, Braunwald E, Fauci AS, et al., eds. *Harrison's principles of internal medicine*. 16th ed. New York: McGraw-Hill; 2006:271–278.

49. Mulcahy JJ, Wilson SK. Current use of penile implants in erectile dysfunction. *Curr Urol Rep*. 2006;7:485–489.

50. Mulligan T, Reddy S, Gular P, et al. Disorders of male sexual function. *Clin Geriatr Med*. 2003. 19:473–481.

51. Nandipati KC, Raina R, Agarwal A, et al. Erectile dysfunction following radical retropubic prostatectomy. Epidemiology, pathophysiology and pharmacological management. *Drugs Aging* 2006;23:101–117.

52. Nappi R, Salonia A, Traish AM, et al. Clinical biologic pathophysiologies of women's sexual dysfunction. *J Sex Med*. 2005;2:4–25.

53. National Institutes of Health Consensus Development Panel on Impotence. Impotence *JAMA*. 1993;270:83–90.

54. Rhoden EL, Ribeiro EP, Reidner CE, et al Glycosylated haemoglobin levels and the severity of erectile function in diabetic men. *BJU Int* 2005;95:615–617.

55. Robinson D, Cardozo LD. The role of estrogen in female lower urinary tract dysfunction. *Urology* 2003;62:45–51.

56. Rodgers RG, Leeman, LL. Postpartum genitourinary changes. *Urol Clin North Am*. 2007;34:13–21

57. Rowland DL, Greenleaf WJ, Dorfman LJ, et al Aging and sexual function in men. *Arch Sex Behav*. 1993;22:545–557.

58. Schuessler B, Baessler K. Pharmacologic treatment of stress urinary incontinence: expectations for outcomes. *Urology*. 2003;62:31–38.

59. Seftel AD, Mack RJ, Secrest AR, et al. Restorative increases in serum testosterone levels are significantly correlated to improvements in sexual functioning. *J Androl*. 2004;25:963–972.

60. Soderdahl DW, Knight RW, Hansberry KL. Erectile dysfunction following transurethral resection of the prostate. *J Urol*. 1996;156: 1354–1356.

61. Steers WD. Pharmacologic treatment of erectile dysfunction. *Rev Urol*. 2002;4[Suppl 3]:517–525.

62. Stewart W, Van Rooyen J, Cundiff G, et al. Prevalence and burden of overactive bladder in the United States. *World J Urol*. 2003;20:327–336.

63. Tanagho EA. Urinary incontinence. In: Tanagho EA, McAninch JW, eds. *Smith's general urology.* 16th ed. New York: McGraw-Hill; 2003:473–491.
64. Tejada IS, Angulo J, Cellek S, et al. Pathophysiology of erectile dysfunction. *J Sex Med.* 2005;2:26–39.
65. Tsitouras PD, Martin CE, Harmen SM. Relationship of serum testosterone to sexual activity in healthy elderly men. *J Gerontol.* 1982; 37:288–293.
66. Walsh PC, Marschke P, Ricker D, et al. Patient-reported urinary continence and sexual function after anatomic radical prostatectomy. *Urology.* 2000;55:58–61.
67. Wein AJ. Pathophysiology and classification of voiding dysfunction. In: Walsh PC, Retik AB, Vaughan ED, et al., eds. *Campbell's urology.* 8th ed. Philadelphia: Saunders; 2002:887–899.
68. Wein AJ, Rackley RR. Overactive bladder: a better understanding of pathophysiology, diagnosis and management. *J Urol.* 2006;175:S5–S10.
69. Wilson MG. Urinary incontinence: selected current concepts. *Med Clin North Am.* 2006; 90:825–836.
70. Witherington R. Vacuum constriction device for management of erectile impotence. *J Urol.* 1989; 141:320–322.
71. Wright PJ. Comparison of phosphodiesterase type 5 (PDE5) inhibitors. *Int J Clin Pract.* 2006; 60:967–975.
72. Zheng H, Bidasee KR, Mayhan WG, et al. Lack of central nitric oxide triggers erectile dysfunction in diabetics. *Am J Physiol Regul Integr Comp Physiol.* 2007;292:R1158–R1164.

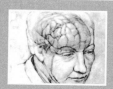

SECTION III

SPECIFIC NEUROLOGICAL CONDITIONS AFFECTING THE OLDER ADULT

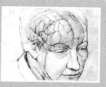

CHAPTER 17

Ischemic Cerebrovascular Disease

Scott E. Kasner, Julio A. Chalela, and Susan L. Hickenbottom

DEFINITION OF TERMS

- *Stroke* is a clinical syndrome characterized by rapidly developing symptoms or signs of focal neurologic dysfunction due to a vascular cause. Therefore, stroke includes both ischemic and hemorrhagic cerebrovascular events.
- *Cerebral infarction* or *ischemic stroke* is used when radiologic or pathologic confirmation of the suspected stroke is obtained.
- The colloquial term *cerebrovascular accident (CVA)* and the classical term *apoplexy* should be avoided because they connote a fortuitous origin, whereas stroke is usually caused by a well-defined pathogenic mechanism.
- *Stroke-in-evolution* is sometimes used to describe stroke characterized by gradual progression of the symptoms over the first few minutes to hours. However, this imprecise term lacks a standard definition.
- *Transient ischemic attack (TIA)* is an abrupt, focal loss of neurologic function caused by temporary ischemia. Although in the past it was thought that TIAs could persist up to 24 hours, modern imaging techniques have shown that deficits lasting more than an hour usually represent irreversible cerebral infarcts and that most true TIAs typically last <15 minutes (55,87). For the same reason, the term *reversible ischemic neurologic deficit (RIND)* referring to symptoms lasting 1 to 7 days has been abandoned.
- *Stroke in the elderly* is applied in many studies to refer to strokes occurring in patients older than 60 years, although certain studies use the term only in patients older than 65 or 75. The term *stroke in the very old* is used in cohorts older than 80 or 85 (19). Regardless of the cutoff point, stroke in the extremes of age has distinct pathophysiologic and prognostic features.

EPIDEMIOLOGY IN OLDER ADULTS

Ischemic stroke affects all age groups but is primarily a disease of older adults. The annual incidence in the United States approaches 750,000 ischemic strokes per year (101) and seems to be increasing as the population ages. Moreover, age is an independent but unmodifiable risk factor for ischemic stroke. The risk of stroke approximately doubles for each successive decade of life, from about three strokes per 1,000 people aged 55 to 64 years to about 25 strokes per 1,000 people over the age of 85 years (106). The risk of stroke is higher among men up to age 75, but over age 75, it is higher among women and is the leading cause of death among women >85 years. African-Americans carry a disproportionate share of the burden of stroke at all ages, with more than double the incidence and mortality of whites. Among patients who have already survived a stroke, a major risk factor for recurrent stroke is age >75 years (45).

RISK FACTORS IN OLDER ADULTS

Many of the recognized risk factors for cerebrovascular disease are overly abundant in the elderly population and contribute to their increased stroke risk (Table 17-1).

Hypertension, the leading risk factor for ischemic stroke, increases with advancing age and is found in more than half of people >65 (20). Furthermore, after the age of 65 years, the risk of stroke depends predominantly on systolic rather than diastolic pressure, which also increases linearly with age. Primary prevention of stroke in older adults should include treatment of hypertension, including treatment of isolated systolic hypertension, since antihypertensive therapy reduces the risk of stroke by more than 30% (92). The

Table 17-1. *Risk Factors for Ischemic Stroke*

Nonmodifiable	Modifiable
Age	Hypertension
Sex	Diabetes
Race/ethnicity	Hyperlipidemia
Family history	Cardiac disease (AF and others)
	Smoking
	Excessive alcohol use
	Physical inactivity

AF, atrial fibrillation.

Seventh Joint National Commission (JNC 7) guidelines currently recommend medical treatment for blood pressure ≥140/90 mm Hg or ≥130/80 mm Hg in patients with diabetes or chronic kidney disease, with ideal blood pressure being 120/80 mm Hg or less (20). The choice of first-line agent for blood pressure treatment remains somewhat controversial.

Based on the results of the Antihypertensive and Lipid-Lowering Treatment to Prevent Heart Attack Trial (ALLHAT) (4), which found the use of a thiazide diuretic to be superior and less expensive than other drug classes in preventing vascular disease, the JNC 7 recommends use of thiazide-type diuretics in most patients with uncomplicated hypertension, either alone or in combination with antihypertensive drugs. The JNC 7 recommendations do acknowledge, however, that most patients will require two or more drugs to reach the target blood pressure goals. On the other hand, recent trials of angiotensin-converting enzyme (ACE) inhibitors and angiotensin receptor blockers (ARBs) in patients with cardiovascular or cerebrovascular disease have also demonstrated reduced risk of stroke with treatment using these types of medications (22,23,83,109). Thus, some clinicians prefer to use ACE inhibitors or ARBs for secondary stroke prevention.

Atrial fibrillation (AF), another risk factor for ischemic stroke, also increases sharply with increasing age. Approximately 0.7% of the general US population is estimated to have AF; this proportion increases to 5% to 8% for persons >65 years old and to 10% to 15% for those >80 years old (94). The median age for patients with AF in the United States is 72 years (94). Multiple epidemiologic studies have demonstrated that AF is an independent risk factor for ischemic stroke and increases the relative risk of stroke approximately fivefold (46). In unselected populations with AF, an annual risk of stroke of about 5% is observed, but patients stratified as "high risk" have stroke rates of up to 12% per year (46). Validated risk factors for stroke in AF include age over 75 years, congestive heart failure or left ventricular fractional shortening <25%, hypertension, diabetes, and history of previous thromboembolism (36,47,97). The use of antiplatelet/anticoagulant therapy for stroke prophylaxis in the elderly with AF is somewhat complicated and will be discussed later in the Treatment Options section.

Diabetes mellitus is a risk factor for ischemic stroke, and stroke is at least twice as common in diabetics than nondiabetics. The prevalence of diabetes increases steadily with age, such that approximately 18% of people aged 65 years or older in the United States have this disorder. Some of the increased risk of stroke appears to be related to concomitant hypertension, but at least some component of risk is independently related to diabetes alone (12). Unfortunately, it remains uncertain whether tight glucose control in diabetics is effective for the prevention of stroke.

The role of hypercholesterolemia as a stroke risk factor remains somewhat controversial. It appears that the effect of total cholesterol seems to wane with increasing age, but high levels of low-density lipoprotein (LDL) and low levels of high-density lipoprotein (HDL) increase the risk of stroke even in elderly populations. The class of lipid-lowering agents known as the 3-hydroxy-3-methylglutaryl coenzyme A (HMG-CoA) reductase inhibitors, or statins, has been studied extensively in patients with vascular disease. It is hypothesized that, in addition to lowering LDL, statins also have "pleiotropic effects" and may stabilize atherosclerotic plaque, reduce platelet aggregation, and decrease inflammation, all of which in turn reduce the risk of vascular events (86). Pooled results of several statin trials involving over 90,000 patients with cardiovascular disease demonstrated a reduction in risk of stroke for patients treated with statins (6). The recently published Stroke Prevention by Aggressive Reduction in Cholesterol Levels (SPARCL) trial confirmed that statins reduce the risk for recurrent stroke in patients who have had a stroke or TIA but who have no established cardiac disease (5). Although these trials did not specifically address lipid management in the elderly, no increase in adverse events associated with statins was noted in this group. Therefore, it is now recommended that stroke and TIA become considered a "coronary heart disease risk equivalent" and that these patients be treated with a statin to bring the LDL cholesterol to <100 mg/dL or to <70 mg/dL in patients considered very high risk, defined as "those who have cardiovascular disease together with either multiple risk factors, especially diabetes, or severe and poorly controlled risk factors (i.e., continued smoking), or metabolic syndrome, or patients hospitalized for acute coronary syndromes" (39). The above studies also demonstrated benefit even in patients with "normal" cholesterol levels, so therapy may also be considered in these patients.

ETIOPATHOGENIC MECHANISMS OF ISCHEMIC STROKE

Ischemia is caused by transient or permanent occlusion of a cerebral blood vessel. The possible causes of cerebrovascular occlusion are myriad and are described individually in the section titled Evaluation of Stroke Etiology. After occlusion, there is impaired cerebral blood flow (CBF), resulting in a central area (core) of severely constrained perfusion and a peripheral area of less constrained perfusion (ischemic penumbra) (52). In the core, CBF is typically

<15 mL/100 g brain tissue/min, and it will invariably succumb to infarction. In the penumbra, CBF averages 18 to 20 mL/100 g/min. The cells in the penumbra lose electrical function but retain structural integrity. The penumbra thus represents a potentially salvageable area, but the time window for intervention appears to be brief. The brain is able to tolerate low CBF only for a limited amount of time, and the threshold for ischemia varies with the duration and the intensity of the ischemic insult. Thus, it is imperative to rapidly re-establish blood flow in acute stroke in order to minimize the cerebral injury.

Impaired cerebral perfusion sets into motion a series of events called the ischemic cascade (67,68,81). Neurons become unable to maintain aerobic respiration, and anaerobic respiration ensues, leading to accumulation of lactic acid. With the change to a less efficient metabolic state, neurons are no longer able to maintain ionic balance. Excitotoxicity occurs, in which glutamate and other excitatory neurotransmitters worsen the neuronal injury via excessive stimulation of neurons during their energy-depleted state. These neurotransmitters depolarize the neuronal cell membrane, which is followed by an influx of sodium, chloride, and water, resulting in cytotoxic edema. Influx of calcium follows and may lead to neuronal death. Several other elements amplify the ischemic cascade. The details of this topic are beyond the scope of this review, but a few key elements deserve attention. Increased intracellular calcium activates several enzymatic pathways that cause proteolysis, destruction of cell wall lipids, free radical formation, further release of intracellular calcium, and increased production of nitric oxide. The enzymatic disturbances and free radical production lead to widespread disruption of neuronal and endothelial integrity. In addition, in the ischemic zone, a series of cytokines are released, some of which may promote an inflammatory response and disrupt the microcirculation, thereby worsening the ischemic injury. Lastly, cell death may occur in a delayed fashion by apoptosis (33), a genetically programmed form of cell death that may be induced by neuronal ischemia. It is distinct from necrosis because it occurs in a delayed manner and may occur in remote areas from the core of infarction.

The sequence of events described in the previous paragraph occurs to a different degree in all subjects exposed to an ischemic injury. However, laboratory experience suggests that age has an impact on these events. Experimental evidence suggests that older animals are less resistant to ischemia than younger ones and that the neurotoxic response may be more robust with advanced age (25,49,90). The ability to neutralize free radicals and extrude calcium from cells is more reduced in older animals compared with younger counterparts. The ability to synthesize proteins is reduced in the elderly and may lead to impaired cerebral reorganization after both trauma and stroke. The blood–brain barrier in the elderly is less efficient than in the young, and toxins normally excluded from the brain may gain access, worsening the ischemic injury (75). Although CBF is lower in older subjects, cerebral metabolism (as measured by the oxygen extraction ratio) is also lower; thus, an imbalance between supply and demand does not exist. Nevertheless, the normal autoregulatory response seen in young subjects in the setting of impaired perfusion is absent in older individuals (93). Collateral circulation may be impaired in the elderly, leading to infarcts of larger volume (66). The inherent elastic properties of intracranial vessels are affected by aging, reducing the efficiency of the compensatory response to ischemia and acidosis. Thus, it is conceivable that, in older patients, comparable vascular insults may result in a more severe injury than in younger patients. Paradoxically, older stroke patients may fare better when they suffer large middle cerebral artery infarcts with significant mass effect because the age-related atrophy may provide additional space for tissue displacement (64).

NATURAL HISTORY OF ISCHEMIC STROKE

Despite significant advances in the treatment of ischemic stroke, the majority of stroke survivors will have some residual neurologic dysfunction. Although most patients have some improvement, it is unfortunately often incomplete. In general, older patients face a worse prognosis than younger patients (56). Mortality due to stroke increases progressively (about 10% below age 65, 20% between ages 65 and 74, 30% between ages 75 and 84, and 40% at age 85 and older) (77). Functional outcome also tends to be worse in older patients, although they have similar neurologic deficits, which suggests that the ability to compensate after stroke is worse in the elderly (56,77). Furthermore, dementia occurs in about one third of elderly stroke survivors, which further adds to the burden of disability (10). A major predictor of outcome after stroke is initial stroke severity, with worse outcomes in patients with more severe deficits (84,91). Recovery depends somewhat on the size and location of the infarction. Small infarctions, particularly subcortical lacunar strokes, may result in little permanent deficit, whereas large hemispheric infarctions may be devastating. The presence of other diseases or medical complications after the stroke also appears to worsen outcome (54), and these tend to be more common among the elderly. Despite these potential prognostic indicators, the marked variability among patients makes prediction for individuals extremely difficult.

Table 17-2. *Major Cerebrovascular Clinical Syndromes*

Artery	Clinical Features
Anterior Circulation	
ACA	Contralateral leg weakness
MCA	Contralateral face + arm >leg weakness, sensory loss, field cut, aphasia/neglect
Posterior Circulation	
PCA	Contralateral field cut
BA	Eye movement abnormalities, ataxia, sensory/motor deficits
VA	Dysarthria, dysphagia, vertigo, ataxia, sensory/motor deficits
Small vessels	Lacunar syndrome (see text) without cortical signs*

ACA, anterior cerebral artery; MCA, middle cerebral artery; PCA, posterior cerebral artery; BA, basilar artery; VA, vertebral artery.
*Cortical signs include aphasia, apraxia, neglect, and other cognitive abnormalities.

Infarcted brain tissue is irreparable, and functional improvement after stroke is believed to occur by recruitment of other neurons to serve new or additional roles. Neurons have been shown to sprout new synapses after stroke in young rodents (17,18,24). Electrical brain mapping in monkeys has demonstrated that the cerebral cortex can be functionally reorganized during recovery after an infarction (24). Similarly, functional magnetic resonance imaging (MRI) in humans has shown increased activity in both hemispheres as patients improve, suggesting recruitment of neighboring cortex and corresponding areas of the contralateral cortex (21). In general, most motor recovery is expected to occur primarily in the first 3 months after stroke. The effect of aging on these reparative processes is unknown in humans, but it is hypothesized that they become less effective with age.

DIAGNOSIS

EMERGENT EVALUATION

The majority of acute stroke patients should be initially evaluated in the emergency department (ED). After attention to the issues of oxygenation and hemodynamic stability, a medical history and physical examination should focus on specific stroke risk factors and etiologies, followed by clinical localization of the ischemic territory (Table 17-2). Other disorders that may resemble ischemic stroke must be considered and excluded if possible given the available information (Table 17-3). Laboratory studies, including a complete blood count, electrolytes, glucose, and coagulation parameters, should be obtained. Electrocardiography (EKG) is needed to assess for evidence of arrhythmia or cardiac ischemia. Emergent computed tomography (CT) is required to identify intracerebral hemorrhage (ICH) and early signs of cerebral ischemia. Recent studies suggest that an MRI is as effective as CT at detecting acute ICH and more effective at detecting subacute and chronic hemorrhage and acute ischemia (60). Furthermore, some studies suggest that the diagnostic yield of noncontrast CT for hospitalized elderly patients with suspected stroke is fairly low (50), suggesting that MRI may be preferable.

Based on these data, which should be obtained in <60 minutes, decisions regarding acute interventions must be reached. These basic emergent diagnostic

Table 17-3. *Differential Diagnosis of Acute Ischemic Stroke*

Disorders That Mimic Stroke	Diagnostic Tools
Intracerebral hemorrhage	CT/MRI
Subarachnoid hemorrhage	CT, lumbar puncture
Subdural/epidural hematoma	History of trauma, CT/MRI
Structural lesion (neoplasm/abscess/etc.)	CT/MRI
Hypo-/hyperglycemia	Finger stick glucose
Other metabolic derangements	Routine chemistry studies
Seizure	Clinical history, EEG
Migraine	Clinical history
Conversion disorder	Clinical history, psychiatric evaluation

CT, computed tomgrapy; MRI, magnetic resonance imaging; EEG, electroencephalography.

issues are the same for young and old because, as described later in Treatment of Acute Ischemic Stroke, age is not a major issue in the acute treatment decision (99). Contrary to popular belief, advanced age is not a contraindication for the administration of thrombolytics, and elderly patients can receive intra-venous and intra-arterial fibrinolytics with reasonable safety. Baseline stroke severity and prior functional status are the most important determinants of out-come after acute stroke (76).

Treatment of the acute stroke patient should ide-ally target the underlying pathophysiology. However, early determination of the stroke mechanism is diffi-cult, and many patients seen within the first 24 hours after onset are incorrectly classified (69). Since ther-apy for acute stroke must be initiated during this window of uncertainty, specific mechanism-directed therapy does not yet exist. Instead, treatment must have broad efficacy for all types of ischemic stroke.

Emergent vascular imaging studies may be useful for some treatment decisions. For determination of vascular anatomy, the "gold standard" is conventional catheter arteriography, which can demonstrate an acute arterial occlusion or embolus lodged at a vascu-lar bifurcation. The vasculature can also be evaluated noninvasively with transcranial Doppler (TCD) ultra-sonography, magnetic resonance angiography (MRA), or CT-angiography (CTA), but these techniques may be less accurate than conventional angiography. Furthermore, conventional angiography provides a route for interventional radiologic therapies, such as intra-arterial thrombolysis or angioplasty, although these are controversial at present.

Physiologic imaging offers the possibility of iden-tifying a viable "ischemic penumbra" around an infarcted core, and this viable tissue may benefit from potential treatments such as reperfusion or neuropro-tection (52). Discussion of these techniques is beyond the scope of this review, but intensive research may bring this type of neuroimaging to the clinical fore-front. A recent study suggested that beyond 3 hours, and possibly before 3 hours, thrombolysis decisions based on MRI findings may be associated with less hemorrhage (61).

EVALUATION OF STROKE ETIOLOGY

After the hyperacute period of the first few hours after stroke onset, secondary prevention therapy should be initiated for all ischemic stroke patients. Diagnostic studies are needed to determine the risk factors and cause of the stroke because specific treatments are available for specific stroke etiologies (see algorithm depicted in Fig. 17-1). There is no true "standard" approach to the evaluation of all stroke patients, and consideration must be given to each patient's medical and neurologic condition, his/her prognosis, and the

possible risks and benefits of the interventions that are being considered. For example, some patients are very poor candidates for carotid revascularization pro-cedures (i.e., endarterectomy or angioplasty/stent) because of their other medical problems and, there-fore, have no need of carotid diagnostic studies. Testing in this situation is costly and inefficient. Similarly, some patients are comatose or moribund due to stroke and are unlikely to survive. In such patients, diagnostic studies should be deferred, at least temporarily, since information regarding etiology is extremely unlikely to alter management. These issues may be particularly important in some elderly patients, and attention should first be paid to the issues of quality of life and level of care.

Characterization of the stroke risk factors is based primarily on the medical history, but the following laboratory investigations are recommended for most patients: complete blood count, prothrombin time (PT), partial thromboplastin time (PTT), serum glu-cose, and fasting lipids. An erythrocyte sedimentation rate (ESR) is also warranted for most elderly patients.

Cardioembolism

Cardioembolism should be considered as a possible cause in virtually all ischemic stroke patients. It is most commonly associated with AF, mural thrombus, focal ventricular akinesis after myocardial infarction, dilated cardiomyopathy, and valvular disease. Embolic events may be multiple and may occur in the territo-ries of any of the major vessels. Cardiac evaluation includes a clinical cardiac history and examination, EKG, and echocardiogram. Either transthoracic echocardiography (TTE) or transesophageal echocar-diography (TEE) may be used as the initial screening test, but TEE is more sensitive to some abnormalities including left atrial appendage thrombus and aortic arch atherosclerosis (74). The superiority of TEE is well established in a wide age range, although its spe-cific superiority in the very old remains to be deter-mined (96). If cardioembolism is suspected but TTE is normal, then TEE should also be performed. Treatment (described later) is aimed toward preven-tion of recurrent clot formation and cerebral embolization, often with anticoagulants.

Large Vessel Atherothromboembolism

Large vessel atherothromboembolism is usually a result of carotid artery stenosis and less commonly a result of stenosis of the vertebral arteries or the intracranial vessels. Stenosis of the internal carotid artery can result in either a thrombotic (acute occlu-sive) or embolic (artery-to-artery embolic) stroke, and in either case, the treatment may include excision of the plaque by endarterectomy. Stenosis in the verte-brobasilar system or in the intracranial circulation

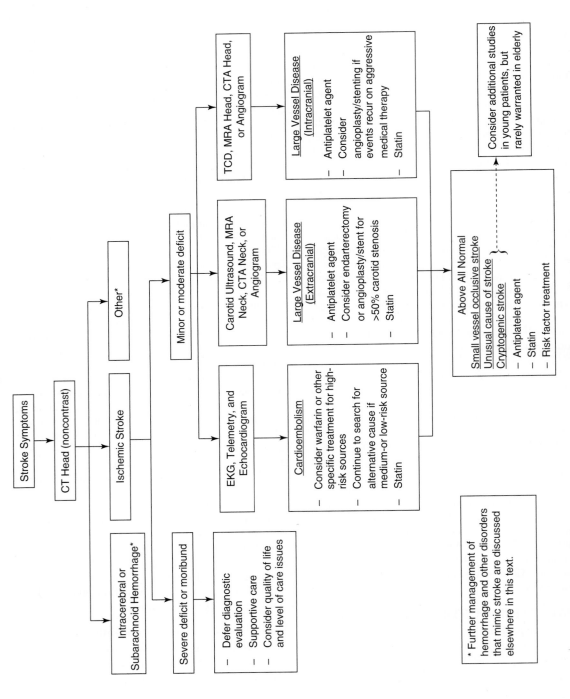

Figure 17-1. Algorithm for the diagnosis of stroke etiology and strategies for secondary prevention.

may cause stroke by the same mechanisms, but these are not amenable to surgery. A hallmark clinical feature is recurrent similar clinical events in the same vascular territory, suggesting the involvement of a single large vessel. Examination of the large vessels should be performed depending on the localization of the stroke. Patients with anterior circulation strokes (Table 17-2) require evaluation of the carotid arteries, whereas patients with posterior circulation strokes (Table 17-2) require evaluation of the vertebral arteries, and both may need evaluation of the intracranial vessels. The extracranial carotid arteries can be evaluated by carotid ultrasonography, whereas both the carotid and vertebral arteries can be reliably imaged with MRA or CTA. The intracranial circulation can be examined by TCD, MRA, or CTA. Conventional cerebral angiography is the definitive study, but because this invasive test carries a 1% risk of stroke and significant expense, it is often reserved for those situations in which treatment decisions require the additional information.

Advanced age in itself should not deter the clinician from pursuing an evaluation for possible carotid stenosis. The outcome of carotid endarterectomy (CEA) in nonagenarians appears to be poor (likely related to stroke severity and frequent need for emergent surgery), but endarterectomy can be performed safely in selected octogenarians (100).

Small Vessel Occlusive Disease

Small vessel occlusive disease is often synonymous with "lacunar infarction." The deep small vessels in the internal capsule, corona radiata, thalamus, and pons seem most susceptible to the process of small vessel occlusive disease. Some of these infarctions may be clinically silent because they are small and may occur in a relatively less important region. However, small lesions do not necessarily cause small deficits. A microvascular infarction in the internal capsule can interrupt the entire corticospinal (motor) tract as it descends, resulting in a severe contralateral motor deficit. The most common lacunar syndromes are pure motor hemiparesis, pure sensory stroke, clumsy hand-dysarthria syndrome, and ataxic hemiparesis (34). The mechanism of the small vessel occlusive process is uncertain, but it is most common in patients with long-standing diabetes or hypertension. The diagnosis of small vessel disease rests on the clinical syndrome, the finding of a small (<1.5 cm) deep infarction on CT or MRI, and the absence of an alternative etiology (1).

Recently, MRI has shown that patients with lacunar infarcts often harbor evidence of small deposits of hemosiderin in the brain. The term "microbleeds" has been used to describe minute, round areas of signal loss, best seen using susceptibility-weighted (also known as gradient echo) images. Microbleeds are likely the result of chronic bleeding due to hypertension or amyloid angiopathy and tend to occur in the basal ganglia and the subcortical region. The association between microbleeds and lacunar infarcts is very strong, and it is hypothesized that the same morphologic changes that cause cerebral infarcts (lipohyalinosis and microaneurysms) cause small ICHs (58).

Other/Unusual Causes of Stroke

There are a number of uncommon causes of stroke, such as arterial dissection, prothrombotic disorders, genetic disorders, drug abuse (such as cocaine), and vasculitis (57). The diagnosis of these other mechanisms may require special laboratory studies, lumbar puncture, cerebral angiography, and even brain biopsy in some circumstances. Although stroke in young patients is disproportionately due to these miscellaneous causes (15), they are quite rare in the elderly, and an extensive evaluation to identify these causes is usually not warranted. However, temporal arteritis (TA) is the one unusual cause that occurs uniquely in older adults and always requires consideration.

TA should be considered in any stroke patient >50 years, and clinical suspicion should be heightened by the presence of jaw or tongue claudication, transient or permanent unilateral visual impairment (amaurosis fugax or ischemic optic neuropathy, respectively), localized headache or scalp tenderness, or temporal artery abnormalities (including diminished pulse, tenderness, induration, or nodules) (65). An ESR is recommended and should be considered abnormal if it exceeds 50 mm/h. If the clinical features are present and/or the ESR is elevated, then a unilateral temporal artery biopsy should be performed. If the level of suspicion is very high but the biopsy is negative, then the other temporal artery should be biopsied. The diagnosis of TA is based on the presence of at least three of the following five criteria: age >50 years, new-onset headache, temporal artery abnormality (tenderness or decreased pulse), ESR above 50 mm/h, and abnormal findings on temporal artery biopsy (89). Steroid therapy can be initiated prior to the biopsy and will not affect the results if performed within approximately 10 to 14 days (65). Treatment with pulsed intravenous (IV) steroids is superior to treatment with oral steroids because it facilitates tapering and leads to better long-term remission (71). Other methods to diagnose TA have been proposed, including ultrasound techniques, but they remain unproven and are not widely available.

Cryptogenic Stroke

Cryptogenic (idiopathic) stroke is diagnosed when all other studies fail to identify any likely stroke mechanism. About half of strokes in young patients are diagnosed as cryptogenic, but this etiology is infrequently invoked in the elderly. Older patients with cryptogenic stroke appear to have a high proportion of aortic atherosclerosis; nevertheless, such a finding is more likely a marker of diffuse vascular disease and not a direct stroke culprit (82).

TREATMENT OPTIONS

In general, treatment of the elderly patient with stroke does not differ much from that of younger patients. This section will discuss treatment options for both acute ischemic stroke and for secondary stroke prevention but will give special attention to areas of controversy in the treatment of elderly stroke patients, including acute stroke treatment with tissue plasminogen activator (tPA), anticoagulation in the setting of AF, and CEA for symptomatic carotid artery stenosis. Treatment of TA is addressed earlier in Other/Unusual Causes of Stroke. A summary of medications typically used in stroke treatment and prevention can be found in Table 17-4.

TREATMENT OF ACUTE ISCHEMIC STROKE

Intravenous tPA, at a dose of 0.9 mg/kg used within 3 hours of symptom onset, is the only Food and Drug Administration (FDA)–approved treatment for acute ischemic stroke. Its approval arose largely as a result of the National Institute of Neurological Disorders and Stroke (NINDS) rt-PA Stroke Study (79). This study documented an 11% to 13% absolute and 30% to 50% relative increase in favorable outcomes on four different outcome scales at 3 months after stroke. Although there was a statistically significant increase in the rate of symptomatic ICH in the tPA-treated group (6.4% vs. 0.6% in the placebo group; $p < 0.0001$), there was no significant difference in mortality at 3 months. The European Cooperative Acute Stroke Study (ECASS I) found no significant benefit for tPA therapy in acute ischemic stroke and high rates of treatment-associated ICH, but this study used a longer time window (6 hours) and higher dose (1.1 mg/kg) than the NINDS tPA trial and was also complicated by a very high rate of protocol violations (109 of 620 patients enrolled) (40). A second European trial, ECASS II, again used a 6-hour time window but used the NINDS dosing regimen of 0.9 mg/kg and required rigorous CT training for its investigators (41). Again, no significant difference in outcome between placebo- and tPA-treated patients was found, but few patients were enrolled with the 0- to 3-hour time window. Symptomatic ICH occurred more frequently in the tPA-treated group (8.8% vs. 3.4% in the placebo group), but there was no difference in mortality at 3 months. In summary, the trials

for IV tPA for acute ischemic stroke demonstrated improved outcome after treatment in selected patients within 3 hours of stroke onset. Although treatment with IV tPA appears to be safe when given up to 6 hours after symptom onset, efficacy has not been proven beyond the 3-hour time window.

It should be noted that the ECASS trial excluded patients over 80 years old. Nevertheless, the initial results from ECASS I did suggest that age was a risk factor for parenchymatous hematoma; this finding was not supported in the subsequent ECASS II trial. Moreover, subgroup analysis of the NINDS t-PA Stroke Study results did not find age to be predictive of ICH (78). Therefore, these studies demonstrated that there was no age-associated increased risk of ICH in the setting of a carefully monitored clinical trial.

An early postmarketing trial of 189 patients treated with IV tPA within 3 hours of stroke onset found no difference in the rates of fatal, symptomatic, or total ICH in patients >80 years old compared with patients <80 years (99). In addition, older and younger patients had equal likelihood of favorable outcome following treatment with tPA (99). In another postmarketing study, the Standard Treatment with Alteplase to Reverse Stroke (STARS) study, the incidence of symptomatic ICH (3.3%) was too low to perform analysis for predictors of ICH; however, age <85 years was a predictor of favorable clinical outcome (3). A more recent meta-analysis of patients >80 years treated with intravenous tPA corroborated such findings. Overall, older patients tended to have worse outcome compared with younger counterparts, but the poor outcomes were explained by greater baseline stroke severity and pre-existing disability. Patients >80 years do not appear to be more prone to tPA-related intracranial hemorrhage than younger patients (30).

The results of these studies indicate that the elderly are not at increased risk for ICH with the use of IV tPA for acute ischemic stroke and that they may be as likely as younger patients to benefit from such treatment. Other therapies for acute ischemic stroke (e.g., intra-arterial thrombolysis, mechanical reperfusion strategies) have been evaluated more recently, but thus far, little data evaluating the specific risks and benefits of these therapies for elderly stroke patients are available. Thrombectomy offers some potential theoretical advantages in the management of acute ischemic stroke because it confirms the presence of a vascular occlusion, may provide information regarding the etiology of the stroke, and, most importantly, may achieve recanalization without the use of thrombolytics. The Mechanical Embolus Removal in Cerebral Ischemia (MERCI) trial studied patients presenting with large vessel occlusions undergoing thrombectomy within 8 hours of symptom onset and

Table 17-4. *Medications Used in Ischemic Stroke*

Medication	Standard Dose	Drug Interactions	Adverse Effects
tPA	0.9 mg/kg (maximum, 90 mg); 10% as IV bolus over 1 minute, then remainder as IV infusion over 1 hour	Anticoagulants, including heparin and warfarin	Systemic and intracranial hemorrhage
Aspirin	50–325 mg qd	Other antiplatelet agents, NSAIDs, heparin, warfarin	Dyspepsia, tinnitus, gastrointestinal bleeding
Ticlopidine	250 mg bid	Aspirin and other antiplatelet agents, NSAIDs, heparin, warfarin, cimetidine, theophylline	Diarrhea, nausea, vomiting, rash, gastrointestinal bleeding, neutropenia, thrombotic thrombocytopenic purpura, aplastic anemia
Clopidogrel	75 mg qd	Aspirin and other antiplatelet agents, NSAIDs, heparin, warfarin; at high concentrations, may inhibit certain hepatic enzymes and decrease metabolism of various medications	Rash, diarrhea, dyspepsia, gastrointestinal bleeding
Dipyridamole	Extended-release formulation (200 mg) given in combination with 25 mg aspirin bid	None	Headache, dizziness, flushing, abdominal distress, diarrhea, vomiting
Warfarin	Individualized according to patient response as measured by international normalized ratio (INR); usual dosages vary from 1–10 mg qd and titrated to keep INR between 2.0 and 3.0	Aspirin and other antiplatelet agents, NSAIDs, ticlopidine, clopidogrel, heparin; interacts with multiple other medications through pharmacokinetic mechanisms; consult literature before initiating therapy	Gastrointestinal and other systemic bleeding, warfarin necrosis syndrome, systemic atheromatous embolization ("purple toe" syndrome)

tPA, tissue plasminogen activator; IV, intravenous; qd, once a day; NSAID, nonsteroidal anti-inflammatory drug; bid, twice a day.

compared the outcomes of those who achieved successful recanalization with the outcome of those who did not recanalize (95). The mean age of patients enrolled onto the study was 67.0 ± 15.5 years, but the exact proportion of patients who were >70 years was not specified. Although age was an independent predictor of poor outcome in the MERCI trial (odds ratio = 0.94 for each decade), the most powerful predictor of good outcome was achievement of recanalization. In the authors' opinion, thrombectomy and intra-arterial thrombolysis are reasonable therapeutic interventions for selected elderly patients with large

vessel occlusion when standard tPA therapy cannot be used (i.e., recent surgery or presentation within 3 to 8 hours).

PREVENTION OF ISCHEMIC STROKE

Strategies for secondary prevention of stroke include risk factor modification, pharmacologic treatment with antiplatelet or anticoagulant therapies, and surgical management of carotid artery disease. Therapies for risk factor modification in hypertension and hyperlipidemia are discussed earlier in the Risk Factors in Older Adults section.

The American College of Chest Physicians (ACCP) has issued practice parameters for stroke prevention in AF (94). In the general AF population, warfarin with dosing adjusted to yield an international normalized ratio (INR) of 2.0 to 3.0 reduces the risk of stroke by about 70% and is recommended for stroke prophylaxis in patients who can be appropriately monitored. Despite this recommendation, warfarin is generally underused, and in elderly populations, underutilization of warfarin may be even more problematic. Several studies designed to assess practice patterns and attitudes about anticoagulation in the elderly with AF have demonstrated decreased willingness on the part of physicians to use warfarin in their older patients (9,72). Some of this hesitance may result from concerns about increased risk for ICH in elderly patients on chronic anticoagulation. The Stroke Prevention in Atrial Fibrillation II (SPAF II) study found that AF patients >75 years old who were treated with adjusted-dose warfarin were at significantly higher risk for ICH than younger patients (98). Unfortunately, a regimen of fixed, low-dose warfarin (INR = 1.2 to 1.5) and aspirin was found to be significantly less effective in preventing stroke than adjusted dose warfarin (INR = 2.0 to 3.0) and cannot be recommended as an alternative (97).

Several validated stroke risk stratification schemes for patients with AF have been developed to assist health care providers in making decisions regarding the need for anticoagulation (36,47,103). The $CHADS_2$ risk index uses a point-based system to assign risk of stroke that is dependent upon clinical characteristics: **C**ongestive heart failure (1 point); **H**ypertention (1 point); **A**ge >75 years (1 point); **D**iabetes (1 point); and prior **S**troke or TIA (**2** points) (36). Stroke rates increase with increasing point total and can be used to assign high, moderate, and low risk of stroke. Based on the use of these risk stratification schemes, the ACCP recommends that patients with persistent or paroxysmal AF at high risk for stroke (those with any of the following features: prior ischemic stroke, TIA, or systemic embolism; age >75 years; moderately or severely impaired left ventricular systolic function and/or congestive heart failure; history of hypertension; or diabetes) be anticoagulated with warfarin with a goal INR of 2.0 to 3.0. Patients aged 65 to 75 years without other risk factors are considered at moderate risk for stroke, and antithrombotic therapy with either warfarin or aspirin is recommended, taking patient preferences and values into account when making this treatment decision (94).

Antiplatelet therapy is also used in secondary prevention of ischemic stroke. To date, clinical trials involving antiplatelet agents for stroke prevention have not focused specifically on treatment of elderly patients. Thus, this section will only briefly outline antiplatelet treatment options that are available for all stroke patients; more detailed discussion of antiplatelet therapy selection can be found elsewhere (2). Aspirin had long been considered the standard initial medical treatment for secondary stroke prevention, and numerous trials and meta-analyses have documented an approximate 25% reduction in the odds of stroke recurrence or vascular death in aspirin recipients compared with placebo (7,8). The best dose of aspirin for stroke prevention has been controversial in the past, but most authors now agree that low to moderate doses of aspirin (50 to 325 mg) are as effective as high doses and have fewer side effects (2). Additional antiplatelet agents have been introduced that have modest benefit for secondary stroke prevention over aspirin, including ticlopidine (48), clopidogrel (16), and an extended-release dipyridamole/low-dose aspirin combination (29,44). The use of ticlopidine has been curtailed because of its adverse safety profile, including the risk of severe neutropenia and thrombotic thrombocytopenic purpura (13). Two recent studies have examined the use of clopidogrel in combination with aspirin for secondary stroke prevention; these studies found increased risk for bleeding complications on combination therapy without increased benefit for stroke prevention (14,28).

Based on the results of these trials, the ACCP has recommended that patients with noncardioembolic stroke or TIA may be treated with any of the following as initial antiplatelet therapy: aspirin 50 to 325 mg daily, clopidogrel 75 mg daily, or the combination of aspirin and extended-release dipyridamole 50/200 mg twice daily.

In addition to pharmacologic agents, surgical intervention with CEA may also be appropriate preventive therapy for selected stroke patients. The North American Symptomatic Carotid Endarterectomy Trial (NASCET) and the European Carotid Surgery Trial (ECST) demonstrated marked benefit for CEA compared with best medical management in symptomatic patients with high-grade carotid stenosis (defined as >70% in NASCET and >80% in ECST) (31,80). NASCET results for symptomatic patients with moderately severe stenosis (50% to 69%) demonstrate a less robust but still significant benefit for CEA in this population (11). Pooled data from both studies was analyzed in a 2004 study and demonstrated an increased benefit from surgery in patients aged 75 years or older (88).

On the other hand, an older study using community hospital discharge data demonstrated that age was a predictor of in-hospital mortality after CEA. The difference may be related to practice variability among the institutions at which the surgery was performed. In NASCET, enrolling centers were required to meet stringent criteria regarding perioperative morbidity and mortality simply to participate in the trial, as compared to CEA performed in community practice. Thus, these data emphasize the importance of knowing the CEA perioperative complication rates of particular surgeons to whom one may refer patients. A recent population-based study from the United Kingdom documented that the incidence of symptomatic carotid disease increases steeply in those >80 years but also that elderly patients with stroke or TIA are less likely to undergo carotid evaluation (32). This underinvestigation results in potential undertreatment of carotid artery disease in the elderly, despite good evidence of major benefit from endarterectomy. In summary, elderly patients with significant symptomatic carotid stenosis can definitely undergo CEA safely in the hands of well-trained surgeons who perform the procedure often and stand to gain increased benefit from the procedure.

Carotid angioplasty/stenting (CAS) has recently emerged as an alternative potential strategy for the management of carotid artery disease in selected elderly patients. The Stenting and Angioplasty with Protection in Patients at High Risk for Endarterectomy (SAPPHIRE) trial randomized patients at high risk for surgical therapy to either CAS with distal embolic protection device or CEA (108). High surgical risk was determined by clinical criteria including age >80 years, serious cardiac or pulmonary disease, contralateral carotid occlusion, and history of previous surgery or radiation or any other factor that might make the surgery more technically difficult. The trial found no significant difference in the risk of major complications (stroke, myocardial infarction, or death) between the two therapies. Based largely on the results of this trial, the FDA recently approved the use of stenting for symptomatic stenosis in patients who are not candidates for conventional surgery due to high surgical risk. However, two more recent trials found stenting to be inferior to endarterectomy (70,85). Additionally, a large randomized trial comparing CAS and CEA in low-risk surgical patients suspended enrollment of patients >80 years old during its lead-in phase due to higher risk of stroke and death in these patients (51). As such, CAS should not be used routinely instead of CEA in elderly patients with symptomatic carotid disease; results from ongoing trials may help to refine recommendations regarding CAS in the elderly.

PSYCHOSOCIAL IMPACT

Stroke is far more often disabling than lethal. It is estimated that stroke currently disables over 4 million Americans. The financial, social, and familial impact of stroke is staggering. The decline in stroke mortality seen in recent years may result in a longer period of disability before death with significant costs for individuals and society. In 2006, the estimated cost of stroke was $57.9 billion. Approximately two thirds of this amount represents the direct cost of hospital care, medical care, and drugs (101). The remainder of the financial burden imposed by stroke is due to long-term care and, to a lesser extent, lost income on the part of patients. The economic impact on family members who become caregivers for stroke survivors is unknown. Older patients are more likely to be discharged to a nursing home and to be handicapped at 3 months, accounting for a significant part of the financial burden of stroke. Older patients also more often tend to be institutionalized prior to the stroke, and that in itself is a predictor of poststroke institutionalization and increased cost. Even after treatment with intravenous tPA, patients older than 80 are more likely to be discharged to a nursing home than younger patients (99).

Stroke impacts significantly the ability to return to work. Of all stroke survivors, only 53% are able to return to work (107). Of those who return to work, 20% do so only on a part-time basis. Advanced age is inversely related to the chance of returning to work. On the other hand, many older stroke survivors are retired or unemployed prior to the stroke, thus confounding the interpretation of poststroke employment status. Stroke severity and cortical involvement also predict inability to return to work. Older patients appear to have more difficulty with instrumental activities of daily living (ambulation outdoors, shopping, public transportation), which hampers their ability to return to work (38).

Depression and anxiety are extremely common after stroke, occurring in approximately 40% of survivors (35,43,53). Major depression occurs in about 25%, and minor depression occurs in 15%. Depression after stroke is not entirely due to the functional deficit because patients with similar deficits due to nonvascular causes do not develop depression with the same frequency. Nevertheless, stroke severity, cognitive impairment, and physical disability correlate with the risk of development of depression (42). The presence of language impairment appears to be correlated with the risk of developing depression (59). Depression may be more frequent in elderly stroke patients than in younger ones. Lack of social support seems to exacerbate poststroke functional and cognitive impairment and may increase the risk of depression in older subjects. The time course of depression after stroke is highly variable. Overall, patients with poststroke depression face a greater mortality during the next few years after the stroke (105). Poststroke cognitive impairment may be aggravated by depression and may manifest as "pseudodementia." Treatment of poststroke depression may improve cognitive performance.

Sexual functioning is affected by stroke and may have a significant psychosocial impact. Up to 50% of stroke survivors and their spouses recommend that sexual counseling should be a part of stroke rehabilitation (62,63). The majority of stroke patients and their partners note diminished libido after stroke. Penile erection decreases in 75% of men. In women, decreased vaginal lubrication occurs in 46%, and anorgasmia occurs in 55%. Older age and severity of deficit seem to be associated with greater dysfunction (37). Sexual dysfunction does not appear to be related to stroke location, stroke etiology, or marital status. Sexual dysfunction is more common among diabetic males and among women taking cardiovascular medicines. A strong correlation exists between impaired sexual performance and depression (37,104).

Finally, stroke takes an enormous toll on the caregivers and family members of the stroke victim. Emotional support, personal hygiene, feeding, ambulation, and nursing care are often under the direct responsibility of the loved ones. Up to half of stroke survivors depend entirely on their family members for assistance with activities of daily living (26). The most common causes for dependency are sphincter incontinence, inability to walk, inability to transfer, inability to feed, and difficulty dressing. Caring for a stroke patient poses constraints upon the social life of the caregiver as well and is particularly burdensome if the caregiver is also elderly or functionally impaired. A significant proportion of stroke victims' family members feel lonely, note a decline in their social activities, experience emotional distress and anxiety, and feel that their role as family member is impaired, with adverse impact on their own quality of life (27,73,102). Furthermore, caregiver anxiety and depression is directly related to stroke severity and functional dependence, which tends to be worse in elderly patients (26). Anxiety and depression also appear to be more common in female caregivers.

REFERENCES

1. Adams HP, Bendixen BH, Kappelle LJ, et al. Classification of subtype of acute ischemic stroke. Definitions for use in a multicenter clinical trial. *Stroke.* 1993;24:35–41.
2. Albers GW, Amarenco P, Easton JD, et al. Antithrombotic and thrombolytic therapy for ischemic stroke: the Seventh ACCP Conference on Antithrombotic and Thrombolytic Therapy. *Chest.* 2004;126[Suppl 3]:483S–512S.
3. Albers GW, Bates VE, Clark WM, et al. Intravenous tissue-type plasminogen activator for treatment of acute stroke: the Standard Treatment with Alteplase to Reverse Stroke (STARS) study. *JAMA.* 2000;283:1145–1150.
4. ALLHAT Officers and Coordinators for the ALLHAT Collaborative Research Group. Major outcomes in high-risk hypertensive patients randomized to angiotensin-converting enzyme inhibitor or calcium channel blocker vs diuretic: the Antihypertensive and Lipid-Lowering Treatment to Prevent Heart Attack Trial (ALLHAT). *JAMA.* 2002;288:2981–2997.
5. Amarenco P, Bogousslavsky J, Callahan A 3rd, et al. High-dose atorvastatin after stroke or transient ischemic attack. *N Engl J Med.* 2006;355:549–559.
6. Amarenco P, Labreuche J, Lavallee P, et al. Statins in stroke prevention and carotid atherosclerosis: systematic review and up-to-date meta-analysis. *Stroke.* 2004;35:2902–2909.
7. Antiplatelet Trialists' Collaboration. Collaborative overview of randomised trials of antiplatelet therapy—I. Prevention of death, myocardial infarction, and stroke by prolonged antiplatelet therapy in various categories of patients. *BMJ.* 1994;308:81–106.
8. Antiplatelet Trialists' Collaboration. Secondary prevention of vascular disease by prolonged antiplatelet treatment. *BMJ.* 1988;296:320–331.
9. Aronow WS. Management of the older person with atrial fibrillation. *J Am Geriatr Soc.* 1999;47:740–748.
10. Barba R, Martinez-Espinosa S, Rodriguez-Garcia E, et al. Poststroke dementia: clinical features and risk factors. *Stroke.* 2000;31:1494–1501.
11. Barnett HJ, Taylor DW, Eliasziw M, et al. Benefit of carotid endarterectomy in patients with symptomatic moderate or severe stenosis. North American Symptomatic Carotid Endarterectomy Trial Collaborators. *N Engl J Med.* 1998;339:1415–1425.
12. Barrett-Connor E, Khaw KT. Diabetes mellitus: an independent risk factor for stroke? *Am J Epidemiol.* 1988;128:116–123.
13. Bennett CL, Weinberg PD, Rozenberg-Ben-Dror K, et al. Thrombotic thrombocytopenic purpura associated with ticlopidine. A review of 60 cases. *Ann Intern Med.* 1998;128:541–544.
14. Bhatt DL, Fox KA, Hacke W, et al. Clopidogrel and aspirin versus aspirin alone for the prevention of atherothrombotic events. *N Engl J Med.* 2006;354:1706–1717.
15. Bogousslavsky J, Pierre P. Ischemic stroke in patients under age 45. *Neurol Clin.* 1992;10:113–124.
16. CAPRIE Steering Committee. A randomised, blinded, trial of clopidogrel versus aspirin in patients at risk of ischaemic events (CAPRIE). *Lancet.* 1996;348:1329–1339.
17. Carmichael ST. Cellular and molecular mechanisms of neural repair after stroke: making waves. *Ann Neurol.* 2006;59:735–742.

18. Carmichael ST, Archibeque I, Luke L, et al. Growth-associated gene expression after stroke: evidence for a growth-promoting region in peri-infarct cortex. *Exp Neurol.* 2005;193:291–311.

19. Chen CI, Iguchi Y, Grotta JC, et al. Intravenous TPA for very old stroke patients. *Eur Neurol.* 2005; 54:140–144.

20. Chobanian AV, Bakris GL, Black HR, et al. The Seventh Report of the Joint National Committee on Prevention, Detection, Evaluation, and Treatment of High Blood Pressure: the JNC 7 report. *JAMA.* 2003;289:2560–2571.

21. Cramer SC, Shah R, Juranek J, et al. Activity in the peri-infarct rim in relation to recovery from stroke. *Stroke.* 2006;37:111–115.

22. Dagenais GR, Pogue J, Fox K, et al. Angiotensin-converting-enzyme inhibitors in stable vascular disease without left ventricular systolic dysfunction or heart failure: a combined analysis of three trials. *Lancet.* 2006;368:581–588.

23. Dahlof B, Devereux RB, Kjeldsen SE, et al. Cardiovascular morbidity and mortality in the Losartan Intervention For Endpoint reduction in hypertension study (LIFE): a randomised trial against atenolol. *Lancet.* 2002;359: 995–1003.

24. Dancause N, Barbay S, Frost SB, et al. Extensive cortical rewiring after brain injury. *J Neurosci.* 2005;25:10167–10179.

25. Davis M, Mendelow AD, Perry RH, et al. The effect of age on cerebral oedema, cerebral infarction and neuroprotective potential in experimental occlusive stroke. *Acta Neurochir Suppl (Wien).* 1994;60:282–284.

26. Dennis M, O'Rourke S, Lewis S, et al. A quantitative study of the emotional outcome of people caring for stroke survivors. *Stroke.* 1998;29: 1867–1872.

27. Dennis M, O'Rourke S, Lewis S, et al. Emotional outcomes after stroke: factors associated with poor outcome. *J Neurol Neurosurg Psychiatry.* 2000;68:47–52.

28. Diener HC, Bogousslavsky J, Brass LM, et al. Aspirin and clopidogrel compared with clopidogrel alone after recent ischaemic stroke or transient ischaemic attack in high-risk patients (MATCH): randomised, double-blind, placebo-controlled trial. *Lancet.* 2004;364:331–337.

29. Diener HC, Cunha L, Forbes C, et al. European Stroke Prevention Study. 2. Dipyridamole and acetylsalicylic acid in the secondary prevention of stroke. *J Neurol Sci.* 1996;143:1–13.

30. Engelter ST, Bonati LH, Lyrer PA. Intravenous thrombolysis in stroke patients of > or = 80 versus <80 years of age—a systematic review across cohort studies. *Age Ageing.* 2006;35:572–580.

31. European Carotid Surgery Trialists' Collaborative Group. MRC European Carotid Surgery Trial: interim results for symptomatic patients with severe (70–99%) or with mild (0–29%) carotid stenosis. *Lancet.* 1991;337:1235–1243.

32. Fairhead JF, Rothwell PM. Underinvestigation and undertreatment of carotid disease in elderly patients with transient ischaemic attack and stroke: comparative population based study. *BMJ.* 2006;333:525–527.

33. Ferrer I. Apoptosis: future targets for neuroprotective strategies. *Cerebrovasc Dis.* 2006;21[Suppl 2]:9–20.

34. Fisher CM. Lacunar strokes and infarcts: a review. *Neurology.* 1982;32:871–876.

35. Fure B, Wyller TB, et al. Emotional symptoms in acute ischemic stroke. *Int J Geriatr Psychiatry.* 2006;21:382–387.

36. Gage BF, van Walraven C, Pearce L, et al. Selecting patients with atrial fibrillation for anticoagulation: stroke risk stratification in patients taking aspirin. *Circulation.* 2004;110:2287–2292.

37. Giaquinto S, Buzzelli S, DiFrancesco L, et al. Evaluation of sexual changes after stroke. *J Clin Psychiatry.* 2003;64:302–307.

38. Grimby G, Andren E, Daving Y, et al. Dependence and perceived difficulty in daily activities in community-living stroke survivors 2 years after stroke: a study of instrumental structures. *Stroke.* 1998;29:1843–1849.

39. Grundy SM, Cleeman JI, Merz CN, et al. Implications of recent clinical trials for the National Cholesterol Education Program Adult Treatment Panel III Guidelines. *J Am Coll Cardiol.* 2004;44: 720–732.

40. Hacke W, Kaste M, Fieschi C, et al. Intravenous thrombolysis with recombinant tissue plasminogen activator for acute hemispheric stroke. *JAMA.* 1995;274:1017–1025.

41. Hacke W, Kaste M, Fieschi C, et al. Randomised double-blind placebo-controlled trial of thrombolytic therapy with intravenous alteplase in acute ischaemic stroke (ECASS II). *Lancet.* 1998;352:1245–1251.

42. Hackett ML, Anderson CS. Predictors of depression after stroke: a systematic review of observational studies. *Stroke.* 2005;36:2296–2301.

43. Hackett ML, Yapa C, Parag V, et al. Frequency of depression after stroke: a systematic review of observational studies. *Stroke.* 2005;36:1330–1340.

44. Halkes PH, van Gijn J, Kappelle LJ, et al. Aspirin plus dipyridamole versus aspirin alone after cerebral ischaemia of arterial origin (ESPRIT): randomised controlled trial. *Lancet.* 2006;367: 1665–1673.

45. Hankey GJ, Jamrozik K, Broadhurst RJ, et al. Long-term risk of first recurrent stroke in the

Perth Community Stroke Study. *Stroke.* 1998; 29:2491–2500.

46. Hart RG, Benavente O, McBride R, et al. Antithrombotic therapy to prevent stroke in patients with atrial fibrillation: a meta-analysis. *Ann Intern Med.* 1999;131:492–501.

47. Hart RG, Halperin JL, Pearce LA, et al. Lessons from the Stroke Prevention in Atrial Fibrillation trials. *Ann Intern Med.* 2003;138:831–838.

48. Hass WK, Easton JD, Adams HP, et al. A randomized trial comparing ticlopidine hydrochloride with aspirin for the prevention of stroke in high-risk patients. *N Engl J Med.* 1989;321:501–507.

49. He Z, Crook JE, Meschia JF, et al. Aging blunts ischemic-preconditioning-induced neuroprotection following transient global ischemia in rats. *Curr Neurovasc Res.* 2005;2:365–374.

50. Hirano LA, Bogardus ST Jr, Saluja S, et al. Clinical yield of computed tomography brain scans in older general medical patients. *J Am Geriatr Soc.* 2006; 54:587–592.

51. Hobson RW 2nd, Howard VJ, Roubin GS, et al. Carotid artery stenting is associated with increased complications in octogenarians: 30-day stroke and death rates in the CREST lead-in phase. *J Vasc Surg.* 2004;40:1106–1111.

52. Hossman K-A. Viability thresholds and the penumbra of focal ischemia. *Ann Neurol.* 1994; 36:557–565.

53. Jia H, Damush TM, Qin H, et al. The impact of poststroke depression on healthcare use by veterans with acute stroke. *Stroke.* 2006;37:2796–2801.

54. Johnston KC, Li JY, Lyden PD, et al. Medical and neurological complications of ischemic stroke: experience from the RANTTAS trial. RANTTAS Investigators. *Stroke.* 1998;29:447–453.

55. Johnston SC, Easton JD. Are patients with acutely recovered cerebral ischemia more unstable? *Stroke.* 2003;34:2446–2450.

56. Jorgensen HS, Reith J, Nakayama H, et al. What determines good recovery in patients with the most severe strokes? The Copenhagen Stroke Study. *Stroke.* 1999;30:2008–2012.

57. Kasner SE. Stroke treatment-specific considerations. *Neurol Clin.* 2000;18:399–417.

58. Kato H, Izumiyama M, Izumiyama K, et al. Silent cerebral microbleeds on T2*-weighted MRI: correlation with stroke subtype, stroke recurrence, and leukoaraiosis. *Stroke.* 2002;33:1536–1540.

59. Kauhanen ML, Korpelainen JT, Hiltunen P, et al. Aphasia, depression, and non-verbal cognitive impairment in ischaemic stroke. *Cerebrovasc Dis.* 2000;10:455–461.

60. Kidwell CS, Chalela JA, Saver JL, et al. Comparison of MRI and CT for detection of acute intracerebral hemorrhage. *JAMA.* 2004;292:1823–1830.

61. Kohrmann M, Juttler E, Fiebach JB, et al. MRI versus CT-based thrombolysis treatment within and beyond the 3 h time window after stroke onset: a cohort study. *Lancet Neurol.* 2006;5:661–667.

62. Korpelainen JT, Kauhanen ML, Kemola H, et al. Sexual dysfunction in stroke patients. *Acta Neurol Scand.* 1998;98:400–405.

63. Korpelainen JT, Nieminen P, Myllyla VV. Sexual functioning among stroke patients and their spouses. *Stroke.* 1999;30:715–719.

64. Krieger DW, Demchuk AM, Kasner SE, et al. Early clinical and radiological predictors of fatal brain swelling in ischemic stroke. *Stroke.* 1999; 30:287–292.

65. Lee AG, Brazis PW. Temporal arteritis: a clinical approach. *J Am Geriatr Soc.* 1999;47:1364–1370.

66. Liebeskind DS. Collateral circulation. *Stroke.* 2003;34:2279–2284.

67. Liebeskind DS, Kasner SE. Neuroprotection for ischaemic stroke: an unattainable goal? *CNS Drugs.* 2001;15:165–174.

68. Lipton SA, Rosenberg PA. Excitatory amino acids as a final common pathway for neurologic disorders. *N Engl J Med.* 1994;330:613–622.

69. Madden KP, Karanjia PN, Adams HP, et al. Accuracy of initial stroke subtype diagnosis in the TOAST study. *Neurology.* 1995;45:1975–1979.

70. Mas JL, Chatellier G, Beyssen B, et al. Endarterectomy versus stenting in patients with symptomatic severe carotid stenosis. *N Engl J Med.* 2006;355: 1660–1671.

71. Mazlumzadeh M, Hunder GG, Easley KA, et al. Treatment of giant cell arteritis using induction therapy with high-dose glucocorticoids: a double-blind, placebo-controlled, randomized prospective clinical trial. *Arthritis Rheum.* 2006;54:3310–3318.

72. McCrory DC, Matchar DB, Samsa G, et al. Physician attitudes about anticoagulation for nonvalvular atrial fibrillation in the elderly. *Arch Intern Med.* 1995;155:277–281.

73. McCullagh E, Brigstocke G, Donaldson N, et al. Determinants of caregiving burden and quality of life in caregivers of stroke patients. *Stroke.* 2005;36:2181–2186.

74. McNamara RL, Lima JA, Whelton PK, et al. Echocardiographic identification of cardiovascular sources of emboli to guide clinical management of stroke: a cost-effectiveness analysis. *Ann Intern Med.* 1997;127:775–787.

75. Mooradian AD, Haas MJ, Chehade JM, et al. Age-related changes in rat cerebral occludin and zonula occludens-1 (ZO-1). *Mech Ageing Dev.* 2003; 124:143–146.

76. Mouradian MS, Senthilselvan A, Jickling G, et al. Intravenous rt-PA for acute stroke: comparing its effectiveness in younger and older patients. *J Neurol Neurosurg Psychiatry.* 2005;76: 1234–1237.

77. Nakayama H, Jorgensen HS, Raaschou HO, et al. The influence of age on stroke outcome. The Copenhagen Stroke Study. *Stroke.* 1994;25: 808–813.

78. National Institute of Neurological Disorders and Stroke rt–PA Stroke Study Group. Intracerebral hemorrhage after intravenous t-PA therapy for ischemic stroke. *Stroke.* 1997; 28:2109–2118.

79. National Institute of Neurological Disorders and Stroke rt-PA Stroke Study Group. Tissue plasminogen activator for acute ischemic stroke. *N Engl J Med.* 1995;333:1581–1587.

80. North American Symptomatic Carotid Endarterectomy Trial Collaborators. Beneficial effect of carotid endarterectomy in symptomatic patients with high-grade carotid stenosis. *N Engl J Med.* 1991;325:445–453.

81. Olney J, Labruyere J, Wang G, et al. NMDA antagonist neurotoxicity: mechanism and prevention. *Science.* 1991;254:1515–1518.

82. Petty GW, Khandheria BK, Meissner I, et al. Population-based study of the relationship between atherosclerotic aortic debris and cerebrovascular ischemic events. *Mayo Clin Proc.* 2006;81:609–614.

83. PROGRESS Collaborative Group. Randomised trial of a perindopril-based blood-pressure-lowering regimen among 6,105 individuals with previous stroke or transient ischaemic attack. *Lancet.* 2001;358:1033–1041.

84. Reith J, Jorgensen HS, Pedersen PM, et al. Body temperature in acute stroke: relation to stroke severity, infarct size, mortality, and outcome. *Lancet.* 1996;347:422–425.

85. Ringleb PA, Allenberg J, Bruckmann H, et al. 30 day results from the SPACE trial of stent-protected angioplasty versus carotid endarterectomy in symptomatic patients: a randomised non-inferiority trial. *Lancet.* 2006;368:1239–1247.

86. Rosenson RS. Biological basis for statin therapy in stroke prevention. *Curr Opin Neurol.* 2000; 13:57–62.

87. Rothwell PM, Buchan A, Johnston SC. Recent advances in management of transient ischaemic attacks and minor ischaemic strokes. *Lancet Neurol.* 2006;5:323–331.

88. Rothwell PM, Eliasziw M, Gutnikov SA, et al. Endarterectomy for symptomatic carotid stenosis in relation to clinical subgroups and timing of surgery. *Lancet.* 2004;363:915–924.

89. Salvarani C, Cantini F, Boiardi L, et al. Polymyalgia rheumatica and giant-cell arteritis. *N Engl J Med.* 2002;347:261–271.

90. Schaller BJ, Graf R. Influence of age on stroke and preconditioning-induced ischemic tolerance in the brain. *Exp Neurol.* 2007;205:9–19.

91. Schlegel D, Kolb SJ, Luciano JM, et al. Utility of the NIH Stroke Scale as a predictor of hospital disposition. *Stroke.* 2003;34:134–137.

92. SHEP Cooperative Research Group. Prevention of stroke by antihypertensive drug treatment in older persons with isolated systolic hypertension. Final results of the Systolic Hypertension in the Elderly Program (SHEP). *JAMA.* 1991; 265:3255–3264.

93. Shinohara Y, Takagi S, Kobatake K. Effect of aging on CBF and autoregulation in normal subjects and CVD patients. *Monogr Neural Sci.* 1984;11:204–209.

94. Singer DE, Albers GW, Dalen JE, et al. Antithrombotic therapy in atrial fibrillation: the Seventh ACCP Conference on Antithrombotic and Thrombolytic Therapy. *Chest.* 2004;126 [Suppl 3]:429S–456S.

95. Smith WS, Sung G, Starkman S, et al. Safety and efficacy of mechanical embolectomy in acute ischemic stroke: results of the MERCI trial. *Stroke.* 2005;36:1432–1438.

96. Sorescu D, Turk RJ, Cain M, et al. Clinical and transthoracic echocardiographic predictors of abnormal transesophageal findings in patients with suspected cardiac source of embolism. *Am J Med Sci.* 2003;326:31–34.

97. Stroke Prevention in Atrial Fibrillation III Investigators. Adjusted-dose warfarin versus low-intensity, fixed-dose warfarin plus aspirin for high-risk patients with atrial fibrillation: Stroke Prevention in Atrial Fibrillation III randomised clinical trial. *Lancet.* 1996;348:633–638.

98. Stroke Prevention in Atrial Fibrillation Writing Committee. Warfarin versus aspirin for prevention of thromboembolism in atrial fibrillation: Stroke Prevention in Atrial Fibrillation II Study. *Lancet.* 1994;343:687–691.

99. Tanne D, Gorman MJ, Bates VE, et al. Intravenous tissue plasminogen activator for acute ischemic stroke in patients aged 80 years and older: the tPA stroke survey experience. *Stroke.* 2000;31:370–375.

100. Teso D, Edwards RE, Frattini JC, et al. Safety of carotid endarterectomy in 2,443 elderly patients: lessons from nonagenarians—are we pushing the limit? *J Am Coll Surg.* 2005;200:734–741.

101. Thom T, Haase N, Rosamond W, et al. Heart disease and stroke statistics—2006 update: a report from the American Heart Association Statistics Committee and Stroke Statistics Subcommittee. *Circulation.* 2006;113:e85–e151.

102. van Exel NJ, Koopmanschap MA, van den Berg B, et al. Burden of informal caregiving for stroke patients. Identification of caregivers at risk of adverse health effects. *Cerebrovasc Dis.* 2005;19:11–17.

103. Wang TJ, Massaro JM, Levy D, et al. A risk score for predicting stroke or death in individuals with

new-onset atrial fibrillation in the community: the Framingham Heart Study. *JAMA*. 2003;290: 1049–1056.

104. Weatherall M. A randomized controlled trial of the Geriatric Depression Scale in an inpatient ward for older adults. *Clin Rehabil*. 2000;14: 186–191.

105. Williams LS, Ghose SS, Swindle RW. Depression and other mental health diagnoses increase mortality risk after ischemic stroke. *Am J Psychiatry*. 2004;161:1090–1095.

106. Wolf PA, D'Agostino RB. Epidemiology of stroke. In: Barnett HJM, Mohr JP, Stein BM, et al., eds. *Stroke: pathophysiology, diagnosis, and management*. New York: Churchill Livingstone; 1998:3–28.

107. Wozniak MA, Kittner SJ, Price TR, et al. Stroke location is not associated with return to work after first ischemic stroke. *Stroke*. 1999;30:2568–2573.

108. Yadav JS, Wholey MH, Kuntz RE, et al. Protected carotid-artery stenting versus endarterectomy in high-risk patients. *N Engl J Med*. 2004;351: 1493–1501.

109. Yusuf S, Sleight P, Pogue J, et al. Effects of an angiotensin-converting-enzyme inhibitor, ramipril, on cardiovascular events in high-risk patients. The Heart Outcomes Prevention Evaluation Study Investigators. *N Engl J Med*. 2000;342:145–153.

SUGGESTED READINGS

Alberts MJ, Hademenos G, Latchaw RE, et al. Recommendations for the establishment of primary stroke centers. Brain Attack Coalition. *JAMA*. 2000;283:3102–3109.

Amarenco P, Bogousslavsky J, et al. High-dose atorvastatin after stroke or transient ischemic attack. *N Engl J Med*. 2006;355:549–559.

Chobanian AV, Bakris GL, et al. The Seventh Report of the Joint National Committee on Prevention, Detection, Evaluation, and Treatment of High Blood Pressure: the JNC 7 report. *JAMA*. 2003;289:2560–2571.

Fairhead JF, Rothwell PM. Underinvestigation and undertreatment of carotid disease in elderly patients with transient ischaemic attack and stroke: comparative population based study. *BMJ*. 2006;333:525–527.

Hart RG, Halperin JL, et al. Lessons from the Stroke Prevention in Atrial Fibrillation trials. *Ann Intern Med*. 2003;138:831–838.

Hobson RW 2nd, Howard VJ, et al. Carotid artery stenting is associated with increased complications in octogenarians: 30-day stroke and death rates in the CREST lead-in phase. *J Vasc Surg*. 2004;40: 1106–1111.

SHEP Cooperative Research Group. Prevention of stroke by antihypertensive drug treatment in older persons with isolated systolic hypertension. Final results of the Systolic Hypertension in the Elderly Program (SHEP). *JAMA*. 1991;265:3255–3264.

WEBSITES OF NATIONAL SUPPORT GROUPS

National Stroke Association: http://www.stroke.org/
American Stroke Association (A Division of American Heart Association): http://www.strokeassociation.org/
The Stroke Network: http://www.strokenetwork.org/

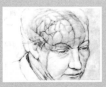

CHAPTER 18

Cognitive Effects of Stroke and Hemorrhage

Henry J. Riordan and Laura A. Flashman

RELATIONSHIP BETWEEN STROKE AND COGNITION

Because the incidence of stroke increases sharply with age, doubling every decade after the age of 55 years, the cognitive and behavioral sequelae of stroke and hemorrhage will undoubtedly become one of the most challenging illnesses that our society must face as this segment of the population grows. Efforts to describe the relationship between cerebrovascular lesions and cognition have guided our understanding of brain-behavior relationships and broader neuropsychological principles with ever mounting evidence of various discrete neurobehavioral disorders following stroke and hemorrhage.

In general, cerebrovascular lesions, including those caused by stroke and hemorrhage, can have three distinct effects on cognition and behavior: a loss of function, a release of function, and a disorganization of function. The most obvious and direct effect of cerebral lesions is a loss of function in which the patient can no longer perform a specific cognitive or behavioral task or set of tasks. A release of function is said to occur when a new behavior appears or the frequency of a behavior is drastically increased subsequent to a brain lesion. When bits or pieces of behavior still occur, but not in the correct order, or when behaviors occur at the wrong time and place, a disorganization of function is said to have occurred.

A number of behavioral changes can be fairly transient following brain damage secondary to stroke or hemorrhage, with a recovery of function taking place over the course of days, weeks, or even years. To date, the processes involved in this recovery are poorly understood, and our understanding is complicated by the variability of recovery across individuals as well as the uncertain onset of cognitive symptoms. It has often been noted that a portion of the cognitive decline recognized following a stroke may have actually been the result of pre-existing cognitive deficits. Pohjasvaara et al. (84) reported that the frequency of prestroke cognitive decline, including dementia, is approximately 9%, with older age, poorer education, and history of prior stroke being the most frequently cited factors. More recent supportive data from the Baltimore Longitudinal Study of Aging (39) suggests that, when cognitive impairment did not exist prior to onset of a stroke, there was no increase in the risk for dementia and that both vascular and Alzheimer pathology can lead to prestroke impairment. Therefore, the possibility of two or more underlying disease processes should be considered in both the diagnosis and treatment of cognitive dysfunction thought to be caused by stroke and hemorrhage.

NEUROBEHAVIORAL CONSEQUENCES OF CEREBRAL VASCULAR LESIONS

Specific cognitive deficits are often viewed as being the direct result of an isolated lesion; however, in clinical practice, rarely do patients present with a cognitive deficit that is caused by an isolated lesion confined to a single functional cerebral region. Additionally, damage to any number of cerebral regions can result in very similar or related patterns of cognitive deficits or even whole constellations of behavioral deficits. To complicate matters even more, very few of the standardized neuropsychological tests commonly used are specifically designed to assess unitary cognitive functions because almost all cognitive tasks rely on a complex networking among various functional cerebral areas. For instance, many neuropsychological tests, even tests that require only a verbal response, involve the visual modality and assume some minimal levels of arousal, attention, and organizational abilities, as well as the ability to make a behavioral response. Thus, few, if any, neuropsychological tests have been devised to elicit a specific functional deficit in a single cognitive domain such as memory, attention, or executive functioning. Therefore, the information presented below is meant to serve as a general guide to some of the more common, if not more interesting, deficits in cognitive and behavioral functioning following stroke and hemorrhage.

Although the extent of lesion is certainly important in the assessment of cognitive dysfunction following stroke, some appreciation of the basic tenants of the localization theory of brain function is also essential. For a much more comprehensive review of the behavioral geography of the human brain, as well as the neurobehavioral consequences of stroke and hemorrhage, please see Lezak (66) or Robinson (88).

COGNITIVE EFFECTS OF CORTICAL LESIONS

Occlusion of the carotid arteries can result in infarction of the border zones between the anterior and middle or middle and posterior cerebral arteries. Clinical presentation in these instances includes primarily cortical deficits, including transcortical aphasia with preserved repetition, visuospatial deficits, and sensorimotor changes involving the proximal arm and leg (100). Occlusion of the anterior, middle, or posterior cerebral artery produces hemisphere-specific deficits related to the role of the affected tissue in the irrigated territory of the artery. Characteristic left hemisphere deficits include aphasia, apraxia, alexia, agraphia, and acalculia, whereas more representative right hemisphere deficits include visuospatial deficits, amusia, and impaired prosody.

FRONTAL CORTEX

Comprising nearly one third of the mass of the cerebral hemispheres, the frontal lobes are the largest of the lobes of the brain and the most recently developed portion of the cerebrum. The frontal lobe has been called the "executor," maintaining control over all other cognitive processes. Although not directly responsible for many overt behaviors, the frontal lobes play an executive role in the planning and performance of many behaviors. Additionally, damage to the prefrontal cortex can result in deficits in self-awareness that, in turn, can affect almost all areas of cognitive function. Damage to selective areas in the frontal lobe can interfere with motor or language functioning as well as relatively higher order cognitive processes such as abstract reasoning, planning, selective attention, complex problem solving, concept formation, and cognitive flexibility (108).

The frontal lobes play an important role in nearly all cognitive processes. Language-mediated tasks tend to be under control of the dominant, usually left, hemisphere, and nonverbal tasks are usually associated with the nondominant hemisphere. Thus, damage to the left frontal lobe can produce deficits in verbal behavior, including naming and fluency, whereas damage to the right frontal lobe can result in deficits in figural or design fluency (25,55). However, verbal fluency deficits, albeit less severe, also have been noted following right frontal lobe lesions, suggesting that the degree of laterality varies among

individuals. Some of the more commonly seen neurobehavioral disorders resulting from damage to the prefrontal cortex include Broca's aphasia, memory deficits, attentional deficits, and volitional deficits (60,66).

Broca's Aphasia

Damage to the opercular and triangular portions of the inferior frontal gyrus (also known as Brodmann area 44) causes a constellation of deficits in expressive language commonly referred to as Broca's aphasia (41). Broca's aphasia is also known as expressive, nonfluent, or motor aphasia, suggesting that most of the deficits are in expressive rather than receptive language processing. In fact, patients with Broca's aphasia tend to have relatively good language comprehension skills. Patients who have a lesion of this area tend to produce very few words orally or in written form, exhibit extreme difficulty in word production, have impaired repetition and naming abilities, tend to leave out articles and qualifiers, and speak and write in a manner best described as "telegraphic."

Memory Deficits

Patients with prefrontal lobe lesions tend to have difficulty with the initial acquisition of new information because of their poor attention and organizational skills. They also tend to make numerous errors of perseveration and commission (e.g., false-positive errors on cued memory recall tasks) because they have difficulty inhibiting inappropriate responses. Working memory, which refers to temporarily holding a limited amount of information in mind for a few seconds while manipulating it, also depends on intact frontal lobe functioning (40). Impairments in working memory can result in diminished declarative memory performance by limiting the amount of material that is acquired initially. Although the frontal cortex plays a role in various memory processes, deficits in retention of new information are more likely to be seen following a lesion of the temporal lobes (see below).

Attentional Deficits

The prefrontal cortex is intrinsically involved in the capacity to focus or shift attention as required by changing task demands (73,74). Damage to the prefrontal cortex can result in numerous types of attentional deficits. For example, patients may be slow to react to stimuli and have attentional difficulties that are characterized by an inability to maintain or sustain focus, an inability to shift mental sets, and poor cognitive flexibility. Patients with prefrontal lesions can be described as having a "rigid" approach to problem solving in general and are often unable to benefit from contextual cues or even direct instructional sets that direct them to the correct solution. Once again, their cognitive style can be characterized by numerous errors of perseveration, a deficit that may be seen across a variety of mental tasks and settings. An extreme example of this is when a patient is unable to stop making the same erroneous perseverative responses even though he or she can accurately state a correct answer.

Related to this "rigid" cognitive style is an inability to overcome literal associations. These patients tend to view events and interactions at face value and are unable to detect more subtle nuances and, therefore, the genuine meaning of events. This concrete approach also results in an inability to generate or appropriately use abstract notions, such as symbols, proverbs, and metaphors.

Volitional Deficits

Finally, many patients with prefrontal lesions tend to have difficulties in both initiating and stopping behavior, a deficit that can dramatically affect cognitive functioning. Difficulties in initiation can be related to apathy, poor spontaneity, and productivity, whereas difficulties in stopping a behavior may be more closely related to poor impulse control or an inability to benefit from feedback suggesting the cessation of a behavior is warranted; difficulties in stopping behavior can also be caused by an inability to overcome perseverative responses. This type of disinhibition is often seen following lesions of the orbitofrontal circuitry, whereas symptoms such as spontaneity and apathy are more likely to follow injury to the anterior cingulate circuitry (25).

TEMPORAL CORTEX

Because of the complex organization and the numerous and diverse tasks mediated by the temporal cortex, both the anatomic boundaries and the functional specialization of the temporal lobes are relatively less well defined than other lobes of the brain (108). The temporal cortex serves various functions related to the primary perception of audition, olfaction, and visual information and serves to integrate all aspects of our senses into a unified and meaningful experience. The temporal cortex also plays a critical role in memory and is intrinsically tied to the limbic system. Thus, the temporal lobe plays a role in associating emotional and motivational aspects of information to various sensory experiences and helps form impressions and knowledge of the world. Although numerous cognitive deficits can arise from stroke or hemorrhage of the temporal neocortex and adjacent medial temporal lobe structures, some of the more commonly observed and interesting neurobehavioral disorders include those of auditory perception, visual perception, and memory.

AUDITORY PERCEPTUAL DEFICITS

One of the most notable, if not the most disabling, disorders of auditory perception is referred to as Wernicke's aphasia (also known as sensory, fluent, or jargon aphasia), which can result from a lesion of the left temporal association cortex (Brodmann area 22). In this disorder, patients typically have very poor language comprehension but relatively intact speech production abilities (41). This pattern of preserved language production but impaired comprehension is at direct odds with Broca's aphasia, in that patients with Wernicke-type aphasia can be characterized as being hyperverbal despite the fact that their speech itself is nonsensical. In fact, these patients may even show signs of an anosognosia or inability to recognize their impaired speech and, therefore, can have difficulties benefiting from feedback in speech therapy. Interestingly, patients with similar lesions of the right temporal cortex may experience similar problems with nonverbal sound recognition and discrimination (71). In some cases, right temporal lesions can result in amusia (i.e., a deficit in music perception where patients are unable to differentiate various musical tones or rhythms) (92).

Visual Perceptual Deficits

Lesions of the temporal cortex can cause deficits in visual discrimination, visual word recognition, pattern recognition, and even object recognition. These visual perceptual deficits can occur despite relatively normal performance on standard visual-spatial tasks. For example, patients with right temporal lobe lesions may have difficulty recognizing objects from incomplete or partially drawn figures, may fail to recognize salient aspects of pictures, and may have relatively poor spatial reasoning abilities (108).

Material-Specific Memory Deficits

Damage to the temporal cortex and medial temporal structures have long been known to result in material-specific memory deficits (32,83). Lesions of the left temporal lobe can result in impairment in the ability to encode and recall a list of aurally presented words, numbers, or letters; semantic memory; and verbal paired-associate learning (108). Patients with left temporal lobe lesions can have difficulty recalling words, which can also adversely affect fluent speech production. When severe, this inability is referred to as anomia. Patients with this disorder can have impaired comprehension of complex information and, therefore, find it difficult to learn new verbal material.

Patients with right temporal lobe lesions are more likely to have memory difficulties involving visual-spatial stimuli such as faces, nonverbalizable designs, and figures. They can also have difficulty with maze learning and any stimuli or task that does not readily lend itself to verbal tagging or labeling. Deficits in material-specific memory caused by unilateral temporal lobe lesions tend to produce relatively mild cognitive dysfunction that may only be noticeable with neuropsychological testing. However, bilateral temporal lobe lesions can result in a global amnesia (i.e., a severe and pervasive deficit in forming new conscious memories for all types of material). Although amnesia has been noted after unilateral temporal lobe lesions (typically of the dominant hemisphere), the most likely cause of an amnestic stroke is bilateral infarction of the posterior cerebral arteries affecting inferomedial structures of the temporal lobe, including the hippocampus and amygdala. This type of bilateral infarction is not exceptional because both posterior cerebral arteries arise from a single basilar artery (108).

PARIETAL CORTEX

Situated between the frontal, temporal, and occipital lobes, the parietal lobe shares many of the functional features of the other lobes. In fact, it could be argued that lesions of the parietal lobes are associated with a greater variety of cognitive and behavioral disorders than any other lobe of the brain. However, unlike other cerebral regions, the cognitive deficits associated with parietal lesions often require specialized neuropsychological and behavioral techniques to be recognized. Some of the more commonly seen neurobehavioral disorders following a stroke or hemorrhage of the parietal lobe include agraphia or acalculia, disorders of spatial orientation, alexia, constructional apraxia, and anosognosia. When lesions are located within the angular gyrus, which is the inferior lobule of the dominant parietal lobe (Brodmann area 39), a constellation of deficits characterized by right-left disorientation, dysgraphia, acalculia, and finger agnosia often occurs and is known as Gerstmann syndrome.

Agraphia

Agraphia, an inability to write, has been associated with lesions in the angular gyrus itself or connections to this region within the left parietal lobe. Less commonly, these deficits can be seen following right hemisphere lesions as well. There are several types of agraphia, but the particular type of agraphia seen following posterior dominant hemisphere lesions tends to be characterized by well-formed letters joined together but with incorrect spellings, abnormal word order, and frequent omissions (11). This is in contrast to the more anterior type of agraphia characterized by large, crude, scrawling output that is poorly constructed and agrammatic. Isolated agraphia (not in the context of aphasia), which can also be seen following lesions of the angular gyrus, can co-occur with acalculia.

Acalculia

Acalculia refers to the inability to perform certain mathematical operations. It can be seen following damage of the left parietal lobe and often co-occurs with agraphia. Several types of agraphia and acalculia

reflect a disruption of more complicated higher order cognitive processes. One form of acalculia, in which patients cannot comprehend or write numbers correctly or even substitute one number for another, can be seen after damage to the dominant hemisphere language areas. Damage to the nondominant parietal-occipital junction can result in a visual-spatial discrimination problem that causes an acalculia that is characterized by poor placement of numbers in space such that the numbers are not aligned properly to allow for complex calculations. In this case, patients can understand numbers, symbols, and computation signs and may even be able to successfully complete most mathematical operations.

Spatial Neglect and Disorders of Spatial Orientation

Disorders of spatial orientation, including contralateral neglect, are seen after right parietal lesions. Contralateral neglect involves the neglect of visual, tactile, and auditory stimulation from the side of the body or hemifield that is contralateral to the site of the lesion. Allegri (3) reported that left-sided neglect after right hemisphere lesions is more common (31% to 46%) than right-sided neglect following lesions in the left hemisphere (2% to 12%). Thus, although unilateral neglect can be seen following left parietal infarcts, this is relatively rare compared with most patients who present with a left neglect corresponding to right parietal damage. Unilateral neglect has also been observed following frontal and subcortical vascular damage as well. Patients with parietal lesions can also experience route-finding problems and an inability to recognize objects that might ordinarily serve as landmarks (i.e., topographic agnosia). Additionally, patients with left parietal lesions can also present with significant right-left spatial disorientation problems.

A more holistic knowledge about landmarks and direction information is a function referred to as "wayfinding." Wayfinding probably involves multiple neural mechanisms, and the exact neural circuitry involved in disorders of wayfinding is controversial. However, a recent study by van Asselen et al. (105) examined the neuroanatomic correlates of wayfinding in 31 patients with known unilateral stroke locations via magnetic resonance imaging (MRI). These patients were tested in a series of tasks including landmark recognition, landmark ordering, route reversal, and even route drawing. The findings suggested that landmark recognition was impaired by right hippocampal formation damage with a relatively weaker association being seen between landmark ordering and dorsolateral prefrontal cortical damage. Route drawing appeared to be related to right temporal damage, whereas route reversal (or tracing a route from end to beginning) was impacted by several cerebral regions including the right hippocampal formation, the right posterior parietal cortex, the right dorsolateral prefrontal cortex, and the right temporal lobe.

Apraxias

Apraxia can be simply defined as an inability to carry out purposeful movement in the absence of some type of motor disturbance such as a paralysis. Many different types of apraxia occur, with one of the most notable forms being constructional apraxia, or the inability to perform familiar sequences of movements when making or preparing something (108). Interestingly, this deficit is seen when patients can still perform all of the individual actions or steps involved in a particular sequence. For example, a patient may be able to perform all of the individual steps needed to mail a letter (e.g., licking the stamp and sealing the envelope) but is unable to make the proper sequence of movements to actually complete the task of mailing the letter. Constructional disorders characterized by an inability to draw or construct objects or shapes have also been observed following lesions to either hemisphere, with qualitative differences in the process and product of the construction providing valuable clues as to lesion laterality. For example, the drawings of patients with right hemisphere lesions are frequently seen as fragmented and characterized by poor spatial relations. These drawings can also be characterized by poor or faulty orientation. Conversely, patients with left hemisphere lesions may produce better spatial orientation and relations, but their drawing can be overly simple, lack detail, and be especially labored to produce. More recently, it has been suggested that there are actually two different but complementary systems for encoding spatial relations (categorical and coordinate). Therefore, there may actually be two qualitatively different forms of constructional apraxia caused by unilateral lesions (64). This may suggest why some authors, such as Sunderland et al. (102), suggest that disorders of constructional apraxia are very resistant to recovery, whereas other authors, such as Nys et al. (80), have posited that they have the best prognosis.

Anosognosias

Anosognosia can be defined generally as the failure to perceive illness. Numerous types of anosognosias exist. Asomatognosia, or loss of knowledge about the body or about a bodily condition, is a disorder that can be seen following damage to the parietal cortex of either hemisphere, of which many varieties exist. Anosodiaphoria refers to a general indifference to a disorder. An inability to name and localize body parts is known as autotopagnosia. These agnosias all stem from lesions to the left parietal cortex. Patients with right parietal or frontal infarcts have been shown to

have significantly fewer introspective capacities and less concern over their illness than patients with infarcts in other regions, despite similar degrees of cognitive impairment (52).

OCCIPITAL CORTEX

Although small lesions of the visual cortex can often produce defects or "blind spots" in the visual field, these types of lesions are unlikely to affect higher cognitive functioning as related to visual perception and comprehension. However, when other subcortical and associative cortices are involved, several neurobehavioral deficits can result. These neurobehavioral disorders include cerebral blindness, Anton syndrome, and the visual agnosias.

Cerebral Blindness and Anton Syndrome

Occlusion of the posterior cerebral artery resulting in bilateral visual cortex damage can lead to a condition known as cerebral or cortical blindness, a condition characterized by an inability to distinguish forms or patterns despite intact responsiveness to light changes (68). Cerebral blindness may be accompanied by a period of confusion, amnesia, or even unconsciousness. Astonishingly, patients who are cerebrally blind (or more commonly referred to as "cortically blind") can exhibit visually responsive behaviors and be able to detect visual stimuli in the blind field without the experience of vision (85), a phenomenon called "blindsight." Hartmann et al. (48) described a patient with cerebral blindness resulting from bioccipital and left parietal lesions who, although denying visual perception, correctly named objects, colors, and famous faces; recognized facial emotions; and read various types of single words with greater than 50% accuracy when they were presented in the upper right visual field. When questioned about his apparent visual abilities, the patient continued to deny visual perceptual awareness, typically stating, "I feel it." The authors suggest that this type of denial of visual perception is best explained as a disconnection of the parietal lobe attention system from regions controlling visual perception. In direct opposition to "blindsight," patients with Anton syndrome fail to appreciate the fact that they are blind and make elaborate confabulations and rationalizations as to their impaired performance. Anton syndrome typically stems from lesions of the bilateral occipital lobe and most likely is caused by the disruption of corticothalamic connections (27).

Visual Agnosias

Visual agnosias are characterized by defective visual perception or distortion of visual stimuli, despite normal visual input, and can be seen following infarction of the visual association areas (10). For example, visual object agnosia is characterized by intact visual perception of

Table 18-1. *Common Neurobehavioral Disorders Associated with Cortical Vascular Lesions*

	Right Hemisphere	Left Hemisphere[a]	Bilateral Hemisphere
Frontal lobe	Figural fluency	Broca's aphasia (area 44)	Working memory
		Verbal fluency	Cognitive flexibility
Temporal Lobe	Visual discrimination	Wernicke's aphasia (area 22)	Amnesia
	Visual reasoning and	Verbal reasoning and	
	memory	memory	
	Amusia	Dysnomia	
Parietal Lobe	Unilateral (left) neglect	Agraphia/acalculia	
	Constructional apraxia	Right-left confusion	
	Anosognosia	Topographic agnosia	
	Anosodiaphoria	Autotopagnosia	
Occipital Lobe	Visual object agnosia	Simultagnosia	Cerebral blindness
	Prosopagnosia	Color anomia	Anton syndrome
	Color agnosia		
	Achromatopsia		

[a]Assumes left hemisphere dominance.

the visual stimulus but an inability to recognize the object. Patients with this neurobehavioral disorder can often draw the object or copy a picture of it, confirming intact visual perceptual abilities. This type of agnosia can be seen after lesions of the dominant occipital lobe (108). Simultagnosia (Balint syndrome) is characterized by an inability to perceive more than one aspect of a stimulus at one time, despite the ability to identify and remember single aspects of features of an object. This neurobehavioral deficit may be partially caused by an inability to shift attentional focus and direct gaze (10). Another more rare type of visual agnosia is characterized by an inability to recognize familiar faces. This disorder is referred to as prosopagnosia, and in severe cases, some patients do not even recognize their own reflection in the mirror. The neuroanatomic underpinnings of this disorder are still in question; however, prosopagnosia has been associated with bilateral, left, and right hemisphere lesions of both the parietal and occipital lobe (67). Some suggestion exists for a relatively greater frequency of bilateral and nondominant lesions to a greater degree (33), as well as for a relatively greater degree of dysfunction seen following right versus left hemisphere lesions (66). Finally, another type of visual agnosia for colors has also been known to follow occipital lobe lesions. This type of neurobehavioral disorder can take on various manifestations, including an inability to distinguish color hues (i.e., achromatopsia), an inability to name colors (i.e., color anomia), and an inability to associate particular colors with objects and vice versa (i.e., color agnosia) (60). Table 18-1 summarizes some of the more common neurobehavioral disorders following cortical stroke

and hemorrhage that have been described in more detail earlier. The anatomic localization of some of these disorders is somewhat equivocal, and deficits assigned solely to left hemisphere lesions assume left hemisphere language dominance.

COGNITIVE EFFECTS OF SUBCORTICAL LESIONS

MULTI-INFARCT DEMENTIA

Vascular dementia can be caused by both white matter ischemia and multiple occlusions of blood vessels (a series of small strokes) that result in focal areas of dead tissue. Hachinski et al. (45) introduced the term multi-infarct dementia (MID) and concluded that most infarctions were secondary to disease of the heart and of extracranial blood vessels. Clinical dementia can be caused by a multi-infarct state, but the neuropathology is often complicated by the presence of more than one disease process. Histopathologic studies have variously concluded that vascular factors are involved in 10% to 40% of cases (93). The prevalence of vascular dementia is difficult to establish because the criteria for diagnosis are inexact, and when diagnosing vascular dementia, it is essential to rule out presence of Alzheimer's disease.

Patients may also have vascular cognitive deficits but not frank dementia. The pattern of neuropsychological deficits in patients who have vascular cognitive impairment-no dementia (CIND) was characterized by Nyenhuis et al. (78) by comparing cognitive and behavioral performance of 41 poststroke CIND patients with that of 62 poststroke patients with no cognitive impairment. Multivariate logic regression models suggested that immediate recall and psychomotor performance predicted group inclusion best. However, since these deficits are also very apparent in vascular dementia, it may be that vascular CIND lies on a continuum between normal cognitive function and vascular dementia.

CEREBRAL AUTOSOMAL DOMINANT ARTERIOPATHY WITH SUBCORTICAL INFARCTS AND LEUKOENCEPHALOPATHY

Cerebral autosomal dominant arteriopathy with subcortical infarcts and leukoencephalopathy (CADASIL) is a model of pure vascular dementia, but its cognitive profile has not been fully described. The most recent analysis was performed by Buffon et al. (17), who assessed 42 consecutive CADASIL patients (ages 35 to 73) across multiple cognitive domains and compared patients with and without dementia. Younger patients presented with disorders in attention (69%), memory (70%), and executive functioning (100%). In contrast, visual-spatial abilities deteriorated with age, mostly after age 60. Although a quarter of the patients had dementia (noted by a relative preservation of encoding in episodic memory), no association was noted with the number of ischemic attacks.

LACUNAR STROKES

Small infarcts deep in the cerebral hemispheres and in the brainstem caused by occlusion of perforating end arteries originating in the circle of Willis and of the proximal middle, posterior cerebral, and basilar arteries are often described as lacunae (36). The most commonly encountered lacunar syndrome is pure motor hemiplegia, which affects the face, arm, and leg as a result of infarction in the internal capsule or in the basis pontis (93). By definition, aphasia, visuospatial neglect, agnosia, apraxia, and visual field defects do not occur in lacunar syndromes but can be present as a result of larger striatocapsular infarcts, which probably have a different cause.

A lacunar state refers to the occurrence of multiple lacunes, which usually results in both motoric and intellectual dysfunction. Most patients who present with a lacunar state describe a series of discrete cognitive or behavioral episodes, each representing a new vascular event that involves the appearance of new symptoms. However, in up to one third of patients with demonstrable lacunar infarctions, the deterioration appears gradual, and the syndrome is often mistaken for a degenerative process (109). The clinical presentation of multiple lacunar infarctions typically involves prominent motor dysfunction with more limited somatosensory and visual impairment. Pyramidal signs are common and include spasticity, gait abnormalities, hyperreflexia, and extensor plantar response.

Pseudobulbar palsy with dysarthria, dysphagia, facial paresis, hyperreflexive gag response, and emotional incontinence can also occur (53). Extrapyramidal symptoms are often intermixed with the upper motor neuron signs.

SUBCORTICAL ISCHEMIC VASCULAR DISEASE

Subcortical ischemic vascular disease (SIVD) is characterized by extensive white matter lesions and multiple lacunes and up until recently has not had a well-characterized pattern of cognitive deficits. Recently, Jokinen et al. (54) assessed 323 consecutive patients with ischemic stroke aged 55 to 85 years with a cognitive battery. Eighty-five patients who met SIVD criteria via MRI were compared with the 238 patients who did not meet SIVD criteria, as well as with 38 healthy controls. They reported that the SIVD group performed more poorly than the healthy control patients on all cognitive domains and that, in comparison to the stroke patients, the SIVD patients exhibited poorer performance on measures of executive functioning and delayed memory recall (with the latter being more related to degree of temporal lobe atrophy). Thus, executive function appears to be the hallmark feature of this poorly characterized subtype of vascular cognitive impairment.

SINGLE INFARCTIONS

Small subcortical infarctions can result in disruption of multiple cognitive domains, depending on their location. Circumscribed damage to the thalamus, caudate nucleus, or globus pallidus can produce multifaceted cognitive deficits because of disruption of specific subcortical-cortical circuits. The caudate nucleus, globus pallidus, and thalamus are neuroanatomically connected to the dorsolateral prefrontal cortex. Damage to any part of this circuit results in deficits, primarily in executive functions and motor programming. The exact nature of the behavioral changes depends on which structure in the circuit is damaged. Single infarctions to the caudate or pallidal nuclei are rare in humans, and therefore, little is known about them. In contrast, many studies have examined the effects of thalamic lesions on neuropsychological functioning.

THALAMIC STROKE

Neuropsychological syndromes resulting from thalamic infarctions vary widely and are largely determined by the specific thalamic nuclei involved. The thalamus contains at least three principal types of cortical projection nuclei (specific sensory, nonspecific, and association), as well as nuclei that project to the limbic system and frontal lobes (1,70,75). Despite the wide range of neurobehavioral features associated with thalamic infarct, three cardinal clinical features of thalamic hemorrhage have been generally reported

(37). In the dominant hemisphere, these are greater sensory than motor loss, oculomotor impairments (particularly abnormalities of vertical gaze with the eyes deviated downward and inward), and moderate dysphasia. Transcortical sensory aphasias and memory impairment can also occur. Given the degree of thalamic-cortical interconnectivity (with almost the entire neocortex and striatum receiving fibers from the thalamus), it is not surprising that many of the neurobehavioral disorders following thalamic lesions are qualitatively similar in nature to some of the neurobehavioral deficits following cortical lesions. Some of the more common of these disorders, including disorders of arousal and attention, executive functioning, language, and memory, are described in the following sections.

Disorders of Arousal and Attention

Disorders of arousal, including loss of consciousness, are commonly observed following thalamic hemorrhage. Although this is seen most commonly after bilateral paramedian thalamic infarction, coma and extreme disturbances of consciousness have been known to occur with unilateral lesions as well (38,42,101). In patients who display an initial disturbance of consciousness, generally, a gradual improvement is seen over time marked by considerable fluctuations in arousal level (8,44,58). As recovery proceeds, patients with thalamic hemorrhage may be fully alert but slow to respond, apathetic, and susceptible to hypersomnolence if not stimulated (58,106). It is believed that the hypersomnolence noted in these patients results from local pressure on the reticular activating system of the rostral brainstem (18,42,58). Individuals with thalamic lesions can have other attentional problems that can be easily seen when they are trying to complete less structured tasks [e.g., digit span may be intact, but maze learning is impaired (101)].

Disorders of Executive Functioning

Patients with lesions of the thalamus often demonstrate behavioral changes consistent with those previously described following lesions to the frontal lobes or to the frontal-limbic circuitry (14,28,98,99). For example, confabulation and reduplicative paramnesia can be present (16,101,103). Various alterations in mood have been described, including apathy, akinesia, lack of concern, and euphoria (58,72,96). Other executive characteristics that have been reported include perseveration, increased susceptibility to interference, problems sequencing information, and inability to maintain sustained interest in a topic or task.

Disorders of Language

Language disorders occur almost universally after damage to the left thalamus (9,57), although controversy exists about the necessary lesion within the thalamus. Most studies suggest that involvement of the pulvinar (23) or the ventrolateral nucleus (30,42) is necessary. The type of language disturbance following thalamic damage can be best described as multifarious and resulting from a disruption of cortical-subcortical integration (24).

Language disturbances following thalamic infarct can be attributable to multiple dysfunctions, including alterations in alerting, arousal, and monitoring. However, in general, mutism may occur initially, followed by poor initiation of speech, with limited output and many pauses. Word list generation can be moderately to severely impaired, and speech can be characterized by diminished volume, impaired prosody, and variable dysarthria. Perseverations, perceptual errors, intrusions, and nonaphasic misnaming have also been observed.

Disorders of Memory

Significant memory dysfunction secondary to thalamic insult is common and is characterized primarily by anterograde memory disturbance (69,111). As with cortical lesions, this memory disturbance appears to be hemisphere specific. Bilateral lesions result in a severe and persistent memory disturbance, whereas unilateral left and right lesions produce verbal and nonverbal memory disturbances, respectively (96,101). In patients with bilateral thalamic damage, a subcortical dementia syndrome also has been reported, with impairment noted in memory, attention, language, and visuospatial ability as well as changes in personality. This syndrome appears to be more consistent with the impairment noted in other "subcortical" dementias, rather than Alzheimer's disease, due to the absence of apraxia, agnosia, or definite aphasia and the presence of slowed information processing speed, inertia, and apathy (26). Unlike other subcortical dementias, however, the dementia syndrome associated with bilateral thalamic insult combines frontal-subcortical dysfunction with a severe memory disorder (101).

CEREBELLAR STROKE

Although it is well established that the cerebellum is essential for the coordination of movement, more recent evidence suggests that the cerebellum is also involved in higher order cognitive functioning (49,91). Studies evaluating patients with damage limited to the cerebellum (either as a result of cerebellar degeneration or cerebellar stroke) indicate neurobehavioral impairment that appears related to the cerebellum itself (7,43,65). Furthermore, recent functional neuroimaging studies have demonstrated cerebellar activation during nonmotor tasks (4,5,35), suggesting that it plays a role in other cognitive functions such as learning and memory, attention, and language.

Cerebellar Cognitive Affective Syndrome

Schmahmann (90) and Schmahmann and Sherman (91) have described a pattern of behavioral and cognitive abnormalities resulting from cerebellar insult, referred to as the cerebellar cognitive affective syndrome (CCAS). The syndrome includes impairment in executive functions that is characterized by perseveration, distractibility or inattention, visual-spatial disturbances, difficulties with language production, and personality changes. Remote episodic and semantic memory is preserved, and new learning is only mildly affected. The net effect of these neurobehavioral disturbances is a general lowering of intellectual functioning, despite the fact that arousal and alertness levels are not affected (91). These core features set this syndrome apart from nonspecific confusional states as well as from other currently accepted notions of dementia. For example, features more typical of cortical dementia (e.g., aphasia, apraxia, and agnosia) are largely absent (91). Dementia also is more often noted in patients with evidence of more widespread central nervous system involvement (i.e., cerebellar signs as well as extrapyramidal and pyramidal tract disorders) than in patients manifesting spinal and cerebellar syndromes exclusively (50).

Behavioral changes related to cerebellar damage have been characterized by personality change, with blunting of affect, disinhibition of behavior or inappropriate behavior, and impairment of a number of executive functions, including planning, impaired ability to shift set, and difficulties with abstract reasoning. Cognitive disturbances associated with lesions of the posterior lobe of the cerebellum and the vermis include other executive abilities [e.g., decreased verbal fluency and impaired working memory; problems with spatial cognition, including visual-spatial organization and memory (15,91); and language deficits including agrammatism, dysprosody, and mild anomia (91,94)].

More recently, Schmahmann (89) has suggested that the cognitive and psychiatric components of CCAS, together with the ataxic motor disability of cerebellar disorders, can be better conceptualized as a "dysmetria of thought." This concept posits that a universal cerebellar transform assists modulation of behavior around a baseline and that the behavior being modulated is determined by the specificity of the anatomic loops within the cerebrocerebellar system. Any damage to the cerebellar component of a distributed neural loop serving sensorimotor, cognitive, and emotional processing disrupts this universal transform. Thus, the universal impairment is characterized by ataxia when the sensorimotor cerebellum is involved and as CCAS when the lesion is in the lateral hemisphere of the posterior cerebellum or in the vermis cerebellum. According to Schmahmann (89), both cognitive and mood disorders can accompany cerebellar impairment or may be their principal clinical presentation, which has implications for both the diagnosis and management of cerebellar dysfunction.

PROGNOSIS, REHABILITATION, AND PHARMACOLOGIC TREATMENT

PROGNOSTIC FACTORS

Improved treatment regimens, coupled with educational efforts designed to reduce the amount of time elapsed between initial stroke symptoms and treatment, have significantly reduced the mortality associated with stroke and hemorrhage. However, this increased survival rate also means that increasingly more patients need a rehabilitation program (95). In response to this, the last decade has seen an increase in research focusing on functional outcomes following stroke and hemorrhage. However, relatively little research has investigated the relationship between cognitive functioning and stroke outcome. This is surprising because cognition and affective functioning are well known to be important contributors to quality of life.

An attempt to discover the clinical factors that predict prognosis of acute cognitive dysfunction following stroke was conducted by Nys et al. (80), who administered two cognitive batteries to 111 stroke survivors and 77 healthy controls (baseline within 3 weeks after stroke and follow-up between 6 and 10 months later). Findings suggested that relatively poorer cognitive recovery was associated with older age, lower pre-existent verbal abilities, lesions in specific lobes (temporal, frontal, and occipital), overall lesion volume, and the presence of diabetes mellitus. This group also noted that the prognosis for higher level visual disturbances in memory and construction was the most encouraging (with better long-term recovery and lower association between acute and long-term domain-specific dysfunction). Cognitive impairment and vascular risk factors also are important predictors of depressive symptoms and quality of life after 6 to 10 months (81).

Other studies support the utility of clearly defining stroke subtypes on admission that are based on cognitive test performance and lesion laterality and suggest that rehabilitation programs can be specifically tailored to meet various stroke subtypes in an effort to maximize functional outcome. In fact, Hajek et al. (46) suggest that rehabilitation outcome could be better predicted if the results of functional assessment were coupled with in-depth cognitive assessment. Therefore, a comprehensive and standardized neuropsychological evaluation of all stroke patients at admission and intermittently during the recovery process is warranted.

Although other researchers (62) have failed to find a significant impact of cognitive impairment on the quality of life of stroke survivors, larger studies (104) suggest that cognitive impairment is a significant independent predictor of functional outcome, after adjusting for age and physical impairment. Specifically, the investigators reported that the degree of cognitive impairment was related to increased functional impairment and that a lack of cognitive impairment was associated with frequency of independent living after discharge. In another study of 59 patients (aged 75 years and older), Kong et al. (61) reported that admission scores on cognitive tests, as well as the Modified Barthel Index (MBI), could predict discharge MBI scores. Feigenson et al. (34) reported that the presence of severe cognitive and perceptual dysfunction or a homonymous hemianopsia, in addition to a motor deficit, has been shown to be related to an unfavorable outcome and longer length of hospital stay in a retrospective analysis of 248 patients with stroke. In another study involving 199 elderly stroke victims who had rehabilitation treatment, Kanemaru et al. (56) examined the effect of various factors on discharge in a multiple regression analysis with discharge place as the dependent variable. They reported that higher scores on the Wechsler Adult Intelligence Scale (performance IQ measures), along with older age and higher levels of activities of daily living (ADLs), were significantly related to the likelihood of home discharge.

In a population-based stroke study, Appelros et al. (6) assessed the effects of living setting, gender, stroke severity, cognitive impairment, and depression on 377 stroke survivors 1 year before and 1 year after a stroke. In addition to all of these factors predicting the need for specialized housing, they reported an increase in nursing home accommodations from 13% to 20% and an increase in help needed to complete ADLs from 21% to 36%. They also noted that female spouses accepted a heavier burden of caregiver responsibilities.

For stroke patients under the age of 65, cognitive function and ADLs show a similar pattern of improvement after 1 year (51). However, 83% of the 58 patients still had cognitive dysfunction, and 20% were still dependent on caregivers to achieve ADL function. Strikingly, very few patients had returned to work, and as much as 3 years later, only 20% had returned to gainful employment. Although neurologic status was a factor in recovery of cognitive function, it was not significant for return to work. This notion was confirmed by Pasquini et al. (82), who reported on 192 consecutive patients living at home before their stroke over the course of 3 years. They found that both age and cognitive impairment are important predictors of institutionalization at 3 years, but not severity of the neurologic deficit.

The importance of longer term risk factors in cognitive recovery following stroke in larger sample sizes was also addressed by del Ser et al. (31) who examined 193 consecutive stroke patients at 3 months and 24 months after stroke. All patients were administered an extensive neuropsychological test battery as well as the Clinical Dementia Rating Scale (in order to classify patients in terms of dementia). They reported that age, prior cognitive decline, polypharmacy, and hypotension at admission were risk factors associated with progression of cognitive decline. However, they reported that cognitive status at 24 months was stable in most cases (78%), with a decline seen in 14% of patients and improvement seen in 7.8% of patients.

Reitz et al. (87) examined the association between stroke and cognitive changes in 1,271 elderly patients without dementia at baseline over a 5-year period. They used generalized estimating equations to relate stroke to the slope of performance across multiple cognitive domains. They concluded that memory performance declined over time, whereas abstract/visuospatial and language performance remained relatively stable. The association between stroke and memory decline was stronger for men and those with no *apolipoprotein ε4* allele.

Given the importance of laterality on cognitive functioning, it is also unexpected that only modest research to date supports the effects of lateralized stroke on functional outcome. Although some researchers have reported that laterality is not an important factor in stroke outcome, others have suggested that, in fact, it is. One such study by Sisson (95) reported that patients with right parietal and temporal lobe stroke had greatest difficulties with memory, concentration, and mental fatigue at four time periods after stroke (10 days, 1 month, 3 months, and 6 months). Sisson (95) also reported a positive association between cognitive functioning and physical abilities that remained over the study period. Chae and Zorowitz (19) examined the effects of cortical and subcortical nonhemorrhagic infarct and lesion laterality on functional outcome of stroke victims and reported that both level of lesion (subcortical vs. cortical) and laterality are important determinants of outcome during inpatient rehabilitation. Specifically, subcortical stroke survivors were reported to have higher self-care, better mobility function, and higher communication and social cognition than cortical stroke survivors. Importantly, this effect was seen only for patients with left hemisphere lesions. Additionally, left hemisphere stroke survivors tended to have relatively poorer communication and social cognitive functioning than right hemisphere stroke survivors.

NEUROIMAGING

More recently, functional neuroimaging has been used to help assess and predict the pattern of cognitive recovery following stroke and hemorrhage. Unlike the numerous standardized neuropsychological tasks that were largely validated on lesion location models in patients with known cerebral deficits, experimental cognitive probes are administered while an individual is being scanned, and activation patterns from patients recovering from stroke and hemorrhage are compared to activation patterns seen in age-matched, healthy controls. Results suggest different patterns of activation that are associated with better cognitive recovery.

For example, Crinion and Price (22) used functional MRI (fMRI) to investigate narrative speech in patients with left hemisphere stroke and a history of aphasia (compared to 18 healthy control subjects). They reported that, irrespective of lesion site, performance on measures of auditory sentence comprehension was correlated with activity just anterior to the primary auditory cortex in the right lateral superior temporal gyrus. This may suggest spatial recruitment of the contralateral hemisphere during the recovery process. This finding is supported by a review of available studies of auditory speech comprehension suggesting that recovery depends on both left and right temporal lobe activation (86). Furthermore, Crinion and Price (22) reported that when the temporal cortex was not involved in the stroke, performance on this task correlated with activity in the left posterior superior temporal cortex (Wernicke area). In contrast, story recognition was associated with left inferior frontal and right cerebellar activation.

Imaging studies of speech production in patients with aphasia after left hemisphere stroke suggest that recovery depends on slowly evolving changes in activation within the left hemisphere. Changes in the right hemisphere do not appear to be correlated with recovery but are the result of transcallosal disinhibition (86).

Strangman et al. (97) investigated the utility of near-infrared spectroscopy in assessing the process of rehabilitation in healthy control subjects over time. They were able to establish adequate test-retest reliability on a motor control task, suggesting that this imaging technique may be a reliable tool in assessing rehabilitation progress and longitudinal recovery from stroke. For a summary of the conceptual issues important in the context of imaging changes in neural function through the recovery process, please see Munoz-Cespedes et al. (76).

PHARMACOLOGIC TREATMENT

Currently, there are no treatments approved by the Food and Drug Administration (FDA) to treat stroke and its sequelae. There have been numerous efforts to develop treatments of the cognitive dysfunction

following stroke, with the latest activity stemming from the FDA's willingness to approve a pharmacologic agent based solely on its ability to improve cognitive functioning. The model of cognitive deficits associated with schizophrenia is likely to be the first one to be evaluated by the FDA and has shown the greatest promise as judged by the volume of drugs designed for this indication and trials in progress. There are also various models to assess cognition secondary to stroke, and most studies to date have been examined via two basic methodologies. The first approach is to use a neuroprotective agent administered within a relatively short time period after the stroke and then to follow patients over time to examine acute outcomes. The second is to examine changes in cognitive functioning over a specified treatment period in patients who have more chronic and stable pattern of cognitive deficits. This model has been more typically employed in patients who have a presumed vascular etiology of their cognitive dysfunction (e.g., vascular dementia).

ACUTE NEUROPROTECTIVE AGENTS

Because excessive activation of the N-methyl-D-aspartate (NMDA) subclass of glutamate receptors appears to be a key mediator of brain injury during acute ischemic stroke, this neurotransmitter has become a target for many novel compounds. Despite promising results in some animal models, severe adverse reactions were seen with early NMDA antagonists (e.g., Selfotel, also known as CGS 19755) in humans (29). Antagonists of glycine at the NMDA receptor, such as aptiganel and gavestinel, were also thought to be promising neuroprotective agents in animal models of focal brain ischemia. Although these compounds have been much better tolerated in clinical trials (2,47), they have failed to show the efficacy needed in terms of more traditional functional outcomes (e.g., Barthel Index, National Institutes of Health Stroke Scale, modified Rankin scores) that take into account overall cognitive functioning but do not measure this precisely. To date, there have been no studies conducted with NMDA-targeted agents that specifically measure cognitive function (as assessed by standardized neuropsychological tests) as the primary or even as a key secondary endpoint in clinical trials of acute or subacute ischemic stroke.

Other compounds, such as the nootropic compound cerebrolysin (Ebewe Pharma, Unterach, Austria), also have shown some promise in preclinical studies. Cerebrolysin is a neuroprotective compound that contains peptides that have a unique biologic activity that protects the nerve cells from the hazards of the ischemic cascade. Cerebrolysin reduces excitotoxic damage, blocks overactivation of calcium-dependent proteases, and scavenges free oxygen radicals and, thus, increases neuronal viability and survival during and after ischemic events. Despite an abundance of positive preclinical evidence, the only placebo-controlled trial in acute stroke patients (63) showed no significant improvement on the Canadian Neurological Scale, the Barthel Index, or the Clinical Global Impression (CGI) scale at time points up to 90 days after stroke. However, a significant improvement in cognitive function of the patients on cerebrolysin was observed on the Syndrome Short Test (a measure of attention and memory) when compared to the placebo.

Another study (79) examined whether intravenous recombinant tissue plasminogen activator (rtPA) treatment given after an acute ischemic stroke has a favorable effect on cognitive and functional outcome at 6 months after stroke. The study was not placebo controlled but, instead, used a cohort of untreated patients as the control group. Unfortunately, although this study suggested a benefit of the drug on functional outcomes, as measured by various ADLs, no effect on neuropsychological test outcomes was noted.

The Women's Estrogen for Stroke Trial (107) followed 664 postmenopausal women after a recent stroke or transient ischemic attack to determine whether estrogen therapy reduced the risk of cognitive decline compared with placebo. Overall, estrogen did not have significant effects on cognitive measures after an average of 3 years of follow-up. However, the study showed that, in a subset of women with normal cognitive function at baseline, there may be a benefit for estrogen therapy in reducing the risk for later cognitive decline (relative risk, 0.46; 95% CI, 0.24 to 0.87).

CHRONIC VASCULAR DEMENTIA AGENTS

Cholinesterase inhibitors have been shown to be helpful in various randomized controlled trials of vascular dementia; however, their use is not licensed yet for this indication. Two identical randomized, double-blind, placebo-controlled studies of donepezil (13,110), involving a combined 1,219 patients enrolled at 109 investigational sites in the United States, Canada, Europe, and Australia, yielded largely positive results. The patients in these studies were randomized 1:1:1 to donepezil 5 mg, donepezil 10 mg, or placebo. Dual primary outcome measures were employed: the Alzheimer's Disease Assessment Scale–Cognitive Subscale (ADAS-cog) and the Clinician's Interview-Based Impression of Change–Plus version (CIBIC-plus). After 24 weeks of treatment, both donepezil-treated groups in both studies showed statistically significant improvements in cognitive function on the ADAS-cog compared with patients receiving placebo. In the Wilkinson et al. (110) study, the CIBIC-plus was also statistically significantly different from placebo for both treatment groups, but in the Black et al. (13) study, the CIBIC-plus results were not as

conclusive. A significant treatment effect was observed in the donepezil 5 mg group but not in the donepezil 10 mg group. It is noteworthy, though, that the group receiving donepezil 10 mg in this study did separate from placebo on other functional outcome measures such as the Sum of the Boxes of the Clinical Dementia Rating (CDR-SB) and the Alzheimer's Disease Functional Assessment and Change Scale (ADFACS). Open-label studies with rivastigmine have suggested some benefit, and larger, prospective, double-blind studies of patients with vascular dementia are currently underway.

Xiao et al. (112) examined the efficacy of cerebrolysin in patients with vascular dementia. This was a double-blind, placebo-controlled study of a 30-mL dose of cerebrolysin given intravenously 5 days per week for 4 weeks. The primary outcomes were the Mini-Mental State Examination (MMSE) and the CGI. A statistically significant improvement was evident for the cerebrolysin group compared with the placebo group after the 4-week treatment period. No significant difference, however, was observed with the CGI. Significant differences in favor of cerebrolysin were also demonstrated on both forms of the Trail Making Test, but no differences were shown on other measures of clinical and functional outcome used in the study.

Several other compounds have also been evaluated for their potential effects on cognition in patients with vascular dementia as confirmed by formal diagnostic criteria or in otherwise stable patients with a history of multiple infarcts. Overall, these studies have failed to provide positive results in terms of the primary analysis, but some ad hoc analyses in various subpopulations have suggested limited benefits. Published reports are available for the following compounds: pentoxifylline, a hemorheologic agent used to treat intermittent claudication (12); vinpocetine (ethyl apovincaminate), a drug that selectively stimulates cerebral circulation and oxygen consumption, inhibits thrombocyte aggregation, and is thought to have a neuroprotective effect as well (59); and citicoline, a form of the B vitamin choline that may reduce ischemic injury in the CNS by preserving membrane phospholipids. In its freebase form, citicoline is marketed as a dietary supplement in the United States and as a drug in Japan. The sodium salt of citicoline, the form used in clinical trials, is sold as a drug in Europe (20,21).

Finally, very interesting data from Nyenhuis et al. (78) suggest that statins may actually lower the risk for cognitive decline following a stroke. These investigators examined 103 consecutive stroke patients (41 with vascular CIND and 62 with no evidence of any cognitive impairment after their stroke). They reported that the three most significant predictors of cognitive impairment were the patient's level of education (cognitive reserve), the presence of heart disease, and a history of hypercholesterolemia. When they controlled for the effects of education, only hypercholesterolemia remained a significant predictor. However, this finding most likely relates to the treatment of hypercholesterolemia rather than any favorable effects of cholesterol.

REFERENCES

1. Aggleton JP, Mishkin M. Visual recognition impairment following medial thalamic lesions in monkeys. *Neuropsychologia*. 1983;21:189–197.
2. Albers GW, Goldstein LB, Hall D. Aptiganel hydrochloride in acute ischemic stroke. *J Am Med Assoc*. 2001;286:2673–2682.
3. Allegri RF. Attention and neglect: neurological basis, assessment and disorders. *Rev Neurol*. 2000;30:491–494.
4. Allen G, Buxton RB, Wong EC, et al. Attentional activation of the cerebellum independent of motor involvement. *Science*. 1997;275:1940–1943.
5. Andreasen NC, O'Leary DS, Arndt S, et al. Neural substrates of facial recognition. *J Neuropsychiatry Clin Neurosci*. 1995;8:139–146.
6. Appelros P, Nydevik I, Terent A. Living setting and utilisation of ADL assistance one year after a stroke with special reference to gender differences. *Disabil Rehabil*. 2006;28:43–49.
7. Appollonio IM, Grafman J, Schwartz V, et al. Memory in patients with cerebellar degeneration. *Neurology*. 1993;43:1536–1544.
8. Archer CR, Ilinsky IA, Goldfader PR, et al. Aphasia in thalamic stroke: CT stereotactic localization. *J Comput Assist Tomogr*. 1981;5:427–432.
9. Barraguer-Bordas L, Illa I, Escartin A, et al. Thalamic hemorrhage. A study of 23 patients with diagnosis by computed tomography. *Stroke*. 1981;12:524–527.
10. Benson DF. Disorders of visual gnosis. In: Brown JW, ed. *Neuropsychology of visual perception*. New York: The IRBN Press; 1989.
11. Benson DF, Geschwind N. Aphasia and related disorders: a clinical approach. In: Mesulam M, ed. *Principles of behavioral neurology*. Philadelphia: FA Davis Co; 1985:193–238.
12. Black RS, Barclay LL, Nolan KA, et al. Pentoxifylline in cerebrovascular dementia. *J Am Geriatr Soc*. 1992;40:237–244.
13. Black S, Román GC, Geldmacher DS, et al. Efficacy and tolerability of donepezil in vascular dementia: positive results of a 24-week, multicenter, international, randomized, placebo-controlled clinical trial. *Stroke*. 2003;34;2323–2330.
14. Bogousslavsky J, Regli F, Uske A. Thalamic infarcts: clinical syndromes, etiology and prognosis. *Neurology*. 1988;38:837–848.
15. Botez-Marquard T, Leveille J, Botez MI. Neuropsychological functioning in unilateral cerebellar damage. *Can J Neurol Sci*. 1994;21:353–357.
16. Brion S, Mikol J, Plas J. Memoire et specialization fonctionnelle hemispherique. Rapport anatomo-clinique. *Rev Neurol*. 1983;139:39–43.
17. Buffon F, Porcher R, Hernandez K, et al. Cognitive profile in CADASIL. *J Neurol Neurosurg Psychiatry*. 2006;77:175–180.
18. Castaigne P, Lhermitte F, Buge A, et al. Paramedian thalamic and midbrain infarcts: clinical and neuropathological study. *Ann Neurol*. 1981;10:127–148.
19. Chae J, Zorowitz R. Functional status of cortical and subcortical nonhemorrhagic stroke survivors and the effect of lesion laterality. *Am J Phys Med Rehabil*. 1998;77:415–420.
20. Cohen RA, Browndyke JN, Moser DJ, et al. Long-term citicoline (cytidine diphosphate choline) use in patients with vascular dementia: neuroimaging and neuropsychological outcomes. *Cerebrovasc Dis*. 2003;16:199–204.
21. Conant R, Schauss AG. Therapeutic applications of citicoline for stroke and cognitive dysfunction in the elderly: a review of the literature. *Altern Med Rev*. 2004;9:17–31.
22. Crinion J, Price CJ. Right anterior superior temporal activation predicts auditory sentence comprehension following aphasic stroke. *Brain*. 2005;128:2858–2871.
23. Crosson B. Role of the dominant thalamus in language: a review. *Psychol Bull*. 1984;96:491–517.
24. Crosson B. Subcortical functions in language: a working model. *Brain Lang*. 1985;25:257–292.
25. Cummings JL. Frontal-subcortical circuits and human behavior. *Arch Neurol*. 1993;50:873–880.
26. Cummings JL, Benson DF. *Dementia: A Clinical Approach*. Boston: Butterworth-Heineman; 1983.
27. Damasio AR. Disorders of complex visual processing: agnosias, achromatopsia, Balint's syndrome, and related difficulties of orientation and construction. In: Mesulam M, ed. *Principles of behavioral neurology*. Philadelphia: FA Davis Co; 1985:259–288.
28. Damasio AR. The frontal lobes. In: Heilman KM, Valenstein E, eds. *Clinical neuropsychology*. New York: Oxford University Press; 1985:339–375.
29. Davis SM, Lees KR, Albers GW, et al. Selfotel in acute ischemic stroke: possible neurotoxic

effects of an NMDA antagonist. *Stroke.* 2000; 31:347–354.

30. Davous P, Bianco C, Duval-Lota AM, et al. Aphasie par infarctus thalamique paramedian gauche. Observation anatomo-clinique. *Rev Neurol.* 1984;140:711–719.

31. del Ser T, Barba R, Morin MM, et al. Evolution of cognitive impairment after stroke and risk factors for delayed progression. *Stroke.* 2005;36: 2670–2675.

32. De Renzi E. Memory disorders following focal neocortical damage. *Philos Trans R Soc Lond B Biol Sci.* 1982;298:73–83.

33. De Romanis F, Benfatto B. Presentazione e discussione di quattro casi di prosopagosia. *Riv Neurol.* 1973;43:111–132.

34. Feigenson JS, McDowell FH, Meese P, et al. Factors influencing outcome and length of stay in a stroke rehabilitation unit. Part 1. Analysis of 248 unscreened patients—medical and functional prognostic indicators. *Stroke.* 1977;8: 651–656.

35. Fiez JA, Raichle ME. Linguistic processing. *Int Rev Neurobiol.* 1997;41:233–254.

36. Fisher CM. Lacunar strokes and infarct: a review. *Neurology.* 1982;32:871–876.

37. Fisher CM. The pathologic and clinical aspects of thalamic hemorrhage. *Trans Am Neurol Assoc.* 1959;84:56–59.

38. Friedman JH. Syndrome of diffuse encephalopathy due to nondominant thalamic infarction. *Neurology.* 1985;35:1524–1526.

39. Gamaldo A, Moghekar A, Kilada S, et al. Effect of a clinical stroke on the risk of dementia in a prospective cohort. *Neurology.* 2006; 67:1363–1369.

40. Goldman-Rakic PS. Specification of higher cortical functions. *J Head Trauma Rehabil.* 1993;8: 13–23.

41. Goodglass H. Phonological factors in aphasia. In: Brookshire RH, ed. *Clinical aphasiology.* Minneapolis: BRK Publishers; 1975:28–44.

42. Graff-Radford NR, Damasio H, Yamada T, et al. Nonhemorrhagic thalamic infarction. Clinical, neuropsychological, and electrophysiological findings in four anatomical groups defined by computed tomography. *Brain.* 1985;108:485–516.

43. Grafman J, Litvan I, Massaquoi S, et al. Cognitive planning deficit in patients with cerebellar atrophy. *Neurology.* 1992;42:1493–1496.

44. Guberman A, Stuss D. The syndrome of bilateral paramedian thalamic infarction. *Neurology.* 1983;33:540–546.

45. Hachinski VC, Iliff LD, Zilhka E, et al. Cerebral blood flow in dementia. *Arch Neurol.* 1975;32: 632–637.

46. Hajek VE, Gagnon S, Ruderman JE. Cognitive and functional assessments of stroke patients: an analysis of their relation. *Arch Phys Med Rehabil.* 1997;78:1331–1337.

47. Haley EC Jr., Thompson JLP, Levin B, et al. Gavestinel does not improve outcome after acute intracerebral hemorrhage: an analysis from the GAIN International and GAIN Americas studies. *Stroke.* 2005;36;1006–1010.

48. Hartmann JA, Wolz WA, Roeltgen DP, et al. Denial of visual perception. *Brain Cogn.* 1991; 16:29–40.

49. Heath RG, Franklin DE, Shraberg D. Gross pathology of the cerebellum in patients diagnosed and treated as functional psychiatric disorders. *J Nerv Ment Dis.* 1979;167:585–592.

50. Hier DB, Cummings JL. Rare acquired and degenerative subcortical dementias. In: Cummings JL, ed. *Subcortical dementia.* New York: Oxford University Press; 1990:199–217.

51. Hofgren C, Bjorkdahl A, Esbjornsson E, et al. Recovery after stroke: cognition, ADL function and return to work. *Acta Neurol Scand.* 2007;115: 73–80.

52. Hutter BO, Gilsbach JM. Introspective capacities in patients with cognitive deficits after subarachnoid hemorrhage. *J Clin Exp Neuropsychol.* 1995;17:499–517.

53. Ishii N, Nishahara Y, Imamura T. Why do frontal lobe symptoms predominate in vascular dementia with lacunes? *Neurology.* 1986;36: 340–345.

54. Jokinen H, Kalska H, Mantyla R, et al. Cognitive profile of subcortical ischaemic vascular disease. *J Neurol Neurosurg Psychiatry.* 2006;77:28–33.

55. Jones-Gotman M, Milner B. Design fluency: the invention of nonsense drawings after focal cortical lesions. *Neuropsychologia.* 1977;15:653–674.

56. Kanemaru A, Takahashi R, Yamanaka T, et al. Relationship between cognitive function and discharge place among stroke patients after rehabilitation. *Nippon Ronen Igakkai Zasshi.* 1998;35:307–312.

57. Karussis D, Leker RR, Abramsky O. Cognitive dysfunction following thalamic stroke: a study of 16 cases and review of the literature. *J Neurol Sci.* 2000;172:25–29.

58. Katz DI, Alexander MP, Mandell AM. Dementia following strokes in the mesencephalon and diencephalon. *Arch Neurol.* 1987;44:1127–1133.

59. Kemeny V, Molnar S, Andrejkovics M, et al. Acute and chronic effects of vinpocetine on cerebral hemodynamics and neuropsychological performance in multi-infarct patients. *J Clin Pharmacol.* 2005;45:1048–1054.

60. Kolb B, Whishaw IQ. *Fundamentals of Human Neuropsychology*. New York: WH Freeman and Company; 1985.

61. Kong KH, Chua KS, Tow AP. Clinical characteristics and functional outcome of stroke patients 75 years old and older. *Arch Phys Med Rehabil*. 1998;79:1535–1539.

62. Kwa VI, Linburg M, de Haan RJ. The role of cognitive impairment in the quality of life after ischaemic stroke. *J Neurol*. 1996;243:599–604.

63. Ladurner G, Kalvach P, Moessler H. Neuroprotective treatment with cerebrolysin in patients with acute stroke: a randomised controlled trial. *J Neural Transm*. 2005;112:415–428.

64. Laeng B. Constructional apraxia after left or right unilateral stroke. *Neuropsychologia*. 2006;44:1595–1606.

65. Levisohn L, Cronin-Golomb A, Schmahmann JD. Neuropsychological sequelae of cerebellar tumors in children. *Soc Neurosci Abstr*. 1997;23:496.

66. Lezak MD. *Neuropsychological Assessment*. New York: Oxford University Press; 1995.

67. Lopera F. Processing of faces: neurological bases, disorders and evaluation. *Rev Neurol*. 2000;30:486–490.

68. Luria AR. *Higher Cortical Functions in Man*. New York: Basic Books; 1966.

69. Markowitsch HJ. Thalamic mediodorsal nucleus and memory: a critical evaluation of studies in animals and man. *Neurosci Biobehav Rev*. 1982;6:351–380.

70. Martin JJ. Thalamic syndromes. In: Vincken PJ, Bruyn GW, eds. *Handbook of clinical neurology*. Vol. 2. Amsterdam: North Holland Press; 1968:469–496.

71. McGlone J, Young B. Cerebral localization. In: Baker AB, ed. *Clinical neurology*. Philadelphia: Harper & Row; 1986.

72. Mills RP, Swanson PD. Vertical oculomotor apraxia and memory loss. *Ann Neurol*. 1978;4:149–153.

73. Milner B. Effects of different brain lesions on card sorting. *Arch Neurol*. 1963;9:90–100.

74. Mirsky AF. The neuropsychology of attention: elements of a complex behavior. In: Perecman E, ed. *Integrating theory and practice in clinical neuropsychology*. Hillsdale, NJ: Laurence Erlbaum; 1989.

75. Mishkin M. A memory system in the monkey. In: Broadbent DE, Weiskrantz L, eds. *The neuropsychiatry of cognitive function*. London: The Royal Society; 1982:85–95.

76. Munoz-Cespedes JM, Rios-Lago M, Paul N, et al. Functional neuroimaging studies of cognitive recovery after acquired brain damage in adults. *Neuropsychol Rev*. 2005;15:169–183.

77. National Stroke Association. Be stroke smart (Newsletter). Englewood, CO: National Stroke Association; 1995.

78. Nyenhuis DL, Gorelick PB, Geenen EJ, et al. The pattern of neuropsychological deficits in vascular cognitive impairment-no dementia (vascular CIND). *Clin Neuropsychol*. 2004;18:41–49.

79. Nys GM, van Zandvoort MJ, Algra A, et al. Cognitive and functional outcome after intravenous recombinant tissue plasminogen activator treatment in patients with a first symptomatic brain infarct. *J Neurol*. 2006;253:237–241.

80. Nys GM, Van Zandvoort MJ, De Kort PL, et al. Domain-specific cognitive recovery after first-ever stroke: a follow-up study of 111 cases. *J Int Neuropsychol Soc*. 2005;11:795–806.

81. Nys GM, van Zandvoort MJ, van der Worp HB, et al. Early cognitive impairment predicts long-term depressive symptoms and quality of life after stroke. *J Neurol Sci*. 2006;247:149–156.

82. Pasquini M, Leys D, Rousseaux M, et al. Influence of cognitive impairment on the institutionalisation rate 3 years after a stroke. *J Neurol Neurosurg Psychiatry*. 2007;78:56–59.

83. Pillon B, Bazin B, Deweer B, et al. Specificity of memory deficits after right or left temporal lobectomy. *Cortex*. 1999;34:561–571.

84. Pohjasvaara T, Mantyla R, Aronen HJ, et al. Clinical and radiological determinants of prestroke cognitive decline in a stroke cohort. *J Neurol Neurosurg Psychiatry*. 1999;67:742–748.

85. Poppel E, Held R, Front D. Residual visual function after brain wounds involving the central visual pathways. *Nature*. 1973;243:295–296.

86. Price CJ, Crinion J. The latest on functional imaging studies of aphasic stroke. *Curr Opin Neurol*. 2005;18:429–434.

87. Reitz C, Luchsinger JA, Tang MX, et al. Stroke and memory performance in elderly persons without dementia. *Arch Neurol*. 2006;63:571–576.

88. Robinson RG. *The Clinical Neuropsychiatry of Stroke: Cognitive, Behavioral, and Emotional Disorders following Vascular Brain Injury*. Cambridge, United Kingdom: Cambridge University Press; 1998.

89. Schmahmann JD. Disorders of the cerebellum: ataxia, dysmetria of thought, and the cerebellar cognitive affective syndrome. *J Neuropsychiatry Clin Neurosci*. 2004;16:367–378.

90. Schmahmann JD. Rediscovery of an early concept. *Int Rev Neurobiol*. 1997;41:3–27.

91. Schmahmann JD, Sherman JC. The cerebellar cognitive affective syndrome. *Brain*. 1998;121:561–579.

92. Schuppert M, Munte TF, Wieringa BM, et al. Receptive amusia: evidence for cross-hemispheric neural networks underlying music processing strategies. *Brain*. 2000;123:546–549.

93. Semple PF. *An Atlas of Stroke*. New York: The Parthenon Publishing Group; 1998.

94. Silveri MC, Leggio MG, Molinari M. The cerebellum contributes to linguistic production: a case of agrammatic speech following a right cerebellar lesion. *Neurology*. 1994;44:2047–2050.

95. Sisson RA. Cognitive status as a predictor of right hemisphere stroke outcomes. *J Neurosci Nurs*. 1995;27:152–156.

96. Speedie LJ, Heilman KM. Amnestic disturbance following infarction of the left dorsomedial nucleus of the thalamus. *Neuropsychologia*. 1982; 20:597–604.

97. Strangman G, Goldstein R, Rauch SL, et al. Near-infrared spectroscopy and imaging for investigating stroke rehabilitation: test-retest reliability and review of the literature. *Arch Phys Med Rehabil*. 2006;87:12–19.

98. Stuss DT, Benson DF. Neuropsychological studies of the frontal lobes. *Psychol Bull*. 1984; 95:3–28.

99. Stuss DT, Benson DF. *The Frontal Lobes*. New York: Raven Press; 1986.

100. Stuss DT, Cummings JL. Subcortical vascular dementias. In: Cummings JL, ed. *Subcortical dementia*. New York: Oxford University Press; 1990:145–163.

101. Stuss DT, Guberman A, Nelson R, et al. The neuropsychology of paramedian thalamic infarcts. *Brain Cogn*. 1988;8:348–378.

102. Sunderland A, Tinson D, Bradley L. Differences in recovery from constructional apraxia after right and left hemisphere stroke? *J Clin Exp Neuropsychol*. 1994;16:916–920.

103. Swanson RA, Schmidley JW. Amnestic syndrome and vertical gaze palsy: early detection of bilateral thalamic infarction by CT and NMR. *Stroke*. 1985;16:823–827.

104. Tatemichi TK, Desmond DW, Stern Y, et al. Cognitive impairment after stroke: frequency, patterns, and relationship to functional abilities. *J Neurol Neurosurg Psychiatry*. 1994;57:202–207.

105. van Asselen M, Kessels RP, Kappelle LJ, et al. Neural correlates of human wayfinding in stroke patients. *Brain Res*. 2006;1067:229–238.

106. Van Der Werf YD, Weerts JG, Jolles J, et al. Neuropsychological correlates of a right unilateral lacunar thalamic infarction. *J Neurol Neurosurg Psychiatry*. 1999;66:36–42.

107. Viscoli CM, Brass LM, Kernan WN, et al. Estrogen therapy and risk of cognitive decline: results from the Women's Estrogen for Stroke Trial (WEST). *Am J Obstet Gynecol*. 2005;192: 387–393.

108. Walsh K. *Neuropsychology: A Clinical Approach*. 2nd ed. New York: Churchill Livingstone; 1987.

109. Weisberg LA. Lacunar infarcts. Clinical and computed tomographic correlations. *Arch Neurol*. 1982;39:37–40.

110. Wilkinson D, Doody R, Helme R, et al. Donepezil in vascular dementia: a randomized, placebo-controlled study. *Neurology*. 2003;61: 479–486.

111. Winocur G, Oxbury S, Roberts R, et al. Amnesia in a patient with bilateral lesions to the thalamus. *Neuropsychologia*. 1984;22:123–143.

112. Xiao S, Yan H, Yao P, et al. The efficacy of cerebrolysin in patients with vascular dementia: results of a Chinese multicentre, randomized, double-blind, placebo-controlled trial. *Hong Kong J Psychiatry*. 1999;9:13–19.

SUGGESTED READINGS

Lezak MD. *Neuropsychological Assessment*. New York: Oxford University Press, 1995.

McCrum R. *My Year Off: Rediscovering Life after a Stroke*. New York: WW Norton; 1998.

Robinson RG. *The Clinical Neuropsychiatry of Stroke: Cognitive, Behavioral, and Emotional Disorders following Vascular Brain Injury*. Cambridge, United Kingdom: Cambridge University Press; 1998.

LISTING OF WEBSITES OF NATIONAL SUPPORT GROUPS

National Stroke Association: http://www.stroke.org/ NS804.0_Recov&Rehab.html

American Heart Association: http://www.american heart.org/

The Stroke Network: http://www.strokenetwork.org/

National Institute of Neurological Diseases and Stroke: http://www.nih.gov/about/almanac/organization/ NINDS.htm

American Society of Neurorehabilitation: http:// www.asnr.com/

Neuropsychology Central is a metasource for neuropsychology information on the Internet: http:// www.neuropsychologycentral.com

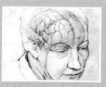

CHAPTER 19

Spontaneous and Traumatic Cerebral Hemorrhage in the Elderly

Eelco F.M. Wijdicks

Cerebral hemorrhage, which is common in the vulnerable elderly population, typically refers to hypertensive cerebral hemorrhage, traumatic lobar contusions, or subdural hematoma. Intracerebral hemorrhage is more frequent in the elderly for several reasons, including falls, amyloid deposition producing brittle cortical arteries, and the long-term effects of hypertension finally leading to a fatal complication. Its management is complicated because of associated morbidity and unexpected responses to pharmacy, nosocomial infections, and in-hospital complications. Age is an important independent and also overpowering risk factor for poor outcome in all types of cerebral hemorrhage. Although the incidence of cerebral infarction is declining, the frequency of intracerebral hemorrhage is increasing both for men and women and is clearly linked to older age. More uplifting is that survivors of cerebral hematomas return to the community (18). Clinical findings, complications, diagnosis, therapeutic modalities, and prognosis of hemorrhagic stroke in the older adult are reviewed in this chapter.

EPIDEMIOLOGY

The elderly population has been growing over the last 30 years, specifically those aged 85 years and older, and this growth has been accompanied by an increased incidence of cerebrovascular disease. This older age group has a two- to threefold greater frequency of both ischemic and hemorrhagic stroke than the group composed of those aged 65 to 74 years (14).

In a study of acute stroke in very old people (≥85 years) by Arboix et al. (2), data were collected on 2,000 patients of all ages between 1986 and 1995. The incidence of stroke was 13% in those 85 years or older, 37% in patients aged 75 to 84 years, and 28% in those 65 to 74 years of age. Stroke was more prevalent in women than in men. The main cardiovascular risk factors were hypertension, atrial fibrillation, and diabetes. More recently, a dramatic several-fold increase in anticoagulation-associated hemorrhages has been noted with no concomitant increase of ischemic stroke in the elderly (age 80 or older). The increase was considered largely due to increase in use

of warfarin during the 10-year study period (8). As expected, hemorrhagic stroke was less frequently present (14%) than ischemic stroke (86%), but the ratio of hemorrhagic versus ischemic stroke remained similar over the years. The elderly population had the worst outcome, with longer hospitalizations and the greatest in-hospital mortality rate. Altered consciousness, limb weakness, sensory deficit, parietal and temporal lobe involvement, internal capsule involvement, intraventricular hemorrhage, and respiratory and cardiac events were considered predictive factors of in-hospital morbidity and mortality.

ETIOLOGY

Cerebral hemorrhages can involve the subcortical (ganglionic) or lobar structures. These localizations are equally prevalent, but the causes are different. Hemorrhage from a ruptured arteriovenous malformation is uncommon. Although the cumulative risk of rupture increases, most patients who experience hemorrhage are between 10 and 35 years of age. Hemorrhage into a metastasis or anticoagulation-associated hemorrhages should also be considered. Hypertension-associated cerebral hemorrhages, in particular isolated systolic hypertension, and cerebral amyloid angiopathy are common causes of intracerebral hemorrhage.

Long-standing hypertension is probably a common cause of intracerebral hemorrhage in the elderly. Its presentation can be biphasic, at the onset of the hypertension or later when long-standing injury to the penetrating arteries has resulted in formation of fibrinoid degeneration and, possibly, microaneurysms. The predilection sites in the basal ganglia, pons, and cerebellum attest to that.

Cerebral amyloid angiopathy is a common cause of hemorrhage in the oldest-old (26). It is usually diagnosed at autopsies, suggested by magnetic resonance imaging (MRI), or found in surgical specimens and more often in the temporal and occipital lobes (23). In many instances, amyloid deposits involve leptomeningeal or cortical vessels and can completely and continuously involve the blood vessel wall. Severe angiopathy can cause lobar cerebral hemorrhage from rupture of a cortical or meningeal vessel and dementia, which is noted by family members. Schutz et al. (24) found that the incidence is 30 to 40 per 100,000 patients 70 years of age and older, which would make cerebral amyloid angiopathy responsible for 30% to 50% of cerebral hemorrhage in this age group. Autopsies have also revealed that the prevalence is 2.3% for those between 65 and 74 years, 8% for those aged 75 to 84 years, and 12% for those older than 85 years (10).

Coagulopathy is an important cause of hemorrhage in this age group, particularly because warfarin is commonly initiated to prevent ischemic stroke in conditions such as atrial fibrillation, prosthetic heart valves, and rheumatic mitral stenosis. When stroke occurs, it has a high morbidity and mortality rate (4). To complicate matters even further, the Massachusetts General Hospital group documented a clear link between cerebral amyloid angiopathy and warfarin-associated lobar hemorrhage.

Trauma can also lead to cerebral hemorrhage and is probably the predominant cause in elderly patients. Hemorrhage caused by trauma is often characterized by frontal and temporal lobe contusions or a blood collection located between the dura and the underlying brain. According to the time interval between the trauma and the onset of symptoms, subdural hematoma is divided into acute (<24 hours), subacute (1 to 10 days), and chronic (>10 days). Subdural hematomas are typically located over the convexity and, in some cases, can be bilateral. Acute subdural hematoma remains a common traumatic cerebral hemorrhage in the elderly.

CLINICAL COURSE

The clinical findings are manifestations of initial tissue destruction and subsequent mass effect. A tendency is seen for progression of the focal neurologic deficits over a few hours.

Patients with intracerebral hemorrhage complain of headaches, vomiting, and a decreased level of consciousness. The headaches are more common with lobar or cerebellar hematomas. Because the location is near to the meningeal surface, meningeal signs may appear.

A decreased level of consciousness is present in large cerebral hematomas causing brainstem shift and when the lesion is located primarily in the posterior fossa compressing the brainstem. Although the decreased level of alertness is considered an adverse prognostic sign, it may simply reflect a larger volume, more tissue shift, or the development of hydrocephalus. Vomiting is also present as a consequence of the increased press or pressure on the vomiting center in the floor of the fourth ventricle. Seizures can be present in cases of a lobar hemorrhage but are rare in putaminal and thalamic hemorrhage. Most often, seizures occur at the time of the bleeding. One recent large study by Bladin et al. (3) found early-onset seizures (within 2 weeks) in 8% and late-onset seizures in 2.6% of patients, with recurrent seizures only in patients with late-onset seizures.

Fever has been significantly associated with intracerebral hemorrhage and with the presence of mass effect, transtentorial herniation, and intraventricular blood on computed tomography (CT) scan. Patients who developed fever were older but also had larger volume hemorrhages.

The physical findings depend on the location of the hemorrhage. Level of consciousness involves arousal and content. Content disturbances can be more prevalent as a premorbid condition in elderly, and diminished attention and lack of integration should not be interpreted as altered state of consciousness. Acute confusional state commonly affects the elderly patient, who also may be susceptible because of underlying dementia. Sleep becomes quickly disturbed, and additional sedative drugs can cause a more profound state. In putaminal hemorrhage, patients present with hemiplegia, homonymous hemianopia, and eye deviation to the side of the hemorrhage. Mild and transient contralateral hemiparesis and a clinical picture similar to subarachnoid hemorrhage characterize a caudate hemorrhage. Hydrocephalus is a common feature because of the early extension of the bleeding to the ventricles. Hemiplegia, hemisensory syndrome, upward gaze paralysis, and small nonreactive pupils are seen in thalamic hemorrhage. Also seen is frequent communication with the ventricular system, and prognosis is related to the size of the hematoma. A poor prognosis is seen in cases of hydrocephalus caused by aqueductal obstruction.

Lobar cerebral hemorrhages are characterized by hemiparesis of upper limb in frontal hematomas, sensory motor deficit and hemianopia in parietal location, fluent aphasia in dominant temporal hematomas, and homonymous hemianopia in occipital hemorrhages. Because of their superficial location, a better prognosis is seen for lobar hemorrhages than for other types of hematomas because they are easily approached surgically.

In cerebellar hemorrhage, patients complain of sudden vertigo, vomiting, headache, and an inability to stand or walk. Ipsilateral limb ataxia, horizontal gaze palsy, and peripheral facial palsy are present. Pontine hemorrhage is typically massive, bilateral, and characterized by quadriplegia, decerebrate posturing, horizontal ophthalmoplegia, pinpoint reactive pupils, respiratory rhythm abnormalities, coma, and hyperthermia. The clinical features are summarized in Table 19-1.

Table 19-1. *Clinical Features of Cerebral Hemorrhage*

Primary Site	Extension	Telltale Signs
Caudate nucleus	Localized intraventricular hemorrhage	Headache, confusion, drowsiness-stupor, abulia
	Capsule, putamen, diencephalon	Hemiparesis, eye deviation, Horner's syndrome
Putamen	Localized	Hemiparesis, eye deviation, global aphasia
	Posterior extension	
Thalamus	Localized	Fluent aphasia
		Paresthesia, hemineglect, nonfluent aphasia (often preserved repetition), disorientation to place
	Mesencephalon	Marked bradykinesia
Cerebellum	Localized	Dysarthria, appendicular ataxia, headache
	Vermis	Deterioration in consciousness, marked gait ataxia
Pons	Localized	Ataxic hemiparesis ophthalmoplegia, ocular bobbing
	Mesencephalon	Hyperthermia, coma, pinpoint pupils

Adapted from Intracerebral hematoma. In: Wijdicks EFM, ed. *Neurologic catastrophies*. Boston: Butterworth-Heineman; 2000:127.

Acute subdural hematomas are usually associated with severe brain damage. Additional contusions not only are found in direct proximity to the subdural hematoma but can be scattered throughout both hemispheres. The mortality rate for acute subdural hematomas in elderly is extremely high. Age older than 65 years and no motor response or eye opening to pain in combination with no verbal response and postoperative intracranial pressure (ICP) greater than 45 mm Hg are poor predictors of outcome. Chronic subdural hematomas are characterized by persistent headaches for several days, followed by decreased consciousness. They can develop after unrecognized trauma, and their clinical picture is similar to subacute processes. Importantly, in the elderly, brain atrophy provokes stretching of cortical veins, making this age group more susceptible even with a seemingly trivial trauma.

However, age has at least one advantage: Shrinkage of the brain allows for accommodation of large clots. Thus, brain shift is less common, and large-volume hemorrhages are more easily tolerated in the posterior fossa. Therefore, the volume needs to be large or the hematoma needs to be located in a strategic location (e.g., pons) to cause immediate permanent damage.

NEUROIMAGING

Although MRI has much better resolution, a CT scan of the brain remains the first mode of imaging in cerebral hemorrhage. Imaging time has been reduced to a matter of minutes, and information about potential life-threatening lesions is quickly available.

Several specific features are evident in the elderly (Table 19-2). These are profound sulci, large ventricles, and, less commonly, brain shift (Fig. 19-1). Commonly, prior lacunar strokes and white matter hypodensity are seen with ganglionic hemorrhages, a reflection of long-standing effects of hypertension. Subdural hematomas can be difficult to detect when they become isodense. A typical CT scan feature is the "supernormal CT" in which the CT scan image looks like it is that of a much younger person (the isodense subdural hematoma effaces the sulci).

Acute subdural hematoma in the elderly is often accompanied by additional contusions, which may determine outcome rather than subdural hematoma itself. These contusions may not be apparent on admission CT scan. The number of contusions, as well as localization, can have a dramatic impact on long-term outcome. An example of a patient with massive subdural hematoma with comparatively little mass effect but multiple contusions resulting in poor outcome in this particular case is shown in Figure 19-2.

Table 19-2. *Neuroimaging Findings in Elderly Patients with Cerebral Hemorrhage*

Leukoaraiosis, silent strokes, and lacunes
Enlarged ventricles
Less brain shift with large-volume hematoma
Isodense subdural hematoma
Hemosiderin associated with prior hemorrhages

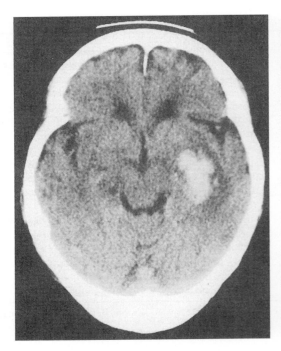 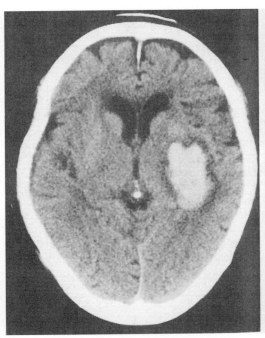

Figure 19-1. CT scan in a 92-year-old man with a putaminal (hypertensive) hemorrhage. Note marked sulci and fissures. Despite large volume of hemorrhage, no shift is seen, and the additional volume is well-tolerated.

MANAGEMENT

Few data exist about specific management of brain hemorrhage in the elderly. Nonetheless, well-recognized aspects in management include the need of mechanical ventilation, management of increased ICP, blood pressure control, a surgical approach, and management of complications.

MECHANICAL VENTILATION

Decreased ICP and airway protection are the main goals of mechanical ventilation. For those patients with midline shift, hyperventilation aiming at a partial pressure of carbon dioxide ($PaCO_2$) between 30 and 35 mm Hg will decrease cerebral blood flow and ICP. This can be better controlled with sedation and the assist control mode. The beneficial effect is transient and usually decreases after 3 to 4 days. Hyperventilation to levels less than 25 mm Hg has not proved to be beneficial.

A retrospective study by Gujjar et al. (11) reviewed indications, timing, and outcome of mechanical ventilation in hemorrhagic and ischemic stroke in 230 patients. The rates of intubation were higher with hemorrhagic strokes, and 75% of patients required intubation at arrival. Older age, intubation on arrival, intubation because of neurologic deterioration rather than primary pulmonary causes, and absence of

corneal, pupillary, and oculocephalic reflexes were considered predictors of high mortality.

It is important to emphasize that aging is associated with changes in pulmonary function such as decrease in elastic recoil, expiratory flow rates, and oxygen-diffusing capacity; increased pulmonary compliance; and ventilation-perfusion mismatch. Furthermore, cardiopulmonary comorbidities, such as chronic obstructive pulmonary disease, congestive heart failure, and coronary artery disease, are much more common in the elderly, which contributes to a high mortality rate.

The incidence of hospital-acquired pneumonia (HAP) increases with age. Risk factors for HAP in the elderly are underlying diseases that decrease immune function (e.g., diabetes, cirrhosis, malnutrition, and malignancy), oropharyngeal colonization with gram-negative organisms, presence of nasogastric tubes, recent antibiotic use, neutralization of gastric pH, and aspiration caused by a neurologic deficit. A study using age-matched elderly control subjects found that endotracheal intubation is also an important risk factor for HAP in elderly. Several studies have identified prognostic factors of mortality. Some found that age could be an independent risk factor for death from pneumonia, but others found that the presence of concomitant cardiopulmonary illnesses contributed to the higher mortality rate.

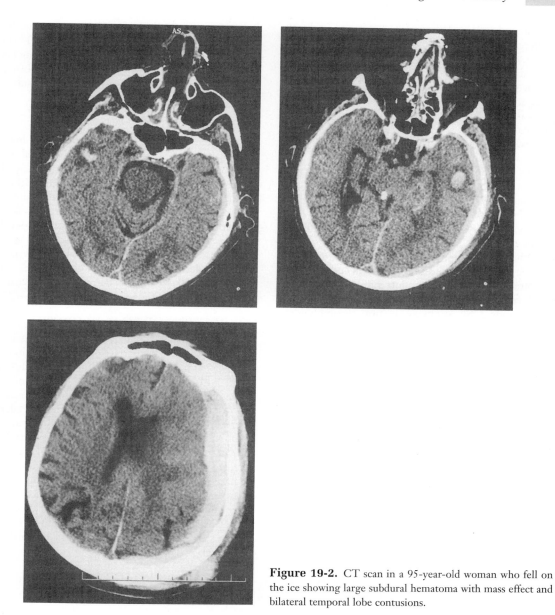

Figure 19-2. CT scan in a 95-year-old woman who fell on the ice showing large subdural hematoma with mass effect and bilateral temporal lobe contusions.

A prospective cohort study was conducted attempting to determine whether age had an independent effect on the outcome of patients treated with mechanical ventilation. Enrolled were 63 patients 75 years of age or older and 237 patients younger than 75 years of age. In-hospital mortality rate, duration of mechanical ventilation, length of stay (intensive care unit and hospital), and cost of care were measured. After adjusting for the severity of illness, elderly patients were found to have a similar length of stay and time with mechanical ventilation.

MANAGEMENT OF INTRACRANIAL PRESSURE

Patients with cerebral hemorrhage may have an ICP causing decreased responsiveness. Monitoring of ICP could provide important information and is required in those patients with multiple contusions. The normal ICP is between 5 and 20 mm Hg, and patients with values of about 20 mm Hg need emergent intervention. The increased ICP compromises cerebral perfusion pressure (CPP), which is obtained after subtracting ICP from mean arterial pressure. Ideal values of CPP above 70 mm Hg should be pursued.

All attempts are directed at decreasing the ICP. Different approaches can be used, such as hyperventilation, osmotic diuretics, and barbiturate coma. Once the patients are mechanically ventilated, they need to be adequately sedated to decrease the ICP.

Mannitol is the most common agent used to decrease ICP. However, it has a transient beneficial effect and sometimes can cause a rebound increase of ICP when discontinued. Using different modes of infusion of mannitol, one study found that when an urgent reduction of ICP is required, a dose of 1 g/kg mannitol should be given in 30 minutes (20). Mannitol has side effects such as hyperosmolarity and renal failure. In addition, theoretical concerns exist that these hypertonic agents could increase the size of the hematoma.

Other approaches used to decrease ICP are elevating the head of the bed to 30 degrees and avoiding endotracheal suctioning and intermittent drainage of cerebrospinal fluid (CSF) with a ventricular catheter. Continuous CSF drainage is not recommended because of inability to measure ICP. No study has documented the benefit of ventriculostomy in patients with cerebral hemorrhage.

Surgical options for increased ICP are subtemporal decompression, subfrontal decompressive craniectomy, internal decompression, or removal of existing bone flaps. In our experiences and that of others, these aggressive measures are of no use, and in virtually all instances, family members object. Corticosteroids do not improve outcome and can increase the risk of nonketotic hyperosmolar coma in an elderly patient. Emergency evacuation of a lobar hematoma in warfarin-associated hemorrhage is particularly unsuccessful in elderly patients (22).

BLOOD PRESSURE CONTROL

Blood pressure management in the elderly after a cerebral hemorrhage is very complicated. One study found that a significantly high blood pressure on admission and inadequate control negatively affected the prognosis of hypertensive cerebral hemorrhage (5). Marked blood pressure reduction may not be tolerated (particularly with use of propofol), and persistent blood pressure elevation can trigger congestive heart failure. Obviously, the goal is to decrease the blood pressure while avoiding hypoperfusion, but target levels are not known. It is recommended to use short-acting agents (e.g., labetalol or esmolol). It is prudent to gradually lower the blood pressure, probably not more than 10% to 20%. Nitroprusside should be avoided in patients with increased ICP because of its possible deleterious effects in the CPP (16).

Much more is known about long-term control of blood pressure. One prospective study investigated blood pressure control and recurrence of brain hemorrhage in 74 patients with hypertensive brain hemorrhage who were followed for 2.8 years (1). They compared different clinical parameters, including blood pressure, between patients with and without rebleeding and found that a higher diastolic blood pressure was associated with an increased rate of rebleeding.

SEIZURE CONTROL

The incidence of seizures with intracerebral hemorrhage is between 5% and 15%. It is the initial manifestation in 30% of patients with hemorrhage, and in the remaining 70%, seizure usually occurs within 72 hours. The seizures are commonly isolated and self-limited events. A higher incidence of seizures is seen with lobar hematomas. Predisposition to develop epilepsy is greater if the seizures present weeks after the ictus. Prophylaxis with anticonvulsants is not recommended in most patients with intracerebral hemorrhage. The concerns with pharmacodynamics in the elderly are outlined elsewhere in this text.

CORRECTION OF COAGULOPATHY

Warfarin-associated intracerebral hemorrhages in the elderly need immediate correction of the coagulopathy. However, treatment may be particularly difficult in the elderly with associated comorbidity. The use of fresh frozen plasma may result in a major osmotic challenge and result in rapidly developing pulmonary edema. Therefore, alternative drugs such as Recombinant factor VII may be safer. Correction of international normalized ratio (INR) with a low dose (40 μg/kg) is noted within an hour and typically safe. However, its use has been associated with thromboembolic complications and acute myocardial infarction. Moreover, a better outcome using recombinant activated factor VII has not been demonstrated. Its use should be considered for both traumatic and nontraumatic hemorrhages (8,15,17,21,28).

SURGICAL APPROACH

Surgical management of acute deep-seated cerebral hematoma does not result in a better outcome than medical supportive care (19). Nonetheless, clear indications for a surgical approach have been developed for superficially located hematoma. Thus, cerebellar and lobar hemorrhages are mostly considered.

In cerebellar hemorrhage, ventriculostomy followed by suboccipital craniotomy is recommended. In a retrospective study, both conscious and comatose patients benefited from immediate surgery because of risk of brainstem compression (7). In comatose patients on arrival, morbidity is greater, but a chance for recovery still exists. Bulbar dysfunction, bilateral gaze paresis, limb weakness, severe hypertension, and moderate to severe hydrocephalus are considered to be predictors of clinical deterioration in conscious patients.

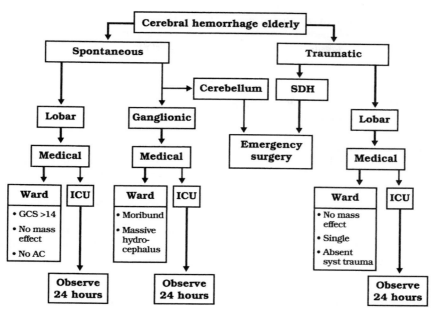

Figure 19-3. Flow chart showing triage and management of cerebral hemorrhage. SDH, subdural hematoma; ICU, intensive care unit; GCS, Glasgow Coma Scale; AC, anticoagulation.

One study suggested that, in lobar hemorrhage, a hematoma less than 20 mL in diameter could be approached conservatively, but those between 20 and 44 mL had better outcomes with surgery (13). In addition, their superficial location has a reduced risk of additional neurologic trauma than the already established deficit.

Cerebral amyloid angiopathy severity fluctuates from asymptomatic amyloid deposition to complete replacement and breakdown of vessel wall. Presumptive diagnosis is made in elderly patients with multiple lobar hemorrhages without apparent cause. The treatment in amyloid angiopathy is not different than any other type of cerebral hemorrhage. Anticoagulant or antiplatelet withdrawal is important for preventing cerebral amyloid angiopathy–related hemorrhage.

A surgical approach is typically needed for acute subdural hematoma. Management of chronic subdural hematoma depends on the size and the patient's reliability. If the hematoma is small and the patient is without neurologic deficits, surgery can be postponed. However, a recent study suggested that delayed deterioration in the elderly occurs, and thus, observation is frequently warranted (12).

The triage and initial management are shown in the flow chart in Figure 19-3.

PROGNOSIS

Prognosis is poor when the initial level of consciousness is reduced or the volume of hematoma exceeds 50 mL. Other important prognostic factors are severe hypertension on admission and failure to control blood pressure. The presence and duration of fever in patients who survive more than 72 hours is also associated with poor prognosis. Diringer et al. (6) recognized that hydrocephalus is an independent predictor of mortality after intracerebral hemorrhage.

A retrospective study was conducted at the Mayo Clinic to identify predictive features for poor neurologic outcome with cerebellar hematomas. In the study, 72 patients were enrolled for clinical and neuroimaging analysis. The presence of systolic pressure greater than 200 mm Hg, pinpoint pupils, abnormal corneal or oculocephalic reflexes, hematoma size more than 3 cm in diameter, hemorrhage extending in the vermis, brainstem distortion, intraventricular hemorrhage, upward herniation, and acute hydrocephalus were considered predictors of neurologic deterioration (25).

Another study recently analyzed patients with deep cerebral hemorrhage (putaminal hemorrhage and thalamic-caudate hemorrhage). Hydrocephalus was present in 40% of these patients, with a 30-day mortality rate of 29%. This trial concluded that a Glasgow Coma Scale score equal to or less than 8 and hydrocephalus were predictors of 30-day mortality. When to withdraw support or defer surgical intervention is determined by a reasonable period of observation (5 to 7 days in coma), expected disability (aphasia or ataxia), intervening systemic medical complication (aspiration pneumonitis or sepsis), and prior expressed wishes. Outcome of surgically managed subdural hematoma in the elderly depends on the ability to rapidly awaken postoperatively and early mobilization. Surprisingly, good results have been reported in anecdotal cases such as a 102-year-old patient (27).

CONCLUSION

The best care and management of intracerebral hematoma in the elderly is not well defined. Only generalizations apply. Prognosis is decisively worse in the elderly because an aggressive approach may not be permitted because of existing living wills. The harsh reality is that prolonged rehabilitation and care may not be adequately provided or funded in these patients who have lived to an old age.

REFERENCES

1. Arakawa S, Saku Y, Ibayashi S, et al. Blood pressure control and recurrence of hypertensive brain hemorrhage. *Stroke*. 1998;29:1806–1809.
2. Arboix A, Garcia-Eroles L, Massons J, et al. Acute stroke in very older people: clinical features and predictors of in-hospital mortality. *J Am Geriatr Soc*. 2000;48:36–41.
3. Bladin C, Alexandrov A, Bellavance A, et al. Seizures after stroke: a prospective multicenter study. *Arch Neurol*. 2000;57:1617–1622.
4. Cantalapiedra A, Gutierrez O, Tortosa J, et al. Oral anticoagulant treatment: risk factors involved in 500 intracranial hemorrhages. *J Thromb Thrombolysis*. 2006;22:113–120.
5. Dandapani B, Suzuki S, Kelley R, et al. Relation between blood pressure and outcome in intracerebral hemorrhage. *Stroke*. 1995;26:21–24.
6. Diringer M, Edwards D, Zazulia A. Hydrocephalus: a previously unrecognized predictor of poor outcome from supratentorial intracerebral hemorrhage. *Stroke*. 1998;29:1352–1357.
7. Dunne J, Chakera T, Kermode S. Cerebellar haemorrhage—diagnosis and treatment: a study of 75 consecutive cases. *Q J Med*. 1987;245:739–754.
8. Flaherty M, Kissela B, Woo D, et al. The increasing incidence of anticoagulant-associated intracerebral hemorrhage. *Neurology*. 2007;68:116–121.
9. Freeman W, Brott T, Barrett K, et al. Recombinant factor VIIa for rapid reversal of warfarin anticoagulation in acute intracranial hemorrhage. *Mayo Clin Proc*. 2004;79:1495–1500.
10. Greenberg S. Cerebral amyloid angiopathy: prospects for clinical diagnosis and treatment. *Neurology*. 1998;51:690–694.
11. Gujjar A, Deibert E, Manno E, et al. Mechanical ventilation for ischemic stroke and intracerebral hemorrhage: indications, timing, and outcome. *Neurology*. 1998;51:447–451.
12. Itshayek E, Rosenthal G, Fraidfeld S, et al. Delayed posttraumatic acute subdural hematoma in elderly patients on anticoagulation. *Neurosurgery*. 2006;58:E851–E856.
13. Kase C. Diagnosis and management of intracerebral hemorrhage in elderly patients. *Clin Geriatr Med*. 1991;7:549–567.
14. Kurtzke J. Epidemiology of cerebrovascular disease. In: McDowell F, Caplan L, eds. *Cerebrovascular survey report for the National Institute of Neurological and Communicative Disorders and Stroke*. Bethesda, MD: National Institute of Neurological and Communicative Disorders and Stroke; 1985:1–34.
15. MacLaren R, Weber L, Brake H, et al. A multicenter assessment of recombinant factor VIIa off-label usage: clinical experiences and associated outcomes. *Transfusion*. 2005;45:1434–1442.
16. Manno E, Atkinson J, Fulgham J, et al. Emerging medical and surgical management strategies in the evaluation and treatment of intracerebral hemorrhage. *Mayo Clin Proc*. 2005;80:420–433.
17. Mayer S. Recombinant activated factor VII for acute intracerebral hemorrhage. *Stroke*. 2007;38:763–767.
18. Mayo N, Nadeau L, Daskalopoulou S, et al. The evolution of stroke in Quebec: a 15-year perspective. *Neurology*. 2007;68:1122–1127.
19. Mendelow A, Gregson B, Fernandes H, et al. Early surgery versus initial conservative treatment in patients with spontaneous supratentorial intracerebral haematomas in the International Surgical Trial in Intracerebral Haemorrhage (STICH): a randomised trial. *Lancet*. 2005;365:389–397.
20. Node Y, Nakazawa S. Clinical study of mannitol and glycerol on raised intracranial pressure and on their rebound phenomenon. *Neurology*. 1990;52:359–363.
21. Park P, Fewel M, Garton H, et al. Recombinant activated factor VII for the rapid correction of coagulopathy in nonhemophilic neurosurgical patients. *Neurosurgery*. 2003;53:34–38.
22. Rabinstein AA, Wijdicks EFM. Determinants of outcome in anticoagulation-associated cerebral hematoma requiring emergency evacuation. *Arch Neurol*. 2007;64:203–206.
23. Rosand J, Muzikansky A, Kumar A, et al. Spatial clustering of hemorrhages in probably cerebral amyloid angiopathy. *Ann Neurol*. 2005;58:459–462.
24. Schutz H, Bodeker R, Damian M, et al. Age-related spontaneous intracerebral hematoma in a German community. *Stroke*. 1990;21:1412.
25. St. Louis E, Wijdicks EFM, Li H. Predicting neurologic deterioration in patients with cerebellar hematomas. *Neurology*. 1998;51:1364–1369.

26. Thanvi B, Robinson T. Sporadic cerebral amyloid angiopathy—an important cause of cerebral haemorrhage in older people. *Age Ageing*. 2006; 35:565–571.
27. Vyas N, Chicoine M. Extended survival after evacuation of subdural hematoma in a 102-year-old patient: case report and review of the literature. *Surg Neurol*. 2007;67:314–316.
28. White C, Schrank A, Baskin T, et al. Effects of recombinant activated factor VII in traumatic nonsurgical intracranial hemorrhage. *Curr Surg*. 2006;63:310–317.

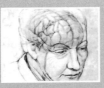

CHAPTER 20

Cognitive Effects of Head Trauma in the Older Adult

Laurie M. Ryan and Judith R. O'Jile

Head injury, a frequent occurrence in the United States and other industrialized nations, is the leading cause of brain injury. Centers for Disease Control and Prevention estimates suggest that at least 1.4 million people sustain a traumatic brain injury (TBI) per year in the United States. Of those, 50,000 result in death, 235,000 result in hospitalizations, and 1,111,000 result in emergency department visits (43). Severity of head injury varies, but most (70% to 90%) are mild (17,41), and most are closed or nonpenetrating (i.e., intact skull with no exposure of brain tissue) (46). Given the greater frequency of nonpenetrating head injury in general and particularly in older adults, this chapter focuses exclusively on the damage associated with closed head trauma. The terms head trauma, TBI, and head injury are used interchangeably.

Research in the area of geriatric head trauma remains somewhat limited. This chapter delineates the known information about geriatric head trauma and provides information regarding possible interventions. The incidence of head injury is related to age and gender, as well as other sociodemographic variables. Three age-related peaks of head injury occurrence seem to exist: ages 1 to 5, 15 to 24, and greater than 65 years; of these, the highest incidence rates are seen among people in the age range of 15 to 24 years (17,41,58). In terms of gender, males have consistently outnumbered females in rates of head injury among the younger age groups, but no gender differences are seen among older adults (11,12). In younger adults, motor vehicle accidents account for most head injuries, whereas in older adults, falls predominate. It has been estimated that over half of all head injuries in those over 65 years of age are the result of falls (13,14). The second most common cause of geriatric head injury appears to be motor vehicle accidents, with a larger proportion involving pedestrian injuries (58,76).

INJURY SEVERITY

Head injury is usually characterized as mild, moderate, or severe and is measured by a number of methods, including loss of consciousness (LOC), posttraumatic amnesia (PTA), and magnetic resonance imaging

(MRI) or computed tomography (CT). The length of LOC at the time of injury is often related to severity; however, it is now well established that brain injury can occur without complete LOC (2). Alteration of consciousness (AOC) or mental status (i.e., being dazed, disoriented, or confused) following head trauma is considered the minimal grade of concussion or cerebral injury (61). The Glasgow Coma Scale (GCS) (77) quantifies level of consciousness, ranging from alert to comatose, with scores of 13 to 15 (of a maximum score of 15) considered mild injury, scores of 9 to 12 considered moderate injury, and scores of 8 or less considered severe injury. PTA presupposes that the patient is alert and functioning and has recovered from the comatose state but has persistent, severe deficits in retaining new information and processing new memories (2). It is generally accepted that the greater the length of PTA, the greater the severity of the head injury. Moreover, patients with injuries classified as mild by GCS, LOC/AOC, or PTA but with evidence of intracranial pathology on neuroimaging are considered to have moderate injuries, although the term complicated mild TBI is also used.

Studies of young TBI patients have demonstrated that these severity markers (GCS score and duration of AOC/LOC and PTA) are related to both the initial degree of cognitive and behavioral deficits and to the level of recovery (44). However, the clinical utility of these severity markers to predict outcome in older adults may be more variable. Goldstein and Levin (24) demonstrated that GCS and the presence of intracranial pathology were more strongly related to outcome than duration of LOC or PTA in older adults. The authors suggest that these results may reflect measurement issues because older adults are more likely to be injured in low-velocity falls and have delayed complications where LOC/PTA may not occur and/or be very brief or may be difficult to assess by the time the older individual gets medical attention. The differential clinical presentation of older adults with head trauma is discussed later in this chapter.

Structural neuroimaging techniques (MRI or CT) can provide additional information to help in the estimation of injury severity. Neuroradiographic evidence of abnormality (i.e., edema, hemorrhage, and any other structural lesion) can suggest a greater level of severity of injury than indicated by PTA or LOC alone (2). Functional neuroimaging methods, including single photon emission CT (SPECT) and positron emission tomography (PET), may be more sensitive to cerebral dysfunction after TBI and identify areas of abnormality that appear intact with structural imaging. McAllister et al. (55) reviewed the literature on neuroimaging and mild TBI and noted that SPECT is more sensitive than structural imaging for the identification of cerebral dysfunction. Similarly, PET may have increased sensitivity over CT or structural MRI. Therefore, it is important to realize that no one neuroimaging technique can identify all of the neuropathophysiologic processes of TBI.

PATHOLOGY

A large body of evidence indicates that neuropathologic changes occur with even mild head injury. Mild head injury represents the low end of a spectrum where pathologic changes increase as the severity of injury increases (10). In all head injuries, mechanical force to the head, either through direct impact or acceleration-deceleration motion, leads to a rapid displacement of the skull, which, if sufficiently severe, can cause differential motion between the brain and skull. The path of head motion, the anatomic surfaces surrounding the brain, and the violence of the motion determine the severity of displacement. Deformation of brain tissue is a result of such displacement and is thought to be the primary factor in traumatic brain damage. Cerebral deformation can result in structural alterations of neurons such as axonal and cytoskeletal injury, vascular changes (e.g., contusions and hemorrhage), generation of oxygen radicals, and excessive neural depolarization causing abnormal neurochemical agonist-receptor interactions related to excitotoxic processes (10). Evidence suggests that changes in muscarinic, nicotinic, and N-methyl-D-aspartic acid (NMDA) glutamate receptors are involved (34,82). Such neurochemical alterations may play a role in the behavioral changes associated with head injury.

Diffuse axonal injury has been demonstrated in clinical and laboratory studies of head injury and seems to be a consistent feature of all injuries, regardless of severity, with the distribution and number of axons involved increasing with injury severity (66). Povlishock et al. (65) found that axonal changes occurred without the presence of focal parenchymal or vascular damage even in mild head injuries. The traditional notion held that axons are physically torn at the time of injury. However, it appears that this is not true in most cases, except in severe injuries with high physical stress (19,67). It is now known that focal

alteration of the axon membrane occurs after TBI. This membrane alteration results in progressive changes that disrupt axonal transport, subsequently leading to focal swelling. This swelling then leads to the collapse and detachment of the axon at the point of swelling and can take from several hours to several days after trauma. Moreover, impaired axonal transport leads to the production and accumulation of toxic proteins, peptides, and their aggregates, some of which have been implicated in the pathology of neurodegenerative disorders including Alzheimer's disease (AD). In particular, the accumulation of amyloid precursor protein (APP) and beta-amyloid peptides found in AD has been observed in damaged axons after TBI in animals and in human brain tissue (74).

Orbitofrontal and anterior temporal regions are particularly vulnerable to contusions, lacerations, abrasions, hematomas, and intercerebral hemorrhages caused by forceful contact with the rough bony surface of the skull in these areas during head injury (47,51,80). In addition, diffuse axonal damage can disrupt frontal pathways to other cortical and subcortical regions, including the limbic system. Damage to these regions has been linked to deficits in complex neurocognitive functioning, including attention, memory, and emotional changes (51).

With aging, a greater risk exists for postinjury neurologic changes, including subdural hematomas, intracranial hemorrhage, and posttraumatic infections. Older adults are at increased risk for subdural hematoma because brain atrophy increases the distance between the brain surface and the venous sinuses. Bridging veins are more vulnerable to rupture, increasing the risk of subdural bleeds, even with less severe or seemingly trivial injuries (1,8,39). Subdural hematomas are also common consequences of falls (12), the most common cause of TBI for those aged 65 years and older. Older adults with head injuries may have a delayed presentation for medical care, even hours to days or weeks to months after a TBI. Acute subdural hematomas (clinically evident within 72 hours) usually occur in younger adults, whereas chronic subdural hematomas (>20 days old) usually occur in older adults, with a peak incidence in the sixth and seventh decades of life (39).

DIFFERENTIAL CLINICAL PRESENTATION IN THE OLDER ADULT

The clinical presentation of older individuals with head trauma can differ from that of younger adults because of differences in demography (e.g., live alone, no close family or friends), etiology, and prevalence of comorbidity (15). The course of the geriatric patient can be further complicated by comorbid medical or neurologic disease (e.g., cardiovascular disease, dementia, diabetes, or chronic obstructive pulmonary disease). Falls are a major cause of morbidity and mortality in older individuals (79). Moreover, falls themselves are often the result of comorbid medical conditions. Coronado et al. (7) found that older adults hospitalized for a TBI-related fall had a greater number of comorbid medical conditions than those with TBI secondary to motor vehicle crashes. Falls were more likely in individuals with gait disturbance, dizziness, history of stroke, decreased visual acuity, cognitive impairment, and postural hypotension. In addition, polypharmacy, which is common in older adults, and medications with psychotropic effects also put individuals at greater risk for falls.

In contrast to younger patients, an older person may fall, lose consciousness, and not be brought for medical treatment until they are found unconscious or confused or they recover enough to call for help themselves. Alternatively, an older patient may gradually develop a subdural hematoma after a relatively minor injury. Such a patient may present as much as 3 months after the onset of mental status changes and even longer after the injury (35,81). As Flanagan et al. (14) noted, clinicians should keep an "index of suspicion" regarding TBI when seeing an older patient with a history of cognitive changes that have occurred over a period of weeks to months. In addition, urgent orthopaedic or other medical problems may supersede or even prevent recognition of the TBI. Common situations include hip fractures with head trauma or head trauma from a fall precipitated by a medical problem such as syncope. Even when head trauma is recognized, severity can be difficult to assess because the medical problems may contribute to the altered mental status. Finally, older individuals may present with a chronic progressive cognitive impairment and disability; for example, an older patient with pre-existing dementia may be brought to medical attention by family or friends because of a rapid change in their ability to perform day-to-day activities. Although evidence of physical trauma may be seen, the patient may be unable to provide details. In such a case, head trauma should be suspected as contributing to or exacerbating the patient's pre-existing cognitive difficulties (e.g., dementia) (15).

OVERALL COGNITIVE OUTCOME

In general, both injury severity and the patient's age at the time of injury influence the cognitive outcome following head injury. With increasing age is seen increasing risk of negative outcome as well as greater risk for mortality (63,68,69,79). The cognitive effects of a closed head injury emerge after resolution of PTA

and have been well documented in younger patients (47,54). Although the deficits observed vary with injury severity, they generally include problems with executive and attention functions (e.g., concentration, speed of information processing, mental flexibility, problem solving), memory, and aspects of language such as naming. These cognitive deficits are found within the overall context of diffuse cerebral injury and, in particular, injury to frontal and temporal areas. Each of the cognitive domains and associated functions is discussed in the following sections.

EXECUTIVE AND ATTENTION FUNCTIONING

Executive functions refer to those higher level cognitive abilities that enable an individual to successfully engage in independent goal-directed behavior and are associated with frontal brain systems. Initiation of action, planning and organization, problem solving, information processing, and self-monitoring are all part of executive functioning. Diffuse injury is often manifested by diminished mental speed, concentration, cognitive efficiency, and higher level reasoning abilities. Related to these decreased abilities, patient complaints include distractibility, difficulty performing more than one task at a time, confusion and perplexity in thinking, irritability, fatigue, and increased effort to perform even simple tasks (20,47). Such problems are easily identified on a neuropsychological examination but otherwise may be misinterpreted as the onset of dementia. For example, slowed speed of mental processing can result in significantly lowered scores on timed tests, despite the capacity to perform the required task accurately (47). In general, patients with diffuse damage perform relatively poorly on measures requiring concentration and working memory (i.e., limited-capacity memory system where material is held temporarily while it is manipulated for complex cognitive tasks such as learning and reasoning). Tasks involving these abilities include mental arithmetic, serial calculations, and reasoning problems (31). In addition, mental inflexibility is problematic, as evidenced by disturbed behavioral or conceptual shifting in response to changing circumstances (45).

It should be noted that patients with mental efficiency problems frequently interpret their slowed processing and attentional deficits as memory problems, even when recall is intact. Although they report memory loss, analysis of their neuropsychological performance often indicates reduced auditory attention span and difficulty with divided attention and verbal retrieval problems rather than true problems retaining information. Many patients are acutely aware of these cognitive difficulties and try to use various strategies to compensate. One such strategy is a continual rechecking of their actions (46).

With the most severe injuries, additional executive deficits often include impaired capacity for self-determination, self-direction, and self-control and regulation, all of which depend on intact awareness of oneself and the environment. Such impairments are often the most crippling and most intractable disorders to remediate. Compromised self-awareness is reflected in diminished insight, which can lead to dysfunctional social interactions but, more importantly, to increased safety risks when unsupervised. For example, geriatric head-injured patients with poor insight and other cognitive dysfunction may leave food cooking unattended on the stove or wander away from familiar places when taking a walk. Perseveration in thoughts and behavioral responses is typical and can compromise both cognitive and social functioning. Often, patients have the ability to perform tasks, but their ability to initiate actions or to plan and choose alternatives is impaired. It is these types of deficits that often account for the poor outcome and lack of independence seen in severely injured patients (47).

MEMORY

Following traumatic head injury, complaints of learning and memory dysfunction are common, with problems usually found in the acquisition and retrieval of information. Patients may have difficulty learning information, but once encoded, the information is generally retained. However, patients may also have problems retrieving material from memory once it has been stored (31). Thus, patients tend to perform better on recognition or with cueing than from free recall. In addition, because of cerebral lateralization of functions, verbal and visual memory can be affected differentially in the presence of focal injuries (e.g., contusion or hematoma) to the brain, depending on the location. Left-sided injuries often result in problems with verbal memory, and right-sided lesions are often associated with nonverbal memory deficits. In very severe injuries, memory can be affected to such an extent that new learning is almost completely disrupted. However, even in these cases, procedural memory (e.g., skill learning) is typically preserved (47).

LANGUAGE

Classic aphasia syndromes are atypical after closed head injury, except when associated with focal lesions (47). However, a decline can be seen in certain language abilities, typically including defective or slowed naming and word-finding problems that lead to circumlocution and semantic word substitutions. Circumlocution involves using an unnecessarily large number of words to express an idea. Semantic word substitution refers to the use of a word that is within the category that one wants to convey but is not the exact word (e.g., using the word "toy" instead of

"ball"). Even with more mild injuries, a breakdown in the ability to effectively communicate and understand thoughts and ideas (i.e., linguistic competence) can also occur and affects the pragmatic aspects of language. Pragmatic language skills include conversational turn taking, gestures, loudness of speech, verbal appropriateness, making inferences, and understanding humor (75).

COGNITIVE SEQUELAE OF HEAD TRAUMA IN THE OLDER ADULT

Compared to the extensive literature on the cognitive sequelae of head injury in younger adults, the data remain relatively limited for older adults. Research to date does suggest that deficits experienced by older individuals after head injury are similar to those of younger adults (12,22,25,36). Goldstein et al. (27) examined the neurocognitive effects of head injury in adults aged 50 years and older who were relatively early in the recovery process (<7 months). Injury severity ranged from mild to moderate. These subjects were found to have deficits in memory, verbal fluency, naming, and reasoning. The pattern of deficits observed in the older subjects was similar to that typically seen in younger TBI survivors. Goldstein et al. (26) also investigated the effect of mild versus moderate TBI on early cognitive outcome in older adults without premorbid histories of neurologic or psychiatric disturbance. These investigators sought to determine whether there was a dose-response relationship between the severity of injury and degree of cognitive deficit. Eighteen patients (mean age, 62.3 years; range, 50 to 79 years) sustained mild head injuries with GCS scores of 13 to 15, LOC <20 minutes, and normal neurologic and neuroimaging findings. Seventeen patients (mean age, 65.2; range, 50 to 78 years) sustained moderate head injuries; four of these patients obtained GCS scores between 9 and 11, and 13 patients had GCS scores of 13 to 15 but with evidence of intracranial contusions and hematomas. A control group of 14 community residents was also tested. The neuropsychological test performance of the mild TBI patients did not significantly differ from the controls except on a measure of verbal fluency. In contrast, the performance of the moderate TBI patients was significantly worse than that of controls and mild TBI patients. Mild TBI patients performed significantly better than the moderate TBI patients on almost all of the cognitive measures assessing attention, executive functioning, memory, and language. These results are consistent with earlier findings by Goldstein et al. (28) that demonstrated that a single uncomplicated mild head injury did not result in clinically significant cognitive deficits at 2 months after injury in a group of high-functioning older individuals without history of previous psychiatric or neurologic conditions.

Prospective studies investigating the long-term cognitive recovery from TBI in older adults are even more lacking. Only recently have the results of a longitudinal study been published. Rapoport et al. (69) examined the effects of TBI 1 year after injury on cognition and functioning in older adults with mild to moderate TBI but without premorbid history of neurologic, psychiatric, or other serious medical illness. The TBI patients were compared with an age-, gender-, and education-matched healthy control group. There were 69 subjects aged 50 years and older with TBI and 79 healthy control subjects. There were significant differences in cognitive functioning between the patients and controls at 1 year. Patients with TBI showed poorer attention, verbal memory, naming, and executive functioning compared with controls. The differences noted were between the moderate TBI patients and controls but not between the mild patients and controls. Thus these investigators also found a dose-response relationship with injury severity.

FUNCTIONAL OUTCOME IN THE OLDER ADULT

On the whole, a negative relationship appears to exist between age and functional and psychosocial outcome after TBI. Advancing age at the time of injury is associated with increased long-term disability (63,76,79). In one sample of head-injured elderly, 72% of survivors had experienced a change in functional status that necessitated increased family involvement and use of community support services (87). Similarly, studies (12,13) have shown that older adults who have sustained a significant head injury are less likely to be discharged from the hospital to their home and are more likely to be placed in a nursing home. Rothweiler et al. (70) found that a significantly greater proportion of older individuals who had been hospitalized for their injuries were rated as disabled compared with younger adults at 1 year after injury. Persons 60 years and older were more disabled than those under 50, and those from 30 to 49 years were more disabled than those under 30 years old. Significantly fewer older adults returned to their former living status 1 year after injury compared with younger adults, with most requiring a more supervised living environment. For those employed before the injury, a smaller percentage of those individuals over 50 returned to work. It is noteworthy that, although increasing dependence is associated with increasing age, variability in functional outcome was marked in the older sample. Older individuals showed

a greater range of outcomes, from good outcome in 20% of the sample to death in 32%. A more recent multicenter prospective study of patients hospitalized for TBI (57) found that, although older patients (aged 65 and older) had a higher mean GCS score (14.1 vs. 12.5 for the younger patients), they required more inpatient rehabilitation and lagged behind the younger patients in rate of recovery. However, the older patients did show continued improvement at 6 months after discharge, and the majority of those with milder injuries were able to live independently.

Individuals sustaining TBI, particularly milder injuries, often report a constellation of physical, cognitive, and emotional/behavioral symptoms referred to as postconcussion symptoms (PCSs). The most commonly reported PCSs are headache, dizziness, decreased concentration, memory problems, irritability, fatigue, visual disturbances, sensitivity to noise, judgment problems, depression, and anxiety. Although PCSs often resolve within a month or so after mild injuries, in some individuals, PCSs can persist from months to years following injury and may even cause permanent disability. Age is a risk factor for persistent PCSs such that older individuals who sustain a head injury are at greater risk of developing persisting problems [see review by Ryan and Warden (71)].

HEAD TRAUMA AND ALZHEIMER'S DISEASE

DIFFERENTIAL COGNITIVE EFFECTS OF HEAD TRAUMA AND ALZHEIMER'S DISEASE

Cognitive deficits observed in head-injured older patients may reflect premorbid dementia, a magnification of such a pre-existing condition, or the sequelae of head trauma. Without a good history, it is often difficult to differentiate the cause of a cognitive disturbance in older individuals. As previously noted, although falls are the primary cause of head injury, cognitive dysfunction (e.g., dementia) itself can be a predisposing factor for falls (49). Differential diagnosis is further complicated by overlap in cognitive symptoms in head injury and dementing disorders, including difficulties with memory, verbal fluency, and naming (22,29). Research comparing the neuropsychological test performance of subjects with dementia and subjects with head injury suggests that the cognitive effects of head injury in older adults can be differentiated from those of dementia.

Older head-injured subjects have been shown to perform better than a group of subjects with mild dementia on measures of verbal memory and executive functioning (90). Furthermore, there are qualitative differences between these groups such that memory deficits appear to be related to retrieval deficits in head injury and encoding problems in AD (29). Thus, individuals who have TBI show an ability to learn and retain newly learned information over time, although at a reduced level, whereas learning and retention are impaired in individuals with AD (14).

HEAD TRAUMA AS A RISK FACTOR FOR ALZHEIMER'S DISEASE

TBI has been shown to be a risk factor for AD and other neurodegenerative disorders and, as noted earlier, is associated with pathologic processes found in AD. However, the exact nature of the relationship between head trauma and AD is still unclear. It has been hypothesized that *apolipoprotein E (ApoE) ε4*, a genetic risk factor for AD, acts synergistically with TBI to increase risk. Mayeux et al. (52) found a 10-fold increase in the risk for AD in individuals with the *ApoE ε4* allele compared with those who lacked both the *ApoE ε4* allele and TBI. A more recent study (40) examined the association between *ApoE ε4* genotype and psychiatric disorders in 60 subjects with a history of TBI (an average of 30 years prior). Dementia was significantly more common in those with the *ApoE ε4* genotype, whereas the occurrence of other psychiatric disorders did not differ. Furthermore, animal studies have demonstrated increased beta-amyloid deposition in mice expressing human *ApoE ε4* (33) after TBI.

Severity of head injury may also play a role in increasing the risk of AD. A large case-controlled study (32) that was part of the Multi-Institutional Research in Alzheimer's Genetic Epidemiology Project (MIRAGE) found that the risk of AD for those with head injury with LOC was double that of those with head injury without LOC. This suggests that the magnitude of risk was proportional to head injury severity. Moreover, even head injury without LOC significantly increased the risk of AD in first-degree relatives of patients with the disease, suggesting a link between head injury without LOC and family history. However, this study did not find an increased risk of AD for those with both a history of head injury and *ApoE ε4*.

Recently, Luukinen et al. (48) completed a large 9-year population-based study among cognitively intact older adults that examined the relationship between the occurrence of fall-related TBI and risk of dementia. A representative sample of 325 persons aged 70 years or older was followed. At the end of the follow-up, 152 persons were examined for dementia. TBI, mild or moderate, was associated with the diagnosis of dementia and with a younger age at the time of detection of the dementia (hazard ratio = 3.56; 95% confidence interval, 1.35 to 9.34) even after adjusting for sex and educational status. Moreover, the effect of TBI and *ApoE ε4* appeared synergistic (hazard ratio = 7.68; 95% confidence interval, 2.32 to 25.3). These results are consistent with earlier findings suggesting reduced time to onset of AD with TBI (18,59).

TREATMENT

COGNITIVE REHABILITATION

Research investigating cognitive rehabilitation of the older head-injured patient remains limited. The rehabilitation studies to date suggest that older persons do demonstrate functional improvement, albeit at a slower rate and subsequently greater cost (6,16,21,57). Even patients with head injury and progressive neurodegenerative disorders such as AD have been found to benefit from cognitive remediation strategies using standard mnemonic techniques (30). Although the data are limited, given the apparent efficacy for even these more impaired individuals, cognitive rehabilitation should be considered for older head-injured persons (Fig. 20-1). For a recent evidence-based review of the cognitive rehabilitation literature, see the article by Cicerone et al. (5).

PHARMACOLOGIC INTERVENTIONS
Psychostimulants

Psychostimulants are probably the most commonly used medication in the treatment of attentional problems following head injury, although no studies have been conducted solely on older head-injured subjects (Table 20-1; Fig. 20-1). A recent evidence-based review of the literature on the pharmacologic treatment of cognitive disorders after TBI (60) recommended the use of methylphenidate at the guideline level for the treatment of deficits in attention and speed of processing. Psychostimulant medications (e.g., methylphenidate) increase activity in the catecholamine system, which is one of the neurotransmitter systems disturbed in TBI (50,88). Placebo-controlled studies suggest that methylphenidate can result in significantly greater improvement in attention and speed of information processing compared with the improvement expected from natural recovery and is generally well tolerated by patients (23,37,85,86). Again, it is important to note that none of these studies focused on older head-injured patients.

Dopaminergic Agents

Dopaminergic agents have also been used to improve cognitive functioning in patients with head injury, although once again, no studies have examined older head-injured subjects as a group (Table 20-1; Fig. 20-1). The rationale for the use of dopaminergic medications is based on the finding of lowered levels of dopamine metabolites following TBI. Moreover, dopamine is important for frontal system functioning, which is often affected in TBI (4,62). Investigations of dopaminergic medications have included amantadine and bromocriptine. Of the studies done, many have been small case series.

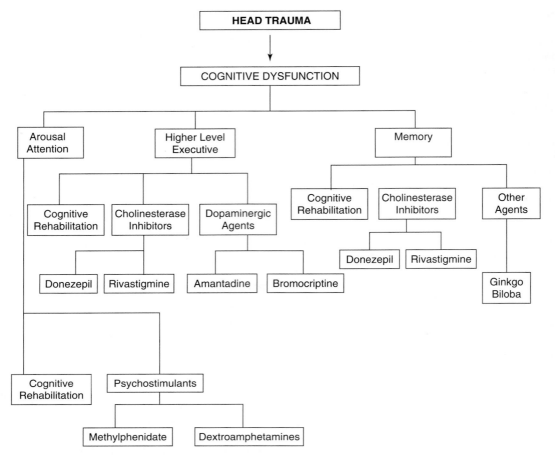

Figure 20-1. Treatment of cognitive dysfunction following head trauma.

In their recent evidence-based review, the Neurobehavioral Guidelines Working Group (60) recommended the use of bromocriptine to enhance aspects of executive functioning. The one randomized controlled trial noted by this group was a study by McDowell et al. (56) that found that bromocriptine was effective in improving executive functioning in severely head-injured patients.

In addition to the dopaminergic effects of amantadine, it is an NMDA glutamate receptor antagonist and, as such, might provide a protective effect against excitotoxic release following head trauma (83). In a study (42) examining the efficacy of amantadine in the treatment of cognitive and behavioral sequelae of brain injury patients at least 1 year after injury, all patients showed some degree of positive response in executive functions to amantadine based on improved neuropsychological test performance. A recent case study by Wu and Garmel (89) reported improved functioning in an 82-year-old woman who sustained a

severe TBI (GCS = 6) after being struck by a motor vehicle while crossing the street.

Cholinesterase Inhibitors
Similar to AD, cholinergic dysfunction has also been found in TBI, raising the question of possible usefulness of cholinesterase inhibitors such as donepezil as a treatment for cognitive dysfunction associated with head injury (Table 20-1; Fig. 20-1) (72). The recent evidence-based review by the Neurobehavioral Guidelines Working Group (60) recommended the use of donepezil to enhance aspects of memory and attention after moderate to severe TBI. A recent randomized, placebo-controlled, cross-over trial (91) demonstrated improvement in memory and attention with donepezil in patients with moderate to severe TBI who were 2 to 24 months post injury. Moreover, patients who received donepezil in the first phase sustained cognitive improvement in the placebo phase. Tenovuo (78) reported that TBI patients with chronic sequelae were treated with

Table 20-1. *Cognitive-Enhancing Medications*

Drug Type	Medication	Cognitive Indications	Medical Contraindications
Psychostimulants:	Methylphenidate	Arousal/attention deficits	Motor tics, Tourette, family history of Tourette, significant anxiety, tension, agitation, glaucoma, hypersensitivity to methylphenidate
	Dextroamphetamines	Same as above	Advanced arteriosclerosis, symptomatic cardiovascular disease, moderate to severe hypertension, hyperthyroidism, hypersensitivity to sympathomimetic amines, glaucoma, agitation, history of drug abuse, MAO inhibitor use. *Cautions:* Mild hypertension, Tourette
Dopaminergic Agents:	Amantadine	Frontal-executive dysfunction	Renal dysfunction, hypersensitivity to amantadine. *Cautions:* Seizures, CHF, peripheral edema, liver disease, orthostatic hypertension, psychosis, CNS stimulant use
	Bromocriptine	Same as above	Uncontrolled hypertension, hypersensitivity to ergot alkaloids, pregnancy. *Cautions:* Renal disease, liver disease
Cholinesterase Inhibitors:	Donepezil	Memory and attention	Hypersensitivity to donepezil or piperidine derivatives. *Cautions:* Supraventricular cardiac conduction conditions, ulcers, asthma, COPD, seizures
	Rivastigmine	Same as above	Hypersensitivity to rivastigmine or carbamate derivatives. *Cautions:* Same as above
Other Cognitive Agents:	Ginkgo biloba	Same as above	No known. *Cautions:* Anticoagulant or NSAID use

MOA, monoamine oxidase; CHF, congestive heart failure; CNS, central nervous system; COPD, chronic obstructive pulmonary disease; NSAID, nonsteroidal anti-inflammatory drug.

cholinesterase inhibitors, donepezil, galantamine, or rivastigmine in a clinical setting. A majority of patients (61%) had a significant positive response, whereas 39% of patients had a modest or no response. Of the responders, most had improved attention. There were no significant differences between the three drugs regarding effect or tolerability. A very recent randomized controlled trial of rivastigmine demonstrated that the drug was safe and well tolerated in patients with TBI and effective in improving aspects of cognition in a subgroup of patients with moderate to severe chronic memory deficits (73).

Other Cognitive Enhancers

Ginkgo biloba, a botanical supplement, has been found in a number of studies to show multiple pharmacologic effects on neuronal functioning, including improved glucose metabolism, antioxidant effects, increased acetylcholine synthesis and release, and an increase in cholinergic receptors (84). Results of initial trials comparing ginkgo biloba extract (EGb 761) and cholinesterase inhibitors, including donepezil, suggest similar efficacy between the treatments on cognitive symptom progression in patients with AD (53,84). A large-scale, placebo-controlled, randomized clinical trial evaluating ginkgo biloba to prevent dementia with over 3,000 subjects aged 75 and older is currently underway (9) (Table 20-1; Fig. 20-1).

Vitamin E is a powerful antioxidant, and preclinical and epidemiology studies suggested that it may be useful in treating and/or preventing cognitive decline/dementia. However, recent randomized placebo-controlled trials have failed to show benefit (38,64), and a recent meta-analysis of randomized antioxidant prevention trials showed increased risk of mortality with vitamin E (3).

REFERENCES

1. Adhiyaman V, Asghar M, Ganeshram KN, et al. Chronic subdural haematoma in the elderly. *Postgrad Med J*. 2002;78:71–75.
2. Bigler ED. Neuropathology of traumatic brain injury. In: Bigler ED, ed. *Traumatic brain injury: mechanisms of damage, assessment, intervention, and outcome*. Austin: Pro-Ed Inc.; 1990:13–49.
3. Bjelakovic G, Nikolova D, Gluud LL, et al. Mortality in randomized trials of antioxidant supplements for primary and secondary prevention: systematic review and meta-analysis. *JAMA*. 2007;297:842–857.
4. Brown RM, Crane AM, Goldman PS. Regional distribution of monoamines in the cerebral cortex and subcortical structures of the rhesus monkey: concentrations and in vivo synthesis rates. *Brain Res*. 1979;168:133–150.
5. Cicerone KD, Dahlberg C, Malec JF, et al. Evidence-based cognitive rehabilitation: updated review of the literature from 1998 through 2002. *Arch Phys Med Rehabil*. 2005;86:1681–1692.
6. Cifu DX, Kreutzer JS, Marwitz JH, et al. Functional outcomes of older adults with traumatic brain injury: a prospective, multicenter analysis. *Arch Phys Med Rehabil*. 1996;77:883–888.
7. Coronado VG, Thomas KE, Sattin RW, et al. The CDC Traumatic Brain Injury Surveillance System: characteristics of persons aged 65 years and older hospitalized with a TBI. *J Head Trauma Rehabil*. 2005;20:215–228.
8. Cummings JL, Benson DF. *Dementia: A Clinical Approach*. 2nd ed. Stoneham, MA: Butterworth-Heinemann; 1992.
9. DeKosky ST, Fitzpatrick A, Ives DG, et al. The Ginkgo Evaluation of Memory (GEM) study: design and baseline data of a randomized trial of ginkgo biloba extract in prevention of dementia. *Contemp Clin Trials*. 2006;27:238–253.
10. Dixon CE, Taft WC, Hayes RL. Mechanisms of mild traumatic brain injury. *J Head Trauma Rehabil*. 1993;8:1–12.
11. Ferell RV, Tanev KS. Traumatic brain injury in older adults. *Curr Psychiatry Rep*. 2002;4:354–362.
12. Fields RB. Geriatric head injury. In: Nussbaum PD, ed. *Handbook of neuropsychology and aging*. New York: Plenum Press; 1997:281–297.
13. Fife D, Faich G, Hollinshead W, et al. Incidence and outcome of hospital-treated head injury in Rhode Island. *Am J Public Health*. 1986;76:773–778.
14. Flanagan SR, Hibbard MR, Reardon B, et al. Traumatic brain injury in the elderly: diagnostic and treatment challenges. *Clin Geriatr Med*. 2006;22:449–468.
15. Fogel BS, Duffy J. Elderly patients. In: Silver J, Udosfky SC, Hales RE, eds. *Neuropsychiatry of traumatic brain injury*. Washington, DC: American Psychiatric Press; 1994:412–441.
16. Frankel JE, Marwitz JH, Cifu DX, et al. A follow-up study of older adults with traumatic brain injury: taking into account decreasing length of stay. *Arch Phys Med Rehabil*. 2006;87:57–62.
17. Frankowski RF. Descriptive epidemiologic studies of head injury in the United States: 1974–1983. *Adv Psychosom Med*. 1986;16:153–172.
18. Gedye A, Beattie BL, Tuokko H, et al. Severe head injury hastens age of onset of Alzheimer's disease. *J Am Geriatr Soc*. 1989;37:970–973.
19. Gennarelli TA, Graham DI. Neuropathology. In: Silver JM, McAllister TW, Yudofsky SC, eds. *Textbook of traumatic brain injury*. Washington, DC: American Psychiatric Publishing; 2005:27–50.
20. Gentilini N, Nichelli P, Schoenhuber R. Assessment of attention in mild head injury.

In: Levin HS, Eisenberg HM, Benton AL, eds. *Mild head injury.* New York: Oxford University Press; 1989:163–175.

21. Gershkoff AM, Cifu DX, Means KM. Geriatric rehabilitation: social, attitudinal, and economic factors. *Arch Phys Med Rehabil.* 1993;74 (suppl):S402–S405.

22. Ginsberg JP, Long CJ. Acceleration of age-related decline in neuropsychological performance after recovery from severe traumatic brain injury. *Arch Clin Neuropsychol.* 1996;11:394.

23. Glenn MB. Methylphenidate for cognitive and behavioral dysfunction after traumatic brain injury. *J Head Trauma Rehabil.* 1998;13:87–90.

24. Goldstein FC, Levin HS. Cognitive outcome after mild and moderate traumatic brain injury in older adults. *J Clin Exp Neuropsychol.* 2001;23:739–753.

25. Goldstein FC, Levin HS, Goldman WP, et al. Cognitive and behavioral sequelae of closed head injury in older adults according to their significant others. *J Neuropsychiatry Clin Neurosci.* 1999; 11:38–44.

26. Goldstein FC, Levin HS, Goldman WP, et al. Cognitive and neurobehavioral functioning after mild and moderate traumatic brain injury. *J Int Neuropsychol Soc.* 2001;7:373–383.

27. Goldstein FC, Levin HS, Presley RM, et al. Neurobehavioral consequences of closed head injury in older adults. *J Neurol Neurosurg Psychiatry.* 1994;57:961–966.

28. Goldstein FC, Levin HS, Roberts VJ, et al. Neurocognitive recovery in older adults with closed head injury. *J Int Neuropsychol Soc.* 2000; 6:183.

29. Goldstein FC, Levin HS, Roberts VJ, et al. Neuropsychological effects of closed head injury in older adults: a comparison with Alzheimer's disease. *Neuropsychology.* 1996;10:147–154.

30. Gouvier WD, Ryan LM, O'Jile JR, et al. Cognitive retraining with brain-damaged patients. In: Wedding D, Horton A, Webster J, eds. *The neuropsychology handbook: clinical and behavioral perspectives.* Vol. 2. 2nd ed. New York: Springer Publishing; 1997:3–46.

31. Gronwall D, Wrightson P. Memory and information processing capacity after closed head injury. *J Neurol Neurosurg Psychiatry.* 1981;44:889–895.

32. Guo Z, Cupples LA, Kurz A, et al. Head injury and the risk of AD in the MIRAGE study. *Neurology.* 2000;54:1316–1323.

33. Hartman RE, Laurer H, Longhi L, et al. Apolipoprotein E4 influences amyloid deposition but not cell loss after traumatic brain injury in a mouse model of Alzheimer's disease. *J Neuosci.* 2002;22:10083–10087.

34. Hayes RL, Jenkins LW, Lyeth BG. Neurotransmitter-mediated mechanisms of traumatic brain injury: acetylcholine and excitatory amino acids. *J Neurotrauma.* 1992;9[Suppl 1]:173–187.

35. Jennett B. Head injuries. In: *Neurological disorders in the elderly.* Littleton, MA: John Wright and Sons; 1982:202–211.

36. Johnstone B, Childers MK, Hoerner J. The effects of normal ageing on neuropsychological functioning following traumatic brain injury. *Brain Inj.* 1998;12:569–576.

37. Kaelin DL, Cifu DX, Matthies B. Methylphenidate effect on attention deficit in the acutely brain-injured adult. *Arch Phys Med Rehabil.* 1996;77:6–9.

38. Kang JH, Cook N, Manson J, et al. A randomized trial of vitamin E supplementation and cognitive function in women. *Arch Intern Med.* 2006;166:2462–2468.

39. Karnath B. Subdural hematoma: presentation and management in older adults. *Geriatrics.* 2004; 58:18–23.

40. Koponen S, Taiminen T, Kairisto V, et al. APOE-ε-4 predicts dementia but not other psychiatric disorders after traumatic brain injury. *Neurology.* 2004;63:749–750.

41. Kraus JF, Chu LD. Epidemiology. In: Silver JM, McAllister TW, Yudofsky SC, eds. *Textbook of traumatic brain injury.* Washington, DC: American Psychiatric Publishing; 2005:3–26.

42. Kraus MF, Maki PM. Effect of amantadine hydrochloride on symptoms of frontal lobe dysfunction in brain injury: case studies and review. *J Neuropsychiatr Clin Neurosci.* 1997;9:222–230.

43. Langlois JA, Rutland-Brown W, Thomas KE. Traumatic brain injury in the United States: emergency department visits, hospitalizations, and deaths. Atlanta: Centers for Disease Control and Prevention, National Center for Injury Prevention and Control; 2006.

44. Levin HS. Prediction of recovery from traumatic brain injury. *J Neurotrauma.* 1995;12:913–922.

45. Levin HS, Goldstein FC, Williams DH, et al. The contribution of frontal lobe lesions to the neurobehavioral outcome of closed head injury. In: Levin HS, Eisenberg HM, Benton AL, eds. *Frontal lobe function and dysfunction.* New York: Oxford University Press; 1991:318–337.

46. Lezak MD. *Neuropsychological Assessment.* 3rd ed. New York: Oxford University Press; 1995.

47. Lezak MD, Howieson DB, Loring DW. *Neuropsychological Assessment.* 4th ed. New York: Oxford University Press; 2004.

48. Luukinen H, Viramo P, Herala M, et al. Fall-related brain injuries and the risk of dementia in elderly people: a population-based study. *Eur J Neurol.* 2005;12:86–92.

49. Luukinen H, Viramo P, Koski K, et al. Head injuries and cognitive decline among older adults: a population-based study. *Neurology.* 1999;52:557–562.

50. Malone MA, Kerschner JR, Swanson JM. Hemispheric processing and methylphenidate effects in attention-deficit hyperactivity disorder. *J Child Neurol.* 1994;9:181–189.

51. Mattson AG, Levin HS. Frontal lobe dysfunction following closed head injury: a review of the literature. *J Nerv Ment Dis.* 1987;178:282–291.

52. Mayeux R, Ottman R, Maestre G, et al. Synergistic effects of traumatic head injury and apolipoprotein-epsilon 4 in patients with Alzheimer's disease. *Neurology.* 1995;45:555–557.

53. Mazza M, Capuano A, Bria P, et al. Ginkgo biloba and donepezil: a comparison in the treatment of Alzheimer's dementia in a randomized placebo-controlled double-blind study. *Eur J Neurol.* 2006;13:981–985.

54. McAllister, TW. Neuropsychiatric sequelae of head injuries. *Psychiatr Clin North Am.* 1992;15:395–413.

55. McAllister TW, Sparling MB, Flashman LA, et al. Neuroimaging findings in mild traumatic brain injury. *J Clin Exp Neuropsychol.* 2001;23:775–791.

56. McDowell S, Whyte J, D'Esposito M. Differential effect of a dopaminergic agonist on prefrontal function in traumatic brain injury patients. *Brain.* 1998;121:1155–1164.

57. Mosenthal AC, Livingston DH, Lavery RF, et al. The effect of age on functional outcome in mild traumatic brain injury: 6-month report of a prospective multicenter trial. *J Trauma.* 2004;56:1042–1048.

58. Naugle RI. Epidemiology of traumatic brain injury in adults. In: Bigler ED, ed. *Traumatic brain injury: mechanisms of damage, assessment, intervention, and outcome.* Austin: Pro-Ed Inc.; 1990:69–103.

59. Nemetz PN, Leibson C, Naessens JM, et al. Traumatic brain injury and time to onset of Alzheimer's disease: a population-based study. *Am J Epidemiol.* 1999;149:32–40.

60. Neurobehavioral Guidelines Working Group, Warden DL, Gordon B, et al. Guidelines for the pharmacologic treatment of neurobehavioral sequelae of traumatic brain injury. *J Neurotrauma.* 2006;23:1468–1501.

61. Ommaya, AK, Gennarelli TA. Cerebral concussion and traumatic unconsciousness. *Brain.* 1974;97:633–654.

62. Pearlson GD, Robinson RG. Suction lesions of the frontal cerebral cortex in the rat induced asymmetrical behavioral and catecholaminergic responses. *Brain Res.* 1981;218:233–242.

63. Pentland B, Jones PA, Roy CW, et al. Head injury in the elderly. *Age Aging.* 1986;15:193–202.

64. Petersen RC, Thomas RG, Grundman M, et al. Vitamin E and donepezil for the treatment of mild cognitive impairment. *N Engl J Med.* 2005;352:2379–2388.

65. Povlishock JT, Becker DP, Cheng CLY, et al. Axonal change in minor head injury. *J Neuropathol Exp Neurol.* 1983;42:225–242.

66. Povlishock JT, Erb DE, Astrug J. Axonal response to traumatic brain injury: reactive axonal change, deafferentation, and neuroplasticity. *J Neurotrauma.* 1992;9[Suppl 1]:189–200.

67. Povlishock JT, Katz DI. Update of neuropathology and neurological recovery after traumatic brain injury. *J Head Trauma Rehabil.* 2005;20:76–94.

68. Rakier A, Guilburd JN, Soustiel JF, et al. Head injuries in the elderly. *Brain Inj.* 1995;9:187–193.

69. Rapoport MJ, Herrmann N, Shammi P, et al. Outcome after traumatic brain injury sustained in older adulthood: a one-year longitudinal study. *Am J Geriatr Psychiatry.* 2006;14:456–465.

70. Rothweiler B, Temkin NR, Dikmen SS. Aging effect on psychosocial outcome in traumatic brain injury. *Arch Phys Med Rehabil.* 1998;79:881–887.

71. Ryan LM, Warden DL. Post concussion syndrome. *Int Rev Psychiatry.* 2003;15:310–316.

72. Salmond CH, Chatfield DA, Menon DK, et al. Cognitive sequelae of head injury: involvement of basal forebrain and associated structures. *Brain.* 2005;128:189–200.

73. Silver JM, Koumaras B, Chen M, et al. Effects of rivastigmine on cognitive function in patients with traumatic brain injury. *Neurology.* 2006;67:748–755.

74. Smith DH, Uryu K, Saatman KE, et al. Protein accumulation in traumatic brain injury. *Neuromolecular Med.* 2003;4:59–72.

75. Sohlberg MM, Mateer CA. Evaluation and treatment of communicative skills. In: Kreutzer JS, Wehman P, eds. *Community integration following traumatic brain injury.* Baltimore: Brooks; 1990.

76. Susman M, DiRusso SM, Sullivan T, et al. Traumatic brain injury in the elderly: increased mortality and worse functional outcome at discharge despite lower injury severity. *J Trauma.* 2002;53:219–224.

77. Teasdale G, Jennett B. Assessment of coma in impaired consciousness: a practical scale. *Lancet.* 1974;2:81–84.

78. Tenovuo O. Central acetylcholinesterase inhibitors in the treatment of chronic traumatic brain injury-clinical experience in 111 patients. *Prog Neuropsychopharmacol Biol Psychiatry.* 2005;29:61–67.

79. Testa JA, Malec JF, Moessner AM, et al. Outcome after traumatic brain injury: effects of aging on recovery. *Am J Phys Med Rehabil.* 2005;86:1815–1823.

80. Varney NR, Menefee L. Psychosocial and executive deficits following closed head injury: implications for orbito-frontal cortex. *J Head Trauma Rehabil.* 1993;8:32–44.

81. Velasco J, Head M, Farlin E, et al. Unsuspected subdural hematoma as a differential diagnosis in elderly patients. *South Med J.* 1995;88:977–979.

82. Verbois SL, Cheffe SW, Pauli JR. Time-dependent changes in rat brain cholinergic receptor expression after experimental brain injury. *J Neurotrauma.* 2002;19:1569–1585.

83. Weller M, Kornhuber J. A rationale for NMDA receptor antagonist therapy for neuroleptic malignant syndrome. *Med Hypotheses.* 1992;38:329–333.

84. Wettstein A. Cholinesterase inhibitors and gingko extracts—are they comparable in the treatment of dementia? Comparison of published placebo-controlled efficacy studies of at least six months' duration. *Phytomedicine.* 2000;6:393–401.

85. Whyte J, Hart T, Schuster K, et al. Effects of methylphenidate on attentional function after traumatic brain injury. A randomized, placebo-controlled trial. *Am J Phys Med Rehabil.* 1997;76:440–450.

86. Whyte J, Hart T, Vaccaro M, et al. Effects of methylphenidate on attention deficits after traumatic brain injury: a multidimensional, randomized, placebo-controlled trial. *Am J Phys Med Rehabil.* 2004;83:401–420.

87. Wilson JA, Pentland B, Currie CT, et al. Outcome after severe head injury in the elderly. *Brain Inj.* 1987;1:183–188.

88. Wroblewski BA, Glenn MB. Pharmacological treatment of arousal and cognitive deficits. *J Head Trauma Rehabil.* 1994;9:19–42.

89. Wu TS, Garmel GM. Improved neurological function after amantadine treatment in two patients with brain injury. *J Emerg Med.* 2005; 28:289–292.

90. Young L, Fields RB, Lovell M. Neuropsychological differentiation of geriatric head injury from dementia. *J Neuropsychiatry Clin Neurosci.* 1995;7:414.

91. Zhang L, Plotkin RC, Wang G, et al. Cholinergic augmentation with donepezil enhances recovery in short-term memory and sustained attention after traumatic brain injury. *Arch Phys Med Rehabil.* 2004;85:1050–1055.

SUGGESTED READINGS

Flanagan SR, Hibbard MR, Reardon B, et al. Traumatic brain injury in the elderly: diagnostic and treatment challenges. *Clin Geriatr Med.* 2006;22:449–468.

Goldstein FC, Levin HS, Goldman WP, et al. Cognitive and neurobehavioral functioning after mild and moderate traumatic brain injury. *J Int Neuropsychol Soc.* 2001;7:373–383.

Neurobehavioral Guidelines Working Group, Warden DL, Gordon B, et al. Guidelines for the pharmacologic treatment of neurobehavioral sequelae of traumatic brain injury. *J Neurotrauma.* 2006;23:1468–1501.

Rapoport MJ, Herrmann N, Shammi P, et al. Outcome after traumatic brain injury sustained in older adulthood: a one-year longitudinal study. *Am J Geriatr Psychiatry.* 2006;14:456–465.

WEBSITES OF NATIONAL SUPPORT GROUPS

Brain Injury Association: http://www.biausa.org/
Alzheimer's Association: http://www.alz.org/
Alzheimer's Disease Education and Referral (ADEAR) Center:http://www.nia.nih.gov/Alzheimers/

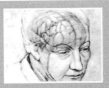

CHAPTER 21.1

Dementia: Risk Factors and Genetics

Richard J. Caselli

ALZHEIMER'S DISEASE

Purported risk factors for Alzheimer's disease (AD) encompass acquired and genetic factors and are summarized in Table 21-1.

ACQUIRED FACTORS

AD is the most common cause of dementia overall, accounting for more than half of all dementia cases. The lifetime risk of developing AD is estimated to be between 12% and 17% (32,60). The single greatest risk factor for AD is advancing age. Epidemiologic age-specific estimates of incidence and prevalence vary somewhat by region and study due to differences in diagnostic criteria and population demographics,

but all show an exponential increase in incidence and prevalence with advancing age at least through the ninth and probably through the tenth decade. The prevalence of severe dementia over the age of 60 years is estimated at 5%, and over the age of 85, it is estimated to be between 20% and 50%.

Diabetes, the metabolic syndrome [defined as three or more of the following: abdominal obesity, hypertriglyceridemia, low high-density lipoprotein cholesterol, hypertension, and hyperglycemia (31)] (74,94), and hyperinsulinemia (23,66) are associated with an increased risk of AD. In the Rotterdam study, diabetes mellitus doubled the risk of incident AD over a follow-up period that averaged slightly over 2 years (74). Prevalence of AD in a Finnish population aged

Table 21-1. *Purported Risk Factors for Alzheimer's Disease*

Risk Factor	References
Acquired	
Age	Farrer and Cupples (32); Kokmen et al. (60)
Diabetes mellitus	Craft (23); Luchsinger et al. (66); Ott et al. (74); Vanhanen et al. (94)
Hypertension	Hayden et al. (45); Luchsinger et al. (65); White and Launer (98)
Hypercholesterolemia	Sparks et al. (88)
Intracranial atherosclerosis	Honig et al. (48); Roher et al. (81)
Lower education	Caamano-Isorna et al. (15)
Depression	Ownby et al. (75)
Female gender	DeRonchi et al. (27); Webber et al. (97)
Estrogen replacement therapy	Espeland et al. (30); Zandi et al. (102)
Head trauma	Fleminger et al. (34); Jellinger (54)
Copper	Sparks et al. (86,87)
Genetic: Alzheimer's disease	
Amyloid precursor protein (chromosome 21)	Wisniewski et al. (100)
Presenilin 1 (chromosome 14)	Sherrington et al. (84)
Presenilin 2 (chromosome 1)	Levy-Lahad et al. (64)
Apolipoprotein E (chromosome 19)	Corder et al. (22); Saunders et al. (82)
Genetic: Other dementias	
Huntington's disease: *huntingtin* (chromosome 4)	Huntington's Disease Collaborative Research Group (52)
Frontotemporal dementia:	
tau (chromosome 17)	Hutton et al. (53)
progranulin (chromosome 14)	Baker et al. (5)

69 to 78 years was 7.2% in those with metabolic syndrome compared with 2.8% in those without metabolic syndrome, but the difference seemed confined to women (94). In addition to diabetes, other vascular risk factors such as hypercholesterolemia (88), hypertension, and hyperhomocysteinemia are correlated with a greater risk for AD (45,65,98). Less clear, however, is the relationship between stroke and AD. Vascular risk factors correlate with increased susceptibility to both AD and vascular dementia (45,47,49,90,98), and some studies have shown a correlation between cerebral atherosclerosis and AD (48,81). Cerebral infarction, whether related to atherosclerosis or amyloid angiopathy, further impairs cognition in patients with AD (46,99) but does not appear to predispose to AD itself (83).

Other purported risk factors have weaker associations, and some are more controversial because not all well-controlled epidemiologic studies have found them to be significant. Some of these factors include limited education (15), depression (75), gender (27,97), estrogen replacement therapy (30,102), and head trauma (34,54). Similarities between dementia pugilistica and AD include abeta deposition (40), neurofibrillary pathology (70), and similar genetic predisposition factors [apolipoprotein E (*ApoE*) *ε4*] (58). Possible protective effects have been claimed and disputed regarding the use of vitamin E (61,78) and the use of anti-inflammatory drugs (2,91). Neither can be strongly encouraged for AD prevention at this time.

Chronic aluminum exposure was once thought to play a role in AD mainly due to encephalopathy occurring in dialysis patients who were exposed to toxic levels of aluminum. The possible mechanisms by which aluminum could lead to AD histopathology include promoting hyperphosphorylation of tau and subsequent formation of neurofibrillary tangles, altering processing of amyloid precursor protein (APP) and then leading to the formation of neuritic plaques, and initiating a local inflammatory response (4). However, at present, aluminum exposure is no longer thought to be a major risk factor for AD. More recently, Sparks et al. (86,87) have proposed that copper exposure from drinking water may play a role in predisposition or progression of AD.

GENETIC FACTORS

There are three levels of genetic susceptibility to AD. The first level is that conferred by autosomal dominant mutations with high penetrance that cause early-onset familial AD (EOFAD). EOFAD strikes patients when they are young, typically ranging from mid-thirties to mid-fifties. To date, more than 100 mutations of three genes have been identified that may cause EOFAD, and all are inherited in an autosomal dominant pattern. The largest number of EOFAD cases are caused by mutations of the *presenilin-1* (*PS1*)

gene, and thus, *PS1* is thought to account for the majority of autosomal dominant kindreds (84). The *PS1* mutation is currently the only autosomal dominant mutation for which there is a commercially available genetic test. A smaller number of mutations have been localized to the *APP* gene on chromosome 21 (100) and the *presenilin-2* (*PS2*) gene on chromosome 1 (64). All result in elevated levels of abeta-amyloid (Aβ), underscoring the pathogenetic importance of Aβ in the evolution of AD (43). Genetic testing of patients with possible EOFAD may confirm the genetic cause in a family, thus allowing preclinical testing of unaffected family members who may be at risk.

The second level of genetic susceptibility is conferred by a common variant of a gene (or genes) not known to be directly related to Aβ. The genetic risk factor that accounts for more cases of AD than any other is the *ApoE ε4* allele located on chromosome 19. *ApoE ε4* is associated with late-onset familial and sporadic AD but not autosomal dominant EOFAD (22,82). *ApoE ε4* has lower penetrance than the autosomal dominant mutations that cause EOFAD, but it is a far more prevalent risk factor, accounting for as many as half of all cases. Positive predictive value of *ApoE ε4* in a patient with dementia is nearly 100%, but negative predictive value is low, making genetic testing for *ApoE ε4* of limited clinical value (71). The *ApoE ε2* allele, in contrast, is associated with reduced susceptibility to AD (22,82).

Although there are regional variations, the prevalence of *ApoE ε4* in North America is approximately 20% (21,38,104). Global regions that are associated with lower AD prevalence, including some Mediterranean and Asian countries, have led to speculation that dietary habits, such as the Mediterranean diet, and green tea may protect against AD. Although nutritional effects are possible, it is an interesting coincidence that *ApoE ε4* prevalence is low and *ApoE ε2* prevalence is high in many of these regions (Table 21-2).

ApoE genotype influences not only susceptibility to AD, but also the age of onset of AD (22,82). Each additional copy of the *ApoE ε4* gene is associated with a slightly younger median age of dementia onset. It is less clear whether *ApoE ε4* influences the rate of cognitive decline in most patients with AD (7,25,39,41,63). *ApoE ε4* homozygotes with AD may have a faster rate of decline than more common *ApoE* subgroups (24), and several studies have suggested that *ApoE* genotype may influence the rate of age-related cognitive decline in nondemented individuals (8,17–19,57). In addition to enhancing risk for AD, the *ApoE ε4* isoform of *ApoE* also correlates with poor neurologic outcome following head trauma (35,58,85) and intracerebral hemorrhage (3,68,69).

Although it is not known how *ApoE* exerts these effects, possible adverse functional consequences of the

Table 21-2. *Prevalence of ApoE in Countries with Low ApoE ε4 Prevalence*

	ApoE ε2	*ApoE ε3*	*ApoE ε4*
Sardinia	0.050	0.898	0.052
Greece	0.054	0.878	0.068
China	0.105	0.824	0.071
Turkey	0.061	0.860	0.079
Morocco	0.065	0.850	0.085
Maya	0.0	0.911	0.089
Spain	0.052	0.856	0.091
Italy	0.060	0.849	0.091
Japan	0.048	0.851	0.101

Derived from Corbo RM, Scacchi R. Apolipoprotein E (APOE) allele distribution in the world. Is APOE*4 a 'thrifty' allele? *Ann Hum Genet*. 1999;63:301–310.

ApoE ε4 isoform compared to the *ApoE ε3* and *ApoE ε2* isoforms include: enhanced rate of cerebral amyloid deposition; reduced protection against oxidative injury; reduced efficiency of synaptic and neuronal repair; reduced neurotrophic properties possibly related to reduced tau binding, causing microtubule destabilization and consequently reduced neurite outgrowth (50); and *ApoE ε4* isoform carboxyl fragment toxicity (14,44,51). These effects are not mutually exclusive, and all may be operational to varying degrees. Several of these possibilities, however, suggest that *ApoE* genotype, apart from its role in senescence and injury, could influence neural development (9,42,72) with potential indirect effects on AD susceptibility related to developmental differences between *ApoE ε4* carriers and noncarriers [such as adult brain myelination patterns (6)].

There may be additional susceptibility genes for late-onset AD with effects similar to *ApoE ε4*. Some studies have raised the possibility of such additional genetic loci accounting for late-onset AD on chromosomes 10 (29) and 12 (101).

The third level of genetic susceptibility reflects not a single gene, but multiple genes that constitute a metabolic pathway. Individually, normal variations of single genes within such a pathway have only a minor effect, but collectively, they may exert an effect equal to that of *ApoE ε4*. Such weaker genetic risk factors have been identified in cholesterol and glucose metabolic pathways, and they may further influence the cumulative genetic risk for late-onset or sporadic AD (56,76,77,96).

NON-ALZHEIMER'S DEMENTIA

Less is known about acquired or environmental factors that may predispose to non-Alzheimer's forms of dementia, but genetic factors have been identified in some cases.

Huntington's disease is caused by an autosomal dominant mutation of the *huntingtin* gene on chromosome 4 in which there is an unstable expansion of a trinucleotide repeat (CAG) region (52). Normal individuals have between 11 and 34 repeats, but individuals with Huntington's disease have between 37 and 86.

Frontotemporal dementia (FTD) and related tauopathies can be caused by autosomal dominantly inherited mutations of the gene for microtubule-associated protein tau (MAPT) on chromosome 17 (53). More recently, familial tau-negative cases have been associated with *progranulin* mutations on chromosome 17 (5). *Tau* or *progranulin* mutations are found in 10% or less of all cases but in a higher proportion of those with a family history of dementia (37,89). FTD associated with amyotrophic lateral sclerosis has been linked instead to a locus on chromosome 9 (93).

Parkinson's disease is associated with dementia in roughly a third of patients either in the form of dementia with Lewy bodies (DLB) or as Parkinson's disease with dementia (PDD) (13,95) and, thus, itself may be considered a risk factor for dementia. Rapid eye movement (REM) sleep behavior disorder, a sleep disorder characterized by dream enactment behavior, is associated with synucleinopathies in general but seems to have a particularly strong association with DLB (10,11,16,33,36,92). Multiple genetic associations have been identified for familial parkinsonism in which dementia sometimes co-occurs including *alpha-synuclein* (79,103), *parkin* (55,67), and *tau* (20,28,53).

Regarding vascular dementia, incidence and prevalence rates are affected by the definition used. The prevalence of poststroke vascular dementia ranges from 11.3% using the National Institute of Neurological Disorders and Stroke–Association Internationale pour la Recherche et l'Enseignement en Neurosciences (NINDS-AIREN) criteria to 20.1% using the International Classification of Diseases to Neurology (ICD-10-NA) criteria, and the incidence ranges from 2.6% with the Alzheimer's Disease Diagnostic and Treatment Centers (ADDTC) criteria to 5.2% with the ICD-10-NA (80). In one longitudinal population-based study, among patients with mild cognitive impairment who progressed to dementia, 60% progressed to AD, and 33% progressed to vascular dementia (12). Others have found that midlife hypercholesterolemia and hypertension increased the risk for AD (26,59), whereas physical exercise such as walking reduced the risk. The incidence rate of AD is higher among individuals with prevalent cardiovascular disease (34.4 per 1,000 person-years) than among those without it (22.2 per 1,000 person-years) (1), so it is difficult to disentangle the role that vascular risk factors play for the development of vascular dementia exclusive of AD (62,73).

REFERENCES

1. Abbott RD, White LR, Ross GW, et al. Walking and dementia in physically capable elderly men. *JAMA.* 2004;292:1447–1453.
2. Aisen PS, Schafer KA, Grundman M, et al. Effects of rofecoxib or naproxen vs placebo on Alzheimer disease progression: a randomized controlled trial. *JAMA.* 2003;289:2819–2826.
3. Alberts MJ, Graffagnino C, McClenny C, et al. ApoE genotype and survival from intracerebral haemorrhage. *Lancet.* 1995;346:575.
4. Armstrong R, Winsper S, Blair J. Aluminum and Alzheimer's disease: review of possible pathogenic mechanisms. *Dementia.* 1996;7:1–9.
5. Baker M, Mackenzie JR, Pickering-Brown SM, et al. Mutations in progranulin cause tau-negative frontotemporal dementia linked to chromosome 17. *Nature* 2006;442:916–919.
6. Bartzokis G, Lu PH, Geschwind DH, et al. Apolipoprotein E genotype and age-related myelin breakdown in healthy individuals: implications for cognitive decline and dementia. *Arch Neurol.* 2006;63:63–72.
7. Basun H, Grut M, Winblad B, et al. Apolipoprotein epsilon 4 allele and disease progression in patients with late-onset Alzheimer's disease. *Neurosci Lett.* 1995;183:32–34.
8. Baxter LC, Caselli RJ, Johnson SC, et al. Apolipoprotein E epsilon 4 affects new learning in cognitively normal individuals at risk for Alzheimer's disease. *Neurobiol Aging.* 2003;24:947–952.
9. Bellosta S, Nathan BP, Orth M, et al. Stable expression and secretion of apolipoproteins E3 and E4 in mouse neuroblastoma cells produces differential effects on neurite outgrowth. *J Biol Chem.* 1995;270:27063–27071.
10. Boeve BF, Silber MH, Ferman TJ, et al. Association of REM sleep behavior disorder and neurodegenerative disease may reflect an underlying synucleinopathy. *Mov Disord.* 2001;16:622–630.
11. Boeve BF, Silber MH, Parisi JE, et al. Synucleinopathy pathology and REM sleep behavior disorder plus dementia or parkinsonism. *Neurology.* 2003;61:40–45.
12. Bowen J, Teri L, Kukull W, et al. Progression to dementia in patients with isolated memory loss. *Lancet.* 1997;349:763–765.
13. Bower JH, Maraganore DM, McDonnell SK, et al. Incidence and distribution of parkinsonism in Olmsted County. *Neurology.* 1999;52:1214–1220.
14. Brecht WJ, Harris FM, Chang S, et al. Neuron-specific apolipoprotein e4 proteolysis is associated with increased tau phosphorylation in brains of transgenic mice. *J Neurosci.* 2004;24:2527–2534.
15. Caamano-Isorna F, Corral M, Montes-Martinez A, et al. Education and dementia: a meta-analytic study. *Neuroepidemiology.* 2006;26:226–232.
16. Caselli RJ, Chen KW, Bandy D, et al. A preliminary fluorodeoxyglucose positron emission tomography study in healthy adults reporting dream-enactment behavior. *Sleep.* 2006;29:927–933.
17. Caselli RJ, Graff-Radford NR, Reiman EM, et al. Preclinical memory decline in cognitively normal apolipoprotein E-epsilon4 homozygotes. *Neurology.* 1999;53:201–207.
18. Caselli RJ, Osborne D, Reiman EM, et al. Preclinical cognitive decline in late middle-aged asymptomatic apolipoprotein E-e4/4 homozygotes: a replication study. *J Neurol Sci.* 2001;189:93–98.
19. Caselli RJ, Reiman EM, Osborne D, et al. Longitudinal changes in cognition and behavior in asymptomatic carriers of the APOE e4 allele. *Neurology.* 2004;62:1990–1995.
20. Clark LN, Poorkaj P, Wszolek Z, et al. Pathogenic implications of mutations in the tau gene in pallido-ponto-nigral degeneration and related neurodegenerative disorders linked to chromosome 17. *Proc Natl Acad Sci USA.* 1998;95:13103–13107.
21. Corbo RM, Scacchi R. Apolipoprotein E (APOE) allele distribution in the world. Is APOE*4 a 'thrifty' allele? *Ann Hum Genet.* 1999;63:301–310.
22. Corder EH, Saunders AM, Strittmatter WJ, et al. Gene dose of apolipoprotein E type 4 allele and the risk of Alzheimer's disease in late onset families. *Science.* 1993;261:921–923.
23. Craft S. Insulin resistance syndrome and Alzheimer's disease: age and obesity-related effects on memory, amyloid, and inflammation. *Neurobiol Aging.* 2005;26[Suppl 1]:65–69.
24. Craft S, Teri L, Edland SD, et al. Accelerated decline in apolipoprotein E-epsilon4 homozygotes with Alzheimer's disease. *Neurology.* 1998;51:149–153.
25. Dal FG, Rasmusson DX, Brandt J, et al. Apolipoprotein E genotype and rate of decline in probable Alzheimer's disease. *Arch Neurol.* 1996;53:345–350.
26. DeCarli C, Miller BL, Swan GE, et al. Cerebrovascular and brain morphologic correlates of mild cognitive impairment in the National Heart, Lung, and Blood Institute Twin Study. *Arch Neurol.* 2001;58:643–647.
27. DeRonchi D, Berardi D, Menchetti M, et al. Occurrence of cognitive impairment and

dementia after the age of 60: a population-based study from Northern Italy. *Demen Geriatr Cogn Disord.* 2005;19:97–105.

28. Dumanchin C, Camuzat A, Campion D, et al. Segregation of a missense mutation in the microtubule-associated protein tau gene with familial frontotemporal dementia and parkinsonism. *Hum Mol Genet.* 1998;7:1825–1829.

29. Ertekin-Taner N, Graff-Radford N, Younkin LH, et al. Linkage of plasma Abeta42 to a quantitative locus on chromosome 10 in late-onset Alzheimer's disease pedigrees. *Science.* 2000;290: 2303–2304.

30. Espeland MA, Rapp SR, Shumaker SA, et al. Conjugated equine estrogens and global cognitive function in postmenopausal women: Women's Health Initiative Memory Study. *JAMA.* 2004; 29:2959–2968.

31. Expert Panel on Detection, Evaluation, and Treatment of High Blood Cholesterol in Adults. Executive Summary of the Third Report of the National Cholesterol Education Program (NCEP) Expert Panel on Detection, Evaluation, and Treatment of High Blood Cholesterol in Adults (Adults Treatment Panel III). *JAMA.* 2001;285:2486–2497.

32. Farrer LA, Cupples LA. Estimating the probability for major gene Alzheimer disease. *Am J Hum Genet.* 1994;54:374–383.

33. Ferini-Strambi L, Di Gioia MR, Castronovo V, et al. Neuropsychological assessment in idiopathic REM sleep behavior disorder (RBD). Does the idiopathic form of RBD really exist? *Neurology.* 2004;62:41–45.

34. Fleminger S, Oliver DL, Lovestone S, et al. Head injury as a risk factor for Alzheimer's disease: the evidence 10 years on; a partial replication. *J Neurol Neurosurg Psychiatry.* 2003;74: 857–862.

35. Friedman G, Froom P, Sazbon L, et al. Apolipoprotein E-epsilon4 genotype predicts a poor outcome in survivors of traumatic brain injury. *Neurology.* 1999;52:244–248.

36. Gagnon JF, Bedard MA, Fantini ML, et al. REM sleep behavior disorder and REM sleep without atonia in Parkinson's disease. *Neurology.* 2002;59:585–589.

37. Gass J, Cannon A, Mackenzie J, et al. Mutations in progranulin are a major cause of ubiquitin-positive frontotemporal lobar degeneration. *Hum Mol Genet.* 2006;15:2988–3001.

38. Gerdes LU, Klausen IC, Sihm I, et al. Apolipoprotein E polymorphism in a Danish population compared to findings in 45 other study populations around the world. *Genet Epidemiol.* 1992;9: 155–167.

39. Gomez-Isla T, West HL, Rebeck GW, et al. Clinical and pathological correlates of apolipoprotein E epsilon 4 in Alzheimer's disease. *Ann Neurol.* 1996;39:62–70.

40. Graham DI, Gentleman SM, Nicoll JA, et al. Altered beta-APP metabolism after head injury and its relationship to the aetiology of Alzheimer's disease. *Acta Neurochir Suppl.* 1996; 66:96–102.

41. Growdon JH, Locascio JJ, Corkin S, et al. Apolipoprotein E genotype does not influence rates of cognitive decline in Alzheimer's disease. *Neurology.* 1996;47:444–448.

42. Handelmann GE, Boyles JK, Weisgraber KH, et al. Effects of apolipoprotein E, beta-very low density lipoproteins, and cholesterol on the extension of neurites by rabbit dorsal root ganglion neurons in vitro. *J Lipid Res.* 1992;33: 1677–1688.

43. Hardy JA, Higgins GA. Alzheimer's disease: the amyloid cascade hypothesis. *Science.* 1992;256: 184–185.

44. Harris FM, Brecht WJ, Xu Q, et al. Carboxyl-terminal-truncated apolipoprotein E4 causes Alzheimer's disease-like neurodegeneration and behavioral deficits in transgenic mice. *Proc Natl Acad Sci USA.* 2003;100:10966–10971.

45. Hayden KM, Zandi PP, Lyketsos CG, et al. Vascular risk factors for incident Alzheimer disease and vascular dementia: the Cache County study. *Alzheimer Dis Assoc Disord.* 2006;20: 93–100.

46. Heyman A, Fillenbaum GG, Welsh-Bohmer KA, et al. Cerebral infarcts in patients with autopsy-proven Alzheimer's disease: CERAD, part XVIII. Consortium to Establish a Registry for Alzheimer's Disease. *Neurology.* 1998;51: 159–162.

47. Hogervorst E, Ribeiro HM, Molyneux A, et al. Plasma homocysteine levels, cerebrovascular risk factors, and cerebral white matter changes (leukoaraiosis) in patients with Alzheimer disease. *Arch Neurol.* 2002;59:787–793.

48. Honig LS, Kukull W, Mayeux R. Atherosclerosis and AD: analysis of data from the US National Alzheimer's Coordinating Center. *Neurology.* 2005;64:494–500.

49. Honig LS, Tang MX, Albert S, et al. Stroke and the risk of Alzheimer disease. *Arch Neurol.* 2003;60:1707–1712.

50. Horsburgh K, McCarron MO, White F, et al. The role of apolipoprotein E in Alzheimer's disease, acute brain injury and cerebrovascular disease: evidence of common mechanisms and utility of animal models. *Neurobiol Aging.* 2000; 21:245–255.

51. Huang Y, Weisgraber KH, Mucke L, et al. Apolipoprotein E: diversity of cellular origins, structural and biophysical properties, and effects in Alzheimer's disease. *J Mol Neurosci.* 2004;23: 189–204.

52. Huntington's Disease Collaborative Research Group. A novel gene containing a trinucleotide repeat that is expanded and unstable on Huntington's disease chromosomes. *Cell.* 1993; 72:971–983.

53. Hutton M, Lendon CL, Rizzu P, et al. Association of missense and 5'-splice-site mutations in tau with the inherited dementia FTDP-17. *Nature.* 1998;393:702–705.

54. Jellinger KA. Head injury and dementia. *Curr Opin Neurol.* 2004;17:719–723.

55. Jellinger KA. Morphological substrates of mental dysfunction in Lewy body disease: an update. *J Neural Transm Suppl.* 2000;59:185–212.

56. Johansson A, Katzov H, Zetterberg H, et al. Variants of CYP46A1 may interact with age and APOE to influence CSF Abeta42 levels in Alzheimer's disease. *Hum Genet.* 2004;114:581–587.

57. Jonker C, Schmand B, Lindeboom J, et al. Association between apolipoprotein E epsilon4 and the rate of cognitive decline in community-dwelling elderly individuals with and without dementia. *Arch Neurol.* 1998;55:1065–1069.

58. Jordan BD, Relkin NR, Ravdin LD, et al. Apolipoprotein E epsilon4 associated with chronic traumatic brain injury in boxing. *JAMA.* 1997;278:136–140.

59. Kivipelto M, Helkala EL, Hanninen T, et al. Midlife vascular risk factors and late-life mild cognitive impairment. A population-based study. *Neurology.* 2001;56:1683–1689.

60. Kokmen E, Beard CM, O'Brien PC, et al. Epidemiology of dementia in Rochester, Minnesota. *Mayo Clin Proc.* 1996;71:275–282.

61. Kontush K, Schekatolina S. Vitamin E in neurodegenerative disorders: Alzheimer's disease. *Ann NY Acad Sci.* 2004;1031:249–262.

62. Korczyn AD. Mixed dementia—the most common form of dementia. *Ann NY Acad Sci.* 2002; 977:129–134.

63. Kurz A, Egensperger R, Haupt M, et al. Apolipoprotein E epsilon 4 allele, cognitive decline, and deterioration of everyday performance in Alzheimer's disease. *Neurology.* 1996; 47:440–443.

64. Levy-Lahad E, Wasco W, Poorkaj P, et al. Candidate gene for the chromosome 1 familial Alzheimer's disease locus. *Science.* 1995;269: 973–977.

65. Luchsinger JA, Reitz C, Honig LS, et al. Aggregation of vascular risk factors and risk of

incident Alzheimer disease. *Neurology.* 2005;65: 545–551.

66. Luchsinger JA, Tang MX, Shea S, et al. Hyperinsulinemia and risk of Alzheimer disease. *Neurology.* 2004;63:1187–1192.

67. Lucking CB, Durr A, Bonifati V, et al. Association between early-onset Parkinson's disease and mutations in the parkin gene. French Parkinson's Disease Study Group. *N Engl J Med.* 2000;342:1560–1567.

68. McCarron MO, Hoffmann KL, DeLong DM, et al. Intracerebral hemorrhage outcome: apolipoprotein E genotype, hematoma, and edema volumes. *Neurology.* 1999;53:2176–2179.

69. McCarron MO, Muir KW, Weir CJ, et al. The apolipoprotein E epsilon4 allele and outcome in cerebrovascular disease. *Stroke.* 1998;29:1882–1887.

70. McKenzie JE, Roberts GW, Royston MC. Comparative investigation of neurofibrillary damage in the temporal lobe in Alzheimer's disease, Down's syndrome, and dementia pugilistica. *Neurodegeneration.* 1996;5:259–264.

71. Nalbantoglu J, Gilfix BM, Bertrand P, et al. Predictive value of apolipoprotein E genotyping in Alzheimer's disease: results of an autopsy series and an analysis of several combined studies. *Ann Neurol.* 1994;36:889–895.

72. Nathan BP, Bellosta S, Sanan DA, et al. Differential effects of apolipoproteins E3 and E4 on neuronal growth in vitro. *Science.* 1994; 264:850–852.

73. Newman AB, Fitzpatrick AL, Lopez O, et al. Dementia and Alzheimer's disease in relationship to cardiovascular disease in the Cardiovascular Health Study cohort. *J Am Geriatr Soc.* 2005;53:1101–1107.

74. Ott A, Stolk RP, van Harskamp F, et al. Diabetes mellitus and the risk of dementia: the Rotterdam study. *Neurology.* 1999;53:1937–1942.

75. Ownby RL, Crocco E, Acevedo A, et al. Depression and risk for Alzheimer disease: systematic review, meta-analysis, and metaregression analysis. *Arch Gen Psychiatry.* 2006;63: 530–538.

76. Papassotiropoulos A, Fountoulakis M, Dunckley T, et al. Genetics, transcriptomics, and proteomics of Alzheimer's disease. *J Clin Psychiatry.* 2006;67:652–670.

77. Papassotiropoulos A, Streffer JR, Tsolaki M, et al. Increased brain beta-amyloid load, phosphorylated tau, and risk of Alzheimer disease associated with an intronic CYP46 polymorphism. *Arch Neurol.* 2003;60:29–35.

78. Petersen RC, Thomas RG, Grundman M, et al. Vitamin E and donepezil for the treatment of

mild cognitive impairment. *N Engl J Med.* 2005; 352:2379–2388.

79. Polymeropoulos MH, Lavedan C, Leroy E, et al. Mutation in the alpha-synuclein gene identified in families with Parkinson's disease. *Science.* 1997;276:2045–2047.

80. Rasquin SM, Lodder J, Verhey FR. The effect of different diagnostic criteria on the prevalence and incidence of post-stroke dementia. *Neuroepidemiology.* 2005;24:189–195.

81. Roher AE, Esh C, Kokjohn TA, et al. Circle of Willis atherosclerosis is a risk factor for sporadic Alzheimer's disease. *Arterioscl Thromb Vasc Biol.* 2003;23:2055–2062.

82. Saunders AM, Strittmatter WJ, Schmechel D, et al. Association of apolipoprotein E allele epsilon 4 with late-onset familial and sporadic Alzheimer's disease. *Neurology.* 1993;43:1467–1472.

83. Schneider JA, Wilson RS, Bienias JL, et al. Cerebral infarctions and the likelihood of dementia from Alzheimer disease pathology. *Neurology.* 2004;62:1148–1155.

84. Sherrington R, Rogaev EI, Liang Y, et al. Cloning of a gene bearing missense mutations in early-onset familial Alzheimer's disease. *Nature.* 1995;375:754–760.

85. Sorbi S, Nacmias B, Piacentini S, et al. ApoE as a prognostic factor for post-traumatic coma. *Nat Med.* 1995;1:852.

86. Sparks DL, Friedland R, Petanceska S, et al. Trace copper levels in the drinking water, but not zinc or aluminum influence CNS Alzheimer-like pathology. *J Nutr Health Aging.* 2006;10: 247–254.

87. Sparks DL, Petanceska S, Sabbagh M, et al. Cholesterol, copper and abeta in controls, MCI, AD and the AD Cholesterol-Lowering Treatment Trial (ADCLT). *Curr Alzheimer Res.* 2005;2:527–539.

88. Sparks DL, Sabbagh MN, Breitner JC, et al. Is cholesterol a culprit in Alzheimer's disease? *Int Psychogeriatr.* 2003;15[Suppl 1]:152–159.

89. Stanford PM, Brooks WS, Teber ET, et al. Frequency of tau mutations in familial and sporadic frontotemporal dementia and other tauopathies. *J Neurol.* 2004;251:1098–1104.

90. Stenset V, Johnsen L, Kocot D, et al. Associations between white matter lesions, cerebrovascular risk factors, and low CSF abeta42. *Neurology.* 2006;67:830–833.

91. Szekely CA, Thorne JE, Zandi PP, et al. Nonsteroidal anti-inflammatory drugs for the prevention of Alzheimer's disease: a systematic review. *Neuroepidemiology.* 2004;23:159–169.

92. Turner RS. Idiopathic rapid eye movement sleep behavior disorder is a harbinger of dementia with Lewy bodies. *J Geriatr Psychiatry Neurol.* 2002;15:195–199.

93. Vance C, Al-Chalabi A, Ruddy D, et al. Familial amyotrophic lateral sclerosis with frontotemporal dementia is linked to a locus on chromosome 9p13.2-21.3. *Brain.* 2006;129:868–876.

94. Vanhanen M, Koivisto K, Moilanen L, et al. Association of metabolic syndrome with Alzheimer disease: a population-based study. *Neurology.* 2006;67:843–847.

95. Wakisaka Y, Furuta A, Tanizaki Y, et al. Age-associated prevalence and risk-factors of Lewy body pathology in a general population: the Hisayama study. *Acta Neuropathol (Berl).* 2003; 106:374–382.

96. Wang B, Zhang C, Zheng W, et al. Association between a T/C polymorphism in intron 2 of cholesterol 24S-hydroxylase gene and Alzheimer's disease in Chinese. *Neurosci Lett.* 2004;369: 104–107.

97. Webber KM, Casadesus G, Perry G, et al. Gender differences in Alzheimer disease: the role of luteinizing hormone in disease pathogenesis. *Alzheimer Dis Assoc Disord.* 2005;19:95–99.

98. White L, Launer L. Relevance of cardiovascular risk factors and ischemic cerebrovascular disease to the pathogenesis of Alzheimer disease: a review of accrued findings from the Honolulu-Asia Aging Study. *Alzheimer Dis Assoc Disord.* 2006;20[Suppl 2]:S79–S83.

99. White L, Petrovitch H, Hardman J, et al. Cerebrovascular pathology and dementia in autopsied Honolulu-Asia Aging Study participants. *Ann NY Acad Sci.* 2002;977:9–23.

100. Wisniewski KE, Wisniewski HM, Wen GY. Occurrence of neuropathological changes and dementia of Alzheimer's disease in Down's syndrome. *Ann Neurol.* 1985;17:278–282.

101. Wu WS, Holmans P, Wavrant-DeVrieze F, et al. Genetic studies on chromosome 12 in late-onset Alzheimer disease. *JAMA.* 1998;280:619–622.

102. Zandi PP, Carlson MC, Plassman BL, et al. Hormonal replacement therapy and incidence of Alzheimer disease in older women: the Cache County study. *JAMA.* 2002;288:2123–2129.

103. Zaranz JJ, Alegre J, Gomez-Esteban JC, et al. The new mutation, E46K, of alpha-synuclein causes Parkinson and Lewy body dementia. *Ann Neurol* 2004;55:164–173.

104. Zekraoui L, Lagarde JP, Raisonnier A, et al. High frequency of the apolipoprotein E *4 allele in African pygmies and most of the African populations in sub-Saharan Africa. *Hum Biol.* 1997;69:575–581.

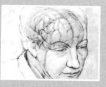

CHAPTER 21.2

Dementia: Diagnostic Evaluation and Treatment

Bryan K. Woodruff

DEFINITION

Dementia is a progressive cognitive disorder that results in disability for affected individuals and an increasing burden for caregivers and the health care system. Formally defined, it is characterized by impairment in at least two or more cognitive domains, including short- and long-term memory, abstract thinking, language, judgment, or other higher cortical functions (4). Patients also frequently exhibit behavioral disturbance such as depression, anxiety, agitation, aggression, and psychosis. These cognitive and behavioral changes impair the affected individual's ability to function normally in their occupation, interpersonal interactions, and eventually self-care. These clinical manifestations must not be due to an underlying psychiatric condition or delirium. After excluding these and other causes of cognitive dysfunction with appropriate diagnostic studies, the clinician can make a clinical diagnosis of dementia. In multiple clinical and pathologic series of dementia, Alzheimer's disease (AD) is the most common cause of dementia and will be the main focus of discussion in this chapter. Table 21-3 lists the most common causes of dementia encountered in one recent autopsy series and their relative frequencies, also illustrating that dementia with mixed underlying pathology is common (9).

Table 21-3. *Frequency of Major Dementia Subtypes in an Autopsy Series*

Dementia Type	Frequency
AD (pure AD)	77% (42%)
LBD (pure LBD)	26% (8%)
VaD (pure VaD)	18% (3%)
FTD (pure FTD)	5% (4%)

AD, Alzheimer's disease; LBD, Lewy body dementia; VaD, vascular dementia; FTD, frontotemporal dementia.

From Barker WW, et al. Relative frequencies of Alzheimer's disease, Lewy body, vascular and frontotemporal dementia, and hippocampal sclerosis in the State of Florida Brain Bank. *Alzheimer Dis Assoc Disord.* 2002;16:203–212.

SIGNIFICANCE

Individuals suffering from dementia require increasing supervision as the disease progresses. The costs of diagnostic evaluation and pharmacotherapy are overshadowed by the costs of skilled care and the emotional burden on caregivers. The economic burden of such care is staggering (25). The cost of such increasing care is particularly concerning considering the aging demographic of the United States and other developed countries. Age-specific prevalence of AD shows a disturbing trend; from age 65 to 69 years, prevalence is approximately 2%, increasing to 35% to 40% in individuals aged 85 and older (55,56). Incidence of AD also increases with age (7). In the United States, the "baby boomer" generation is entering retirement and also, unfortunately, the age of increased risk for development of dementia. Assuming these observations of increased prevalence of dementia with increased age persist in this population, the cost of care may be insurmountable unless more effective preventive or symptomatic treatments are developed.

RISK FACTORS FOR DEMENTIA

The greatest risk factor for the development of dementia is increasing age. Other risk factors include a history of stroke (65), midlife hypertension (46), diabetes mellitus (6), head injury (39), and education level (15). There are genetic causes and risk factors specific to different forms of dementia, and these will be discussed in the following sections.

MILD COGNITIVE IMPAIRMENT

Given increasing life expectancy due to improvements in prevention and treatment of many common general medical conditions, more individuals are living to ages where the prevalence of cognitive dysfunction increases. However, cognitive dysfunction is not encountered uniformly in older individuals, and attempts to differentiate between normal cognitive performance and cognitive impairment can be challenging in some circumstances. The "gray" zone between normal cognition and dementia has been a subject of

Table 21-4. *Clinical Criteria for Amnestic Mild Cognitive Impairment*

- Memory complaint, preferably corroborated by an informant
- Essentially normal general cognition
- Largely normal activities of daily living
- Objective memory impairment for age
- Not demented

From Petersen RC, et al. Practice parameter: early detection of dementia: mild cognitive impairment (an evidence-based review). Report of the Quality Standards Subcommittee of the American Academy of Neurology. *Neurology*. 2001;56: 1133–1142.

intense research interest, prompting establishment of a practice parameter for evaluation and management of such patients, with the clinical designation of mild cognitive impairment (MCI) (97). Current clinical criteria for MCI are outlined in Table 21-4. Patients with MCI do not meet clinical criteria for dementia but suffer from memory or other cognitive dysfunction of sufficient degree to be recognized by the patient and ideally corroborated by a reliable informant. The cognitive dysfunction should not significantly interfere with the affected individual's functional status.

Amnestic MCI is the best characterized subtype and is associated with a high risk of conversion to AD over time, with approximately 10% to 12% of affected individuals converting to AD per year (95) and approximately 80% of patients converting to AD by 6 years (99). Neuroimaging of patients with amnestic MCI demonstrates patterns of medial temporal lobe atrophy that are predictive of conversion to AD (53). Pathologic studies of patients with a clinical diagnosis of amnestic MCI support these clinical observations, with demonstration of intermediate neuropathologic findings between neurofibrillary changes of normal aging and early AD (96). Although there are no approved treatments for MCI, a recent study suggests that a subset of patients may benefit from treatment with a cholinesterase inhibitor (ChEI) (98). Other subtypes of MCI are not as clearly characterized as amnestic MCI but, in some cases, represent early stages of other non-AD dementias (132). For example, isolated mild impairment of language function may be a precursor to the clinical syndrome of primary progressive aphasia. Further longitudinal studies of the various subtypes of MCI and their clinical outcomes are needed to clarify these relationships.

ALZHEIMER'S DISEASE

CLINICAL FEATURES

Clinical manifestations of AD are typically insidious in onset, with patients demonstrating short-term memory problems such as difficulty recalling recent conversations or events or a tendency to repeat themselves excessively (94). This is clearly linked to the location of the early pathology of the disease (described in the following section). Patients often have limited or no awareness of their memory loss; to put it simply, they forget that they forget (113). Family members or close companions are often the impetus for evaluation of the initial symptoms, and therefore, information from a reliable informant is essential when obtaining a meaningful history. Several criteria have been proposed for the clinical diagnosis of AD, including those outlined in the *Diagnostic and Statistical Manual of Mental Disorders, 4th Edition* (4) and also those presented by the National Institute of Neurological and Communicative Disorders and Stroke and the Alzheimer's Disease and Related Disorders Association (NINCDS-ADRDA) (78), summarized in Table 21-5.

Atypical presentations of AD are also recognized, including those manifesting primarily with a behavioral disturbance (70), language dysfunction (38), and visuospatial deficits (37,122). The patterns of atrophy and distribution of AD pathology in these cases correlate with the clinical symptomatology (e.g., prominent posterior cortical atrophy in "visual variant" of AD).

Disease course is variable among patients with AD. Typically, the time from disease diagnosis to placement in a skilled care facility is 3 to 6 years (44). Placement is typically dictated by an individual's support network, with some patients able to remain in a home environment throughout the course of their illness. Structured counseling on caregiver strategies may delay nursing home placement in some cases (83). However, most families lack the resources to provide sufficient care in the home in advanced stages of the disease. The presence or absence of disruptive behavioral symptoms often dictates the need for placement. After placement in a skilled care facility, most patients survive for approximately 3 years (126); death usually is secondary to intercurrent illness such as pneumonia or vascular disease (11,68).

PATHOLOGY

Gross examination of a brain with AD typically demonstrates generalized cerebral atrophy with a predilection for temporal and parietal regions. The medial temporal lobes may be particularly atrophic. Focal atrophy of other brain regions may be seen in atypical clinical presentations of AD. Histopathologically, there are characteristic findings of neuronal loss and gliosis, extracellular amyloid plaques, and intraneuronal neurofibrillary tangles, and their distribution throughout the brain correlates with severity of illness. Various staging methods have been developed for the description of AD pathology (14,82,88). Modern immunostaining techniques have identified beta-amyloid peptide as a major constituent of the insoluble senile plaques (90),

Table 21-5. *Clinical Criteria for Alzheimer's Disease (AD)*

DSM-IV[a]

- Gradual onset and continuing decline of cognitive function from a previously higher level, resulting in impairment of social and occupational function
- Impairment of recent memory and at least one of the following:
  - Language disturbances
  - Word-finding difficulties
  - Disturbances of praxis
  - Disturbances of visual processing
  - Visual agnosia
  - Constructional disturbances
  - Disturbances of executive function, including abstract reasoning and concentration
- Cognitive deficits are not due to other psychiatric, neurologic, or systemic diseases
- Cognitive deficits do not exclusively occur in the setting of delirium

NINCDS-ADRDA[b]
Probable AD

- Criteria for the clinical diagnosis of probable AD
  - Dementia established by clinical examination, documented by mental status testing, and confirmed by neuropsychological tests
  - Deficits in two or more areas of cognition
  - Progressive worsening of memory and other cognitive functions
  - No disturbance of consciousness
  - Onset between ages 40 and 90
  - Absence of systemic or other brain diseases that could account for dementia
- Diagnosis of probable AD is supported by:
  - Progressive deterioration of specific cognitive functions such as language (aphasia), motor skills (apraxia), and perception (agnosia)
  - Impaired activities of daily living and altered patterns of behavior
  - Family history of similar disorders, particularly if confirmed neuropathologically
  - Laboratory results of:
    - Normal lumbar puncture as evaluated by standard techniques
    - Normal pattern or nonspecific changes in EEG, such as increased slow-wave activity
    - Evidence of progressive cerebral atrophy on CT by serial observation
- Features consistent with diagnosis of probable AD:
  - Plateaus in the course of progression of the illness
  - Associated symptoms of depression; insomnia; incontinence; delusions; illusions; hallucinations; catastrophic verbal, emotional, or physical outbursts; sexual disorders; and weight loss
  - Other neurologic abnormalities, especially with more advanced disease and including motor signs such as increased muscle tone, myoclonus, or gait disorder
  - Seizures in advanced disease
  - CT normal for age
- Features that make diagnosis of probable AD unlikely:
  - Sudden onset
  - Focal neurologic findings
  - Seizures or gait disturbances early in the course of the illness

Possible AD

- Criteria for the clinical diagnosis of possible AD:
  - Atypical onset, presentation, or clinical course of dementia in the absence of other neurologic, psychiatric, or systemic causes
  - Presence of second systemic or brain disorder sufficient to produce dementia but not considered to be the cause of the dementia
  - Single, gradually progressive, severe cognitive deficit identified in the absence of other identifiable cause

Definite AD

- Criteria for the diagnosis of definite AD:
  - Clinical criteria for probable AD
  - Histopathologic evidence obtained from a biopsy or autopsy

[a]American Psychiatric Association. *Diagnostic and Statistical Manual of Mental Disorders*. 4th ed. Washington, DC: American Psychiatric Association; 1994.
[b]McKhann G, et al. Clinical diagnosis of Alzheimer's disease: report of the NINCDS–ADRDA Work Group under the auspices of Department of Health and Human Services Task Force on Alzheimer's Disease. *Neurology*. 1984;34:939–944.

whereas the microtubule-associated protein tau is the main component of tangles and other neurofibrillary pathology (133). Of particular interest is the presence of these and other pathologic findings in elderly individuals without evidence of clinical dementia (61), suggesting a window of opportunity for interventions aimed at arresting pathologic progression before the actual clinical manifestation of dementia develops.

GENETICS

The greatest risk factor for the development of AD is increasing age. Clearly, there are genetic factors that influence risk, demonstrated by an increased risk to first-degree relatives of patients with AD. The most well-defined genetic risk factor for AD is the *apolipoprotein E (ApoE)* gene (19), although linkage studies suggest that other genes also contribute to risk (26). The *ApoE ε4* allele confers increased risk of developing AD, especially in homozygotes (28). Although testing for *ApoE* genotype is available clinically, the presence or absence of an ε4 allele does not confirm or refute the presence of AD pathology in demented patients. Similarly, individuals without cognitive impairment desiring such testing should be counseled that their *ApoE* genotype cannot predict with certainty whether they will ultimately develop AD. Rare autosomal dominant hereditary forms of AD also exist, accounting for a minority of early-onset AD cases, and are related to mutations in three identified genes: *presenilin 1 (PS1)* on chromosome 14 (52,114), *presenilin 2 (PS2)* on chromosome 1 (102), and the *amyloid precursor protein (APP)* on chromosome 21 (119). In patients with a family history suspicious for familial AD, the option of genetic testing should be discussed, typically screening initially for *PS1* because it is more common than the other two mutations. Similar to protocols used for other genetic conditions such as Huntington's disease, it is recommended that patients and families interested in testing be referred to a genetic counselor to discuss the implications of positive or negative test results before proceeding. This is particularly important in the setting of testing for untreatable degenerative conditions that are uniformly fatal.

LEWY BODY DISEASE

After AD, dementia with Lewy bodies (DLB) is felt to be one of the most common causes of degenerative dementia, accounting for up to 15% to 25% of cases of dementia (77). Increasing recognition of this distinct presentation of dementia has yielded consensus criteria for the clinical and neuropathologic diagnosis of DLB (2,77). The core clinical diagnostic features of DLB are shown in Table 21-6. Key clinical features of DLB include cognitive impairment, neuropsychiatric disturbance, parkinsonism, sleep disorders, and autonomic dysfunction. Although cognitive dysfunction in DLB can resemble that of AD, often there are prominent executive and visuospatial deficits that can be identified in the office or on formal neuropsychological assessment (29,85). Fluctuations consisting of dramatic changes in level of arousal or cognitive function are also typical of DLB, but the basis for these fluctuations is not well understood. The most prominent neuropsychiatric feature of DLB is vivid, formed visual hallucinations (1), but depression and delusions can also occur. The parkinsonism of DLB can be identical to that encountered in idiopathic PD, but some patients exhibit a more prominent postural tremor, and others exhibit myoclonus. REM sleep behavior disorder commonly occurs in DLB as well as

Table 21-6. *Clinical Criteria for Dementia with Lewy Bodies (DLB)*

Core features
- Progressive cognitive decline that interferes with normal social and occupational functioning
- Deficits on tests of attention/concentration, verbal fluency, psychomotor speed, and visuospatial functioning often prominent
- Prominent or persistent memory loss may not be present early in the course of illness
- Two of the following core features necessary for the diagnosis of clinically probable DLB, and one necessary for the diagnosis of clinically possible DLB:
  ° Fluctuating cognition or alertness
  ° Recurrent visual hallucinations
  ° Spontaneous features of parkinsonism

Supportive features
- Repeated falls
- Syncope
- Transient loss of consciousness
- Neuroleptic sensitivity
- Systematized delusions
- Tactile or olfactory hallucinations
- REM sleep behavior disorder
- Depression

Features suggesting disorder other than DLB
- Cerebrovascular disease evidenced by focal neurologic signs and/or cerebral infarct(s) present on neuroimaging study
- Findings on examination or on ancillary testing that another medical, neurologic, or psychiatric disorder sufficiently accounts for clinical features

Adapted from McKeith IG, et al. Consensus guidelines for the clinical and pathologic diagnosis of dementia with Lewy bodies (DLB): report of the consortium on DLB international workshop. *Neurology.* 1996;47:1113–1124.

other synucleinopathies (12). This often dramatic condition involves loss of normal muscle atonia during REM sleep, resulting in the patient acting out their dreams, sometimes violently. Other sleep disturbances such as obstructive sleep apnea, restless legs syndrome, and periodic limb movement in sleep can also occur (13). Autonomic dysfunction, including orthostatic hypotension, urinary incontinence, and sexual dysfunction, is also common in DLB (8).

Gross pathology in DLB is often unremarkable, aside from pallor of the substantia nigra similar to that seen in PD. The histopathologic hallmark of DLB is the presence of cortical and subcortical Lewy bodies, readily visible with alpha-synuclein immunohistochemical staining (118). Lewy bodies identified in the intermediolateral column of the spinal cord may be related to the autonomic dysfunction frequently observed in DLB patients (45). One important aspect of the neuropathology of DLB is the frequent coexistence of AD pathology, estimated in approximately 80% of cases with limbic and neocortical Lewy body pathology (67). The genetics of DLB are not well understood, but the clinical features have been reported in a kindred carrying an alpha-synuclein mutation (69) and in several other families (32,124). A family history of dementia also appears to be associated with risk of developing DLB, similar to that observed in AD (113).

VASCULAR DEMENTIA

Because risk of cognitive impairment and vascular disease both increase with age, it is not surprising that these two conditions often coexist. Although less common than AD, it is estimated that vascular dementia (VaD) represents close to 18% of incident dementia (31). Prevalence estimates of VaD vary widely in the literature, likely due to the use of different diagnostic criteria. A community-based autopsy series estimates that pure VaD is the cause of approximately 13% of dementia cases and an additional 12% with coexistent AD (64). There is little doubt that cerebrovascular disease can result in cognitive dysfunction, either alone or in combination with neurodegenerative conditions. Clearly large or multiple infarcts involving eloquent cortex can result in cognitive impairment. Strategically located smaller infarcts affecting hippocampal formations, thalamus, and other subcortical structures have been implicated in significant cognitive dysfunction (73), as has widespread lacunar cerebrovascular disease (130). These observations led to the development of consensus diagnostic criteria for diagnosis of probable VaD (104), which are summarized in Table 21-7.

Known risk factors for cardiovascular disease such as hypertension and diabetes also appear to confer risk for VaD (46). As in AD, the *ApoE ε4* genotype appears to confer risk for VaD (117), but because coexistent AD pathology is quite common in the setting of a clinical diagnosis of VaD, the genotype may simply be contributing to the risk of the AD pathology. Disease course is variable, as in other forms of dementia, but a definite relationship between the onset of dementia and a defined stroke confers worse survival (63). Neuropathologic findings of cerebrovascular disease can vary from large-vessel infarction to microvascular pathology only noted on histologic examination, and the neuropathologist must make a judgment regarding the significance of the burden of vascular disease to the clinical diagnosis of dementia. Although inflammatory disorders such as primary central

Table 21-7. *Clinical Criteria for Vascular Dementia (NINDS-AIREN)*

Probable Vascular Dementia
- Dementia defined by cognitive decline from a previously higher level of functioning and manifested by impairment of memory and of two or more cognitive domains
- Evidence of cerebrovascular disease by focal signs on neurologic examination consistent with stroke
- Evidence of relevant cerebrovascular disease by brain imaging including multiple large-vessel infarcts or a single strategically placed infarct as well as multiple basal ganglia and white matter lacunes or extensive periventricular white matter lesions or combinations thereof
- A relationship between the dementia and the cerebrovascular disease manifested or inferred by one or more of the following:
  ° Onset of dementia abruptly or within 3 months of a recognized stroke
  ° Abrupt deterioration in cognitive function
  ° Fluctuating, stepwise progression of cognitive deficits

Adapted from Roman GC, et al. Vascular dementia: diagnostic criteria for research studies. Report of the NINDS-AIREN International Workshop. *Neurology.* 1993;43:250–260.

nervous system (CNS) vasculitis could cause a VaD, such conditions are rare and typically have a more fulminant presentation (127). Also, rare hereditary forms of VaD, such as cerebral autosomal dominant arteriopathy with subcortical infarcts and leukoencephalopathy (CADASIL) (20) or mitochondrial disorders (93), should be considered in patients with a strong family history of dementia, especially with a young age of onset.

FRONTOTEMPORAL DEMENTIA

Although much less common than AD, DLB, and VaD, the disorders collectively referred to as frontotemporal dementia (FTD) are important causes of degenerative dementia and are notable for their often dramatic clinical presentations. As a group, they accounted for approximately 5% of dementia cases in a large autopsy series (9) and a more substantial percentage of dementia cases with age of onset before 65 (60). There are two major clinical presentations recognized: the behavioral presentation characterized by prominent euphoria, disinhibition, apathy, or repetitive behaviors, and the language presentation characterized by progressive nonfluent or fluent aphasia. The term primary progressive aphasia is generally used to describe the nonfluent presentation (80), whereas the term semantic dementia is often applied to the fluent form. Less common presentations involving progressive prosopagnosia and FTD with associated motor neuron disease (121) and parkinsonism (35) are also recognized. Given the wide array of

clinical presentations encompassed by FTD, consensus criteria for FTD were developed by a group of specialists (89) and are outlined in Table 21-8.

Similar to the varied clinical characteristics, FTD can be associated with a number of different underlying

Table 21-8. *Clinical Features of Frontotemporal Dementia (FTD)*

- Frontal Lobe Dementia
  - ° Core diagnostic features
    - Insidious onset and gradual progression
    - Early decline in social interpersonal conduct
    - Early impairment in regulation of personal conduct
    - Early emotional blunting
    - Early loss of insight
  - ° Supportive diagnostic features
    - Behavioral disorder
      - Decline in personal hygiene and grooming
      - Mental rigidity and inflexibility
      - Distractibility and impersistence
      - Hyperorality and dietary changes
      - Perseverative and stereotyped behavior
      - Utilization behavior
    - Speech and language
      - Altered speech output
        - ° Aspontaneity and economy of speech
        - ° Press of speech
      - Stereotypy of speech
      - Echolalia
      - Perseveration
      - Mutism
        - ° Brain imaging (structural and/or functional): dominant frontal and/or anterior temporal lobe abnormality
- Progressive Nonfluent Aphasia
  - ° Core diagnostic features
    - Insidious onset and gradual progression
    - Nonfluent spontaneous speech with at least one of the following: agrammatism, phonemic paraphasias, anomia
  - ° Supportive diagnostic features
    - Speech and language
      - Stuttering or oral apraxia
      - Impaired repetition
      - Alexia, agraphia
      - Early preservation of word meaning
      - Late mutism
    - Behavior
      - Early preservation of social skills
      - Late behavioral changes similar to FTD

  - ° Brain imaging (structural and/or functional): asymmetric abnormality predominantly affecting dominant hemisphere
- Progressive Fluent Aphasia/Semantic Dementia
  - ° Core diagnostic features
    - Insidious onset and gradual progression
    - Language disorder characterized by:
      - Progressive, fluent, empty spontaneous speech
      - Loss of word meaning, manifest by impaired naming and comprehension
      - Semantic paraphasias
  - ° Supportive diagnostic features
    - Press of speech
    - Idiosyncratic word usage
    - Surface dyslexia and dysgraphia
  - ° Brain imaging (structural and/or functional): asymmetric abnormality predominantly affecting dominant (left) anterior temporal lobe
- Prosopagnosia
  - ° Core diagnostic features
    - Insidious onset and gradual progression
    - Perceptual disorder characterized by:
      - Prosopagnosia: impaired recognition of identity of familiar faces and/or
      - Associative agnosia: impaired recognition of object identity
  - ° Supportive diagnostic features
    - Press of speech
    - Idiosyncratic word usage
    - Surface dyslexia and dysgraphia
  - ° Brain imaging (structural and/or functional): asymmetric abnormality predominantly affecting nondominant (right) anterior temporal lobe
- Other Supportive Clinical Features Common to FTD Syndromes
  - ° Onset before 65 years
  - ° Positive family history of similar disorder in first-degree relative
  - ° Bulbar palsy, muscular weakness, and wasting; fasciculations

Adapted from Neary D, et al. Frontotemporal lobar degeneration: a consensus on clinical diagnostic criteria. *Neurology.* 1998;51:1546–1554.

pathologic changes. All FTDs typically exhibit lobar atrophy that preferentially affects frontal and temporal lobes and may be striking in some cases. The affected regions demonstrate neuronal loss, microvacuolation and astrocytic gliosis. Immunohistochemistry allows subdivision of FTD into groups based on the presence or absence of different intracellular inclusions. Tau-positive inclusions are seen in Pick's disease (Pick bodies), FTD with parkinsonism linked to chromosome 17 (FTDP-17), and other tauopathies that may present with an FTD clinical syndrome such as corticobasal ganglionic degeneration and progressive supranuclear palsy (36). The presence of ubiquitin inclusions is the defining feature of another subset of FTD cases (FTD-U), sometimes associated with clinical or pathologic features of motor neuron disease (FTD-MND) (87). Finally, some FTD cases lack any distinguishable pathologic inclusions and have been referred to as "dementia lacking distinctive histology" (59).

The majority of FTD cases are sporadic, but kindreds with autosomal dominant FTD have been studied extensively, leading to identification of mutations in the genes coding for the microtubule-associated protein tau (*MAPT*) (51) and, more recently, progranulin (*PGRN*) (34). Linkage studies point to other candidate genes causing familial FTD on chromosomes 3 and 9 (48,116). Clinical screening for *MAPT* mutations is available, but genetic counseling prior to testing is recommended as for familial AD.

NORMAL PRESSURE HYDROCEPHALUS

Normal pressure hydrocephalus (NPH) has received increased public attention, in part due to media advertising for newer programmable valves for ventriculoperitoneal (VP) shunting. Classically, patients present with the clinical triad of gait disturbance, urinary incontinence, and cognitive dysfunction (40). The gait difficulties can resemble those of PD, with shortened stride length and freezing (125), but often exhibit a wider base (120). Urinary urgency typically predates frank incontinence but is somewhat insensitive given the common occurrence of urinary difficulties in older individuals. The cognitive dysfunction is not typical of AD and is characterized by a "subcortical" pattern of impaired working memory and slowed processing speed (125), similar to the pattern seen in VaD with extensive subcortical ischemic changes. Brain imaging with computed tomography (CT) or magnetic resonance imaging (MRI) should demonstrate ventriculomegaly not attributable to generalized cerebral atrophy. Although other techniques, such as magnetic resonance flow imaging and radioisotope cisternography, have been proposed to

aid in the diagnosis of NPH, they cannot successfully predict outcome of a shunting procedure (42).

When NPH is clinically suspected, a number of approaches to the diagnosis can be used. The most common approach is high-volume lumbar puncture (30 to 50 mL), with assessment of clinical improvement in gait disturbance. This can most reliably be assessed by same-day video documentation of gait before and after shunting, with quantifiable measures such as gait velocity and stride length before and after lumbar puncture (120). Serial lumbar punctures may improve accuracy of diagnosis. Continuous lumbar CSF drainage is another approach (75) but generally requires hospitalization and may pose a greater risk of complications such as infection or cerebrospinal fluid (CSF) leak. If patients have a favorable response to such procedures, a definitive VP shunt procedure can be performed, although there are no randomized controlled trials evaluating the efficacy of this technique (27). Approximately 59% of patients have improvement following shunting, although sustained improvement is observed in only 29%, and complications occur in 38% (42). Given the relatively high complication rate, patients and families should be carefully counseled before proceeding with a shunt procedure. Another concern is the possible coexistence of degenerative disorders contributing to the cognitive or motor dysfunction that would not respond to shunting and may account for some patients who later decline after an initial beneficial response. Biomarkers such as CSF beta-amyloid and tau levels may have utility in counseling patients about possible coexistent AD before proceeding with a shunt procedure.

RAPIDLY PROGRESSIVE DEMENTIA

Most degenerative dementias are characterized by insidious onset and gradual progression. More fulminant presentations of dementia may be difficult to distinguish from other conditions associated with rapid onset of cognitive and behavioral disturbance. Delirium due to metabolic derangement such as hyponatremia or thiamine deficiency, hypoxemia, or occult infection should be excluded, but if cognitive dysfunction persists, more detailed evaluation for rare conditions should be pursued. Prion diseases such as Creutzfeldt-Jakob disease (CJD) and variant CJD should be considered in the setting of rapidly progressive dementia, especially when accompanied by myoclonus, seizures, or gait disturbance (33). Periodic sharp wave complexes may be present on EEG, and diffusion-weighted abnormalities may be seen in the basal ganglia, thalamus, and cortical ribbon (18). Unfortunately, there is no effective treatment for prion disorders, and they are invariably fatal. Other entities to consider when faced with a rapidly progressive dementia syndrome include paraneoplastic limbic encephalitis (71) or autoimmune encephalopathies such as Hashimoto encephalopathy (16). These conditions are important to recognize because identification and treatment of the underlying malignancy in the paraneoplastic syndromes or institution of prompt immunosuppressant therapy in inflammatory encephalopathies may be curative.

EVALUATION

A practice parameter submitted by the American Academy of Neurology outlines a rational approach to the diagnosis of dementia (62). The initial evaluation of a patient with suspected cognitive impairment/dementia should include a careful history regarding the presenting symptoms, preferably corroborated by a reliable informant because many patients with dementia have limited insight into their deficits. Psychiatric illness such as depression may masquerade as dementia, but careful questioning when obtaining the clinical history typically will identify such cases. A standard neurologic examination including a mental status examination, such as the Folstein Mini-Mental State exam (30) or the Kokmen Short Test of Mental Status (66), should be conducted. Physical examination findings such as focal deficits or parkinsonism may suggest particular entities such as VaD or DLB, respectively. Disinhibition or other unusual behaviors may suggest FTD, and striking language disturbance could indicate one of the progressive aphasias.

Routine laboratory evaluations should be obtained to exclude comorbid medical conditions that may contribute to cognitive dysfunction, including hepatic or renal dysfunction, thyroid dysfunction, and vitamin B_{12} deficiency. These conditions are generally readily recognizable due to other clinical manifestations and do not present with an isolated dementia syndrome. Routine laboratory testing for neurosyphilis is not recommended in the evaluation of dementia, unless patients have an identifiable risk factor (62).

Structural brain imaging with CT or MRI should be pursued as part of the initial evaluation of a patient with suspected dementia, primarily to exclude conditions that may mimic dementia including neoplasms, subdural hematoma and other cerebrovascular diseases, and hydrocephalus. Functional neuroimaging with single photon emission CT (SPECT) and positron emission tomography (PET) shows promise in the evaluation and differentiation of the major dementia syndromes, but SPECT and PET require further study before their routine use can be advocated. Figure 21-1 demonstrates typical imaging findings in patients with normal cognition, MCI, and AD.

Neuropsychological assessment is an important tool in the evaluation of patients with cognitive complaints. Not only can it provide a quantitative measure of cognitive performance in multiple cognitive domains essential for an accurate diagnosis of dementia, but it can also yield patterns of dysfunction that may be suggestive of particular dementia syndromes. For example, patients with FTD may have intact performance on memory measures typically abnormal in AD patients and, instead, demonstrate difficulties on tasks of executive function and cognitive flexibility. Perhaps more importantly, neuropsychological assessment can be helpful to differentiate between MCI and dementia, which has significant implications for clinical management. Also, monitoring progression or stability of impairment can readily be accomplished using serial neuropsychological assessments. Appropriate normative data should be applied to the

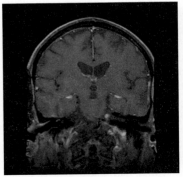 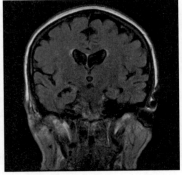 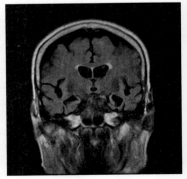

Figure 21-1. Coronal MRI images in **(A)** normal cognition (T1 with gadolinium), **(B)** mild cognitive impairment [fluid-attenuated inversion recovery (FLAIR)], and **(C)** Alzheimer's disease (FLAIR). Note progression of medial temporal lobe atrophy with degree of cognitive impairment.

interpretation of neuropsychological data in older patients to control for age-related changes in cognition that may be misinterpreted as impairment (41). Similarly, caution should be used when interpreting such data in special populations, such as individuals speaking English as a second language, or in minority populations (74).

TREATMENT

Although treatment for the cognitive symptoms of dementia are limited, the ChEIs donepezil, rivastigmine, and galantamine all demonstrate efficacy for the treatment of mild to moderate AD (103,105,123). An important effect of these agents is to delay progression of symptoms by a median of 5 months (84), but because they do not appear to directly impact the underlying pathology of AD or other dementias, clinicians should counsel patients and their caregivers to have realistic expectations about the benefits of these agents. There are data to suggest that some patients may derive neuropsychiatric benefit from ChEIs as well (47). More recent studies suggest that ChEIs may be of benefit in the setting of VaD (24,128) and DLB (106). Donepezil has also been demonstrated to show efficacy for moderate to severe AD (129). Memantine demonstrates benefit for the treatment of moderate to severe AD (101), but like the ChEIs, it appears to primarily delay, rather than arrest, symptomatic progression. The exact mechanism of action is not well understood but appears to involve modulation of glutamatergic transmission by antagonism at *N*-methyl-D-aspartic acid (NMDA) receptors.

Treatment of behavioral symptoms of dementia is unfortunately less well defined. Agents commonly used include atypical and typical neuroleptics, antidepressants, mood-stabilizing agents such as valproic acid, and benzodiazepines. A recent black box warning about the use of atypical neuroleptics for the management of behavioral manifestations of dementia in elderly patients called into question the safety of such agents, citing concerns about increased cardiovascular morbidity (112). Further analysis of these agents in a large multicenter prospective trial suggested benefit of atypical neuroleptics for a minority of patients with behavioral symptoms of dementia, with limiting side effects and lack of efficacy being commonly cited reasons for discontinuation (111). In particular, caution must be used when considering neuroleptic use in patients with suspected DLB because these patients often exhibit exquisite neuroleptic sensitivity (2). In the absence of an approved therapeutic guideline for treatment of these troubling symptoms, clinicians must use a trial and error approach, counseling patients and their caregivers about potential risks of each treatment option.

Another clinical scenario that deserves comment is abrupt decline in a patient with an established diagnosis of dementia. In general, this is not related to a change in the trajectory of the clinical course of their dementia, but rather heralds the presence of a comorbid illness with associated delirium. Infectious causes such as urinary tract infections, pneumonia, or cellulitis should be excluded. Polypharmacy or recent medication changes may be contributing factors as well. Repeat assessment for changes in pulmonary, hepatic, renal, or endocrine function should be considered. Repeat brain imaging may be indicated, especially when confronted with alteration in level of consciousness or history of trauma. Electroencephalography (EEG) may be helpful if there is suspicion of subclinical seizure activity, and spinal fluid exam should be pursued if there are any signs of meningeal irritation or the initial evaluations are unrevealing.

SAFETY

Once a diagnosis of dementia is established, certain issues must be discussed with patients and their family/caregivers. Supervision of medications is imperative, especially for medications with potentially life-threatening complications if taken improperly such as anticoagulants. A family member or other designated individual should also supervise all complex legal, medical, or financial decision making to ensure that the affected individual does not fall victim to scams or other nefarious activity. Driving safety must also be discussed given the potential for injury to the patient or others if poor judgment while driving results in an accident. A practice parameter from the American Academy of Neurology outlines recommendations for driving cessation in patients with dementia (22). There are no specific driving guidelines for patients with MCI, but baseline and periodic driving assessment is one suggested approach to ensure that cognitive dysfunction is not adversely affecting performance.

Later stages of dementia are associated with a different set of safety concerns. In particular, wandering behavior can lead to tragic outcomes (107). Increased supervision and identity bracelets, such as those available through the Safe Return program of the Alzheimer's Association, may be helpful. Potentially dangerous tools or firearms should not be accessible to patients with dementia. Any use of household appliances must be supervised to reduce risk of fires or other accidents. The thermostat may need to be adjusted on the water heater to reduce risk of scalding. As the degree of supervision required increases with progression of disease, ultimately placement in an assisted living or skilled care facility may be necessary.

PREVENTION

No proven therapy exists that provides protection against the development of dementia. Past data have suggested a potential protective benefit from hormone replacement therapy (57) and use of nonsteroidal anti-inflammatory drugs (NSAIDs) (76) with respect to risk of developing AD, but subsequent studies cast doubt on these observations (43,86,109). Flurbiprofen shows promise in preliminary studies and is felt to have a lower likelihood of gastrointestinal toxicity compared to other NSAIDs due to its unique stereochemical properties (23). High-dose vitamin E was also proposed as a potential therapy for reducing oxidative damage and thereby risk of development of AD (108), but recent data suggest potential for risk of such treatment (81). Use of vitamin C in combination with vitamin E was associated with decreased incidence and prevalence of AD, but the data are limited (134). Lowering plasma homocysteine levels with vitamin B_{12} and B_6 and folate supplements did not improve cognition in a recent randomized trial (79). Supplements such as ginkgo biloba (72) and acetyl-L-carnitine (92) lack sufficient data to recommend their use for prevention or treatment of dementia.

ON THE HORIZON: DIAGNOSTIC AND THERAPEUTIC APPROACHES

There is great interest in the use of CSF biomarkers of AD, and CSF levels of beta-amyloid 1-42 and tau proteins show predictable patterns in AD patients (50). CSF beta-amyloid 1-42 levels are reduced in AD patients relative to elderly controls, but it is unclear what factors may influence these levels, especially in very early dementia cases or those with atypical features (54). Elevated CSF tau is present in AD but is also seen in other dementias, reducing diagnostic specificity (5). Until these techniques are refined, CSF biomarkers for AD are not recommended for clinical practice (62). Neuroimaging advances show great promise in identification of individuals either suffering from or at risk for development of AD. The Pittsburgh Compound B shows significant promise as a tool for the in vivo imaging of amyloid pathology using PET (58). Also, PET imaging shows distinct regions of altered brain metabolism in *ApoE ε4* carriers with no evidence of dementia (100), a potentially useful biomarker for presymptomatic cognitive decline in individuals at high risk for later cognitive decline.

An exciting novel approach to AD treatment via vaccination against the beta-amyloid peptide itself was pursued after promising results in animal studies of transgenic mice carrying the *APP 717* mutation (110). Unfortunately, a significant number of patients participating in the multicenter international trial of amyloid vaccination for AD developed an inflammatory meningoencephalitis that was fatal in some cases (91). With modification of the vaccination technique, hopefully additional vaccine trials will be more successful. Given prominent gliosis in the neuropathology of AD and past epidemiologic studies suggesting benefit of anti-inflammatory drugs, further treatment trials have been pursued, including a negative study of prednisone (3) and ongoing studies of intravenous immunoglobulin (IVIG) (21). Therapies specifically targeting the biochemical basis of AD are of particular interest, including modulation of the secretases responsible for cleavage of *APP* and generation of the toxic species of amyloid that lead to plaque formation (17,115). One concern with this approach is the inadvertent disruption of other necessary cellular functions of the secretases, including Notch cleavage (10). Targeting *ApoE* itself for the treatment or prevention of AD is of interest, given the clear differential risk of developing AD conferred to an individual based on their *ApoE* genotype. Preliminary studies suggest that, by directly targeting the functions or conformation of *ApoE ε4*, pathologic processing of amyloid may be suppressed (49).

Eventually, more effective treatments will be identified for the treatment of AD and other forms of dementia. In the future, identification of presymptomatic individuals with a combination of genetic, imaging, and laboratory markers will hopefully allow early intervention and prevent, or at least significantly delay, the development of these devastating diseases.

ACKNOWLEDGMENTS

This work was supported in part by funding from grant P30 AG19610-01 from the Arizona Alzheimer's Disease Consortium.

DISCLOSURE

Dr. Woodruff has served as a paid consultant to GlaxoSmithKline in the past 5 years.

REFERENCES

1. Aarsland D, et al. A comparative study of psychiatric symptoms in dementia with Lewy bodies and Parkinson's disease with and without dementia. *Int J Geriatr Psychiatry.* 2001;16: 528–536.
2. Aarsland D, et al. Neuroleptic sensitivity in Parkinson's disease and parkinsonian dementias. *J Clin Psychiatry.* 2005;66:633–637.
3. Aisen PS, et al. A randomized controlled trial of prednisone in Alzheimer's disease. Alzheimer's

Disease Cooperative Study. *Neurology*. 2000;54: 588–593.

4. American Psychiatric Association. *Diagnostic and Statistical Manual of Mental Disorders*. 4th ed. Washington, DC: American Psychiatric Association; 1994.

5. Arai H, Higuchi S, Sasaki H. Apolipoprotein E genotyping and cerebrospinal fluid tau protein: implications for the clinical diagnosis of Alzheimer's disease. *Gerontology*. 1997;43[Suppl 1]: 2–10.

6. Arvanitakis Z, Wilson RS, Bennett DA. Diabetes mellitus, dementia, and cognitive function in older persons. *J Nutr Health Aging*. 2006; 10:287–291.

7. Bachman DL, et al. Incidence of dementia and probable Alzheimer's disease in a general population: the Framingham Study. *Neurology*. 1993; 43:515–519.

8. Ballard C, et al. High prevalence of neurovascular instability in neurodegenerative dementias. *Neurology*. 1998;51:1760–1762.

9. Barker WW, et al. Relative frequencies of Alzheimer disease, Lewy body, vascular and frontotemporal dementia, and hippocampal sclerosis in the State of Florida Brain Bank. *Alzheimer Dis Assoc Disord*. 2002;16: 203–212.

10. Barten DM, et al. Gamma-secretase inhibitors for Alzheimer's disease: balancing efficacy and toxicity. *Drugs R D*. 2006;7:87–97.

11. Beard CM, et al. Cause of death in Alzheimer's disease. *Ann Epidemiol*. 1996;6:195–200.

12. Boeve BF, et al. Association of REM sleep behavior disorder and neurodegenerative disease may reflect an underlying synucleinopathy. *Mov Disord*. 2001;16:622–630.

13. Boeve BF, Silber MH, Ferman TJ. Current management of sleep disturbances in dementia. *Curr Neurol Neurosci Rep*. 2002;2:169–177.

14. Braak H, Braak E. Staging of Alzheimer's disease-related neurofibrillary changes. *Neurobiol Aging*. 1995;16:271–284.

15. Callahan CM, et al. Relationship of age, education, and occupation with dementia among a community-based sample of African Americans. *Arch Neurol*. 1996;53:134–140.

16. Castillo P, et al. Steroid-responsive encephalopathy associated with autoimmune thyroiditis. *Arch Neurol*. 2006;63:197–202.

17. Citron M. Emerging Alzheimer's disease therapies: inhibition of beta-secretase. *Neurobiol Aging*. 2002;23:1017–1022.

18. Collie DA, et al. MRI of Creutzfeldt-Jakob disease: imaging features and recommended MRI protocol. *Clin Radiol*. 2001;56:726–739.

19. Corder EH, et al. Gene dose of apolipoprotein E type 4 allele and the risk of Alzheimer's disease in late onset families. *Science*. 1993;261: 921–923.

20. Dichgans M. et al. The phenotypic spectrum of CADASIL: clinical findings in 102 cases. *Ann Neurol*. 1998;44:731–739.

21. Dodel RC, et al. Intravenous immunoglobulins containing antibodies against beta-amyloid for the treatment of Alzheimer's disease. *J Neurol Neurosurg Psychiatry*. 2004;75:1472–1474.

22. Dubinsky RM, Stein AC, Lyons K. Practice parameter: risk of driving and Alzheimer's disease (an evidence-based review): report of the Quality Standards Subcommittee of the American Academy of Neurology. *Neurology*. 2000;54:2205–2211.

23. Eriksen JL, et al. NSAIDs and enantiomers of flurbiprofen target gamma-secretase and lower Abeta 42 in vivo. *J Clin Invest*. 2003;112:440–449.

24. Erkinjuntti T, et al. Efficacy of galantamine in probable vascular dementia and Alzheimer's disease combined with cerebrovascular disease: a randomised trial. *Lancet*. 2002;359:1283–1290.

25. Ernst RL, Hay JW. Economic research on Alzheimer disease: a review of the literature. *Alzheimer Dis Assoc Disord*, 1997;11[Suppl 6]: 135–145.

26. Ertekin-Taner N, et al. Linkage of plasma Abeta42 to a quantitative locus on chromosome 10 in late-onset Alzheimer's disease pedigrees. *Science*. 2000;290:2303–2304.

27. Esmonde T, Cooke S. Shunting for normal pressure hydrocephalus (NPH). *Cochrane Database Syst Rev*. 2002;3:CD003157.

28. Farrer LA, et al. Effects of age, sex, and ethnicity on the association between apolipoprotein E genotype and Alzheimer disease. A meta-analysis. APOE and Alzheimer Disease Meta Analysis Consortium. *JAMA*. 1997;278:1349–1356.

29. Ferman TJ, et al. Neuropsychological differentiation of dementia with Lewy bodies from normal aging and Alzheimer's disease. *Clin Neuropsychol*. 2006;20:623–636.

30. Folstein MF, Folstein SE, McHugh PR. Mini-mental state. A practical method for grading the cognitive state of patients for the clinician. *J Psychiatr Res*. 1975;12:189–198.

31. Fratiglioni L, et al. Incidence of dementia and major subtypes in Europe: a collaborative study of population-based cohorts. Neurologic Diseases in the Elderly Research Group. *Neurology*. 2000; 54[Suppl 5]:S10–S15.

32. Galvin JE, et al. Familial dementia with Lewy bodies: clinicopathologic analysis of two kindreds. *Neurology*. 2002;59:1079–1082.

33. Gambetti P, et al. Sporadic and familial CJD: classification and characterisation. *Br Med Bull.* 2003;66:213–239.

34. Gass J, et al. Mutations in progranulin are a major cause of ubiquitin-positive frontotemporal lobar degeneration. *Hum Mol Genet.* 2006;15:2988–3001.

35. Ghetti B, Hutton M, Wszolek Z. Frontotemporal dementia and parkinsonism linked to chromosome 17 associated with tau gene mutations (FTDP–17T). In: Dickson D, ed. *Neurodegeneration: the molecular pathology of dementia and movement disorders.* Basel: ISN Neuropath Press; 2003:86–102.

36. Goedert M. Introduction to the tauopathies. In: Dickson D, ed. *Neurodegeneration: the molecular pathology of dementia and movement disorders.* Basel: ISN Neuropath Press; 2003:82–85.

37. Graff-Radford NR, et al. Simultanagnosia as the initial sign of degenerative dementia. *Mayo Clin Proc.* 1993;68:955–964.

38. Green J, et al. Progressive aphasia: a precursor of global dementia? *Neurology.* 1990;40:423–429.

39. Guo Z, et al. Head injury and the risk of AD in the MIRAGE study. *Neurology.* 2000;54:1316–1323.

40. Hakim S, Adams RD. The special clinical problem of symptomatic hydrocephalus with normal cerebrospinal fluid pressure. Observations on cerebrospinal fluid hydrodynamics. *J Neurol Sci.* 1965;2:307–327.

41. Harris ME, Ivnik RJ, Smith GE. Mayo's Older Americans Normative Studies: expanded AVLT Recognition Trial norms for ages 57 to 98. *J Clin Exp Neuropsychol.* 2002;24:214–220.

42. Hebb AO, Cusimano MD. Idiopathic normal pressure hydrocephalus: a systematic review of diagnosis and outcome. *Neurosurgery.* 2001;49:1166–1184.

43. Henderson VW, et al. Estrogen for Alzheimer's disease in women: randomized, double-blind, placebo-controlled trial. *Neurology.* 2000;54:295–301.

44. Heyman A, et al. Predictors of time to institutionalization of patients with Alzheimer's disease: the CERAD experience, part XVII. *Neurology.* 1997;48:1304–1309.

45. Hishikawa N, et al. Clinical and neuropathological correlates of Lewy body disease. *Acta Neuropathol (Berl).* 2003;105:341–350.

46. Hofman A, et al. Atherosclerosis, apolipoprotein E, and prevalence of dementia and Alzheimer's disease in the Rotterdam Study. *Lancet.* 1997;349:151–154.

47. Holmes C, et al. The efficacy of donepezil in the treatment of neuropsychiatric symptoms in Alzheimer disease. *Neurology.* 2004;63:214–219.

48. Hosler BA, et al. Linkage of familial amyotrophic lateral sclerosis with frontotemporal dementia to chromosome 9q21-q22. *JAMA.* 2000;284:1664–1669.

49. Huang Y, et al. Apolipoprotein E: diversity of cellular origins, structural and biophysical properties, and effects in Alzheimer's disease. *J Mol Neurosci.* 2004;23:189–204.

50. Hulstaert F, et al. Improved discrimination of AD patients using beta-amyloid (1-42) and tau levels in CSF. *Neurology.* 1999;52:1555–1562.

51. Hutton M. Molecular genetics of chromosome 17 tauopathies. *Ann NY Acad Sci.* 2000;920:63–73.

52. Hutton M, et al. Complete analysis of the presenilin 1 gene in early onset Alzheimer's disease. *Neuroreport.* 1996;7:801–805.

53. Jack CR Jr., et al. Prediction of AD with MRI-based hippocampal volume in mild cognitive impairment. *Neurology.* 1999;52:1397–1403.

54. Jensen M, et al. Cerebrospinal fluid A beta42 is increased early in sporadic Alzheimer's disease and declines with disease progression. *Ann Neurol.* 1999;45:504–511.

55. Jorm AF, Jolley D. The incidence of dementia: a meta-analysis. *Neurology.* 1998;51:728–733.

56. Kawas C, et al. Age-specific incidence rates of Alzheimer's disease: the Baltimore Longitudinal Study of Aging. *Neurology.* 2000;54:2072–2077.

57. Kawas C, et al. A prospective study of estrogen replacement therapy and the risk of developing Alzheimer's disease: the Baltimore Longitudinal Study of Aging. *Neurology.* 1997;48:1517–1521.

58. Klunk WE, et al. Imaging brain amyloid in Alzheimer's disease with Pittsburgh Compound-B. *Ann Neurol.* 2004;55:306–319.

59. Knopman DS. Overview of dementia lacking distinctive histology: pathological designation of a progressive dementia. *Dementia.* 1993;4:132–136.

60. Knopman DS, et al. Dementia lacking distinctive histologic features: a common non-Alzheimer degenerative dementia. *Neurology.* 1990;40:251–256.

61. Knopman DS, et al. Neuropathology of cognitively normal elderly. *J Neuropathol Exp Neurol.* 2003;62:1087–1095.

62. Knopman DS, et al. Practice parameter: diagnosis of dementia (an evidence-based review). Report of the Quality Standards Subcommittee of the American Academy of Neurology. *Neurology.* 2001;56:1143–1153.

63. Knopman DS, et al. Survival study of vascular dementia in Rochester, Minnesota. *Arch Neurol.* 2003;60:85–90.

64. Knopman DS, et al. Vascular dementia in a population-based autopsy study. *Arch Neurol.* 2003;60:569–575.

65. Kokmen E, et al. Dementia after ischemic stroke: a population-based study in Rochester, Minnesota (1960-1984). *Neurology.* 1996;46:154–159.

66. Kokmen E, et al. The short test of mental status. Correlations with standardized psychometric testing. *Arch Neurol.* 1991;48:725–728.

67. Kosaka K. Diffuse Lewy body disease. *Neuropathology.* 2000;20(suppl):S73–S78.

68. Kukull WA, et al. Causes of death associated with Alzheimer disease: variation by level of cognitive impairment before death. *J Am Geriatr Soc.* 1994;42:723–726.

69. Langston JW, et al. Novel alpha-synuclein-immunoreactive proteins in brain samples from the Contursi kindred, Parkinson's, and Alzheimer's disease. *Exp Neurol.* 1998;154:684–690.

70. Larner AJ. Frontal variant Alzheimer's disease: a reappraisal. *Clin Neurol Neurosurg.* 2006;108:705–708.

71. Lawn ND, et al. Clinical, magnetic resonance imaging, and electroencephalographic findings in paraneoplastic limbic encephalitis. *Mayo Clin Proc.* 2003;78:1363–1368.

72. Le Bars PL, et al. A placebo-controlled, double-blind, randomized trial of an extract of ginkgo biloba for dementia. North American EGb Study Group. *JAMA.* 1997;278:1327–1332.

73. Leys D, et al. Vascular dementia: the role of cerebral infarcts. *Alzheimer Dis Assoc Disord.* 1999;13[Suppl 3]:S38–S48.

74. Lucas JA, et al. Mayo's Older African Americans Normative Studies: normative data for commonly used clinical neuropsychological measures. *Clin Neuropsychol.* 2005;19:162–183.

75. Marmarou A, et al. Diagnosis and management of idiopathic normal-pressure hydrocephalus: a prospective study in 151 patients. *J Neurosurg.* 2005;102:987–997.

76. McGeer PL, Schulzer M, McGeer EG. Arthritis and anti-inflammatory agents as possible protective factors for Alzheimer's disease: a review of 17 epidemiologic studies. *Neurology.* 1996;47:425–432.

77. McKeith IG, et al. Consensus guidelines for the clinical and pathologic diagnosis of dementia with Lewy bodies (DLB): report of the consortium on DLB international workshop. *Neurology.* 1996;47:1113–1124.

78. McKhann G, et al. Clinical diagnosis of Alzheimer's disease: report of the NINCDS–ADRDA Work Group under the auspices of Department of Health and Human Services Task Force on Alzheimer's Disease. *Neurology.* 1984;34:939–944.

79. McMahon JA, et al. A controlled trial of homocysteine lowering and cognitive performance. *N Engl J Med.* 2006;354:2764–2772.

80. Mesulam MM. Primary progressive aphasia. *Ann Neurol.* 2001;49:425–432.

81. Miller ER 3rd, et al. Meta-analysis: high-dosage vitamin E supplementation may increase all-cause mortality. *Ann Intern Med.* 2005;142:37–46.

82. Mirra SS, et al. The Consortium to Establish a Registry for Alzheimer's Disease (CERAD). Part II. Standardization of the neuropathologic assessment of Alzheimer's disease. *Neurology.* 1991;41:479–486.

83. Mittelman MS, et al. Improving caregiver well-being delays nursing home placement of patients with Alzheimer disease. *Neurology.* 2006;67:1592–1599.

84. Mohs RC, et al. A 1-year, placebo-controlled preservation of function survival study of donepezil in AD patients. *Neurology.* 2001;57:481–488.

85. Mori E, et al. Visuoperceptual impairment in dementia with Lewy bodies. *Arch Neurol.* 2000;57:489–493.

86. Mulnard RA, et al. Estrogen replacement therapy for treatment of mild to moderate Alzheimer disease: a randomized controlled trial. Alzheimer's Disease Cooperative Study. *JAMA.* 2000;283:1007–1015.

87. Munoz DG, et al. The neuropathology and biochemistry of frontotemporal dementia. *Ann Neurol.* 2003;54[Suppl 5]:S24–S28.

88. National Institute on Aging–Reagan Institute Working Group. Consensus recommendations for the postmortem diagnosis of Alzheimer's disease. The National Institute on Aging, and Reagan Institute Working Group on Diagnostic Criteria for the Neuropathological Assessment of Alzheimer's Disease. *Neurobiol Aging.* 1997;18[Suppl 4]:S1–S2.

89. Neary D, et al. Frontotemporal lobar degeneration: a consensus on clinical diagnostic criteria. *Neurology.* 1998;51:1546–1554.

90. Ogomori K, et al. Beta-protein amyloid is widely distributed in the central nervous system of patients with Alzheimer's disease. *Am J Pathol.* 1989;134:243–251.

91. Orgogozo JM, et al. Subacute meningoencephalitis in a subset of patients with AD after Abeta42 immunization. *Neurology.* 2003;61:46–54.

92. Passeri M, et al. Acetyl-L-carnitine in the treatment of mildly demented elderly patients. *Int J Clin Pharmacol Res.* 1990;10:75–79.

93. Pavlakis SG, et al. Mitochondrial myopathy, encephalopathy, lactic acidosis, and strokelike episodes: a distinctive clinical syndrome. *Ann Neurol.* 1984;16:481–488.

94. Petersen RC, et al. Memory function in very early Alzheimer's disease. *Neurology.* 1994;44: 867–872.

95. Petersen RC, et al. Mild cognitive impairment: clinical characterization and outcome. *Arch Neurol.* 1999;56:303–308.

96. Petersen RC, et al. Neuropathologic features of amnestic mild cognitive impairment. *Arch Neurol.* 2006;63:665–672.

97. Petersen RC, et al. Practice parameter: early detection of dementia: mild cognitive impairment (an evidence-based review). Report of the Quality Standards Subcommittee of the American Academy of Neurology. *Neurology.* 2001;56: 1133–1142.

98. Petersen RC, et al. Vitamin E and donepezil for the treatment of mild cognitive impairment. *N Engl J Med.* 2005;352:2379–2388.

99. Petersen RC, Morris JC. Clinical features. In: Petersen RC, ed. *Mild cognitive impairment: aging to Alzheimer's disease.* New York: Oxford University Press; 2003:15–40.

100. Reiman EM, et al. Declining brain activity in cognitively normal apolipoprotein E epsilon 4 heterozygotes: a foundation for using positron emission tomography to efficiently test treatments to prevent Alzheimer's disease. *Proc Natl Acad Sci USA.* 2001;98:3334–3339.

101. Reisberg B, et al. Memantine in moderate-to-severe Alzheimer's disease. *N Engl J Med.* 2003; 348:1333–1341.

102. Rogaev EI, et al. Familial Alzheimer's disease in kindreds with missense mutations in a gene on chromosome 1 related to the Alzheimer's disease type 3 gene. *Nature.* 1995;376:775–778.

103. Rogers SL, et al. A 24-week, double-blind, placebo-controlled trial of donepezil in patients with Alzheimer's disease. Donepezil Study Group. *Neurology.* 1998;50:136–145.

104. Roman GC, et al. Vascular dementia: diagnostic criteria for research studies. Report of the NINDS-AIREN International Workshop. *Neurology.* 1993;43:250–260.

105. Rosler M, et al. Efficacy and safety of rivastigmine in patients with Alzheimer's disease: international randomised controlled trial. *BMJ.* 1999;318:633–638.

106. Rowan E, et al. Effects of donepezil on central processing speed and attentional measures in Parkinson's disease with dementia and dementia with Lewy bodies. *Dement Geriatr Cogn Disord.* 2006;23:161–167.

107. Rowe MA, Bennett V. A look at deaths occurring in persons with dementia lost in the community. *Am J Alzheimers Dis Other Dement.* 2003;18:343–348.

108. Sano M, et al. A controlled trial of selegiline, alpha-tocopherol, or both as treatment for Alzheimer's disease. The Alzheimer's Disease Cooperative Study. *N Engl J Med.* 1997;336: 1216–1222.

109. Scharf S, et al. A double-blind, placebo-controlled trial of diclofenac/misoprostol in Alzheimer's disease. *Neurology.* 1999;53:197–201.

110. Schenk D, et al. Immunization with amyloid-beta attenuates Alzheimer-disease-like pathology in the PDAPP mouse. *Nature.* 1999;400:173–177.

111. Schneider LS, et al. Effectiveness of atypical antipsychotic drugs in patients with Alzheimer's disease. *N Engl J Med.* 2006;355:1525–1538.

112. Schneider LS, Dagerman KS, and Insel P. Risk of death with atypical antipsychotic drug treatment for dementia: meta-analysis of randomized placebo-controlled trials. *JAMA.* 2005;294: 1934–1943.

113. Seltzer B, et al. Awareness of deficit in Alzheimer's disease: relation to caregiver burden. *Gerontologist.* 1997;37:20–24.

114. Sherrington R, et al. Cloning of a gene bearing missense mutations in early-onset familial Alzheimer's disease. *Nature.* 1995;375:754–760.

115. Siemers ER, et al. Effects of a gamma-secretase inhibitor in a randomized study of patients with Alzheimer disease. *Neurology.* 2006;66:602–604.

116. Skibinski G, et al. Mutations in the endosomal ESCRTIII-complex subunit CHMP2B in frontotemporal dementia. *Nat Genet.* 2005;37: 806–808.

117. Slooter AJ, et al. Apolipoprotein E epsilon4 and the risk of dementia with stroke. A population-based investigation. *JAMA.* 1997;277:818–821.

118. Spillantini MG, et al. Filamentous alpha-synuclein inclusions link multiple system atrophy with Parkinson's disease and dementia with Lewy bodies. *Neurosci Lett.* 1998;251:205–208.

119. St George-Hyslop PH, et al. The genetic defect causing familial Alzheimer's disease maps on chromosome 21. *Science.* 1987;235:885–890.

120. Stolze H, et al. Gait analysis in idiopathic normal pressure hydrocephalus—which parameters respond to the CSF tap test? *Clin Neurophysiol.* 2000;111:1678–1686.

121. Strong MJ, et al. Cognitive impairment, frontotemporal dementia, and the motor neuron diseases. *Ann Neurol.* 2003;54[Suppl 5]:S20–S23.

122. Tang-Wai DF, et al. Clinical, genetic, and neuropathologic characteristics of posterior cortical atrophy. *Neurology.* 2004;63:1168–1174.

123. Tariot PN, et al. A 5-month, randomized, placebo-controlled trial of galantamine in AD. The Galantamine USA-10 Study Group. *Neurology.* 2000;54:2269–2276.

124. Tsuang DW, et al. Familial dementia with Lewy bodies: a clinical and neuropathological study of 2 families. *Arch Neurol.* 2002;59:1622–1630.

125. Vanneste JA. Diagnosis and management of normal-pressure hydrocephalus. *J Neurol.* 2000;247:5–14.

126. Welch HG, Walsh JS, Larson EB. The cost of institutional care in Alzheimer's disease: nursing home and hospital use in a prospective cohort. *J Am Geriatr Soc.* 1992;40:221–224.

127. West SG. Central nervous system vasculitis. *Curr Rheumatol Rep.* 2003;5:116–127.

128. Wilkinson D, et al. Donepezil in vascular dementia: a randomized, placebo-controlled study. *Neurology.* 2003;61:479–486.

129. Winblad B, et al. Donepezil in patients with severe Alzheimer's disease: double-blind, parallel-group, placebo-controlled study. *Lancet.* 2006;367:1057–1065.

130. Wolfe N, et al. Frontal systems impairment following multiple lacunar infarcts. *Arch Neurol.* 1990;47:129–132.

131. Woodruff BK, et al. Family history of dementia is a risk factor for Lewy body disease. *Neurology.* 2006;66:1949–1950.

132. Yaffe K, et al. Subtype of mild cognitive impairment and progression to dementia and death. *Dement Geriatr Cogn Disord.* 2006;22:312–319.

133. Yen SH, et al. Alzheimer's neurofibrillary tangles contain unique epitopes and epitopes in common with the heat-stable microtubule associated proteins tau and MAP2. *Am J Pathol.* 1987;126:81–91.

134. Zandi PP, et al. Reduced risk of Alzheimer disease in users of antioxidant vitamin supplements: the Cache County Study. *Arch Neurol.* 2004;61:82–88.

CHAPTER 21.3

Dementia: Behavioral and Cognitive Aspects

Barbara L. Malamut and Laurie M. Ryan

Recognition that a person is experiencing a decline in mental status can often be obvious, especially to the physician who is well acquainted with the patient over a period of years; however, determining the cause of the mental decline is often more challenging and frequently requires a multidisciplinary approach. Some mental status changes such as depression, anxiety, metabolic disorders, and adverse drug interactions are reversible if properly diagnosed and treated, but they can resemble dementia; therefore, if they are not carefully assessed, they can lead to misdiagnosis and improper management. Similarly, there are many different forms of dementia, each with its own cognitive profile and behavioral manifestation, and as new medications that mediate the progression of illness are developed, diagnostic accuracy will become essential to inform treatment decisions. Neuropsychology contributes greatly to the diagnosis of dementia by helping to determine the subtype, nature, and severity of cognitive changes and by characterizing the impact of these deficits on functional aspects of a person's behavior.

In this chapter, the neuropsychological and behavioral aspects of the most common neurodegenerative dementing illnesses are discussed. Particular emphasis is placed on Alzheimer's disease (AD) because of the prevalence of this disorder.

According to the American Psychiatric Association's *Diagnostic and Statistical Manual of Mental Disorders*, 4th Edition (DSM-IV) (7), the cognitive manifestations of dementia must include impairment in at least two or more of the following domains: short- and long-term memory, abstract thinking, impaired judgment, language or other disturbances of higher cortical functioning, or personality change. Dementia affects an individual's social and occupational skills as well as the ability for self-care. The cognitive and behavioral disturbances must not be caused by psychiatric mental disorders. Once the physician suspects mental status changes, performs a screening test of mental status, and runs the appropriate battery of medical tests to rule out a reversible process, the patient should be referred for a neuropsychological assessment.

THE ROLE OF THE NEUROPSYCHOLOGIST

Distinguishing between age-related decline, mild cognitive impairment (MCI), and dementia such as AD can be difficult, requiring careful evaluation within and across many cognitive functions. There is significant overlap in symptoms among conditions, and it is only by looking at the pattern of functioning within various cognitive and behavioral domains that one can begin to understand the etiology of the disorder. For example, impairment in memory is not specific to any one dementing disorder and should be viewed as a sign of cognitive dysfunction rather than a diagnostic certainty. Problems in free recall can be characteristic of confusional states, depression, or attentional disorders, thereby reflecting a deficit in activating encoding processes. Other memory problems observed in depression, frontal lobe dementias, or a frontal lobe–related deficit can be caused by impairment in retrieval of information. Alternatively, poor performance on a free recall measure could be a symptom of a pure amnestic disorder caused by hippocampal or temporal lobe damage.

Because different cognitive functions subserve functional activities, it is also the role of the neuropsychologist to address functional issues related to a person's ability to safely carry out instrumental activities of daily living (IADL), such as driving, medication management, and handling finances, as well as basic activities of daily living (BADL), such as bathing, toileting, and dressing. By definition, dementia interferes with a person's ability to function normally in everyday life. Skills needed for self-care, social and occupational functioning, and financial management are greatly affected, but the degree and pattern of functional impairment vary widely according to the type and stage of dementia.

In the early and middle stages of a dementing process, evaluation of cognitive status is critical to help ensure the individual's day-to-day safety, as IADLs and BADLs are strongly associated with changes in executive functioning and memory (72). When a cognitively impaired person lives alone, they can be at even greater risk for harm due to self-neglect or disorientation. In an 18-month prospective study examining cognitive predictors of harm in 130 elderly people, 21% of the people had an incident of harm. The study found that three neuropsychological tests that measured executive functioning, recognition memory, and conceptualization were independent risk factors for harm (146). In the later stages of dementia, a neuropsychological evaluation is usually requested to help with problematic behaviors such as wandering, screaming, or verbal abuse to determine what, if any, behavioral or environmental interventions would be effective in arresting or minimizing such behavior, thereby reducing the use of psychotropic medication to control these behaviors.

DIAGNOSIS

A first step in determining a diagnosis is to understand the nature of the cognitive disturbance and to narrow the causes for the change in mental status. Other than medical and psychiatric history, four key features are important when forming a diagnosis: information regarding when the problems began (i.e., time of onset of initial symptoms); the course of the symptomatology (i.e., insidious, acute presentation with little change, or step-wise); rate of progression of the disorder (i.e., slow or rapidly progressing); and presenting symptoms. Demographic information (e.g., education, occupation) and social history (e.g., living situation, hobbies, alcohol and drug consumption) are also pertinent variables so that test results may be placed within a context. Tables 21-9 and 21-10 illustrate differences between the pattern of presentation and rate of progression among the various dementing syndromes.

When obtaining the history, even in the early stages of dementia, it is general practice to obtain independent collateral information about cognitive and functional capabilities from a person who knows the patient well. Individuals with dementia often are unaware of their deficits, and self-reports are often not consistent with cognitive performance on testing (28,44). Despite the inconsistency between a patient's self-report and objective test data, it is still important to interview patients because, in the early phase of AD, the patient's lack of awareness of their functional deficits has been shown to strongly predict a future diagnosis of AD (144). However, Loewenstein et al. (88) found that informant reports were not always reliable with regard to functional capacity. They found that caregivers were accurate in predicting the functional performance of patients with AD who were not impaired on objective tests of functional status, but they overestimated the functional abilities of AD patients who were impaired on objective testing. Higher Mini-Mental State Examination (MMSE) (47) scores were associated with caregivers' overestimation of functional capacities (e.g., ability to tell time, identify currency, make change for a purchase, and use eating utensils).

Table 21-9. *Patterns of Onset and Progression of Dementing Disorders*

Onset	Disease Progression		
	Progressive (Slow)	Step-Wise	Rapid
Insidious			
	AD	AD + VaD	Pick's disease
	VaD		Jakob-Creutzfeldt disease
	FTD-lv (PPA); -bv; -mv		Lewy body disease
	CSH		
	Alcoholism		
	Parkinson's disease		
	NPH, HD, PSP		
Acute			
	Vitamin B deficiency	MID, stroke	Herpes encephalitis
		Head trauma	Meningitis
		Encephalitis	
		Anoxia	

AD, Alzheimer's disease; CSH, chronic subdural hematoma; FTD-lv, -bv, -mv, frontal temporal dementia language variant, behavioral variant, motor variant; HD, Huntington's disease; MID, multi-infarct dementia; NPH, normal pressure hydrocephalus; PPA, primary progressive aphasia; PSP progressive supranuclear palsy; VaD, vascular dementia.

Table 21-10. *Comparison of Neuropsychological Findings in the Early Stages of Different Dementing Disorders and Depression*

Domain	AD	DLB	VaD	FTD-lv (PPA)	DFT-bv	PD	Depression
Attention	Distractible	Fluctuating	Distractible	Normal	Distractible	Normal	Poor
Digit Span Forward	Normal	Unknown	Variable	Normal	Impaired	Normal	Variable
Executive	Mild imp	Variable	[Impaired]	Intact	[Impaired]	Impaired	Slowed
Reasoning	Mild imp	Impaired	Variable	Intact	Impaired	Impaired	Slowed
Info Processing Speed	Variable	Variable	[Slow]	Variable	Fast	[Impaired]	[Slow]
Language							
Naming	[Impaired]	Intact	Intact	[Impaired]	Intact	Intact	Intact
Fluency	[Impaired]	Intact	Slow	[Impaired]	Mild, echolalia	Slow	Slow
Comprehension	Normal	Intact	Intact	[Impaired]	Intact	Intact	Intact
Praxis	Mild imp	Intact	Intact	Impaired	Unknown	Intact	Intact
Memory							
Acquisition	[Impaired]	Intact	[↓Initiating strategies]	Impaired	Mild	Impaired	Poor
Storage	[Impaired]	Intact	Mild	Impaired	Intact	Impaired	Intact
Free Recall	[Impaired]	↓ Retrieval	Variable	Impaired	Variable	Impaired	Impaired
Recognition	[Impaired]	Preserved	Nml/mild	Impaired	Variable	Impaired	Intact
Remote	Variable	Unknown	Intact	Unknown	Intact	Intact	Intact
Motor	Intact	[EPS]	Impaired	Intact	Intact	[Impaired]	Slow
Handwriting	Intact	Impaired	Intact/tremor	Intact	Intact	[Small/tremor]	Intact
Visuoperception	Normal	[Agnosia]	Variable	Intact	Intact	Intact	Intact
Visual Constructional	Impaired	[Severely impaired]	Variable	Intact	Intact	Impaired	Intact
Affect	Variable, apathetic	Variable	Blunted, apathetic	No change	[Hyperoral, blunt]	Flattened	Blunted, apathetic
Psychiatric	Paranoid, depressed, anxious	[Visual hallucinations, depression, delusions]	Depression	None	↓ Insight ↓ Social conduct	Depressed	Depressed

Symptoms contained in a box ☐ represent the most common presenting signs for the type of dementia.
AD, Alzheimer's disease; DLB, dementia with Lewy bodies; VaD, vascular dementia due to small-vessel disease; FTD-lv, frontotemporal degeneration language variant; PPA, primary progressive aphasia; FTD-bv, frontotemporal dementia behavioral variant; PD, Parkinson's disease; EPS, extrapyramidal signs; Imp, impaired; Nml, normal.

SCREENING MEASURES

The most commonly used clinical screening tool for the presence of dementia in medical and psychological settings is the Folstein MMSE (133), which is easily administered in about 5 to 10 minutes. Although it has proved to be highly sensitive to changes in mental status in people over 65, it is most helpful for amnestic forms of dementia. The MMSE is not a good screening test for individuals with other illnesses that primarily involve language dysfunction. One reason for its lack of specificity is that the MMSE does not measure long-term memory, recognition memory, or executive functions (91). Another drawback to the MMSE is that it is not informative about the level of care needed for patients with mild to moderate levels of dementia. The MMSE has a total score of 30 points, with a score of 23 or lower usually considered indicative of organic dysfunction. However, when age (>80 years) and education (<9 years) are taken into account, the cutoff score suggestive of dementia decreases. It has been suggested that, for people with fewer than 9 years of education, a score of 17 should be considered as the cutoff (148), whereas a cutoff score of 26 or less has been suggested as optimum to detect mild to moderate dementia in people with higher education (151). Cultural background has also been shown to affect MMSE scores; Hispanics performed worse than non-Hispanics on the serial subtraction subtest when both groups were matched on education, age, and overall level of dementia. Similar results were found when spelling a word in reverse was substituted for serial subtraction (67).

Another quick screening test that is often administered along with the MMSE is the Clock Drawing Test. Together with MMSE scores, Clock Drawing Test performance has been shown to be sensitive to the presence of dementia, especially in those with very mild disease, but, on its own, it is not useful in discriminating between different forms of dementia (61,133). There are multiple steps involved in executing this task, and several diverse skills are required, including planning, visual attention, spatial conceptualization, and graphomotor control. In this test, the person is asked to draw the face of a clock, put all the numbers in the correct location, and set the clock to a specific time, either 10 minutes after 11:00 or 20 minutes after 8:00 (Fig. 21-2). These two times are most sensitive to dementia because they are sensitive to hemi-inattention and spatial conceptualization (49). Several different scoring systems of the clock have been devised to objectively quantify the presence and level of impairment (49,86,120), one of which (132) was found to be the most effective in detecting AD when combined with the MMSE.

The Mattis Dementia Rating Scale-2 (DRS-2) (74) is another frequently used screening measure that takes somewhat longer to administer than the MMSE and Clock Drawing Test but is useful for early detection, differential diagnosis, and staging of dementia for individuals at the lower end of functioning. The DRS-2 is more comprehensive than the MMSE and looks at attention, initiation/perseveration, construction, conceptualization, and memory in greater depth. The second version of the DRS uses the same test

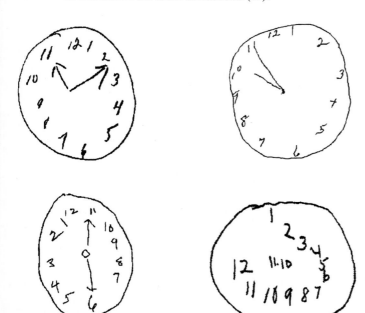

Figure 21-2. Top row from left to right, clocks drawn by: a normal elderly woman and a patient with mild AD. Second row from left to right, clocks drawn by: a patient with moderate AD and a patient with moderate to severe AD.

questions as the first version, but in collaboration with the Mayo Older Americans Normative Studies, the normative data were revised to take age and education into account when interpreting test results. Because the normative data were drawn mostly from white samples in rural or suburban settings, another set of normative data has been developed for older African-Americans to allow for greater diagnostic accuracy (121).

The Alzheimer's Disease Assessment Scale (ADAS) is used mostly in research settings, but it is mentioned here because of its wide use in drug trials (127). It is designed to evaluate the severity of both cognitive and noncognitive functions that are characteristic of AD. The scale is comprised of 21 items tapping memory, language and praxis, mood, and behavioral changes (e.g., depression, agitation, psychosis, and vegetative symptoms). It is administered in an interview format and takes about 45 minutes.

NEUROPSYCHOLOGICAL PROFILES OF DEMENTING DISORDERS

ALZHEIMER'S DISEASE

AD is the most common form of dementia, affecting an estimated 7% to 8% of people over 65 years of age and 30% to 40% of people over the age of 85 (138). The initial presentation for most patients with AD often involves memory lapses with an insidious onset. Families often report that a holiday meal was burned or a parent became lost while driving a familiar route. Often, relatives of the affected individual will realize in hindsight that certain episodes that occurred several years earlier were actually the beginning signs of the dementia.

Three diagnostic categories for AD are definite, probable, and possible. Table 21-5 in Chapter 21.2 outlines the National Institute of Neurological and Communicative Disorders and Stroke and the Alzheimer's Disease and Related Disorders Association (NINCDS-ADRDA) criteria for diagnosing probable, possible, and definite AD. A diagnosis of definite AD can be made only postmortem because, in addition to meeting criteria for probable AD, specific histopathologic findings are required.

Neuropsychological Profile of Presymptomatic Alzheimer's Disease Patients

Although patients with AD most often present to their physicians in the mild to moderate stages of the disease, more and more individuals complain of memory loss before any other signs of disease are evident, including normal performance on the MMSE. It is now understood that AD can have a long preclinical period during which subtle difficulties are detectable on neuropsychological testing and a diagnosis of MCI

is given (see Chapter 21.4). On neuropsychological testing, problems in delayed recall memory of a word list and executive functioning as measured by the Trail Making Test B (118) in individuals who were clinically presymptomatic at the time of neuropsychological testing could discriminate those who would manifest AD 18 months later from those who would remain normal (29). In another population-based prospective study, recall memory distinguished those who would remain healthy from those individuals who would develop AD from 3 to 6 years in advance of a diagnosis (9). No differences were noted in digit span forward and reverse between those who remained healthy and those who developed the disease.

Olfactory dysfunction also has been found in patients diagnosed with AD very early in the disease process (4,103,104). Patients with normal MMSE scores who were unaware of their deficit were more likely to develop AD than those with olfactory deficits who were aware of their poor performance on the test (40). Research is ongoing to determine whether impairment in olfactory identification is a reliable indicator of early AD.

Imaging has also been helpful in diagnosing AD. Magnetic resonance imaging (MRI) studies in AD show atrophy in the same brain areas where AD neuropathology is seen, and over time, these atrophic changes mirror the progression of the neuropathology. Specifically, in MCI/early AD, atrophy is observed in the entorhinal cortex and hippocampus, progressing to the temporal and parietal lobes and finally the frontal lobes in the late stages (101,136). Neuron loss and atrophy are not specific to AD and are found in other neurodegenerative disorders and normal aging. However, both longitudinal and cross-sectional studies have demonstrated differences in the pattern and rate of atrophy between AD and normal aging, particularly in the hippocampus and entorhinal cortex (42,71,101). Despite some overlap in brain areas affected, the degree of atrophy and the pattern of affected brain areas is different enough to allow discrimination between AD and other types of dementia including dementia with Lewy bodies (DLB) and frontotemporal dementia (FTD) (19,24,101). For example, in contrast to AD, marked atrophy of the amygdala has been found in FTD (155).

An advanced MRI technique, magnetic resonance spectroscopy (MRS), measures brain metabolites including N-acetylaspartate (NAA), which is a marker of neuronal activity; myoinositol (mI), which is a marker of gliosis; and creatine (Cr), which is a marker of intracellular energy use. Studies are very limited but suggest abnormalities in these metabolites in patients with AD in many of the same regions that show atrophy (8,101). Single photon emission computed tomography (SPECT) and positron emission tomography (PET) findings correlate with the degree of cognitive dysfunction and the progression of cognitive dysfunction in patients with AD (5). SPECT, however, has a lower spatial resolution than PET, and studies comparing both techniques show greater sensitivity with PET in terms of correlation with dementia severity and in differentiating controls and AD patients (31,101).

Presenting Neuropsychological Signs

The core features of individuals who were shown to have only AD pathology determined at autopsy are a progressive decline in explicit memory, anomia, executive function difficulties, visuospatial deficits, and a variety of other behavioral features discussed below. The rate and order in which these functions decline are variable among patients and reflect the differential competencies premorbidly and differences in the progressive accumulation of neuritic plaques and NFTs within the various association cortices (139).

Most patients with AD present initially with the greatest problems in episodic memory, but great variability is seen in the *pattern* of decline among the other neuropsychological domains such that some skills remain preserved longer than others. Consistent with the pattern of cognitive changes, studies with PET, specifically 18F-flurodeoxyglucose (FDG) PET, show a related pattern of glucose hypometabolism in parietal, temporal, and posterior cingulate areas with later involvement of frontal areas (101,137). In the largest PET study of mildly impaired patients with dementia to date, not only was this pattern of regional brain metabolism a highly sensitive indicator of AD, but the initial pattern was also strongly associated with the subsequent overall course of disease progression (134).

Memory

Verbal and visual episodic memory loss is the hallmark of AD. On tests of episodic memory (e.g., story recall or list learning), AD patients demonstrate a rapid rate of forgetting and often do not recall or recognize the new information after 10 to 20 minutes (16,81,147). Furthermore, the normal pattern of learning a list of words known as the serial position effect (i.e., better immediate recall of items from the beginning and end of a word list, with poorest recall of words in the middle of the list) is also disrupted early in the disease process (15,135). In contrast to normal elderly people, AD patients tend to recall the last few words of a supraspan word list immediately after it is read aloud. Patients with AD also tend to make more intrusion and perseverative errors on memory tests when compared with normal elderly controls (26). In addition to new learning, the disease also affects memories from the remote past but to a much lesser degree. In the early stages of the disease,

patients perform worse than normal control subjects in their ability to recall and recognize famous faces, public events, and autobiographical information, but some memories from the past remain preserved.

Executive Functioning

The term "executive functioning" refers to the capacity to plan and carry out complex goal-oriented behaviors and allows a person to independently adapt his or her behavior to changing contingencies, which is necessary for the performance of all independent goal-directed activities including IADLs. Due to the variety of cognitive processes involved in executive functioning, it must be evaluated with a series of tasks looking at different variables. The most commonly used tests involve problem solving (e.g., Wisconsin Card Sorting) (63), planning and organization, working memory (e.g., digit span backward), mental flexibility (e.g., Trail Making Test B) (118), and response inhibition (e.g., Color Word Interference Test) (37). Changes in executive functioning appear very early in the disease process and have even been found in nondemented older adults who were at genetic risk for AD by having the *apolipoprotein E ε4* allele (153). Although executive dysfunction is evident in the early stages of AD, it is usually not as prominent as episodic memory loss. In patients with mild or moderate AD, deficits in executive functioning have been related to a decline in IADL and, therefore, have important implications for safety issues such as medication management and driving (22), as well as medical decision making and financial management capacities.

Language and Semantic Memory

Early in the course of AD, patients demonstrate impairments in the linguistic aspects of speech. Conversations are often vague, and discourse is filled with circumlocutions and overlearned phrases. On formal testing, AD patients have deficits on tests of word list generation (52) and naming, and they tend to make more lexical and semantic naming errors on fluency and naming tests compared with normal elderly controls (13,26,36,143). With disease progression, paraphasic errors and impairment in written and oral comprehension develop. In the late stages, dysarthria and mutism may occur.

Typically, the linguistic aspects of speech are examined through category fluency tests (i.e., rapidly name items within a specific category) and letter fluency tests (i.e., rapidly name words beginning with specific letters). Many neuropsychological and imaging studies have shown that differences in performance between these tests can be of diagnostic significance. At one time, having better category than letter fluency was thought to be evidence of cortical dementia, such as AD, whereas the reverse pattern was thought to indicate a subcortical dementia such as in Parkinson's disease, Huntington's disease, or vascular dementia (VaD) (25,126). However, several studies have disputed these findings and found no difference in performance on category and letter fluency tests between patients with dementia due to different causes (130,143). It is now well recognized that both fluency tasks involve executive functions mediated by the frontal lobe such as attention, search strategies, initiation, and retrieval, and differences in test results may be due to differential impairment in functions other than linguistic processes. The impact of executive dysfunction on different verbal fluency tasks was illustrated in a study looking at two cortical dementia groups: autopsy-confirmed AD and FTD (115). In this study, letter fluency was more impaired in the FTD group compared to the AD group, whereas semantic fluency was more impaired in patients with AD. For both groups, the disparity between fluency tests increased with increasing severity of dementia.

Semantic memory refers to knowledge of words (vocabulary) and factual information and is affected in the beginning stages of AD as noted by consistent impairments in naming and fluency tasks. The level of the semantic memory impairment is related to the level of dementia. Semantic memory for generic knowledge (e.g., how many days are there in a week?) is impaired relatively early in the course of the disease and declines further as the disease progresses (105). One possible explanation for the semantic memory impairment is that a degradation of the organization and content of semantic knowledge causes the impairment. An alternative argument is that the patient has problems in accessing information from an intact semantic store (14,48,129,145). In either case, studies have shown that task difficulty that requires active searches of semantic memory and greater attentional resources is one of the intervening variables.

Praxis

Ideomotor apraxia is a disorder of skilled movement or gestural behavior to verbal command or imitation in the absence of motor impairment. It is thought to be caused by disruption in the access to stored memories of familiar action patterns. Apraxia usually emerges in AD after memory and language disturbances, but it can be seen in the early stages of the disease (33). Ideomotor praxis can be evaluated in many ways. When the four types of movements listed in Table 21-11 were evaluated in a group of patients with moderate to severe disease, transitive limb movements to command were found to decline before intransitive limb, buccofacial, and axial actions (113). The most common errors on transitive limb praxis testing involved patients using their body part as the object (e.g., using a finger to demonstrate teeth

Table 21-11. *Sample Apraxia Battery*

Buccofacial
Show me how you . . .
1. Cough
2. Stick out your tongue
3. Suck through a straw
4. Blow out a match
5. Sniff a flower

Limb intransitive
Show me how you . . .
1. Wave goodbye
2. Beckon "come here"
3. Hitchhike
4. Salute
5. Signal "stop"

Limb transitive
Show me how you . . .
1. Brush your teeth
2. Stir coffee with a spoon
3. Comb your hair
4. Saw a board
5. Use a screwdriver

Ideational
1. Fold the paper, place it in an envelope, and seal and address it
2. Prepare a cup of instant coffee with sugar
3. Put a candle in the holder, light it, and blow it out

brushing). Deficits are also found in ideational praxis where a person is asked to perform a series of actions using objects to accomplish a goal, such as, "Fold a paper, put it in the envelope, seal it, and address it." In ideational praxis, the deficits are usually a result of sequencing errors (e.g., sealing the envelope before putting the paper in). Evaluation of praxis is an important part of a dementia evaluation in patients suspected of having AD because it has been shown to differentiate depressed elderly patients with cognitive impairment from those with probable disease (33).

Visuospatial

Visuospatial functioning is often impaired early in AD and declines further as the disease progresses. Visual agnosia (i.e., trouble recognizing a well-known object) usually does not appear until the middle to late stages of the disorder, whereas visuospatial constructional apraxia can be seen early in the disease process. This is usually tested with tasks involving graphomotor skills, such as drawing a clock or copying simple and complex drawings, and tasks involving manipulation of materials (i.e., constructing a design with blocks to look like a model). When drawing a clock to command, patients with AD often fail to include the numbers or clock hands, or they have problems in spatial conceptualization. In the moderate to severe stages of the disease, patients often will write the time rather than draw clock hands (Fig. 21-2). Their performance often reflects a loss of knowledge or a deficit in accessing the attributes of a clock. Usually, their copy of a clock is much better than their spontaneous drawing. In other drawing tasks, patients are usually asked to copy geometric forms that increase in complexity (e.g., circle, Red Cross sign, diamond, cube). In AD, as the disease progresses, patients' performance will often decline in the reverse order of the developmental sequence (125). Thus, in the mild stages of the disease, patients may demonstrate problems copying a cube but have no difficulty copying a diamond or circle. As the disease progresses, problems develop when copying the diamond. In the moderate to severe stages, patients often draw over the shape or use part of the form in their drawing (i.e., closing in) rather than draw in the space provided.

Motor

Extrapyramidal signs (e.g., bradykinesia, rigidity, gait disturbance, tremor, postural instability) appear more frequently in the later stages of AD, but when present early in the disease, they are important predictors of decline in patients with the disease. Patients who have at least one extrapyramidal sign at baseline evaluation are reported to demonstrate a more rapid cognitive and functional decline than those with AD and no extrapyramidal signs (119).

Atypical Neuropsychological Presentations

Although the three subtypes discussed earlier are the most common patterns of presentation of AD, atypical presentations involving circumscribed deficits related to other cognitive functions have also been reported. The neurobiologic basis for this clinical heterogeneity is related to variations in the distribution of the pathogenic changes occurring with the disease. Neuropathologic studies have shown that differences in the distribution of pathogenic changes associated with AD account for some of the variability in cognitive profiles. When a group of patients who presented with disproportionate frontal lobe impairments on neuropsychological testing while in the mild stages of dementia were followed to autopsy, there was as much as a 10-fold increase in neurofibrillary tangles (NFTs), but not plaques, in the frontal lobes when compared with individuals with typical AD neuropsychological presentations (66). Both groups had the expected NFT hippocampal pathology, but of the five regions sampled, the patients with neuropsychological frontal impairment had the greatest proportion of NFT in the frontal region. The patients with initial frontal presentations eventually demonstrated

memory and visuospatial deficits characteristic of AD, but their performance was worse on tests sensitive to frontal lobe functioning. Similarly, subgroups of patients have presented with isolated visual disturbances early in the disease without memory impairments (50). In another subgroup of patients demonstrating a selective impairment of episodic and semantic memory, SPECT showed focal temporal lobe dysfunction. In contrast, the group with typical disease demonstrated bilateral mesial temporal hypoperfusion but also posterior parietal and temporal parietal hypoperfusion. The authors suggested that focal temporal lobe dysfunction is a rare but distinct anatomoclinical form of AD with a slower rate of cognitive decline (27).

Behavioral Manifestations

Many patients with AD have concomitant psychiatric symptoms at some point in their illness (35). Early in the disease process, decreased spontaneity and increased passivity are the most common behavioral changes, although not noted in all individuals. Other patients demonstrate restlessness, hyperactivity, and disinhibited behavior. Agitation is also seen, which often increases with disease severity. Hallucinations are most common toward the end stages of the disease. Estimates of the incidence of psychosis in AD (i.e., hallucinations and delusions) range from 10% to 75%, with delusions occurring more often than hallucinations (109). Psychotic symptoms in earlier stages of AD have been associated with increased rates of aggression, cognitive impairment, and functional decline (90,93,109,114,140). In a 5-year longitudinal study examining the relationship between the course of psychopathological features and level of cognitive functioning in AD in 236 patients, wandering/agitation and delusions were noted throughout the disease course and, when present, increased as a function of cognitive decline until later in the disease course when they decreased (68). Hallucinations were less prevalent than delusions but remained relatively stable despite cognitive changes. Physical aggression was less prevalent and also increased with decline in cognitive status. It persisted in the more severely cognitively impaired patients.

LEWY BODY

DLB is thought to be the second most frequent type of dementia in the elderly, affecting as many as 20% to 30% of people with dementia (73). Lewy bodies are intraneuronal inclusions in the neocortex and subcortical regions of the brain that can be found in individuals with Parkinson's disease and, less often, AD, but DLB is a distinct dementing illness with specific clinical and pathologic features (23,53,54,97). As in AD, where the severity of dementia is related to the density of cortical neuritic plaques and NFTs, in DLB, the density of Lewy bodies appears to be strongly related to dementia severity (60).

According to the criteria established by the Consortium on Dementia with Lewy Bodies (see Table 21-6 in Chapter 21.2), the clinical presentation usually has an insidious onset, with progressive and disabling mental impairment that develops into a dementia within months to several years (96,97). To make a diagnosis of possible DLB, one of the following three core features must by present: fluctuation in the level of cognitive functioning, prominent visual hallucinations, or extrapyramidal motor features of parkinsonism. Fluctuation in cognition, as measured by choice reaction time tests and vigilance reaction time tests, has been shown to be more common and severe in DLB than in AD or VaD (152).

Neuropsychological Profile

Very few autopsy-confirmed neuropsychological studies have been performed on individuals who had DLB without some Alzheimer, vascular, or parkinsonian pathology. The reports of pure DLB indicate that the core neuropsychological features evident early in the disease involve attention and visuospatial difficulties (131). Problem-solving and executive functioning deficits have also been reported but do not appear as prominent as attentional and visuospatial difficulties. Memory impairment is also reported in DLB, but it is not as severe as in AD (10), and the characteristics of the memory problems differ between groups. In comparison to AD, DLB is associated with more favorable performance on measures of sustained attention, phonemic fluency, spatial judgment, psychomotor speed, working memory, word list free recall, and recognition (34). In DLB, the memory dysfunction may be caused by problems in retrieval of information rather than problems with memory acquisition and consolidation that are characteristic of AD. Conversely, visuoconstructive and psychomotor impairments are more severe in DLB than in AD (34,128).

Although language problems are generally not reported in the early stages, one case study of autopsy-confirmed pure DLB reported that the patient presented with distinctive verbal fluency deficits in the context of mild language impairment, intact recognition memory, and impaired paragraph recall (58). Similar to AD, people with DLB demonstrate global impairment across all neuropsychological domains as the disease progresses.

Behavioral Manifestations

In the early stages, DLB is associated with psychiatric morbidity such as visual and auditory hallucinations, depression, delusions, and delusional misidentification (11). A number of psychiatric symptoms were found in common when DLB was compared with AD,

but visual hallucinations were found to be more persistent in DLB (12). Hirono et al. (65) found that most of their DLB subjects had visual hallucinations, but the frequency and severity of visual hallucinations did not differ between DLB and AD. Instead, the type of delusion distinguished the two groups such that misidentification delusions were more common in DLB than in AD. Shimomura et al. (131) suggested that defective visual perception plays a role in the development of visual hallucinations, delusional misidentifications, visual agnosias, and visuoconstructive disability.

In individuals who have both Lewy body and AD pathology, the clinical presentation is different than the presentation characteristic of either condition alone. This is especially true at the beginning stages of the disease process. When patients with mixed disease pathologies were compared with individuals with AD pathology only, delusions and hallucinations were more frequent, greater impairment was noted on visuospatial and executive tasks, and lesser impairment was noted on memory and praxis tasks (32,38,51).

VASCULAR DEMENTIA

It is estimated that dementia caused solely by cerebral vascular disease can account for 2% to 18% of all dementias (77,82,154). Because VaD can result from cerebral ischemic episodes, multiple infarction, cerebral hemorrhages, or vascular-induced periventricular white matter changes, ischemia, and hypoxia secondary to cardiac arrest, the neuropsychological findings depend upon the location and extent of pathologic disruption. For the purpose of this chapter, VaD refers to dementia caused by subcortical small-vessel disease resulting in ischemic injury or small subcortical lacunar infarct(s) in the basal ganglia, pons, and white matter of the centrum ovale (i.e., lacunar state). These types of brain lesions are noted in the periventricular region and subcortical structures on MRI. They usually present subacutely with an insidious onset and negative neurologic examination (46). As such, cognitive changes in these patients are often progressive rather than the step-wise course noted in larger vessel disease. This clinical entity represents the most frequent type of subcortical dementia, particularly among people older than 75 years of age.

Although white matter hyperintensities (WMH) are commonly found on MRI in the elderly, some individuals demonstrate cognitive decline or a dementia, whereas others appear cognitively intact. Several studies have shown that it is the extent of white matter involvement that determines the development of dementia (57,107,112). A very recent study by Hentschel et al. (64) examined white matter lesions (WMLs) on MRI in normal control and dementia subjects, including those with MCI, AD, and VaD.

The investigators developed a visual rating scale and demonstrated that WMLs can be reliably quantified and that WML scores correlate with age and level of cognitive decline. Moreover, WML scores differentiated VaD from the other groups. Specifically, global WML scores and frontal WML scores were significantly increased in VaD compared to normal control, MCI, and AD groups.

Neuropsychological Profile

Specific DSM-IV criteria for a diagnosis of VaD are listed in Table 21-12, and National Institute of Neurological Disorders and Stroke–Association Internationale pour la Recherche et l'Enseignement en Neurosciences (NINDS-AIREN) International Workgroup criteria for probable and possible VaD can be found in Chapter 21.2, Table 21-7.

In a meta-analysis of 23 studies examining the relationship between WMH and cognitive functioning in nondemented elderly, processing speed, executive functioning, and immediate and delayed explicit memory were sensitive to WMH, whereas intelligence and

Table 21-12. *DSM-IV Diagnostic Criteria for Vascular Dementia*

The development of multiple cognitive deficits manifested by both:

1. Memory impairment (impaired ability to learn new information or to recall previously learned information)
2. One (or more) of the following cognitive disturbances:
   a. aphasia
   b. apraxia
   c. agnosia
   d. disturbance in executive functioning

The cognitive deficits in criteria 1 and 2 above each cause significant impairment in social or occupational functioning and represent a significant decline from a previous level of functioning.

Focal neurologic signs and symptoms (e.g., exaggeration of deep tendon reflexes, extensor plantar response, pseudobulbar palsy, gait abnormalities, weakness of an extremity) or laboratory evidence indicative of cerebrovascular disease (e.g., multiple infarctions involving cortex and underlying white matter) that are judged to be etiologically related to the disturbance.

The deficits do not occur exclusively during the course of a delirium.

From American Psychiatric Association. *Diagnostic and Statistical Manual of Mental Disorders.* 4th ed. Washington, DC: American Psychiatric Association; 1994.

fine motor functioning did not appear related to the presence or extent of WMH (57).

Although there is general consensus of whether a person fulfills criteria of dementia, a clear neuropsychological profile for VaD has proven to be more elusive. When compared to AD, some studies have reported greater executive functioning deficits in VaD (89), whereas others have not (117). It has also been suggested that VaD patients may be more impaired than AD patients in some aspects of executive function (i.e., retrieval search strategies), whereas AD patients are more impaired in self-monitoring (158). The discrepancy in results could be due to the fact that most studies relied on clinical diagnoses and the subjects were not examined at autopsy, raising the possibility that many of the subjects also had some pathology consistent with AD.

In other studies, it was suggested that the neuropsychological profile of patients with significant white matter ischemic disease is similar to that of other subcortical dementias such as Parkinson's or Huntington's disease (41,85) and is characterized by impairment in executive functions, greater perseverative errors, and slowed mental processing speed compared to normal controls (41,80,84,122). The nature of the perseverative errors in VaD might be different than in AD; VaD perseverations are more motor related, whereas perseverations are more conceptual and language mediated in AD (80).

Patients with extensive subcortical cerebrovascular disease often demonstrate memory deficits, but the nature of the memory impairment usually differs from AD or other disease states affecting the temporal lobe. In contrast to the poor memory consolidation/storage that is characteristic of AD, patients with VaD show less forgetting and demonstrate better recognition memory (84,85,89,158). In mild to moderate VaD, patients usually demonstrate problems in initiating strategies to more efficiently acquire and retrieve the new material (150). Once information is acquired, however, there is some retention of the learned information that can best be demonstrated on recognition tests. Thus, the pattern of memory deficits in VaD is consistent with the interruption of frontal-subcortical circuits rather than temporal lobe dysfunction. Functional imaging has supported these distinctions in memory functioning. In one FDG-PET study, during a continuous verbal memory task, performance in VaD patients correlated with prefrontal hypometabolism, whereas in AD, memory correlated with left hippocampal and temporal lobe metabolism (116).

Diffusion-weighted MRI (DWI) and diffusion tensor imaging (DTI), a more sophisticated form of DWI, are newer MRI techniques that are sensitive to white matter changes (69,83). In AD, abnormalities have been found in the corpus callosum, hippocampus, posterior cingulate, and parietal, temporal, and occipital lobes (62,101). A very recent study by Mayzel-Oreg et al. (94) used high *b*-value DWI, a technique that may have increased sensitivity over conventional DWI, to compare AD and VaD patients and normal controls. The results indicated that VaD patients had very significant white matter changes, whereas AD patients demonstrated greater gray matter changes. In addition, the pattern of white matter changes was different, with the AD patients showing frontal and temporal changes and the VaD patients showing widespread changes.

Behavior

Behavioral changes, such as depression, apathy, delusions, hallucinations, and aggression, have frequently been reported in patients with VaD, regardless of the severity of cognitive decline. In patients with small infarct volumes (<15 mL), the combination of microinfarction, diffuse white matter disease, and perivascular changes was found to be associated with depression (12). Frontal WMLs have been associated with high depression scores in nondemented elderly and in patients with all types of dementia (VaD, AD, and DLB), suggesting that it is caused by a common pathophysiology such as a disturbance in the frontostriatal pathways (20,106). Although similar types of changes were also noted in AD without vascular changes, they were usually related to the level of dementia and were most prevalent during the later stages of the disease. In VaD, behavioral changes are thought to be more common than in AD and independent of level of severity of dementia (3,56,59). In cases where AD and microvascular changes were present, patients were particularly vulnerable to depression (12).

FRONTOTEMPORAL DEMENTIA

FTD is much less common than AD in older adults but may comprise as much as 50% of dementia cases before age 60 years (55). Compared with neuropsychological studies in AD, relatively few studies have been conducted on patients with FTD. However, there has been much greater interest in this population in the last 10 years, and prospective studies with imaging and larger sample sizes have clearly established that there are several FTD subtypes, each with specific behavioral profiles. Furthermore, the differences in behavioral presentations appear due to differences in the specific anatomic regions involved.

Two FTD classification systems have emerged. One clarifies the various terms used in the past (98), and the other describes three clinical syndromes that are incorporated into one label (i.e., frontal temporal lobar dementia) (102). There is general consensus that, early in the disease process, the presenting

feature of FTD involves either behavioral disturbances (FTD-bv), disruption in language (FTD-lv), or extrapyramidal signs (FTD-mv) (see Chapter 21.2, Table 21-8) and that there are distinct clinicopathologic findings on MRI or computed tomography (CT) imaging that differentiate these disorders. However, although the biggest changes occur within the frontal and temporal lobes, adjacent cortical regions can also contribute to the various clinical presentations of the disorders (55). Moreover, with progression of the disease, the patients frequently develop at least one of the other syndromes to varying degrees.

For the FTD-bv group, changes in personality and behavior are the initial presenting symptoms, and patients usually demonstrate poor insight, distractibility, stereotyped perseverative behavior, and profound changes in social conduct. Decreased speech output, reduced conversational initiation, echolalia, and weaknesses in pragmatic speech have been associated with FTD-bv (18). In terms of other nonlanguage cognitive functions, deficits are noted early in the disease in attention, reasoning, and abstraction and many aspects of executive functions such as cognitive flexibility, planning, and problem solving (111). Many language functions (e.g., naming and comprehension), memory, and visual spatial skills remain intact initially. Similar to AD, semantic fluency is often more impaired than phonemic fluency in FTD-bv. The psychiatric characteristics include lack of empathy, emotional blunting, deterioration of social comportment, and problems in self-regulation of behavior. These patients demonstrate increased risk-taking behavior rather than mere impulsivity. Because there is so much overlap in these behavioral characteristics between late-onset schizophrenia and FTD-bv, neuropsychological testing is often helpful in making the differential diagnosis (159). Sociopathic behaviors (e.g., stealing, indecent exposure, sexual disinhibition) can be present and are more prevalent in FTD-bv than in other dementing illnesses but are not present in all people with FTD-bv (99). These behaviors appear to be dependent upon the location and pattern of cortical degeneration and are most evident when the affected brain region is localized to the right frontotemporal region.

When FTD-bv patients with sociopathy were compared to those without sociopathy, the only difference in their neuropsychological test results was impairment in the sociopathic group on motor tasks involving Alternate Tapping and Go/No-Go tests. Mendez et al. (99) opined that the sociopathic acts result from a combination of diminished concern for their acts and disinhibition. Unfortunately, due to the nature of their social impropriety, patients with FTD-bv and sociopathy are often in legal trouble; however, because they are aware of their actions, know that they are wrong but do not care or have remorse, they do not pass legal criteria for insanity in many jurisdictions within the United States.

FTD-lv is also known as primary progressive aphasia (PPA); impairment in speech and language is the hallmark of PPA. Diagnostic criteria for PPA require disruption of language as the prominent symptom for 2 years before other symptoms appear (100). In the early stages, results of MRI indicate asymmetric atrophy in the left temporal lobe. In contrast to FTD-bv, reasoning and cognitive flexibility, skills usually associated with frontal lobe functioning, have been shown to be intact early in the course of the illness (156). These findings have significant positive implications for PPA patients with regard to IADLs and capacity judgments early in the disease course.

Three clinical variants of PPA have been identified and are known as semantic dementia (SEMD), which refers to the progressive loss of knowledge about words and objects; progressive nonfluent aphasia, which is characterized by hesitant, effortful speech and agrammatism; and logopenic progressive aphasia, which is characterized by decreased speech output, anomia, and problems with short-term verbal memory (124). These language deficits appear to be caused by a progressive breakdown in semantic memory, including loss of general knowledge that results in impairment on tests of both nonverbal and verbal semantic knowledge. Areas of preserved neuropsychological functioning include visuospatial and perceptual abilities often measured by Judgment of Line Orientation and Rey Figure Copy tests, nonverbal problem solving (Wisconsin Card Sorting Test), working memory, and intact day-to-day episodic memory (66).

Disruptions in behavior similar to FTD-bv are also noted in FTD-lv but at a later stage in the disease. Only SEMD has been associated with behaviors similar in quality to FTD-bv and characterized by disinhibition, aberrant motor behavior, and eating disorders. The behavioral disturbances in the other two variants of PPA did not occur any more often than in AD.

The last group within the FTD grouping initially presents with changes in motor functioning (FTD-mv) and includes FTD with parkinsonism, FTD with motor neuron disease, corticobasal degeneration (CBD), and progressive supranuclear palsy (PSP). For a full description of the specific neuropsychological consequences associated with these various FTD movement disorders, see Chapter 23.

When determining a diagnosis, it is important to consider all phenotypes of FTD. Individual well-studied cases have reported some patients who presented with clinical symptoms consistent with PPA and FTD but had underlying primary pathology consistent with CBD and PSP.

DEMENTIA SYNDROME OF DEPRESSION

Depression in the elderly can cause cognitive changes that are often misinterpreted as early signs of a dementia; however, in depression, cognitive functioning improves once a person is effectively treated. Although depressed patients demonstrate improvement with treatment, not all of these individuals return to their baseline level of cognitive functioning. This has led some researchers to conclude that, in a subset of elderly patients in whom depression is associated with residual cognitive dysfunction, their depression may actually be a prodromal phase of irreversible dementia (6,78). Others have argued that, with longer follow-up spanning 8 to 10 years, depressed patients with residual cognitive decline have a poorer prognosis in terms of global psychiatric morbidity (123). This remains an area of ambiguity, and further prospective neuropsychological and neuropsychiatric longitudinal studies are ongoing.

The reversible decline accompanying depression is known as dementia syndrome of depression (DSD). Reports of the neuropsychological profile in DSD vary widely, with no clear consensus regarding whether depression affects separate functions (e.g., memory or attention) or all cognitive domains equally. Neuropsychological studies have reported that, in depression, elderly patients often demonstrate intact speech but limited spontaneous elaboration. Impairment is also noted in psychomotor speed, speed of information processing, attention, and memory efficiency (secondary to attentional problems). Conversely, deficits in language, visuospatial abilities, and mathematical skills are often observed in dementia (1,142). Furthermore, depressed patients often have heightened awareness of their memory problems in contrast with patients with AD who are usually unaware of their memory decline (21). When patients demonstrate depression and impairment in language, recognition memory, and visual constructional praxis, consider diagnoses of depression and dementia.

DIFFERENTIATING THE DEMENTIAS

Differentiating the various cortical dementias can be challenging without further evaluation because family members often voice the same complaints (i.e., memory problems). Although a decline in memory is usually the most frequent complaint about individuals with AD, people often confuse word-finding difficulty with memory problems, making it difficult to initially differentiate the various phenotypes of FTD from AD or other progressive dementias. More rapidly progressive language deterioration distinguishes all forms of FTD from AD, and a change in personality early in the course of a disease is usually more indicative of FTD-bv than the other syndromes (17,18,99). However, two studies have shown that some patients with pathologically confirmed FTD initially presented with amnesia as the prominent symptom, with more typical FTD behavioral changes developing later (76). In general, AD patients demonstrate impairment or decline in several cognitive domains. When patients with AD and the three phenotypes of FTD were individually compared on a battery of neuropsychological tests using principal components analysis, AD patients performed worse on tests of declarative memory, whereas patients diagnosed with SEMD did worse on tests of semantic memory (87). Patients with FTD-bv were faster than the other groups on tests of processing speed/mental flexibility, although they made more errors on some of the tests. Patients with CBD and progressive nonfluent aphasia were impaired on tests of working memory. When FTD was compared to AD on the Clock Drawing Test, drawings from the FTD patients were significantly better than drawings from the AD group. AD was associated with more global impairment, and the AD group had more errors, whereas the FTD group had fewer stimulus-bound responses, conceptual deficits, and spatial or planning errors (18).

With regard to the cognitive profile over time, studies reported that results of initial testing of the FTD group were worse than the results of normal controls on all neuropsychological tests, except on a measure of visuospatial function (108). The AD group performed worse than controls on all measures. Patients with FTD were superior on visuospatial functioning. During the course of the disease, measures of explicit memory and visuospatial and reasoning skills worsened equally. Demented Parkinson's disease patients have been shown to decline faster than those with dementia due to AD on language tests (i.e., category fluency, naming), global measures of dementia severity, and ADLs (70,141).

IMAGING

FDG-PET has been shown to provide greater diagnostic accuracy when added to the clinical assessment of dementia because patterns of hypometabolism on FDG-PET can help differentiate neurodegenerative disorders. For example, FDG-PET patterns for FTD demonstrate frontal hypometabolism, whereas patterns for LBD demonstrate temporal, parietal, occipital, and cerebellar hypometabolism (137). Silverman et al. (134) found that FDG-PET identified AD and other neurodegenerative disorders with 94%

sensitivity and 73% and 78% specificities among patients with histopathologic diagnoses. Cerebral hypometabolism was associated with disease progression, and a negative initial PET scan indicated that progression of cognitive dysfunction during the 3-year follow-up was unlikely. A study of MCI patients found that FDG-PET patterns of patients who progressed to AD showed greater hypometabolism in the temporal-parietal regions compared with those who did not progress over 18 months (30). The usefulness of FDG-PET in the diagnosis of dementia has been recognized by the Centers for Medicare and Medicaid Services (CMS). In 2004, CMS approved Medicare reimbursement for FDG-PET used to assist with the differential diagnosis of AD versus FTD (136).

Another imaging technique, functional MRI (fMRI), combines high-speed image acquisition with blood oxygen level–dependent (BOLD) contrast (nonradioactive) to show changes in blood flow over time (8). Studies of fMRI in AD and other dementias are limited to date but have shown decreased activation in the hippocampal region in patients with AD (79).

Only recently have PET imaging techniques been developed that allow for visualization of neuropathologic lesions associated with AD. Specifically, tracers have been identified that bind to beta-amyloid and tau aggregates in the living brain. Researchers from the University of Pittsburgh identified a thioflavin-T analog tracer that has a high affinity for fibrillar beta-amyloid, ^{11}C-labeled Pittsburgh Compound-B (^{11}C-PIB), also known as the Pittsburgh Compound B (PIB). PIB-PET has been shown to bind specifically to fibrillar beta-amyloid in postmortem AD brains but has low binding in postmortem brains from healthy controls or dementias that are not associated with beta-amyloid such as FTD (75). A very recent study by Rabinovici et al. (110) found that all of the AD patients demonstrated positive PIB scans, and most of the FTD patients had negative PIB scans. The investigators speculate that the four positive FTD patients may have had comorbid AD and FTD pathology or underlying AD pathology mimicking FTD. They note that three of these four patients had cognitive test profiles more or equally suggestive of AD.

Researchers at the University of California, Los Angeles (UCLA) have developed a small-molecule tracer, 2-(1-{6-[(2-[F-18]fluoroethyl)(methyl)amino]-2-naphthyl}ethylidene) malononitrile ([18F]FDDNP), that binds to fibrillar beta-amyloid and tau aggregates/NFT (31,136). Higher [18F]FDDNP binding has been seen with [18F]FDDNP-PET in temporal, parietal, and frontal regions in AD patients compared to healthy controls (136). The UCLA group has recently shown that global [18F]FDDNP binding is significantly lower in healthy controls compared to MCI patients and significantly lower in MCI patients compared to AD patients. Moreover, lower [^{18}F]FDDNP binding was inversely correlated with cognitive test scores (137). These investigators have also examined [^{18}F]FDDNP-PET in dementias with prominent tauopathies, including FTD (137). Higher [^{18}F]FDDNP binding was noted in frontal regions compared to controls. Comparison of the images between FTD and AD revealed a prominent frontal/temporal signal in FTD compared to a prominent parietal/medial temporal signal in AD.

In summary, the field of neuroimaging in dementia is rapidly evolving, and there are a number of promising techniques that may aid early diagnosis of AD and other dementias. Currently, structural imaging with CT/MRI is recommended to assist with diagnosis, as is FDG-PET when AD and FTD are being considered.

PSYCHOSOCIAL ASPECTS OF DEMENTIA

MEDICATION MANAGEMENT

Overall level of cognitive dysfunction in dementia, as assessed by global screening measures, is associated with impairment in the ability to carry out IADL, with an increase in functional problems typically seen in individuals with greater cognitive impairment (2,95). In AD and VaD, changes in executive functioning and memory were predictive of IADL and BADL changes, respectively (22,72).

Determining whether a person is able to self-manage medication is an important consideration in deciding whether a person can safely live alone. To date, no specific neuropsychological test has been shown to be associated with medication compliance. This is probably because taking medication involves diverse skills such as telling time, memory, sequencing, and motor skills, and impairment in any one skill can result in problems with taking medication. One study reported that level of global cognitive dysfunction as measured by MMSE was strongly correlated with the inability to take medications independently in a group of geriatric medical outpatients (45). However, these results are skewed because of the inclusion of severely demented patients who perform poorly on the MMSE and have problems taking medications on their own. It is generally accepted that multiple neuropsychological measures are needed to maximize the prediction of functional skills. The most common situation where medication management is discussed occurs in patients who are in the early stages of a disease and are likely to be living on their own.

DRIVING

With the growing numbers of people developing dementing disorders, determining a person's fitness to drive has become an increasingly important issue.

A decline in response time, sensory and perceptual changes, and a decline in some cognitive functions that are associated with aging are just a few reasons why some normal healthy elderly individuals become unfit to drive. In people with a dementia, normal age-related changes can increase their vulnerability to problems when driving because the affected individuals may no longer be able to compensate for their deficits. Furthermore, in many cases, they may not even be aware of these changes. For example, in a driving simulation task, FTD patients committed many more offenses (e.g., speeding tickets, ran stop signs, off-road crashes) than matched nondemented control subjects (39).

In one study, individuals with dementia had 2.5 times the crash rate of other age-matched nondemented residents randomly selected from their community (149). Another group who were not demented but had medical problems had a crash rate that was 2.2 times that of healthy elderly community residents.

Since the late 1980s, an increasing number of studies have tried to determine what factors distinguish safe from unsafe drivers. Early studies were inconclusive in finding specific cognitive variables that predict a person's driving fitness; some later studies have reported that visual perceptual and attentional aspects are likely to correlate with unsafe driving. Trails B test from the Trail Making Test (118), a test requiring the conceptual shifting between two alternating sequences of numbers and letters, was the only neuropsychological test that was repeatedly related to traffic violations or crashes (157). These results led to the conclusion, however, that people with mild dementia who have intact visual perceptual skills and normal performance on the Trails B test may still be safe drivers. Therefore, a diagnosis of dementia alone may not justify terminating a person's driving privileges.

To develop a practice parameter regarding driving and AD, the Quality Standards Subcommittee of the American Academy of Neurology reviewed literature regarding automobile accident frequency among drivers with the disease and concluded that level of dementia was an important factor (43). Specifically, driving was found to be mildly impaired in those drivers with probable AD and a clinical dementia rating (CDR) of 0.5, but AD drivers with a CDR severity of 1 were found to pose a significant traffic safety problem, both from crashes and from driving performance measurements. The committee recommended that patients and their families be told that those with AD whose CDR is 1 should not drive because of a substantially increased risk of crashing and that patients with possible disease and a CDR of 0.5 pose a significant traffic problem compared with other elderly drivers. It was also recommended that driving performance of the milder group be evaluated by a qualified examiner, with a re-evaluation of dementia severity and driving privileges every 6 months. In the future, it is imperative to develop a better understanding of the variables that make a person unfit to drive so that a person's independence can be maximized while minimizing the risk of accidents. Important ethical and legal considerations related to decisions about driving competency are discussed in Chapter 35.

FINANCIAL COMPETENCY

The ability to manage financial affairs involves a broad continuum of activities and specific skills. Marson (92) has developed a conceptual model whereby financial competency (FC) can be divided into *conceptual*, *pragmatic*, and *judgment* abilities that involves a complex set of cognitive functions ranging from using established crystallized knowledge (i.e., basic monetary skills, checkbook management, and bank statement management) to understanding of basic concepts, such as a loan or savings account, to the application of concepts and knowledge (i.e., selecting interest rates). Financial judgment involves an even more cognitively complex set of activities and consists of tasks related to detection/awareness of financial fraud and to making informed investment choices. There is a hierarchy to the development and decline of these abilities. Impairments in these higher order financial skills and judgment have been demonstrated by patients with mild dementia and even some patients with MCI. Furthermore, impairments in less complex activities such as checkbook and bank statement management are often a characteristic of mild AD. In fact, mild AD patients are at significant risk for impairment in most financial activities, but most moderate AD patients cannot manage any of their financial affairs.

CONCLUSION

Although researchers have made great progress in identifying and defining the various dementing syndromes over the past 30 years, problems with diagnostic criteria continue to exist. Results from genetic studies appear very promising in further elucidating clinical subtypes and course of dementing diseases. More prospective, longitudinal neuropsychological studies with radiologic and genetic testing are needed to better elucidate similarities and differences among various dementing disorders. Further work must be done to refine these criteria and develop diagnostic tools that are more sensitive early in the disease process so that the effects of potential therapies can be accurately measured.

REFERENCES

1. Abas MA, Sahakian BJ, Levy R. Neuropsychological deficits and CT scan changes in elderly depressives. *Psychol Med*. 1990;20:507–520.
2. Agüero-Torres H, Fratiglioni L, Guo Z, et al. Dementia is the major cause of functional dependence in the elderly: 3-year follow-up data from a population-based study. *Am J Public Health*. 1998;88:1452–1456.
3. Aharon-Peretz J, Kliot D, Tomer R. Behavioral differences between white matter lacunar dementia and Alzheimer's disease: a comparison of the neuropsychiatric inventory. *Dement Geriatr Cogn Disord*. 2000;11:294–298.
4. Albers MW, Tabert MH, Devanand DP. Olfactory dysfunction as a predictor of neurodegenerative disease. *Curr Neurol Neurosci Rep*. 2006;6:379–386.
5. Alexander GE, Chen K, Pietrini P, et al. Longitudinal PET evaluation of cerebral metabolic decline in dementia: a potential outcome measure in Alzheimer's disease treatment studies. *Am J Psychiatry*. 2002;159:738–745.
6. Alexopoulos GS, Meyers BS, Young RC, et al. The course of geriatric depression with "reversible dementia": a controlled study. *Am J Psychiatry*. 1993;150:1693–1699.
7. American Psychiatric Association. *Diagnostic and Statistical Manual of Mental Disorders*. 4th ed. Washington, DC: American Psychiatric Association; 1994.
8. Anderson VC, Litvack ZN, Kaye JA. Magnetic resonance approaches to brain aging and Alzheimer's disease-associated neuropathology. *Top Magn Reson Imaging*. 2005;16:439–452.
9. Backman L, Small BJ, Fratiglioni L. Stability of the preclinical episodic memory deficit in Alzheimer's disease. *Brain*. 2001;124:96–102.
10. Ballard C, Ayre G, O'Brien J, et al. Simple standardized neuropsychological assessments aid in the differential diagnosis of dementia with Lewy bodies from Alzheimer's disease and vascular dementia. *Dement Geriatr Cogn Disord*. 1999;10:104–108.
11. Ballard C, Holmes C, McKeith I, et al. Psychiatric morbidity in dementia with Lewy bodies: a prospective clinical and neuropathological comparative study with Alzheimer's disease. *Am J Psychiatry*. 1999;156:1039–1045.
12. Ballard CG, O'Brien J, Swann AG, et al. The natural history of psychosis and depression in dementia with Lewy bodies and Alzheimer's disease: persistence and new cases over 1 year of follow-up. *J Clin Psychiatry*. 2001;62:46–49.

13. Bayles KA, Tomoeda CK. Confrontation naming impairment in dementia. *Brain Lang.* 1983;19:98–114.

14. Bayles KA, Tomoeda CK, Cruz RF. Performance of Alzheimer's disease patients in judging word relatedness. *J Int Neuropsychol Soc.* 1999;5:668–675.

15. Bayley PJ, Salmon DP, Bondi MW, et al. Comparison of the serial position effect in very mild Alzheimer's disease, mild Alzheimer's disease, and amnesia associated with electroconvulsive therapy. *J Int Neuropsychol Soc.* 2000;6:290–298.

16. Becker JT, Boller F, Saxton J, et al. Normal rate of forgetting of verbal and non-verbal material in Alzheimer's disease. *Cortex.*1987;23:59–72.

17. Binetti G, Locascio JJ, Corkin S, et al. Differences between Pick disease and Alzheimer disease in clinical appearance and rate of cognitive decline. *Arch Neurol.* 2000;57:225–232.

18. Blair M, Kertesz A, McMonagle P, et al. Quantitative and qualitative analyses of clock drawing in frontotemporal dementia and Alzheimer's disease. *J Int Neuropsychol Soc.* 2006;12:159–165.

19. Boccardi M, Laakso MP, Bresciani L, et al. The MRI pattern of frontal and temporal brain atrophy in fronto-temporal dementia. *Neurobiol Aging.* 2003;24:95–103.

20. Boland RJ. Depression in Alzheimer's disease and other dementias. *Curr Psychiatry Rep.* 2000;2:427–433.

21. Bolla KI, Lindgren KN, Bonaccorsy C, et al. Memory complaints in older adults. Fact or fiction? *Arch Neurol.* 1991;48:61–64.

22. Boyle PA, Malloy PF, Salloway S, et al. Executive cognitive dysfunction and apathy predict functional impairment in Alzheimer's disease. *Am J Geriatr Psychiatry.* 2003;11:214–221.

23. Brown DF. Lewy body dementia. *Ann Med.* 1999;31:188–196.

24. Burton EJ, Karas G, Paling SM, et al. Patterns of cerebral atrophy in dementia with Lewy bodies using voxel-based morphometry. *Neuroimage.* 2002;17:618–630.

25. Butters N, Granholm E, Salmon DP, et al. Episodic and semantic memory: a comparison of amnestic and demented patients. *J Clin Exp Neuropsychol.* 1987;9:585–589.

26. Cahn DA, Salmon DP, Bondi MW, et al. A population-based analysis of qualitative features of the neuropsychological test performance of individuals with dementia of the Alzheimer type: implications for individuals with questionable dementia. *J Int Neuropsychol Soc.* 1997;3:387–393.

27. Cappa A, Calcagni ML, Villa G, et al. Brain perfusion abnormalities in Alzheimer's disease: comparison between patients with focal temporal lobe dysfunction and patients with diffuse cognitive impairment. *J Neurol Neurosurg Psychiatry.* 2001;70:22–27.

28. Carr DB, Gray S, Baty J, et al. The value of informant versus individual's complaints of memory impairment in early dementia. *Neurology.* 2000;55:1724–1727.

29. Chen P, Ratcliff G, Belle SH, et al. Cognitive tests that best discriminate between presymptomatic AD and those who remain nondemented. *Neurology.* 2000;55:1847–1853.

30. Chetelat G, Desgranges B, de la Sayette V, et al. Mild cognitive impairment: can FDG-PET predict who is to rapidly convert to Alzheimer's disease? *Neurology.* 2003;60:1374–1377.

31. Coimbra A, Williams DS, Hostetler ED. The role of MRI and PET/SPECT in Alzheimer's disease. *Curr Topics Med Chem.* 2006;6:629–647.

32. Connor DJ, Salmon DP, Sandy TJ, et al. Cognitive profiles of autopsy-confirmed Lewy body variant vs. pure Alzheimer disease. *Arch Neurol.* 1998;55:994–1000.

33. Crowe SF, Hoogenraad K. Differentiation of dementia of the Alzheimer's type from depression with cognitive impairment on the basis of a cortical versus subcortical pattern of cognitive deficit. *Arch Clin Neuropsychol.* 2000;15:9–19.

34. Crowell TA, Luis CA, Cox DE, et al. Neuropsychological comparison of Alzheimer's disease and dementia with Lewy bodies. *Dement Geriatr Cogn Disord.* 2007;23:120–125.

35. Cummings JL, Benson DF. Dementia of the Alzheimer's type: an inventory of diagnostic clinical features. *J Am Geriatr Soc.* 1986;34:12–19.

36. Cummings JL, Benson DF, Hill MA, et al. Aphasia in dementia of the Alzheimer's type. *Neurology.* 1985;29:394–397.

37. Delis DC, Kaplan E, Kramer JH. *Delis-Kaplan Executive Function System (DKEFS).* San Antonio: The Psychological Corporation; 2001.

38. Del Ser T, Hachinski V, Merskey H, et al. Clinical and pathological features of two groups of patients with dementia with Lewy bodies: effect of coexisting Alzheimer-type lesion load. *Alzheimer Dis Assoc Disord.* 2001;15:31–44.

39. De Simone V, Kaplan L, Patronas N, et al. Driving abilities in frontotemporal dementia patients. *Dement Geriatr Cogn Disord.* 2007;23:1–7.

40. Devanand DP, Michaels-Martson KS, Liu X, et al. Olfactory deficits in patients with mild cognitive impairment predict Alzheimer's disease

at follow-up. *Am J Psychiatry*. 2000;157: 1399–1405.

41. Doody RS, Massman PJ, Mawad M, et al. Cognitive consequences of subcortical magnetic resonance imaging changes in Alzheimer's disease: comparison to small vessel ischemic vascular dementia. *Neuropsychiatry Neuropsychol Behav Neurol*. 1998;11:191–199.

42. Du AT, Schuff N, Kramer JH, et al. Higher atrophy rate of entorhinal cortex then hippocampus in AD. *Neurology*. 2004;62:422–427.

43. Dubinsky RM, Stein AC, Lyons K. Practice parameter: risk of driving and Alzheimer's disease (an evidence-based review). Report of the Quality Standards Subcommittee of the American Academy of Neurology. *Neurology*. 2000;54:2205–2211.

44. Ecklund-Johnson E, Torres I. Unawareness of deficits in Alzheimer's disease and other dementias: operational definitions and empirical findings. *Neuropsychol Rev*. 2005;15:147–166.

45. Edelberg HK, Shallenberger E, Wei JY. Medication management capacity in high functioning community-living older adults: detection of early deficits. *J Am Geriat Soc*. 1999;47:592–596.

46. Erkinjuntti T, Inzitari D, Pantoni L, et al. Research criteria for subcortical vascular dementia in clinical trials. *J Neural Transm*. 2000;59 (suppl):23–30.

47. Folstein MF, Folstein SE, McHugh PR. "Mini-mental state." A practical method for grading the cognitive state of patients for the clinician. *J Psychiatr Res*. 1975;12:189–198.

48. Ford JM, Askari N, Gabrieli JD, et al. Event-related brain potential evidence of spared knowledge in Alzheimer's disease. *Psychol Aging*. 2001;16:161–176.

49. Freedman M, Leach L, Kaplan E, et al. *Clock Drawing: A Neuropsychological Analysis*. New York: Oxford University Press; 1994.

50. Furey-Kurkjian ML, Pietrini P, Graff-Radford NR, et al. Visual variant of Alzheimer disease: distinctive neuropsychological features. *Neuropsychology*. 1996;10:294–300.

51. Galasko D, Katzman R, Salmon DP, et al. Clinical and neuropathological findings in Lewy body dementias. *Brain Cogn*. 1996;31: 166–175.

52. Gomez RG, White DA. Using verbal fluency to detect very mild dementia of the Alzheimer type. *Arch Clin Neuropsychol*. 2006;21:771–775.

53. Gomez-Isla T, Growdon WB, McNamara M, et al. Clinicopathologic correlates in temporal cortex in dementia with Lewy bodies. *Neurology*. 1999;53:2003–2009.

54. Gomez-Tortosa E, Irizarry MC, Gomez-Isla T, et al. Clinical and neuropathological correlates of dementia with Lewy bodies. *Ann NY Acad Sci*. 2000;920:9–15.

55. Graff-Radford NR, Woodruff BK. Frontotemporal dementia. *Semin Neurol*. 2007;27: 48–57.

56. Groves WC, Brandt J, Steinberg M, et al. Vascular dementia and Alzheimer's disease: is there a difference? A comparison of symptoms by disease duration. *J Neuropsychiatry Clin Neurosci*. 2000;12:305–315.

57. Gunning-Dixon FM, Raz N. The cognitive correlates of white matter abnormalities in normal aging: a quantitative review. *Neuropsychology*. 2000;14:224–232.

58. Gurd JM, Herzberg L, Joachim C, et al. Dementia with Lewy bodies: a pure case. *Brain Cogn*. 2000;44:307–323.

59. Hargrave R, Reed B, Mungas D. Depressive syndromes and functional disability in dementia. *J Geriatr Psychiatry Neurol*. 2000;13:72–77.

60. Haroutunian V, Serby M, Purohit DP, et al. Contribution of Lewy body inclusions to dementia in patients with and without Alzheimer disease neuropathological conditions. *Arch Neurol*. 2000;57:1145–1150.

61. Harvan JR, Cotter V. An evaluation of dementia screening in the primary care setting. *J Am Acad Nurse Pract*. 2006;18:351–360.

62. Head D, Buckner RL, Shimony JS, et al. Differential vulnerability of anterior white matter in nondemented aging with minimal acceleration in dementia of the Alzheimer's type: evidence from diffusion tensor imaging. *Cereb Cortex*. 2004;14:410–423.

63. Heaton RK, Chelune GJ, Talley JL, et al. *Wisconsin Card Sorting Test Manual, Revised and Expanded*. Odessa, FL: Psychological Assessment Resources; 1993.

64. Hentschel F, Damian M, Krumm B, et al. White matter lesions-age adjusted values for cognitively healthy and demented subjects. *Acta Neurol Scand*. 2007;115:174–180.

65. Hirono N, Mori E, Tanimukai S, et al. Distinctive neurobehavioral features among neurodegenerative dementias. *J Neuropsychiatry Clin Neurosci*. 1999;11:498–503.

66. Hodges JR, Patterson K, Ward R, et al. The differentiation of semantic dementia and frontal lobe dementia (temporal and frontal variants of frontotemporal dementia) from early Alzheimer's disease: a comparative neuropsychological study. *Neuropsychology*. 1999;13:31–40.

67. Hohl U, Grundman M, Salmon DP, et al. Mini-mental examination and Mattis dementia rating

scale performance differs in Hispanic and non-Hispanic Alzheimer's disease patients. *J Int Neuropsychol Soc.* 1999;5:301–307.

68. Holtzer R, Tang MX, Devanand DP, et al. Psychopathological features in Alzheimer's disease; course and relationship with cognitive status. *J Am Geriat Soc.* 2003;51:953–960.

69. Horsfield MA, Jones DK. Application of diffusion-weighted and diffusion tensor MRI to white matter diseases: a review. *NMR Biomed.* 2002;15:570–577.

70. Huber SJ, Shuttleworth EC, Freidenberg DL. Neuropsychological differences between the dementias of Alzheimer's and Parkinson's diseases. *Arch Neurol.* 1989;46:1287–1291.

71. Jack CR, Shiung MM, Gunter JL, et al. Comparison of different MRI brain atrophy rate measures with clinical disease progression in AD. *Neurology.* 2004;62:591–600.

72. Jefferson AL, Cahn-Weiner D, Boyle P, et al. Cognitive predictors of functional decline in vascular dementia. *Int J Geriatr Psychiatry.* 2006;21:752–754.

73. Jellinger KA. Morphological substrates of mental dysfunction in Lewy body disease: an update. *J Neural Transm.* 2000;59(suppl):185–212.

74. Jurica PJ, Leitten CL, Mattis S. *Dementia Rating Scale-2 Professional Manual.* Lutz, FL: Psychological Assessment Resources, Inc.; 2001.

75. Klunk WE, Wang Y, Huang GF, et al. The binding of 2-(4'-methylaminophenyl) benzothiazole to postmortem brain homogenates is dominated by the amyloid component. *J Neurosci.* 2003;23:2086–2092.

76. Knibb JA, Kipps CM, Hodges JR. Frontotemporal dementia. *Curr Opin Neurol.* 2006;19:565–571.

77. Knopman DS, Parisi JE, Boeve BF, et al. Vascular dementia in a population-based autopsy study. *Arch Neurol.* 2003;60:569–575.

78. Kral VA, Emery OB. Long-term follow-up of depressive pseudodementia of the aged. *Can J Psychiatry.* 1989;34:445–446.

79. Krishnan S, Talley BD, Slavin MJ, et al. Current status of functional MR imaging, perfusion-weighted, and diffusion-tensor imaging in Alzheimer's disease diagnosis and research. *Neuroimaging Clin N Am.* 2005;15:853–868.

80. Lamar M, Podell K, Carew TG, et al. Perseverative behavior in Alzheimer's disease and subcortical ischemic vascular dementia. *Neuropsychology.* 1997;11:523–534.

81. Larrabee GJ, Youngjohn JR, Sudilovsky A, et al. Accelerated forgetting in Alzheimer-type dementia. *J Clin Exp Neuropsychol.* 1993;15:701–712.

82. Larson EB, Reifler BV, Sumi SM, et al. Diagnostic evaluation of 200 elderly outpatients with suspected dementia. *J Gerontol.* 1985;40:536–543.

83. LeBihan D, van Zijl P. From the diffusion coefficient to the diffusion tensor. *NMR Biomed.* 2002;15:431–434.

84. Libon DJ, Bogdanoff B, Bonavita J, et al. Neuropsychological deficits associated with ischemic vascular dementia caused by periventricular and deep white matter alterations. *Arch Clin Neuropsychol.* 1997;12:239–250.

85. Libon DJ, Bogdanoff B, Leopold N, et al. Neuropsychological profile associated with subcortical white matter alterations and Parkinson's disease—implications for the diagnosis of dementia. *Arch Clin Neuropsychol.* 2001;16:19–32.

86. Libon DJ, Malamut BL, Swenson R, et al. Further analyses of clock drawings among demented and nondemented older subjects. *Arch Clin Neuropsychol.* 1996;11:193–205.

87. Libon DJ, Xie SX, Moore BS, et al. Patterns of neuropsychological impairment in frontotemporal dementia. *Neurology.* 2007;68:369–375.

88. Loewenstein DA, Arguelles S, Bravo M, et al. Caregivers' judgments of the functional abilities of the Alzheimer's disease patient: a comparison of proxy reports and objective measures. *J Gerontol B Psychol Sci Soc Sci.* 2001;56:78–84.

89. Looi JC, Sachdev PS. Differentiation of vascular dementia from AD on neuropsychological tests. *Neurology.* 1999;53:670–678.

90. Lopez OL, Becker JT, Brenner RP, et al. Alzheimer's disease with delusions and hallucinations: neuropsychological and electroencephalographic correlates. *Neurology.* 1991;41:906–912.

91. Malloy PF, Cummings JL, Coffey CE, et al. Cognitive screening instruments in neuropsychiatry: a report of the Committee on Research of the American Neuropsychiatric Association. *J Neuropsychiatry Clin Neurosci.* 1997;9:189–197.

92. Marson DC. Loss of financial capacity in dementia: conceptual and empirical approaches. *Aging Neuropsychol Cogn.* 2001;8:164–181.

93. Mayeux R, Stern Y, Spanton S. Heterogeneity in dementia of the Alzheimer type: evidence of subgroups. *Neurology.* 1985;35:453–461.

94. Mayzel-Oreg O, Assaf Y, Gigi A, et al. High *b*-value diffusion imaging of dementia: application to vascular dementia and Alzheimer disease. *J Neurol Sci.* 2007;10:1–9.

95. McCue M. The relationship between neuropsychology and functional assessment in the elderly. In: Nussbaum P, ed. *The handbook of*

neuropsychology and aging. New York: Plenum Press; 1996:394–408.

96. McKeith IG, Galasko D, Kosaka K, et al. Consensus guidelines for the clinical and pathologic diagnosis of dementia with Lewy bodies (DLB): report of the Consortium on DLB International Workshop. *Neurology.* 1996;47: 1113–1124.

97. McKeith IG, Perry EK, Perry RH. Report of the second dementia with Lewy body international workshop: diagnosis and treatment. Consortium on Dementia with Lewy Bodies. *Neurology.* 1999;53:902–905.

98. McKhann GM, Albert MS, Grossman M, et al. Clinical and pathological diagnosis of frontotemporal dementia; report of the Work Group on Frontotemporal Dementia and Pick's Disease. *Arch Neurol.* 2001;58:1803–1809.

99. Mendez MF, Selwood A, Mastri AR, et al. Pick's disease versus Alzheimer's disease: a comparison of clinical characteristics. *Neurology.* 1993;43: 289–292.

100. Mesulam MM. Primary progressive aphasia. *Ann Neurol.* 2001;49:425–432.

101. Mueller SG, Weiner MW, Thal LJ, et al. Ways toward an early diagnosis in Alzheimer's disease: the Alzheimer's Disease Neuroimaging Initiative (ADNI). *Alzheimers Dement.* 2005;1: 55–66.

102. Neary D, Snowden JS, Gustafson L, et al. Frontotemporal lobar degeneration: a consensus on clinical diagnostic criteria. *Neurology.* 1998;51:1546–1554.

103. Nordin S, Murphy C. Impaired sensory and cognitive olfactory function in questionable Alzheimer's disease. *Neuropsychology.* 1996;10: 113–119.

104. Nordin S, Murphy C. Odor memory in normal aging and Alzheimer's disease. *Ann NY Acad Sci.* 1998;885:686–693.

105. Norton LE, Bondi MW, Salmon DP, et al. Deterioration of generic knowledge in patients with Alzheimer's disease: evidence from the Number Information Test. *J Clin Exp Neuropsychol.* 1997;19:857–866.

106. O'Brien JT, Metcalfe S, Swann A, et al. Medial temporal lobe width on CT scanning in Alzheimer's disease: comparison with vascular dementia, depression and dementia with Lewy bodies. *Dement Geriatr Cogn Disord.* 2000;11: 114–118.

107. O'Brien MD. How does cerebrovascular disease cause dementia? *Dementia.* 1994;5:133–136.

108. Pachana NA, Boone KB, Miller BL, et al. Comparison of neuropsychological functioning in Alzheimer's disease and frontotemporal dementia. *J Clin Exp Neuropsychol Soc.* 1996;2: 505–510.

109. Paulson JS, Salmon DP, Thal LJ, et al. Incidence of and risk factors for hallucinations and delusions in patients with probable AD. *Neurology.* 2000;54:1965–1971.

110. Rabinovici GD, Furst AJ, O'Neil JP, et al. ^{11}C-PIB PET imaging in Alzheimer disease and frontotemporal lobar degeneration. *Neurology.* 2007;68:1205–1212.

111. Rahman S, Sahakian BJ, Hodges JR, et al. Specific cognitive deficits in early frontal variant frontotemporal dementia. *Brain.* 1999;122: 1469–1493.

112. Rao SM, Mittenberg W, Bernardin L, et al. Neuropsychological test findings on subjects with leukoaraiosis. *Arch Neurol.* 1989;46:40–47.

113. Rapcsak SZ, Croswell SC, Rubens AB. Apraxia in Alzheimer's disease. *Neurology.* 1989;39:664–668.

114. Rapoport MJ, van Reekum R, Freedman M, et al. Relationship of psychosis to aggression, apathy and function in dementia. *Int J Geriatr Psychiatry.* 2001;16:123–130.

115. Rascovsky K, Salmon DP, Hansen LA, et al. Disparate letter and semantic category fluency deficits in autopsy-confirmed frontotemporal dementia and Alzheimer's disease. *Neuropsychology.* 2007;21:20–30.

116. Reed BR, Eberling JL, Mungas D, et al. Memory failure has different mechanisms in subcortical stroke and Alzheimer's disease. *Ann Neurol.* 2000;48:275–284.

117. Reed BR, Mungas D, Kramer JHY, et al. Clinical and neuropsychological features in autopsy-defined vascular dementia. *Clin Neuropsychol.* 2004;18:63–74.

118. Reitan RM. Validity of the Trailmaking test as an indicator of organic brain damage. *Percept Mot Skills.* 1958;8:271–276.

119. Richards M, Bell K, Dooneief F, et al. Patterns of neuropsychological performance in Alzheimer's disease patients with and without extrapyramidal signs. *Neurology.* 1993;43:1708–1711.

120. Richardson HE, Glass JN. A comparison of scoring protocols on the Clock Drawing Test in relation to ease of use, diagnostic group, and correlations with Mini-Mental State Examination. *J Am Geriatr Soc.* 2002;50:169–173.

121. Rillings LM, Lucas JA, Ivnik RJ, et al. Mayo's Older African American Normative Studies: Norms for the Mattis Dementia Rating Scale. *Clin Neuropsychol.* 2005;19:229–242.

122. Roman GC, Royall DR. Executive control function: a rational basis for the diagnosis of vascular dementia. *Alzheimer Dis Assoc Disord.* 1999;13 [Suppl 3]:S69–S80.

123. Ron MA, Toone BK, Garralda ME, et al. Diagnostic accuracy in presenile dementia. *Br J Psychiatry*. 1979;34:161–168.

124. Rosen HJ, Allison BS, Ogar MS, et al. Behavioral features in semantic dementia vs other forms of progressive aphasias. *Neurology*. 2006;67:1752–1756.

125. Rosen WG. Neuropsychological patterns with focus on constructional apraxia. In: *Symposium, longitudinal studies of dementia of the Alzheimer type: neuropsychological and neurophysiological patterns*. Houston: International Neuropsychological Society; 1984.

126. Rosen WG. Verbal fluency in aging and dementia. *J Clin Neuropsychol*. 1980;2:135–146.

127. Rosen WG, Mohs RC, Davis KL. A new rating scale for Alzheimer disease. *Am J Psychiatry*. 1984;141:1356–1364.

128. Salmon DP, Galasko D, Hansen LA, et al. Neuropsychological deficits associated with diffuse Lewy body disease. *Brain Cogn*. 1996;31:148–165.

129. Salmon DP, Heindel WC, Lange KL. Differential decline in word generation from phonemic and semantic categories during the course of Alzheimer's disease: implications for the integrity of semantic memory. *J Int Neuropsychol Soc*. 1999;5:692–703.

130. Sherman AM, Massman PJ. Prevalence and correlates of category versus letter fluency discrepancies in Alzheimer's disease. *Arch Clin Neuropsychol*. 1999;14:411–418.

131. Shimomura ME, Fujimora M, Hirono N, et al. Visuoperceptual impairment in dementia with Lewy bodies. *Arch Neurol*. 2000;57:489–493.

132. Shulman KI, Gold D, Cohen C, et al. Clock drawing and dementia in the community: a longitudinal study. *Int J Geriatr Psychiatry*. 1993;8:487–496.

133. Shulman KI, Herrmann N, Brodaty H, et al. IPA survey of brief cognitive screening instruments. *Int Psychogeriatr*. 2006;18:281–294.

134. Silverman DHS, Small GW, Chang CY, et al. Positron emission tomography in evaluation of dementia: regional brain metabolism and long-term outcome. *JAMA*. 2007;286:2120–2127.

135. Simon E, Leach L, Winocur G, et al. Intact primary memory in mild to moderate Alzheimer disease: indices from the California Verbal Learning Test. *J Clin Exp Neuropsychol*. 1994;16:414–422.

136. Small GW. Diagnostic issues in dementia: neuroimaging as a surrogate marker of disease. *J Geriatr Psychiatry Neurol*. 2006;19:180–185.

137. Small GW, Kepe V, Barrio JR. Seeing is believing: neuroimaging adds to our understanding of cerebral pathology. *Curr Opin Psychiatry*. 2006;19:564–569.

138. Small GW, Rabins PV, Barry PP, et al. Diagnosis and treatment of Alzheimer disease and related disorders. Consensus statement of the American Association for Geriatric Psychiatry, the Alzheimer's Association, and the American Geriatrics Society. *JAMA*. 1997;278:1363–1371.

139. Stern Y, Albert M, Tang MX, et al. Rate of memory decline in AD is related to education and occupation: cognitive reserve? *Neurology*. 1999;53:1942–1947.

140. Stern Y, Mayeux R, Sano M, et al. Predictors of disease course in patients with probable Alzheimer's disease. *Neurology*. 1987;37:1649–1653.

141. Stern Y, Ming-Xin T, Jacobs DM, et al. Prospective comparative study of the evolution of probable Alzheimer's disease and Parkinson's disease dementia. *J Int Neuropsychol Soc*. 1998;4:279–284.

142. Stoudemire A, Hill C, Gulley L, et al. Neuropsychological and biomedical assessment of depression-dementia syndromes. *J Neuropsychiatry Clin Neurosci*. 1989;1:347–361.

143. Suhr JA, Jones RD. Letter and semantic fluency in Alzheimer's, Huntington's, and Parkinson's dementias. *Arch Clin Neuropsychol*. 1998;13:447–454.

144. Tabert MH, Albert SM, Borukhova-Milov L, et al. Functional deficits in patients with mild cognitive impairment: prediction of AD. *Neurology*. 2002;58:758–764.

145. Thompson-Schill SL, Gabrieli JD, Fleischman DA. Effects of structural similarity and name frequency of picture naming in Alzheimer's disease. *J Int Neuropsychol Soc*. 1999;5:659–667.

146. Tierney MC, Snow WG, Charles J, et al. Neuropsychological predictors of self-neglect in cognitively impaired older people who live alone. *Am J Geriatr Psychiatry*. 2007;15:140–148.

147. Troster AI, Butters N, Salmon DP, et al. The diagnostic utility of savings scores: differentiating Alzheimer's and Huntington's diseases with the logical memory and visual reproduction tests. *J Clin Exp Neuropsychol*. 1993;15:773–788.

148. Tuokko H, Hadjistavropoulos T. Screening instruments for cognitive impairment. In: *An assessment guide to geriatric neuropsychology*. Mahwah, NJ: Lawrence Erlbaum; 1998:28–43.

149. Tuokko H, Tallman K, Beattie BL, et al. An examination of driving records in a dementia clinic. *J Gerontol B Psychol Sci Soc Sci*. 1995;50:S173–S181.

150. Vanderploeg RD, Yuspeh RL, Schinka JA. Differential episodic and semantic memory

performance in Alzheimer's disease and vascular dementias. *J Int Neuropsychol Soc.* 2001;7:563–573.

151. Van Gorp WG, Marcotte TD, Sultzer D, et al. Screening for dementia: comparison of three commonly used instruments. *J Clin Exp Neuropsychol.* 1999;21:29–38.

152. Walker MP, Ayre GA, Cummings JL, et al. Quantifying fluctuation in dementia with Lewy bodies, Alzheimer's disease, and vascular dementia. *Neurology.* 2000;25:1616–1625.

153. Wetter SR, Delis DC, Houston WS, et al. Deficits in inhibition and flexibility are associated with the APOE-e4 allele in nondemented older adults. *J Clin Exp Neuropsychol.* 2005;27:943–952.

154. White L, Petrovitch H, Ross GW, et al. Prevalence of dementia in older Japanese-American men in Hawaii: the Honolulu-Asia Aging Study. *JAMA.* 1996;276:955–960.

155. Whitwell JL, Sampson EL, Watt HC, et al. A volumetric magnetic resonance imaging study of the amygdala in frontotemporal lobar degeneration and Alzheimer's disease. *Dement Geriatr Cogn Disord.* 2005;20:238–244.

156. Wickland AH, Johnson N, Weintraub S. Preservations of reasoning in primary progressive aphasia: further differentiation from Alzheimer's disease and the behavioral presentation of frontotemporal dementia. *J Clin Exp Neuropsychol.* 2004;26:347–355.

157. Withaar FK, Brouwer WH, Van Zomeren AH. Fitness to drive in older drivers with cognitive impairment. *J Int Neuropsychol Soc.* 2000;6:480–490.

158. Yuspeh RL, Vanderploeg RD, Crowell TA, et al. Differences in executive functioning between Alzheimer's disease and subcortical ischemic vascular dementia. *J Clin Exp Neuropsychol.* 2002;24:745–754.

159. Zakzanis KK, Kielar A, Young DA, et al. Neuropsychological differentiation of late onset schizophrenia and frontotemporal dementia. *Cogn Neuropsychiatry.* 2001;6:63–77.

WEBSITES

Alzheimer's Association: http://www.alz.org/

The Association for Frontotemporal Dementias: http://ftd-picks.org/

National Parkinson Foundation: http://www.parkinson.org

Internet Mental Health: http://www.mentalhealth.com

U.S. Public Health Service: http://www.surgeongeneral.gov/library/mentalhealth

American Psychiatric Association: http://www.psych.org/

Alzheimer's Weekly: http://www.alzheimersweekly.com

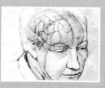

CHAPTER 21.4

Mild Cognitive Impairment and the Role of Imaging

Laura A. Flashman, Barbara L. Malamut, and Andrew J. Saykin

Recent research continues to advance our understanding of the boundary between normal aging and dementia. In addition to identifying changes associated with both normal and abnormal aging, researchers have identified a group of individuals whose cognitive deficits place them in an intermediate position on this continuum. The diagnosis of mild cognitive impairment (MCI) is given when older individuals have greater than expected memory impairment for their age but do not meet criteria for dementia (132). Thus, MCI denotes a transitional state between the cognitive changes associated with normal aging and the earliest clinical features of dementia (137,200). This "preclinical" phase is associated with neuropathologic and cognitive disturbances, which gradually rise to a level sufficient for a diagnosis of probable dementia (154). The original formal MCI criteria (56,136) include: (a) significant memory complaints, such as a chronic forgetting of important information, corroborated by an informant; (b) memory impairment on standardized tests relative to age- and education-matched healthy controls (at least 1.5 standard deviation below the mean); (c) otherwise normal cognitive function; (d) normal activities of daily living (ADLs); and (e) failure to meet criteria for dementia. This profile is now considered to indicate the amnestic subtype of MCI (132).

Compared to age-matched peers, individuals with a diagnosis of MCI generally present with subjective memory difficulties of insidious onset. In fact, subjective cognitive complaints can be a harbinger of dementia even before the development of demonstrable cognitive deficits, particularly in highly educated individuals (90). As time progresses, the memory problem becomes more frequent and significant. Despite increasing memory problems, social and occupational functioning is relatively preserved. Nonmemory cognitive domains are relatively spared in MCI, as originally defined, but in practice, they may fall slightly below age- and education-based normative data. For example, speed of processing and cognitive flexibility may be subtly impaired (132).

As more researchers have become involved in studying MCI, it has become clear that it is not a homogeneous disorder, and there appear to be several cognitive subtypes (148). Currently, there are four classifications of MCI, which are based on the presence or absence of memory problems and difficulties in other cognitive domains. These are amnestic MCI–single domain, amnestic MCI–multiple domains, nonamnestic MCI–single domain, and nonamnestic MCI–multiple domains (24). At one time, it was believed that the amnestic variant of MCI would progress to Alzheimer's disease (AD), whereas the other MCI forms would progress to other forms of dementia such as Lewy body or vascular dementia (136). However, more recent studies have shown that cognitive subtypes of MCI are not necessarily predictive of conversion to specific types of dementia, and both amnestic MCI and nonamnestic MCI frequently develop into AD (53,114). In a community-based study of 980 dementia-free people with diagnoses of all four cognitive subtypes of MCI, many of the individuals continued to demonstrate cognitive decline and eventually dementia. All forms of MCI, except nonamnestic MCI–multiple domains, converted to AD within 6 years of follow-up, whereas many individuals in the nonamnestic MCI–multiple domains group progressed to non-AD forms of dementia (24). More longitudinal studies of the various MCI clinical profiles are needed to diagnose individuals as early as possible in the disease course so that, when further treatments become available, they can be used before there is too much irreversible brain damage.

This chapter will focus on the amnestic variant of MCI. Current estimates indicate conversion rates from MCI to AD of between 6% and 25% per year (133), with most studies falling in the 10% to 15% per year range (19,46,56,133,136,188). This is significantly greater than the 1% to 2% per year rate at which AD develops in the normal elderly population. Petersen et al. (136) report that up to 50% of individuals diagnosed with MCI will convert to AD within 4 years, and Morris et al. (124) report a conversion rate of >80% in individuals followed for 9.5 years.

Given the likelihood of progression to AD in individuals with MCI, early identification and diagnosis have important implications for treatment (2).

Although it is not yet clear who will or will not convert to AD, several potential risk factors have been identified. Prominent among the risk factors is the presence of the *apolipoprotein (ApoE) ε4* allele. *ApoE* is a marker initially studied as a risk factor for cardiovascular disease. It is involved in the normal regulation of phospholipid metabolism and cholesterol and may play a role in neural repair. Identified cognitive correlates of *ApoE* genotype include subtle decreases on verbal memory tested over time in longitudinal studies (33) and failure to benefit from cueing at recall (134). Neuroimaging associations with *ApoE* include mesial temporal lobe changes such as decreased volume of the hippocampus (82) and entorhinal cortex (58,82,95,96,103), as well as decreased medial temporal gray matter (201). The use of magnetic resonance imaging (MRI) or other imaging techniques such as functional neuroimaging may be useful to distinguish MCI patients who will develop AD from those who will not (27).

COGNITION

Given the heightened risk for dementia in patients with MCI as compared to cognitively intact older adults, researchers are closely examining the neuropsychological profiles of these individuals. The diagnoses of MCI and AD both require the presence of memory impairment. To distinguish between MCI and AD, it is important to determine not only the degree and course of memory impairment, but also, in particular, the presence or absence of additional domains of cognitive dysfunction and the impact of cognitive problems on the individual's daily functioning (32,132,135,136).

The initial memory impairment exhibited in AD is the most distinguishing early feature of the disease. Specific components of memory are differentially affected as a function of stage of AD. Episodic and semantic memory are impaired early in AD, with episodic memory perhaps showing the earliest changes. In contrast, other components such as procedural memory may remain relatively unaffected until later in the disease (14,25,102,140,166,167).

Diagnosis of MCI is complicated by disagreements about its definition and classification process and by research indicating that many MCI patients show subtle nonamnestic difficulties and other clinical problems (115,117,118,146,183,200). Although the primary cognitive deficit identified in MCI is impairment in episodic memory, individuals also may demonstrate relative weaknesses in other areas of cognition, with performance falling below expected levels of functioning. Research indicates that mild declines in executive functioning are present in preclinical dementia and that neuropsychological measures of

executive function can be useful in predicting later conversion to AD (1,28,38,49,124,146). Furthermore, patients who present with primary complaints about recent memory also frequently voice concern about aspects of executive functioning (38,112). These findings suggest that changes in executive functioning may be a subtle manifestation of incipient AD, along with memory dysfunction.

Additionally, although initial conceptualizations of MCI excluded changes in ADL and instrumental ADL (IADL) functioning, research suggests that tests of IADL skills may be helpful in the differential diagnosis. Recent work suggests that some MCI patients may present with mild impairments in higher order activities, such as financial capacity (70,123). Research also shows that, even at the early stages of cognitive impairment, caregivers of MCI patients take on new responsibilities including medication administration, medical decision making, meal preparation, transportation, and managing finances (63). These IADL deficits have been related to brain structure and function in patients with AD (177). Furthermore, consideration of mood through measures of depression (e.g., Geriatric Depression Scale or Beck Depression Inventory) and vascular involvement (72) are also likely to help with differential diagnosis.

NEUROANATOMY

Normal aging is associated with a 7% to 8% decrease in brain weight (113,191), as well as subtle changes in brain structure, including generally mild cortical atrophy and ventricular enlargement. Region-specific studies show greater neuronal decreases in some areas, including the superior frontal and temporal gyrus, precentral gyrus, visual cortex, locus ceruleus, substantia nigra, nucleus basalis of Meynert, and cerebellar Purkinje cells (113). In primary degenerative dementia, the decrease in brain weight is as much as 10% more than that seen in normal aging (186). As with normal aging, atrophy and eventual cell loss are region specific in AD. Structural brain changes have also been reported in patients with MCI. Medial temporal structures, including the hippocampus and entorhinal cortex, are particularly vulnerable.

STRUCTURAL IMAGING

A relatively recent advance in the evaluation of people with suspected AD is the use of structural imaging to assess *in vivo* neuroanatomic changes. This noninvasive technique can also be used in conjunction with neuropsychological test data to better understand the relationship between the structural brain changes and the cognitive deficits that characterize the disease.

HIPPOCAMPUS

Integrity of the hippocampus has been strongly implicated in episodic memory (61). MRI studies indicate substantial hippocampal atrophy in AD, even in the very early stages of the disease (80,87,104,111,162). In contrast, the hippocampus is spared significant aging effects through the seventh decade of life in healthy normal people (13). Studies of hippocampal atrophy in patients and healthy controls have reported age-related volume changes (i.e., greater volume loss with increased age) only in healthy controls; in contrast, in patients with MCI and AD, volume reductions were not related to age (40,45). Although minimal longitudinal data are available, Jack et al. (83,84) reported significant annual decline in hippocampal volume in healthy older adults; MCI patients showed somewhat greater rates of decline, whereas patients with AD showed the greatest decline. Furthermore, within the control and MCI groups, clinical decline was related to greater rates of hippocampal atrophy. Using an innovative surface-based hippocampal analytic technique on structural MRI data, Apostolova et al. (5) have demonstrated that hippocampal atrophy spreads in a pattern that follows the known trajectory of neurofibrillary tangle dissemination, with the main group differences between AD and MCI participants in the CA1 region bilaterally and the CA2 and CA3 region on the right. Age, race, gender, education, and Mini-Mental State Examination (MMSE) were significant predictors of hippocampal volume, and hippocampal volume was a significant predictor of clinical diagnosis.

Wang et al. (195) measured cerebrovascular volume and blood–brain barrier permeability in the hippocampus and cerebellum of 11 patients with MCI relative to 11 elderly normal control subjects using dynamic contrast-enhanced MRI (DCE-MRI). They found that the enhancement kinetics measured from hippocampus of MCI individuals demonstrated a lower magnitude and slower decay than healthy controls, suggesting that they had a smaller vascular volume in the right side.

Several studies have examined the relationship between hippocampal volume and cognitive functioning. For example, in the above study, Wang et al. (195) found that the vascular volume index was significantly correlated with naming ability in individuals with MCI and normal controls. de Leon et al. (40) found that, after controlling for age, education, and immediate memory, a significant correlation was found between delayed memory and hippocampal atrophy in normal controls but not in individuals with MCI. In contrast, Convit et al. (35) found that there was a relationship between delayed memory function and hippocampal volume in both healthy controls and patients with MCI. This may reflect the degree of impairment in the MCI population in the de Leon study, since these relations become harder to detect as cognitive impairment becomes more severe. General cognitive measures, such as the MMSE, did not distinguish between normal controls and participants with MCI and had no relationship to hippocampal volumes. This lack of association has also been reported in patients with AD (45). Wilson et al. (199) reported that hippocampal formation volume was associated with a delayed recall measure, but not with immediate recall, and with an object naming test in patients with AD. Medial temporal region volumes have been found to be correlated with delayed memory performance in patients with AD (108) and in nondemented elderly individuals (35,66).

ENTORHINAL CORTEX

Recent evidence strongly suggests that one of the earliest changes in AD is neurofibrillary tangles in the entorhinal cortex (EC) (21). MRI studies show significant reductions of EC volume in AD (43,95,110,129). Juottonen et al. (95) reported a significant correlation between left EC volume (corrected for whole brain size) and MMSE scores in patients with AD. Measurement of the EC also appears to be a useful marker for early diagnosis (15), and more recent studies have shown that EC volume is reduced in MCI patients compared to controls on MRI (204) and postmortem evaluation (109). Furthermore, baseline volumes of the EC appear to predict conversion from MCI to AD (58,82,103).

OTHER STRUCTURAL CHANGES

Other important limbic system structures have also been examined to further understand where there are structural changes in the early stages of dementia. Copenhaver et al. (36) examined the volumes of the fornix and mammillary bodies in nondepressed older patients with mild AD or MCI and demographically matched healthy controls. After adjustment for total intracranial volume (ICV), significant volume reductions were observed in the fornix and mammillary bodies, which are two structures known to be involved in episodic memory (61,62,98,99,126,184,206). When patients with AD were compared with controls and MCI participants, there was relative preservation of these structures in preclinical disease stages, indicating that atrophy of the fornix and mammillary bodies becomes apparent at the point of conversion from MCI to AD.

Studies examining the corpus callosum have yielded variable results. Wang et al. (197) reported that individuals with AD had significantly smaller callosum areas than healthy controls. Both the AD and the MCI group demonstrated a significant reduction of the posterior region (isthmus and splenium) of the corpus callosum relative to controls. However, Thomann et al. (187) reported that the corpus callosum was significantly smaller in patients with MCI and AD in rostral parts of the corpus callosum. In contrast, Wang and Su (196) found that hippocampal volume, but not corpus callosum volume, was significantly reduced in MCI patients relative to healthy controls. Using diffusion-weighted imaging analysis, however, they reported that apparent diffusion coefficient (ADC) values for both hippocampus and corpus callosum were increased in MCI to a similar extent. They concluded that alterations in water diffusivity may precede corpus callosum atrophy during the development of MCI, whereas diffusion changes may occur simultaneously in allocortex and neocortex.

Of clinical importance is the identification of markers that can be used routinely to help predict which patients with MCI will actually progress to dementia. One study (64) found that use of standardized visual assessment of medial temporal atrophy (MTA) was an accurate predictor of progression in patients with MCI with memory disturbance only or with MCI with memory and other neuropsychological deficits compared to nonamnestic MCI patients. Other investigators have demonstrated the importance of measuring whole brain volume (57,58) to differentiate AD patients from healthy controls. White matter (WM) lesions (9,39,51,202) and metabolite changes [for review, see Valenzuela and Sachdev (192)] may also be helpful to distinguish between healthy controls and individuals with MCI and AD. These measures may prove to be useful early indicators of conversion from MCI to AD.

Normal aging, MCI, and AD have been associated with loss of gray matter (GM) and WM (136,145,193). For example, van Es et al. (193) recently evaluated whether structural brain damage in AD and MCI, as detected by magnetization transfer imaging (MTI), is located in the GM and/or WM. Their results indicated that participants with AD had a lower GM volume than controls, whereas both MCI and AD patients demonstrated more structural changes in both GM and WM than healthy controls. Furthermore, in MCI and AD, cerebral lesion load in both GM and WM was associated with the degree of cognitive impairment, indicating that cerebral changes are present in GM and WM even before individuals are clinically demented. In other work examining GM and WM differences, higher ADCs were found in hippocampus, temporal lobe GM, and corpus callosum of patients with MCI compared with control subjects (144). With all subjects pooled together, an elevated hippocampal ADC was significantly correlated with worse memory performance scores in 5-minute and 30-minute delayed word list recall tasks.

Similarly, there are reports of a hierarchical change in cortical thickness (168), with the thickness of the cortex significantly decreased when healthy elderly brains were compared to those with MCI. A reduction of cortical thickness was found mainly in the medial temporal lobe region and in some regions of the frontal and parietal cortices. With the progression of disease from MCI to AD, a general thinning of the entire cortex with significant extension into the lateral temporal lobe was found. Interestingly, in all cases, the results were more pronounced in the left hemisphere.

RECENT ADVANCES

Voxel-based morphometry (VBM) is a recent method for looking at structural images that may be sensitive to the earliest stages of dementia, before the onset of cognitive changes measurable on comprehensive neuropsychological evaluation. VBM assesses GM and WM tissue compartments on a voxel-by-voxel basis and has the advantages of automation, reliability, and unbiased comprehensive sampling across the brain (7,67). Regional decline in GM volume has been reported in healthy adults as a function of age (68,182,189), with more pronounced reductions reported in patients with MCI (29,101,130) and AD (10,23,29,59,69,71,100). Consistent with more traditional reports, the regions most frequently implicated include medial temporal lobe structures (including the EC) and cingulate, as well as diffuse cortical association regions (10,23,29,59,69,71,100,101). GM density changes in the temporal, frontal, and parietal lobes have also been reported (20), with volumes in the MCI group frequently falling intermediate between the AD and healthy control group.

Researchers have attempted to assess whether different patterns of regional GM loss in patients with MCI are associated with different risks of conversion to AD (20,30) and found that MCI-to-AD converters show more widespread areas of reduced GM density than nonconverters, particularly in the hippocampal region, inferior and middle temporal gyri, posterior cingulate, and precuneus, with a pattern of abnormalities similar to that seen in patients with AD. This appears to be a promising technique for identification of relevant patterns of GM density distribution in patients with MCI who may be more likely to convert to AD. The boundary shift index (152) has been similarly employed to examine regional atrophy.

Magnetic resonance diffusion tensor imaging (DTI) has also shown promise for early detection. DTI can measure, in vivo, the directionality of diffusion of water molecules and estimate the integrity of WM tracts. Significant statistical differences in diffusivity measurements between groups are determined on a voxel-by-voxel basis. Several studies have examined WM integrity in individuals with MCI (52,120,150). Studies have found changes in WM integrity in multiple posterior WM regions (120), as well as in the left temporal area and in the left hippocampus (52), in participants with MCI and AD compared to controls. Rose et al. (150) assessed differences in the brains of participants with MCI relative to an age-matched control group and found significantly raised mean diffusivity measurements in the left and right ECs (BA28), posterior occipital-parietal cortex (BA18 and BA19), right parietal supramarginal gyrus (BA40), and right frontal precentral gyri (BA4 and BA6) in participants with MCI. Significant correlations were found between neuropsychological assessment scores and regional measurements of mean diffusivity and fractional anisotropy.

SUMMARY

Quantitative structural neuroimaging has revealed prominent and progressive cortical atrophy in AD starting in the earliest stages of the disease, with particular involvement of mesial temporal structures including EC and hippocampus observed in individuals with amnestic MCI. In clinical practice, detailed evaluation of MRI findings in very mild cases may be of particular interest for early diagnosis (34,35,45, 81,128,176), and brain changes, while correlating with neuropsychological performance, may occur even before measurable cognitive performance changes. Work attempting to identify differences in MCI-to-AD converters versus nonconverters has implicated regions including the hippocampal area and ECs, as well as regions in the frontal, temporal, and parietal lobes, confirming that both local and global changes occur very early in the dementing process. VBM and DTI may increase the clinical applicability of volumetric assessment in the early detection of at-risk individuals and those with early stages of dementia. Other promising techniques include functional and molecular neuroimaging methods, as described in the following sections.

FUNCTIONAL IMAGING

Functional imaging methods used in research on aging, MCI, and AD include single photon emission computed tomography (SPECT), positron emission tomography (PET), and functional MRI (fMRI). PET and SPECT use radioisotope tracers to detect brain metabolism or blood flow. fMRI is a noninvasive method that indicates regions of activation by detecting changes in blood oxygenation in capillaries. Normally, brain metabolism, blood flow, and neuronal activity are tightly coupled. The extent to which this relationship is altered in normal aging, MCI, and AD requires further investigation (44,88,151).

Functional imaging research can involve several types of study design. Resting state studies are those that examine brain metabolism in various regions of the brain without engaging the participants in a particular activity or cognitive task. Other studies correlate resting state activation with neuropsychological status on tests completed outside of the scanner. Finally, activation studies examine patterns of brain activity associated with cognitive activities in which the participant engages during scanning.

RESTING STATE SPECT AND PET STUDIES

Numerous resting state PET studies of regional cerebral metabolic rates for glucose and oxygen indicate hypometabolism in all association cortices in AD, with temporal-parietal regions generally most affected early in the disease (31,75,139). Bilateral hippocampal hypometabolism has also been reported in some (131) but not all (78) studies. By contrast, primary sensory and motor areas and subcortical GM show relative metabolic preservation (75,139). In patients with MCI, a similar pattern of regional hypometabolism has been demonstrated (74) [see Almkvist and Winblad (2) for review]. DeSanti et al. (42) have shown metabolic reductions in both MCI and AD relative to healthy age-matched controls using PET. Metabolic reductions in the hippocampus and anterior parahippocampal gyrus discriminated MCI patients from controls, whereas more widespread reductions in temporal regions of interest discriminated AD patients from those with MCI. The general pattern of affected brain regions on PET remains relatively stable over time. The degree of hypometabolism is modestly correlated with disease severity (127). Herholz et al. (76) showed a relation between the degree of glucose hypometabolism at baseline and subsequent progression in AD. In patients with MCI at study entry, the presence of severely impaired metabolism predicted a significantly greater rate of progression relative to individuals whose metabolism was intact or only mildly impaired.

Near-infrared spectroscopy (NIRS) measures changes in cortical hemoglobin oxygenation. In one study, participants with AD and MCI and healthy controls were assessed with NIRS during a verbal fluency task (6). The amplitude of changes in the waveform, quantitatively calculated by a signal-processing method, was significantly lower in the frontal and bilateral parietal areas in the AD group but only in the right parietal area for participants with MCI relative to healthy controls.

SPECT scanning has been used by researchers to help identify various perfusion abnormalities in patients with MCI who show progression versus those who remain stable (79). The investigators found that those individuals who showed progression in their illness demonstrated asymmetric perfusion reductions in the parahippocampus (5%), lateral parietal (8%), and posterior cingulate (11%) cortices; these reductions were consistent with those found in patients with mild AD. In addition, using multiple modalities to help identify profiles has been examined. For example, Borroni et al. (18) evaluated the platelet amyloid precursor protein ratio, a peripheral measure of neurodegeneration and development of senile plaques, and ⁹⁹ᵐTc-ethylcysteine dimer SPECT perfusion profiles in subjects with MCI who progressed to AD and in those who did not. The combined evaluation was reported to increase the discriminative power of the analysis in identifying presymptomatic AD.

FUNCTIONAL ACTIVATION STUDIES

Functional activation studies examine patterns of brain activation that occur during task performance. There are few functional activation studies of memory in AD or MCI. One hypothesis that has been addressed in some PET activation studies posits a shift in activation from expected foci to a more widespread cortical distribution during cognitive task performance in patients with AD compared to healthy controls (12,203). This may reflect compensatory recruitment of remaining neural resources; however, studies to date have not ruled out loss of inhibitory neural processing leading to abnormally widespread activation (155). The pattern in MCI with regard to activation is still under investigation and may vary as a function of task type and difficulty.

Several studies have shown abnormalities of mesial temporal activation on fMRI in individuals with early AD and MCI. In a study by Small et al. (171), elderly subjects with and without memory complaints and AD patients participated in a visual memory encoding task. Whereas AD patients showed strongly reduced task-related activation across all investigated regions of the hippocampal formation, participants with isolated memory complaints showed reductions either in the subiculum or in the EC. The authors of this study suggested that the subgroup that revealed underactivation in the EC might represent preclinical AD because of the early involvement of this area in AD pathology. Similarly, the hippocampal formation was found to be less active in MCI subjects and AD patients during memory encoding when compared with age-matched healthy elderly subjects (119). Petrella et al. (138) used 4-T fMRI imaging to study patients with MCI and healthy elderly controls during a novel versus familiar face-name encoding-retrieval task. Brain regions activated by the task (prefrontal, medial temporal, and parietal regions) during encoding were similar to those activated

during retrieval, with larger areas activated during retrieval. Subjects with MCI showed decreased magnitude of activation in bilateral frontal cortex regions (during both encoding and retrieval conditions), the left hippocampus (during the retrieval condition), and the left cerebellum (during the encoding condition) compared with activation in control subjects and showed increased activation in the posterior frontal lobes during the retrieval condition only. Lower hippocampal activation during retrieval was the most significant correlate of clinical severity of memory loss in participants with MCI.

Celone et al. (26) used multivariate analytic techniques to investigate memory-related fMRI activity in individuals across the continuum of normal aging, MCI, and mild AD. Independent component analyses revealed specific memory-related networks that activated or deactivated during an associative memory paradigm. Across all subjects, hippocampal activation and parietal deactivation demonstrated a strong reciprocal relationship. Furthermore, there was evidence of a nonlinear trajectory of fMRI activation across the continuum of impairment. Less impaired MCI subjects showed paradoxical hyperactivation in the hippocampus compared with controls, whereas more impaired MCI subjects demonstrated significant hypoactivation, similar to the levels observed in the mild AD subjects. There was a parallel curve observed in the pattern of memory-related deactivation in medial and lateral parietal regions, with greater deactivation in the less impaired MCI subjects and loss of deactivation in more impaired MCI and mild AD subjects. The failure to deactivate in these regions was associated with increased positive activity in a neocortical attentional network in MCI and AD. That is, loss of functional integrity of the hippocampal-based memory system may be directly related to alterations of neural activity in parietal regions seen over the course of MCI and AD.

Functional connectivity (FC) analyses provide a means of analyzing fMRI or PET data to examine disruption in normal patterns of coactivation of brain regions within a functional circuitry (60). Antuono et al. (4) reported preliminary evidence of disrupted FC within the hippocampus of individuals with AD. The degree of FC disruption was greater than that in healthy controls, whereas MCI patients had an intermediate level. Bokde et al. (16) investigated changes in FC of the right middle fusiform gyrus in subjects with MCI during performance of a face-matching task, since the right middle fusiform gyrus is considered a key area for processing face stimuli. There were no statistical differences found in task performance between groups, but there were different patterns of correlation between the right middle fusiform gyrus and related structures (visual cortex, inferior and superior parietal lobules, dorsolateral prefrontal cortex, and anterior cingulate) in the MCI and control groups. Compensatory processes in individuals with MCI appeared initially in parietal lobe regions. These results demonstrate that FC can be an effective marker for the detection of changes in brain function in MCI subjects.

Studies of working memory in patients with AD and MCI (205) indicate an increased extent of activation and recruitment of additional areas (including the right superior frontal gyrus and bilateral middle temporal, middle frontal, anterior cingulate, and fusiform gyri) in both groups.

ACTIVATION-PERFORMANCE RELATIONSHIPS

Research in young healthy controls has indicated that, during memory encoding, higher activation in the medial temporal lobe and frontal regions strongly correlates with rate of successful retrieval (22,105,194). Work in healthy elderly subjects has indicated that bilateral prefrontal activation is associated with successful encoding in older adults (122). Increased temporal lobe activations were not observed with successful encoding in these older adults, although we (156) found that healthy controls did show greater right medial temporal activation when listening to items they would later correctly recognize compared to items they did not remember. By contrast, early AD patients failed to show the same degree of differential activity in this area. Johnson et al. (86) reported, in healthy individuals, that greater activation during encoding of words was correlated with higher performance on the California Verbal Learning Test (CVLT). Heun et al. (77) investigated this relationship in elderly subjects in various stages of cognitive decline (AD and MCI patients and elderly controls) and found that successful verbal retrieval was significantly correlated with concurrent activation of the left hippocampus and posterior cingulate gyrus. Similarly, Johnson et al. (89) reported that individuals with MCI exhibited less activity in the posterior cingulate during recognition of previously learned items and in the right hippocampus during encoding of novel items, despite comparable task performance to healthy controls.

Dickerson et al. (48) measured functional activation patterns during episodic memory encoding in individuals with MCI and demonstrated that the extent of activation in the medial temporal lobe correlated with better memory performance. Additionally, they found that activation was most extended in patients with more severe clinical status at baseline and in those who showed the fastest cognitive decline during follow-up. This finding may result from higher task demand in the more impaired subjects who, in turn, revealed additional compensatory recruitment of adjacent neuronal tissue in order to maintain task performance. Similarly, healthy subjects at genetically increased risk to develop AD (17,173) and even AD patients (203) showed a higher extent of functional activation than healthy controls when they maintained good task performance.

PHARMACOLOGIC CHALLENGES

fMRI is also being used to measure changes in regional brain activation during cognitive task performance after pharmacologic manipulation [see Dickerson (47) for review]. In MCI, recent reports demonstrate alterations in neocortical activation after acute and prolonged administration of various acetylcholinesterase inhibitors. These functional changes may relate to both behavioral performance and measures of brain structure (e.g., hippocampal volume). For example, Goekoop et al. (65) compared effects of cholinergic stimulation on brain function between AD and MCI patients by examining brain function during recognition of familiar and unfamiliar information after exposure to galantamine, a cholinesterase inhibitor used for treating memory deficits in AD. In participants with MCI, acute exposure led to increased activation in posterior cingulate, left inferior parietal, and anterior temporal lobe, whereas prolonged exposure resulted in decreased activation in similar posterior cingulate areas and in bilateral prefrontal areas. Effects were stronger for familiar than for unfamiliar decisions, suggesting that the primary effect was specific to *memory retrieval*. In patients with AD, acute exposure increased activation bilaterally in hippocampal areas; prolonged exposure decreased activation in these areas. Effects were more pronounced for unfamiliar than for familiar decisions, suggesting a preferential effect on *memory encoding*.

Saykin et al. (158) examined the effects of donepezil hydrochloride (Aricept) on cognition and brain activity in participants with MCI. At baseline, participants with MCI showed reduced activation of frontoparietal regions relative to controls during a working memory task. After stabilization on donepezil, participants with MCI showed increased frontal activity relative to unmedicated age-matched healthy controls, which was positively correlated with improvement in task performance as well as baseline hippocampal volume. In this study, short-term treatment with a cholinesterase inhibitor enhanced frontal circuitry activation in patients with MCI and was related to improved cognition and to baseline integrity of the hippocampus.

MOLECULAR IMAGING

Klunk et al. (106) introduced amyloid imaging as a new principle, enabling direct visualization of amyloid plaques in the living human brain. Using a novel

PET tracer called Pittsburgh Compound-B (PIB), the authors found marked retention of the molecule in patients with AD in areas of the brain known to contain large amounts of beta-amyloid (Aβ) plaques. Several lines of evidence support PIB as a marker for fibrillar Aβ, including its high binding affinity for both plaque and cerebrovascular amyloid (but not neurofibrillary tangles) (107) in neuropathologic specimens and the close correlation between PIB binding and levels of insoluble Aβ in AD (50). Interestingly, some MCI cases show PIB binding, and some cognitively normal elderly individuals show both marked retention of PIB and low levels of $Aβ_{42}$ in the cerebrospinal fluid (CSF) (50). This may be indicative of Aβ deposition and plaque pathology early in the disease, even in asymptomatic cases. These promising data suggest that PIB may be useful as a biomarker for MCI. Finally, PIB may be used in clinical trials with participants with MCI and AD to increase the possibility of identifying a drug effect on the conversion rate from MCI to AD.

Other tracers have been developed for molecular imaging in dementia. Small et al. (169) examined both 2-(1-{6-[(2-[F-18]fluoroethyl)(methyl)amino]-2-naphthyl}ethylidene) malononitrile (FDDNP) and 2-deoxy-2-[F-18]fluoro-D-glucose (FDG) PET in patients with AD, individuals with MCI, and healthy controls and found that global values for FDDNP-PET binding (average of the values for the temporal, parietal, posterior cingulate, and frontal regions) were lower in the control group than in the group with MCI and lower in the MCI group than in the AD group. FDDNP-PET binding differentiated among the diagnostic groups better than FDG-PET or MRI structural findings.

SUMMARY

Findings evaluating brain activation patterns in patients with MCI and AD have been contradictory and have resulted in reports of increases, decreases, and shifts in activation location and extent, even within the same studies. Altered functional activation responses that occur in patients with MCI or AD may result in elevated or extended activation (accompanying unaffected or mildly impaired performance) or in activation deficits (more often with severely impaired performance). Whether the more widespread activation is due to a compensatory mechanism, a loss of inhibitory neural processing, or some other as yet unidentified process remains unanswered. Consideration of task demands and performance should be considered when evaluating results and may account for the conflicting findings of hyperactivation and hypoactivation in individuals with MCI and dementia (141). Pharmacologic challenges are able to measure differential response to treatment in individuals with MCI based on type of administration and type of memory process assessed. Both structural and functional neuroimaging have provided rich insights into the neuroanatomic and neurophysiologic changes in the brain in MCI and early AD (Table 21-13). Future research integrating analyses of brain structure, brain activation patterns, and cognitive performance is likely to further illuminate brain-behavior relations and mechanisms of impairment and compensation in this population.

IDENTIFICATION OF INDIVIDUALS WITH PRE-MCI

Our group has been studying individuals with MCI and AD as well, and we have also identified a cohort of individuals who only partially meet the Peterson criteria for MCI. That is, they endorse significant memory complaints, which are often corroborated by an informant, but they do not demonstrate significant memory or other cognitive deficits on neuropsychological testing. In an attempt to further understand these individuals with cognitive complaints (CCs) and whether they may represent a cohort of individuals who are at greater risk for developing MCI, we have included these individuals in our research protocols and assessed these individuals using neuropsychological evaluation and structural and functional imaging (159).

Our working hypothesis is that significant CCs in the absence of measurable cognitive deficits may signify a very early stage of the dementing process for some individuals and may constitute a pre-MCI stage. However, models suggesting a continuum from normal aging to AD have been questioned based on neuropathologic evidence of changes characteristic of AD in some individuals with MCI (123). Only limited data are presently available for CC cohorts. Longitudinal research on older adults with CCs has yielded inconsistent findings (55,91,93,94,163,164,185,190), although a range of associated factors including *ApoE* genotype, depression, somatic concerns, female sex, and older age have been identified (11,41,90,92,157,174,180,181). We briefly describe our work to date exploring this potential group of patients with pre-MCI. For all of the studies presented, participants from all groups were excluded if they had medical, psychiatric, or neurologic conditions (other than MCI), history of head trauma, or substance dependence. No participant was clinically depressed, as determined by a participating geropsychiatrist and scores on the Geriatric Depression Scale. No participant was taking medication that could affect cognition.

COGNITION

As noted, although the primary cognitive deficits in MCI involve episodic memory, individuals may demonstrate relative weaknesses and complaints

Table 21-13. *Summary of Findings*

	Alzheimer's Disease (AD)	Amnestic Mild Cognitive Impairment (MCI)	Cognitive Complaint Group
Memory impairment	Yes	Yes	No
Impairment in other cognitive domains	Yes	May be subtle executive deficits	No
Subjective complaints	Variable	Yes	Yes
Instrumental activities of daily living	Impairment	May be very subtle problems	No impairment
Reduced hippocampal volume	Yes	Yes	Yes; intermediate between MCI and healthy controls
Reduced entorhinal cortex volume	Yes	Yes	Not examined
Reduced fornix/ mammillary body volume	Yes	No	No
Reductions in corpus callosal volumes	Yes	Mixed findings	Yes in posterior region
Gray matter changes	Yes	Yes	Intermediate between MCI and controls
Cortical thinning	Yes	Yes; on a continuum between AD and healthy controls	Not examined
White matter integrity changes	Yes	Yes	Intermediate pattern between MCI and controls
Resting state hypometabolism	Yes	Yes	Not examined
Near-infrared spectroscopy changes	Yes	Yes; more selective	Not examined
Functional MRI changes	Yes; increases, decreases, and shifts in activation location	Yes; increases, decreases, and shifts in activation location	Yes; to lesser degree, increases, decreases, and shifts in activation location
Pharmacologic challenges	Leads to increases and decreases in activation	Leads primarily to increases in activation	Not examined
Molecular imaging	Greater changes than in healthy controls	Greater changes than in healthy controls; intermediate between AD and controls?	Not examined

regarding other areas of cognition, including executive functioning. In addition, as described earlier, structural imaging has revealed reduced GM density in distributed brain regions, including frontal areas, relative to cognitively intact elders (29,130,161), and functional neuroimaging studies have shown abnormal brain activation of frontal lobe systems during MCI patients' performance on executive function tasks (149,160).

We (142) recently conducted a study evaluating executive functions in individuals with MCI and CCs and in healthy controls using the Behavioral Rating Inventory of Executive Function–Adult Version (BRIEF-A) (153), a newly developed self- and informant report questionnaire. The BRIEF-A contains 75 items and yields an overall score that is a composite of two index scores (i.e., the Behavioral Regulation Index and the Metacognitive Index). The Behavioral Regulation Index is comprised of four scales: Inhibit, Shift, Emotional Control, and Self-Monitor. The Metacognitive Index is comprised of five scales: Initiation, Working Memory, Planning/Organization, Task Monitoring, and Organization of Materials. Mean and standard scores (*T*) were calculated for each of the clinical scales and indices and for the summary. Higher scores reflect greater difficulties experienced by the individual.

Although individuals with MCI and CC did not show clinically meaningful difficulties on formal neuropsychological tests of executive function, consistent with the diagnostic criteria, they did self-report difficulties with selective aspects of executive functioning on the BRIEF-A. The MCI group reported statistically significant elevations on eight of nine BRIEF-A clinical scales, whereas patients with CCs showed an intermediate pattern of results with elevations on six of nine scales. Informants of participants with MCI showed a slightly attenuated pattern of findings, reporting elevations on seven of nine clinical scales; in contrast, informants of the CC participants reported an elevation on only one of the scales. Of note, both participants with MCI and CC and their informants indicated concern about working memory abilities, and this domain showed the strongest effect size. BRIEF-A self-reports and informant reports for corresponding scales were moderately correlated (average correlation, $r = 0.42$, standard deviation = 0.15), with higher relations generally observed on scales within the Metacognitive Index.

Finally, although little research has investigated awareness of deficit or difficulty in MCI or CC patients, some recent research suggests that MCI and/or CC patients may be "hyperaware" of certain cognitive difficulties (i.e., report a greater degree of dysfunction compared to their informants) (97,125). This is in contrast to the sizable literature indicating that patients with AD often show unawareness of their cognitive and behavioral deficits (37,73,116). Inspection of data showing the percentage of cases within each participant group exhibiting clinically elevated BRIEF-A scores (defined as $T \geq 65$) further confirmed that MCI and CC participants were more likely to report clinically meaningful executive problems than their informants, although informants identify a similar pattern of difficulty. Although considerable research has shown that patients with dementia lack awareness or insight about their cognitive and behavioral deficits, these results suggest that individuals in preclinical disease stages can and do identify areas of executive weakness in themselves and confirm that many individuals with MCI and CC are concerned about their own executive functions before others notice or before problems become demonstrable on formal assessment.

Our results complement recent neuropsychological studies documenting subtle executive problems in older adults with MCI (149,158) and CCs (85,159) and are consistent with other behavioral, cognitive, and neuroimaging research suggesting that subclinical executive deficits precede or exist alongside

memory declines and may be a common feature of MCI and pre-MCI. These findings have implications for everyday functioning and treatment planning. For example, even mild deficiencies in abilities such as working memory, task initiation, and planning and organizing can be associated with functional difficulties in older adults. Subtle executive decline may affect performance in a variety of domains, such as social and occupational activities, emotional responses, adherence to treatment recommendations, or management of important medical, legal, and financial issues (146). The subtle executive difficulties elucidated by the BRIEF-A in older adults with complaints about cognition may provide useful information to guide thinking about current psychosocial functioning, intervention efforts, and long-term outcome for both patients and caregivers.

STRUCTURAL IMAGING

In the Copenhaver et al. (36) study described earlier, which examined the volumes of the fornix and mammillary bodies in individuals with MCI and healthy controls, a group of patients with CCs was included as well. No volume differences were observed between healthy controls and CC and MCI participants, suggesting that there is relative preservation of these structures in preclinical disease stages. Work examining whether there are global or regionally specific decreases in callosal area in early AD, MCI, and CC (197) found that all three groups showed a significant reduction of the posterior region (isthmus and splenium) of the corpus callosum relative to healthy controls. This suggests that callosal changes occur very early in the dementing process and that these earliest changes may be too subtle for detection by neuropsychological assessment, including memory tests.

We (158,159) have also examined the neural basis of CCs in healthy older adults to determine whether there are medial temporal lobe GM changes, as have been reported in AD and MCI. We hypothesized that participants with CCs would show decreased GM density in medial temporal lobe and other cortical regions, as well as an intermediate level of hippocampal volume reduction, between MCI and controls. We also hypothesized that subjective and objective measures of memory would be related to GM density. There were 40 participants in each group. Structural brain MRI scans of the participants with CC were compared to those of patients with MCI and healthy controls using VBM and hippocampal volume (region of interest) analysis.

Results indicated that the MCI and CC groups showed a similar pattern of reduced GM density in bilateral medial temporal, frontal, and other distributed brain regions relative to the healthy control group, indicating that structural brain changes similar to those seen in MCI are present even in cognitively intact, nondepressed older adults with significant memory concerns. As hypothesized, these GM reductions were more extensive in the MCI group than the CC group. Furthermore, manually segmented hippocampal volumes, adjusted for age and ICV, were significantly reduced only in the MCI group relative to healthy controls, with the CC group showing an intermediate level.

Looking at the combined sample of older adults, reduction of GM density in medial temporal and other regions was correlated with both subjective memory complaints and verbal learning performance, providing support for the idea that the structural brain changes seen in the CC and MCI groups have functional significance in terms of memory ability. Together with prior research relating frontal metabolism to subjective memory ratings in older adults (170), these findings highlight the importance of CCs in the clinical evaluation of older adults and suggest that those who present with significant CCs warrant evaluation and close monitoring over time, since CCs in older adults may indicate underlying neurodegenerative changes, even when unaccompanied by deficits on formal testing.

DTI studies have shown increased diffusivity of water in the hippocampus of older adults with AD and MCI compared to healthy controls, suggesting possible early structural breakdown in the medial temporal region. We (198) compared trace diffusivity (TD) and fractional anisotropy (FA) in individuals with MCI and in our CC group, as well as in a sample of healthy controls. The MCI group showed increased TD in the cingulate, hippocampus, and surrounding WM pathways relative to controls and a pattern of decreased FA in the WM pathways, and the CC group showed a similar but intermediate pattern. These findings indicate the sensitivity of DTI to early preclinical degenerative changes in regions associated with AD.

Summary

Our observations indicate that, in many instances, the volume reductions seen in MCI are seen to a lesser degree in individuals with CC. This suggests that, despite lack of neuropsychological evidence of memory impairment, the CC group shows structural brain changes that fall on a continuum between healthy controls and individuals with MCI. Longitudinal study of these individuals will yield a cohort of individuals who develop MCI and ultimately AD and will provide us with information about the best earliest predictors to use for early detection, selection of participants in clinical trials, and treatment monitoring.

FUNCTIONAL IMAGING

As described earlier, functional imaging studies of memory-related processes demonstrate altered patterns of brain activity in patients with or at risk for AD. These alterations include both increases and decreases in activity relative to healthy controls, depending on the disease stage and memory system being investigated (17,172). For example, Saykin et al. (158) reported areas of decreased activity and also compensatory frontal and hippocampal increases during semantic, episodic, and working memory in patients with MCI relative to controls, with a strikingly similar pattern of functional neuroimaging results in the CC group relative to that observed in the MCI group.

Novelty detection and repetition suppression are basic components of memory that rely on neuroanatomic systems implicated in the early stages of dementia, but they have yet to be examined using fMRI in AD or preclinical disease stages such as MCI. Rabin et al. (143) examined fMRI activation after participants were instructed to listen carefully to a list of words but not to respond. We hypothesized that the MCI group would show an altered pattern of activation relative to healthy controls and that the CC group would show an intermediate pattern of activation. Three words were then repeatedly presented at 1-second intervals for 3 minutes (habituation phase). For the remaining 8 minutes, novel words were interspersed pseudo-randomly between habituated words. The contrast of interest was the novel greater than habituated stimuli, which may represent novelty detection. Both the MCI and CC groups showed increased brain activation relative to the healthy controls in medial temporal and frontal regions. This may indicate a compensatory process similar to that seen in AD during episodic and semantic memory tasks. It is notable that, contrary to our hypothesis, the CC group showed significant increases in activation relative to healthy controls, whereas MCI patients showed an intermediate pattern in similar brain regions. Recent work from our lab using VBM has revealed bilateral MTA in the CC group similar to, but less extensive than, that associated with MCI (161). Expanded activation/compensation in the CC group may be related to their greater structural integrity of crucial task-related brain regions compared with MCI patients.

In addition, across the entire combined sample, the relationship between activation and episodic memory performance (using learning across trials of the CVLT-Second Edition) was examined (N = 75), and expanded activation in memory-related circuitry was negatively correlated with verbal learning scores in distributed temporal, frontal, and parietal regions. This suggests that compensatory activity may have functional significance in terms of novelty detection.

Overall, these findings suggest that brain systems involved in memory, novelty detection, and habituation may be sensitive to preclinical stages of disease and may be useful markers for early diagnosis and treatment monitoring. It will be important to follow the MCI and CC participants longitudinally using neuropsychological and neuroimaging methods to determine their cognitive trajectory, progression of brain activation changes, and diagnostic outcome.

Summary

As new treatments and preventive strategies for MCI and AD are developed and refined, the earliest possible accurate detection of people at increased risk of dementia will take on critical importance. Our recent work with individuals with significant CCs in the absence of any cognitive impairments supports the idea that, although subtle cognitive anomalies may be present many years before dementia onset (3,8,175), incorporating information on CCs (54) and structural and functional changes in these individuals may be important for prognosis (Table 21-13). However, a potential limitation in terms of the generalizability of our results is that the majority of participants in our studies, including those in the CC group, had high education and estimated baseline intellect. High baseline functioning or cognitive reserve may buffer the effects of brain pathology on cognition (147,179), and individuals with a high baseline level of cognition may be more likely to express subjective complaints before objective measures can detect decline in this group. Our studies warrant replication in cohorts with lower levels of baseline functioning given the potential implications for early diagnosis.

CONCLUSION

With life expectancy increasing continuously, the effects of neurodegeneration on brain function are a topic of ever increasing importance. Thus, there is a need for tools and models that probe both the functional consequences of neurodegenerative processes and compensatory mechanisms that might occur. To date, there has been a substantial body of literature dealing with predictors of dementia in patients with MCI (121). These predictors range from a simple delayed recall task on the MMSE to sophisticated radiologic techniques and CSF biomarkers. The presence of the *ApoE ε4* allele has been associated with increased risk of conversion, but the sensitivity is quite low. CSF biochemical markers are being developed with encouraging results. Hippocampal or entorhinal atrophy on MRI is one of the most used radiologic markers of conversion, but quantification

of atrophy is not simple because it is subject to artifacts and anatomic variations. Until an accurate marker is developed, a combined use of cognitive tests, *ApoE* genotype, and neuroradiologic techniques is probably the best option for prediction purposes depending on availability and experience.

Advances in in vivo imaging methods are providing the tools for identifying different trajectories of normal and abnormal aging, and better understanding of and knowledge about these brain changes may promote opportunities for treatment. Healthy aging appears to primarily affect a frontal-striatal system that is responsible for executive control of cognition, while minimally affecting medial temporal lobe structures. Functional imaging studies suggest that enhanced prefrontal engagement may offer compensatory plasticity that minimizes age-related cognitive losses. MCI appears to affect medial temporal lobe structures, including the EC in particular, with functional consequences in other brain regions. AD is characterized by severe impact on the hippocampal system, although early-stage AD may relatively spare some cortical regions. Current data suggest that regional damage to the medial temporal lobes underlies initial MCI, whereas more global brain changes, such as whole brain atrophy and WM changes, contribute to further progression of cognitive decline. In general, deficits in individuals with MCI tend to fall on a continuum between healthy aging and AD. It is important to keep in mind that neurodegenerative burden and compensatory mechanisms may change over time.

Research aimed at identifying the earliest identifiable manifestations of memory impairment has led to investigation of individuals who endorse subjective complaints of memory deficit that are not reflected in performance on neuropsychological assessment. However, detailed study using structural and functional imaging techniques suggests that, in at least a subgroup of these patients, there are changes in brain morphology and activation patterns that fall intermediate between individuals with MCI and healthy controls. Further characterization of cohorts of both individuals with CCs and those with MCI who progress to the next stage of impairment may help us to recognize important markers that will allow for early intervention and remediation.

ACKNOWLEDGMENT

Supported in part by grants from the National Institute on Aging (R01 AG19771), Alzheimer's Association (IIRG-99-1653 sponsored by the Hedco Foundation), Hitchcock Foundation, Ira DeCamp Foundation, National Science Foundation, New Hampshire Hospital, and NAMIC (U54 EB005149).

REFERENCES

1. Albert MS, Moss MB, Tanzi R, et al. Preclinical prediction of AD using neuropsychological tests. *J Int Neuropsychol Soc.* 2001;7:631–639.
2. Almkvist O, Winblad B. Early diagnosis of Alzheimer dementia based on clinical and biological factors. *Eur Arch Psychiatry Clin Neurosci.* 1999;249[Suppl 3]:3–9.
3. Amieva H, Jacqmin-Gadda H, Orgogozo J-M, et al. The 9 year cognitive decline before dementia of the Alzheimer type: a prospective population-based study. *Brain.* 2005;128: 1093–1101.
4. Antuono P, Li S-J, Jones J. A functional MRI index as a biological marker for Alzheimer's disease. Presented at the 52nd Annual Meeting of the American Academy of Neurology, San Diego, CA, April 29-May 6, 2000.
5. Apostolova LG, Dinov ID, Dutton RA, et al. 3D comparison of hippocampal atrophy in amnestic mild cognitive impairment and Alzheimer's disease. *Brain.* 2006;129:2867–2873.
6. Arai H, Takano M, Miyakawa K, et al. A quantitative near-infrared spectroscopy study: a decrease in cerebral hemoglobin oxygenation in Alzheimer's disease and mild cognitive impairment. *Brain Cogn.* 2006;61:189–194.
7. Ashburner J, Friston KJ. Why voxel-based morphometry should be used. *Neuroimage.* 2001;14:1238–1243.
8. Backman L, Jones S, Berger A-K, et al. Cognitive impairment in preclinical Alzheimer's disease: a meta-analysis. *Neuropsychology.* 2005; 19:520–531.
9. Barber R, Scheltens P, Gholkar A, et al. White matter lesions on magnetic resonance imaging in dementia with Lewy bodies, Alzheimer's disease, vascular dementia, and normal aging. *J Neurol Neurosurg Psychiatry.* 1999;67:66–72.
10. Baron JC, Chetelat G, Desgranges B, et al. In vivo mapping of gray matter loss with voxel-based morphometry in mild Alzheimer's disease. *Neuroimage.* 2001;14:298–309.
11. Baxter LC, Caselli RJ, Johnson SC, et al. Apolipoprotein E e4 affects new learning in cognitively normal individuals at risk for Alzheimer's disease. *Neurobiol Aging.* 2003;24: 947–952.
12. Becker JT, Mintun MA, Aleva K, et al. Compensatory reallocation of brain resources supporting verbal episodic memory in Alzheimer's disease. *Neurology.* 1996;46: 692–700.
13. Bigler ED, Blatter DD, Anderson CV, et al. Hippocampal volume in normal aging and traumatic brain injury. *Am J Neuroradiol.* 1997;18:11–23.
14. Birren JE, Schaie KW. *Handbook of the Psychology of Aging.* 3rd ed. San Diego: Academic Press; 1990.
15. Bobinski M, de Leon MJ, Convit A, et al. MRI of entorhinal cortex in mild Alzheimer's disease. *Lancet.* 1999;353:38–40.
16. Bokde AL, Lopez-Bayo P, Meindl T, et al. Functional connectivity of the fusiform gyrus during a face-matching task in subjects with mild cognitive impairment. *Brain.* 2006;129: 1113–1124.
17. Bookheimer SY, Strojwas MH, Cohen MS, et al. Patterns of brain activation in people at risk for Alzheimer's disease. *N Engl J Med.* 2000;343: 450–456.
18. Borroni B, Perani D, Broli M, et al. Pre-clinical diagnosis of Alzheimer disease combining platelet amyloid precursor protein ratio and rCBF SPECT analysis. *J Neurol.* 2005;252: 1359–1362.
19. Bowen J, Teri L, Kukull W, et al. Progression to dementia in patients with isolated memory loss. *Lancet.* 1997;349:763–765.
20. Bozzali M, Filippi M, Magnani G, et al. The contribution of voxel-based morphometry in staging patients with mild cognitive impairment. *Neurology.* 2006;67:453–460.
21. Braak H, Braak E, Bohl J. Staging of Alzheimer-related cortical destruction. *Eur Neurol.* 1993; 33:403–408.
22. Brewer JB, Zhao Z, Desmond JE, et al. Making memories: brain activity that predicts how well visual experience will be remembered. *Science.* 1998;281:1185–1187.
23. Busatto GF, Garrido GE, Almeida OP, et al. A voxel-based morphometry study of temporal lobe gray matter reductions in Alzheimer's disease. *Neurobiol Aging.* 2003;24:221–231.
24. Busse A, Hensel A, Guhne U, et al. Mild cognitive impairment: long-term course of four clinical subtypes. *Neurology.* 2006;67:2176–2185.
25. Carlesimo GA, Oscar-Berman M. Memory deficits in Alzheimer's patients: a comprehensive review. *Neuropsychol Rev.* 1992;3:119–169.
26. Celone KA, Calhoun VD, Dickerson BC, et al. Alterations in memory networks in mild cognitive impairment and Alzheimer's disease: an independent component analysis. *J Neurosci.* 2006;26:10222–10231.
27. Celsis P. Age-related cognitive decline, mild cognitive impairment or preclinical Alzheimer's disease? *Ann Med.* 2000;32:6–14.
28. Chen P, Ratcliff G, Belle SH, et al. Cognitive tests that best discriminate between presymptomatic

AD and those who remain nondemented. *Neurology.* 2000;55:1847–1853.

29. Chetelat G, Desgranges B, De La Sayette V, et al. Mapping gray matter loss with voxel-based morphometry in mild cognitive impairment. *Neuroreport.* 2002;13:1939–1943.

30. Chetelat G, Landeau B, Eustache F, et al. Using voxel-based morphometry to map the structural changes associated with rapid conversion in MCI: a longitudinal MRI study. *Neuroimage.* 2005;27:934–946.

31. Coleman RE. Positron emission tomography in the evaluation of dementia. Presented at the 48th Annual Meeting of the Society of Nuclear Medicine, Toronto, Ontario, Canada, June 23–27, 2001.

32. Collie A, Maruff P. The neuropsychology of preclinical Alzheimer's disease and mild cognitive impairment. *Neurosci Biobehav Rev.* 2000; 24:365–374.

33. Collie A, Maruff P, Shafiq-Antonaci R, et al. Memory decline in healthy older people: implications for identifying mild cognitive impairment. *Neurology.* 2001;56:1533–1538.

34. Convit A, de Asis J, de Leon MJ, et al. Atrophy of the medial occipitotemporal, inferior, and middle temporal gyri in non-demented elderly predict decline to Alzheimer's disease. *Neurobiol Aging.* 2000;21:19–26.

35. Convit A, de Leon MJ, Tarshish C, et al. Specific hippocampal volume reductions in individuals at risk for Alzheimer's disease. *Neurobiol Aging.* 1997;18:131–138.

36. Copenhaver BR, Rabin LA, Saykin AJ, et al. The fornix and mammillary bodies in older adults with Alzheimer's disease, mild cognitive impairment, and cognitive complaints: a volumetric MRI study. *Psychiatry Res.* 2006;147: 93–103.

37. Cotrell V. Awareness deficits in Alzheimer's disease: issues in assessment and intervention. *J Appl Gerontol.* 1997;16:71–90.

38. Crowell TA, Luis CA, Vanderploeg RD, et al. Memory patterns and executive functioning in mild cognitive impairment and Alzheimer's disease. *Aging Neuropsychol Cogn.* 2002;9: 288–297.

39. DeCarli C, Miller BL, Swan GE, et al. Cerebrovascular and brain morphologic correlates of mild cognitive impairment in the National Heart, Lung, and Blood Institute Twin Study. *Arch Neurol.* 2001;58:643–647.

40. de Leon MJ, George AE, Golomb J, et al. Frequency of hippocampal formation atrophy in normal aging and Alzheimer's disease. *Neurobiol Aging.* 1997;18:1–11.

41. Derouesne C, Lacomblez L, Thibault S, et al. Memory complaints in young and elderly subjects. *Int J Geriatr Psychiatry.* 1999;14:291–301.

42. DeSanti S, deLeon MJ, Rusinek H, et al. Hippocampal formation glucose metabolism and volume losses in MCI and AD. *Neurobiol Aging.* 2001;22:529–539.

43. Desmond PM, O'Brien JT, Tress BM, et al. Volumetric and visual assessment of the mesial temporal structures in Alzheimer's disease. *Aust N Z J Med.* 1994;24:547–553.

44. D'Esposito M, Zarahn E, Aguirre GK, et al. The effect of pacing of experimental stimuli on observed functional MRI activity. *Neuroimage.* 1997;6:113–121.

45. de Toledo-Morrell L, Sullivan MP, Morrell F, et al. Alzheimer's disease: in vivo detection of differential vulnerability of brain regions. *Neurobiol Aging.* 1997;18:463–468.

46. Devanand DP, Folz M, Gorlyn M, et al. Questionable dementia: clinical course and predictors of outcome. *J Am Geriatr Soc.* 1997; 45:321–328.

47. Dickerson BC. Functional magnetic resonance imaging of cholinergic modulation in mild cognitive impairment. *Curr Opin Psychiatry.* 2006; 19:299–306.

48. Dickerson BC, Salat DH, Bates JF, et al. Medial temporal lobe function and structure in mild cognitive impairment. *Ann Neurol.* 2004;56:27–35.

49. Elias MF, Beiser A, Wolf PA, et al. The preclinical phase of Alzheimer disease: a 22-year prospective study of the Framingham Cohort. *Arch Neurol.* 2000;57:808–813.

50. Fagan AM, Mintun MA, Mach RH, et al. Inverse relation between in vivo amyloid imaging load and cerebrospinal fluid Aβ42 in humans. *Ann Neurol.* 2006;59:512–519.

51. Farkas E, Luiten PG. Cerebral microvascular pathology in aging and Alzheimer's disease. *Prog Neurobiol.* 2001;64:575–611.

52. Fellgiebel A, Wille P, Muller MJ, et al. Ultrastructural hippocampal and white matter alterations in mild cognitive impairment: a diffusion tensor imaging study. *Dement Geriatr Cogn Disord.* 2004;18:101–108.

53. Fischer P, Jungwirth A, Zehetmayer S, et al. Conversion from subtypes of mild cognitive impairment to Alzheimer's dementia. *Neurology.* 2007;68:288–291.

54. Fisk JD, Rockwood K. Outcomes of incident mild cognitive impairment in relation to case definition. *J Neurol Neurosurg Psychiatry.* 2005;76:1175–1177.

55. Flicker C, Ferris SH, Reisberg B. A longitudinal study of cognitive function in elderly persons

with subjective memory complaints. *J Am Geriatr Soc.* 1993;41:1029–1032.

56. Flicker C, Ferris SH, Reisberg B. Mild cognitive impairment in the elderly: predictors of dementia. *Neurology.* 1991;41:1006–1009.

57. Fox NC, Rossor MN. Diagnosis of early Alzheimer's disease. *Rev Neurol (Paris).* 1999; 155[Suppl 4]:S33–S37.

58. Fox NC, Warrington EK, Stevens JM, et al. Atrophy of the hippocampal formation in early familial Alzheimer's disease. A longitudinal MRI study of at-risk members of a family with an amyloid precursor protein 717Val-Gly mutation. *Ann NY Acad Sci.* 1996;777:226–232.

59. Frisoni G, Testa C, Zorzan A, et al. Detection of grey matter loss in mild Alzheimer's disease with voxel based morphometry. *J Neurol Neurosurg Psychiatry.* 2003;73:657–664.

60. Friston KJ, Frith CD, Liddle PF, et al. Functional connectivity: the principal-component analysis of large (PET) data sets. *J Cereb Blood Flow Metab.* 1993;13:5–14.

61. Gaffan D. The role of the hippocampus-fornix-mammillary system in episodic memory. In: Squire LR, Butters N, eds. *Neuropsychology of memory.* 2nd ed. New York: Guilford Press; 1992:336–346.

62. Gaffan D. What is a memory system? Horel's critique revisited. *Behav Brain Res.* 2001;127: 5–11.

63. Garand L, Dew MA, Eazor LR, et al. Caregiving burden and psychiatric morbidity in spouses of persons with mild cognitive impairment. *Int J Geriatric Psychiatry.* 2005;20:512–522.

64. Geroldi C, Rossi R, Calvagna C, et al. Medial temporal atrophy but not memory deficit predicts progression to dementia in patients with mild cognitive impairment. *J Neurol Neurosurg Psychiatry.* 2006;77:1219–1222.

65. Goekoop R, Scheltens P, Barkhof F, et al. Cholinergic challenge in Alzheimer patients and mild cognitive impairment differentially affects hippocampal activation—a pharmacological fMRI study. *Brain.* 2006;129:141–157.

66. Golomb J, Kluger A, deLeon MJ, et al. Hippocampal formation size in normal human aging: a correlate of delayed secondary memory performance. *Learn Mem.* 1994;1:45–54.

67. Good CD, Ashburner J, Frackowiak RS. Computational neuroanatomy: new perspectives for neuroradiology. *Rev Neurol (Paris).* 2001;157: 797–806.

68. Good CD, Johnsrude IS, Ashburner J, et al. A voxel-based morphometric study of ageing in 465 normal adult human brains. *Neuroimage.* 2001;14:21–36.

69. Good CD, Scahill RI, Fox NC, et al. Automatic differentiation of anatomical patterns in the human brain: validation with studies of degenerative dementias. *Neuroimage.* 2002;17:29–46.

70. Griffith HR, Belue K, Sicola A, et al. Impaired financial abilities in mild cognitive impairment. *Neurology.* 2003;60:449–457.

71. Grossman M, McMillan C, Moore P, et al. What's in a name: voxel-based morphometric analyses of MRI and naming difficulty in Alzheimer's disease, frontotemporal dementia and corticobasal degeneration. *Brain.* 2004;127: 628–649.

72. Hachinski VC. The decline and resurgence of vascular dementia. *Can Med Assoc J.* 1990;142: 107–111.

73. Harwood DG, Sultzer DL, Wheatley MV. Impaired insight in Alzheimer disease: association with cognitive deficits, psychiatric symptoms, and behavioral disturbances. *Neuropsychiatry Neuropsychol Behav Neurol.* 2000; 13:83–88.

74. Haxby JV, Grady CL, Koss E, et al. Longitudinal study of cerebral metabolic asymmetries and associated neuropsychological patterns in early dementia of the Alzheimer type. *Arch Neurol.* 1990;47:753–760.

75. Herholz K. FDG PET and differential diagnosis of dementia. *Alzheimer Dis Assoc Disord.* 1995; 9:6–16.

76. Herholz K, Nordberg A, Salmon E, et al. Impairment of neocortical metabolism predicts progression in Alzheimer's disease. *Dement Geriatr Cogn Disord.* 1999;10:494–504.

77. Heun R, Freymann K, Erb M, et al. Successful verbal retrieval in elderly subjects is related to concurrent hippocampal and posterior cingulate activation. *Dement Geriatr Cogn Disord.* 2006;22:165–172.

78. Ishii K, Sasaki M, Yamaji S, et al. Relatively preserved hippocampal glucose metabolism in mild Alzheimer's disease. *Dement Geriatr Cogn Disord.* 1998;9:317–322.

79. Ishiwata A, Sakayori O, Minoshima S, et al. Preclinical evidence of Alzheimer changes in progressive mild cognitive impairment: a qualitative and quantitative SPECT study. *Acta Neurol Scand.* 2006;114:91–96.

80. Jack CR Jr., Petersen RC, O'Brien PC, et al. MR-based hippocampal volumetry in the diagnosis of Alzheimer's disease. *Neurology.* 1992;42:183–188.

81. Jack CR Jr., Petersen RC, Xu Y, et al. Medial temporal atrophy on MRI in normal aging and very mild Alzheimer's disease. *Neurology.* 1997;49:786–794.

82. Jack CR Jr., Petersen RC, Xu Y, et al. Prediction of AD with MRI-based hippocampal volume in mild cognitive impairment. *Neurology.* 1999;52: 1397–1403.

83. Jack CR Jr., Petersen RC, Xu Y, et al. Rate of medial temporal lobe atrophy in typical aging and Alzheimer's disease. *Neurology.* 1998;51: 993–999.

84. Jack CR Jr., Petersen RC, Xu Y, et al. Rates of hippocampal atrophy correlate with change in clinical status in aging and AD. *Neurology.* 2000;55:484–489.

85. Jessen F, Feyen L, Freymann K, et al. Volume reduction of the entorhinal cortex in subjective memory impairment. *Neurobiol Aging.* 2006;27: 1751–1756.

86. Johnson SC, Saykin AJ, Flashman LA, et al. Brain activation on fMRI and verbal memory ability: functional neuroanatomical correlates of CVLT performance. *J Int Neuropsychol Soc.* 2001;7:55–62.

87. Johnson SC, Saykin AJ, Flashman LA, et al. Reduction of hippocampal formation in Alzheimer's disease and correlation with memory: a meta-analysis. *J Int Neuropsychol Soc.* 1998; 4:22.

88. Johnson SC, Saykin AJ, Flashman LA, et al. Similarities and differences in semantic and phonological processing with age: patterns of functional MRI activation. *Aging Neuropsychol Cogn.* 2001;8:307–320.

89. Johnson SC, Schmitz TW, Moritz CH, et al. Activation of brain regions vulnerable to Alzheimer's disease: the effect of mild cognitive impairment. *Neurobiol Aging.* 2006;27: 1604–1612.

90. Jonker C, Geerlings MI, Schmand B. Are memory complaints predictive for dementia? A review of clinical and population-based studies. *Int J Geriatr Psychiatry.* 2000;15:983–991.

91. Jorm AF. Alzheimer's disease: risk and protection. *Med J Aust.* 1997;167:443–446.

92. Jorm AF, Butterworth P, Anstey KJ, et al. Memory complaints in a community sample aged 60-64 years: associations with cognitive functioning, psychiatric symptoms, medical conditions, ApoE genotype, hippocampus and amygdala volumes, and white-matter hyperintensities. *Psychol Med.* 2004;34:1495–1506.

93. Jorm AF, Christensen H, Korten AE, et al. Memory complaints as a precursor of memory impairment in older people: a longitudinal analysis over 7-8 years. *Psychol Med.* 2001;31: 441–449.

94. Jorm AF, Masaki K, Davis D, et al. Memory complaints in nondemented men predict future

95. Juottonen K, Laakso MP, Insausti R, et al. Volumes of the entorhinal and perirhinal cortices in Alzheimer's disease. *Neurobiol Aging.* 1998;19:15–22.

96. Juottonen K, Laakso MP, Partanen K, et al. Comparative MR analysis of the entorhinal cortex and hippocampus in diagnosing Alzheimer disease. *Am Soc Neuroradiol.* 1999;20: 139–144.

97. Kalbe E, Salmon E, Perani D, et al. Anosognosia in very mild Alzheimer's disease but not in mild cognitive impairment. *Dement Geriatr Cogn Disord.* 2005;19:349–356.

98. Kapur N, Crewes H, Wise R, et al. Mammillary body damage results in memory impairment but not amnesia. *Neurocase.* 1998;4:509–517.

99. Kapur N, Scholey K, Moore E, et al. The mammillary bodies revisited. Their role in human memory functioning. In: Cermak LS, ed. *Neuropsychological explorations of memory and cognition: essays in honor of Nelson Butters.* New York: Plenum Press; 1994:159–189.

100. Karas GB, Burton EJ, Rombouts SA, et al. A comprehensive study of gray matter loss in patients with Alzheimer's disease using optimized voxel-based morphometry. *Neuroimage.* 2003;18:895–907.

101. Karas GB, Scheltens P, Rombouts SA, et al. Global and local gray matter loss in mild cognitive impairment and Alzheimer's disease. *Neuroimage.* 2004;23:708–716.

102. Kaszniak AW. The neuropsychology of dementia. In: Grant I, Adams K, eds. *Neuropsychological assessment of neuropsychiatric disorders.* New York: Oxford University Press; 1986.

103. Killiany RJ, Gomez-Isla T, Moss M, et al. Use of structural magnetic resonance imaging to predict who will get Alzheimer's disease. *Ann Neurol.* 2000;47:430–439.

104. Killiany RJ, Moss MB, Albert MS, et al. Temporal lobe regions on magnetic resonance imaging identify patients with early Alzheimer's disease. *Arch Neurol.* 1993;50:949–954.

105. Kirchhoff BA, Wagner AD, Maril A, et al. Prefrontal-temporal circuitry for episodic encoding and subsequent memory. *J Neurosci.* 2000;20:6173–6180.

106. Klunk WE, Engler H, Nordberg A, et al. Imaging brain amyloid in Alzheimer's disease with Pittsburgh Compound-B. *Ann Neurol.* 2004;55:306–319.

107. Klunk WE, Wang Y, Huang GF, et al. The binding of 2-(4'-methylaminophenyl)benzothiazole to postmortem brain homogenates is

dominated by the amyloid component. *J Neurosci.* 2003;23:2086–2092.

108. Kohler S, McIntosh AR, Moscovitch M, et al. Functional interactions between the medial temporal lobes and posterior neocortex related to episodic memory retrieval. *Cereb Cortex.* 1998;8:451–461.

109. Kordower JH, Chu Y, Stebbins GT, et al. Loss and atrophy of layer II entorhinal cortex neurons in elderly people with mild cognitive impairment. *Ann Neurol.* 2001;49:202–213.

110. Krasuski JS, Alexander GE, Horwitz B, et al. Volumes of medial temporal lobe structures in patients with Alzheimer's disease and mild cognitive impairment (and in healthy controls). *Biol Psychiatry.* 1998;43:60–68.

111. Laakso MP, Soininen H, Partanen K, et al. Volumes of hippocampus, amygdala and frontal lobes in the MRI-based diagnosis of early Alzheimer's disease: correlation with memory functions. *J Neural Transm Park Dis Dement Sect.* 1995;9:73–86.

112. Lafleche G, Albert MS. Executive function deficits in mild Alzheimer's disease. *Neuropsychology.* 1995;3:313–320.

113. Lauter H. What do we know about Alzheimer's disease today? *Danish Med Bull.* 1985;32 [Suppl 1]: 1–21.

114. Loewenstein DA, Acevedo A, Agron J, et al. Stability of neurocognitive impairment in different subtypes of mild cognitive impairment. *Dement Geriatr Cogn Disord.* 2007;23:82–86.

115. Loewenstein DA, Acevedo A, Ownby R, et al. Using different memory cutoffs to assess mild cognitive impairment. *Am J Geriatr Psychiatry.* 2006;14:911–919.

116. Lopez OL, Becker JT, Somsak D, et al. Awareness of cognitive deficits and anosognosia in probable Alzheimer's disease. *Eur Neurol.* 1994;34:277–282.

117. Lopez OL, Becker JT, Sweet RA. Non-cognitive symptoms in mild cognitive impairment subjects. *Neurocase.* 2005;11:65–71.

118. Lyketsos CG, Lopez O, Jones B, et al. Prevalence of neuropsychiatric symptoms in dementia and mild cognitive impairment: results from the cardiovascular health study. *JAMA.* 2002;288:1475–1483.

119. Machulda MM, Ward HA, Borowski B, et al. Comparison of memory fMRI response among normal, MCI, and Alzheimer's patients. *Neurology.* 2003;61:500–506.

120. Medina D, DeToledo-Morrell L, Urresta F, et al. White matter changes in mild cognitive impairment and AD: a diffusion tensor imaging study. *Neurobiol Aging.* 2006;27:663–672.

121. Modrego PJ. Predictors of conversion to dementia of probable Alzheimer type in patients with mild cognitive impairment. *Curr Alzheimer Res.* 2006;3:161–170.

122. Morcom AM, Good CD, Frackowiak RS, et al. Age effects on the neural correlates of successful memory encoding. *Brain.* 2003;126:213–229.

123. Morris JC. Mild cognitive impairment is early-stage Alzheimer disease: time to revise diagnostic criteria. *Arch Neurol.* 2006;63:15–16.

124. Morris JC, Storandt M, Miller JP, et al. Mild cognitive impairment represents early-stage Alzheimer disease. *Arch Neurol.* 2001;58:397–405.

125. Nutter-Upham KE, Flashman LA, Rabin LA, et al. Awareness of cognitive impairment in MCI and controls with cognitive complaints: dimension variability and relationship to neuropsychological deficits and brain volume. Proceedings of the 32nd Annual Meeting of the International Neuropsychological Society, Baltimore, MD, 2004:3.

126. Parker A, Gaffan D. Mammillary body lesions in monkeys impair object-in-place memory: functional unity of the fornix-mammillary system. *J Cogn Neurosci.* 1997;9:512–521.

127. Parks RW, Haxby JV, Grady CL. Positron emission tomography in Alzheimer's disease. In: Parks RW, Zec RF, Wilson RS, eds. *Neuropsychology of Alzheimer's disease and other dementias.* Oxford: Oxford University Press; 1993.

128. Parnetti L, Lowenthal DT, Presciutti O, et al. 1H-MRS, MRI-based hippocampal volumetry, and 99mTc-HMPAO-SPECT in normal aging, age-associated memory impairment, and probable Alzheimer's disease. *J Am Geriatr Soc.* 1996;44:133–138.

129. Pearlson GD, Harris GJ, Powers RE, et al. Quantitative changes in mesial temporal volume, regional cerebral blood flow, and cognition in Alzheimer's disease. *Arch Gen Psychiatry.* 1992;49:402–408.

130. Pennanen C, Testa C, Laakso MP, et al. A voxel based morphometry study on mild cognitive impairment. *J Neurol Neurosurg Psychiatry.* 2005;76:11–14.

131. Perani D, Bressi S, Cappa SF, et al. Evidence of multiple memory systems in the human brain. A [18F]FDG PET metabolic study. *Brain.* 1993;116:903–919.

132. Petersen RC. Aging, mild cognitive impairment, and Alzheimer's disease. *Neurol Clin.* 2000; 18:789–806.

133. Petersen RC, Doody R, Kurz A, et al. Current concepts in mild cognitive impairment. *Arch Neurol.* 2001;58:1985–1992.

134. Petersen RC, Smith GE, Ivnik RJ, et al. Memory function in very early Alzheimer's disease. *Neurology*. 1994;44:867–872.

135. Petersen RC, Smith GE, Waring SC, et al. Aging, memory, and mild cognitive impairment. *Int Psychogeriatr*. 1997;9[Suppl 1]:65–69.

136. Petersen RC, Smith GE, Waring SC, et al. Mild cognitive impairment: clinical characterization and outcome. *Arch Neurol*. 1999;56:303–308.

137. Petersen RC, Stevens JC, Ganguli M, et al. Practice parameter: early detection of dementia: mild cognitive impairment (an evidence-based review): report of the Quality Standards Subcommittee of the American Academy of Neurology. *Neurology*. 2001;56:1133–1142.

138. Petrella JR, Krishnan S, Slavin MJ, et al. Mild cognitive impairment: evaluation with 4-T functional MR imaging. *Radiology*. 2006;240: 177–186.

139. Pietrini P, Alexander GE, Furey ML, et al. The neurometabolic landscape of cognitive decline: in vivo studies with positron emission tomography in Alzheimer's disease. *Int J Psychophysiol*. 2000;37:87–98.

140. Poon LW, Gurland B, Eisdorfer C, et al, eds. *Handbook for Clinical Memory Assessment of Older Adults*. Washington, DC: American Psychological Association; 1986.

141. Prvulovic D, Van de Ven V, Sack AT, et al. Functional activation imaging in aging and dementia. *Psychiatry Res*. 2005;140:97–113.

142. Rabin LA, Roth RM, Isquith PK, et al. Self and informant reports of executive functions on the BRIEF-A in MCI and older adults with cognitive complaints. *Arch Clin Neuropsychol*. 2006;21:721–732.

143. Rabin LA, Saykin AJ, Wishart HA, et al. Compensatory brain activity associated with novelty detection and habituation in MCI and cognitive complaints. Presented at the 9th International Conference on Alzheimer's Disease and Related Disorders, Philadelphia, PA, July 17–22, 2004.

144. Ray KM, Wang H, Chu Y, et al. Mild cognitive impairment: apparent diffusion coefficient in regional gray matter and white matter structures. *Radiology*. 2006;241:197–205.

145. Raz N, Gunning FM, Head D, et al. Selective aging of the human cerebral cortex observed in vivo: differential vulnerability of the prefrontal gray matter. *Cereb Cortex*. 1997;7:268–282.

146. Ready RE, Ott BR, Grace J, et al. Apathy and executive dysfunction in mild cognitive impairment and Alzheimer disease. *Am J Geriatr Psychiatry*. 2003;11:222–228.

147. Rentz DM, Huh TJ, Faust RR, et al. Use of IQ-adjusted norms to predict progressive cognitive decline in highly intelligent older individuals. *Neuropsychology*. 2004;18:38–49.

148. Ritchie K, Artero S, Touchon J. Classification criteria for mild cognitive impairment: a population-based validation study. *Neurology*. 2001; 56:37–42.

149. Rosano C, Aizenstein HJ, Cochran JL, et al. Event-related functional magnetic resonance imaging investigation of executive control in very old individuals with mild cognitive impairment. *Biol Psychiatry*. 2005;57:761–767.

150. Rose SE, McMahon KL, Janke AL, et al. Diffusion indices on magnetic resonance imaging and neuropsychological performance in amnestic mild cognitive impairment. *J Neurol Neurosurg Psychiatry*. 2006;77:1122–1128.

151. Ross MH, Yurgelun-Todd DA, Renshaw PF, et al. Age-related reduction in functional MRI response to photic stimulation. *Neurology*. 1997; 48:173–176.

152. Rossor MN, Fox NC, Freeborough PA, et al. Slowing the progression of Alzheimer disease: monitoring progression. *Alzheimer Dis Assoc Disord*. 1997;11[Suppl 5]:S6–S9.

153. Roth RM, Isquith PK, Gioia GA. *Behavioral Rating Inventory of Executive Function—Adult Version*. Lutz, FL: Psychological Assessment Resources, Inc.; 2005.

154. Salmon D, Hodges JR. Introduction: mild cognitive impairment—cognitive, behavioral, and biological factors. *Neurocase*. 2005;11:1–2.

155. Saykin AJ, Flashman LA, Frutiger S, et al. Neuroanatomic substrates of semantic memory impairment in Alzheimer's disease: patterns of functional MRI activation. *J Int Neuropsychol Soc*. 1999;5:377–392.

156. Saykin AJ, Johnson S, Flashman L, et al. Event-related fMRI during recently learned and novel words shows hippocampal and differentially lateralized insular change. *Neuroimage*. 1998;7:814.

157. Saykin AJ, Wishart HA. Mild cognitive impairment: conceptual issues and structural and functional brain correlates. *Semin Clin Neuropsychiatry*. 2003;8:12–30.

158. Saykin AJ, Wishart HA, Rabin LA, et al. Cholinergic enhancement of frontal lobe activity in mild cognitive impairment. *Brain*. 2004;127: 1574–1583.

159. Saykin AJ, Wishart HA, Rabin LA, et al. Older adults with cognitive complaints show brain atrophy similar to that of amnestic MCI. *Neurology*. 2006;67:834–42.

160. Saykin AJ, Wishart HA, Rabin LA, et al. Pre-MCI and MCI changes on structural and functional MRI. Presented at the 9th International Conference on Alzheimer's

Disease and Related Disorders, Philadelphia, PA, July 17–22, 2004.

161. Saykin AJ, Wishart HA, Santulli R, et al. Relation of decreased gray matter volume to verbal learning and subjective memory complaints in healthy older adults and patients with mild cognitive impairment. *J Neuropsychiatry Clin Neurosci.* 2003;15:263.

162. Scheltens P, Leys D, Barkhof F, et al. Atrophy of medial temporal lobes on MRI in "probable" Alzheimer's disease and normal ageing: diagnostic value and neuropsychological correlates. *J Neurol Neurosurg Psychiatry.* 1992;55:967–972.

163. Schmand B, Jonker C, Geerlings MI, et al. Subjective memory complaints in the elderly: depressive symptoms and future dementia. *Br J Psychiatry.* 1997;171:373–376.

164. Schmand B, Jonker C, Hooijer C, et al. Subjective memory complaints may announce dementia. *Neurology.* 1996;46:121–125.

165. Schroder J, Buchsbaum MS, Shihabuddin L, et al. Patterns of cortical activity and memory performance in Alzheimer's disease. *Biol Psychiatry.* 2001;49:426–436.

166. Shimamura AP. Aging and memory disorders: a neuropsychological analysis. In: Howe ML, Stones MJ, Brainerd CJ, eds. *Cognitive and behavioral performance factors in atypical aging.* New York: Springer-Verlag; 1990.

167. Shimamura AP. Disorders of memory: the cognitive science perspective. In: Boller F, Grafman J, eds. *Handbook of neuropsychology.* Amsterdam: Elsevier Science Publishers; 1989.

168. Singh V, Chertkow H, Lerch JP, et al. Spatial patterns of cortical thinning in mild cognitive impairment and Alzheimer's disease. *Brain.* 2006;129:2885–2893.

169. Small GW, Kepe V, Ercoli LM, et al. PET of brain amyloid and tau in mild cognitive impairment. *N Engl J Med.* 2006;355:2652–2663.

170. Small GW, Okonek A, Mandelkern MA, et al. Age-associated memory loss: initial neuropsychological and cerebral metabolic findings of a longitudinal study. *Int Psychogeriatr.* 1994; 6:23–44.

171. Small SA, Perera GM, DeLaPaz R, et al. Differential regional dysfunction of the hippocampal formation among elderly with memory decline and Alzheimer's disease. *Ann Neurol.* 1999;45:466–472.

172. Smith CD, Andersen AH, Kryscio RJ, et al. Altered brain activation in cognitively intact individuals at high risk for Alzheimer's disease. *Neurology.* 1999;53:1391–1396.

173. Smith CD, Andersen AH, Kryscio RJ, et al. Women at risk for AD show increased parietal

174. Smith GE, Petersen RC, Ivnik RJ, et al. Subjective memory complaints, psychological distress, and longitudinal change in objective memory performance. *Psychol Aging.* 1996;11: 272–279.

175. Snowdon DA, Greiner LH, Markesbery WR. Linguistic ability in early life and the neuropathology of Alzheimer's disease and cerebrovascular disease: findings from the Nun Study. *Ann NY Acad Sci.* 2000;903:34–38.

176. Soininen HS, Partanen K, Pitkanen A, et al. Volumetric MRI analysis of the amygdala and the hippocampus in subjects with age-associated memory impairment: correlation to visual and verbal memory. *Neurology.* 1994;44:1660–1668.

177. Souder E, Saykin AJ, Alavi A. Multi-modal assessment in Alzheimer's disease. ADL in relation to PET, MRI and neuropsychology. *J Gerontol Nurs.* 1995;21:7–13.

178. Stern CE, Corkin S, Gonzalez RG, et al. The hippocampal formation participates in novel picture encoding: evidence from fMRI. *Proc Natl Acad Sci USA.* 1996;93:8660–8665.

179. Stern Y. What is cognitive reserve? Theory and research application of the reserve concept. *J Int Neuropsychol Soc.* 2002;8:448–460.

180. Stewart R. Cerebral white matter lesions and subjective cognitive dysfunction: the Rotterdam Scan Study. *Neurology.* 2001;57:2149.

181. Stewart R, Russ C, Richards M, et al. Depression, APoE genotype and subjective memory impairment: a cross-sectional study in an African-Caribbean population. *Psychol Med.* 2001;31:431–440.

182. Taki Y, Goto R, Evans A, et al. Voxel-based morphometry of human brain with age and cerebrovascular risk factors. *Neurobiol Aging.* 2004; 25:455–463.

183. Tales A, Haworth J, Nelson S, et al. Abnormal visual search in mild cognitive impairment and Alzheimer's disease. *Neurocase.* 2005;11:80–84.

184. Tate D, Bigler ED. Fornix and hippocampal atrophy in traumatic brain injury. *Learn Mem.* 2000;7:442–446.

185. Taylor JL, Miller TP, Tinklenberg JR. Correlates of memory decline: a 4-year longitudinal study of older adults with memory complaints. *Psychol Aging.* 1992;7:185–193.

186. Terry RD, Davies P. Some morphologic and biochemical aspects of Alzheimer's disease. In: Samuel D, ed. *Aging of the brain.* New York: Raven Press; 1983.

187. Thomann PA, Wustenberg T, Pantel J, et al. Structural changes of the corpus callosum in

mild cognitive impairment and Alzheimer's disease. *Dement Geriatr Cogn Disord*. 2006;21: 215–220.

188. Tierney MC, Szalai JP, Snow WG, et al. Prediction of probable Alzheimer's disease in memory-impaired patients: a prospective longitudinal study. *Neurology*. 1996;46:661–665.

189. Tisserand DJ, van Boxtel MP, Pruessner JC, et al. A voxel-based morphometric study to determine individual differences in gray matter density associated with age and cognitive change over time. *Cereb Cortex*. 2004;14:966–973.

190. Tobiansky R, Blizard R, Livingston G, et al. The Gospel Oak Study stage IV: the clinical relevance of subjective memory impairment in older people. *Psychol Med*. 1995;25:779–786.

191. Tomlinson BE. The neuropathology of dementia. In: Wells CE, ed. *Dementia*. Philadelphia: FA Davis; 1977.

192. Valenzuela MJ, Sachdev P. Magnetic resonance spectroscopy in AD. *Neurology*. 2001;56: 592–598.

193. van Es AC, van der Flier WM, Admiraal-Behloul F, et al. Magnetization transfer imaging of gray and white matter in mild cognitive impairment and Alzheimer's disease. *Neurobiol Aging*. 2006;27:1757–1762.

194. Wagner AD, Schacter DL, Rotte M, et al. Building memories: remembering and forgetting of verbal experiences as predicted by brain activity. *Science*. 1998;281:1188–1191.

195. Wang H, Golob EJ, Su MY. Vascular volume and blood-brain barrier permeability measured by dynamic contrast enhanced MRI in hippocampus and cerebellum of patients with MCI and normal controls. *J Magn Reson Imaging*. 2006;24:695–700.

196. Wang H, Su MY. Regional pattern of increased water diffusivity in hippocampus and corpus callosum in mild cognitive impairment. *Dement Geriatr Cogn Disord*. 2006;22:223–229.

197. Wang PJ, Saykin AJ, Flashman LA, et al. Regionally specific atrophy of the corpus callosum in AD, MCI and cognitive complaints. *Neurobiol Aging*. 2006;27:1613–1617.

198. West JD, Saykin AJ, Arfanakis K, et al. Diffusion tensor MRI in preclinical AD: diffusivity and anisotropy in MCI and older adults with cognitive complaints. Presented at the Alzheimer's Association International Conference on the Prevention of Dementia, Washington, DC, 2005.

199. Wilson RS, Sullivan M, deToledo-Morrell L, et al. Association of memory and cognition in Alzheimer's disease with volumetric estimates of temporal lobe structures. *Neuropsychology*. 1996; 10:459–463.

200. Winblad B, Palmer K, Kivipelto M, et al. Mild cognitive impairment—beyond controversies, towards a consensus: report of the International Working Group on Mild Cognitive Impairment. *J Intern Med*. 2004;256:240–246.

201. Wishart HA, Saykin AJ, Rabin LA, et al. Increased brain activation during working memory in cognitively intact adults with the APOE ε4 allele. *Am J Psychiatry*. 2006;163:1603–1610.

202. Wolf H, Ecke GM, Bettin S, et al. Do white matter changes contribute to the subsequent development of dementia in patients with mild cognitive impairment? A longitudinal study. *Int J Geriatr Psychiatry*. 2000;15:803–812.

203. Woodard JL, Grafton ST, Votaw JR, et al. Compensatory recruitment of neural resources during overt rehearsal of word lists in Alzheimer's disease. *Neuropsychology*. 1998;12: 491–504.

204. Xu Y, Jack CR Jr., O'Brien PC, et al. Usefulness of MRI measures of entorhinal cortex versus hippocampus in AD. *Neurology*. 2000;54: 1760–1767.

205. Yetkin FZ, Rosenberg RN, Weiner MF, et al. fMRI of working memory in patients with mild cognitive impairment and probable Alzheimer's disease. *Eur Radiol*. 2006;16:193–206.

206. Zahajszky J, Dickey CC, McCarley RW, et al. A quantitative MR measure of the fornix in schizophrenia. *Schizophr Res*. 2001;47:87–97.

WEBSITES OF NATIONAL SUPPORT GROUPS

Facts about Dementia: http://www.alzheimers.org .uk/Facts_about_dementia/What_is_dementia/ info_MCI.htm

ClinicalTrials.gov: http://www.clinicaltrials.gov/

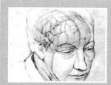

CHAPTER **22**

Movement Disorders in the Older Adult

Nabila A. Dahodwala and Howard I. Hurtig

Several movement disorders increase in incidence and prevalence with old age. However, normal aging is associated with changes (e.g., slowed motor speed) that can resemble common findings of movement disorders. Also, older adults are more likely to take multiple prescription medications and, therefore, are at risk for developing drug-induced movement disorders (81). Thus, the clinician caring for the older adult must distinguish between age-related, normative findings and true movement disorders as well as target therapeutic interventions to the specific needs of the elderly patient.

HYPOKINETIC MOVEMENT DISORDERS: PARKINSONISM

For clinical purposes, movement disorders can be divided into hypokinetic and hyperkinetic disorders. Parkinsonism, the most common of the hypokinetic disorders, is a "syndrome" of slowed movements, rigidity, postural instability, and tremor. Idiopathic parkinsonism or Parkinson's disease (PD) is the most common parkinsonian syndrome, accounting for approximately 75% of the total number of patients with a parkinsonian diagnosis (78). Of the select group of patients that present to autopsy, idiopathic PD represents about 55% of patients with parkinsonism seen at specialty clinics (40). PD is a progressive, degenerative disease of the brain with distinctive clinical features; a specific histopathology characterized by degeneration of neurons throughout the brain, especially pigmented, dopamine-producing neurons in the substantia nigra (SN) of the midbrain; and a strongly positive response to dopamine replacement therapy with levodopa by most patients. Parkinsonism caused by other degenerative disorders such as progressive supranuclear palsy (PSP), multiple system atrophy (MSA), corticobasal degeneration (CBD), adverse effects of drugs (mainly neuroleptics), stroke, and other rare miscellaneous causes comprise the other 25% of cases.

Parkinsonism is a disorder of aging. PD is uncommon before the age of 40, and incidence and prevalence increase steadily until the ninth or 10th decades (96). Although PD can begin in childhood or early adulthood (juvenile PD), the mean age of symptom onset is about 70 years of age (100).

PATHOGENESIS

The cause of PD is unknown. However, the leading hypothesis of causation holds that the pathogenesis in the majority of cases represents a complex interaction of genetic and environmental factors. In the last decade, several genes and genetic loci have been identified that are both dominantly and recessively inherited with varying degrees of penetrance. Thus far, these genes and their corresponding loci include *α-synuclein/PARK1* and *4* (dominant), *LRRK2/PARK8* (dominant), *parkin/PARK2* (recessive), *PINK1/PARK6* (recessive), and *DJ-1/PARK7* (recessive). Understanding the normal function of these proteins and how the altered protein structures lead to PD will help to shed light on the pathophysiology of PD in both genetic and nongenetic cases (35).

The pathology of PD, on the other hand, has been well described for almost a century. Patients with PD who are autopsied are usually severely disabled. At postmortem examination in such a patient, the gross brain sliced transversely at the level of the midbrain shows pallor compared to the dark, linear, mustache-shaped stripe that marks the presence of a population of the approximately 400,000 pigmented neurons in the normal SN. A microscopic view of the SN in PD shows marked depletion of these neurons. The severity of the clinical disability in PD is usually proportional to the loss of dopaminergic neurons in the SN. The histopathologic hallmark of the disease is the eosinophilic, intraneuronal, intracytoplasmic inclusion known as the Lewy body (LB), named for Frederick Lewy, the German neuropathologist who first described the inclusion in 1912. LBs can be found in the SN, locus ceruleus, dorsal motor nucleus of the vagus nerve, thalamus, hypothalamus, substantia innominata (nucleus basalis of Meynert), and cerebral cortex, especially in older patients with a long history of PD who develop dementia (1,59).

LBs consist of the accumulation of a protein called alpha-synuclein whose normal function is believed to involve modulation of synaptic vesicle turnover and synaptic plasticity (14). Several hypotheses exist that explain how these protein aggregates develop and how they may then lead to neuronal death. These include exposure to neurotoxins and oxidative stress and genetic mutations that lead to altered protein folding, polymerization, and degradation (27). There is no single biochemical pathway to date that explains the development of LBs. However, active investigation continues in the field because it provides hope for more targeted and potentially curative therapies.

CLINICAL MANIFESTATIONS

The diagnosis of PD is based on a clinical impression of PD because there are no tests currently available to validate what a doctor finds after interviewing and examining a patient. Computerized imaging techniques, such as computed tomography (CT) and magnetic resonance imaging (MRI), usually are normal in the setting of PD or show only nonspecific changes. Computed isotopic imaging, such as positron emission tomography (PET) and single photon emission CT (SPECT) have shown promise in differentiating patients with PD or another parkinsonian syndrome from patients whose illness has a nonparkinsonian cause, but these techniques are not widely available.

The cardinal features of PD—rest tremor, rigidity, and bradykinesia—usually appear in the limbs asymmetrically, often affecting only one side of the body in the early stages of the disease. Most movement disorder specialists believe that a patient must have two of the three cardinal features and a strongly positive response to levodopa before a clinical diagnosis of PD can be considered definite (39). Patients with other parkinsonian syndromes (e.g., PSP, MSA, and CBD) rarely respond as well to levodopa as do patients with PD. Postural instability (tendency to fall) is a relatively late feature of PD, in contrast to the other parkinsonian syndromes, in which it appears relatively early in the course.

Tremor, often the initial symptom, is eventually present in 75% of patients with PD. It has a frequency of 5 to 7 Hz and usually starts on one side in a hand or foot (24). Tremor is typically most prominent when the affected part is at rest, but it can also be evident with sustention and action. As the disease progresses, the tremor may involve both sides as well as the lips and chin. Rigidity (increased tone) or "stiffness" is a common complaint and can be detected when an examiner observes resistance to passive movement in a relaxed limb that occurs throughout the whole range of movement. Increased tone that starts and stops as the limb is moved passively back and forth is called "cogwheeling." Rigidity is an inconstant finding but can occur in all stages of disease. Bradykinesia refers to slowness of initiating and sustaining movement; it is different from rigidity and can be distinguished from it through a careful examination because rigidity is often not present in a patient who is noticeably slow. Bradykinesia and tremor are the most noticeable and constant physical signs of parkinsonism.

Bradykinesia underlies many of the symptoms of PD, including difficulty with dexterity, fine motor movements, and gait.

Gait dysfunction in PD reflects a composite of bradykinesia, rigidity, and impairment of postural righting reflexes. Stride length is shortened, and the feet shuffle. Arm swing is decreased, more so on the more affected side. Posture is stooped, and the arms assume a flexed and adducted position. Turning in the act of walking is done en bloc, without pivoting or twisting the torso and with multiple small steps that describe a wide arc. As the disease progresses, the gait is interrupted by transient freezing of the feet, as though they were glued to the ground, especially on initiating the first step, when entering a narrow space such as a doorway, or when turning at an acute angle.

Loss of balance and falling tend to occur later in the course of PD. Patients who present with postural instability or frequent falls early in the course of illness should be evaluated for other causes of parkinsonism such as PSP or MSA. A modest backward pull on the patient's shoulders can be used to test postural instability. The patient should be instructed to take only one step back if necessary to prevent going backward. If more than two steps are required to regain balance after a reasonably forceful tug (not too hard!), postural reflexes are impaired. More severely affected patients may fall like solid objects (95), and the examiner must be prepared to catch the patient. Stooped posture and a loss of postural reflexes can lead to an accelerated speed of walking, forward leaning of the patient's torso, and a tendency to fall, as the patient "chases his or her center of gravity." This type of accelerated forward locomotion is referred to as a "festinating gait."

There are many secondary manifestations of PD (Table 22-1), which are classified as "nonmotor" symptoms but are not sufficient by themselves to confirm a diagnosis of the disease. However, some secondary symptoms may be the presenting complaint and may be more debilitating than the primary features of PD.

PD remains a clinical diagnosis, despite recent advances in brain imaging. Computerized isotopic brain imaging (PET and SPECT) and transcranial sonography make it possible to visualize the abnormalities in the basal ganglia caused by PD. The University of Pennsylvania Smell Identification Test (UPSIT) can detect the hyposmia (loss of the sense of smell) that is often seen in the earliest stage of clinical PD. These diagnostic tests are primarily used in research with the goal of detecting early or preclinical PD (92), but PET or SPECT imaging can be useful in the right setting to confirm or refute an uncertain clinical diagnosis.

Table 22-1. *Secondary Symptoms of Parkinson's Disease*

Cognitive and Behavioral	Craniofacial	Autonomic	Other
Dementia	Masked facies	Orthostatic hypotension	Cramps
Anxiety	Decreased blinking	Impaired gastric motility	Paresthesias
Depression	Decreased sense of smell	Urinary bladder dysfunction	Seborrhea
Sleep disturbance	Dysphagia	Abnormal thermoregulation	Micrographia
	Dysarthria	Sexual dysfunction	
	Sialorrhea		

DIAGNOSING PARKINSON'S DISEASE IN THE ELDERLY

Some signs of parkinsonism can be a part of normal aging. In one study, bradykinesia was present in 37% of normal elderly community residents (81). No increase was noted in tone in normal elderly subjects, but joint stiffness caused by arthritis can limit mobility and be confused with increased tone. Similarly, posture tends to become flexed at the neck and trunk as part of normal aging. Dizziness can lead to gait instability, and stride length is shorter in the elderly (71). In a community sample of older adults, 15% of people 65 to 74 years of age and almost 30% of people 75 to 84 years of age had some evidence of parkinsonism (7). This, however, was also associated with a twofold increased risk of mortality and more likely represents a complex interaction of aging, neurologic disease, medication effects, and vascular disease as the etiology of parkinsonism. The descriptive terms "senile gait" and "old person's gait" are two of the many default labels used to define the nonspecific but sometimes incapacitating Parkinson-like abnormality of walking by the elderly when no obvious other cause can be found. Rest tremor does not occur as a manifestation of normal aging and is one of the more specific indicators of PD in the elderly. If bradykinesia and postural instability alone were used in the diagnosis of the disease, many normal elderly patients might be misdiagnosed. Therefore, to make a diagnosis of PD, all patients, young or old, should meet the standard criteria of two of the three cardinal features and a good response to levodopa.

OTHER CAUSES OF PARKINSONISM IN THE ELDERLY

Most cases of parkinsonism are ultimately classified as PD, although the differential diagnosis of secondary parkinsonism is broad (Fig. 22-1). Structural lesions of

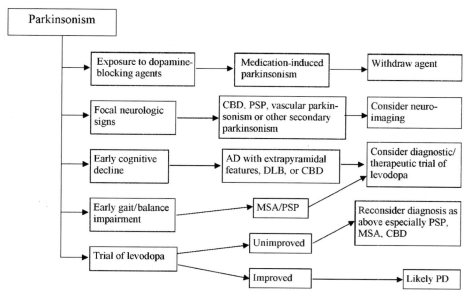

Figure 22-1. Approach to the parkinsonian patient.

the basal ganglia (stroke, hydrocephalus, and tumor), drugs, infections, or metabolic disorders can rarely mimic typical PD. In general, these patients do not have a rest tremor and do not respond to levodopa (66).

Vascular Parkinsonism

Parkinsonism can occur rarely after a single stroke in the basal ganglia or brainstem or as the cumulative result of several strokes. Patients with vascular parkinsonism tend to have a long history of hypertension and a stepwise progression of symptoms that may correlate with each acute clinical stroke. Evidence for stroke may be noted on examination. Gait may be shuffling or magnetic, a term used synonymously with transient freezing. Patients should have evidence of cerebrovascular disease on CT scan or MRI, although asymptomatic ischemic changes are common in older patients and do not independently make the diagnosis of vascular parkinsonism (43).

Hydrocephalus

Hydrocephalus can cause parkinsonian signs and symptoms. Normal pressure hydrocephalus (NPH) is a syndrome characterized by the triad of gait instability, urinary incontinence, and cognitive dysfunction (55,89). As with vascular parkinsonism, gait in NPH is classically magnetic, but other gait disturbances, especially "gait ignition failure" and "frontal gait" (67), have been described in NPH. Brain imaging (CT or MRI) shows communicating hydrocephalus with ventricles enlarged out of proportion to atrophy of the cerebral cortical sulci. This is an important disorder to consider in any patient with a parkinsonian gait, cognitive impairment, and urinary frequency or incontinence because ventriculoperitoneal shunting may lead to the dramatic reversal of a severe disability. For this reason, every patient with parkinsonism deserves to have a computed imaging study of the brain, either CT or MRI, at some time during the course of illness; the sooner it is performed the better to get the question out of the way.

Drug-Induced Parkinsonism

Drug-induced parkinsonism is a critically important entity because it is one of the few reversible causes of parkinsonism. The most common offenders are the antipsychotics, also known as neuroleptics, which as a class can cause parkinsonism because of their dopamine receptor–blocking properties. These include phenothiazines, butyrophenones, and thioxanthenes (45). The antiemetic prochlorperazine (Compazine) and the gastrointestinal promotility agent metoclopramide (Reglan) are also dopamine receptor blockers that have the potential to induce parkinsonism and other "extrapyramidal" involuntary movements, such as dystonia and tardive dyskinesia (TD) (44). Clozapine (Clozaril), the first "atypical" neuroleptic, was introduced to the American market in 1990 after prior experience in Europe as a major breakthrough for treating schizophrenia because its antipsychotic effect is mediated by nondopaminergic neural circuits. Therefore, it relieves symptoms of psychosis without causing parkinsonism or other extrapyramidal side effects. Several other atypical neuroleptics have followed, including olanzapine (Zyprexa), risperidone (Risperdal), ziprasidone (Geodon), and aripiprazole (Abilify), although each has greater affinity for the dopamine receptor than clozapine and can, therefore, produce varying degrees of extrapyramidal side effects. Quetiapine (Seroquel) is one of the more recently developed atypical neuroleptics with an extrapyramidal side effect profile similar to clozapine. Other drugs with a tendency to induce parkinsonism include the antihypertensives methyldopa, verapamil (38), reserpine, and the antiepileptic valproic acid (Depakote). Reserpine can induce signs of parkinsonism by depleting dopamine storage vesicles presynaptically instead of blocking postsynaptic dopamine receptors. Treatment of parkinsonism in this setting consists of a combination of a high index of suspicion and prudent withdrawal of the offending drug.

Alzheimer's Disease and Dementia with Lewy Bodies

Neurodegenerative diseases other than PD often have clinical parkinsonian features. Alzheimer disease (AD), the most common cause of dementia, may be accompanied by varying degrees of parkinsonism in up to 50% of patients (13), usually late in the course of the dementia. In AD, the dementia precedes the parkinsonian signs and is disproportionately more severe. Dementia and parkinsonism also co-occur in the pathologic entity diffuse LB disease, also known clinically as dementia with LB (DLB), which is associated pathologically with widespread distribution of LBs throughout the cerebral cortex. The clinical presentation in DLB consists of prominent and early cognitive decline, fluctuations in cognitive function, spontaneous visual hallucinations that have no other cause, and parkinsonism (62). The parkinsonian signs consist of bradykinesia, rigidity, and a prominent gait disorder; rest tremor is seen less frequently than in PD (26,64). A diagnosis of DLB may be difficult to differentiate from AD or from typical PD with dementia (PDD). However, in PDD, the interval between the onset of parkinsonism and onset of the cognitive disturbance is usually more than a year (62).

Progressive Supranuclear Palsy, Multiple System Atrophy, and Corticobasal Degeneration

PSP, MSA, and CBD closely resemble PD and may be clinically indistinguishable in the early stages of progression, but they usually emerge as distinct clinical entities as the disease evolves. Each has a distinctive neuropathology. PSP presents as an akinetic-rigid syndrome with a prominent gait disorder early in the course of illness. In contrast, walking is usually not a major issue in PD until late in the course. Truncal posture in PSP tends to be upright instead of stooped, and axial and asymmetric limb dystonia may be present (29). Tremor is much less common in PSP than in PD (29). Cognitive impairment occurs earlier than in PD, but the dementia of PSP is usually not as severe as it is in PD, CBD, and some of the other parkinsonian syndromes. Many patients demonstrate a pseudobulbar affect, marked by uncontrollable and inappropriate laughing or crying. Several characteristic eye movement abnormalities are seen, the most important of which is a supranuclear paresis of conjugate gaze, beginning with symptomatic slowing of gaze in the vertical plane. Patients often complain of having trouble looking up, looking at their food during meals, or hitting a golf ball. Examination may reveal impaired voluntary gaze, spontaneous mini-myoclonic jerks of the eyes (square wave jerks), and loss of optokinetic nystagmus, which can be elicited in the normal subject by passing a sequence of stripes or other similar repetitively occurring graphic objects horizontally or vertically across the field of vision (29). Reflex eye movements are preserved because the pathology of PSP interrupts the neural circuits descending from the centers of voluntary gaze in the frontal lobe before they damage the oculomotor nuclei in the brainstem; hence, the term "supranuclear" to the paresis of voluntary gaze in PSP. These relatively well-preserved reflexive eye movements may be demonstrated using the doll's head maneuver, in which the patient is asked to visually fixate a target while the examiner passively moves the patient's head in the horizontal or vertical plane. Preserved reflexive eye movements allow patients to hold their eyes on target despite the head movements. In the late stages of PSP, voluntary and reflexive eye movements in all directions, including the horizontal plane, are severely impaired. MRI may show atrophy of the dorsal midbrain (85).

MSA is a diagnostic grouping of three disorders that are distinguished by parkinsonism, cerebellar ataxia, and autonomic insufficiency in combination with one of the three as the primary presenting deficit. Pyramidal tract deficits can also be seen as part of the mix. By convention, the most prominent neurologic theme determines the subclassification within the overarching domain of MSA, although any assortment of the four types of signs can occur in the same patient. Thus, a mix of parkinsonism and severe autonomic dysfunction (orthostatic hypotension, atonic bladder, and impotence) would be called autonomic MSA or the Shy-Drager syndrome. Pure parkinsonism is called striatonigral MSA or MSA-p; and cerebellar ataxia without a family history is called cerebellar MSA, MSA-c, or olivopontocerebellar atrophy in the old terminology (57). Cerebellar ataxia with a family history is included in the large and growing classification of the spinocerebellar ataxias (88). Autonomic failure and postural instability are early findings. As in PSP, tremor is rare. The MRI scan, which is normal in PD and in most cases of MSA, may sometimes show a combination of shrinkage of the brainstem and cerebellum and an abnormally large area of low signal in the putamen (28). The course of MSA is generally faster than that of PD. In most patients with MSA, especially the parkinsonian form, cognitive function is preserved.

CBD is characterized by highly asymmetric parkinsonism that is associated early on with cognitive impairment and pathognomonic signs that may escape the notice of the naive observer. An early and common sign of CBD is a clumsy or "useless arm" due to rigidity, dystonia, akinesia, or motor apraxia in some combination. Other early features include gait impairment, if onset is in the leg, due to lateralized stiffness or apraxia (60). In addition to dementia, other manifest higher cortical signs are ideational apraxia, aphasia, cortical sensory abnormalities (e.g., loss of spatial orientation), and alien-limb phenomenon. Additional hyperkinetic movements include coarse action tremor and myoclonus (53). Tremor is less likely to be present in CBD than in PD, but when it does manifest, it can be differentiated from Parkinson tremor because it occurs mainly with action, is coarser and higher in frequency, and is associated with marked rigidity of the affected limb or limbs. In cases of suspected CBD, MRI scan may show asymmetric shrinkage of one half of the parietofrontal cortex. The diagnosis of CBD early in its course can be difficult due to the overlap of symptoms with other neurodegenerative diseases, especially PSP, MSA, DLB, and AD.

PSP, MSA, and CBD usually respond poorly to levodopa and other anti-Parkinson drugs. However, a trial of levodopa of as much as 1,000 mg per day may be needed to exclude PD with a high response threshold. Failure to respond is strong evidence that MSA, not PD, is the probable diagnosis. The therapeutic response in patients with PSP, MSA, or CBD is not only disappointing, but the effect may be counterproductive because of aggravation of orthostatic hypotension, particularly in MSA. If patients fail to respond to levodopa, there is no reason to try other dopaminergic agents because they have less therapeutic potency and usually cause more side effects than levodopa. Botulinum toxin (BTX) injections may be useful for focal dystonia, such as eyelid opening apraxia, in PSP and MSA. Autonomic insufficiency, particularly orthostatic hypotension, can be treated with specific drugs. Nonpharmacologic therapies, such as speech therapy, swallowing therapy for dysphagia, and physical therapy, are also an important part of patient care.

TREATMENT OF PARKINSON DISEASE

The objective of treating PD is to suppress symptoms and improve neurologic function. No disease-modifying treatment has yet been proved to slow or reverse the underlying progression of the disease. Some therapeutic strategies, however, may avert or delay the complications that are associated with long-term dopaminergic therapy. The first decision for doctor and patient after the diagnosis is whether the symptoms require treatment. As a general rule, pharmacotherapy should be considered when symptoms begin to interfere with a patient's ability to function at home or work. Once initiated, treatment should be individualized, taking the patient's age, stage of disease, mental state, and tolerance of side effects into account. The algorithm shown in Figure 22-2 outlines a common approach to treatment.

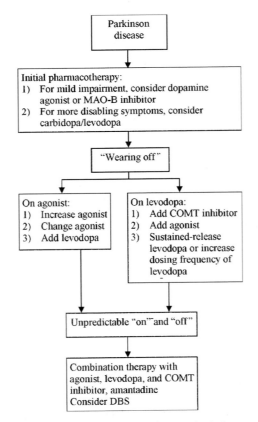

Figure 22-2. Approach to the pharmacological management of Parkinson's disease.

Nonpharmacologic Therapies

The care of patients with PD is best accomplished through a multidisciplinary approach, which should include access to psychological counseling; occupational, physical, and speech therapy; and support groups. Nonpharmacologic intervention can be as important as medications and should be started early in the course of PD. Aerobic and strengthening exercise is vitally important as a health maintenance routine and as a method of exerting psychological control over a chronic, variably progressive disease. Many patients benefit from the mantra, "I have PD but it doesn't have me."

Pharmacotherapy

Levodopa Levodopa was shown to be the first truly effective drug for treating parkinsonism 40 years ago, a distinction that has not been eclipsed by the half dozen or more drugs introduced to the marketplace since then (Table 22-2). Levodopa, the inert precursor of dopamine, was developed as an anti-Parkinson drug because it has long been known that dopamine does not cross the blood–brain barrier, whereas levodopa does. Hence, levodopa enters the brain, where it is decarboxylated by dopa decarboxylase to the therapeutically active dopamine. Levodopa works most efficiently and with fewest side effects when administered in combination with carbidopa, an inhibitor of peripheral dopa decarboxylase, which greatly diminishes the amount of "unprotected" levodopa available to cross the blood–brain barrier into the central nervous system for conversion to dopamine. Carbidopa is joined with levodopa in different ratios (10/100, 25/100, or 25/250) in short-acting and controlled-release formulations. A typical starting dose of carbidopa/levodopa (Sinemet) is one half of a 25/100-mg tablet three times a day (with meals to prevent nausea). Once tolerance is established at a low dose, the amount of carbidopa/levodopa per dose can be slowly increased, usually in half-tablet increments, to an optimal therapeutic level compatible with realistic expectations for the individual patient. Average daily consumption in early stages of disease ranges between 300 and 600 mg/day in three divided doses. The total required daily dose of levodopa tends to increase as the disease progresses, and closer spacing of doses is required to combat the "wearing-off effect" (10). Most patients with typical PD will have a gratifying and smooth initial response to levodopa. Many symptoms improve, but most patients will observe that bradykinesia improves the most. Tremor suppression often lags behind, but it, too, can be well controlled by levodopa.

One of the major drawbacks of levodopa is its short half-life of 90 minutes, which has a major impact on patient satisfaction as the disease progresses. In the

Table 22-2. *Selected Medications for Parkinson's Disease*

Medication	Action	Usual Dose Range	Common Side Effects	Warnings and Contraindications
Carbidopa/levodopa (Sinemet)	Dopamine replacement	Carbidopa ≥ 75 mg, levodopa 300–1,000 mg divided tid	Orthostasis, nausea, vomiting, confusion/hallucinations, dyskinesia	Do not use with nonselective MAO inhibitor
Pramipexole (Mirapex)	Nonergot dopamine agonist	0.375–4.5 mg divided tid	Similar to levodopa + somnolence, swelling of legs	Dopamine agonists more likely to cause adverse effects in elderly than levodopa; known sensitivity to drug or its ingredients; use with caution in patients who drive
Ropinirole (Requip)	Nonergot dopamine agonist	0.75–24 mg/day divided tid	Similar to pramipexole	Similar to pramipexole
Entacapone (Comtan)	Inhibits dopamine metabolism	200 mg with carbidopa/each levodopa dose to maximum of 1,600 mg/day	Similar to levodopa + diarrhea	Known sensitivity to drug or its ingredients
Selegiline (Eldepryl)	Selective MAO-B inhibitor in doses up to 10 mg/day	5 mg/day once-daily dosing	Similar to levodopa	Risk of hypertensive crisis with doses >10 mg/day; do not use with meperidine and other opioids; caution with concomitant use of antidepressants
Rasagiline (Azilect)	Selective MAO-B inhibitor	1 mg daily	Similar to levodopa	Similar to selegiline

tid, three times a day; MAO, monoamine oxidase.

early phase of PD when patients with typical PD first begin using levodopa, the overall response is positive and smooth throughout the day. Few doses per 24 hours are required because of the brain's ability to store the drug in the axon terminals of the still adequate supply of nigrostriatal neurons that have not been decimated by the underlying degenerative process. As more neurons degenerate, the brain's storage capacity declines, and at some point, which varies with the individual's inherent rate of progression, the physiologi-

cally smooth long-duration response (LDR) to levodopa gives way to the physiologically short-duration response (SDR). Clinical expression of the SDR occurs in the form of motor fluctuations, which are characterized by a "wearing off" of the benefit of a dose of carbidopa/levodopa, usually 3 to 4 hours after a dose is taken. The patient will notice a gradual re-emergence of parkinsonian symptoms during this interlude, which at its nadir is called the "off" period. The reciprocal "on" response is gradually re-established (usually within 30 minutes) after the next dose of levodopa is swallowed and transported by gastric contraction to the absorption site in the proximal duodenum or jejunum. Levodopa-induced choreiform or dystonic involuntary movements, called "dyskinesia," commonly begin to occur at the stage of the disease when motor fluctuations start to appear, usually at peak effect 1 to 2 hours after a dose (20). In most patients, dyskinesias are dose related and can be so severe and disabling that they greatly interfere with all activities of daily living. They can be abolished by lowering the dose of levodopa but often at the expense of the benefit provided.

Fluctuations of one sort or another occur as a matter of course in more than half of all patients with typical PD who use levodopa for more than 5 years. Initially, this complication can be remedied by shortening the interval between doses and lowering individual doses. In extreme cases, however, the SDR will contract so much that it will conform to the actual 90-minute half-life of levodopa, and patients will be forced to use levodopa as frequently as every 2 hours. Controlled-release carbidopa/levodopa was developed in the 1980s as a practical approach to combat the motor complications of the SDR, namely the hyperkinetic dyskinesia of the "on" period and the bradykinesia of the "off" period. Controlled-release levodopa is more slowly released into the small intestine by the stomach than is regular carbidopa/levodopa, has a lower peak blood level following absorption, and tends to have a longer pharmacokinetic curve. Unfortunately, the benefit attributable to controlled release has been modest at best, although some patients can reduce the frequency of dosing and experience a partial restoration of the LDR as well as a lessening of the intensity of peak dose dyskinesia. Many patients find its effect disappointing because of its slow onset of action and the tendency for it to cause an increase in the intensity of dyskinesia at the end of the day.

Active debate occurs in the neurologic literature over when to start using levodopa in a patient with advancing symptoms because of its alleged potential for accelerating the progression of PD. Although no clear clinical evidence exists, some investigators and authors claim that levodopa is toxic to nigral neurons because of its in vitro ability to induce oxidant stress, a process that can destroy the lipid membrane of the cell wall (69). According to this hypothesis, early use of levodopa not only increases the rate of nigral cell death, but also hastens the onset of motor fluctuations and the associated disabilities. A recent randomized, double-blind, controlled trial comparing the effects of low, medium, and high doses of levodopa with placebo on the progression of PD in three groups of early-stage patients was conducted to address the question of levodopa toxicity and accelerated neurodegeneration (the ELLDOPA study). The clinical outcome of all

groups when compared with one another at the end of 9 months of observation supported the null hypothesis that levodopa is not toxic. In fact, those patients in the high-dose group did better than those in the other groups, with the placebo group scoring the worst on clinical measures. The only evidence suggesting that levodopa might be toxic was the appearance on a companion isotopic neuroimaging study of a disproportionate depletion of the dopamine transporter, a potential marker of nigrostriatal degeneration, in the levodopa-treated patients compared with those on placebo (76). This finding is still being debated because of its highly theoretical import and uncertain relevance to the long clinical course of PD.

The ELLDOPA study added further support to the notion that chronic use of levodopa is not toxic (i.e., it does not accelerate the variable pace of neurodegeneration in PD), but it did not answer the fundamental question that neurologists must ask themselves when confronting a patient in the office who needs symptomatic treatment: Which drug should be started first? A consensus has probably evolved at the time of this writing to support a practical approach, based on age of the patient, degree of disability, and the presence or absence of comorbidities, particularly cognitive dysfunction. In the young (<60 years), healthy patient with relatively mild disability, pharmacotherapy can be initiated with a dopamine agonist (DA) or one of the several other drugs on the market, which, although generally less effective than levodopa, may work well enough to remedy symptoms and allow the patient to postpone the use of levodopa to a time of greater therapeutic need. In the older patient (>60 years), levodopa becomes a stronger option because of the greater risk of cognitive impairment associated with the use of DAs. In the final analysis of each patient's individual needs, any patient, young or old, with advancing disability that threatens occupational and social stability should be treated with levodopa, the best drug available for the symptomatic relief of the most bothersome symptoms of PD.

Dopamine Agonists DAs are a class of drugs that directly stimulate dopamine receptors and require no metabolism to the active form. Bromocriptine, the first agent of this class, was developed and introduced in the early 1970s to complement and enhance the effect of levodopa. Although not as clinically effective as levodopa, DAs have the advantages of a longer pharmacologic half-life and no need for conversion from precursor to active agent. Four DAs are available in the United States. Two are ergot derivatives: bromocriptine (Parlodel), and cabergoline (Dostinex; approved for use as treatment for pituitary prolactinomas but not for PD). Two nonergot DAs [pramipexole (Mirapex) and ropinirole (Requip)] were introduced to the American pharmaceutical market in the United States in 1997. DAs initially were used as adjuncts to levodopa for patients with motor complications (10), but more recently, they have been studied in early stages of PD as monotherapy in an effort to postpone the initiation of levodopa to prevent the occurrence of motor complications (wearing off and dyskinesia). For example, two recent randomized, controlled trials comparing pramipexole or ropinirole with levodopa as initial monotherapy showed a significantly lower incidence of motor complications in the group of patients taking a DA, although levodopa supplements were required by many in the DA monotherapy groups because of declining therapeutic response to DA monotherapy over time (77,82). For this reason, many patients and doctors have chosen to use DA as the first line of treatment, particularly in young people, and to save levodopa for later when DA monotherapy is no longer sufficient and must be supplemented. Although the side effects of levodopa and DAs are similar, many patients, especially the elderly and cognitively impaired, do not tolerate DAs because of drug-induced confusion, hallucinations, orthostasis, and excessive daytime somnolence (23,87). Two of the three ergot-derived DAs (pergolide and cabergoline) have been linked to increased risk of valvular heart disease because of the potency of these drugs as stimulants of the 5HT2D serotonin receptor (86,105). Pergolide has recently been withdrawn from the market. If patients are on these medications, they should be monitored with an annual visit to a cardiologist for echocardiograms and careful clinical examination. An injectable form, apomorphine (Apokyn), the oldest of the DAs (first used in 1950), is also available and may be useful as a quick "rescue" drug in patients whose off periods occur suddenly and severely (19). Because of the many drug options, it cannot be overstated that drug treatment of patients with PD must be individualized.

Anticholinergics and Monoamine Oxidase-B Inhibitors

Drugs with a primary dopaminergic effect—levodopa and DAs—are the mainstay of treatment for PD, but other, secondary drugs can complement and augment the primary impact of the dopaminergics. Anticholinergics, such as trihexyphenidyl (Artane) and benztropine (Cogentin), may be useful in treating tremor, mainly in young patients. They are less effective in alleviating rigidity and bradykinesia. These agents are usually not well tolerated by older patients because of the high potential for causing short-term memory dysfunction, confusion, prostatism, and blurred vision. Amantadine, a drug with anticholinergic, dopaminergic, and putative glutamate-blocking properties, is inconsistently effective in relieving mild symptoms of PD. It is useful in practice for suppressing levodopa-induced dyskinesias (65). Selegiline (Deprenyl, Eldepryl) and rasagiline

(Azilect) are selective monoamine oxidase-B (MAO-B) inhibitors. They have well-documented, mild symptomatic benefits in treating PD (72,73,75,94). Both selegiline and rasagiline have been studied as potential neuroprotective agents (68,73,74), although the ability of either to delay disease progression has not been proven. A delayed-start, double-blind, placebo-controlled trial of rasagiline is underway to address the potential for neuroprotection. MAO-B inhibitors can be used as initial pharmacotherapy in minimally or mildly symptomatic patients, whereas DAs are appropriate to use in more impaired patients because of the greater potency. However, DAs also have a greater potential for psychiatric and cognitive adverse effects and, as with anticholinergics, should be avoided in older patients with any degree of cognitive impairment.

Catechol-O-Methyltransferase Inhibition

Catechol-O-methyltransferase (COMT) inhibitors work by reducing the peripheral metabolism of levodopa and increasing its availability for transport into the brain for conversion to dopamine. These agents, tolcapone (Tasmar) and entacapone (Comtan), augment and prolong the response to levodopa and are used in patients who are experiencing wearing off. COMT inhibitors decrease "off" time by approximately an hour per day (2). Tolcapone has been removed from the pharmaceutical market in Europe and Canada because of potential hepatotoxicity, but it is still available in the United States under the condition of mandatory biweekly monitoring of liver function tests. Three European patients with PD who were taking tolcapone, among other drugs, died of liver failure, although the exact role of tolcapone was not established (4). Mild, transient, asymptomatic elevations of transaminase were reported in clinical trials before tolcapone received unrestricted U.S. Food and Drug Administration (FDA) approval. A convenient formulation combining entacapone with carbidopa/levodopa (Stalevo) is available. Tolcapone dosing is three times a day, whereas entacapone is generally given with each dose of carbidopa/levodopa, which can be frequent in patients with advanced PD and wearing off who require six to eight doses per day to control symptoms.

Natural substances, vitamins, and other "alternative" therapies for PD are popular but largely unproved. A single double-blind, placebo-controlled trial of high-dose vitamin E (2,000 U/day) showed no effect on symptom relief or the natural history of disease progression when compared with placebo in patients with early PD (75). A small double-blind, placebo-controlled trial of coenzyme Q10 in 80 otherwise untreated patients with early PD (three dose levels plus placebo) showed a significant protective effect in users of the highest of the three doses (1,200 mg/day) but not in doses lower than 1,200 mg/day (90). The results of this study are promising but inconclusive because of the small sample size and are being validated by a planned new trial with larger sample. A major National Institutes of Health (NIH) research initiative has been testing a variety of possible neuroprotective compounds, but after 5 years of experience, only one has been selected for further study.

Surgical Therapies

The neurosurgical treatment of PD has a long and uneven history. The earliest efforts in the 1930s and 1940s targeted various cortical and subcortical regions for ablation without notable success, but it was only in the 1950s that surgeons settled on the motor region of the thalamus for ablation, particularly in patients with severe tremor. Although serious complications were frequent, many patients who survived the procedure experienced satisfactory and sustained tremor suppression. With the introduction of levodopa in the late 1960s, neurosurgical treatment of patients with PD was reserved for those few patients with medically intractable tremor. However, the development of computerized imaging and improved neurosurgical techniques brought about a revival in the 1990s of ablative lesioning of the internal globus pallidus (GPi) (pallidotomy) and thalamus (thalamotomy) with better success than in the earlier technology-poor era of the 1950s and 1960s. More recently, deep brain stimulation (DBS) of the subthalamic nucleus (STN) and GPi has replaced the more destructive and riskier ablative approach. DBS has proved to be relatively safe and effective in numerous short- and long-term studies and is being used worldwide, especially in medical centers that have comprehensive movement disorder programs to guarantee proper patient selection for surgery and good long-term care. However, it is important to note that patients older than 75 and those with significantly impaired cognitive function were excluded in most studies. Also, in two major studies, there was a 13% chance of a serious adverse event with surgery, including one fatal intracerebral hemorrhage (17,54). Thalamic DBS is useful for treating essential tremor, but the thalamus is no longer the preferred site for treating PD because of the superiority of GPi or STN DBS. Target selection remains controversial (34), but the choice of GPi versus STN is being addressed in a randomized controlled trial jointly sponsored by the NIH and Veterans Administration. Also currently under investigation are clinical trials of cell implantation and gene therapy in patients with advanced PD.

PARTICULAR PROBLEMS OF PARKINSON'S DISEASE IN THE ELDERLY

Cognitive impairment and psychiatric symptoms (e.g., depression and psychosis) may be prominent features of PD, especially in the elderly. The neuropsychiatric complications of this disease are discussed in Chapter 23.

Prominent autonomic dysfunction is usually a hallmark of MSA, but mild autonomic insufficiency is common in PD. Findings can include abnormal thermoregulatory responses, with hyperhidrosis, orthostatic hypotension, constipation, urinary frequency and urge incontinence, and impotence. In the elderly, urinary symptoms and syncope caused by orthostatic hypotension are the most clinically troublesome. Urinary tract infection and outflow obstruction caused by prostatic hypertrophy must be considered as causes of disturbed bladder function. Urodynamic studies of the bladder in PD have shown that detrusor hyperreflexia is the most common finding (79). Peripheral anticholinergic drugs (e.g., oxybutynin, tolterodine) may effectively relax the detrusor, but central side effects, especially confusion, are a potential risk in the elderly. Consultation with a urologist or gynecologist is essential (and usually helpful) in this setting.

Orthostatic hypotension occurs in PD because of degenerative changes in the neurons of the autonomic nervous system of the brain and spinal cord and because anti-Parkinson drugs tend to aggravate this already compromised state of blood pressure control. Even without symptoms of orthostatic hypotension, blood pressure in patients with PD is low, often in the range of 90 to 100 mm Hg systolic. Therefore, it is important to monitor brachial blood pressure while sitting and standing when adjusting medications for patients with PD. Many patients with a history of hypertension who later develop PD find that they are able to discontinue taking antihypertensive drugs as the blood pressure drops in response to the autonomic insufficiency of neurodegeneration. Mild orthostasis (e.g., light-headedness) can often be controlled by increasing fluid and salt intake or by using simple compression stockings. Severe symptoms (e.g., recurrent syncope or near syncope) may require the use of the mineralocorticoid, fludrocortisone (Florinef), in a single daily dose of 0.1 mg with salt supplements or with the alpha-adrenergic agonist midodrine (ProAmatine) (63) either singly or in combination.

HYPERKINETIC MOVEMENT DISORDERS: TREMOR, CHOREA, TARDIVE SYNDROMES, AND DYSTONIA

TREMOR

Tremor is the most common hyperkinetic involuntary movement in adults (83). This topic is discussed in Chapter 11.

CHOREA

Chorea consists of irregular, continuous, rapid, usually low-amplitude, involuntary movements that flow randomly from one body part to another. In contrast to tremor, choreiform movements are not predictable. The word chorea is derived from the Greek "to dance." Numerous causes of chorea can manifest during childhood or early adulthood; this chapter focuses on those that predominate among the elderly.

Huntington's disease (HD), the most common hereditary cause of chorea, is transmitted in an autosomal dominant pattern with complete penetrance. In general, the chorea in HD afflicts young and middle-aged adults (fourth to sixth decade), but it can appear for the first time in the elderly. The gene for HD is located on the short arm of chromosome 4; the abnormality is an excessively long repetition of the trinucleotide sequence CAG (normal is <34 repeats). Age of onset is inversely related to the length of the trinucleotide repeat; paternal transmission is often associated with onset in the late teens or early twenties. Instability of repeat size in the male sperm is thought to be responsible for the link between paternal transmission and younger onset of the clinical syndrome. The phenomenon of earlier onset of illness in subsequent generations is known as genetic anticipation (41). The main manifestations of the disease are choreiform, dystonic and slow, twisting (athetoid) movements accompanied by cognitive and behavioral changes, eventually evolving to severe dementia over an average course of 20 years. The onset of the dementia in HD is variable, and if the disease begins late in life, dementia may not occur at all because of age-related shortened life expectancy. Other symptoms gradually accumulate, such as dysarthria, dysphagia, ataxia, rigidity, dystonia (47), and supranuclear gaze problems (80). Behavioral symptoms typically consist of agitation, anxiety, depression, mania, and psychosis (58). Although there is no curative therapy for HD, a recent randomized controlled trial showed symptomatic improvement in the severity of chorea with administration of tetrabenazine, a presynaptic dopamine-depleting agent that works by inducing mild parkinsonism to counterbalance the hyperkinetic state typical of HD (42). However, it has not been approved by the FDA and is not readily available in the United States. There have been conflicting reports of the effect of amantadine in controlling the chorea seen in HD (70,101).

Late-onset idiopathic chorea is an uncommon, insidious, generalized disorder that occurs among patients over 60 years of age. Patients have no family history and lack the cognitive and behavioral changes seen in HD. The pathogenesis and pathophysiology of idiopathic chorea are poorly understood; no specific pathology has been demonstrated based on findings in the few cases that have come to autopsy. Choreiform or dyskinetic movements of unknown cause restricted to the mouth and tongue can be seen in the elderly and are more common among edentulous patients. The movements improve with proper dental appliances (61).

Generalized chorea, hemichorea, and hemiballism can be caused by vascular disease. Ischemic and hemorrhagic strokes and vascular malformations have been implicated as causes of sudden-onset chorea (61). The pathologic anatomy of vascular chorea is located in the basal ganglia, particularly the STN and GP, where small arterioles damaged by chronic hypertension either occlude (ischemic stroke) or rupture (hemorrhagic stroke) (25,102). Although the onset of vascular chorea is abrupt, it can follow the acute insult by weeks or months. The symptoms can resolve spontaneously or persist. Small-artery occlusion or rupture in the basal ganglia can also occur in patients with diabetes, patients with erythematosus, and, rarely, young women taking oral contraceptives with high estrogen content. When treatment is required, drugs that deplete dopamine from the presynaptic terminals (reserpine or tetrabenazine) or block postsynaptic receptors (neuroleptics) can be effective.

TARDIVE DYSKINESIA

The syndrome of TD, which is characterized by choreic and athetoid movements of the face, tongue, limbs, and trunk in isolation or in combination, results from treatment with dopamine receptor–blocking agents (DRBA), most often the older, traditional neuroleptics—the antipsychotics—and the progastrointestinal motility drug metoclopramide (Reglan). Chronic exposure to any dose of a DRBA, including the antinausea drug prochlorperazine (Compazine), for any length of time imposes a risk of TD. In contrast to acute dystonia or subacute parkinsonism associated with the use of these agents, tardive syndromes occur later in the course of treatment or in the setting of drug withdrawal (22). Tardive syndromes can also present with other types of involuntary movements, including akathisia (pathologic restlessness or inability to sit still), dystonia, parkinsonism, myoclonus, and tics (21). The most common manifestation is a pattern of repetitive, stereotyped movements of the mouth and tongue that are suppressed by action. Typically, classic TD consists of repetitive chewing, thrusting, or writhing movements of the mouth and tongue, all of which are relatively suppressed by action, such as talking. Similar movements can occur in the limbs, trunk, and respiratory muscles.

A diagnosis of a tardive syndrome requires exposure to one or more DRBA, with onset of symptoms within 6 months of use of a DRBA and persistence of symptoms for 1 month after withdrawal of the agent

(93). Additionally, patients should have no other clear cause for a movement disorder (5). Because older adults are at increased risk for developing TD, the *Diagnostic and Statistical Manual of Mental Disorders, Fourth Edition, Text Revision* (DSM IV-TR) allows for a diagnosis of TD to be considered in people older than 60 if all other criteria are in place and exposure to an offending drug is less than 1 month (3).

Among the atypical neuroleptics, clozapine and quetiapine appear to be least likely to induce tardive syndromes. Olanzapine and risperidone are atypical neuroleptics (104) with a theoretically lower tendency to cause a tardive movement disorder than the typical neuroleptics, but experience over the decade since they were introduced has shown a higher frequency than expected (33).

The pathogenesis of TD is unclear. The most popular hypothesis is that the dopamine receptor blockade induced by the neuroleptics creates a chemical denervation hypersensitivity with increased production of presynaptic dopamine as a result of interruption of the normal regulatory feedback loop that maintains a homeostatic steady-state of dopamine synthesis and catabolism. Support for this hypothesis is offered by the clinical observation that tardive involuntary movements frequently emerge when the causative drug is being tapered after long-term use. Withdrawal of the drug removes the dopamine receptor blockade, but the increased production of dopamine caused by the postsynaptic chemical denervation persists. Absolute proof for this pathologic mechanism is lacking (11,52).

Epidemiologic studies of TD have been hampered by discrepancies in diagnostic criteria and biased study samples. Data in one study suggest an incidence rate of approximately 5% per year for the 4 years studied (12). Older age and female gender have been consistent risk factors (51). Prevalence rates in a study of patients above 54 years of age using neuroleptics were 25%, 34%, and 53% at 1, 2, and 3 years, respectively (103). Longer duration of exposure and higher total cumulative dose also appear to increase the risk of TD (51).

The treatment of patients with TD is always challenging and often unsatisfactory. Once the involuntary movements appear, the offending agent should be slowly withdrawn or, if the offending drug is an antipsychotic necessary for the treatment of mental illness, substituted with a safer drug, such as clozapine or quetiapine. Increasing the dose of the DRBA may suppress the movements but at the expense of perpetuating or even aggravating the underlying process. If the offending agent is withdrawn reasonably soon after onset of the tardive movements, remission can occur but can take several years. Remissions are more likely in younger patients (91). The risk of TD associated

with the gastric dysmotility drug metoclopramide can be minimized by short-term use (12 weeks or less), as advised by the package insert. The same principle applies to the use of other neuroleptics, such as prochlorperazine for nausea, which have the hidden potential for causing TD in any user.

Dopamine-depleting agents (e.g., reserpine and tetrabenazine) have shown the most consistent results in the treatment of TD and have not been reported to aggravate the involuntary movements with long-term use. Reserpine has been shown to be beneficial in a randomized clinical trial at doses of 0.75 to 1.5 mg/day (37). Side effects include hypotension, parkinsonism, and depression. Atypical neuroleptics, particularly clozapine, have also been reported to improve the symptoms of TD (6). The mechanism of action is unclear because the atypical neuroleptics have a low affinity for dopamine receptors.

DYSTONIA

Dystonia is a syndrome of sustained muscle contractions, causing twisting, repetitive movements, and abnormal postures. Dystonic movements are distinguished from chorea by the sustained nature of the movements and postures. Dystonia is classified etiologically as primary or secondary and anatomically by affected body region—generalized or focal. Primary generalized dystonia (PGD) typically starts in the leg with onset before age 25 and is often hereditary, with autosomal dominant transmission, variable expression, and a 30% penetrance (97). At least 13 genes have been identified that are transmitted mostly as autosomal dominant clinical disorders in families with primary generalized and focal dystonia. The most common of these, but present only in a minority of patients with early-onset PGD, is a mutation at the *DYT1* locus on chromosome 9. Approximately 80% of patients who are *DYT* positive have an Ashkenazi Jewish ancestry. This autosomal dominant disorder is caused by a guanine-adenosine-guanine (GAG) deletion in the *torsin A* gene, a brain protein whose function is yet to be determined. Focal dystonias, in contrast, usually involve the arms, neck, and head; start after the age of 25; and are sporadic (31). Several secondary causes of dystonia are seen in the adult, including focal lesions of the brain (e.g., stroke of the basal ganglia, usually the putamen) and peripheral nervous system, degenerative disorders such as PD and PSP, and drugs. The same drugs that cause classic TD can also cause tardive dystonia. Patients with primary dystonia should have no findings on neurologic examination except for dystonia and, possibly, essential tremor, which frequently coexists with the dystonia. Dystonic tremor tends to be less regular than essential tremor (50). The workup for primary dystonia is negative, by definition, including a normal CT or MRI scan. Dystonia is considered focal if one body area is affected (a hand or the neck), segmental if two contiguous areas are affected (neck and arm), and generalized if both legs and another body area are affected or if both legs and the trunk are involved. The "sensory trick" is a characteristic feature of dystonia. Patients may be able to alleviate the dystonic movement by tactile or proprioceptive input, such as touching or supporting the affected body part against gravity.

Primary Segmental Dystonia

The head and neck are the most common sites for primary segmental dystonia (99). Examples include cervical dystonia (also known as spasmodic torticollis), blepharospasm, oromandibular dystonia (OMD), and spasmodic dysphonia. Cervical dystonia can present with rotation, flexion, extension, tilting of the head, or a combination of these. Sudden spasms of head jerking or head tremor are frequently associated. Blepharospasm can manifest as increased blinking or forced episodic eye closure. Blepharospasm is often exacerbated by reading, driving, or other visual triggers. Meige syndrome is the combination of blepharospasm and OMD. OMD involves the muscles of facial expression causing grimacing, puckering, lip smacking, and several other movements, including jaw opening, jaw closing, or bruxism (98). OMD must be distinguished from TD, which tends to have more regular movements, but the overlap can be considerable. Spasmodic dysphonia is a form of dystonia causing muscles in and around the larynx to assume excessively adducted or abducted positions. Patients with adduction dysphonia tend to have choked or staccato speech, whereas those with abduction dysphonia tend to have breathy, whispered speech (36).

Focal Limb Dystonia

Focal limb dystonias can affect the leg or, more commonly in adults, the arm. Primary limb dystonias are frequently task specific, such as writer's dystonia. In writer's dystonia, the force of the grip may be exaggerated, and the wrist and forearm can assume a flexed or extended posture. Writing becomes shaky and laborious. Several other task-specific dystonias have been described, including dystonias in string musicians, typists, and sportsmen (e.g., golfer's dystonia) (99). Dystonias that are initially task specific rarely generalize to other activities at a later time or spread to the homologous opposite limb.

Pathogenesis

The pathogenesis of dystonia is unknown. The physiologic hallmark of dystonia is sustained contraction of agonist and antagonist muscle pairs (84). In primary dystonia, the cortex and basal ganglia may be involved, according to one study using PET, which showed a relative metabolic overactivity of the lentiform nucleus and premotor cortices (18). This suggests that a relative imbalance or metabolic dissociation within the basal ganglia may be responsible for the hyperkinetic movements. Primary dystonia is not associated with any known histopathologic or biochemical lesion, although the volume of the putamen is increased by about 10% in one report (9).

TREATMENT

Nonpharmacologic treatments (e.g., physical therapy) may be useful in preventing contractures and increasing range of motion, particularly in cervical dystonia. In some cases, braces can be fitted to provide moderating sensory input similar to a sensory trick. The pharmacologic treatment of dystonia is largely based on empiric and anecdotal evidence. However, several randomized clinical trials have reported that anticholinergic agents (e.g., trihexyphenidyl and benztropine) are effective in young-onset generalized dystonia (32). Most older adults are unable to tolerate the relatively high doses required to relieve symptoms and signs. Benzodiazepines (e.g., clonazepam and lorazepam) and gamma-aminobutyric acid (GABA)–ergic agents such as baclofen (Lioresal) can also be helpful, and these agents can be used in combination.

The introduction of BTX in the 1980s revolutionized the treatment of dystonia, and BTX is now the first line of treatment in most cases. The primary effect of BTX is to induce a transient paralysis of skeletal muscles by inhibiting presynaptic release of acetylcholine across the neuromuscular junction (48). BTX type A (Botox) has been well studied and has been proved effective and safe in numerous types of focal dystonia, especially cervical dystonia and blepharospasm. Approximately 85% to 90% of patients will achieve satisfactory and sustained improvement, lasting 3 to 4 months in most cases (46,49). BTX type B (Myobloc) has been studied in the treatment of cervical dystonia and has similar efficacy as BTX type A. However, a trial comparing the two subtypes showed that BTX type B had more side effects and a shorter clinical response time (15). Repeat injections are needed as symptoms return. Adverse effects are uncommon and mild, depending on the toxin type, site injected, and dose delivered. For patients who are unresponsive to BTX, a variety of surgical procedures, including rhizotomy (intradural sectioning of the nerve root) and ramisectomy (extradural sectioning of a nerve division), have been attempted with mixed results (8). DBS has been shown to be effective in selected cases of generalized and focal dystonia (16). A recent randomized, blinded trial comparing neurostimulation or sham stimulation showed bilateral pallidal stimulation to be effective in controlling symptoms in patients with both primary generalized and segmental dystonia (56).

SUMMARY

The diagnosis of movement disorders in the elderly is particularly challenging because clinicians must distinguish between features of normal aging and true disease states. Movement disorders encompass a wide array of clinical phenomena, and clinical impression remains the basis for the most accurate diagnosis because neuroimaging and other technologies, despite advances in the last decade, are helpful in a small minority of cases. Effective treatment of movement disorders in the elderly depends entirely on the accuracy of the diagnosis and can be gratifying for both patient and clinician. Recent therapeutic innovations, such as BTX and DBS, have dramatically brightened the horizons of patients with chronic neurologic disabilities. Treatment strategies must, however, be tailored to the individual patient, with particular attention to medication side effects.

REFERENCES

1. Aarsland D, Perry R, Brown A, et al. Neuropathology of dementia in Parkinson's disease: a prospective, community-based study. *Ann Neurol.* 2005;58:773–776.
2. Adler CH, Singer C, O'Brien C, et al. Randomized, placebo-controlled study of tolcapone in patients with fluctuating Parkinson's disease treated with levodopa-carbidopa. *Arch Neurol.* 1998;55:1089–1095.
3. American Psychiatric Association. *Diagnostic and Statistical Manual of Mental Disorders.* 4th ed. Washington, DC: American Psychiatric Association; 2000.
4. Assal F, Spahr L, Hadengue A, et al. Tolcapone and fulminant hepatitis. *Lancet.* 1998;352:958.
5. Baldessarini RJ, Cole JO, Davis JM, et al. Tardive dyskinesia. Summary of a task force report of the American Psychiatric Association. *Am J Psychiatry.* 1980;137:1163–1172.
6. Bassitt DP, Neto MRL. Clozapine efficacy in tardive dyskinesia in schizophrenia patients. *Eur Arch Psychiatry Clin Neurosci.* 1998;248:209–211.
7. Bennett DA, Beckett LA, Murray AM, et al. Prevalence of parkinsonian signs and associated mortality in a community population of older adults. *N Engl J Med.* 1996;334:71–76.
8. Bertrand CM, Molina-Negro P. Selective peripheral denervation in 111 cases of spasmodic torticollis: rationale and results. *Adv Neurol.* 1987;50:637–643.
9. Black K, Ongur D, Perlmutter JS. Putamen volume in idiopathic focal dystonia. *Neurology.* 1998;51:819–824.
10. Calne DB. Treatment of Parkinson's disease. *N Engl J Med.* 1993;329:1021–1027.
11. Casey DE. Pathophysiology of antipsychotic drug-induced movement disorders. *J Clin Psychiatry.* 2004;65(suppl):25–28.
12. Chakos MH, Alvir JMJ, Woerner MG, et al. Incidence and correlates of tardive dyskinesia in first episode schizophrenia. *Arch Gen Psychiatry.* 1996;53:313–319.
13. Chen JY, Stern Y, Sano M, et al. Cumulative risks of developing extrapyramidal signs, psychosis, or myoclonus in the course of Alzheimer's disease. *Arch Neurol.* 1991;48:1141–1143.
14. Clayton DF, George JM. The synucleins: a family of proteins involved in synaptic function, plasticity, neurodegeneration and disease. *Trends Neuroci.* 1998;21:249–254.
15. Comella, CL, Jankovic J, Shannon KM. Comparison of botulinum toxin serotypes A and B for the treatment of cervical dystonia. *Neurology.* 2005;65:1423–1429.
16. Coubes P, Roubertie A, Vayssiere N, et al. Treatment of DYT-1—generalized dystonia by bilateral stimulation of the internal globus pallidus. *Lancet.* 2000;355:2220–2221.
17. Deuschl G, Schade-Brittinger C, Krack P, et al. A randomized trial of deep-brain stimulation for Parkinson's disease. *N Engl J Med.* 2006;355:896–908.
18. Eidelberg D, Moeller JR, Ishikawa T, et al. The metabolic topography of idiopathic torsion dystonia. *Brain.* 1995;118:1473–1484.
19. Factor SA. Literature review: intermittent subcutaneous apomorphine therapy in Parkinson's disease. *Neurology.* 2004;62:S12–S17.
20. Fahn S. The varied clinical expressions of dystonia. *Neurol Clin.* 1984;2:541–554.
21. Fahn S, Bressman SB. Should levodopa therapy for Parkinsonism be started early or late? Evidence against early treatment. *Can J Neurol Sci.* 1984;11:200–205.
22. Faurbye A, Rasch PJ, Peterson PB, et al. Neurological symptoms in pharmacotherapy of psychosis. *Acta Psychiatr Scand.* 1964;40:10–27.
23. Ferreira JJ, Galitzky M, Montrastruc JL, et al. Sleep attacks and Parkinson's disease treatment. *Lancet.* 2000;355:1333–1334.
24. Findley LJ, Gresty MA, Halmagyi GM. Tremor, the cogwheel phenomenon and clonus in Parkinson's disease. *J Neurol Neurosurg Psychiatry.* 1981;44:534–546.
25. Fukui T, Hasegawa Y, Seriyama S, et al. Hemiballism-hemichorea induced by subcortical ischemia. *Can J Neurol Sci.* 1993;20:324–328.

26. Galasko D, Katzman R, Salmon DP, et al. Clinical and neuropathological findings in Lewy body dementias. *Brain Cogn.* 1996;31:166–175.

27. Giasson BI, Lee VM. Parkin and the molecular pathways of Parkinson's disease. *Neuron.* 2001; 31:885–888.

28. Gillman S. Multiple system atrophy. In: Jankovic J, Tolosa E, eds. *Parkinson's disease and movement disorders.* 3rd ed. Baltimore: Williams & Wilkins; 1998:245–262.

29. Golbe LI. Progressive supranuclear palsy. In: Watts RL, Koller WC, eds. *Movement disorders, neurologic principles and practice.* New York: McGraw-Hill; 1997:279–296.

30. Golbe LI. Young-onset Parkinson's disease: a clinical review. *Neurology.* 1991;41:168–173.

31. Greene P, Kang UJ, Fahn S. Spread of symptoms in idiopathic torsion dystonia. *Mov Disord.* 1995;10:143–152.

32. Greene P, Shale H, Fahn S. Analysis of open label trials in torsion dystonia using high dosage anticholinergics and other drugs. *Mov Disord.* 1988;3:46–60.

33. Gutierrez-Esteinou R, Grebb JA. Risperidone: an analysis of the first three years in general use. *Int Clin Psychopharmacol.* 1997;12:S3–S10.

34. Hallett M, Litvan I. Evaluation of surgery for Parkinson's disease: a report of the Therapeutics and Technology Assessment Subcommittee of the American Academy of Neurology. The Task Force on Surgery for Parkinson's Disease. *Neurology.* 1999;53:1910–1921.

35. Hardy J, Cai H, Cookson MR, et al. Genetics of Parkinson's disease and parkinsonism. *Ann Neurol.* 2006;60:389–398.

36. Hartman DE, Aronson AE. Clinical investigations of intermittent breathy dysphonia. *J Speech Hear Disord.* 1991;46:428–432.

37. Huang CC, Wang RIH, Hasegawa A, et al. Evaluation of reserpine and alpha-methyldopa in the treatment of tardive dyskinesia. *Psychopharmacol Bull.* 1980;16:41–43.

38. Hubble J. Drug-induced parkinsonism. In: Stern MB, Koeller WC, eds. *Parkinsonian syndromes.* New York: Marcel Dekker; 1993:111–122.

39. Hughes AJ, Daniel SE, Kilford L, et al. Accuracy of the clinical diagnosis of idiopathic Parkinson's disease: a clinico-pathological study of 100 cases. *J Neurol Neurosurg Psychiatry.* 1992;55:181–184.

40. Hughes AJ, Daniel SW, Ben-Schlomo Y, et al. The accuracy of diagnosis of parkinsonian syndromes in a specialist movement disorders service. *Brain.* 2002;125:861–870.

41. Huntington's Disease Collaborative Research Group. A novel gene containing a trinucleotide repeat that is expanded and unstable on Huntington's disease chromosomes. *Cell.* 1993;72:971–982.

42. Huntington Study Group. Tetrabenazine as antichorea therapy in Huntington disease. *Neurology.* 2006;66:366–372.

43. Hurtig HI. Vascular parkinsonism. In: Stern MB, Koeller WC, eds. *Parkinsonian syndromes.* New York: Marcel Dekker; 1993:81–93.

44. Indo T, Ando K. Metoclopramide-induced parkinsonism. *Arch Neurol.* 1982;39:494–496.

45. Jankovic J. Tardive syndromes and other drug induced movement disorders. *Clin Neuropharmacol.* 1995;18:197–214.

46. Jankovic J. Treatment of dystonia. In: Watts RL, Koller WC, eds. *Movement disorders, neurologic principles and practice.* New York: McGraw-Hill; 1997:443–454.

47. Jankovic J, Ashizawa T. Huntington's disease. In: Appel SH, ed. *Current neurology.* Chicago: Mosby-Year Book; 1995:29–60.

48. Jankovic J, Brin MF. Therapeutic uses of botulism toxin. *N Engl J Med.* 1991;324:1186–1194.

49. Jankovic J, Schwartz K, Donovan DT. Botulism toxin treatment of cranial-cervical dystonia, spasmodic dysphonia, other focal dystonias, and hemifacial spasm. *J Neurol Neurosurg Psychiatry.* 1990;53:633–639.

50. Jednyak CP, Bonnet AM, Agid Y. Tremor and idiopathic dystonia. *Mov Disord.* 1991;6:230–236.

51. Kane JM, Woerner MW, Lieberman J. Tardive dyskinesia: prevalence, incidence and risk factors. *J Clin Psychopharmacol.* 1988;8:S52–S56.

52. Klawans HL, Rubovitz R. An experimental model of tardive dyskinesia. *J Neural Transm.* 1972;33:235–246.

53. Kompoliti K, Goetz CG, Boeve BF, et al. Clinical presentation and pharmacological therapy in corticobasal degeneration. *Arch Neurol.* 1998;55:957–961.

54. Krack P, Batir A, Van Blercom N. Five-year follow-up of bilateral stimulation of the subthalamic nucleus in advanced Parkinson's disease. *N Engl J Med.* 2003;349:1925–1934.

55. Krauss JK, Regel JP, Droste DW, et al. Movement disorders in adult hydrocephalus. *Mov Disord.* 1997;12:53–60.

56. Kupsch A, Benecke R, Müller J, et al. Pallidal deep-brain stimulation in primary generalized or segmental dystonia. *N Engl J Med.* 2006; 355:1978–1990.

57. Litvan I, Goetz CG, Jankovic J, et al. What is the accuracy of the clinical diagnosis of multiple system atrophy? *Arch Neurol.* 1997;54:937–944.

58. Litvan I, Paulsen JS, Mega MS, et al. Neuropsychiatric assessment of patients with hyperkinetic

and hypokinetic movement disorders. *Arch Neurol.* 1998;55:1313–1319.

59. Lowe J, Lennox G, Leigh PN. Disorders of movement and system degenerations. In: Graham DI, Lantos PL, eds. *Greenfield's neuropathology.* 6th ed. Vol 2. London: Arnold; 1997:281–366.

60. Mahapatra RK, Edwards MJ, Schott JM, et al. Corticobasal degeneration. *Lancet Neurol.* 2004;3:736–743.

61. Mark HM. Other choreatic disorders. In: Watts RL, Koller WC, eds. *Movement disorders, neurologic principles and practice.* New York: McGraw-Hill; 1997:527–539.

62. McKeith IG, Dickson DW, Lowe J, et al. Diagnosis and management of dementia with Lewy bodies: third report of the DLB Consortium. *Neurology.* 2005;65:1863–1873.

63. McTavish D, Goa KL. Midodrine: a review of the pharmacological properties and therapeutic use in orthostatic hypotension and secondary hypotensive disorders. *Drugs.* 1989;38:757–777.

64. Mega MS, Masterman DL, Benson DF, et al. Dementia with Lewy bodies: reliability and validity of clinical and pathologic criteria. *Neurology.* 1996;47:1403–1409.

65. Metman LV, Del Dotto P, van den Munckhof P, et al. Amantadine as treatment for dyskinesias and motor fluctuations in Parkinson's disease. *Neurology.* 1998;50:1323–1326.

66. Murrow RW, Schweiger GD, Kepes JJ, et al. Parkinsonism due to basal ganglia lacunar state: clinicopathologic correlation. *Neurology.* 1990; 40:897–900.

67. Nutt JG. Classification of gait and balance disorders. *Adv Neurol.* 2001;87:135–141.

68. Olanow CW, Hauser RA, Gauger L, et al. The effect of deprenyl and levodopa on the progression of Parkinson's disease. *Ann Neurol.* 1995; 38:771–777.

69. Olanow CW, Koller WC. An algorithm (decision tree) for the management of Parkinson's disease: treatment guidelines. *Neurology.* 1998; 50[Suppl 3]:S5–S7.

70. O'Suilleabhain P, Dewey RB. A randomized trial of amantadine in Huntington disease. *Arch Neurol.* 2003;60:996–998.

71. Parker SW. Dizziness in the elderly. In: Albert ML, Knoefel JE, eds. *Clinical neurology of aging.* 2nd ed. New York: Oxford University Press; 1994:569–579.

72. Parkinson Study Group. A controlled trial of rasagiline in early Parkinson disease. *Arch Neurol.* 2002;59:1937–1943.

73. Parkinson Study Group. A controlled, randomized, delayed-start study of rasagiline in early Parkinson disease. *Arch Neurol.* 2004;61: 561–566.

74. Parkinson Study Group. Effect of deprenyl on the progression of disability in early Parkinson's disease. *N Engl J Med.* 1989;321:1364–1371.

75. Parkinson Study Group. Impact of deprenyl and tocopherol treatment on Parkinson's disease in DATATOP patients requiring levodopa. *Ann Neurol.* 1996;39:37–45.

76. Parkinson Study Group. Levodopa and the progression of Parkinson's disease. *N Engl J Med.* 2004;351:2498–2508.

77. Parkinson Study Group. Pramipexole vs levodopa as initial treatment for Parkinson disease: a 4-year randomized controlled trial. *Arch Neurol.* 2004;61:1044–1053.

78. Paulson H, Stern MB. Clinical manifestations of Parkinson's disease. In: Watts RL, Koller WC, eds. *Movement disorders, neurologic principles and practice.* New York: McGraw-Hill; 1997:181–199.

79. Pavlakis AJ, Siroky MB, Goldstein I, et al. Neurologic findings in Parkinson's disease. *J Urol.* 1983;129:80–83.

80. Penny JB, Young AB, Snodgrass SR, et al. Huntington's disease in Venezuela: 7 years of follow-up on symptomatic and asymptomatic individuals. *Mov Disord.* 1990;5:93–99.

81. Rajput AH. Movement disorders and aging. In: Watts RL, Koller WC, eds. *Movement disorders, neurologic principles and practice.* New York: McGraw-Hill; 1997:674–686.

82. Rascol O, Brooks DJ, Korczyn AD, et al. A five-year study of the incidence of dyskinesia in patients with early Parkinson's disease who were treated with ropinirole or levodopa. *N Engl J Med.* 2000;342:1484–1491.

83. Rautakorpi I, Marttila RJ, Takal J, et al. Occurrences and causes of tremors. *Neuroepidemiology.* 1982;1:209–215.

84. Rothwell JC, Obeso JA. The anatomical and physiological basis of torsion dystonia. In: Marsden CD, Fahn S, eds. *Movement disorders.* London: Butterworths; 1987:313–331.

85. Savoiardo M, Strada L, Girotti F, et al. MR imaging in progressive supranuclear palsy and Shy-Drager syndrome. *J Comput Assist Tomogr.* 1989;13:555–560.

86. Schade R, Andersohn F, Suissa S, et al. Dopamine agonists and the risk of cardiac-valve regurgitation. *N Engl J Med.* 2007;356:29–38.

87. Schapira AHV. Sleep attacks (sleep episodes) with pergolide. *Lancet.* 2000;355:1332–1333.

88. Schöls L, Bauer P, Schmidt T, et al. Autosomal dominant cerebellar ataxias: clinical features, genetics and pathogenesis. *Lancet Neurol.* 2004;3:291–304.

89. Shannon KM. Hydrocephalus and parkinsonism. In: Stern MB, Koeller WC, eds. *Parkinsonian syndromes*. New York: Marcel Dekker; 1993:123–136.

90. Shults CW, Oakes D, Kieburtz K, et al. Effects of coenzyme Q10 in early Parkinson disease. *Arch Neurol*. 2002:59;1541–1550.

91. Smith JM, Baldessarini RJ. Changes in prevalence, severity, and recovery in tardive dyskinesia with age. *Arch Gen Psychiatry*. 1980;37:1368–1373.

92. Spiegel J, Storch A, Jost WH. Early diagnosis of Parkinson's disease. *J Neurol*. 2006:253:IV/2–IV/7.

93. Stacy M, Jankovic J. Tardive dyskinesia. *Curr Opin Neurol Neurosurg*. 1991;4:343–349.

94. Stern MB, Marek KL, Friedman J, et al. Monotherapy in early Parkinson's disease patients. *Mov Disord*. 2004;19:916–923.

95. Sudarsky L. Geriatrics: gait disorders in the elderly. *N Engl J Med*. 1990;322:1441–1446.

96. Tanner C, Hubble JP, Chan P. Epidemiology and genetics of Parkinson's disease. In: Watts RL, Koller WC, eds. *Movement disorders, neurologic principles and practice*. New York: McGraw-Hill; 1997:137–152.

97. Tarsy D, Simon DK. Dystonia. *N Engl J Med*. 2006;355:818–829.

98. Tolosa E, Kulisevsky J, Fahn S. Meige syndrome: primary and secondary forms. *Adv Neuol*. 1988;50:509–515.

99. Tolosa E, Marti JFM. Adult-onset idiopathic torsion dystonia. In: Watts RL, Koller WC, eds. *Movement disorders, neurologic principles and practice*. New York: McGraw-Hill; 1997:429–442.

100. Van Den Eeden SK, Tanner CM, Bernstein AL, et al. Incidence of Parkinson's disease: variation by age, gender and race/ethnicity. *Am J Epidemiol*. 2003;157:1015–1022.

101. Verhagen Metman L, Morris MJ, Farmer C, et al. Huntington's disease: a randomized, controlled trial using the NMDA-antagonist amantadine. *Neurology*. 2002;59:694–699.

102. Vidakovic A, Dragasevic N, Kostic VS. Hemiballism: report of 25 cases. *J Neurol Neurosurg Psychiatry*. 1994;57:945–949.

103. Woerner MG, Alvir JMJ, Saltz BL, et al. Prospective study of tardive dyskinesia in the elderly: rates and risk factors. *Am J Psychiatry*. 1998;155:1521–1528.

104. Wood A. Clinical experience with olanzapine, a new atypical antipsychotic. *Int Clin Psychopharmacol*. 1998;13:S59–S62.

105. Zanettini R, Antonini A, Gatto G, et al. Valvular heart disease and the use of dopamine agonists for Parkinson's disease. *N Engl J Med*. 2007;356:39–46.

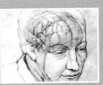

CHAPTER 23

Cognitive Aspects of Parkinson's Disease and Other Neurodegenerative Movement Disorders

Joshua R. Steinerman, Enrique Noé Sebastián, and Yaakov Stern

Although Parkinson's disease (PD), progressive supranuclear palsy (PSP), corticobasal ganglionic degeneration (CBGD), multiple system atrophy (MSA), and Huntington's disease (HD) have traditionally been described as neurodegenerative processes preserving mental functions, cognitive impairment is now fully accepted as part of the clinical presentation of these diseases (Table 23-1). Furthermore, cognitive dysfunction is a common source of disability for patients with degenerative movement disorders. Together with neurobehavioral disturbance, impaired cognition results in significant caregiver burden and is a powerful predictor of institutionalization. Because of their prevalence and impact, such nonmotor disease manifestations should be recognized and treated in conjunction with motor symptoms.

PARKINSON'S DISEASE

PD represents between 70% and 75% of all the parkinsonisms. It is the most common movement disorder in the elderly and one of the most common causes of disability in this population. The prevalence of PD is up to 1% of the population over 65 years of age, and this percentage increases with age. In fact, aging is the most consistent recognized risk factor for the disease. The age of onset varies between 40 and 70 years, with an incidence peak above 60 years of age. Less than 20% of cases have onset before 50 years of age. The progression and evolution of PD vary from patient to patient, with a mean survival time of approximately 10 to 15 years. The impact of the disease is clear if we consider that the risk for death or developing dementia in this disease is

Table 23-1. *Neuropsychological Pattern in Patients with Movement Disorders*

	PD	PD-D	CBGD	PSP	MSA	HD	AD
Orientation	−	++	−	−	−	−/+	+++
Language							
Naming	−/+	+	−/+	−/+	−/+	−/+	++
Fluency	++	+++	++	++	++	+++	+
Aphasia/paraphasia	−	−/+	++	−	−	−/+	+
Visuospatial function							
Visual memory	−/+	++	−/+	−/+	−/+	+	+++
Spatial reasoning	+	+++	+	++	+	++	++
Visuoconstructive	+	++	++	+	+	++	++
Memory							
Immediate recall	+	++	−/+	−/+	+	+	++
Delayed recall	−/+	++	−/+	−/+	−/+	+	+++
Recognition	−	+	−	−	−	−/+	+++
Praxis	−	++	+++	−/+	−	−/+	++
Executive function	++	+++	++	+++	++	++	+
Attention	+	+++	+	++	+++	++	++

(−) Normal function; (+) mild impairment; (++) moderate impairment; (+++) severe impairment.
AD, Alzheimer's disease; CBGD, corticobasal ganglionic degeneration; HD, Huntington's disease; MSA, multiple system atrophy; PD, Parkinson's disease; PD-D, Parkinson's disease with dementia; PSP, progressive supranuclear palsy.
Shading underlines the principal symptoms of each disease.

more than twofold greater than in an age-adjusted population (75).

PSYCHOSOCIAL ASPECTS AND HEALTH CARE

Since the advent of levodopa therapy, the mortality rate for patients with PD is not different compared with age- and sex-matched controls. Today, approximately 60% of patients are over 75 years at death, and the prevalence of the disease is as high as 3% among individuals older than 85 years of age. The decrease in elderly mortality and the improvement in treatment for early PD are generating an increasing number of families living with affected relatives and a greater percentage of patients living to experience the advanced stages of this disease.

The combination of the progressive course of the disease, the prolonged survival, and the broad range of impairment suggests that a high proportion of patients with PD may eventually need long-term care. European and American studies have estimated that the prevalence of patients with PD in nursing homes is about 5% to 10% and that up to 20% of older patients with the disease will eventually be institutionalized. Risk factors for nursing home placement are old age, living alone, motor disability, impairment of activities of daily living, dementia, and psychosis (3,85). A proactive treatment approach, focusing on optimization of general health, stress education, and disease education, is advisable from the time of diagnosis and may mitigate the need for auxiliary care.

PD markedly reduces patients' health-related quality of life, generates an important dysfunction on family roles and activities, and places a major socioeconomic impact on society. The economic costs of PD, including both direct health care costs (for drugs, physician services, and hospitalization) and indirect costs (for lost worker productivity), have been estimated to be around $25 billion per year (108). The total mean societal burden per individual with PD in the United States is more than $6,000/year ($4,000 for drugs, physician services, and hospitalization, and $2,000 for earnings loss) (123). The largest components of family burden are not direct health care costs, but providing informal care giving and earnings loss. The caregiver, usually the spouse, provides an average of 22 hours of care per week. After income loss ($12,000/patient/year), informal care giving is the single most expensive element of burden attributable to PD ($5,000/patient/year) (123).

CIRCUMSCRIBED COGNITIVE DEFICITS

Typical cognitive alterations present in PD include circumscribed deficits in memory, visuospatial, attention, and executive functions. Although mild cognitive deficits can be present in nearly all patients with the disease, they do not invariably progress to dementia. However, a clear progression was shown in approximately 20% of community-based PD patients over 2 years, with a relative risk of 1.7 compared to control subjects (77).

Executive Function

The broad set of abilities that comprise executive function include initiating and planning activities, attentional shifts, concept formation, problem solving, implementing behavior, self-control, and maintenance of socially appropriate behavior. Impairment in these processes has been associated with damage to the frontal lobes or frontal-subcortical circuitry. Numerous authors have reported executive deficits in patients with PD assessed with different tests. Set-shifting deficits have been reported in PD patients who have been tested using the Wisconsin Card Sorting Test (WCST), a conditional associative learning task based on three categorical sorting rules (number-color-shape). Patients with PD show a diminished number of categories and an increased number of perseverative errors. These deficits are present even in de novo patients, regardless of the age of onset, and especially if they are depressed (62,67,118). Similarly, set-shifting and set-maintenance difficulties (Odd-Man-Out Test, Stroop Test) have been reported, even at the beginning of the disease (48,103). Many other attentional and executive tasks are also altered in patients with PD (27,118), including:

- Working memory [Digit Span and Arithmetic subtests of the Wechsler Adult Intelligence Scale (WAIS)]
- Problem solving (Tower of London/Hanoi)
- Verbal or visuospatial abstract reasoning (Raven Progressive Matrices, Similarities and Comprehension subtests of the WAIS)
- Switching or planning (Trail Making Test, WCST)

Results of these tests taken by patients with PD suggest that these patients initially have difficulties in focusing attention and mental flexibility, which are necessary to shift and maintain mental sets. Deficits in initiation and in planning strategies needed to solve problems can occur later in the evolution of the disease.

Visuospatial Function

Visuospatial impairments are among the most common deficits described in PD for tasks including visual recognition, visual analysis and synthesis, spatial planning and attention, visual orientation, and visuoconstructive praxis. Deficits in facial recognition, which can appear 2 to 3 years after the diagnosis of the disease, may be the earliest affected visuospatial function in patients with PD (66). This impairment might not be noted in juvenile forms, suggesting that age might influence performance on this test (118). Deficits in perception, construction, and mental management of objects and figures and alterations in judgment of direction, orientation, and distance can appear later in the evolution of the disease, whatever the age of onset (94,118). Patients show deficits in almost all the performance subtests of the WAIS, including Picture Completion, Block Design, and Object Assembly. These deficits usually appear some years after the diagnosis of the disease, even in the juvenile onset, and are not related to motor dysfunction (66). Other studies have reported deficits in visuoconstructive graphomotor tasks, including difficulties copying complex figures (Rey-Osterrieth Figure) and impairments in copying simple designs (e.g., a house or a clock) with the evolution of the disease (28,56).

Most of the visuospatial tests studied in patients with PD demand manual dexterity or require active planning and strategy formation. However, visuoperceptual impairments have been reported even when motoric task demands are minimized. These impairments were not correlated with the duration of the disease or the severity of motor dysfunction (12,50). A significant correlation between executive and visuospatial tasks has been described, as have beneficial effects of problem-solving clues in visuospatial tasks in patients with PD (14). Qualitative analysis of visuoconstructive test performance shows figures reduced in size, distortions, poor organization, and significant omissions. These data suggest that impoverished performance on visuospatial function in patients with this disease is more related to difficulties in executive tasks and shifting attention than to pure visuospatial difficulties (18).

Memory and Learning

Explicit (declarative) memory deficits and implicit (procedural) memory impairments have consistently been reported in nondemented patients with PD. Explicit memory refers to the conscious recollection (free recall and cued recall) or recognition of a previous event or experience, whereas implicit memory includes perceptual or motor skills learned during life and not readily accessible to conscious recollection. Semantic explicit material (memory for conceptual knowledge and relations that are context free) is usually preserved compared with episodic explicit memory (memory for personally experienced events or episodes). However, some aspects of episodic memory, especially immediate memory, are more affected than long-term memory, cued retrieval, and recognition tasks. Verbal learning and working memory are also commonly affected.

Verbal memory is usually affected later than visuospatial memory because visuospatial material is not semantically related and the recall process requires a greater cognitive effort. As less external supports (fewer cues) are offered and more cognitive demand or self-initiated activities are required, more difficulties appear. For example, conditional associative learning would be more impaired than cue-dependent, paired associative learning because the former requires learning by trial and error. Also, recall of a text or a paragraph that has a semantic structure sufficient to guide memory is less affected than word list learning tasks in which organization must be self-elaborated (27,95). This factor could also explain the superior performance of patients with PD on recognition (which relies on external cues) as opposed to free recall tasks (relying on internal cues) and their ability to benefit from cueing (5). Long-term memory is generally less (and later) impaired than immediate memory, reflecting a problem in acquisition of information (immediate organization) more than a genuine storage, retention, and retrieval deficit (long-term recall) (19). Remote memory is generally preserved.

Although some controversial results have been seen, performance on implicit memory tasks can be affected in patients with PD (13). Because implicit memory refers to a form of remembering that can be expressed only through the performance of task operations, these deficits represent a slowness in the acquisition of new motor, perceptual, and cognitive skills. Some authors have also reported patients having difficulty maintaining these skills against a competing stimulus, suggesting, again, an attentional deficit (35).

Language and Communication

Typically, PD affects mechanical aspects of speech, especially articulatory components (e.g., speed, tone, and volume). These alterations generate monotonous, hypophonic, and dysarthric speech that can compromise communication with these patients. Repetitive speech disorders such as stuttering and palilalia are observed, especially in long-standing PD (8). Handwriting is commonly limited by motor impairments, typically manifest as small, cramped script (micrographia).

Patients with PD without dementia have been shown to be only slightly impaired in syntax and grammar tests and in lexical and semantic tasks. Lack of spontaneous speech, delayed responses, single-word answers, and reduction in the length of the phrases can reflect difficulty planning linguistic sentences and an effort to generate as much information as possible in single sentences (32,53). Vocabulary and naming tasks are usually preserved in nondemented patients with PD at the beginning of the disease, and they become affected with the evolution of the disease (45). Verbal fluency can be affected, even at early stages of the disease, especially if loosely defined categories (e.g., objects) or alternating categories (e.g., birds/colors) are included. Letter verbal fluency tasks are usually affected later than category tasks, suggesting that a "letter" rather than a "category" might act as a cueing device to facilitate semantic retrieval (26,28). Perseverative intrusions in fluency tasks suggest a difficulty shifting between letter categories under a time constraint. Similar to visuospatial and memory dysfunction, it is not clear whether verbal fluency deficits represent a specific language dysfunction or are the expression of an impairment in planning and initiating a systematic search in semantic memory (executive dysfunction).

DEMENTIA IN PARKINSON'S DISEASE

Cross-sectional studies of prevalence of dementia in PD have yielded varied results. Incidence is a better estimate than prevalence of the frequency of dementia in PD because dementia significantly reduces survival in this disease (75). There is an estimated dementia incidence of 3% new cases per year in patients under 60 years of age and up to 14% new cases per year in patients older than 80 years of age (77,80). A longitudinal study of 224 subjects with mean illness duration of 9 years revealed a baseline prevalence of 26% and a cumulative dementia prevalence of 78% after an 8-year follow-up period (1).

Risk factors for PD with dementia (PDD) include increased age, a lower educational background, older age at onset, depression, and longer duration or more severe disease (Table 23-2). Additionally, individuals presenting with PD motor subtypes such as akinetic-dominant (1) and postural instability gait disorder (PIGD) (20) have been shown to be at significantly increased risk for cognitive decline and dementia. Thus, their parkinsonism is more likely to consist of rigidity, bradykinesia, and postural instability instead of tremor (77,115). Demented patients respond poorly to levodopa and are more likely to have adverse psychiatric effects (depression and psychosis) related to dopaminergic therapy.

Neuropsychological studies in nondemented PD subjects have generally associated impairment in executive functions with increased risk for dementia; some have found memory or visuospatial impairment to be predictive as well. One study found that impairment in letter and category fluency tests increased the likelihood of later incident dementia (55). A follow-up study from the same group using an expanded cohort and longer follow-up demonstrated that, in addition to tests of executive function, impaired verbal memory was a significant predictor of incident dementia (68). A separate report related increased dementia risk to impairments in a visuospatial task and the Stroop interference task, in addition to verbal fluency (76). A recent study found that performance on the Stroop interference task was the only significant neuropsychological predictor of dementia in their sample (57).

As in nondemented patients, almost all patients with PDD show prominent executive dysfunction that includes difficulties with planning, problem solving, concept formation, and abstract reasoning when evaluated with frontal-executive tests previously

Table 23-2. *Risk Factors for Dementia in Parkinson's Disease*

Risk Factors	Risk Ratio
Demographic factors	
Age	1.06
Education	1.01
Gender (female)	0.73
Clinical factors	
Age of onset of Parkinson's disease (>60 years)	4.1
Duration of Parkinson's disease (years)	1.01
Unified Parkinson's Disease Rating Scale-Motor Scale (>25)	1.04–3.56
Hamilton Depression Scale (>10)	1.11–3.55
Neuropsychological factors	
Picture Completion of the Wechsler Adult Intelligent Scale (<10)	4.9
Stroop Test (interference <21)	3.8
Letter fluency (CFL <27, M <9)	3.3–2.7
Category fluency (animal, food, clothing <42)	6.01

Data from Jacobs DM, Marder K, Cote LJ, et al. Neuropsychological characteristics of preclinical dementia in Parkinson's disease. *Neurology.* 1995;45:1691–1696; Marder K, Tang MX, Cote L, et al. The frequency and associated risk factors for dementia in patients with Parkinson's disease. *Arch Neurol.* 1995;52:695–701; and Mahieux F, Fenelon G, Flahault A, et al. Neuropsychological prediction of dementia in Parkinson's disease. *J Neurol Neurosurg Psychiatry.* 1998;64:178–183, with permission.

described (73). Visuospatial, visuoperceptual, and visuoconstructive problems are common, even when patients are evaluated with tasks requiring minimal motor demands. Demented patients with PD demonstrate difficulties recognizing faces, assembling objects, drawing figures, mentally assembling puzzles, formulating line and angular judgments, and identifying embedded figures. Most of these deficits are similar to those found in Alzheimer's disease (AD); however, patients with PD performed significantly better on visuospatial memory tasks and had worse visual abstract reasoning when compared with patients with AD. Both declarative and procedural memory may be affected in a similar pattern described previously in nondemented patients with PD.

Cross-sectional studies comparing demented patients with PD with AD patients have shown that the former perform worse on verbal fluency tasks and show better recognition memory (despite equally impaired recall) and a slower rate of forgetting from immediate to delayed recall. Longitudinal studies have confirmed these results and have reported a more rapid decline in naming, delayed recall, and category verbal fluency in PDD. They also described how patients with AD had a poorer performance on delayed recognition memory (47,52,116,117).

Although aphasia is rare, language deficits are present in PDD and include naming and word-finding difficulties, perseverations, decreased phrase length, diminished verbal fluency, and impaired strategies in sentence comprehension (32,52). Compared with AD patients, patients with PD are less likely to have poorer semantic than phonemic fluency.

There remain outstanding questions regarding the overlap and boundary issues between PDD and dementia with Lewy bodies (DLB), although a consensus statement and research agenda have recently been put forth (69). The traditional clinical distinction between the two syndromes reflects the timing of the cognitive decline relative to the motor symptoms (≤1 year in DLB vs. >1 year in PDD). The clinical and cognitive profiles of the two disorders are much the same, and no single feature distinguishes between them. Where there are differences, they are subtle and not qualitatively distinct: DLB patients may make more conceptual and attentional errors, have more pronounced hallucinations and psychosis, and display more frequent adverse reactions to antipsychotic medications; PDD patients tend to have more cardinal signs of parkinsonism and motor asymmetry.

PSYCHIATRIC FEATURES

Up to 60% of patients with PD experience psychiatric complications. The most frequent are mood disorders, anxiety syndromes, and drug-induced psychosis (Table 23-3) (3).

Depression

The prevalence rate of depression in PD is unclear, ranging from 5% to 90%, a percentage significantly higher than in age-matched control groups. Depression in PD may be difficult to recognize because many of the traditional symptoms associated with the diagnosis of depression may be present because of motor disability. Major depression is present in 20% of the cases, whereas others experience adjustment disorders, dysthymia, or bipolar disorders (30). Depression in PD shares symptoms of primary affective depressive disorders, including feelings of poor self-esteem and loss of social, family, and interpersonal relationships. Other atypical features include comorbid anxiety and panic attacks (40% of the cases), irritability and disinhibition (30%), and psychosis (10%) (109).

Depressive symptoms in PD are a combination of endogenous and exogenous factors. Depression can antedate any recognizable motor symptoms and occur independently of disease duration and motor impairment. These data suggest that the depressive syndrome may be caused by endogenous deficiency in monoamines, especially serotonin, more than a reaction to physical impairment. On the other hand, some studies have shown that successful treatment of depression can be associated with better motor function, and motor improvement may be associated with improved mood. So, reactive depression in response to having an inexorably progressive and debilitating disease can predominate at some point in the evolution of the disease (112).

Apathy can be present in PD as a symptom of major depression, delirium, or dementia or as an independent syndrome. Emotional lability is present in 40% of patients from the onset of the disease.

Anxiety

Generalized anxiety disorders occur in 20% to 40% of patients with PD; social phobia or panic disorder is seen in up to 25% of the patients; and mania or euphoria can appear in 10% of the patients. These symptoms may precede the onset of motor features, accompany a major depressive syndrome, and persist after the depressive illness is treated (23,114). Commonly, anxiety appears in fluctuating patients ("on-off" motor fluctuations) during "off" periods, when the patient experiences worsening of parkinsonian symptoms. Anxiety syndromes have to be differentiated from the understandable psychological response to motor impairment, the somatic complaints related to autonomic symptoms, and akathisia (the necessity to be in constant motion), which is a frequent feature of PD.

Table 23-3. *Neuropsychiatric Disturbances in Movement Disorders*

	PD %	CBGD %	PSP %	MSA %	HD %	AD %
Depression	5–90	38–75	18	30–50	9–44	20–50
Apathy	41	40	91	90	34–50	70–90
Anxiety	20–66	13	18	8	34	40–60
Delusions	10–20	7	0	15	6–25	20–50
Hallucinations	4–40	0	0	15	10	5–40
Irritability	30	20	9	?	38–50	42
Euphoria	2–33	0	0	?	10–17	3–17
Disinhibition	12–30	20	36	?	24	36
Agitation	30	20	5	?	50	48–70
Sleep disorders	67–88	?	?(Most)	?(Most)	20	45

AD, Alzheimer's disease; CBGD, corticobasal ganglionic degeneration; HD, Huntington's disease; MSA, multiple system atrophy; PD, Parkinson's disease; PSP, progressive supranuclear palsy.
Shading underlines the principal symptoms of each disease. (?) means that no epidemiologic studies are published yet.
Data are from: Aarsland D, Larsen JP, Lim NG, et al. Range of neuropsychiatric disturbances in patients with Parkinson's disease. *J Neurol Neurosurg Psychiatry*. 1999;67:492–496; Burns A, Folstein S, Brandt J, et al. Clinical assessment of irritability, aggression, and apathy in Huntington's and Alzheimer's disease. *J Nerv Ment Dis*. 1990;178:20–26; Celesia GG, Barr AN. Psychosis and other psychiatric manifestations of levodopa therapy. *Arch Neurol*. 1970;23:193–200; Chokroverty S. Sleep and degenerative neurologic disorders. *Neurol Clin*. 1996;4:807–826; Cummings JL. Depression and Parkinson's disease: a review. *Am J Psychiatry*. 1992;149:443–454; Cummings JL, Cunningham K. Obsessive-compulsive disorder in Huntington's disease. *Biol Psychiatry*. 1992;31:263–270; Dubois B, Pillon B, Lhermitte F, et al. Cholinergic deficiency and frontal dysfunction in Parkinson's disease. *Ann Neurol*. 1990;28:117–121; Esmonde T, Giles E, Gibson M, et al. Neuropsychological performance, disease severity, and depression in progressive supranuclear palsy. *J Neurol*. 1996;243:638–643; Fetoni V, Soliveri P, Monza D, et al. Affective symptoms in multiple system atrophy and Parkinson's disease: response to levodopa therapy. *J Neurol Neurosurg Psychiatry*. 1999;66:541–544; Folstein SE, Folstein MF. Psychiatric features of Huntington's disease: recent approaches and findings. *Psychiatr Dev*. 1983;1:193–205; Inzelberg R, Kipervasser S, Korczyn AD. Auditory hallucinations in Parkinson's disease. *J Neurol Neurosurg Psychiatry*. 1998;64:533–535; Litvan I, Cummings JL, Mega M. Neuropsychiatric features of corticobasal degeneration. *J Neurol Neurosurg Psychiatry*. 1998;65:717–721; Litvan I, Mega MS, Cummings JL, et al. Neuropsychiatric aspects of progressive supranuclear palsy. *Neurology*. 1996;47:1184–1189; Livtan I, Paulsen JS, Mega MS, et al. Neuropsychiatric assessment of patients with hyperkinetic and hypokinetic movement disorders. *Arch Neurol*. 1998;55:1313–1319; Pilo L, Ring H, Quinn N, et al. Depression in multiple system atrophy and in idiopathic Parkinson's disease: a pilot comparative study. *Biol Psychiatry*. 1996;39:803–807; Sanchez-Ramos JR, Ortoll R, Paulson GW. Visual hallucinations associated with Parkinson's disease. *Arch Neurol*. 1996;53:1265–1268; Stein MB, Heuser IJ, Juncos JL, et al. Anxiety disorders in patients with Parkinson's disease. *Am J Psychiatry*. 1990;147:217–220.

Sleep Disorders

Sleep disturbances occur in more than 75% of patients with PD, especially in those with advanced disease and older onset. These patients may experience difficulty falling asleep because of anxiety, but fragmentation of nocturnal sleep is more commonly seen, with frequent awakenings and sleepiness in the morning (24). Circadian rhythm disturbances, with daytime sleepiness and sudden urge to sleep ("sleep attacks"), may be related to the disease itself, although they have also been associated with dopamine agonist use (89). Rapid eye movement (REM) sleep behavior disorder, characterized by loss of physiologic atonia and prominent abnormal movements and vocalizations during REM sleep, is a common cause of disrupted sleep in PD patients and their bed partners.

Psychosis

Psychosis, which occurs in up to 40% of patients with PD, is generally drug related and a major precipitant of nursing home placement. Psychosis can occur in up to 80% of demented patients with PD but also in up to 20% of cognitively intact patients (54,107). Although psychoses are often considered a levodopa effect, they occur with all dopaminergic drugs. Prevalence rates of psychosis increase with the presence of cognitive impairment, depressive symptoms, sleep-wake disturbances, older age, and longer duration of the disease (29).

Hallucinations usually occur as a late complication of antiparkinsonian medication in the context of a clear sensorium but can also be present as features of major depressive episodes or mania syndromes or as a part of a drug-induced toxic delirium. Polymodal, disturbing, and vague in content hallucinations are more common during delirium. Visual, well-formed, not frightening, and nocturnal hallucinations are more common in the context of a clear mental sensorium (106). In these cases, the most frequent types of hallucinations are the vivid sensation of the presence of somebody, brief visions of a person or an animal passing sideways, and elaborate visual hallucinations (79).

Illusions (10% to 20%) and auditory hallucinations (10%) are less common and usually accompany visual hallucinations. Delusions are present in approximately 10% of patients after some years of dopaminergic treatment. They are usually accompanied or preceded by vivid dreams, nightmares, or visual hallucinations. Delusions are complex in content and well structured. Paranoid, grandiosity, erotomanic, and auto-referential contents are common (29). Although a decrease in sexual activity with loss of libido is present in the early stages of PD, hypersexuality and altered sexual behavior (e.g., paraphilia, exhibitionistic thoughts, voyeurism, pedophilia) have also been reported in 1% to 13% of the patients after initiating dopaminergic treatment (119).

PATHOLOGY

The pathologic hallmark of PD is the progressive loss of dopaminergic cells in the substantia nigra, with associated intraneuronal aggregates of the protein α-synuclein, termed Lewy bodies. The prominent impairment on executive tasks described in the disease and most of the psychiatric complications associated with it have been attributed to degeneration of frontosubcortical circuits. These systems link specific areas of the frontal cortex involved in executive function (dorsolateral cortex), motivation (orbitofrontal cortex), and social behavior (anterior cingulate cortex) with the striatum, globus pallidus, and thalamus (4). It has been suggested that the decreased dopaminergic nigrostriatal stimulation induces cognitive and behavior abnormalities, reflecting interruption of these circuits.

Degeneration of the medial substantia nigra, with associated loss of dopaminergic nigral projections to the limbic cortex (mesolimbic pathway) and frontal areas (mesocortical pathway), has also been implicated in cognitive dysfunction. In addition to the predominant dopaminergic deficiency, degeneration of subcortical ascending systems with neuronal losses in serotonergic, cholinergic, and noradrenergic nuclei has also been reported in PD. Involvement of these neurotransmitter systems has been related to depression and cognitive dysfunction in some patients with the disease.

PDD is characterized pathologically by the spread of Lewy bodies to the cerebral cortex. Concurrent

pathologies may variously contribute to the dementia syndrome and can include neuronal loss, cholinergic deficit, vascular injury, and AD-associated amyloid plaques and neurofibrillary tangles.

TREATMENT

The most important consideration when prescribing a medication for patients with parkinsonian symptoms is that the underlying brain disease and older age renders them especially vulnerable to adverse effects. Often, patients respond to low doses of medicine. Increasing the dose runs the risk of aggravating motor and cognitive symptoms. Before adding any new treatment, a careful review of antiparkinsonian and other medications should be done in an effort to reduce polypharmacy and drug interactions. Systemic and other causes of cognitive or behavioral symptoms should be ruled out (e.g., infections, metabolic alterations, and endocrine imbalances). Finally, when prescribing any new drug, increase the dosage slowly, and taper over a long period when discontinuing (120).

Cognitive Impairment

There are now effective drug therapies for PD associated dementia (86). There have been several randomized, placebo-controlled trials of cholinesterase inhibitors initially approved for use in AD. A small, 20-week crossover trial of donepezil demonstrated improvements on MMSE and a Clinician's Global Impression of Change (CGI) Scale without worsening of PD motor scores (2). Another small study of donepezil in PD dementia used a 10-week crossover design with a 6-week washout period. Again, there was a significant improvement among the donepezil arm in the secondary outcomes of MMSE and CGI. There was a trend toward improvement of the primary outcome, the Alzheimer's Disease Assessment Scale–Cognitive Subscale (ADAS-cog); similar to the previous study, no worsening in parkinsonism or tremor was noted (100). Subsequently, a large, 24-week trial of rivastigmine demonstrated a significant mean improvement of 2.1 on the 70-point ADAS-cog scale compared to a 0.7-point decline in the placebo arm; worsened tremor was reported in 10% of the rivastigmine group and 4% of the placebo group (36). In 2006, largely on the basis of this study, rivastigmine was approved by the Food and Drug Administration (FDA) for mild to moderate dementia associated with PD. In summary, modest cognitive improvements have been observed with treatment with cholinesterase inhibitors in PD dementia. Gastrointestinal side effects are common with these agents; patients should also be monitored for worsened tremor.

Anticholinergic drugs, which are sometimes used to treat tremor, have a recognized negative effect on memory [Wechsler Memory Scale (WMS)], executive (WCST), and attentional (Digit Span) tasks in PD (27,35). Cognitive side effects of anticholinergic drugs are more likely to occur in older and demented patients, so this kind of treatment should be reserved for younger nondemented patients. Short-term memory may recover, at least partly, after withdrawal of long-term anticholinergic medication.

Deep brain stimulation (DBS) is an increasingly used treatment option for control of motor symptoms in PD. The cognitive sequelae of this intervention are not yet established, due in part to its novelty and methodologic shortcomings of early studies. Two recent studies reported declines in select neuropsychological variables but relatively favorable outcomes in the context of improved motor function and quality of life (25,110). Nevertheless, some individuals experience a dramatic cognitive decline, highlighting the need for further study and optimized patient selection for this surgical treatment (111).

Psychiatric Symptoms

Antidepressants Depression treatment should not be delayed because early treatment of depressed patients can result in a less severe cognitive decline. The use of classic nonselective monoamine oxidase inhibitors and the combination of these drugs with other antidepressants should be avoided because of the high prevalence of side effects. The overall efficacy of most antidepressants is similar, but the selective serotonin reuptake inhibitors (SSRIs) have advantages over tricyclic antidepressants (TCA) because of the absence of anticholinergic features. The doses of SSRIs for depression in patients with PD are the same as for depression in the general population. Some reported cases have suggested that SSRIs worsen the motor condition for patients with this disease. Electroconvulsive therapy is another effective treatment for depression in patients with PD (30).

Anxiolytics and Hypnotics Anxiety associated with *off periods* should be managed by strategies designed to lessen the severity of the motor symptoms and to increase the *on time*. If this does not control the anxiety, benzodiazepines, buspirone, and antidepressants can be used in the management of these symptoms. Short-acting benzodiazepines—alprazolam and lorazepam—are better tolerated (less confusion) in older populations but have the disadvantage of their repeated administration. Buspirone does not have the sedative side effects of benzodiazepines and seems to be effective in reducing aggressive and anxiety symptoms. Sedative TCAs can be used as anxiolytics, whereas stimulating SSRIs may be useful in apathy.

However, because of the anticholinergic and orthostatic hypotensive properties of TCAs, SSRIs are preferred for the treatment of anxiety associated with agitated depression.

Levodopa can cause sleep disruption in patients with mild to moderate disease but has a beneficial effect on those nocturnal disabilities that cause sleep disruption in more severely affected patients. Hypnotic agents, as well as trazodone, or atypical antipsychotics can help with insomnia.

Antipsychotics Traditional antipsychotic agents (e.g., haloperidol) block dopaminergic D_2 receptors and have long been associated with drug-induced parkinsonism; they should be avoided in the patient with PD. Atypical antipsychotic agents such as clozapine and quetiapine are unlikely to worsen parkinsonism, either because of their affinities for non–D_2 dopamine receptors or their preferential action on mesocortical and mesolimbic systems. They are preferred agents if drug treatment is necessary to address psychosis or other disturbing behavioral symptoms in PD. Sedation is the most frequent side effect of clozapine (20%), whereas granulocytopenia (1% to 3%) is the most serious and requires regular hematologic monitoring. Quetiapine may be a less potent antipsychotic, but its safety profile and ease of use often make this a preferred first-line therapy. Drowsiness, orthostatic hypotension, and weight gain are potential adverse effects. It should be noted that atypical antipsychotics are not FDA approved for psychosis in dementia and are thought to lead to small increases in mortality. Thus, detailed discussion with caregivers, behavioral approaches, and consideration of other behavior-modifying drug classes should precede the initiation of an antipsychotic drug. Anecdotal evidence and the results of small open-label trials suggest that the cholinesterase inhibitors rivastigmine, donepezil, and galantamine may improve psychotic symptoms in PD (1,11,101).

CORTICOBASAL GANGLIONIC DEGENERATION

CBGD represents approximately 5% of all the parkinsonisms. The age of onset is between 60 and 70 years, but earlier onset has been reported. The mean evolution is around 7 years. The major features of the disease are cortical (e.g., aphasia, apraxia, and agnosia) and subcortical (e.g., parkinsonism, limb dystonia, and bulbar abnormalities). The parkinsonism responds poorly to levodopa; it is usually asymmetric, with rigidity and bradykinesia more common than tremor, and is frequently associated with atypical signs (e.g., myoclonus or a Babinski sign) (43,104).

CIRCUMSCRIBED COGNITIVE DEFICITS

Aphasia occurs in up to 53% of patients with CBGD. Aphasia is typically nonfluent and associated with dysnomia, perseverations, and paraphasias. Speech is almost always abnormal, especially as the disease progresses, and has been described as slow, slurred, dysphonic, mute, echolalic (involuntary repetition of words and phrases spoken by others), or palilalic (repetition of a phrase involuntarily with increasing rapidity) (42).

Apraxia, defined as the inability to carry out purposeful movements despite intact comprehension, muscular power, sensibility, and coordination, can occur in more than 70% of patients with CBGD. *Ideomotor* apraxia is when the implementation of a gesture in a motor program is disrupted such that the patient uses an incorrect gesture but can imitate a movement. *Ideational* apraxia is when the gesture is lacking so the patient does not know how to do or imitate a movement. *Constructive* apraxia is an inability to represent graphically geometric patterns. Dressing apraxia, apraxia of gaze, apraxia of eyelids, buccofacial apraxia, apraxia of speech, and apraxia of gait have all been reported as well. Limb apraxia, the most common form, can be asymmetric, frequently affecting the right upper extremity; it is sometimes difficult to evaluate because of other coexisting motor disturbances (64,96). Both aphasia and apraxia can be symptoms of the disease, but nearly all cases presenting with progressive aphasia eventually evolve to show impairment in other cognitive spheres (Table 23-1).

Although neglect syndromes have been noted in a few patients, "alien limb phenomenon" (limb movements without patient awareness) is reported to occur in 50% of patients with CBGD. Alien limb phenomena include levitation and posturing of the arm when attention is diverted or the eyes are closed, mechanical movement against patient's wishes, and a tendency to "forget" the limb while walking. Cortical sensory loss (impaired stereognosis, graphesthesia, two-point discrimination, and double simultaneous stimulation) has also been reported (104).

DEMENTIA

Approximately 25% to 45% of patients with CBGD become demented as the disease evolves (104). The clinical characteristics of dementia accompanying CBGD are similar to those found in other parkinsonisms, with the exception of an increased number of cortical symptoms (e.g., aphasia, apraxia, agnosia) and a high prevalence of visuospatial and constructional deficits accompanying the executive difficulties. Immediate and delayed recall of verbal material is generally preserved compared with patients with AD, whereas praxis, motor programming, sustained attention, and mental control tasks are moderately impaired (78). Frontotemporal dementia is the principal clinical differential diagnosis, which can be difficult to differentiate in the absence of typical motor features (59). Impaired attention, acalculia, difficulties in recall and learning, abstract reasoning deficits, and left-right confusion have been noted in a number of patients.

PSYCHIATRIC FEATURES

More than 75% of patients with CBGD manifest neuropsychiatric features, mostly depressive symptoms (73%) and personality changes including irritability (20%), increased aggression (20%), apathy (40%), and, less commonly, anxiety, disinhibition, or drug-induced psychoses (Table 23-3) (70).

PATHOLOGY

The characteristic combination of both cortical and subcortical cognitive changes in CBGD is mirrored by similar mixed neuropathologic changes. Subcortical pathology includes neuronal loss and gliosis in the substantia nigra, locus ceruleus, thalamus, subthalamic nucleus, red nucleus, and midbrain tegmentum (43). Similar to PD, degeneration of multiple subcortical ascending systems may be responsible for some of the cognitive dysfunction found in these patients, especially the executive deficits.

On the other hand, cortical changes include cell loss, gliosis, and the presence of *tau*-positive astrocytic plaques, especially in frontoparietal regions contralateral to the side of the body with pronounced motor symptoms. The hippocampus is typically spared. Involvement of these cortical areas has been related to the presence of ideomotor apraxia, ideational apraxia, visuospatial and constructional disorders, and neglect syndromes (88). Both cortical and subcortical changes contribute to aphasic syndromes.

PROGRESSIVE SUPRANUCLEAR PALSY

PSP is a rare neurodegenerative disorder accounting for approximately 5% of all the parkinsonisms. The age of onset (50 to 75 years) and the clinical symptoms resemble PD, although the presence of early gait disturbances with falls, pseudobulbar palsy, nuchal dystonia, and supranuclear gaze palsy may help in the differential diagnosis. The prevalence is approximately one in 10,000 and increases with age. The mean interval from onset of symptoms to diagnosis is approximately 3 to 4 years, and the median survival time from onset to death is 6 years (71). The presence of cognitive and behavioral abnormalities in PSP was first described by Steele et al. (113) in 1964. The prominent features they reported included emotional and personality disturbances associated with mild cognitive deficits early in the clinical course of the disease.

CIRCUMSCRIBED COGNITIVE DEFICITS

More than half of patients with newly diagnosed disease and almost all long-term patients show some kind of cognitive impairment on neuropsychological assessment (Table 23-1).

Visuospatial Function

The performance subtests of the WAIS and other visuoconstructive tests are impaired in patients with PSP (84). These deficits should be interpreted cautiously because most patients present with oculomotor abnormalities and motor disabilities, which may interfere with their task performance. This is especially true in cases where the evaluation includes tasks relying heavily on visual search and scanning ability (digit symbol), timed tests (block design, picture completion, and picture arrangement), or graphomotor abilities (drawing tests) (37).

Memory

Although complaints of forgetfulness are common, the memory disorder of PSP is generally mild and affects semantic more than episodic memory (121). Most of the recall difficulties are relayed in the executive component of memory tasks, which generates abnormally rapid forgetting, increased sensitivity to interference, and difficulty using strategic mechanisms when searching information. This can also explain why most of these abnormalities are considerably alleviated or even normalized by controlled encoding associated with cued recall.

Language

Semantic and syntactic components of language are often preserved, but motor components are severely affected. Dysarthria associated with a severe reduction of spontaneous speech often impairs communicative ability. Letter and semantic verbal fluency tasks are equally affected (105). Reading difficulties, visual dyslexia, constructional dysgraphia, an increased rate of self-corrections, misnaming, and disturbances of handwriting have also been reported (99).

Executive Function

Comparative studies of patients with PD, striatonigral degeneration (SND), and PSP have shown that the latter presents the earliest and most severe deficits on tasks sensitive to frontal lobe function (91,96). Neuropsychologically, this represents problems in response initiation (verbal fluency tasks are impoverished), planning (decreased motor speed and information process on Trail Making Tests), shifting of attention (increased interference effect on Stroop Test), or problem solving (failure to develop logical strategies to solve the WCST). This produces an abnormal regulation of behavior that is associated with a loss of interest in the environment, inertia, lack of initiative, and a marked reduction in spontaneous activity.

DEMENTIA

Estimates of the prevalence of dementia in PSP range from 20% to 70%. The term "subcortical dementia" was originally used to describe this condition, although the overlap with frontal executive deficits led to the term "frontosubcortical dementia" being proposed (82). This pattern can be useful in distinguishing patients with PSP who are demented from other cortical dementias (e.g., AD). On the other hand, dementia in PSP is more frequent, is more severe (especially in frontal tasks), and appears earlier than dementia in other parkinsonisms.

PSYCHIATRIC FEATURES

Apathy is the dominant behavior change found in PSP (91%) and is only occasionally accompanied by depression (18%). Disinhibition, obsessive disorders, inappropriate sexual behavior, aggressiveness, and impulsive behavior occur in one third of patients with this disease. Lability of mood, emotional incontinence, perseverative responses, and grasping, imitation, and utilization behaviors have also been reported. Sleep disorders are present in almost all cases of PSP (Table 23-3) (24,72).

PATHOLOGY

Pathologic changes in PSP occur in diffuse regions of the basal ganglia (caudate, globus pallidus, and subthalamic nucleus), thalamus, and brainstem (substantia nigra, red nucleus, reticular formation, locus ceruleus, superior colliculus, third and fourth cranial nerve nuclei, and vestibular and dentate nuclei), with minimal changes in the frontal cerebral cortex (33). Involvement of the dopaminergic nigrostriatal pathway, associated with damage in several output nuclei (striatum, thalamus) and afferent areas (frontal cortex), has been related to the greater dysexecutive syndrome found in PSP. Dementia has been attributed to a disruption of the subcorticofrontal connections needed to activate frontal lobe function as well as a dysfunction of cholinergic substantia innominata cortical and septohippocampal systems involved in memory processes. Uncontrolled behaviors are considered to result from the lack of inhibitory frontal lobe control.

MULTIPLE SYSTEM ATROPHY

MSA includes three different entities considered to be different manifestations of a single disease process: olivopontocerebellar atrophy (OPCA), SND, and

Shy-Drager syndrome (SDS). Autopsy studies show that 7% to 20% of patients diagnosed with PD have pathologic evidence of MSA. The median age of onset is 60 years, and the median survival time from onset of motor symptoms is 7.5 years. Although motor symptoms are the prominent and distinguishing features of MSA, cognitive changes are commonly associated symptoms (Table 23-1) (9).

CIRCUMSCRIBED COGNITIVE DEFICITS AND DEMENTIA
Olivopontocerebellar Atrophy

Dementia has been reported in up to 60% of the familial and 40% of the sporadic forms of OPCA. Dementia tends to occur both in mild to late disease and also in the early course of the disease (3%) (9). Although WAIS and WMS quotients may be normal, mild but definite cognitive abnormalities affecting memory (Logical Memory of the WMS), visuospatial (Block Design of the WAIS, Rey Complex Figure, and Visual Hooper Organization Test), and predominantly executive tasks (WCST, Verbal Fluency, Tower Tests, and Similarities and Comprehension of the WAIS) have been described consistently in patients with OPCA (6,10,15,16). Almost all patients show mixed dysarthria, with combinations of hypokinetic, ataxic, and spastic components (61).

Striatonigral Degeneration and Shy-Drager Syndrome

Patients with MSA (SND-SDS) rarely develop dementia. The cognitive profile of these patients is similar to that found in other forms of parkinsonisms. Specifically, there is a recall memory deficit solved with cues or recognition, a reduced speed of processing information, and increasing difficulty depending on the "effort-demanding" gradient of the tasks. A recent comparative study showed no disturbance of apraxic functions in patients with MSA compared with patients with PSP and PD (65).

Executive impairment (Verbal Fluency, Trail Making Test), even in the absence of intellectual deterioration, is the most consistent finding described in patients with SND and SDS. The dysexecutive syndrome found in SND is far less dramatic than in PSP and more selective than in PD because performance in the WCST seems to be preserved in patients with SND compared with those with PD. However, consistent greater impairment is seen in attentional resources (Stroop Test) in patients with SND than in patients with PD (83). Other language, memory, or perceptual tasks are relatively preserved. Mild visuospatial organizational abnormalities and memory deficits (Buschke Selective Reminding Test) have also been reported in SND and are thought to be due to an inefficient planning of visuospatial or memory processes.

PSYCHIATRIC FEATURES

Patients with MSA were reported to exhibit depression similar to that seen in patients with PD (Table 23-3). A few descriptive studies have reported a high prevalence of apathy (90%), a low percentage of anxiety (8%), and dopaminergic-induced psychotic features (15%) (39,97).

PATHOLOGY

Pathologic features of MSA vary among patients. In patients with prominent cerebellar symptoms (OPCA), prominent atrophy of the cerebellum and brainstem nuclei is seen, whereas striatal degeneration predominates in patients with prominent parkinsonism symptoms (SND and SDS). As described, corticosubcortical deafferentation processes may explain some cognitive deficits found in patients with MSA. Besides, cerebellar pathology can interfere with visuospatial and executive tasks because of defective cerebellocortical (cerebelloparietal and cerebellofrontal) and cerebello-brainstem-cortical loops (6).

HUNTINGTON'S DISEASE

HD is a progressive neurodegenerative disease determined by an excessive number of CAG repeats in the *huntingtin* gene in the short arm of chromosome 4 with an autosomal dominant transmission. Although HD typically begins in midlife (30 to 55 years), late-onset forms (>50 years) occur in up to 25% of the cases. The prevalence of HD is about five to 10 in 10,000. The average life span is 15 to 20 years from onset, with the worst course in early-onset cases. The presentation of HD can be variable. The onset is generally insidious and can be manifested by different combinations of hyperkinetic (choreic) movements (although a small percentage of patients may have parkinsonian features), cognitive impairment, and neuropsychiatric disturbances.

CIRCUMSCRIBED COGNITIVE DEFICITS

Cognitive abnormalities, which usually begin with psychomotor skills, are among the earliest indicators of functional decline (Table 23-1) (81). In fact, neuropsychological impairment can be even more disabling than motor symptoms, especially when the disease progresses and dementia appears (7). Cognitive disturbances have been described in gene carriers with motor symptoms and also in self-reported asymptomatic gene carriers. Psychomotor retardation has also been recognized in medically reported unaffected gene carriers (34,41,60).

Intelligence

Patients with HD present with a decrement in the Full-Scale Intelligence Quotient and in both verbal and, predominantly, performance subtests of the WAIS (22).

Impairment is seen in motor, problem-solving, memory, and concentration skills of the Halstead-Reitan battery, as are difficulties in the initiation/perseveration and construction subscales of the Mattis Dementia Rating Scale (MDRS) (90). The gradual decline in global measures of cognitive function has been associated with longer disease duration, greater severity of motor impairment (akinesia), more trinucleotide repeats, and later onset of motor symptoms (>51 years) (17,44,46,58).

Memory

Memory problems may be the initial symptom of the disease and tend to worsen as the disease progresses. Registration of information is usually normal, but verbal or visual acquisition is slowed and vulnerable to interference effects. Most memory scores are well correlated with performance on tests of executive functions, suggesting that memory impairment in patients with HD results primarily from an inability to initiate systematic retrieval strategies. In accordance with this hypothesis, recent memory is impaired particularly in those tasks that require the ability to spontaneously generate efficient strategies and to use internally guided behavior (92). This failure of retrieval with normal encoding and storing mechanisms also accounts for the deficits in remote memory found in patients with HD.

Language

Motor, syntactical (grammar and syntax), and semantic (vocabulary and naming) components of language are affected. Dysarthria may be present even in the early stages and can make the speech unintelligible as the disease evolves. Verbal fluency is reduced, and the grammatical form, the length of the phrases, and the syntactical complexity of speech are reduced (102). Paraphasic errors and naming difficulties have been described, especially late in the disease course, but at lesser frequency and intensity than in other cortical dementias (49). Comprehension is remarkably well preserved. Motor disturbances can make patients' writing slow, difficult, or even impossible, but dysgraphic errors and perseverations have also been described (98).

Visuospatial Function

Graphomotor visuospatial deficits (Rey-Osterrieth Complex Figure, Clock Drawing), visual memory impairments (Benton Visual Retention Tests), visuoconstructional disturbances (Block Design and Object Assembly of the WAIS), and spatial disorientation (Road Map Test of Direction) have been identified in HD (87) A deficit in visual tracking tasks (Trail Making Test, Digit Symbol) should be interpreted cautiously because eye movements are frequently disturbed in these patients.

Executive Function

Even at early stages of the disease, patients with HD present with deficits in planning and organizing activities (Tower of London/Hanoi), perseverative tendencies (WCST), and an inability to shift mental sets (WCST, Trail Making Test, Stroop Test) (63,122). Abstract reasoning and concept formation can be preserved at early stages but decline as the disease progresses (Similarities, Comprehension, and Calculation subtests of the WAIS). In general, patients with HD present with more difficulties when the task includes novel material, timed tasks, manipulation, or reasoning. As mentioned, slowed mental processing and set-shifting or set-maintenance difficulties can also contribute to performance failures in visuospatial, language, and memory tasks.

DEMENTIA

The prevalence rate of dementia varies from 15% to 95% among studies (93). Sample differences and the method for assessing dementia may be partially responsible for these discrepancies. Cognitive decline seems to be related to the number of years affected more than to age at onset. Dementia is consistently present at the final stages of the disease if survival is long enough, although the time of its onset is difficult to determine precisely.

The dementia of HD is classified as subcortical, so apraxia, agnosia, and aphasia are not common symptoms. Attentional disorders, retrieval deficits, and executive impairments are present at early stages of the dementing process. As described, free recall of information from both episodic and semantic memory is impaired at this stage. Although cued recall and recognition are generally normal, these mechanisms can also be affected with disease progression (51).

PSYCHIATRIC FEATURES

The prevalence of psychiatric symptoms in HD varies between 35% and 75% (Table 23-3). Psychiatric symptoms may be the presenting manifestation of the disease in up to 50% of the cases and may precede the onset of motor or cognitive symptoms by as much as 10 years, so they cannot readily be ascribed to declining cognitive or motor abilities (124).

Globally, irritability (50%), agitation (50%), apathy (50%), depression (30%), psychosis (20%), and mania (10%) are the most common symptoms (21,40). A gradient is seen, with anxiety, impulsivity, lability, irritability, and aggressiveness more commonly associated with suicidal and homicidal behavior in the early stages of the illness. Depression, dysthymia, mania, dysphoria, and psychosis (persecutory delusions and auditory hallucinations) are seen in the middle phases, with apathy, abulia, and dementia appearing in the late stages.

Depression may antedate the onset of neurologic symptoms in up to 75% of the cases, suggesting that it is not simply a reaction to motor disabilities. The risk of suicide is eight to 20 times higher than in the general population, especially in the middle-aged group. Obsessions and compulsions are present in most patients (31). Sleep disturbances have been reported in about 20% of patients with late-onset HD (24). Paraphilias and altered sexual behavior have also been reported, especially in the early phases of the disease, and have also been associated with mania or hypomania (38).

PATHOLOGY

The core pathologic feature of HD is the selective loss of inhibitory gamma-aminobutyric acidergic striatal neurons projecting to the globus pallidus and substantia nigra pars reticulata. This process generates an increase in the activity of the excitatory neurotransmitters, which can have neurotoxic effects. The degenerative process may also involve the cerebellum, thalamic nuclei, subthalamic nucleus, and frontal and prefrontal cortex. Most of the early cognitive and psychiatric deficits reported in HD have been related to an increased excitatory subcortical output flow to the dorsolateral (executive impairment), orbitofrontal (mania and obsessive-compulsive disorder), and anterior cingulate cortex (abulia and apathy). At later stages, depression, apathy, and other cognitive impairment may be secondary to more widespread frontal or caudate degeneration (74).

REFERENCES

1. Aarsland D, Andersen K, Larsen JP, et al. Prevalence and characteristics of dementia in Parkinson disease: an 8-year prospective study. *Arch Neurol.* 2003; 60:387–392.
2. Aarsland D, Laake K, Larsen JP, et al. Donepezil for cognitive impairment in Parkinson's disease: a randomised controlled study. *J Neurol Neurosurg Psychiatry.* 2002;72:708–712.
3. Aarsland D, Larsen JP, Lim NG, et al. Range of neuropsychiatric disturbances in patients with Parkinson's disease. *J Neurol Neurosurg Psychiatry.* 1999;67:492–496.
4. Alexander GE, DeLong MR, Strick PL. Parallel organization of functionally segregated circuits linking basal ganglia and cortex. *Annu Rev Neurosci.* 1986;9:357–381.
5. Appollonio I, Grafman J, Clark K, et al. Implicit and explicit memory in patients with Parkinson's disease with and without dementia. *Arch Neurol.* 1994;51:359–367.
6. Arroyo-Anllo EM, Botez-Marquard T. Neurobehavioral dimensions of olivopontocerebellar atrophy. *J Clin Exp Neuropsychol.* 1998;20:52–59.
7. Bamford KA, Caine ED, Kido DK, et al. A prospective evaluation of cognitive decline in early Huntington's disease: functional and radiographic correlates. *Neurology.* 1995;45:1867–1873.
8. Benke T, Hohenstein C, Poewe W, et al. Repetitive speech phenomena in Parkinson's disease. *J Neurol Neurosurg Psychiatry.* 2000;69:319–324.
9. Berciano J. Olivopontocerebellar atrophy. A review of 117 cases. *J Neurol Sci.* 1982;53:253–272.
10. Berent S, Giordani B, Gilman S, et al. Neuropsychological changes in olivopontocerebellar atrophy. *Arch Neurol.* 1990;47:997–1001.
11. Bergman J, Lerner V. Successful use of donepezil for the treatment of psychotic symptoms in patients with Parkinson's disease. *Clin Neuropharmacol.* 2002;25:107–110.
12. Boller F, Passafiume D, Keefe NC, et al. Visuospatial impairment in Parkinson's disease. Role of perceptual and motor factors. *Arch Neurol.* 1984;41:485–490.
13. Bondi MW, Kaszniak AW. Implicit and explicit memory in Alzheimer's disease and Parkinson's disease. *J Clin Exp Neuropsychol.* 1991;13:339–358.
14. Bondi MW, Kaszniak AW, Bayles KA, et al. Contribution of frontal system dysfunction to memory and perceptual abilities in Parkinson's disease. *Neuropsychology.* 1993;7:89–102.
15. Botez-Marquard T, Botez MI. Cognitive behavior in heredodegenerative ataxias. *Eur Neurol.* 1992;33:351–357.
16. Botez-Marquard T, Botez MI. Olivopontocerebellar atrophy and Friedreich's ataxia: neuropsychological consequences of bilateral versus unilateral cerebellar lesions. *Int Rev Neurobiol.* 1997;41:387–410.
17. Brandt J, Strauss ME, Larus J, et al. Clinical correlates of dementia and disability in Huntington's disease. *J Clin Neuropsychol.* 1984;6:401–412.
18. Brown RG, Marsden CD. Visuospatial function in Parkinson's disease. *Brain.* 1986;109:987–1002.
19. Brown RG, Marsden CD. Cognitive function in Parkinson's disease: from description to theory. *Trends Neurosci.* 1990;13:21–29.
20. Burn DJ, Rowan EN, Allan LM, et al. Motor subtype and cognitive decline in Parkinson's disease, Parkinson's disease with dementia, and dementia with Lewy bodies. *J Neurol Neurosurg Psychiatry.* 2006;77: 585–589.
21. Burns A, Folstein S, Brandt J, et al. Clinical assessment of irritability, aggression, and apathy in Huntington and Alzheimer disease. *J Nerv Ment Dis.* 1990;178:20–26.
22. Caine ED, Hunt RD, Weingartner H, et al. Huntington's dementia. Clinical and neuropsychological features. *Arch Gen Psychiatry.* 1978; 35:377–384.

23. Celesia GG, Barr AN. Psychosis and other psychiatric manifestations of levodopa therapy. *Arch Neurol.* 1970;23:193–200.

24. Chokroverty S. Sleep and degenerative neurologic disorders. *Neurol Clin.* 1996;4:807–826.

25. Contarino MF, Daniele A, Sibilia AH, et al. Cognitive outcome 5 years after bilateral chronic stimulation of subthalamic nucleus in patients with Parkinson's disease. *J Neurol Neurosurg Psychiatry.* 2007;78: 248–252.

26. Cools AR, van den Bercken JH, Horstink MW, et al. Cognitive and motor shifting aptitude disorder in Parkinson's disease. *J Neurol Neurosurg Psychiatry.* 1984;47:443–453.

27. Cooper JA, Sagar HJ, Doherty SM, et al. Different effects of dopaminergic and anticholinergic therapies on cognitive and motor function in Parkinson's disease. A follow-up study of untreated patients. *Brain.* 1992;115: 1701–1725.

28. Cooper JA, Sagar HJ, Jordan N, et al. Cognitive impairment in early, untreated Parkinson's disease and its relationship to motor disability. *Brain.* 1991;114:2095–2122.

29. Cummings JL. Behavioral complications of drug treatment of Parkinson's disease. *J Am Geriatr Soc.* 1991;39:708–716.

30. Cummings JL. Depression and Parkinson's disease: a review. *Am J Psychiatry.* 1992;149: 443–454.

31. Cummings JL, Cunningham K. Obsessive-compulsive disorder in Huntington's disease. *Biol Psychiatry.* 1992;31:263–270.

32. Cummings JL, Darkins A, Mendez M, et al. Alzheimer's disease and Parkinson's disease: comparison of speech and language alterations. *Neurology.* 1988;38:680–684.

33. Daniel SE, de Bruin V, Lees AJ. The clinical and pathological spectrum of Steele-Richardson-Olszewski syndrome (progressive supranuclear palsy): a reappraisal. *Brain.* 1995;118:759–770.

34. De Boo GM, Tibben A, Lanser JB, et al. Early cognitive and motor symptoms in identified carriers of the gene for Huntington disease. *Arch Neurol.* 1997;54:1353–1357.

35. Dubois B, Pillon B, Lhermitte F, et al. Cholinergic deficiency and frontal dysfunction in Parkinson's disease. *Ann Neurol.* 1990;28: 117–121.

36. Emre M, Aarsland D, Albanese A, et al. Rivastigmine for dementia associated with Parkinson's disease. *N Engl J Med.* 2004;351: 2509–2518.

37. Esmonde T, Giles E, Gibson M, et al. Neuropsychological performance, disease severity, and depression in progressive supranuclear palsy. *J Neurol.* 1996;243:638–643.

38. Fedoroff JP, Peyser C, Franz ML, et al. Sexual disorders in Huntington's disease. *J Neuropsychiatry Clin Neurosci.* 1994;6:147–153.

39. Fetoni V, Soliveri P, Monza D, et al. Affective symptoms in multiple system atrophy and Parkinson's disease: response to levodopa therapy. *J Neurol Neurosurg Psychiatry.* 1999;66: 541–544.

40. Folstein SE, Folstein MF. Psychiatric features of Huntington's disease: recent approaches and findings. *Psychiatr Dev.* 1983;1:193–205.

41. Foroud T, Siemers E, Kleindorfer D, et al. Cognitive scores in carriers of Huntington's disease gene compared to noncarriers. *Ann Neurol.* 1995;37:657–664.

42. Frattali CM, Grafman J, Patronas N, et al. Language disturbances in corticobasal degeneration. *Neurology.* 2000;54:990–992.

43. Gibb WR, Luthert PJ, Marsden CD. Corticobasal degeneration. *Brain.* 1989;112: 1171–1192.

44. Girotti F, Marano R, Soliveri P, et al. Relationship between motor and cognitive disorders in Huntington's disease. *J Neurol.* 1988;235:454–457.

45. Globus M, Mildworf B, Melamed E. Cerebral blood flow and cognitive impairment in Parkinson's disease. *Neurology.* 1985;35: 1135–1139.

46. Gomez-Tortosa E, del Barrio A, Garcia Ruiz PJ, et al. Severity of cognitive impairment in juvenile and late-onset Huntington disease. *Arch Neurol.* 1998;55:835–843.

47. Heindel WC, Salmon DP, Shults CW, et al. Neuropsychological evidence for multiple implicit memory systems: a comparison of Alzheimer's, Huntington's, and Parkinson's disease patients. *J Neurosci.* 1989;9:582–587.

48. Henik A, Singh J, Beckley DJ, et al. Disinhibition of automatic word reading in Parkinson's disease. *Cortex.* 1993;29:589–599.

49. Hodges JR, Salmon DP, Butters N. The nature of the naming deficit in Alzheimer's and Huntington's disease. *Brain.* 1991;114:1547–1558.

50. Hovestadt A, de Jong GJ, Meerwaldt JD. Spatial disorientation as an early symptom of Parkinson's disease. *Neurology.* 1987;37:485–487.

51. Huber SJ, Paulson GW. Memory impairment associated with progression of Huntington's disease. *Cortex.* 1987;23:275–283.

52. Huber SJ, Shuttleworth EC, Freidenberg DL. Neuropsychological differences between the dementias of Alzheimer's and Parkinson's diseases. *Arch Neurol.* 1989;46:1287–1291.

53. Illes J, Metter EJ, Hanson WR, et al. Language production in Parkinson's disease: acoustic and

linguistic considerations. *Brain Lang*. 1988;33: 146–160.

54. Inzelberg R, Kipervasser S, Korczyn AD. Auditory hallucinations in Parkinson's disease. *J Neurol Neurosurg Psychiatry*. 1998;64:533–535.

55. Jacobs DM, Marder K, Cote LJ, et al. Neuropsychological characteristics of preclinical dementia in Parkinson's disease. *Neurology*. 1995;45:1691–1696.

56. Jagust WJ, Reed BR, Martin EM, et al. Cognitive function and regional cerebral blood flow in Parkinson's disease. *Brain*. 1992;115: 521–537.

57. Janvin CC, Aarsland D, Larsen JP, et al. Cognitive predictors of dementia in Parkinson's disease: a community-based, 4-year longitudinal study. *J Geriatr Psychiatry Neurol*. 2005;18:149–154.

58. Jason GW, Suchowersky O, Pajurkova EM, et al. Cognitive manifestations of Huntington disease in relation to genetic structure and clinical onset. *Arch Neurol*. 1997;54:1081–1088.

59. Kertesz A, Davidson W, Munoz DG. Clinical and pathological overlap between frontotemporal dementia, primary progressive aphasia and corticobasal degeneration: the Pick complex. *Dement Geriatr Cogn Disord*. 1999;10[Suppl 1]: 46–49.

60. Kirkwood SC, Siemers E, Stout JC, et al. Longitudinal cognitive and motor changes among presymptomatic Huntington disease gene carriers. *Arch Neurol*. 1999;56:563–568.

61. Kluin KJ, Gilman S, Lohman M, et al. Characteristics of the dysarthria of multiple system atrophy. *Arch Neurol*. 1996;53:545–548.

62. Kuzis G, Sabe L, Tiberti C, et al. Cognitive functions in major depression and Parkinson disease. *Arch Neurol*. 1997;54:982–986.

63. Lawrence AD, Sahakian BJ, Hodges JR, et al. Executive and mnemonic functions in early Huntington's disease. *Brain*. 1996;119:1633–1645.

64. Leiguarda RC, Lees AJ, Merello M, et al. The nature of apraxia in corticobasal degeneration. *J Neurol Neurosurg Psychiatry*. 1994;57:455–459.

65. Leiguarda RC, Pramstaller PP, Merello M, et al. Apraxia in Parkinson's disease, progressive supranuclear palsy, multiple system atrophy and neuroleptic-induced parkinsonism. *Brain*. 1997; 120:75–90.

66. Levin BE, Llabre MM, Reisman S, et al. Visuospatial impairment in Parkinson's disease. *Neurology*. 1991;41:365–369.

67. Levin BE, Llabre MM, Weiner WJ. Cognitive impairments associated with early Parkinson's disease. *Neurology*. 1989;39:557–561.

68. Levy G, Jacobs DM, Tang MX, et al. Memory and executive function impairment predict dementia in Parkinson's disease. *Mov Disord*. 2002;17: 1221–1226.

69. Lippa CF, Duda JE, Grossman M, et al. DLB and PDD boundary issues: diagnosis, treatment, molecular pathology, and biomarkers. *Neurology*. 2007;68:812–819.

70. Litvan I, Cummings JL, Mega M. Neuropsychiatric features of corticobasal degeneration. *J Neurol Neurosurg Psychiatry*. 1998;65: 717–721.

71. Litvan I, Mangone CA, McKee A, et al. Natural history of progressive supranuclear palsy (Steele-Richardson-Olszewski syndrome) and clinical predictors of survival: a clinicopathological study. *J Neurol Neurosurg Psychiatry*. 1996; 60:615–620.

72. Litvan I, Mega MS, Cummings JL, et al. Neuropsychiatric aspects of progressive supranuclear palsy. *Neurology*. 1996;47:1184–1189.

73. Litvan I, Mohr E, Williams J, et al. Differential memory and executive functions in demented patients with Parkinson's and Alzheimer's disease. *J Neurol Neurosurg Psychiatry*. 1991;54:25–29.

74. Litvan I, Paulsen JS, Mega MS, et al. Neuropsychiatric assessment of patients with hyperkinetic and hypokinetic movement disorders. *Arch Neurol*. 1998;55:1313–1319.

75. Louis ED, Marder K, Cote L, et al. Mortality from Parkinson disease. *Arch Neurol*. 1997;54: 260–264.

76. Mahieux F, Fenelon G, Flahault A, et al. Neuropsychological prediction of dementia in Parkinson's disease. *J Neurol Neurosurg Psychiatry*. 1998;64:178–183.

77. Marder K, Tang MX, Cote L, et al. The frequency and associated risk factors for dementia in patients with Parkinson's disease. *Arch Neurol*. 1995;52:695–701.

78. Massman PJ, Kreiter KT, Jankovic J, et al. Neuropsychological functioning in cortical-basal ganglionic degeneration: differentiation from Alzheimer's disease. *Neurology*. 1996;46:720–726.

79. Masterman D, DeSalles A, Baloh RW, et al. Motor, cognitive, and behavioral performance following unilateral ventroposterior pallidotomy for Parkinson disease. *Arch Neurol*. 1998;55: 1201–1208.

80. Mayeux R, Chen J, Mirabello E, et al. An estimate of the incidence of dementia in idiopathic Parkinson's disease. *Neurology*. 1990;40:1513–1517.

81. Mayeux R, Stern Y, Herman A, et al. Correlates of early disability in Huntington's disease. *Ann Neurol*. 1986;20:727–731.

82. Mayeux R, Stern Y, Rosen J, et al. Is "subcortical dementia" a recognizable clinical entity? *Ann Neurol*. 1983;14:278–283.

83. Meco G, Gasparini M, Doricchi F. Attentional functions in multiple system atrophy and Parkinson's disease. *J Neurol Neurosurg Psychiatry.* 1996;60:393–398.

84. Milberg W, Albert M. Cognitive differences between patients with progressive supranuclear palsy and Alzheimer's disease. *J Clin Exp Neuropsychol.* 1989;11:605–614.

85. Mitchell SL, Kiely DK, Kiel DP, et al. The epidemiology, clinical characteristics, and natural history of older nursing home residents with a diagnosis of Parkinson's disease. *J Am Geriatr Soc.* 1996;44:394–399.

86. Miyasaki JM, Shannon K, Voon V, et al. Practice parameter: evaluation and treatment of depression, psychosis, and dementia in Parkinson disease (an evidence-based review): report of the Quality Standards Subcommittee of the American Academy of Neurology. *Neurology.* 2006;66: 996–1002.

87. Mohr E, Brouwers P, Claus JJ, et al. Visuospatial cognition in Huntington's disease. *Mov Disord.* 1991;6:127–132.

88. Okuda B, Tachibana H, Kawabata K, et al. Slowly progressive limb-kinetic apraxia with a decrease in unilateral cerebral blood flow. *Acta Neurol Scand.* 1992;86:76–81.

89. Ondo WG, Dat Vuong K, Khan H, et al. Daytime sleepiness and other sleep disorders in Parkinson's disease. *Neurology.* 2001;57:1392–1396.

90. Paulsen JS, Butters N, Sadek JR, et al. Distinct cognitive profiles of cortical and subcortical dementia in advanced illness. *Neurology.* 1995; 45:951–956.

91. Pillon B, Blin J, Vidailhet M, et al. The neuropsychological pattern of corticobasal degeneration: comparison with progressive supranuclear palsy and Alzheimer's disease. *Neurology.* 1995; 45:1477–1483.

92. Pillon B, Deweer B, Agid Y, et al. Explicit memory in Alzheimer's, Huntington's, and Parkinson's diseases. *Arch Neurol.* 1993;50:374–379.

93. Pillon B, Dubois B, Agid Y. Severity and specificity of cognitive impairment in Alzheimer's, Huntington's, and Parkinson's diseases and progressive supranuclear palsy. *Ann NY Acad Sci.* 1991;640:224–227.

94. Pillon B, Ertle S, Deweer B, et al. Memory for spatial location in 'de novo' parkinsonian patients. *Neuropsychologia.* 1997;35:221–228.

95. Pillon B, Ertle S, Deweer B, et al. Memory for spatial location is affected in Parkinson's disease. *Neuropsychologia.* 1996;34:77–85.

96. Pillon B, Gouider Khouja N, Deweer B, et al. Neuropsychological pattern of striatonigral degeneration: comparison with Parkinson's disease and progressive supranuclear palsy. *J Neurol Neurosurg Psychiatry.* 1995;58:174–179.

97. Pilo L, Ring H, Quinn N, et al. Depression in multiple system atrophy and in idiopathic Parkinson's disease: a pilot comparative study. *Biol Psychiatry.* 1996;39:803–807.

98. Podoll K, Caspary P, Lange HW, et al. Language functions in Huntington's disease. *Brain.* 1988;111:1475–1503.

99. Podoll K, Schwarz M, Noth J. Language functions in progressive supranuclear palsy. *Brain.* 1991;114:1457–1472.

100. Ravina B, Putt M, Siderowf A, et al. Donepezil for dementia in Parkinson's disease: a randomised, double blind, placebo controlled, crossover study. *J Neurol Neurosurg Psychiatry.* 2005;76:934–939.

101. Reading PJ, Luce AK, McKeith IG, et al. Rivastigmine in the treatment of parkinsonian psychosis and cognitive impairment: preliminary findings from an open trial. *Mov Disord.* 2001;16:1171–1174.

102. Rich JB, Troyer AK, Bylsma FW, et al. Longitudinal analysis of phonemic clustering and switching during word-list generation in Huntington's disease. *Neuropsychology.* 1999;13: 525–531.

103. Richards M, Cote LJ, Stern Y. Executive function in Parkinson's disease: set-shifting or set-maintenance? *J Clin Exp Neuropsychol.* 1993;15: 266–279.

104. Riley DE, Lang AE, Lewis A, et al. Cortical-basal ganglionic degeneration. *Neurology.* 1990;40: 1203–1212.

105. Rosser A, Hodges JR. Initial letter and semantic category fluency in Alzheimer's disease, Huntington's disease, and progressive supranuclear palsy. *J Neurol Neurosurg Psychiatry.* 1994;57: 1389–1394.

106. Saint Cyr JA, Taylor AE, Lang AE. Neuropsychological and psychiatric side effects in the treatment of Parkinson's disease. *Neurology.* 1993;43[Suppl 6]:47–52.

107. Sanchez-Ramos JR, Ortoll R, Paulson GW. Visual hallucinations associated with Parkinson disease. *Arch Neurol.* 1996;53:1265–1268.

108. Scheife RT, Schumock GT, Burstein A, et al. Impact of Parkinson's disease and its pharmacologic treatment on quality of life and economic outcomes. *Am J Health Syst Pharm.* 2000;57: 953–962.

109. Schiffer RB, Kurlan R, Rubin A, et al. Evidence for atypical depression in Parkinson's disease. *Am J Psychiatry.* 1988;145:1020–1022.

110. Smeding HM, Speelman JD, Koning-Haanstra M, et al. Neuropsychological effects of bilateral STN stimulation in Parkinson disease: a controlled study. *Neurology.* 2006;66:1830–1836.

111. Speelman JD, Smeding HM, Schmand B, et al. Does chronic subthalamic nucleus stimulation in advanced Parkinson's disease cause invalidating cognitive and behavioural dysfunctions? *J Neurol Neurosurg Psychiatry.* 2007;78:221.

112. Starkstein SE, Mayberg HS, Leiguarda R, et al. A prospective longitudinal study of depression, cognitive decline, and physical impairments in patients with Parkinson's disease. *J Neurol Neurosurg Psychiatry.* 1992;55:377–382.

113. Steele JC, Richardson JC, Olzewski J. Progressive supranuclear palsy: a heterogeneous degeneration involving the brain stem, basal ganglia, and cerebellum with vertical gaze and pseudobulbar palsy, nuchal dystonia and dementia. *Arch Neurol.* 1964;10:333–359.

114. Stein MB, Heuser IJ, Juncos JL, et al. Anxiety disorders in patients with Parkinson's disease. *Am J Psychiatry.* 1990;147:217–220.

115. Stern Y, Marder K, Tang MX, et al. Antecedent clinical features associated with dementia in Parkinson's disease. *Neurology.* 1993;43:1690–1692.

116. Stern Y, Richards M, Sano M, et al. Comparison of cognitive changes in patients with Alzheimer's and Parkinson's disease. *Arch Neurol.* 1993;50:1040–1045.

117. Stern Y, Tang MX, Jacobs DM, et al. Prospective comparative study of the evolution of probable Alzheimer's disease and Parkinson's disease dementia. *J Int Neuropsychol Soc.* 1998;4:279–284.

118. Tsai CH, Lu CS, Hua MS, et al. Cognitive dysfunction in early onset parkinsonism. *Acta Neurol Scand.* 1994;89:9–14.

119. Uitti RJ, Tanner CM, Rajput AH, et al. Hypersexuality with antiparkinsonian therapy. *Clin Neuropharmacol.* 1989;12:375–383.

120. Valldeoriola F, Nobbe FA, Tolosa E. Treatment of behavioural disturbances in Parkinson's disease. *J Neural Transm.* 1997;51(suppl):175–204.

121. Van der Hurk PR, Hodges JR. Episodic and semantic memory in Alzheimer's disease and progressive supranuclear palsy: a comparative study. *J Clin Exp Neuropsychol.* 1995;17:459–471.

122. Watkins LH, Rogers RD, Lawrence AD, et al. Impaired planning but intact decision making in early Huntington's disease: implications for specific fronto-striatal pathology. *Neuropsychologia.* 2000;38:1112–1125.

123. Whetten-Goldstein K, Sloan F, Kulas E, et al. The burden of Parkinson's disease on society, family, and the individual. *J Am Geriatr Soc.* 1997;45:844–849.

124. Zappacosta B, Monza D, Meoni C, et al. Psychiatric symptoms do not correlate with cognitive decline, motor symptoms, or CAG repeat length in Huntington's disease. *Arch Neurol.* 1996;53:493–497.

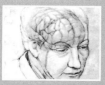

CHAPTER 24

Diseases of the Spinal Cord and Vertebrae

H. Gordon Deen, Jr.

A wide range of disease processes may affect the vertebral column of the older adult. The spinal cord, cauda equina, and spinal nerve roots may also be involved. This chapter will provide an overview of these diseases, with an emphasis on the more common disorders that the primary care practitioner or neurologist will be more likely to encounter in clinical practice.

OSTEOPOROSIS

Osteoporosis is a very common problem in the elderly, with an estimated 700,000 new cases per year in the United States alone. Although osteoporosis has received much recent attention in medical publications and in the lay press, this disorder is sometimes under-recognized and undertreated. Osteoporosis is seen more frequently in women but can also occur in men. From a conceptual standpoint, osteoporosis can be defined as a systemic skeletal disease characterized by low bone mass and microarchitectural deterioration with a consequent increase in bone fragility and susceptibility to fracture. From an operational standpoint, osteoporosis is defined as a bone mineral density (T-score) that is 2.5 standard deviations (SD) below the mean peak value in young adults. Patients with osteoporosis can sustain fractures with minimal trauma. The vertebral column, proximal femur, and distal forearm are most commonly involved, but fracture of any bone can occur. Vertebral compression fractures are the most common manifestation of osteoporosis of the spine. The lower thoracic and upper lumbar vertebrae are the most common sites of involvement. A compression fracture above the T7 level is rarely caused by osteoporosis, and the diagnosis of tumor or infection should be considered in such cases.

Osteoporotic spinal compression fractures cause back pain, with or without radiculopathy. Symptoms often respond poorly to treatment. Multiple vertebral fractures occurring over time may lead to secondary spinal disorders such as spinal stenosis, scoliosis, or kyphotic deformity.

"Benign" osteoporotic compression fracture should be a diagnosis of exclusion (Fig. 24-1). The physician should always consider the possibility that an acute spinal compression fracture may be caused by neoplasm or infection. Magnetic resonance imaging (MRI) usually provides some clues in this regard. In osteoporotic spinal compression fractures, the adjacent epidural and paraspinal soft tissues are normal, and the pedicle is not involved. There is usually only one acute fracture; however, there may be old, healed compression fractures in other vertebral bodies. In cases where the fracture is due to metastatic tumor, there are often abnormalities of the adjacent epidural and paraspinal soft tissues and in the pedicle. There are often acute lesions at other levels of the spinal column. In cases where the fracture is due to infection, the abnormalities are centered in the intervertebral disk space. There is abnormal T1 signal in the vertebral bodies, adjacent to the disk. The epidural and paraspinal soft tissues are often involved. In most cases, the MRI, coupled with clinical findings, enables the physician to determine whether the patient has a benign osteoporotic compression fracture or whether a more ominous diagnosis is present. A few patients, initially felt to have benign spinal compression fractures, have persistent or worsening pain or indeterminate MRI findings. These individuals should have a follow-up MRI examination in 6 weeks to 3 months.

When the diagnosis of osteoporosis is suspected, the physician should inquire about risk factors, including family history, cigarette smoking, alcohol abuse, sedentary lifestyle, low body weight, inadequate dietary calcium, low exposure to sunlight, early menopause, and chronic medication therapy with steroids, certain anticonvulsants (phenytoin), and anticoagulants. The physician should also be aware that a variety of endocrine diseases (e.g., Cushing's syndrome), hematologic diseases (e.g., multiple myeloma), rheumatologic diseases (e.g., rheumatoid arthritis), and gastrointestinal diseases (e.g., malabsorption syndromes) may be associated with osteoporosis. Radiotherapy that includes the spinal column in the treatment fields may also predispose to loss of skeletal bone mass.

Osteoporosis is now viewed as having primary and secondary forms (7). The typical osteoporosis seen in

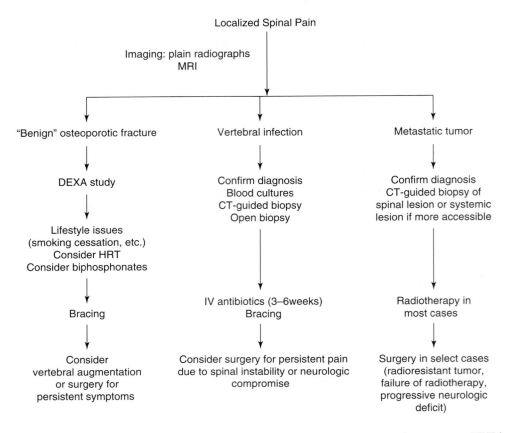

Localized Spinal Pain

Imaging: plain radiographs
MRI

| "Benign" osteoporotic fracture | Vertebral infection | Metastatic tumor |

DEXA study

Confirm diagnosis
Blood cultures
CT-guided biopsy
Open biopsy

Confirm diagnosis
CT-guided biopsy of
spinal lesion or systemic
lesion if more accessible

Lifestyle issues
(smoking cessation, etc.)
Consider HRT
Consider biphosphonates

Bracing

IV antibiotics (3–6weeks)
Bracing

Radiotherapy in
most cases

Consider
vertebral augmentation
or surgery for
persistent symptoms

Consider surgery for persistent pain
due to spinal instability or neurologic
compromise

Surgery in select cases
(radioresistant tumor,
failure of radiotherapy,
progressive neurologic
deficit)

Figure 24-1. Diagnosis algorithm for spinal compression fracture. DEXA, dual-energy X-ray absorptiometry; HRT, hormone replacement therapy; IV, intravenous.

elderly women with no other risk factors is referred to as primary osteoporosis. Patients with risk factors such as liver or kidney failure, chronic steroid therapy, and early menopause are said to have secondary osteoporosis. Patients with secondary osteoporosis develop earlier and more severe bony disease than patients with primary osteoporosis.

Management of osteoporosis involves both prevention and treatment. The physician should first focus on lifestyle issues, emphasizing the importance of smoking cessation and avoidance of excessive alcohol, while encouraging an adequate level of physical exercise and dietary calcium. Patients should be counseled to avoid heavy lifting and to take care to avoid falls. The risk of falling can be decreased by eliminating sedating medications. Some patients may benefit from using a cane or walker. Estrogen replacement therapy is the treatment of choice for women with postmenopausal osteoporosis. Other pharmacologic options include bisphosphonates, raloxifene, and calcitonin nasal spray.

An acute osteoporotic spinal compression fracture is managed with short-term activity reduction, analgesics,

and bracing. A lightweight corset is better tolerated and less expensive and appears to be as effective as more rigid, custom-made orthoses. Narcotics may be necessary for short-term pain control.

For patients with painful compression fractures, percutaneous vertebral augmentation with either vertebroplasty or balloon kyphoplasty has emerged as a very effective treatment. These procedures involve the percutaneous injection of methylmethacrylate bone cement, under fluoroscopic guidance, into the symptomatic, compressed vertebral body. The difference between the two techniques is that balloon kyphoplasty involves inflation of a balloon tamp in the compressed vertebral body. This creates a cavity in the bone, which permits a low-pressure injection of bone cement with less risk of cement extravasation and embolus. In some cases, balloon inflation also helps restore spinal alignment. Local anesthesia plus intravenous sedation or a light general anesthetic may be used. The procedures typically require just an overnight stay in the hospital and may sometimes be performed on an outpatient basis.

Experience accumulated over the last decade indicates that the procedure can be done safely, with excellent short-term pain relief. Patients are still at risk for fractures at other levels, and this possibility should be kept in mind if a patient develops new pain after a successful vertebral augmentation procedure. Refracture of a treated level is uncommon. Vertebral augmentation is contraindicated if there is significant compromise of the spinal canal from retropulsion of compressed bone fragments.

Open surgery is usually not needed for osteoporotic spinal compression fractures. An occasional patient with significant spinal canal compromise and myelopathy or cauda equina syndrome will need to be considered for spinal canal decompression and stabilization via anterior and/or posterior surgical approaches. Unfortunately, these surgical procedures are often lengthy and complex, with the potential for significant blood loss and other complications. Prolonged hospital care and rehabilitation may be required. Furthermore, the patients who harbor osteoporotic compression fractures are often elderly and debilitated. Therefore, a decision to intervene with major reconstructive surgery should not be taken lightly by the physician or the patient.

SPINAL METASTATIC TUMOR

The diagnosis of spinal metastatic tumor should be strongly considered in the older adult who presents with acute, severe spinal pain. The patient typically reports intense, localized, persistent pain at the level of the lesion. The pain is often worse at night. There may be a wide range of neurologic involvement. The patient may have a monoradiculopathy, myelopathy, or cauda equina syndrome from neural compression. Some patients have no neurologic symptoms or signs, whereas others present with a rapidly progressive, severe neurologic deficit. Some patients have an established diagnosis of systemic cancer, whereas many others do not. The physician should be aware that the metastatic component of a tumor may cause symptoms before the primary tumor. For example, a patient with carcinoma of the lung may present with spinal metastasis, with the primary lesion being discovered only during subsequent evaluation. The physician will also encounter an occasional patient with spinal metastatic cancer, in whom a primary tumor is never identified despite aggressive workup. Metastases account for 70% of all tumors of the spine. The most common primary tumor types are carcinoma of the breast, carcinoma of the lung, lymphoma, and carcinoma of the prostate. Carcinoma of the kidney and colon and a wide range of less common tumors may also have metastatic involvement of the spinal column.

Plain radiographs of the spine still play a useful role in the evaluation of spinal metastatic disease. The first radiographic evidence of spinal metastasis is the "winking owl" sign caused by obliteration of the pedicle. Spinal compression fractures may be seen. These lesions may be osteolytic, osteoblastic, or mixed. Carcinoma of the prostate and Hodgkin's disease are known to cause osteoblastic bony changes with the so-called "ivory vertebrae." MRI is more sensitive than plain radiographs and should be performed whenever spinal metastasis is a diagnostic possibility. MRI shows bony lesions before they become apparent on plain radiographs and also reveals their soft tissue components, epidural spread, and neural compromise. Patients with spinal metastatic disease often have involvement of multiple spinal segments. Therefore, if one lesion is identified, the clinician must diligently search for lesions at other levels.

Spinal metastatic tumors are almost always extradural in location. Intradural metastases from primary brain tumors, such as glioblastoma multiforme and medulloblastoma, are uncommon. These so-called "drop metastases" have a characteristic MRI appearance of multiple nodules on the spinal cord and cauda equina. Intramedullary metastasis of non–central nervous system tumors into the substance of the spinal cord is rare. The lesion is usually well seen on MRI. These cases are characterized by rapid neurologic deterioration. Prognosis is poor.

The mainstay of treatment is radiotherapy of the involved spinal segments. Surgery is reserved for patients harboring tumors known to be radiotherapy resistant, patients with a rapidly progressive neurologic deficit or severe pain, and patients who have failed radiation therapy. A surgical approach may also be necessary to obtain diagnostic tissue in the occasional patient in whom the diagnosis is uncertain. Laminectomy as a stand-alone procedure is seldom indicated. Surgical treatment usually involves both decompression and stabilization from anterior or posterior (or combined) surgical approaches.

Vertebral augmentation may be a useful option for patients with pathologic compression fractures secondary to metastatic disease (5). Similar to benign fractures, pain relief is generally excellent in patients with pathologic fractures. Vertebral augmentation has the added advantage of permitting prompt radiotherapy after the procedure, in contrast to open surgery that mandates several weeks of wound healing before radiotherapy can be started.

Prognosis depends on the biologic activity of the underlying neoplasm. For example, spinal metastasis from carcinoma of the prostate often pursues an indolent course with little morbidity. In contrast, spinal metastasis from carcinoma of the lung carries a poorer prognosis. Outcome is variable with multiple myeloma.

Some patients with this disease have a rapidly progressive downhill course, whereas others have prolonged survival for 5 years or more. Prognosis also depends on whether the spinal lesions are single or multiple and on whether there is any neurologic involvement. An isolated spinal metastatic lesion without neurologic compromise can generally be controlled with radiotherapy and surgery, provided the malignancy is not progressing elsewhere in the body. In contrast, the prognosis is much worse in patients with multiple spinal metastases and significant cord compression and in patients with rapidly progressive extraspinal disease.

PRIMARY BONE TUMORS AFFECTING THE SPINE

A number of primary bone tumors can be found in the spinal column. In contrast to metastatic tumors, primary bone tumors of the spine are uncommon and are seen infrequently, even by spinal surgeons. These lesions may be benign or malignant. Benign tumors include osteochondroma, osteoid osteoma, aneurysmal bone cyst, hemangioma, giant cell tumor, and eosinophilic granuloma. Malignant tumors include chordoma, sarcoma, and chondrosarcoma.

Similar to spinal metastases, the hallmark of primary bone tumors of the spine is intractable pain. Neurologic deficits due to neural compression may also be present. Treatment usually involves radical surgery using anterior or posterior or combination approaches. Postoperative radiotherapy may be needed in selected cases.

SPINAL INTRADURAL TUMORS

A wide variety of tumors and other mass lesions can occur within the spinal dura. Most are uncommon in the elderly and will rarely be encountered by the primary care physician. Even a neurologist or neurosurgeon will see only a handful of these cases each year.

Lesions arising within the substance of the spinal cord are referred to as intramedullary tumors (4). All other intradural tumors are considered to be intradural, extramedullary in location. This includes tumors of the spinal nerve roots, cauda equina, and meninges.

The most common intramedullary tumors are ependymoma and astrocytoma. Less common lesions include hemangioblastoma, lipoma, and metastasis. Nonneoplastic mass lesions are occasionally seen in the cord, including cavernoma, epidermoid cyst, neuroglial cyst, and sarcoid granuloma.

The most common intradural, extramedullary tumors are meningioma and Schwannoma. Both are benign lesions.

Although a wide range of pathologic processes may occur within the spinal dura, the clinical presentation, evaluation, and treatment are similar for each type of lesion.

Intradural tumors usually present with localized pain and progressive neurologic deficit that may include radiculopathy, myelopathy, or cauda equina syndrome. Symptoms usually develop insidiously, but lesions that hemorrhage may cause acute, even catastrophic, neurologic deterioration. Examples of cord lesions that may be associated with hemorrhage include cavernoma and true arteriovenous malformations.

MRI is the imaging modality of choice for patients with intradural tumors. MRI accurately demonstrates the level of the lesion and whether the lesion is intramedullary or extramedullary. Cord expansion, cystic and solid components of the tumor, and presence of an associated syrinx can be identified.

Surgical excision, usually via a posterior (laminectomy) approach, is the treatment of choice. Prognosis depends on the histology of the lesion and the extent of the preoperative neurologic deficit. Postoperative radiotherapy may be recommended in selected cases.

One of the most difficult decisions facing the neurologist or neurosurgeon is whether to recommend a spinal cord biopsy in the patient with an unexplained intramedullary cord lesion (3). In rare cases, such as lymphoma, cord biopsy plays a crucial role in patient management by yielding a treatable diagnosis and guiding subsequent therapy. However, biopsy carries a significant risk of neurologic deterioration and often yields findings that are abnormal but not diagnostic.

Tumors are typically associated with a slow progression of neurologic findings and expansion of the cord and significant contrast enhancement on MRI. In contrast, inflammatory lesions usually cause rapid and profound neurologic deficits, with an absence of cord expansion and only minimal contrast enhancement on MRI.

In some cases, a period of observation, with follow-up imaging in 3 to 6 months, before making a decision on a cord biopsy may be prudent. Lesions that wax and wane on serial imaging are most likely inflammatory.

DURAL ARTERIOVENOUS FISTULA

A rare but treatable cause of myelopathy in the elderly is dural arteriovenous fistula (1). These lesions usually occur in the thoracic region and are characterized by progressive neurologic deterioration. The pathophysiology is venous hypertension of the spinal cord due to an arterialized vein arising from a radicular artery at the neural foramen. These lesions may not be diagnosed promptly because they are uncommon and the clinical picture may mimic the more common condition of neurogenic claudication and spinal stenosis in its early stages. Characteristic imaging findings include T2 signal changes in the cord on MRI and evidence of abnormal vasculature on computed tomography (CT)/myelogram, MRI/magnetic resonance angiography (MRA), or conventional spinal angiography. Surgical treatment consists of division of the arterialized vein at the fistula site and disconnection of the fistula from the venous system of the spinal cord.

SPINAL INFECTIONS

Spinal infections are uncommon but must be considered in the older adult with back pain. These infections may be pyogenic, tuberculous, or fungal. The term spinal infection encompasses a spectrum of specific entities, including intervertebral diskitis, osteomyelitis of the vertebral bodies, epidural abscess, infection of the paravertebral structures (e.g., psoas abscess), or some combination of these. The patient often presents with intense, localized pain, similar to spinal metastatic disease. Neurologic involvement is variable. Patients often have no neurologic symptoms or signs but may have radiculopathy, myelopathy, or cauda equina syndrome.

Spinal infections can be divided into two groups. The first group includes spinal infections that occur as a complication of spinal surgery. These typically present within 2 to 3 weeks of surgery, although more indolent infections may not manifest for 6 to 8 weeks.

The second group includes patients who have not had recent spinal surgery. In these patients, spinal infection is presumably caused by hematogenous spread of bacteria from some distant site. A wide range of infections can lead to secondary involvement of the spinal column. Urinary tract infection, subacute bacterial endocarditis, septic arthritis, and sinusitis are frequent antecedent sources of infection. The physician should also be aware that infections of the skin, respiratory system, and gastrointestinal tract may also lead to spinal infection. The physician should inquire about recent invasive procedures that can cause bacteremia, such as cystoscopy and dental work. Diabetes mellitus, advancing age, and intravenous drug abuse are risk factors associated with spinal infection. Other factors that may play a contributing role include alcoholism, long-term steroid therapy, rheumatoid arthritis, immunosuppression, coexisting malignancy, and osteoporosis.

The physician should strongly consider the possibility of spinal infection in the patient with fever and back pain; however, most patients harboring spinal infections are afebrile. Thus, the presence of a fever can help establish the diagnosis of spinal infection, but the absence of fever in no way excludes this diagnosis. Surprisingly, the white blood cell count and differential are often normal, even in the face of active spinal infection, and provide little guidance in establishing this diagnosis. In contrast, the erythrocyte sedimentation rate (ESR) is quite helpful. An elevated ESR suggests the presence of infection, whereas a normal ESR strongly suggests that a spinal infection is not present. The ESR is also a good way to follow the disease and the response to antibiotic treatment. C-reactive protein (CRP) is also sensitive for spinal infection but may not be widely available in some centers. Blood cultures should be obtained in all cases where spinal infection is suspected.

Early in the course of the illness, plain radiographs and even MRI may be completely normal. The radiographic hallmark of infection is that the epicenter of involvement of the spinal column is the disk space, with secondary spread to the adjacent vertebral bodies. In contrast, metastatic tumor usually starts in the vertebral body and spares the disk space, at least initially. The MRI can help define whether the patient has diskitis, osteomyelitis, epidural abscess, paraspinal infection (e.g., psoas abscess), or some combination of these processes. MRI is also useful in assessing the response to antibiotic treatment.

It is important to obtain an accurate microbiologic diagnosis before proceeding with treatment. If blood cultures are positive and the clinical and imaging findings support the diagnosis of vertebral osteomyelitis/diskitis, antibiotic treatment can be initiated. If blood cultures are negative, a CT-guided percutaneous biopsy of the involved spinal segment should be performed. If the CT-guided biopsy is negative, an open surgical biopsy should be performed. With each biopsy procedure, a full range of aerobic, anaerobic, fungal, and mycobacterial cultures and stains should be obtained.

The most common organisms found in spinal infections are coagulase-positive and coagulase-negative staphylococci. *Escherichia coli* and other gram-negative organisms, tuberculosis, and fungi can be seen in intravenous drug abusers and immunocompromised individuals.

Antibiotics represent the primary treatment for spinal infection. Spinal infections are typically treated with 3 to 6 weeks of intravenous antibiotics, often followed by a course of oral therapy.

Early surgery is sometimes needed for patients with spinal cord or cauda equina compression, and late surgery is occasionally needed for patients who develop spinal instability or deformity as a result of the infectious process. It is uncommon to find a localized collection of purulent fluid that is amenable to drainage. Dural enhancement usually just represents a secondary inflammatory response but is often overdiagnosed as representing an epidural abscess. Thus, the MRI diagnosis of epidural abscess must be interpreted cautiously and in the context of the clinical findings.

Bracing, usually with a lightweight corset, is helpful for symptomatic relief. Patients may continue with their usual physical activities as tolerated. Much of the treatment of these patients can be conducted in the outpatient setting. Hospitalization is needed only for surgical procedures and occasionally for pain control.

LUMBAR SPINAL STENOSIS

Degenerative lumbar spinal stenosis is a very common spinal disorder in older adults. In its more advanced forms, lumbar spinal stenosis causes neurogenic claudication, which refers to leg pain and paresthesia that is precipitated by standing and walking and relieved by sitting down. This diagnosis is being made with increasing frequency, partly as a result of the widespread availability of MRI and partly as a result of increased recognition of the clinical syndrome of neurogenic claudication. Patients may present with varying degrees of low back pain, but intervention usually depends on whether leg symptoms are present.

A careful history is essential to establish the diagnosis. Patients with neurogenic claudication give varying descriptions of their lower extremity symptoms. Some patients report true leg pain, whereas others describe tingling, heaviness, or a sensation that their legs are going to "give out." The leg symptoms may be unilateral or bilateral.

The physician should be aware that lumbar spinal stenosis, vascular occlusive disease, degenerative joint disease of the hip, and peripheral neuropathy are all common in the elderly and can cause similar symptoms. Patients with vascular claudication develop leg pain with walking but gain relief by standing still. In contrast, patients with neurogenic claudication must sit down in order to gain relief. Patients with degenerative joint disease of the hip describe hip and groin pain, without distal radiation. Patients with peripheral neuropathy typically describe painless numbness affecting both legs symmetrically in a stocking distribution.

In patients with lumbar spinal stenosis, the neurologic examination is usually normal or may reveal mild abnormalities. If the patient has a moderate or severe neurologic deficit, a second diagnosis may be present. For example, the patient might have lumbar spinal stenosis with a superimposed acute disk herniation. It is important to check distal pulses to assess vascular status and also to do the Fabere maneuvers to assess for degenerative joint disease of the hip.

MRI or myelogram/CT should be used to establish the diagnosis of lumbar spinal stenosis. These studies may reveal stenosis of the central canal, lateral recess, or neural foramina. A degenerative spondylolisthesis or scoliosis may be present. Plain radiographs with flexion and extension views should also be obtained.

Symptoms may wax and wane early in the course of the disease process; however, the natural history of lumbar spinal stenosis is one of gradual progression of discomfort and functional limitation over time.

Conservative treatment, including physical therapy with or without modalities and lumbar epidural steroid injections, may help in selected cases. Patients with disabling neurogenic claudication, coupled with severe spinal stenosis, usually require surgical treatment.

Before making a surgical referral, it is important for the physician to ask how much the patient is limited in his or her usual activities of daily living. For example, the patient who develops mild leg aching after walking 3 miles in 30 minutes probably does not need any active treatment, even if there is radiographic evidence of lumbar spinal stenosis. In contrast, the patient who consistently develops severe leg pain after walking 50 meters in 2 minutes should be considered for surgery.

Surgical treatment involves a lumbar decompressive laminectomy of the stenotic spinal segments. A fusion may be required for some patients with spondylolisthesis or scoliosis. A good or excellent result can be expected in 70% to 90% of cases at 1 year of follow-up. With longer follow-up, a few patients who had good or excellent outcomes at 1 year will develop recurrent symptoms and will require further investigation and treatment. Despite this, surgical results are superior to patients treated nonoperatively at long term follow-up.

Risk factors for poor outcome after decompressive laminectomy include coexisting illness (severe arthritis at sites other than the spine, rheumatoid arthritis, or cardiac disease), single-interspace laminectomy, female gender, and presence of a preoperative neurologic deficit. Advanced age does not appear to be a risk factor for poor outcome.

SPINAL SYNOVIAL CYST

Synovial cysts can occur in the spine and can cause neurologic symptoms as they enlarge. These cysts arise from the lining of the facet joint and can be viewed as a subset of degenerative spinal stenosis. They are most common in the lumbar region but can occur in the cervical spine. Synovial cysts are typically solitary but can be multiple. Conservative treatment is usually not helpful. MRI is the imaging procedure of choice, although myelogram/CT can also be used.

Synovial cysts usually cause radicular pain and paresthesias due to compression of the underlying spinal nerve root(s). Symptoms usually develop gradually; however, patients occasionally present with the sudden onset of severe pain if there has been acute hemorrhage into the cyst.

Clinical indications for surgery are similar to those for other lumbar spinal operations. The ideal candidate for surgery has intractable leg pain (rather than back pain) as the primary symptom. The imaging studies should demonstrate a synovial cyst in a location that correlates well with the clinical findings.

The surgical procedure consists of a lumbar laminectomy and cyst removal. A concomitant fusion is occasionally needed if there is a spondylolisthesis at the level of the cyst. Surgical results are excellent, and the cyst recurrence rate is low.

HERNIATED INTERVERTEBRAL DISK

Intervertebral disk herniations are most common in middle-aged adults but are also frequently seen in the elderly. Disk herniations occur most commonly in the lumbar region, somewhat less frequently in the cervical spine, and occasionally in the thoracic spine. MRI is the imaging procedure of choice; however, the myelogram/CT remains a superb diagnostic tool for those patients in whom MRI is contraindicated. The natural history of disk herniation at any level of the vertebral column is one of spontaneous improvement. Most patients will improve without any active treatment. Conservative treatment, including physical therapy (exercises and/or modalities) and epidural steroid injections, may be of benefit in selected patients. Surgery is needed in only a small percentage of cases. The management of intervertebral disk disease is discussed in more detail in Chapter 15.

INFLAMMATORY SPINAL DISORDERS

The most common inflammatory spinal disorders are ankylosing spondylitis and rheumatoid arthritis. The spine may also be affected by other rheumatologic processes, including gout, pseudogout, acromegaly, amyloidosis, lupus, and diffuse idiopathic skeletal hyperostosis.

Ankylosing spondylitis is a chronic inflammatory disease that chiefly affects the spine. This disease is characterized by involvement of the sacroiliac joint and spinal column and has an association with the histocompatibility antigen HLA-B27. The disease typically has its onset between puberty and age 45. Men are affected more often than women. The pathologic picture includes inflammation, bony erosion, and ankylosis. Over time, complete ossification of the anterior longitudinal ligament occurs, and bridging osteophytes develop. The radiographic appearance is described as a "bamboo" spine.

Patients with ankylosing spondylitis usually present with the insidious onset of low back pain and stiffness. Symptoms are usually worse in the morning and improve with exercise. There may be buttock pain that spreads diffusely to the posterior thighs. Leg pain with ankylosing spondylitis usually does not radiate below the knee and does not represent sciatica due to nerve root compression.

Ankylosing spondylitis is a chronic disease with a variable course, most often characterized by spontaneous remissions and exacerbations. Symptoms typically begin in the lumbosacral region and progress rostrally over time to involve the thoracic and cervical regions. Patients may have extraspinal involvement as well. Constitutional symptoms, peripheral arthritis, ocular disease, cardiovascular disease, and pulmonary complications may occur.

The primary goals of management are to optimize functional status and minimize pain and stiffness. Physical therapy and exercise are important for maintaining good functional status and joint mobility. Standard pharmacologic treatment includes nonsteroidal anti-inflammatory drugs (NSAIDs), analgesics, and muscle relaxants for symptomatic relief. There has been recent interest in using disease-modifying antirheumatic drugs such as sulfasalazine, methotrexate, or corticosteroids. These agents may be helpful in selected patients with an active inflammatory component manifested by acute pain and an elevated ESR. Unfortunately, none of these antirheumatic drugs has been shown to prevent disease progression.

Spinal fracture represents a frequent complication of ankylosing spondylitis. These fractures can occur after minor trauma and often remain undiagnosed. Some of these cases can be managed nonoperatively with bracing, whereas others require surgical treatment. Surgery is also needed in a limited number of cases for correction of severe spinal deformity (for example, the "chin-on-chest" deformity) or for management of progressive myelopathy.

Rheumatoid arthritis is another inflammatory disorder that often affects the spine. In contrast to ankylosing spondylitis, rheumatoid arthritis has a female preponderance and more significant polyarticular joint involvement. Patients typically present with pain and stiffness of multiple joints, fatigue, and low-grade fever. Extra-articular manifestations include ocular involvement, pericarditis, myocarditis, pleural effusions, and pulmonary nodules, which may be difficult to distinguish from malignancies. Neurologic involvement includes peripheral neuropathy, mononeuritis multiplex, and compression neuropathies, such as carpal tunnel syndrome. Patients may also develop cervical myelopathy from cord compression.

A wide range of spinal abnormalities is seen in patients with rheumatoid arthritis, including cervical spine instability with subluxation. Atlantoaxial subluxation is the most common spinal deformity seen in rheumatoid arthritis; however, subluxations can occur at any level of the cervical spine.

The overall management of rheumatoid arthritis involves a team approach including internists, rheumatologists, neurologists, physiatrists, and orthopaedic specialists. Social and psychological support is essential. The overall goals of therapy include pain relief and maintaining or improving functional capacity. These patients often have neck pain due to rheumatoid involvement of the cervical spine. Conservative management with physical therapy, exercises, NSAIDs, and various types of cervical collars is usually helpful. Surgery may be required if the cervical spine is unstable or if there is a significant neurologic deficit.

SPINAL TRAUMA

Spinal injury should be suspected in patients with severe systemic trauma, patients with minor trauma who report spinal pain or have sensory or motor symptoms, and patients with an impaired level of consciousness after trauma (2). Patients with acute spinal injury will usually present to a hospital emergency department but may also be seen at urgent care centers or other outpatient facilities. The cervical spine is the most mobile segment of the spinal column and is the most common site of spinal cord injury. The thoracic spine from T1 to T10 has intrinsic stability due to the rib cage and is relatively immobile. Injuries to this region are uncommon. The thoracolumbar junction (T11 to L2) is a transition zone between the rigid thoracic spine and the more mobile lumbar spine and is the second most common site of spinal fractures and dislocations. Fractures of the lower lumbar spine are less common.

Patients with acute spinal trauma report pain at the site of injury. The unconscious patient should be considered to have a cervical spine injury until proven otherwise with appropriate imaging studies. General physical examination may reveal bruising, tenderness, and muscle spasm at the site of injury. A detailed neurologic examination should include motor testing, sensory testing (light touch, pinprick, joint position sense) of the entire body including the perianal region, deep tendon reflexes, rectal tone, and bulbocavernosus reflex.

The neurologic assessment can reveal a wide spectrum of findings from a completely normal examination to a severe spinal cord injury. It is important to distinguish between complete and incomplete spinal cord injury. Patients with complete cord injuries rarely improve, whereas patients with incomplete spinal cord injuries may experience substantial neurologic recovery.

Incomplete spinal cord injury syndromes can occur and should be carefully documented. The central cord syndrome is characterized by weakness that is more profound in the upper extremities than the lower extremities. Elderly patients are at particular risk for this syndrome, which typically occurs with acute hyperextension of the neck in patients with cervical spinal canal stenosis on a congenital or acquired basis. Brown-Sequard syndrome is a unilateral spinal cord injury, usually caused by penetrating trauma. These patients have loss of motor function and joint position sense ipsilateral to the injury and loss of pain and temperature sensation contralateral to the injury.

The physician should be aware that patients with acute spinal injury may have other severe injuries, including head injury, that require rapid diagnosis and treatment.

Guidelines for the imaging requirements in patients with possible cervical spine injury continue to evolve. Current recommendations are that low-risk patients can be cleared without any imaging studies. Patients in this category must meet the following five criteria: no midline cervical tenderness, no focal neurologic deficit, normal alertness, no intoxication, and no painful, distracting injury (8).

For patients with intermediate and high risk of cervical spine injury, helical CT scanning has replaced plain film radiography as the imaging modality of choice (6). CT has a sensitivity of 96% in the detection of cervical spine fracture, compared with 64% for plain radiography. The advantage of CT is even more significant in the elderly, in whom advanced degenerative changes may mask findings of acute trauma on plain radiographs.

MRI is used in select cases. MRI can demonstrate compression, edema, or hemorrhage of the cord; traumatic disk herniations; and ligamentous injuries. Major disadvantages of this technique include prolonged scanning times and difficulty in imaging patients on advanced life support. These factors may preclude MRI in the unstable, multiple trauma patient.

Lateral flexion–extension radiographs, performed with physician supervision, may be needed to exclude ligamentous instability.

The basic principles of management of acute spinal injury include immobilization, airway management, and cardiovascular resuscitation. Pharmacologic treatment is indicated for acute spinal cord injury. For patients seen within 3 hours of injury, high-dose methylprednisolone is administered intravenously, with an initial bolus of 30 mg/kg, followed by a continuous infusion of 5.4 mg/kg for 23 hours. For patients seen between 3 and 8 hours following injury, the methylprednisolone infusion is continued for 48 hours. For patients seen more than 8 hours following injury, methylprednisolone should not be given.

Patients with acute, unstable fractures of the cervical spine should be placed in traction to immobilize the spine. Some spinal injuries can be managed nonoperatively with bracing, whereas others require surgery to decompress neural elements and to realign and stabilize the spinal column. An active rehabilitation program is needed for patients with spinal cord injury. The acute management of the injury should be carried out as expeditiously as possible, so that the patient can be mobilized and get into rehabilitation as soon as possible. This is especially important in the elderly. Rapid mobilization will help minimize the complications of bed rest, including deep venous thrombophlebitis, skin breakdown, and pneumonia.

Steady progress has been made in the management of spinal cord injury, and mortality has been significantly reduced. Despite these improvements, traumatic spinal cord injury remains a devastating condition that alters every aspect of the victim's life.

CONCLUSIONS

Many spinal disorders may be encountered in the older adult. Some affect the bony structures of the spinal column primarily. Examples include osteoporosis, metastatic cancer, and vertebral infection. Neurologic symptoms or signs may occur if there is compression of the spinal cord, cauda equina, or spinal nerve roots due to pathologic fracture of the vertebral body or extension of the disease process into the spinal canal itself. Degenerative spinal disorders, including spinal canal stenosis and disk herniations, are very common in the elderly. Inflammatory arthropathies are chronic illnesses that develop in young and middle-aged adults and present in more advanced forms in the elderly. Acute spinal injury is most common in young adult males but can be seen at any age. A wide range of primary intradural tumors can occur in the elderly. Most are uncommon and will be rarely encountered by the primary care physician. Prompt, accurate diagnosis of each of these disorders is essential. Treatment is individualized, based on the underlying disease process.

REFERENCES

1. Atkinson JLD, Miller GM, Krauss WE, et al. Clinical and radiographic features of dural arteriovenous fistula, a treatable cause of myelopathy. *Mayo Clin Proc.* 2001;76:1120–1130.
2. Chiles BW, Cooper PR. Acute spinal injury. *N Engl J Med.* 1996;334:514–520.
3. Cohen-Gadol AA, Zikel OM, Miller GM, et al. Spinal cord biopsy: a review of 38 cases. *Neurosurgery.* 2003;52:806–816.
4. Fischer G, Brotchi J. *Intramedullary Spinal Cord Tumors.* New York: Thieme Medical Publishers; 1996:21–23.
5. Fourney DR, Schomer DF, Nader R, et al. Percutaneous vertebroplasty and kyphoplasty for painful vertebral body fractures in cancer patients. *J Neurosurg.* 2003;98[Suppl 1]:21–30.
6. Grogan EL, Morris JA, Dittrus RS, et al. Cervical spine evaluation in urban trauma centers: lowering institutional costs and complications through helical CT scan. *J Am Coll Surg.* 2005;200:160–165.
7. Harrop JS, Prpa B, Reinhardt MK, et al. Primary and secondary osteoporosis: incidence of subsequent vertebral compression fractures after kyphoplasty. *Spine.* 2004;29:2120–2125.
8. Hoffman JR, Mower WR, Wolfson AB, et al. Validity of a set of clinical criteria to rule out injury to the cervical spine in patients with blunt trauma. *N Engl J Med.* 2000;343:94–99.

SUGGESTED READINGS

Hazzard WR, Blass JP, Ettinger WH, et al. *Principles of Geriatric Medicine and Gerontology.* 4th ed. New York: McGraw-Hill; 1999:1174–1190.

Popp AJ, ed. *A Guide to the Primary Care of Neurological Disorders.* Park Ridge, IL: American Association of Neurological Surgeons; 1998:101–120.

Ropper AH, Brown RH, eds. *Adams and Victor's Principles of Neurology.* 8th ed. New York: McGraw-Hill; 2005.

Winn HR, ed. *Youman's Neurological Surgery.* 5th ed. Philadelphia: Saunders; 2004.

LISTING OF WEBSITES OF NATIONAL SUPPORT GROUPS AND OTHER RESOURCES.

Arthritis Foundation: http://www.arthritis.org/

National Institutes of Health/National Institute of Arthritis and Musculoskeletal and Skin Diseases: http://www.niams.nih.gov/

National Osteoporosis Foundation: http://www.nof.org/

National Scoliosis Foundation: http://www.scoliosis.org/

National Spinal Cord Injury Association: http://www.spinalcord.org/

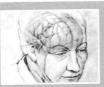

CHAPTER 25.1

Common Peripheral Neuropathies in the Older Adult

Charlene R. Hoffman Snyder and Benn E. Smith

Age influences several morphologic and functional features of the peripheral nervous system (PNS). Axonal atrophy and loss of myelinated and unmyelinated nerve fibers occur in the older adult, contributing to the functional and electrophysiologic reduction of the PNS. These aging changes include a decline in nerve conduction velocity, muscle strength, sensory discrimination, autonomic responses, and endoneurial blood flow. The capacity for axonal regeneration and reinnervation is constant throughout life but tends to be delayed and less effective with aging (37). Normal aging itself does not generate changes in clinical signs, symptoms, or functional status. When the presence of common age-related conditions (e.g., cancer, renal disease, diabetes, infection, and increased polypharmacy) combines with age-related neurologic changes, the outcome can be the expression of common peripheral neuropathies of the older adult (25).

DEFINITIONS

Peripheral neuropathy (PN) refers to a group of disorders (polyneuropathy, single and multiple mononeuropathies, and radiculopathy) that result in deranged function and structure of the peripheral motor, sensory, and autonomic systems. The definition of PN is somewhat arbitrary in anatomic terms because any disorder that causes damage to the nerve fibers within the PNS is technically a neuropathy. Therefore, the common definition is limited in topographic terms. It is helpful to distinguish two broad topographic categories in the definition of PN: polyneuropathy or mononeuropathy. These categories represent a pattern of involvement in the PNS that provides a guide to causation (35). *Polyneuropathies* are processes that result in bilaterally symmetric disturbance of function. *Polyradiculopathy* and *polyradiculoneuropathy* suggest a course of involvement of the spinal roots or involvement of both the roots and the peripheral nerve trunks, respectively. The second pattern of PN is focal or single-nerve disorders, termed *mononeuropathy*. A common example is nerve entrapment (carpal tunnel or peroneal nerve injury). Multiple mononeuropathies are sequential involvement of noncontiguous nerve

trunks, as may occur within the multiple nerve infarcts of vasculitis. The term *neuronopathy* describes diseases that affect neuron cell bodies. The diseases are usually pure sensory or pure motor and encompass ganglionopathies (sensory and/or autonomic) and motor neuron disease (motor) (3).

Further classification of PN (Table 25-1) depends on analysis of the temporal course (acute or chronic), anatomic pattern (distal sensorimotor, polyradiculopathy, or multiple mononeuropathies), pathology (axonal, demyelinating, or mixed), modality specificity (motor neuronopathy, sensory neuronopathy, or autonomic), functional class (small- or large-fiber type), and severity of the disorder at hand (21). The information gathered from the history, physical, and electrodiagnostic studies helps to classify the neuropathies by their pathophysiology (metabolic, inflammatory, toxic, infectious, vasculitic, paraneoplastic, or hereditary) and guide further laboratory studies and treatment (35).

EPIDEMIOLOGY

Although the complaints of "burning toes" and "numb feet" are common in clinical practice, epidemiologic data on polyneuropathy are relatively limited in the older adult. This scarcity of data may be due in part to the fact that PN frequently occurs as a component of several common and rare diseases that are diverse, multifactorial, sometimes obscure, and often idiopathic (21).

There are approximately 10 million people with neuropathy in the U.S. population, 3.4 million of whom are Centers for Medicare and Medicaid Services beneficiaries (20). Estimates are that between 3% and 8% of adults over the age of 50 suffer from acquired chronic axonal sensory or sensorimotor polyneuropathies (21,38). An estimated 23% of patients with symptoms of PN have chronic idiopathic sensory polyneuropathy (38). Finding the pathologic cause of PN is accomplished about 75% of the time with careful evaluation (7). Hereditary neuropathy is found one third of the time, with inflammatory demyelinating disorder [chronic inflammatory demyelinating polyradiculoneuropathy (CIDP)]

Table 25-1. *Classification of Common Peripheral Neuropathies in the Older Adult*

Pathophysiology	Disorders	Temporal Course	Anatomical Pattern	Functional Class	Modality Specificity	Pathology
Unknown	Idiopathic	Chronic	DSSP	Small fiber/large fiber	S, SM	Axonal
Acquired						
Metabolic states	Impaired glucose Diabetes mellitus	Chronic/subacute	DSSP, PSMP, MM, PRN	Small fiber	S, M, A	Axonal/mixed
	End-stage renal failure (uremic neuropathy)	Chronic	DSSP	Small fiber/large fiber	S	Axonal
	Nutritional deficiencies Vitamin B$_{12}$ deficiency Copper	Subacute/chronic	DSSP	Small fiber/large fiber	S > M	Axonal
Immune-mediated	Guillain–Barré syndrome	Acute/relapsing-remitting course	PSMP, PRN	Large fiber > small fiber	M > S, A	Demyelinating > axonal
	Chronic inflammatory demyelinating polyneuropathy	Subacute/chronic Relapsing-remitting	PSMP, PRN, MM	Large fiber > small fiber	M > S, A	Demyelinating > mixed
	Vasculitic Systemic or nonsystemic	Acute/subacute	PSMP, PRN, MM	Small fiber/large fiber	M, S, A	Mixed
	Connective tissue-related: rheumatoid arthritis, sarcoidosis, systemic lupus erythematosus, Sjögren's syndrome, systemic sclerosis, trigeminal sensory neuropathy	Acute/chronic	DSSP, PRN	Large fiber > small fiber	S > M	Axonal
Malignancies	Cancer-related paraneoplastic, lymphoproliferative disorders, lymphoma, myeloma, primary amyloidosis	Subacute	S > DSSP, PSMP, MM	Small fiber/large fiber	S > M	Axonal

(Continued)

Table 25-1. *(Continued)*

Pathophysiology	Disorders	Temporal Course	Anatomical Pattern	Functional Class	Modality Specificity	Pathology
Paraproteinemic	Monoclonal gammopathy of undetermined significance (MGUS), Waldenström	Subacute/chronic	PSMP, PRN, MM	Large fiber > small fiber	S = M	Mixed
Infections	Varicella zoster, HIV-related, Lyme disease, Hanson's disease, bacterial Parasitic, Creutzfeldt-Jakob	Acute/subacute/relapsing-remitting	DSSP, PSMP, PRN, MM	Small fiber/large fiber	S, A	Axonal
Toxins	Industrial and environmental	Subacute	DSSP, PSMP, PRN	Small fiber/large fiber	S = M	Axonal
	Drug-induced; chemotherapy, other drugs, Alcohol Vitamin B$_6$	Acute/relapsing-remitting	DSSP, PSMP	Small fiber/large fiber	S > M, A	Axonal
Critical illness	Intensive care	Acute	DSSP	Large fiber > small fiber	M = S	Mixed
Hereditary	Charcot-Marie-Tooth Hereditary neuropathy with predisposition to pressure palsies, familial amyloidosis, porphyria, Fabry, leukodystrophies	Chronic	DSSP, MM	Large fiber > small fiber	M = S	Mixed
Mononeuropathies	Carpal tunnel syndrome, fibular (peroneal) mononeuropathy	Acute to subacute	—	Large fiber/small fiber	S = M	Mixed

DSSP, distal symmetric sensorimotor polyneuropathy; PSMP, proximal symmetric motor polyneuropathies; MM, multiple mononeuropathies; PRN, polyradiculoneuropathy; SN, sensory neuronopathy or ganglionopathy; S, sensory neuropathy; M, motor neuropathy; A, autonomic neuropathy; HIV, human immunodeficiency virus.

Modified after Bosch EP, Smith BE. Disorders of peripheral nerves. In: Bradley WG, Daroff RB, Fenichel GM, et al., eds. *Neurology in clinical practice.* Woburn, MA: Butterworth-Heinemann; 2000:2106–2109.

occurring at a rate of 13% to 21% and a remaining 13% to 15% being found to have systemic, toxic, or malignant causes (3,7). Of the systemic causes, diabetic neuropathy is the acquired neuropathy of greatest frequency in Western populations.

PATHOLOGY

Although there are more than 100 different causes for neuropathies, the peripheral nerve has a limited repertoire of responses to injury or metabolic insults. Wallerian degeneration is the response to axonal disruption and results in degeneration of the axon and myelin sheath distal to the site of injury. In axonal degeneration or axonopathy, the most distal portion of the axons degenerates along with breakdown of the myelin sheath, resulting in a "dying-back" or length-dependent neuropathy. Primary neuronal (perikaryal) degeneration or neuronopathy occurs at the level of the motor neuron or dorsal root ganglion cells with subsequent degeneration of their peripheral and central processes. Even if the inciting cause can be removed, recovery is often incomplete. Segmental demyelination occurs at the level of the myelin sheath but spares axons, allowing recovery to be more rapid (5).

Although the cause of the nerve damage does not dictate whether a neuropathy will be painful, pain is common and a prominent symptom with many of the PNs. Although the specific pathologic lesions responsible for neuropathic pain are unknown, theories suggest that ectopic spontaneous impulses may result in the sensation we associate with pain. In the older adult, the most common type of painful neuropathy is believed to be caused by damage to small myelinated and nociceptive C (unmyelinated) nerve fibers. However, large nerve fibers can be affected as well (22).

NEUROPATHY OF UNKNOWN ETIOLOGY

CHRONIC IDIOPATHIC SENSORY NEUROPATHY

The most commonly seen PN in general adult practice is the painful, distal, sensory neuropathy that is further unclassified because its pathophysiologic origin is unknown. Estimates are that more than one third of the 15 to 20 million adults over 40 years old with PN have chronic idiopathic axonal polyneuropathy (CIAP). This condition presents as a chronic, slowly evolving loss of sensation in the distal extremities associated with or without pain. Eventually, pain is the complaint that usually brings the patient to the office. Pain is often the most disabling feature, even though progression to a nonambulatory disability is very rare. Diagnostic findings by electromyography

(EMG), quantitative sudomotor axon reflex test (QSART), and/or sensory testing show predominantly mild, distal sensory dysfunction. Emerging evidence suggests that impaired glucose tolerance is associated with idiopathic neuropathy (12,33). The association of impaired glucose metabolism as a component of an overall metabolic syndrome is well known, but how this contributes to peripheral nerve disease remains obscure. In addition to treating the pain associated with CIAP, addressing the underlying impaired glucose metabolism through diet and exercise is highly recommended (32).

NEUROPATHIES OF ACQUIRED ETIOLOGIES

METABOLIC POLYNEUROPATHIES
Diabetic Neuropathy

There are over 14.7 million Americans with diabetes mellitus; of these, an estimated 50% have diabetic PN (2). Diabetic neuropathy is not a homogeneous entity but may present with several different neuropathic patterns, including distal symmetric neuropathy, small-fiber neuropathy, and mononeuropathy. Although diabetes mellitus is one of the most common causes of PN, the true prevalence is unknown. Several pathophysiologic factors are thought to explain the findings of neuropathy, including metabolic alterations, microvascular pathology, and inflammatory changes. Diabetic nerves have an increased susceptibility to compression injury and to inflammatory vasculopathy. This may account for the broad spectrum of multifocal neuropathies seen as diabetic lumbosacral, radiculoplexus neuropathy, truncal neuropathy, cranial neuropathy, mononeuropathy, and multiplex mononeuropathy. Over 11% of patients with diabetic neuropathy are said to have neuropathic pain. Diabetic neuropathy is both a clinical diagnosis and a diagnosis of exclusion, remembering that diabetics may have additional comorbid factors that may contribute to the PN (renal failure). In addition to EMG (which focuses on abnormalities of large-diameter nerve fibers), testing that assesses small-diameter nerve fibers, such as autonomic testing, is often helpful. Management focuses on a combination of symptom relief (pain management, foot care, fall prevention, gait training, and conditioning) and glycemic control. Multiple therapies are under investigation including aldolase reductase inhibitors, gamma-linolenic acid, alpha-lipoic acid, and immunotherapy (10,15).

Uremic Neuropathy

At least 80% of patients with end-stage renal failure requiring dialysis develop PN. However, when the renal failure is effectively treated, the incidence is much less. The accumulation of systemic toxins and possibly ethylene oxide from dialysate solutions is a proposed pathogenesis, but nothing specific has been conclusively identified. Symptoms present as a slowly emerging chronic, predominantly sensory polyneuropathy. Cramps, unpleasant dysesthesias, distal foot muscle weakness, and restless legs syndrome occur frequently. When renal failure develops in the context of diabetes, a more severe polyneuropathy can occur. The diagnosis of uremic polyneuropathy is contingent on the presence of chronic end-stage renal failure (creatinine clearance <10mL/min) of at least several months in duration. The early recognition and reatment of renal failure will often result in the stabilization and/or reversal of nerve dysfuncion. Chronic dialysis, whether hemodialysis or peritoneal dialysis, is similar effective on nerve function, whereas renal transplantation provides the greatest benefit (5).

Nutritional Deficiencies and Neuropathy

Vitamin B_{12} deficiency develops in 7% to 16% of individuals, and population surveys estimate that 2% of persons 60 years and older have undiagnosed pernicious anemia. PN is a part of the clinical picture of vitamin B_{12} deficiency. The associated PN results in paresthesias in the hands and feet, as well as large-fiber modality sensory loss on physical examination. There is often an associated complaint of unsteadiness. The examination reveals absent or diminished Achilles reflexes, hyperactive or normoactive patellar reflexes, bilateral Babinski signs, and loss of vibratory and joint position sense. Electrophysiologic studies may demonstrate distal axonal degeneration. A low or low-normal serum vitamin B_{12} level and elevated methylmalonic acid and/or homocysteine levels support the diagnosis. The two-stage Schilling test may confirm the deficiency, but it is no longer considered necessary. The natural course of this reversible PN is about 50% improvement in symptoms if treatment begins soon enough to correct the anemia. Life-long cobalamin replacement will usually stabilize the neuropathy (5).

IMMUNE-MEDIATED POLYNEUROPATHIES

These disorders involve an acute, subacute, or chronic process of inflammatory immune attack on the PNS, namely Schwann cells, myelin, and axons. Although these neuropathies are not unique to the older adult, the largest peak incidence occurs between the fifth and eighth decades, and severity of the disease and prognosis are age related.

Guillain-Barré Syndrome

Guillain-Barré syndrome (GBS) is an acute, acquired, inflammatory polyradiculoneuropathy hallmarked by flaccid areflexic ascending paralysis. It is the most common acute anterior paralytic disease in Western countries since the decline of acute poliomyelitis. The occurrence rate is higher in persons in the fifth through eighth decades than in young individuals. The pathogenesis of GBS is incompletely defined, but expert thinking believes that one prominent mechanism is autoimmune attack prompted by preceding infection. The infections linked to GBS include *Campylobacter jejuni*, cytomegalovirus, Epstein-Barr virus, varicella-zoster virus, hepatitis A and B, human immunodeficiency virus (HIV), *Mycoplasma*, and West Nile virus. *Campylobacter jejuni* is the most common identifiable bacterial organism linked to GBS, particularly the axonal forms.

Differential diagnostic considerations in GBS include other conditions associated with subacute motor weakness. The hallmarks of GBS are symmetrical weakness and paresthesias in the hands or feet (or both) progressing rapidly in an ascending manner over a relatively short time (<4 weeks to nadir). Low pain and autonomic dysfunction (hypo- or hypertension or cardiac arrhythmias) may be attending findings. Neurologic signs include hyporeflexia or areflexia. Key to the diagnosis is the cerebrospinal fluid (CSF) examination. Serial electrophysiologic studies may prove helpful. The natural history of the disease is that of an acute reversible course with progression of symptoms ending 1 to 4 weeks into the illness. Continuation of progression beyond 4 weeks may lead to a diagnosis of subacute inflammatory demyelinating polyradiculoneuropathy or CIDP. Modern critical care facilities have dramatically changed the outcomes in GBS. The current mortality rates are between 5% and 10%. Studies have shown an age-related poorer prognosis with increased incidence of ventilatory support, rapid progression of deficits, and less probability of walking independently in 6 months (14).

In treating GBS patients with rapidly worsening deficits until the maximum extent of the syndrome is established, the most favorable outcomes occur with supportive care in modern intensive care units (ICUs) where many complications can be prevented. The recognition and avoidance of respiratory, bulbar, and autonomic complications are critical to improving outcomes. Therapeutic interventions aimed at mitigating the effects of serum autoantibodies, including plasma exchange and high-dose intravenous immunoglobulin (IVIG), have been shown to be similarly effective. Data from controlled clinical trials do not show an advantage to using both together. Corticosteroids have not been proven to be effective. Physical therapy is an integral part of the prevention strategy to prevent contracture disability, venous stasis, and joint immobilization. Attention to psychological support is valuable and required by both the patient and family members, considering that recovery may take several months (14).

Chronic Inflammatory Demyelinating Polyradiculoneuropathy

Unlike GBS, CIDP has a chronic protracted clinical course with no clear association to antecedent infection. Respiratory failure is an unusual occurrence. The temporal profile of CIDP takes two forms: a stepwise progressive course over months to years or a relapsing-remitting course. The chronic progressive course is more age related (mean, 51 years), with the fifth and sixth decades being the peak incidence ages for the disease. Diagnostic criteria include insidious onset of proximal and distal limb weakness in both upper and lower limbs over at least 2 months with little muscle wasting. Hyporeflexia and areflexia are distinguishing neurologic signs with sensory deficits in a "stocking glove" pattern suggesting large-fiber neuropathy, often without pain. The combination of history, neurologic examination, CSF evaluation, electrodiagnostic studies suggesting demyelination, and sural nerve biopsy supports the diagnosis. The natural history of disease shows a chronic relapsing-remitting pattern with lingering neurologic deficits; less than 10% of patients will have spontaneous remission. Modulation of the immune response with plasmapheresis, prednisone, and/or human immunoglobulin, with resulting reduction of deficits, is the primary treatment goal. Long-term treatment is often required due to relapses (20).

Vasculitic Neuropathy

Many forms of vasculitis may affect the PNS. Vasculitic neuropathy generally presents with an acute or subacute onset of multiple painful mononeuropathies or as an asymmetric polyneuropathy. The classification scheme for the various forms of vasculitic neuropathy divides them into systemic or nonsystemic vasculitis with further categorization designating primary (Wegener's granulomatosis, Churg-Strauss syndrome, polyarteritis nodosa, and microscopic polyangiitis) and secondary (rheumatoid, hepatitis C, mixed cryoglobulinemia, HIV, cytomegalovirus, and paraneoplastic) forms. Systemic necrotizing vasculitis is an acute potentially life-threatening syndrome affecting multiple organ systems that is often reversible, whereas nonsystemic (multiple mononeuropathies) vasculitis is a much more benign condition, typically following a nonfatal course. Diabetic lumbosacral radiculoplexus neuropathy is an acute microscopic vasculitis that is in a category by itself; this unique monophasic condition is confined to the lumbosacral plexus and root, sparing other systemic organs (29).

The initial presentation of vasculitic neuropathy is usually an acute or subacute painful sensory or sensorimotor neuropathy, asymmetric polyneuropathy, or multiple mononeuropathies. Most patients have initial symptoms in the lower extremities (fibular or tibial divisions of the sciatic nerve). Accompanying constitutional symptoms may include myalgias, arthralgias, weight loss, respiratory symptoms, hematuria, abdominal pain, rash, or night sweats. Electrodiagnostic studies reveal acute or subacute axonal loss of both sensory and motor nerve fibers, usually in a patchy multifocal distribution. Laboratory markers of inflammation are helpful in the systemic form but less so in the nonsystemic form. Because of the need for long-term treatment with potentially toxic agents, a full-thickness sural nerve biopsy is needed for histologic confirmation. This is most feasible when the disease process has clearly involved the sural territory. Rapidly suppressing the course of the illness to limit ongoing nerve and organ damage is the main goal of treatment with adequate immunosuppressive therapy (prednisone and/or cytotoxic agents). New treatments showing promise include IVIG and a variety of biologic agents (29).

Connective Tissue Neuropathies

Rheumatoid arthritis, systemic lupus erythematosus, systemic sclerosis, and Sjögren's syndrome are diseases associated with peripheral nerve involvement. Patterns of involvement include distal sensorimotor neuropathy, mononeuropathy, multiple mononeuropathies, trigeminal sensory neuropathy, sensory ganglionopathy, and polyradiculoneuropathy. The diagnostic approach includes assessing inflammatory markers and obtaining a nerve biopsy if vasculitis is suspected. Treatment is directed at the underlying disease process (26).

NEUROPATHIES ASSOCIATED WITH MALIGNANCIES

There are several mechanisms related to cancer or its treatment that leads to PN. They are as follows: nerve compression or destruction by the tumor mass; metastasis with involvement of adjacent transiting nerves; autoimmune paraneoplasia with generation of antineuronal antibodies; entrapment neuropathies caused by loss of supporting muscle and adjacent tissue around nerve trunks as a result of severe malignancy-associated cachexia; and neurotoxic chemotherapy. It is common for cancer patients to have distal symmetrical sensorimotor polyneuropathy. Clinically, these are slow in onset, chronic, and often indistinguishable from distal axonal neuropathies in persons without a malignancy. Lung, stomach, breast, colon, pancreas, and testes are the most common sites of neoplasms with the comorbidity of PN (5).

Paraneoplastic neurologic syndromes, although less common disorders, often present in middle age and beyond and, therefore, are worth mentioning. A subacute onset of numbness, painful paresthesias, and piercing pain in an asymmetric distribution evolving to symmetric distribution are the presenting complaints and are suggestive of a sensory polyganglionopathy.

The most common underlying neoplasm is small-cell carcinoma, followed in decreasing frequency by breast cancer, ovarian cancer, and lymphoma. These patients harbor a characteristic antibody in serum and spinal fluid termed antineuronal nuclear antibody type 1 (ANNA-1) or "anti-HU." The prognosis for paraneoplastic sensory neuronopathy is poor. The neuropathic symptoms respond poorly to treatment. The disorder often tracks an unremitting course despite treatment with corticosteroids, immunosuppressive agents, plasmapheresis, or high-dose IVIG. Management of the neoplasm may stabilize but does not usually reverse the nerve dysfunction and symptoms (5,11,13).

Paraproteinemic Neuropathy

The existence of a monoclonal protein [immunoglobulin (Ig) G, IgA, or IgM] in the serum of a person with PN introduces the possibility of underlying primary amyloidosis, multiple or osteosclerotic myeloma, Waldenström macroglobulinemia, lymphoma, or lymphoproliferative disease. Approximately two thirds of the time after exclusion of these diseases, no identifiable cause is found, and the neuropathy is classified as being associated with monoclonal gammopathy of undetermined significance (MGUS). MGUS occurs in approximately 5% to 10% of adult patients with CIAP, which represents a sixfold increase over the general population. MGUS is more frequent in older adults, with higher rates in males compared with females and with greater occurrences in black compared with white populations (16,18).

The typical clinical presentation of MGUS-associated chronic polyneuropathy (also called paraproteinemic neuropathy) begins in the sixth decade and progresses in a slow insidious pattern as a distal symmetrical sensorimotor polyneuropathy. Sensory deficits of the lower limbs are initially involved and to a greater extent than the upper extremities. Muscle stretch reflexes are globally diminished or absent with sparing of cranial nerves. Paresthesias, ataxia, and pain may be significant. Electrophysiologic studies often demonstrate demyelination or both demyelination and axonal degeneration.

A serum protein electrophoresis (SPEP) identifies many monoclonal gammopathies but lacks the sensitivity to detect small M proteins. Immunoelectrophoresis or immunofixation is necessary to identify small amounts of M protein, confirm the monoclonal nature of the disorder, and characterize the heavy- and light-chain types. All patients with neuropathy and an M protein should have a 24-hour urine collection for the detection of Bence Jones protein, a complete blood count, a radiologic bone survey to detect lytic lesions, bone marrow aspirate and biopsy to differentiate malignant plasma cell dyscrasias from MGUS, and a fat biopsy to rule out possible amyloidosis.

Although MGUS is a common finding in clinical practice, determining whether it will remain stable or progress to multiple myeloma is a significant challenge. Patients with MGUS need indefinite monitoring with repeat SPEP every 6 to 12 months. Although the natural history of evolution of the MGUS to malignancy is unknown, genetic changes, bone marrow angiogenesis, various cytokines related to myeloma bone disease, and possibly infectious agents may all play a part. The size of the M protein value is the most important predictor, with the risk of progression with a serum M protein value of 15 g/L being twice the risk of progression with a value of 5 g/L.

The treatment for MGUS neuropathy is unclear. The decision to treat depends on the severity and temporal path of the neuropathy. An indolent course and minor deficits may mandate watchful waiting. However, if the neuropathy is severe and meets diagnostic criteria for CIDP, the patient may respond to immunomodulatory therapies. The response to plasmapheresis, IVIG, prednisone, or combinations has been promising (5). When there is a rapid clinical deterioration of the neuropathy despite treatment, re-evaluation for underlying malignant lymphoproliferative disorders or amyloidosis is prudent (16,18,19).

NEUROPATHIES ASSOCIATED WITH INFECTIONS

Prion, viral, bacterial, and parasitic infections have all been associated with neuropathy. Associated viral agents include HIV type 1, cytomegalovirus, Epstein-Barr virus, herpes simplex virus, varicella-zoster virus, hepatitis B and C, and human T-cell lymphotropic virus type 1. At least 50% of the population will have immunogenic exposure to one varicella-zoster virus by the age of 80 years, occurring most frequently in the elderly. Although usually self-limiting, there is an associated increased risk of developing postherpetic pain or neuralgia with increasing age (8). Hansen's disease (leprosy) is the most common worldwide bacterial cause of neuropathy. Other infectious diseases associated with neuropathy include HIV infection, Lyme disease, and Chagas disease (28). The prion-caused Creutzfeldt-Jakob disease primarily affects the central nervous system, but a demyelinating PN has been described (24).

TOXINS ASSOCIATED WITH NEUROPATHIES

In the older adult, increasing polypharmacy not only contributes to iatrogenic health risks, but may also be the most common offender in chemical nervous system toxicity. Numerous medications and toxins have been identified as causing neuropathy, although clear empirical evidence is limited (Table 25-2). Estimates are that medication- and toxin-induced neuropathies may

Table 25-2. *Toxic Drugs Most Often Associated with Peripheral Neuropathy*[a]

Chemotherapeutic Agents	Cardiovascular Agents	Antibiotics	Central Nervous System Agents	Miscellaneous
Bortezomib	Amiodarone	Nucleoside analogs	Nitrous oxide	Colchicine
Cisplatin, oxaliplatin, and platinum derivatives	Hydralazine	Dapsone		Dichloroacetate[b]
Misonidazole	Perhexiline[b]	Isoniazid		Disulfiram
Suramin[b]	Statins	Metronidazole		Ethanol
Taxanes		Nitrofurantoin		Gold salts
Thalidomide		Podophyllin resin		Leflunomide
Vinca alkaloids				Penicillamine
				Pyridoxine
				Tacrolimus

[a]This is not an exhaustive list.
[b] Not currently approved by the Food and Drug Administration or unavailable in the United States.
Adapted with permission from Pratt RW, Weimer LH. Medication and toxin-induced peripheral neuropathy. *Semin Neurol.* 2005;25:204–216.

account for 2% to 4% of the estimated cases of neuropathy; because these neuropathies are potentially reversible, clinical recognition is crucial. Neurotoxic agents (chemotherapeutic drugs, alcohol, and vitamin B_6) may produce axonopathy, myelinopathy, or ganglionopathy or a symmetrical, dying-back pattern. Toxin-induced axonal degeneration can follow a neuronopathy or ganglionopathy (pyridoxine, cisplatin) or, less often, primary demyelination (amiodarone). The following key factors should be present before presuming that a particular drug is the offending agent: (a) there is evidence that the drug causes PN in humans or animals; (b) exposure to the drug is verified and temporally related to the clinical course; (c) neurologic signs and symptoms with abnormal electrodiagnostic study results support the involvement of the PNS; (d) susceptibility factors are present, such as pre-existing neuropathy, simultaneous use of other neurotoxic drugs, or metabolic dysfunction; and (e) cessation of the drug results in stabilization or improvement of symptoms (5).

Diagnosis begins with a high degree of clinical suspicion during the history, the presence of an abnormal neurologic sensory and/or motor examination, and the presence of electrophysiologic features of axonal neuropathy. The natural history of neuropathies associated with these toxins is often dose related, with insidious progression over weeks or months. A "coasting" phenomenon often occurs, with symptoms continuing to evolve and worsen up to 6 months after discontinuation of certain neurotoxic chemotherapy agents. Symptoms may be more severe if the individual has an underlying neuropathy. Treatment involves discontinuation of the drug and, if necessary, instituting neuropathic pain treatment (5,8)

Alcohol accounts for as much as 15% of the neuropathies occurring in the elderly and, therefore, is one of the most common toxins associated with the development of PN. This chronic neuropathy presents with sensory and motor deficits and with other features of distal axonal degeneration. Whether it is a combination of thiamine deprivation and B-complex vitamin deprivation or a direct neurotoxic effect of alcohol, the exact biochemical pathophysiology is uncertain. The most important steps in treatment are recognition of the offending agent and eliminating the alcohol use (27).

Critical Illness Polyneuropathy

Critical illness polyneuropathy is an acute, acquired, relatively common problem in ICUs. It is the major cause of difficulty weaning patients from a ventilator. Investigations show that approximately 50% of ICU patients with sepsis and multisystem organ failure have electrodiagnostic features of an axonal neuropathy. Acute myopathy may be present and may predominate. Although the pathophysiology of the syndrome is unknown, it appears likely that the systemic inflammatory syndrome results from sepsis, severe trauma, or burns. The clinical diagnosis relies heavily on electrodiagnostic studies because clinical evaluation of neuromuscular weakness is frequently difficult in the ICU setting due to concomitant sedation and encephalopathy. CSF usually shows normal protein levels; the demonstration of normal CSF protein levels is helpful in excluding GBS. The natural history of the syndrome is one of slow recovery in weeks to months after discharge from the ICU. There is no specific treatment once GBS and CIDP are excluded (4).

HEREDITARY NEUROPATHIES

Hereditary neuropathies are a large group of heterogeneous disorders that are unrecognized in many patients. This as-yet nonreversible group of neuropathies presents with a chronic, indolent pattern affecting myelinated motor and sensory axons in a length-dependent pattern. The symptom course can take decades to appear, making inherited neuropathy a relatively peripheral disorder of the older adult. Some of these neuropathies are caused by metabolic abnormalities including amyloid neuropathies, Refsum disease, Fabry disease, porphyria, and hypolipoproteinemias. Charcot-Marie-Tooth type 2 (CMT-2) is the most common inherited PN, with symptoms frequently appearing in middle age. Often patients are unaware of neurologic deficits or their "funny walk," particularly if they have had insidious painless loss of distal sensation. Detailed questioning leads to a positive family history. Classic findings include pes cavus, hammer or claw toes, and symmetric atrophy affecting the muscles of the feet and the anterior more than the posterior leg compartment muscles, giving the appearance of "inverted champagne bottles." Sensory examination reveals distal impairment of afferent modalities bilaterally in hands and feet, with enlargement of nerves seen in some CMT-1 or CMT-3 patients. Electrophysiologic findings and histologic studies serve to distinguish CMT-1 and CMT-2 (30). At present, DNA testing is evolving, and CMT-1A is the only widely available test. CMT-2A has recently been linked to a mutation in the *mitofusin 2* gene. The natural history of CMT-2 is slow, with disability typically presenting from early adulthood to late in life. Management is primarily supportive, including meticulous foot care, review of neurotoxic drug risks due to increased susceptibility to these agents, and evaluation for gait aids when needed.

Familial amyloid polyneuropathy is a group of autosomal dominant neuropathies that results in the extracellular deposition of amyloid in peripheral nerves and other tissues. Sensory complaints of loss of pain and thermal sensation may bring the patient to the clinician, but the history and examination can reveal hints of autonomic dysfunction, including distal anhidrosis, abnormal pupils with scalloped margins, orthostatism, gastrointestinal symptoms, and accompanying weight loss. Systemic involvement includes the ocular vitreous, heart, and kidneys. In addition to the neurologic examination, an abnormal EMG showing distal axonal neuropathy (sensory fibers affected earlier than motor fibers) and an abdominal fat aspirate test revealing positive Congo red staining characterize the presence of amyloid deposition. DNA diagnosis requires a blood or tissue sample in which antibodies raised against one of the three aberrant proteins of interest or a DNA blood test identifying a mutation in the genes for transthyretin apolipoprotein A1 or gelsolin is present. Genetic counseling is the standard of care. The natural course is a relentless progression of systemic organ failure, with cardiac or renal failure occurring 10 to 15 years after onset. Treatment consists of supportive care for the neuropathy and may include cardiac pacing, dialysis, parenteral nutrition, and physical therapy (30). Liver transplantation is considered in some cases.

MONONEUROPATHIES

The most vulnerable nerves to entrapment are the median, ulnar, and fibular (peroneal) nerves. The incidence of entrapment mononeuropathies from compression increases with age due in part to multiple factors, including repeated traumatic loss of protective subcutaneous tissue, prolonged periods of immobility, and coexistence of metabolic disorders (diabetes, renal insufficiency, and thyroid dysfunction), which increases susceptibility. Carpal tunnel is the most common entrapment syndrome and is often found to be greater in severity in the older population. Prolonged sitting or immobilization in bed appears to increase the risk of fibular (peroneal) neuropathy.

Multiple mononeuropathies are associated with diabetes mellitus and vasculitis but may occur in inherited tendency to pressure palsies, amyloidosis, sarcoidosis, HIV infection, Lyme disease, and leprosy (5).

DIFFERENTIAL DIAGNOSIS

A logical approach to common disorders of PN begins with a directed history, a comprehensive neurologic examination, electrophysiologic studies, and further laboratory investigations. This allows for the objective establishment of the presence of neuropathy and its categorization by clinical and pathologic criteria in an organized and cost-effective manner. It is possible to establish a specific neuropathy diagnosis in up to 75% of patients evaluated in tertiary referral centers by experts in neuromuscular disease (Fig. 25-1).

CONSIDER THE ONSET AND COURSE OF THE NEUROPATHY

Determine the temporal course (onset, duration, and evolution) of symptoms. Acute onset is days to weeks and suggests GBS, a metabolic event, or toxic exposure. More common in PN is a slow chronic or insidious progression. A history of clearing or remission suggests CIDP or other immune-related

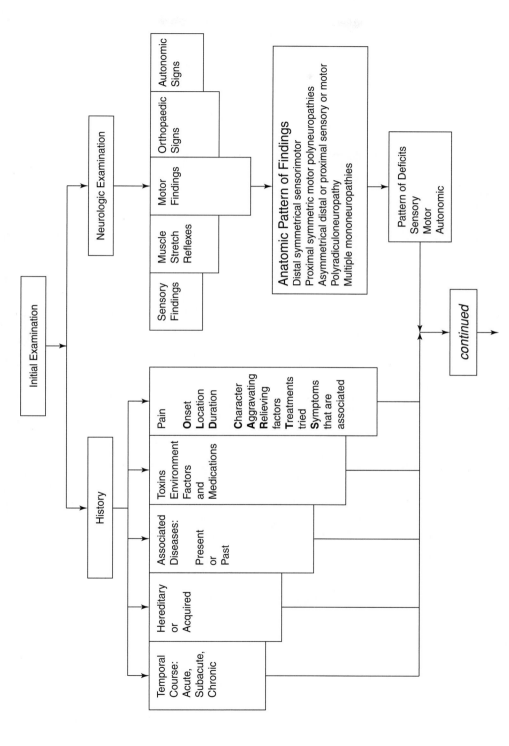

Figure 25-1. Approach to evaluation of peripheral neuropathies.

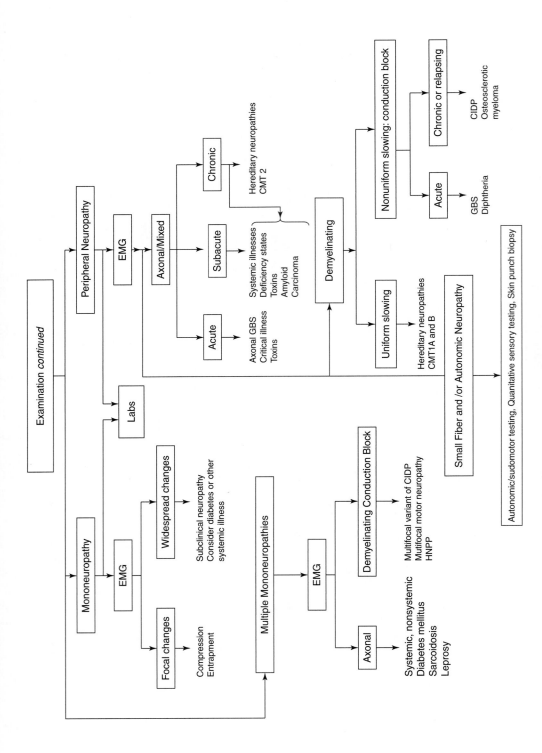

Figure 25-1. (Continued) CIDP, chronic inflammatory demyelinating polyradiculoneuropathy; CMT, Charcot-Marie-Tooth disease 1A and B, 2; GBS, Guillain-Barré syndrome; HNPP, hereditary neuropathy with liability to pressure palsies; NP, neuropathy. (Adapted with permission from Bosch EP, Smith BE. Disorders of peripheral nerves. In: Bradley WG, Daroff RB, Fenichel GM, et al., eds. *Neurology in clinical practice.* Woburn, MA: Butterworth-Heinemann; 2000:2106–2109.)

neuropathy. The patient's lack of awareness of the evolving symptoms suggests a hereditary neuropathy.

CHECK FOR ASSOCIATIONS WITH PRESENT OR PAST DISEASE

There are a variety of systemic, infectious, inflammatory, and malignant diseases as well as toxins that are associated with neuropathy. The presence of constitutional symptoms, such as weight loss, malaise, and anorexia, or associated infections as well as disease patterns are important clues that may point to associated disease conditions.

DECIDE WHETHER THE DISORDER IS LIKELY TO BE INHERITED OR ACQUIRED

Questions uncovering whether family members had high-arched feet, hammer or claw toes, or wasting muscles; complained about foot pain; had difficulty walking on heels; used foot braces; or had difficulty rising from a kneeling position are all pertinent in uncovering a hereditary link.

CLASSIFY THE ANATOMIC–PATHOLOGIC PATTERN OF INVOLVEMENT

Identification of the positive (pain, tingling, cramps, fasciculations, hyperhidrosis, and diarrhea) and negative (numbness, lack of feeling, weakness, orthostatic hypotension, and constipation) neurologic symptoms conveys information as to the pathology (axonal, demyelinating, or mixed), and when combined with the history, the pathophysiology (metabolic, inflammatory, inherited, toxic, or vascular) begins to emerge. The physical examination establishes the anatomic pattern, which is narrowed to specific modalities (motor, sensory, or autonomic). Unilateral motor and sensory sign are associated with single root (monoradiculopathy), brachial, or lumbar plexopathies and imply a local process. Multiple mononeuropathies or mononeuropathy multiplex denotes sequential damage to multiple noncontiguous nerves.

Distal sensorimotor polyneuropathy is characterized by symmetrical, distal motor and sensory deficits with a graded increase in severity distally and distal reduction of reflexes. Sensory deficits present a stocking glove pattern, involving the tips of the fingers as the dysesthesias (unpleasant sensation in response to an ordinary stimulus) reach the level of the knees. In most polyneuropathies, the lower extremities are more severely affected than the upper extremities. When the examination reveals motor deficits (weakness, muscle twitches, atrophy), the identification of additional pattern features, including asymmetry, the number of muscles involved, and distal versus proximal weakness, provides additional

diagnostic clues. Polyradiculopathies are length dependent, with moderate to severe weakness of proximal and distal muscles and sensory loss in proximal and distal areas.

Changes in blood pressure (>30 mm Hg systolic blood pressure decrease at 2 minutes) recorded after doing orthostatic blood pressure recordings suggest an autonomic involvement.

CONFIRM THE ANATOMIC–PATHOLOGIC PATTERN BY USING CHARACTERIZING TESTS

EMG is a valuable tool in providing objective evidence to support the diagnosis of PN. Nerve conduction studies (NCS) are helpful to make deductions about pathologic alterations of fibers (axonal degeneration or demyelination) and about distribution and severity of deficits, which are important distinctions in establishing the diagnosis of PN. The complimentary needle examination determines whether abnormal conduction results are due to muscle or nerve disease.

Quantitative sensory testing, although dependent on subjective responses from the patient, is useful to detect or confirm sensory loss and to identify the modality and class of fibers affected. This investigation can be helpful in identifying small-fiber neuropathy.

Autonomic testing is beneficial in the categorization of various types of sympathetic and parasympathetic dysfunction and may help to localize the disorder as either central or peripheral in origin. An additional test available in a few academic centers is the thermoregulatory sweating test, which may reveal quite striking neurologic impairment not readily apparent by clinical or other diagnostic tests (6).

PERFORM HEMATOLOGIC, BIOCHEMICAL, AND SEROLOGIC TESTING AND IMAGING

There are a few blood tests that are initially ordered in the evaluation of PN (Table 25-3). A second group of studies can be ordered in selective cases when uncommon etiologies are considered. Lumbar puncture for spinal fluid analysis is warranted if there is a suspicion for an acquired demyelinating neuropathy (GBS or CIDP) or leptomeningeal malignancy.

Diagnostic radiography, myelography, computed tomography (CT), and magnetic resonance imaging (MRI) may provide additional information for anatomic localization (lesions in roots, ganglia, or nerves or a variety of structures impinging on nerves).

PERFORM A NERVE BIOPSY

This is most useful in multiple mononeuropathies when vasculitis is suspected. Before committing a patient to the prospect of long-term corticosteroid treatment, it is

Table 25-3. *Common Biochemical Studies Useful in the Diagnosis of Peripheral Neuropathy*

Obtained in Most Patients with Unknown Etiology	Additional Studies Obtained in Selective Patients
CBC	Methylmalonic acid and homocysteine
Sedimentation rate	Thyroid function test
Metabolic profile	Antinuclear antibodies
Serum protein electrophoresis and immunofixation electrophoresis	Paraneoplastic panel, Antineuronal nuclear antibody type 1 (ANNA-1 or anti-HU)
Vitamin B_{12}	Rheumatoid factor
2-hour oral glucose tolerance test	Lyme, antibody, HIV antibody, West Nile
	Myelin-associated glycoprotein (MAG) antibody
	Copper
	Blood and urine for heavy metals
	Gliadin antibodies

CBC, complete blood cell count; HIV, human immunodeficiency virus. Adapted (1998) with permission from Barohn RJ. Approach to peripheral neuropathy and neuronopathy. *Semin Neurol.* 1998;18:7–18.

important to document a pathologic diagnosis of necrotizing vasculitis. The sural nerve biopsy may provide a specific diagnosis in amyloidosis, leprosy, sarcoidosis, tumor infiltration, and hereditary neuropathy with predisposition to pressure palsies. A skin punch biopsy is effective in documenting the density of epidermal nerve fibers and is considered a sensitive indicator of small-fiber neuropathy.

MANAGEMENT

The most effective treatment of PN is correction of the underlying disease. When this is not possible, symptomatic relief becomes the therapeutic goal by addressing pain, gait instability and quality-of-life issues. For patients with painful PN, regardless of the underlying pathophysiology, the symptomatic treatment is the same, relief of pain. Another important observation is that symptoms of numbness and tingling without pain will not benefit from use of medications. Initially, simple analgesics (acetaminophen and nonsteroidal anti-inflammatory drugs) may provide relief. Topical anesthetic agents have the advantage of providing some relief with minimum side effects when a small patch of skin is affected. Four broad categories of drugs are available to the clinician, including serotonin-norepinephrine reuptake inhibitors, tricyclic analgesics, anticonvulsants, and opiates (9). Recently, consensus guidelines based on evidence from well-designed clinical trials offer guidance in using a tiered approach when selecting treatment agents (Table 25-4). No agent has been shown to be effective for all patients (1). Those who do not respond to monotherapy after all single agents have received an adequate trial may respond to combination therapy. Narcotic analgesic treatment, although

considered by some as a first-tier treatment agent based on its effectiveness in pain relief, is still reserved for refractory treatment by most authorities (23). The clinician's choice must include consideration of adverse effects, individual patient factors, comorbidities, and cost. Treating concomitant sleep disorders, depression, and social withdrawal frequently adds to the quality of life of patients with chronic neuropathic pain syndromes. Studies of patients with diabetic neuropathic pain revealed greater impairment on measures of emotional reactions, energy, pain, physical mobility, sleep, and interference with enjoyment of life (2). Gait aids and training are important to aid mobility and reduce the risks of falls. Therapies such as acupuncture and transcutaneous electrical nerve stimulation sometimes show benefits.

For immune-mediated PNs (acute or chronic CIDP, vasculitis) a wide range of immunosuppressive therapies is available (Table 25-5). Autonomic neuropathies can be treated first with lifestyle changes (increased salt intake, compression stockings or belt, elevation of the head of the bed, and intake of frequent small meals vs. large meals). Additional medications for therapy include fludrocortisone, midodrine, and pyridostigmine (17,31,34,36).

For those patients with hereditary neuropathy, addressing life issues, such as loss of independence, emotional pain, stress over the guilt of passing along a gene mutation to their children, and fear of progressive disability, can benefit by discussion with an experienced genetic counselor (2). Addressing disease modification, neuropathic pain, disabilities, and psychosocial and emotional issues specific to the individual at different life and disease stages usually requires a multidisciplinary team approach to provide appropriate management to the older adult with PN.

Table 25-4. *Consensus Guidelines for First- and Second-Tier Agents for the Symptomatic Treatment of Neuropathic Pain*[a]

Class of Drug	Drug	Recommended Dose	Adverse Effects	Comments
First tier				
SNRI	Duloxetine	30 mg/day up to 120 mg/day	Sedation, ataxia, nausea, dry mouth, constipation, hyperhidrosis, anorexia	Titrate dose. Avoid concomitant use of MAOIs.
Anticonvulsants	Pregabalin	75 mg/day up to 600 mg/day	Sedation, ataxia, edema, diplopia, weight gain, dry mouth	Titrate dose. Dose adjustment in patients with renal dysfunction.
TCAs	Nortriptyline	10 mg/day to 150 mg/day	Dry mouth, urinary retention, sedation	Titrate dose.
	Desipramine	10 mg/day to 200 mg/day	Insomnia	Titrate dose. May be taken every morning.
	Amitriptyline	25 mg/day to 150 mg/day	Cardiac conduction block, orthostatic hypotension, sedation, confusion (increased in elderly)	Titrate dose. Contraindicated in older adults and patients with cardiovascular disease and glaucoma or taking MAOIs.
Opioids	Oxycodone CR	10 mg/day up to 60 mg/day	Respiratory depression, ataxia, sedation, nausea, constipation, cognitive dysfunction	Titrate dose. Advise patient to avoid concomitant use of ethanol and benzodiazepines. Screen for potential drug abuse.
Second tier				
Anticonvulsants	Gabapentin	100 mg/day up to 3600 mg/day	Sedation, ataxia, edema, weight gain, diplopia, nystagmus.	Titrate dose. Dose adjustment in patients with renal dysfunction.
	Lamotrigine	200 mg/day up to 400 mg/day	Rash, sedation, fatigue, dizziness, headache, Stevens-Johnson syndrome/toxic epidermal necrolysis	Requires strict titration regimen to reduce risk of serious cutaneous reactions.
	Carbamazepine	50 mg/day up to 600 mg/day	Sedation, ataxia, rash, diplegia, hyponatremia, agranulocytosis, nausea, diarrhea, hepatotoxicity, aplastic anemia, Stevens-Johnson syndrome	Requires slow titration. Contraindicated in patients with porphyria or atrioventricular block or taking MAOIs. Monitor CBC, LFTs.

(Continued)

Table 25-4. *(Continued)*

Class of Drug	Drug	Recommend Dose	Adverse Effects	Comments
Analgesic	Tramadol	25 mg/day up to 400 mg/day	Respiratory depression, ataxia, sedation, constipation, seizures, nausea, orthostatic hypotension	Use with caution in patients with epilepsy.
	Venlafaxine ER	75 mg/day up to 225 mg/day	Hypertension, ataxia, sedation, insomnia, nausea, hyperhidrosis, dry mouth, constipation, anxiety, anorexia	Contraindicated in patients taking MAOIs. Adjust dose in patients with renal dysfunction.
Topical agents	5% Lidocaine patch EMLA (lidocaine and prilocaine)	3 patches every 12 hours Every 24–72 hours	Skin erythema, rash	Patch must be applied to painful area.
	Capsaicin cream	Apply cream four times daily	Local skin irritation	Advise patient to apply a thin film over affected area. Will take >1 week to have a noted effect.

SNRI, serotonin-norepinephrine reuptake inhibitor; CR, controlled release; TCA, tricyclic antidepressant; MAOI, monoamine oxidase inhibitor; CBC, complete blood count; LFT, liver function test.

a This is a nonexhaustive list.

From Argoff CE, Backonja MM, Belgrade MJ, et al. Consensus guidelines: treatment planning and options. Diabetic peripheral neuropathic pain. *Mayo Clin Proc.* 2006;81[Suppl 4]:S12–S25.

Table 25-5. *Immunosuppressive Therapy for Immune-Mediated Neuropathies*

Therapy	Indications	Dose	Adverse Effects	Comments
Prednisone	CIDP, VN, MMN +/–	100 mg/day PO for 2–4 weeks, then 100 mg every other day; single AM dose	Hypertension, fluid and weight gain, hyperglycemia, hypokalemia, cataracts, gastric irritation, osteoporosis	Close monitoring
Intravenous immunoglobulin (IVIG)	GBS, CIDP, MMN	Intravenous 0.4g/kg/day over 5 days, or 1 g/kg/day over 2 days; then single doses of 0.4 g/kg every 4–8 weeks as needed	Hypotension, arrhythmias, diaphoresis, flushing, nephrotoxicity, headache, aseptic meningitis, anaphylaxis	Monitor heart rate, blood pressure, creatinine/BUN
Methylprednisone	CIDP, VN +/– MMN	Intravenous 1 g in 100 mL normal saline over 1–2 hours, 3–6 doses, daily or every other day	Arrhythmia, flushing, dysgeusia, anxiety, insomnia, fluid and weight gain	Monitor heart rate, blood pressure, serum glucose/potassium
Azathioprine	CIDP	2–3 mg/kg/day PO; single AM dose	Flulike illness, hepatotoxicity, leukopenia, macrocytosis, neoplasia	Monitor monthly blood counts and LFTs
Cyclophosphamide	VN, CIDP, MMN	1.5–2 mg/kg/day PO; single am dose. Intravenous 0.5–3 g/m² (maximum, 85 mg/kg)	Leukopenia, hemorrhagic cystitis, alopecia, infections, neoplasia; when given intravenously, symptoms can be more severe	Monitor monthly blood count and urinalysis
Cyclosporine	CIDP	3–6 mg/kg/day PO twice a day	Nephrotoxicity, hypertension, hepatotoxicity, tremor, gum hyperplasia, hirsutism	Blood pressure, weekly or monthly cyclosporine level, creatinine/BUN, liver enzymes
Plasmapheresis	GBS, CIDP, MMN	Intravenous therapy, Remove total of 200–250 cm³/kg plasma over 7–14 days; may require periodic exchanges	Hypotension, arrhythmias, electrolyte imbalance anemia, coagulation disorders	Monitor heart rate, blood pressure, blood count, electrolytes, PT/PTT, volume removed and replaced

BUN, blood urea nitrogen; CIDP, chronic inflammatory denyelinating polyneuropathy; GBS, Guillain-Barré syndrome; LFTs, liver function test; MMN, multifocal motor neuropathy; PO, oral; PT, prothrombin time; PTT, partial thromboplastin time; VN, vasculitic neuropathy. Modified and used with permission from Barohn RJ. Approach to peripheral neuropathy and neuronopathy. *Semin Neurol.* 1998;18:7-18.

REFERENCES

1. Argoff CE, Backonja MM, Belgrade MJ, et al. Consensus guidelines: treatment planning and options. Diabetic peripheral neuropathic pain. *Mayo Clin Proc.* 2006;81[Suppl 4]:S12–S25.

2. Argoff CE, Cole BE, Fishbain DA, et al. Diabetic peripheral neuropathic pain: clinical and quality-of-life issues. *Mayo Clin Proc.* 2006;81[Suppl 4]: S3–S11.

3. Barohn RJ. Approach to peripheral neuropathy and neuronopathy. *Semin Neurol.* 1998;18:7–18.

4. Bolton CF. Neuromuscular manifestations of critical illness. *Muscle Nerve.* 2005;32:140–163.

5. Bosch EP, Smith BE. Disorders of peripheral nerves. In: Bradley WG, Daroff RB, Fenichel GM, et al., eds. *Neurology in clinical practice.* Woburn, MA: Butterworth-Heinemann; 2000:2045–2130.

6. Dyck PJ, Dyck PJ, Grant IA, et al. Ten steps in characterizing and diagnosis patients with peripheral neuropathy. *Neurology.* 1996:47(1): 10–17.

7. Dyck PJ, Oviatt KF, Lambert EH. Intensive evaluation of referred unclassified neuropathies yields improved diagnosis. *Ann Neurol.* 1981;10: 222–226.

8. Freimer ML. Peripheral neuropathy. In: Pathy MSJ, ed. *Principles and practice of geriatric medicine.* 3rd ed. Hoboken, NJ: John Wiley and Sons; 1998:865–872.

9. Gilron I, Watson CP, Cahill CM, et al. Neuropathic pain: a practical guide for the clinician. *CMAJ.* 2006;175:265–275.

10. Gooch C, Podwall D. The diabetic neuropathies. *Neurologist.* 2004;10:311–322.

11. Graus F, Delattre JY, Antoine JC, et al. Recommended diagnostic criteria for paraneoplastic neurological syndromes. *J Neurol Neurosurg Psychiatry.* 2004;75:1135–1140.

12. Hoffman-Snyder C, Smith BE, Ross MA, et al. Value of the oral glucose tolerance test in the evaluation of chronic idiopathic axonal polyneuropathy. *Arch Neurol.* 2006;63:1075–1079.

13. Honnorat J. Onconeural antibodies are essential to diagnose paraneoplastic neurological syndromes. *Acta Neurol Scand Suppl.* 2006;183:64–68.

14. Hughes RA, Cornblath DR. Guillain-Barré syndrome. *Lancet.* 2005;366:1653–1666.

15. Kelkar P. Diabetic neuropathy. *Semin Neurol.* 2005;25:168–173.

16. Kissel JT, Mendell JR. Neuropathies associated with monoclonal gammopathies. *Neuromuscul Disord.* 1996;6:3–18.

17. Koski CL. Therapy of CIDP and related immune-mediated neuropathies. *Neurology.* 2002;59[Suppl 6]:S22–S27.

18. Kyle RA, Rajkumar SV. Monoclonal gammopathy of undetermined significance. *Br J Haematol.* 2006;134:573–589.

19. Kyle RA, Therneau TM, Rajkumar SV, et al. Prevalence of monoclonal gammopathy of undetermined significance. *N Engl J Med.* 2006;354: 1362–1369.

20. Latov N. Diagnosis of CIDP. *Neurology.* 2002; 59[Suppl 6]:S2–S6.

21. Martyn CN, Hughes RA. Epidemiology of peripheral neuropathy. *J Neurol Neurosurg Psychiatry.* 1997;62:310–318.

22. Mendell JR, Sahenk Z. Clinical practice. Painful sensory neuropathy. *N Engl J Med.* 2003; 348:1243–1255.

23. Namaka M, Gramlich CR, Ruhlen D, et al. A treatment algorithm for neuropathic pain. *Clin Ther.* 2004;26:951–979.

24. Niewiadomska M, Kulczycki J, Wochnik-Dyjas D, et al. Impairment of the peripheral nervous system in Creutzfeldt-Jakob disease. *Arch Neurol.* 2002; 59:1430–1436.

25. Olney RK. The neurology of aging. In: Aminoff MJ, ed. *Neurology and general medicine.* 3rd ed. Philadelphia: Churchill Livingstone; 2001: 939–953.

26. Olney RK. Neuropathies associated with connective tissue disease. *Semin Neurol.* 1998;18:63–72.

27. Pratt RW, Weimer LH. Medication and toxin-induced peripheral neuropathy. *Semin Neurol.* 2005;25:204–216.

28. Said G. Infectious neuropathies. *Neurol Clin.* 2007;25:115–137.

29. Schaublin GA, Michet CJ, Dyck PJ, et al. An update on the classification and treatment of vasculitic neuropathy. *Lancet Neurol.* 2005;4:853–865.

30. Shy ME, Lupski JR, Chance PF, et al. Hereditary motor and sensory neuropathies: an overview of clinical, genetic, electrophysiologic and pathologic features. In: Dyck PJ, Thomas PK, eds. *Peripheral Neuropathy.* 4th ed. Philadelphia, PA Saunders, 2005:1623–1658.

31. Singer W, Sandroni P, Opfer-Gehrking TL, et al. Pyridostigmine treatment trial in neurogenic orthostatic hypotension. *Arch Neurol.* 2006;63: 513–518.

32. Singleton JR, Smith AG. Therapy insight: neurological complications of prediabetes. *Nat Clin Pract Neurol.* 2006;2:276–282.

33. Singleton JR, Smith AG, Bromberg MB. Painful sensory polyneuropathy associated with impaired glucose tolerance. *Muscle Nerve.* 2001;24: 1225–1228.

34. Sutton IJ, Winer JB. Immunosuppression in peripheral neuropathy: rationale and reality. *Curr Opin Pharmacol.* 2002;2:291–295.

35. Thompson PD, Thomas PK Differential diagnosis and epidemiology. In: Dyck PJ, Thomas PK, eds. *Peripheral Neuropathy*. 4th ed. Philadelphia: Elsevier Saunders: 2005:Vol 1:1137–1161.

36. Van Doorn PA, Garssen MP. Treatment of immune neuropathies. *Curr Opin Neurol.* 2002;15: 623–631.

37. Verdú E, Ceballos D, Vilches JJ, et al. Influence of aging on peripheral nerve function and regeneration. *J Peripher Nerv Syst.* 20000; 5:191–208.

38. Wolfe GI, Barohn RJ. Cryptogenic sensory and sensorimotor polyneuropathies. *Semin Neurol.* 1998;18:105–111.

SUGGESTED READINGS

Dyck PJ, Thomas PK, eds. *Peripheral Neuropathy*. 4th ed. Philadelphia: Elsevier Saunders; 2005.

Noseworthy JH, ed. *Neurological Therapeutics Principles and Practice*. 2nd ed. Boca Raton: Informa Healthcare; 2006.

WEBSITES

The Neuropathy Association is a public, charitable, nonprofit organization that was established in 1995 by people with neuropathy and their families or friends to help those who suffer from disorders that affect the peripheral nerves. http://www.neuropathy.org/site/PageServer

A National Institute of Neurological Disorders and Stroke (NINDS) website designed for patient information on peripheral neuropathy. http://www.ninds.nih.gov/disorders/peripheralneuropathy/peripheralneuropathy.htm

A National Institute of Neurological Disorders and Stroke website designed to provide patient information on diabetic neuropathy. http://www.ninds.nih.gov/disorders/diabetic/diabetic.htm

A Mayo Clinic website developed for patient information and with tools to help patients manage their disease or chronic conditions. http://www.mayoclinic.com/health/peripheral-neuropathy/DS00131

The American Diabetes Association is the nation's leading nonprofit health organization providing diabetes research, information, and advocacy. http://www.diabetes.org/home.jsp

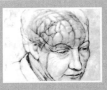

CHAPTER 25.2

Neuromuscular Diseases of the Older Adult

Janaka K. Seneviratne and Mark A. Ross

MOTOR NEURON DISEASE

DEFINITION OF TERMS

Motor neuron disease (MND) refers to a group of disorders resulting from dysfunction and death of motor neurons. Although the pathologic changes in MND are well known, the underlying etiology remains poorly understood. It is likely that common pathogenetic mechanisms cause the different forms of MND and other neurodegenerative diseases. The clinical manifestations of MND depend on the degree of upper motor neuron (UMN) and lower motor neuron (LMN) involvement and the specific regions of the nervous system involved. There are four main clinical categories seen in MND (22).

1. Amyotrophic lateral sclerosis (ALS): UMN and LMN findings
2. Primary lateral sclerosis (PLS): Only UMN findings
3. Progressive muscle atrophy (PMA): Only LMN findings
4. Progressive bulbar palsy (PBP): Only bulbar findings

CLINICAL FEATURES

Clinical features define the different categories of MND. ALS is the most common form of MND. The diagnosis of ALS requires both UMN and LMN findings. The other types of MND, which do not meet the definition of ALS, are initially viewed as tentative diagnostic considerations because of the high likelihood that additional clinical signs will develop as the disease progresses over time. Patients with only LMN findings are diagnosed with PMA, and those with purely UMN findings are diagnosed with PLS. Patients with PBP can have either UMN or LMN findings but do not have sufficient abnormalities to meet the criteria for ALS.

Amyotrophic Lateral Sclerosis

ALS is by far the most common form of MND. The diagnosis is established by clinical criteria that require progressive muscle weakness with both UMN and LMN findings on examination and no alternative explanation after a thorough investigation. The disease typically begins with slowly progressive focal muscle weakness.

Early in the diagnostic evaluation, the motor manifestations may be exclusively UMN, exclusively LMN, or any combination of both. However, both UMN and LMN signs must be present to meet the criteria for diagnosis. As the illness progresses, there is worsening of motor function in affected regions and spread to previously unaffected regions (3).

The LMN signs are muscle weakness, atrophy, and fasciculations. Muscle atrophy is a major contributing factor to the weight loss that regularly occurs in ALS patients. Careful inspection of muscles may be necessary to observe fasciculations. Obesity or edema may completely obscure fasciculations and may even mask muscle atrophy. Muscle cramps are common and may precede other symptoms.

The UMN signs are weakness, spasticity, hyperreflexia, and pathologic reflexes. The pattern of UMN muscle weakness typically affects antigravity muscles. Prominent spasticity can significantly impair motor function despite relatively preserved strength. Many patients do not develop severe spasticity and may simply have hyperreflexia or pathologic reflexes as UMN manifestations. Reflexes that are considered pathologic include the Babinski sign and either clonus or spread of reflexes to other muscles. Reflex spread may be vertical, as with the brachioradialis reflex spreading to the biceps, or horizontal, such as the crossed adductor reflex. Other pathologic reflexes include the jaw jerk, hyperactive gag reflex, and the presence of the superficial abdominal reflex.

Weakness begins in the limbs in 60% to 75% of cases. Either the arms or legs may be initially involved. The weakness often begins asymmetrically in a single limb. Rarely, it may affect the arm and leg on one side at onset, creating a hemiparetic pattern.

Onset with bulbar muscle weakness is the second most common presentation, which may occur in 25% to 40% of patients. Bulbar involvement can begin with dysarthria or dysphagia, but dysarthria is much more common as an initial symptom. Dysarthric speech may result from either UMN or LMN dysfunction or a combination of both. Dysarthric speech due to UMN disease is often characterized as strained or strangulated speech. Dysarthria due to LMN disease is described as slurred speech. Dysphagia is usually first noted as difficulty swallowing liquids. As dysphagia progresses, patients develop difficulty swallowing solid foods. Patients observe choking on thin liquids and foods with particulate consistencies. UMN bulbar signs include hyperactive gag reflex and jaw jerk. Clinical manifestations of LMN bulbar dysfunction include tongue atrophy and tongue fasciculations.

Another common feature of ALS patients with bulbar involvement is emotional lability. This has been called pseudobulbar palsy or pseudobulbar affect. This term refers to a change in emotional expression, such that patients lose the ability to inhibit strong emotions. Consequently, patients display either crying or laughing in situations that formerly would not have prompted such emotional release. This may be an important clue to the illness because this emotional lability is not seen in other neuromuscular disorders causing bulbar dysfunction.

Rarely, respiratory muscle weakness causing dyspnea can be the initial manifestation of ALS. More often, respiratory muscle weakness develops gradually as the patient develops progressive limb weakness. Respiratory muscle failure is the usual cause of death and the reason for the poor prognosis with ALS. There is great variability of survival in ALS, with some patients progressing rapidly to death within 1 year of symptom onset and others surviving for 10 to 20 years. The average survival ranges from 3 to 4 years from the time of diagnosis.

Although ALS is often considered to be a purely motor disorder, some patients develop additional neurologic manifestations. Dementia may occur, and recent studies have suggested that frontotemporal type dementia may be much more common than previously recognized. Sensory symptoms are never a prominent feature of the illness, but many patients may have minor sensory complaints. Autonomic involvement is uncommon, but many patients have problems with constipation, and occasionally, patients develop urinary incontinence.

Primary Lateral Sclerosis

PLS is a gradually progressive form of MND with UMN findings. Some patients develop limited electromyographic evidence of LMN involvement but not sufficient evidence of LMN involvement to meet criteria for ALS. As in ALS, the diagnosis requires thorough investigation to exclude other conditions that could cause UMN disease. Many patients with an initial provisional diagnosis of PLS later develop progressive LMN disease and meet the criteria for ALS (4,31). The most common initial presentation of PLS is asymmetrical spastic leg weakness. The second most common clinical presentation is bulbar dysfunction. Patients with PLS may develop upper extremity weakness and spasticity as the illness progresses, but upper extremity onset is uncommon. Bladder function is usually preserved in PLS. Cognitive function is generally preserved in PLS, although some studies have indicated mild frontal lobe dysfunction (5). The progression of PLS is much slower than ALS, and consequently, the prognosis is much better. In reported series, patients with PLS have died from causes other than PLS.

Progressive Muscular Atrophy

PMA is the term used to describe MND when only LMN involvement is present. Patients with progressive LMN disease require thorough evaluation for other conditions that might cause this clinical presentation. Examples include spinal root disorders, multifocal motor neuropathy, inflammatory myopathy, and viral disorders such as West Nile virus and poliomyelitis. Patients with PMA generally have a slower course than patients with ALS and are less likely to develop bulbar involvement. Most patients initially diagnosed as having PMA will later develop UMN signs and meet criteria for ALS.

Progressive Bulbar Palsy

PBP is a form of MND primarily affecting the bulbar muscles. The disorder begins with bulbar dysfunction with symptoms of dysarthria or dysphagia. Most patients who begin with bulbar disease ultimately go on to develop the typical clinical picture of ALS. Those rare patients who remain with an exclusively bulbar illness without progression to ALS are regarded as having PBP.

EPIDEMIOLOGY IN OLDER ADULTS

The annual incidence of ALS is one to two per 100,000 population, with a prevalence rate of four to six cases per 100,000. ALS is an adult illness, with the average age of onset in the mid-50s and the peak age of incidence in the age range of 50 to 75 years (22,26). The male-to-female ratio is 1.5:1 up to age 70 and 1:1 afterwards. Due to progression of muscle weakness leading to respiratory failure, the average period of survival from diagnosis is 3 to 4 years. Rarely, patients may survive for >10 years. Factors that favor relatively longer survival include young age of onset (<45 years), onset in limb muscles, male gender, and a longer period from symptom onset to diagnosis (33). Of the different categories of MND, ALS has the worst prognosis. Although the other categories of MND have a better prognosis than ALS, it is not possible to be certain of the prognosis or estimate survival for an individual patient with one of the other forms of MND.

The frequency of PLS has been estimated to be roughly 2% to 10% of all cases of MND, with most series showing a rate of <5%. Onset is usually in the fifth decade or later. Both PMA and PBP are infrequent, with each category making up <5% of all cases of MND.

PATHOLOGY

The primary pathology of MND involves degeneration and death of motor neurons. The pathology is similar in the different clinical subtypes of MND. The major pathologic change is loss of motor neurons and resultant gliosis. In forms of MND with UMN involvement, there is evidence of corticospinal tract degeneration. Even some patients with PMA who have no clinical evidence of UMN involvement have been found to have corticospinal tract degeneration at postmortem examination. Such findings have reinforced the concept that the different forms of MND are all variations within the broad spectrum of neurodegenerative disease (4,31).

Neuronal pathology in MND includes chromatolysis, increased lipofuscin, neurofilament accumulation, and ubiquitinated inclusions. Additional pathologic findings include Bunina bodies (34), Lewy-like inclusions, and Hirano bodies.

ETIOLOGY

The cause of MND remains undetermined. Hereditary forms of MND provide evidence that genetic factors can either cause or contribute to the illness. Roughly 10% of ALS cases are familial, with most having an autosomal dominant inheritance pattern. Roughly 20% of familial cases are due to mutations in the *superoxide dismutase 1 (SOD1)* gene. The sporadic and familial forms have similar pathology and clinical features, although several unique clinical presentations are associated with specific *SOD1* mutations.

The most common *SOD1* mutation variant seen in North America is the *A4V* variant. This name describes an alanine substitution for valine at codon 4. This variant accounts for roughly half of the *SOD1* cases in North America and is clinically characterized by an exclusively LMN illness. This disorder is rapidly progressive, with a survival time of 1 year or less. Another important *SOD1* mutation is the *D90A* variant, which manifests as a predominantly UMN illness with survival >10 years.

The precise mechanisms by which *SOD1* mutations lead to MND remain unknown. However, studies from the transgenic mouse model have indicated that the fundamental problem is a gain of an undetermined toxic function rather than an inability to scavenge free radicals (10).

In addition to a genetic basis for MND, other pathogenetic mechanisms that have been considered include toxin exposure (25), viral illness (18), and autoimmune illness. Multiple pathogenic processes have been considered, including mitochondrial dysfunction, protein aggregation (35), oxidative stress (30), disrupted cytoskeleton and impaired axonal transport, and glutamate excitotoxicity (29).

Exposure to toxins may play a role in MND pathogenesis. Several studies have demonstrated an association between exposure to heavy metals such as lead and mercury and MND (23). Although motor neuron degeneration has been associated with significant exposure to heavy metals, this does not appear to be a contributing factor in typical cases of ALS or other forms of MND.

Disorders such as poliomyelitis and West Nile virus complicated by encephalomyelitis provide examples in which motor neuron loss clearly occurs as a complication of a viral illness. Although theoretically attractive, no conclusive association between viral infection and MND has been determined. Efforts to detect viral pathogens including polio virus have not been successful. MND has been reported to occur as a rare consequence of HIV infection (18), but such an association is not clearly established in the majority of cases.

DIAGNOSIS

No specific diagnostic test exists for ALS or the other categories of MND. Consequently, the diagnosis of MND is established by clinical criteria, with diagnostic tests performed primarily to exclude other conditions that may have similar features. It is standard clinical practice to perform thorough diagnostic testing before reaching the conclusion that a patient has MND. Routine tests include laboratory studies, electromyography (EMG), and selected imaging studies of the central nervous system. The purpose of such testing is to determine whether any alternative condition or combination of conditions could possibly account for the clinical phenotype of MND. If an alternative condition can be identified, then the clinician must weigh the evidence for the alternative condition against the possibility of MND.

Laboratory Studies

Laboratory studies are primarily obtained to search for conditions that may, at times, mimic ALS or other forms of MND. Another reason for obtaining laboratory studies is that MND is a chronic progressive illness and there may be systemic complications that need to be monitored with laboratory studies.

Laboratory studies that are commonly assessed for patients suspected of having ALS include complete blood count, chemistry panel, sedimentation rate, thyroid-stimulating hormone, vitamin B_{12} level, rapid plasma reagent, antinuclear antibody, and serum immunofixation electrophoresis. For patients with disease onset at age <40 years, it is common to evaluate the hexosaminidase A level. For patients with a history of exposure to heavy metals, a 24-hour urine collection for heavy metal testing is preformed. A variety of other laboratory tests may be ordered depending on individual case circumstances.

Electromyography

EMG studies are routinely performed as part of the diagnostic evaluation of patients suspected of having MND. The results of EMG studies are integrated with the information obtained through clinical history, physical examination, laboratory studies, and radiologic studies.

EMG studies are critically important for the diagnosis of MND for several reasons. First, EMG studies can reveal evidence of a pathophysiologic process other than motor neuron degeneration, which would completely change the suspected diagnosis. Examples include peripheral neuropathy, such as multifocal motor neuropathy (20); a myopathic process, such as inflammatory myopathy; or a neuromuscular junction transmission disorder, such as myasthenia gravis (MG) or Lambert-Eaton myasthenic syndrome (LEMS). Each of these conditions can mimic ALS, and in some cases, EMG studies may provide the critical clue when the diagnosis is not otherwise suspected.

The EMG studies also provide information about the degree and distribution of LMN abnormalities. There may be times when LMN involvement is not readily apparent on the clinical examination and EMG studies resolve this question. Finding widespread fibrillation potentials can substantiate the diagnosis of ALS or PMA, and the absence of widespread fibrillation potentials can support a diagnosis of PLS or PBP.

Nerve conduction studies may be normal in MND or may show low-amplitude compound muscle action potentials (CMAPs) reflecting loss of motor axons. Repetitive nerve stimulation (RNS) studies may show a decremental response in some patients with ALS.

The EMG findings on needle examination in ALS include fibrillation potentials, fasciculation potentials, and neurogenic motor unit potential changes. Reduced recruitment of motor unit potentials is common. If reinnervation of muscle fibers has occurred, the motor unit potentials become complex with large-amplitude, long-duration, and excessive polyphasia. Such motor unit potentials often show instability with variation in amplitude while firing. This reflects blocking or failure of action potentials from some muscle fibers due to recently formed and immature neuromuscular junctions.

If EMG studies are performed relatively early in the course of the patient's symptomatic illness, there

may not be sufficient LMN abnormalities to be certain of the diagnosis. In this case, it is best to repeat the studies in several months because more abnormalities develop with time.

Neuroimaging Evaluation

Magnetic resonance imaging (MRI) studies of the brain and cervical spinal cord are frequently performed when the diagnosis of MND is suspected. The main purpose of these studies is to exclude other diseases of the central nervous system that could explain UMN findings. In most patients with MND, the brain and cervical spine MRI studies do not reveal abnormalities that can explain the clinical features. MRI studies of the cervical spine are commonly performed to evaluate for cervical spine abnormalities, which at times may mimic ALS. The combination of cervical spinal stenosis and multi-level cervical radiculopathies can produce both UMN and LMN signs that mimic ALS. Brain MRI studies are performed to evaluate for structural abnormalities or diseases of the brain that could explain the patient's UMN signs.

Conventional MRI studies using long T2-weighted or fluid-attenuated inversion recovery (FLAIR) sequences may show hyperintense signal changes in the corticospinal tract at the level of the posterior limb of the internal capsule or cerebral peduncles in some ALS patients (11).

Newer MRI techniques, such as magnetization transfer and diffusion tensor imaging, are being investigated for the potential of better demonstration of abnormal signal within the corticospinal tracts in patients with MND.

DIAGNOSTIC CRITERIA

Despite the lack of specific diagnostic tests for MND, diagnostic criteria for ALS have been developed based on clinical features. The criteria commonly used for research studies are the Revised El Escorial Criteria. These criteria require the basic features of UMN and LMN signs, progression of the illness as manifested by spread of physical signs over time, and exclusion of other disorders that could mimic ALS.

The El Escorial Criteria are based on division of the central nervous system into four anatomic regions: the brainstem and cervical, thoracic, and lumbosacral spinal regions. Each region is assessed for UMN and LMN signs, and the combination of findings is used to place the patient into a category of diagnostic certainty (Table 25-6). The criteria were created for the purpose of standardizing enrollment of ALS patients onto research studies. The current standard for clinical trials in ALS is to limit eligibility for enrollment to those patients with

Table 25-6. *Revised El Escorial Criteria for ALS*

ALS Diagnostic Category	Criteria
Definite ALS	UMN and LMN signs in 3 regions
Definite Familial ALS	UMN and LMN signs in 1 region plus DNA evidence of familial ALS
Probable ALS	UMN and LMN signs in 2 regions (with some UMN signs rostral to LMN signs)
Probable ALS, laboratory supported	UMN and LMN signs in 1 region or UMN signs in ≥ 1 region *plus* EMG evidence of LMN signs in ≥ 2 limbs
Possible ALS	UMN and LMN signs in 1 region

From Brooks BR, Miller RG, Swash M, et al. El Escorial revisited: revised criteria for the diagnosis of amyotrophic lateral sclerosis. *Amyotroph Lateral Scler Other Motor Neuron Disord.* 2000;5:293–299.

definite and probable ALS. Although these categories require clinical evidence of more extensive disease, the term "diagnostic certainty" may be somewhat misleading. There is no evidence that patients who do not meet criteria for definite or probable ALS are less likely to have the diagnosis. Furthermore, there is no evidence that the category of diagnostic certainty is predictive of prognosis. The fact that roughly 10% of ALS patients die of the illness without ever having documented clinical signs to meet criteria for probable or definite ALS underscores the limitations of these criteria.

DIFFERENTIAL DIAGNOSIS

A number of disorders may at times have clinical features that mimic ALS. These can be divided into conditions known to produce a UMN clinical presentation and those that cause an LMN presentation. Usually, the clinical history and physical examination serve to differentiate most of these disorders from ALS. For example, prominent sensory symptoms, bladder dysfunction, and eye findings are features that would allow multiple sclerosis to be readily distinguished from ALS, even though UMN findings may overlap.

UMN Disorders

Disorders commonly causing UMN signs need to be excluded. Examples include multiple sclerosis, cerebrovascular disease, structural abnormalities of the brain, craniovertebral junction or cervical spine disorders (e.g., brain tumors, Chiari malformation, cervical spinal stenosis), vitamin B_{12} deficiency, copper deficiency, human T-lymphotropic virus 1 (HTLV-1) myelopathy, tropical spastic paraparesis, hereditary spastic paraparesis, adrenomyeloneuropathy, and hyperparathyroidism.

LMN Disorders

Some LMN disorders may superficially resemble ALS due to the overlap of LMN findings. These conditions generally are readily distinguished from ALS because of the absence of UMN findings and the associated symptoms or signs that usually do not occur in ALS. For example, sensory symptoms are common in demyelinative polyneuropathies, EMG findings typical of myopathy occur in patients with inflammatory myopathy, and eye muscle weakness is common in patients with MG. The search for disorders with LMN features includes careful review of clinical findings through history and physical examination, EMG, and laboratory testing.

Disorders that need to be excluded include polyneuropathy or polyradiculoneuropathy, myopathy such as polymyositis, neuromuscular transmission disorders such as MG or LEMS, and metabolic disorders such as hyperparathyroidism.

TREATMENT OPTIONS

Presently, there is no effective treatment for stopping or reversing MND. Riluzole has been approved by the Food and Drug Administration for treating ALS because two studies have shown that it has prolonged survival by approximately 3 months compared to placebo (15). The major focus of treatment for ALS is symptomatic care, and many therapies are available for treating the symptoms associated with ALS.

RESPIRATORY INSUFFICIENCY

Respiratory muscle weakness is the most serious complication of ALS because respiratory muscle failure is the ultimate cause of death for most patients. In addition to dyspnea, symptoms of chronic respiratory insufficiency may include morning headache, daytime drowsiness, fatigue, poor concentration, insomnia, nervousness, depression, and anxiety. Examination may reveal tachypnea, use of accessory respiratory muscles, and difficulty sustaining speech due to dyspnea.

Assessment of respiratory function in ALS patients involves clinical history and a number of measurements of respiratory function. Clinical history should include assessment of respiratory symptoms as listed earlier and upper airway symptoms such as excessive secretions and the ability to clear secretions with cough. Patients should be asked if they have difficulty breathing when lying supine. The benefit of gravity aiding the diaphragm's descent is lost in the supine position, and this is often an early symptom of diaphragm weakness.

Pulmonary function tests are performed to provide quantitative measurements of respiratory function. Measurements of inspiratory function include forced vital capacity (FVC), maximal inspiratory pressure (MIP), and sniff nasal pressure (SNP). Measurements of expiratory function include the maximal expiratory pressure (MEP) and the peak cough flow. Measuring the FVC in the upright and supine positions helps provide additional information regarding the degree of diaphragm weakness. Measurement of nocturnal oxygen saturation is helpful to detect hypoventilation that often occurs at night.

Treatment of respiratory symptoms involves many different techniques. The most helpful intervention is noninvasive ventilation, in which a ventilator device delivers pressurized air via a face mask or other interface. The delivery of pressurized air reduces the patient's work of breathing and allows better ventilation than the patient can accomplish with weak respiratory muscles. Noninvasive ventilation requires considerable patient education and follow-up by a pulmonologist or knowledgeable respiratory therapist who can respond to patients' questions and make adjustments in the ventilator settings.

An important aspect of respiratory therapy includes control of oral secretions. This is usually accomplished with medications or use of a hand-held suction device. Medications that may help to dry secretions include tricyclic antidepressants, anticholinergic agents, and glycopyrrolate. Other options include botulinum toxin injection of the parotid glands or radiation treatment of the salivary glands.

NUTRITIONAL STATUS

Impaired swallowing in patients with bulbar muscle weakness often leads to decreased oral intake and compromised nutrition. A speech pathologist conducts an assessment of swallowing function. Video fluoroscopy of swallowing helps to determine the degree of impairment for different consistencies and if the patient is at risk of aspiration of food substances. When aspiration is apparent or patients cannot maintain adequate oral nutrition, a feeding tube is recommended to bypass the oral route. There are several techniques for placing a feeding tube. It is generally recommended that patients have a feeding tube placed before the FVC drops below 50% of the predicted value because the procedure is better tolerated with better respiratory function (12). Evaluation by a dietician is necessary to plan appropriate nutritional supplementation.

SPEECH PROBLEMS

Dysarthric speech may be initially improved with speech therapy exercises. As the illness progresses, the patient's speech may become unintelligible and ultimately lost entirely. Many forms of alternative communication are available, ranging from a simple writing pad to computerized augmented communication devices. The speech therapist works with the patient to select the most appropriate device to meet the patient's needs.

PSYCHOSOCIAL IMPACT

Patients diagnosed with MND encounter many challenges in their personal lives. The knowledge that ALS will progress to incapacitating weakness and that death from respiratory failure can be anticipated in roughly 3 to 4 years forces patients to alter their future plans drastically. All aspects of life need to be reconsidered including relationships with family members, the home environment, the ability to work, the ability to communicate, finances, retirement, and medical care. Patients must make complicated medical decisions regarding interventions that may affect survival such as a feeding tube and ventilation assistance. Some patients initially experience denial and seek a different diagnosis from alternative care providers who are not familiar with ALS. Patients may also experience depression related to the circumstances surrounding their illness. Some patients have impaired cognitive function, which further complicates decision making.

Because of the multiple psychosocial issues that patients face, there is usually benefit from consultation with a clinic specializing in ALS care. Typically, the function of such a clinic is to assemble the group of key health care providers that can answer questions and provide practical solutions to common problems. This group typically consists of the following specialists: occupational therapist, physical therapist, speech therapist, respiratory therapist, dietician, social worker, and a nurse and physician experienced with ALS patients.

KENNEDY'S DISEASE (X-LINKED SPINOBULBAR MUSCULAR ATROPHY)

DEFINITION OF TERMS

Kennedy's disease is an adult-onset, X-linked recessive hereditary disorder characterized by LMN degeneration affecting limb and bulbar muscles and a sensory neuronopathy.

CLINICAL FEATURES

This disorder is characterized by gradual onset of muscle weakness in limb and bulbar muscles. Patients may have fatigability and muscle cramps, and fasciculations are common. Despite the fact that a sensory neuronopathy is a major feature of the disorder, sensory complaints are not prominent. Endocrine abnormalities include diabetes or glucose impairment, gynecomastia, testicular atrophy, and infertility later in life.

The neurologic examination reveals muscle weakness and atrophy with fasciculations. The cranial nerve examination shows tongue and facial muscle weakness, atrophy, and fasciculations. The muscle stretch reflexes are reduced or absent, whereas the sensory examination is normal. The general physical examination shows gynecomastia and may show testicular atrophy.

EPIDEMIOLOGY

In the United States, the estimated incidence is approximately one case in 40,000 men. The average age of onset is 40 to 60 years. The inheritance pattern predicts that only males are affected; however, females who carry the gene may at times show some clinical manifestations.

PATHOPHYSIOLOGY

The genetic defect causing Kennedy's disease is an expanded trinucleotide repeat (CAG) in the first exon of the androgen receptor gene located on the proximal long arm of the X chromosome (14). The precise cellular mechanisms leading to degeneration of both LMNs and dorsal root sensory ganglia are unknown. Abnormal function of the androgen receptor likely contributes to associated endocrine abnormalities including glucose intolerance, gynecomastia, and infertility.

NATURAL HISTORY

The disorder is characterized by gradually progressive muscle weakness and atrophy affecting limb and bulbar muscles, with onset in the fifth to sixth decade. Rarely, clinical features can occur as early as the second decade (1). The progression of the disease is slow, and the life expectancy is not significantly reduced compared to the general population.

DIAGNOSIS

The diagnosis is suspected on the basis of clinical and EMG findings and confirmed with DNA testing. The EMG studies show abnormalities that reflect the LMN disorder and sensory neuronopathy. On nerve conduction studies, the motor and sensory responses show reduced amplitudes. Often the sensory responses are absent. The needle examination demonstrates fibrillation potentials and chronic neurogenic motor unit potential changes. Taken together, the results of nerve conduction studies and EMG examination can give the appearance of a chronic axonal sensorimotor

polyneuropathy. One must interpret the EMG in the context of the clinical setting to realize that this represents a motor and sensory neuronopathy. The diagnosis is confirmed by obtaining commercially available DNA testing.

TREATMENT

Treatment for Kennedy's disease is primarily supportive. Physical therapy, occupational therapy, and speech therapy are used as necessary to treat impairments secondary to muscle weakness. Genetic counseling is recommended to help the patient and family understand the hereditary pattern and risks to family members.

NEUROMUSCULAR TRANSMISSION DISORDERS

MYASTHENIA GRAVIS

Definition of Terms

MG is an autoimmune disorder in which antibodies directed at the acetylcholine receptor (AChR) lead to cross-linking and destruction of AChRs on the postsynaptic muscle membrane. Myasthenic crisis refers to an emergency situation when weakness resulting from MG is severe enough to require intubation for mechanical ventilation or airway protection.

Epidemiology

MG has a prevalence of 77 to 150 cases per million and an annual incidence of four to 11 cases per million (21). The age of onset reveals two peaks. The first peak is between 20 and 40 years and occurs predominantly in women. The second peak is between 60 and 80 years and is roughly equal between men and women.

Late-onset MG (age of onset ≥50 years) results in more frequent involvement of bulbar and neck muscles and relatively less problems with limb weakness. Because the thymus gland typically involutes with age, pathologic assessment is more likely to show atrophy than the hyperplastic changes seen in early-onset disease.

Although MG is not a hereditary disorder, relatives of patients with MG have an increased risk of developing other autoimmune disorders. Certain human leukocyte antigen (HLA) types (cHLA B8, DRW3) are more common in patients with MG, and a high concordance rate in monozygotic twins supports the concept that a genetic component may predispose to MG.

Pathology

The major pathologic change in MG is simplification of the postsynaptic muscle membrane in association with loss of AChRs. In severe cases, there is complete loss of the normal convoluted folding of the postsynaptic membrane. Thymus gland abnormalities occur in approximately 75% of patients. Thymic hyperplasia is the most common abnormality, and about 10% of patients have a thymoma. Thymoma occurs equally in men and women, with a peak onset of around 50 years.

Pathogenesis

The immune-mediated pathogenesis of MG has been clearly established (24). Antibody-mediated destruction of the nicotinic AChR results in a reduced number of AChRs and loss of the complex folding of the postsynaptic skeletal muscle membrane. AChR antibodies may interfere with neuromuscular transmission by several mechanisms including blockade of receptors, cross-linking of receptors, and complement-mediated lysis of receptors.

Natural History

The natural history of MG is variable. Although complex grading systems have been established, it is easiest to think of MG as having ocular and generalized forms.

Patients with strictly ocular MG have a better prognosis than those with generalized MG. Patients who begin with ocular MG may remain ocular or progress to generalized MG. This transformation usually takes place within the first 3 years of the illness, but occasionally, a patient will transition from ocular to generalized MG at a later time.

MG can be a fatal illness, and this was often the case before the availability of immune-modulating therapies. The many therapies for MG have improved the prognosis. In a Danish population-based survival study, the overall survival at 3, 5, 10, and 20 years was quite good at 85%, 81%, 69%, and 63%, respectively (6).

Up to 27% of patients with MG may experience myasthenic crisis at some point in their illness. In roughly 18% of MG patients, myasthenic crisis is the initial manifestation of the illness. Generalized weakness is the most common initial manifestation leading to crisis, and this usually develops rapidly in a matter of several days. The most common cause of myasthenic crisis is worsening of MG. This may be caused by reducing prednisone too quickly. Occasionally, this is precipitated by introduction of prednisone or other medications known to worsen neuromuscular transmission. Respiratory infection and surgery are other situations that may predispose to myasthenic crisis.

Diagnosis

History and Physical Findings The diagnosis of MG is usually considered on the basis of typical clinical history and findings on examination. The typical history is that of fluctuating weakness, such that muscle weakness and fatigue develop with sustained physical activity and improve with rest. Specific muscle groups are commonly involved in MG. These include ocular, bulbar, proximal limb, and respiratory muscles. Ocular muscle weakness causes diplopia or ptosis. Bulbar muscle weakness causes dysarthria and dysphagia. Respiratory muscle weakness causes dyspnea, which can progress to respiratory failure. Proximal limb muscle weakness causes difficulty raising the arms and difficulty rising from a seated position. Weakness of the neck extensor paraspinal muscles may cause head drop. Some patients with MG also develop distal muscle weakness, although this is uncommon.

In addition to sustained physical activity, other factors may precipitate or exacerbate muscle weakness in patients with MG. These include infection, certain drugs (Table 25-7), and surgery.

Diagnostic Tests When patients initially present with symptoms suggesting MG, it is necessary to confirm the diagnosis. This is accomplished with several diagnostic tests. One or more positive tests are

Table 25-7. *Drugs That May Worsen Neuromuscular Transmission*

Antibiotics	Cardiac	Psychiatric	Antiepileptic	Rheumatologic	Endocrine
Clindamycin	Beta-blockers	Chlorpromazine	Phenytoin	Chloroquine	ACTH
Colistin	Lidocaine	Lithium	Trimethadione	D-penicillamine	Prednisone
Gentamicin	Procainamide	Phenelzine			Thyroid
Kanamycin	Quinidine	Promazine			
Lincomycin	Quinine				
Neomycin	Trimethaphan				
Netilmicin	Verapamil				
Polymyxin B					
Streptomycin					
Tetracyclines					
Tobramycin					

ACTH, adrenocorticotropic hormone.

generally required to confirm the diagnosis. The tests most commonly used are AChR antibodies and electrophysiologic tests to evaluate neuromuscular transmission. Other tests include the edrophonium test (19), the ice pack test (2), and the sleep test.

Serologic Studies Serologic studies can help with the diagnosis of MG. AChR antibodies are routinely included in the initial diagnostic evaluation. Several AChR antibodies can be measured, including binding, blocking, and modulating antibodies. AChR antibodies are found in 80% of patients with generalized MG and 55% of patients with ocular MG. Although the specificity of AChR antibodies for MG is very high, it is not 100%. Therefore, clinicians must interpret positive results in the context of the patient's clinical presentation. The titer of AChR antibodies does not correlate with disease severity.

Roughly 20% of patients with MG do not have measurable AChR antibodies. These patients have been referred to as having seronegative MG. Recently, some of these patients have been found to have a different antibody called anti-MuSK antibody. Anti-MuSK antibody is directed against a protein in the neuromuscular junction called muscle-specific protein kinase (MuSK).

Patients with MG and thymoma frequently have high titers of anti-striated muscle antibody. However, many patients with MG who do not have thymoma also have anti-striated muscle antibodies.

Patients with MG may at times have an additional autoimmune disease. Depending on the clinical features, there may a role for testing for other antibodies that may be associated with connective tissue disorders. Examples include antinuclear antibody, rheumatoid factor, and extractable nuclear antigen antibodies.

Electrophysiologic Tests Electrophysiologic studies used to assess neuromuscular transmission in patients suspected of having MG include RNS studies and single-fiber EMG (SFEMG) studies. RNS studies are commonly performed, whereas SFEMG studies are less readily available due to the demanding technical aspects of the study. RNS studies involve recording the CMAP following four to five serial electrical stimuli given at a rate of 2 to 5 Hz. In normal individuals, the size of the CMAP remains unchanged. Patients with MG often show a decline in the CMAP amplitude referred to as a decremental response. RNS studies are most likely to reveal a decremental response when recorded from weak muscles. Consequently, RNS studies recorded from cranial or proximal muscles have a much higher yield of abnormality than recordings from distal muscles (7).

SFEMG studies involve using an intramuscular needle electrode to record pairs of muscle action potentials belonging to the same motor unit and analyzing the variation in action potential firing time between the two potentials. The mean interpotential difference between the two firing action potentials is referred to as "jitter" (23). Jitter is a normal phenomenon resulting from variation in the rise time of endplate potentials in different muscle fibers belonging to the same motor unit. An endplate potential refers to a localized depolarization of the muscle fiber endplate membrane that precedes initiation of the muscle fiber action potential. In patients with MG, the jitter is increased beyond the normal range. In MG patients with weakness, some of the endplate potentials fail to reach the threshold level necessary to generate an action potential. This results in failure of the action potential, called "blocking."

Other Tests The other tests used to facilitate the diagnosis of MG are tests that involve reversal of muscle weakness. The edrophonium test (2) is a pharmacologic test in which an intravenous dose of edrophonium is administered to determine whether this reverses an objective neurologic examination finding such as ptosis, extraocular muscle weakness, or dysarthria. Edrophonium is a rapidly acting cholinesterase inhibitor, meaning that it inhibits the enzyme that breaks down acetylcholine (Ach). This permits the patient's ACh to have a longer duration of action and thus improves neuromuscular transmission. The test can only be performed if there is an objective abnormality on the physical examination that can be monitored. The test cannot be performed if the only complaint is subjective, such as fatigue. Because of the potential for developing a bradyarrhythmia during the test, it is necessary to have a syringe containing atropine available at the time the edrophonium test is conducted.

The ice pack test (7) involves placing an ice pack over the eyes and, after a period of cooling, checking to see whether ptosis or ophthalmoparesis has improved. The test is based on the fact that cooling improves neuromuscular transmission and this might temporarily correct ptosis or ophthalmoparesis. The use of this test is limited to patients with weakness of the eye muscles.

The sleep test involves observing the effect of a 30-minute nap on a patient's ptosis or ophthalmoparesis. Immediately following the nap, there may be improvement or resolution of ptosis or ophthalmoparesis. These signs may then reappear over the subsequent 30 seconds to 5 minutes.

Treatment Options

Treatment of MG is planned according to the severity of the illness and individual patient circumstances. Treatment options include use of a cholinesterase inhibitor to improve neuromuscular transmission and a variety of medications or procedures to reduce the patient's autoimmune attack on the neuromuscular junction.

The cholinesterase inhibitor most often used is pyridostigmine. It is usually tolerated, but side effects that may limit its use include diarrhea, abdominal cramps, and skeletal muscle cramps. Patients with ocular MG or mild generalized MG may at times be successfully managed with pyridostigmine alone. Often, pyridostigmine alone is not sufficient to improve the patient's weakness, and it may be necessary to add some form of immune-modulating therapy.

There are multiple immune-modulating therapies available to treat MG. These include prednisone, immunosuppressive drugs, plasmapheresis, intravenous immunoglobulin (IVIG), and thymectomy. Prednisone therapy typically works well to improve the symptoms of MG. The disadvantages of prednisone are significant side effects associated with long-term use and a delay of several months from initiation until improvement occurs. In addition, when prednisone is introduced, it may cause initial worsening of neuromuscular transmission before improvement occurs from immune suppression. Thus, it is necessary to carefully monitor a patient for worsening of symptoms when prednisone is introduced. This is of greatest concern when the patient has bulbar or respiratory muscle weakness because worsening weakness in these muscle groups can lead to life-threatening complications.

The side effects of prednisone vary from patient to patient. Generally, more prominent side effects occur with higher doses and longer use. The multiple potential side effects of prednisone should be reviewed with the patient before initiating treatment. A complete review of steroid side effects is beyond the scope of this work. There are several options for initiating prednisone therapy. One approach is to initiate a low dose and gradually increase the dose as necessary. The other option is to initiate a high dose and gradually reduce the dose once the patient has started to improve. Beginning with a high dose is likely to result in more rapid improvement but also may be more likely to precipitate transient worsening of MG symptoms.

Once the patient has improved, prednisone is gradually transitioned from daily dosing to every other day because this is believed to be associated with fewer side effects. Prednisone must be tapered gradually because too rapid tapering may precipitate an exacerbation of MG. Rapid tapering of prednisone may also precipitate myasthenic crisis.

Other immunosuppressive agents are often used in the treatment of MG. Specific agents include azathioprine, mycophenolate mofetil, cyclosporine, and methotrexate. These agents are often used to reduce the need for prednisone. In some patients, other immunosuppressive drugs may be used as the main immune-modulating treatment without use of prednisone.

For patients with myasthenic crisis or those with severe generalized muscle weakness, plasmapheresis is usually recommended because the removal of harmful antibodies typically induces improvement in a relatively short time. Patients are usually given five exchanges on an every-other-day schedule. Depending on the clinical course, additional exchanges may be required. IVIG has also been used to treat exacerbations of MG.

Thymectomy has been considered a potentially beneficial treatment for selected patients with MG. Thymectomy has been felt to offer the possibility of either inducing remission of MG or reducing the patient's long-term commitment to immune-modulating therapies. Thymectomy has been recommended for patients under the age of 60 years, especially when the illness is severe and the patient requires chronic immunosuppressive treatment. The retrospective evidence supporting thymectomy has been questioned, and a prospective controlled trial comparing thymectomy and medical management is ongoing.

Psychosocial Impact

MG is a chronic illness requiring regular medical care. Because of the availability of effective therapies, many patients are able to have fairly good control of symptoms. Patients with more severe forms of the illness may struggle to function with disabling weakness and fatigue and side effects of chronic therapies. In addition, severe worsening of the illness with myasthenic crisis causes some patients to deal with long intensive care unit hospitalizations and realize the life-threatening severity of the illness. These factors can interfere with all aspects of daily life and thus may affect the patient's psychological state. The possibility of depression needs to be considered as yet another complication of the illness.

LAMBERT-EATON MYASTHENIC SYNDROME

Definition of Terms

LEMS is an immune-mediated neuromuscular transmission disorder typically presenting as a gait disturbance with proximal lower extremity weakness. In this disorder, antibodies directed against P/Q-type voltage-gated calcium channels (VGCCs) in the motor nerve terminal lead to cross-linking and destruction of VGCCs. The damage to VGCCs prevents binding of ACh vesicles to the presynaptic membrane and interferes with normal ACh release. LEMS is most often associated with small-cell lung cancer (SCLC) or other malignancy, and 40% of presentations are idiopathic (17).

Clinical Features

The major symptom is impaired walking with proximal leg weakness and generalized fatigue. The weakness may improve after exercise. Bulbar and ocular muscles are occasionally involved, but usually the degree of involvement is minor compared to patients with MG. Respiratory failure is extremely rare. Patients may have some evidence of autonomic dysfunction such as postural hypotension, dry mouth, or impotence in males. An unusual symptom is a complaint of a metallic taste in the mouth.

Examination reveals proximal leg weakness, which may fluctuate. There may be some initial improvement in strength with repeated testing. Muscle stretch reflexes are usually reduced but can be facilitated by serial tapping over the tendon. Sensory examination and coordination can be normal or show additional abnormalities.

Some patients with LEMS and underlying SCLC may have other paraneoplastic syndromes such as syndrome of inappropriate antidiuretic hormone secretion, sensorimotor neuropathy, or cerebellar degeneration (13).

Epidemiology

LEMS usually begins in mid to late life. Only rare cases have been reported in children (27). The prevalence is estimated at one per 100,000 (9). The male-to-female ratio is 1:1. Roughly 60% of cases are paraneoplastic, with SCLC being the most common malignancy. Symptoms usually begin insidiously, and the diagnosis may be delayed for months to years. In some patients, a microscopic lung cancer may only be detected at autopsy. It has been estimated that up to 3% of patients with SCLC have LEMS.

Pathology

The pathology in LEMS is in the presynaptic nerve terminal (8). Ultrastructural studies reveal that active zone particles, which represent VGCCs, become clustered and reduced in number due to antibody-mediated injury. There is also pathology involving the underlying malignancy, which is most often an SCLC.

Etiology

LEMS is an antibody-mediated immune disorder in which antibodies directed against P/Q-type VGCCs in the motor nerve terminal lead to cross-linking and destruction of VGCCs. The damage to VGCC interferes with the normal release of ACh quanta associated with a nerve action potential.

The frequent association with SCLC is explained by the fact that SCLC cells are of neuroectodermal

origin and contain high concentrations of VGCCs. The immune response to the SCLC results in production of VGCC antibodies, which then cause injury to the patient's VGCCs on the presynaptic motor nerve terminal. There has also been an association with LEMS and other autoimmune disorders.

Diagnosis

The diagnosis is made by the combination of clinical features, the results of EMG studies, and serologic confirmation of VGCC antibodies.

Electrophysiologic Studies A characteristic feature of LEMS is that the amplitude of CMAPs is reduced. With RNS studies at 2 Hz, a baseline decrement is typically seen. When the CMAP is reassessed immediately following 10 seconds of maximal voluntary exercise, there is usually a marked increase in the CMAP amplitude. The explanation for this is that muscle fiber action potentials are blocked initially due to impaired release of ACh. The exercise increases the presynaptic calcium concentration, which transiently facilitates release of ACh. Consequently, the CMAP increases, a process called facilitation. Occasionally, exercise does not provide a great enough stimulus, and it may be necessary to perform high-frequency RNS studies. In these studies, the CMAP amplitude is monitored while the patient receives high-frequency RNS. It is necessary to use a frequency in the range of 20 to 50 Hz, which can be quite uncomfortable. Facilitation of more than 100% is highly suggestive of LEMS in the correct clinical setting.

Conventional needle EMG in LEMS demonstrates markedly unstable motor unit action potentials, which vary in shape and amplitude. This variability is detected as "jitter" in SFEMG. The jitter is markedly increased in LEMS, and there is frequent impulse blocking.

Calcium Channel Antibodies VGCC antibodies of P/Q type are detected in LEMS patients with lung cancer and close to 90% of patients without a cancer. Low titers of these antibodies are detected in connective tissue disorders and MG (16). The titer of VGCC antibodies does not correlate with disease severity but improves with immunosuppressive therapy.

Investigating an Underlying Malignancy Whenever LEMS is suspected, investigations should be performed to detect an underlying neoplasm. This typically involves computerized tomography images of chest, abdomen, and pelvis. A paraneoplastic antibody panel should be obtained when LEMS is suspected. Consultation with a pulmonologist may be necessary to consider bronchoscopy to investigate for lung cancer.

Treatment Options

The first step in planning therapy for LEMS is to attempt to identify an underlying malignancy and begin treatment. If no tumor can be found, re-evaluation is necessary at some interval such as 3 to 6 months. For patients who do have an underlying malignancy, successful treatment of the tumor may result in improvement of LEMS. However, improvement of LEMS with treatment of the tumor is not consistent.

There are many options for treating LEMS. Pyridostigmine may help improve neuromuscular transmission through the same mechanism described earlier for MG. Improvement of neuromuscular transmission may also occur by blocking the potassium-dependent potassium channel with 3,4-diaminopyridine (DAP) (28). This therapy prolongs the period of depolarization following a nerve action potential. This leads to increased presynaptic calcium concentration, which facilitates release of ACh. LEMS may also respond to treatment with a variety of immune-modulating therapies including steroids, immunosuppressive drugs, and IVIG.

Psychosocial Impact

Patients should be advised regarding the prognosis of their underlying malignancy. The problems associated with chronic disease described earlier for MG are similar in LEMS.

REFERENCES

1. Barkhaus PE, Kennedy WR, Stern LZ, et al. Hereditary proximal spinal and bulbar motor neuron disease of late onset. A report of six cases. *Arch Neurol*. 1982;39:112–116.
2. Benatar M. A systematic review of diagnostic studies in myasthenia gravis. *Neuromuscul Disord*. 2006;16:459–467.
3. Bradley WG. Overview of motor neuron disease: classification and nomenclature. *Clin Neurosci*. 1995–1996;3:323–326.
4. Brownell B, Oppenheimer DR, Hughes JT. The central nervous system in motor neuron disease. *J Neurol Neurosurg Psychiatry*. 1970;33:338–357.
5. Caselli RJ, Smith BE, Osborne D. Primary lateral sclerosis: a neuropsychological study. *Neurology*. 1995;45:2005–2009.
6. Christensen PB, Jensen TS, Tsiropoulos I, et al. Mortality and survival in myasthenia gravis: a Danish population based study. *J Neurol Neurosurg Psychiatry*. 1998;64:78–83.
7. Costa J, Evangelista T, Conceicao I, et al. Repetitive nerve stimulation in myasthenia gravis—relative sensitivity of different muscles. *Clin Neurophysiol*. 2004;115:2776–2782.
8. Elmqvist D, Lambert EH. Detailed analysis of neuromuscular transmission in a patient with the myasthenic syndrome sometimes associated with bronchogenic carcinoma. *Mayo Clin Proc*. 1968;43:689–713.
9. Elrington GM, Murray NM, Spiro SG, et al. Neurological paraneoplastic syndromes in patients with small cell lung cancer: a prospective survey of 150 patients. *J Neurol Neurosurg Psychiatry*. 1991;54:764–767.
10. Gurney ME, Pu H, Chiu AY, et al. Motor neuron degeneration in mice that express a human Cu, Zn superoxide dismutase mutation. *Science*. 1994;264:1772–1775.
11. Jack CR Jr, Lexa FJ, Trojanowski JQ, et al. Normal aging, dementia, and neurodegenerative disease: amyotrophic lateral sclerosis. In: Atlas SW, ed. *Magnetic resonance imaging of the brain and spine*. Philadelphia: Lippincott Williams & Wilkins; 2002: 1227–1229.
12. Kasaskis EJ, Scarlata D, Hill R, et al. A retrospective study of percutaneous endoscopic gastrostomy in ALS patients during the BDNF and CNTF trials. *J Neurol Sci*. 1999;169:118–125.
13. Kobayashi H, Matsuoka R, Kitamura S, et al. Bronchogenic carcinoma with subacute cerebellar degeneration and Eaton-Lambert syndrome: an autopsy case. *Jpn J Med*. 1988;27:203–206.
14. La Spada AR, Wilson EM, Lubahn DB, et al. Androgen receptor gene mutations in X-linked spinal and bulbar muscular atrophy. *Nature*. 1991;35:77–79.
15. Leigh PN, Abrahams S, Al-Chalabi A, et al. The management of motor neuron disease. *J Neurol Neurosurg Psychiatry*. 2003;74[Suppl IV]:32–47.
16. Lennon VA. Serological profile of myasthenia gravis and distinction from the Lambert-Eaton myasthenic syndrome. *Neurology*. 1997;48: S23–S27.
17. Mareska M, Gutmann L. Lambert-Eaton myasthenic syndrome. *Semin Neurol*. 2004;24: 149–153.
18. Moulignier A, Moulonguet A, Pialoux G, et al. Reversible ALS-like disorder in HIV infection. *Neurology*. 2001;57:995–1001.
19. Nicholson GA, McLeod JG, Griffiths LR. Comparison of diagnostic tests in myasthenia gravis. *Clin Exp Neurol*. 1983;19:45–49.
20. Olney RK, Lewis RA, Putnam TD, et al. Consensus criteria for the diagnosis of multifocal motor neuropathy. *Muscle Nerve*. 2003;27:117–121.
21. Robertson NP, Deans J, Compston DAS. Myasthenia gravis: a population based epidemiological study in Cambridgeshire, England. *J Neurol Neurosurg Psychiatry*. 1998;65:492–496.

22. Rocha JA, Reis C, Simois F, et al. Diagnostic investigation and multidisciplinary management in motor neuron disease. *J Neurol.* 2005;252:1435–1447.

23. Roelofs-Iverson RA, Mulder DW, Elveback LR, et al. ALS and heavy metals: a pilot case-control study. *Neurology.* 1984;34:393–395.

24. Romi F, Skeie GO, Aarli JA, et al. Muscle autoantibodies in subgroups of myasthenia gravis patients. *J Neurol.* 2000;247:369–375.

25. Roos PM, Vesterberg O, Nordberg M. Metals in motor neuron disease. *Exp Biol Med.* 2006;231:1481–1487.

26. Ross MA. Acquired motor neuron disorders. *Neurol Clin.* 1997;15:481–500.

27. Sanders DB. Lambert-Eaton myasthenic syndrome: clinical diagnosis, immune-mediated mechanisms, and update on therapy. *Ann Neurol.* 1995;37[Suppl 1]:S63–S73.

28. Sanders DB. Lambert-Eaton myasthenic syndrome. Diagnosis and treatment. *Ann NY Acad Sci.* 2003;998:500–508.

29. Shaw PJ. Molecular and cellular pathways of neurodegeneration in motor neuron disease. *J Neurol Neurosurg Psychiatry.* 2005;76:1046–1057.

30. Shaw PJ, Ince PG, Falkous G, et al. Oxidative damage to protein in sporadic motor neuron disease spinal cord. *Ann Neurol.* 1995;38:691–695.

31. Short CL, Scott G, Blumbergs PC, et al. A case of presumptive primary lateral sclerosis with upper and lower motor neuron pathology. *J Clin Neurosci.* 2005;12:706–709.

32. Stalberg E, Trontelj JV. The study of normal and abnormal neuromuscular transmission with single fibre electromyography. *J Neurosci Methods.* 1997;74:145–154.

33. Stambler N, Charatan M, Cedarbaum JM. Prognostic indicators of survival in ALS. ALS CNTF Treatment Study Group. *Neurology.* 1998;50:66–72.

34. Strong MJ, Kesavapany S, Pant HC. The pathobiology of amyotrophic lateral sclerosis: a proteinopathy? *J Neuropathol Exp Neurol.* 2005;64:649–664.

35. Wood JD, Beaujeux TP, Shaw PJ. Protein aggregation in motor neuron disorders. *Neuropathol Appl Neurobiol.* 2003;29:529–545.

WEBSITES

The ALS Association, USA National Office: http://www.alsa.org/

Muscular Dystrophy Association's ALS Division: http://www.als.mdausa.org

ALS Survival Guide: http://www.alssurvivalguide.com

ALS Therapy Development Foundation: http://www.als-tdf.org

Kennedy's Disease Association: http://www.kennedysdisease.org/

National Organization for Rare Disorders: http://www.rarediseases.org/

This association addresses some uncommon or orphan neurologic disorders for which no dedicated organization exists.

Myasthenia Gravis Foundation of America: http://www.myasthenia.org

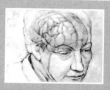

CHAPTER 26

Nonviral Infectious Diseases of the Nervous System

Karen L. Roos

An acquired immunodeficiency occurs with aging that increases an individual's susceptibility to infection. The older adult is at risk for disseminated disease that, in a younger person, may remain localized to the primary site of infection. The older adult is at risk for reactivation of latent infection in the central nervous system (CNS) that has remained latent for years because of intact cell-mediated immunity. The increased risk for shingles with aging is a classic example of this. The older adult may also have chronic illness (diabetes mellitus, cardiopulmonary disease, or chronic renal insufficiency) or cancer or be treated with immunosuppressive therapy or corticosteroid therapy, all of which contribute to impaired cell-mediated immunity. For these reasons, the older adult is at risk for CNS infections that are classically associated with an immunocompromised state.

This chapter reviews the nonviral infectious diseases of the nervous system, which include bacterial, fungal, and tuberculous meningitis and brain abscess. A concise discussion of the infectious etiologies of stroke and the infectious etiologies of dementia is provided. An understanding of the acquired immunodeficiency that occurs with aging is needed in order to prevent the reactivation of latent CNS infections and the acquisition of opportunistic CNS infections in the older adult. Until then, a high degree of suspicion for the possibility of these infectious diseases in the older adult should be maintained.

MENINGITIS

BACTERIAL MENINGITIS

Bacterial meningitis is an acute purulent infection in the subarachnoid space that is associated with an inflammatory reaction in the brain parenchyma and cerebral blood vessels that causes decreased consciousness, seizure activity, raised intracranial pressure (ICP), and stroke.

Epidemiology in Older Adults

The most common etiologic organisms of bacterial meningitis in older adults are *Streptococcus pneumoniae*, *Listeria monocytogenes*, and gram-negative bacilli

(*Escherichia coli*, *Klebsiella* species, *Pseudomonas aeruginosa*, and *Enterobacter* species). *Streptococcus agalactiae* is a leading cause of bacterial meningitis and sepsis in neonates and is increasingly seen in older adults with underlying diseases. *Haemophilus influenzae* type b, once the most common causative organism of bacterial meningitis in children, is now rarely seen in children but remains a causative organism of bacterial meningitis in older adults, especially those with chronic lung disease, those who have had a splenectomy, and patients who are immunocompromised. The most common causative organisms of bacterial meningitis in patients who have had a neurosurgical procedure are gram-negative bacilli and staphylococci.

Clinical Presentation

The classic triad of symptoms of meningitis is fever, headache, and stiff neck. An altered level of consciousness ranging from lethargy to stupor or coma and seizure activity can accompany or follow the initial symptoms. The combination of fever, headache, stiff neck, and an altered level of consciousness is highly suggestive of bacterial meningitis. Nuchal rigidity is the pathognomonic sign of meningeal irritation and is present when the neck resists passive flexion. Neck stiffness is sometimes difficult to interpret in the older adult. In this age group, resistance to passive movement of the neck may be due to meningeal infection or inflammation, cervical spondylosis, parkinsonism, or paratonic rigidity. When neck stiffness is due to meningitis, the neck resists flexion but can usually be passively rotated from side to side. When neck stiffness is due to cervical spondylosis, parkinsonism, or paratonic rigidity, any passive movement of the neck (lateral rotation, extension, or flexion) meets with resistance. The possibility that nuchal rigidity is due to meningeal infection or inflammation is supported by a positive Brudzinski and/or Kernig sign. Brudzinski sign is elicited with the patient in the supine position and is positive when passive flexion of the neck results in spontaneous flexion of the hips and knees. Kernig sign is elicited with the patient in the supine position, and the thigh is flexed on the abdomen with the knee flexed. Passive extension of the leg is limited by pain when meningeal irritation is present.

Seizures occur as part of the initial presentation of bacterial meningitis or during the course of the illness in up to 40% of patients. The majority of seizures have a focal onset, suggesting that focal arterial ischemia or infarction is a major cause of seizure activity in bacterial meningitis. Focal seizures may also be due to cortical venous thrombosis with hemorrhage or focal edema. Generalized seizure activity and status epilepticus are due to fever, anoxia from decreased cerebral perfusion, spread from a focal onset to a generalized tonic-clonic convulsion, or, less commonly, toxicity from antimicrobial agents.

Raised ICP is an expected complication of bacterial meningitis and is the major cause of obtundation and coma in this disease. Signs of increased ICP include an altered or deteriorating level of consciousness, papilledema, dilated poorly reactive pupils, sixth-nerve palsies, decerebrate posturing, and the Cushing reflex (bradycardia, hypertension, and irregular respirations).

Diagnosis

When the clinical presentation is suggestive of bacterial meningitis, Gram's stain and blood cultures should be immediately obtained, and empiric antimicrobial therapy should be initiated without delay (Fig. 26-1). The diagnosis of bacterial meningitis is made by examination of the cerebrospinal fluid (CSF) (Table 26-1). As stated earlier, raised ICP is an expected complication of bacterial meningitis and is the major cause of obtundation and coma in this disease. The role of lumbar puncture as a causative factor for cerebral herniation in patients with acute bacterial meningitis has been debated for years and remains unresolved. The risk of cerebral herniation from acute bacterial meningitis independent of lumbar puncture is approximately 6% to 8%. When the possibility of increased ICP exists because of a decreased level of consciousness, lumbar puncture should either be delayed (but empiric antimicrobial therapy should be initiated) until the increased ICP can be treated or performed with a 22-gauge needle 30 to 60 minutes after mannitol 1 g/kg has been administered intravenously. The patient can also be intubated and hyperventilated, in addition to being treated with mannitol, to decrease ICP prior to lumbar puncture. CSF should be obtained for cell count (1.0 mL), glucose and protein concentrations (1.0 mL), Gram's stain and bacterial culture (1.0 mL), latex agglutination test (0.5 mL), and/or polymerase chain reaction (PCR) for bacterial nucleic acid. CSF should also be examined for viral DNA because herpes simplex virus encephalitis is the leading disease in the differential diagnosis of bacterial meningitis.

The classic CSF abnormalities in bacterial meningitis are as follows: (a) increased opening pressure; (b) a pleocytosis of polymorphonuclear leukocytes (10 to 10,000 cells/mm^3); (c) decreased glucose concentration (<45 mg/dL and/or CSF:serum glucose ratio of <0.31); and (d) an increased protein concentration. CSF bacterial cultures are positive in >80% of patients, and CSF Gram's stain demonstrates organisms in >60%.

Opening pressure should be measured with the patient in the lateral recumbent position. The normal opening pressure for adults is <180 mm H$_2$O. In obese adults, however, the normal opening pressure is <250 mm H$_2$O. In adults, in uninfected CSF, the normal white blood cell (WBC) count ranges from 0 to 5 mononuclear cells (lymphocytes and monocytes)/mm^3. In normal uninfected CSF in the adult, there should be no polymorphonuclear leukocytes; however, a rare polymorphonuclear leukocyte can be found in concentrated CSF specimens. If the total WBC count is <5 cells/mm^3, the presence of a single polymorphonuclear leukocyte may be considered normal. The latex particle agglutination (LA) test for the detection of bacterial antigens of *S. pneumoniae*, *Neisseria meningitidis*, *H. influenzae* type b, *S. agalactiae*, and *E. coli* K1 strains in the CSF can be used to make a rapid diagnosis of bacterial meningitis and to make a diagnosis of bacterial meningitis in those patients who have been pretreated with antibiotics in whom Gram's stain and CSF culture are negative. The LA test has a rapid turnaround time, usually less than a few hours, but a negative LA test does not rule out bacterial meningitis. A broad-range PCR can detect small amounts of viable and nonviable organisms in CSF. When the broad-range PCR is positive, a PCR that uses specific bacterial primers to detect the nucleic acid of *S. pneumoniae*, *N. meningitidis*, *E. coli*, *L. monocytogenes*, *H. influenzae*, or *S. agalactiae* should be done based on the clinical suspicion of the meningeal pathogen. However, the turnaround time for PCR may be several days. The *Limulus* amebocyte lysate assay is a rapid diagnostic test for the detection of gram-negative endotoxin in CSF and thus for making a diagnosis of gram-negative meningitis.

All patients with bacterial meningitis should have neuroimaging performed, either before or after lumbar puncture. Indications for performing neuroimaging prior to lumbar puncture are an altered level of consciousness, papilledema, a focal neurologic deficit, focal or generalized seizure activity, or an immunocompromised state. Magnetic resonance imaging (MRI) is preferred over computed tomography (CT) because of its superiority in demonstrating areas of cerebral edema and ischemia.

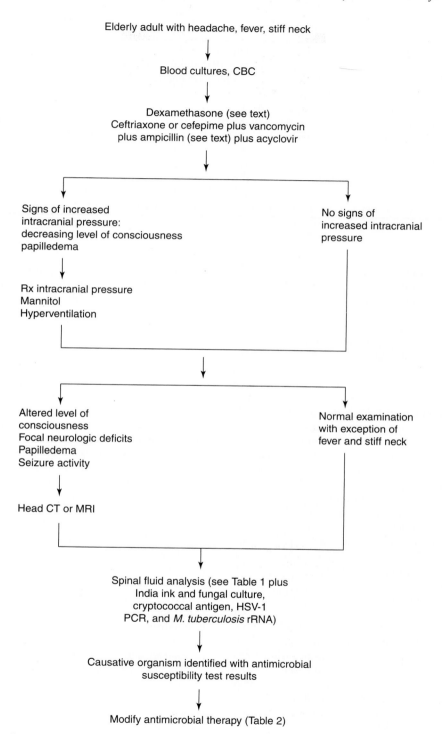

Figure 26-1. Algorithm for management of older adult with headache, fever, and stiff neck.

Treatment

Antimicrobial therapy should be initiated immediately in every older adult with fever, headache, and stiff neck. There is a heightened sense of urgency in initiating antimicrobial therapy when these symptoms are accompanied by an altered level of consciousness. The choice of antimicrobial therapy should be based on the predisposing conditions for bacterial meningitis. There are a

Table 26-1. *Cerebrospinal Fluid (CSF) Analysis in Bacterial Meningitis*

Opening pressure	>180 mm H_2O
White blood cells	>10 to <10,000/mm^3 – neutrophils predominate
Red blood cells	Absent unless traumatic tap
Glucose	<40 mg/dL
CSF:serum glucose ratio	<0.40
Protein	>50 mg/dL
Gram's stain	Positive in 70% to 90% of untreated cases
Culture	Positive in 80% of cases
PCR	Detects bacterial nucleic acid
Latex agglutination	Specific for antigens of *S. pneumoniae, N. meningitidis, E. coli*, Hib and group B *streptococcus*
Limulus amebocyte lysate assay	Positive in gram-negative meningitis

number of predisposing conditions that increase the risk of pneumococcal meningitis in the older adult, the most important of which is pneumococcal pneumonia. Due to the emergence of penicillin- and cephalosporin-resistant *Streptococcus pneumoniae*, empiric therapy of community-acquired bacterial meningitis in the older adult should include a third- or fourth-generation cephalosporin, vancomycin, and acyclovir. Acyclovir is added to the initial empiric regimen because herpes simplex virus encephalitis is the leading disease in the differential diagnosis. Ampicillin should be added to the empiric regimen for coverage of *L. monocytogenes* in older adults. In hospital-acquired meningitis and, particularly, meningitis following neurosurgical procedures, staphylococci and gram-negative organisms, including *P. aeruginosa*, are the most common etiologic organisms. In these patients, empiric therapy should include a combination of vancomycin and ceftazidime, cefepime, or meropenem. If a third-generation cephalosporin is chosen for empiric therapy of meningitis in neurosurgical patients and in neutropenic patients in whom *P. aeruginosa* is a possible meningeal pathogen, ceftazidime should be substituted for ceftriaxone or cefotaxime because ceftazidime is the only third-generation cephalosporin with sufficient activity against *P. aeruginosa* in the CNS. Once the organism has been identified by Gram's stain or by bacterial culture of CSF and the results of antimicrobial susceptibility tests are known, antimicrobial therapy can be modified accordingly (Table 26-2). Some strains of pneumococci are sensitive to penicillin, but in clinical practice, few physicians use penicillin to treat pneumococcal meningitis. A CSF isolate of *S. pneumoniae* is considered to be susceptible to penicillin with a minimal inhibitory concentration (MIC) <0.06 μg/mL, to have intermediate resistance when the MIC is 0.1 to 1.0 μg/mL, and to be highly resistant when the MIC is >1.0 μg/mL. Isolates of *S. pneumoniae* that have

cephalosporin MICs ≤0.5 μg/mL are considered sensitive to the cephalosporins (cefotaxime, ceftriaxone, cefepime). Those with MICs equal to 1 μg/mL are considered to have intermediate resistance, and those with MICs ≥2 μg/mL are considered resistant (11). For meningitis due to pneumococci with cefotaxime or ceftriaxone MICs of 0.5 μg/mL or less, treatment with cefotaxime or ceftriaxone is usually adequate. If the MICs are ≥1 μg/mL, vancomycin is the antibiotic of choice. Patients with *S. pneumoniae* meningitis should have a repeat lumbar puncture performed 24 to 36 hours after the initiation of antimicrobial therapy to document sterilization of the CSF unless findings on the neurologic examination are worrisome for a risk of herniation. Use of intraventricular vancomycin should be considered when intravenous vancomycin fails to sterilize the CSF after 24 to 36 hours of therapy. The intraventricular route of administration is preferred over the intrathecal route because adequate concentrations of vancomycin in the cerebral ventricles are not always achieved with intrathecal administration. Intrathecal administration of vancomycin is safe and is not associated with a risk of seizure activity. Cefepime is a broad-spectrum fourth-generation cephalosporin that is increasingly seen on the medication charts of hospitalized patients. Cefepime has in vitro activity similar to that of cefotaxime or ceftriaxone against *S. pneumoniae* and greater activity against *Enterobacter* species and *P. aeruginosa*. The dose of cefepime is 3 g intravenously every 8 hours in adults. In clinical trials, cefepime has been demonstrated to be equivalent to cefotaxime in the treatment of pneumococcal meningitis, but its efficacy in bacterial meningitis caused by penicillin- and cephalosporin-resistant pneumococcal organisms, *Enterobacter* species, and *P. aeruginosa* has not been established. A 2-week course of intravenous antimicrobial therapy is recommended for pneumococcal meningitis.

Table 26-2. *Antimicrobial Therapy of Bacterial Meningitis*

Organism	Antibiotic	Total Daily Adult Dose (dosing interval)
Streptococcus pneumoniae		
Sensitive to penicillin	Penicillin G	24 million U/day (every 4 hours)
Relatively resistant to penicillin	Ceftriaxone or	4 g/day (every 12 hours)
	cefotaxime or	12 g/day (every 4 hours)
	cefepime	6 g/day (every 8 hours)
Resistant to penicillin	Vancomycin plus	30–45 mg/kg/day (every 8 hours)
	cefepime, ceftriaxone,	
	or cefotaxime	
	± intraventricular	
	vancomycin	20 mg/day
Gram-negative bacilli	Ceftriaxone or	
(except *P. aeruginosa*)	cefotaxime or	
	cefepime	
Pseudomonas aeruginosa	Ceftazidime or	8 g/day (every 8 hours)
	meropenem	6 g/day (every 8 hours)
Staphylococci		
Methicillin-sensitive	Nafcillin	9–12 g/day (every 4 hours)
Methicillin-resistant	Vancomycin	30–45 mg/kg/day (every 8 hours)
Listeria monocytogenes	Ampicillin ±	12 g/day (every 4 hours)
	gentamicin	6 mg/kg/day (every 8 hours)
Haemophilus influenzae	Ceftriaxone or	4 g/day (every 12 hours)
	cefotaxime	12 g/day (every 4 hours)
Streptococcus agalactiae	Ampicillin or	12 g/day (every 4 hours)
	penicillin G	20–24 million U/day (every 4 hours)

All antibiotics are administered intravenously. Doses indicated are for patients with normal renal function.

The third-generation cephalosporins—cefotaxime, ceftriaxone, and ceftazidime—are equally efficacious for the treatment of gram-negative bacillary meningitis, with the exception of meningitis due to *P. aeruginosa*. Ceftazidime or meropenem is recommended for meningitis due to this organism. A 3-week course of intravenous antimicrobial therapy is recommended for meningitis due to gram-negative bacilli. Meningitis due to *S. aureus* or coagulase-negative staphylococci is treated with nafcillin or oxacillin. Vancomycin is the drug of choice for methicillin-resistant staphylococci. The CSF should be monitored during therapy, and if the spinal fluid continues to yield viable organisms after 48 hours of intravenous therapy, then intraventricular vancomycin 20 mg once daily can be added.

A 3- to 4-week course of ampicillin is recommended for *L. monocytogenes* meningitis. Gentamicin should be added to ampicillin in critically ill patients because the combination of ampicillin and gentamicin has greater bactericidal activity than ampicillin alone in experimental models of meningitis (15).

Adjunctive Therapy The neurologic complications of bacterial meningitis (raised ICP, seizure activity, stroke) continue long after the CSF has been sterilized by antimicrobial therapy (20). The pathophysiology of the neurologic complications of bacterial meningitis is shown in Figure 26-2. The release of bacterial cell wall components by the multiplication of bacteria and the lysis of bacteria by bactericidal antibiotics leads to the production of the inflammatory cytokines, interleukin-1 (IL-1) and tumor necrosis factor (TNF), in the subarachnoid space, which initiates a cascade of events that ultimately leads to increased ICP, coma, stroke, seizures, and obstructive and communicating hydrocephalus. Dexamethasone has a beneficial effect by inhibiting the synthesis of IL-1 and TNF at the level of mRNA and by decreasing CSF outflow resistance and stabilizing the blood–brain barrier. IL-1 and TNF are produced by microglia, astrocytes, monocytes, and macrophages. The rationale for giving dexamethasone before antibiotic therapy is that dexamethasone inhibits the production of TNF if administered to macrophages and microglia before they are activated by bacterial cell wall components. A meta-analysis of randomized, concurrently controlled trials of dexamethasone therapy in childhood bacterial meningitis

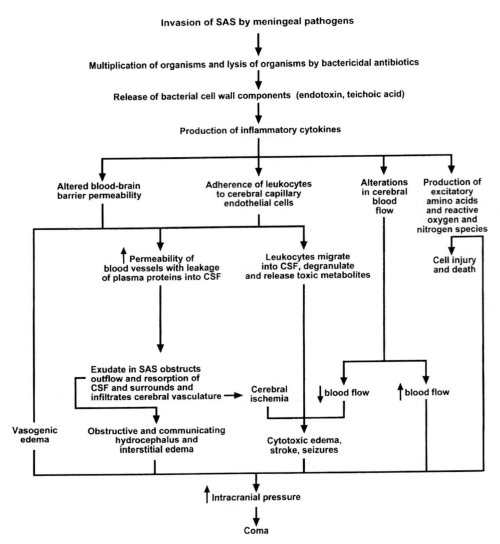

Figure 26-2. The neurologic complications of bacterial meningitis are the result of this inflammatory cascade. (© Roos KL, Tyler KL. Meningitis, encephalitis, brain abscess, and empyema. In: Kasper DL, Braunwald E, Fauci AS, et al., eds. *Harrison's principles of internal medicine.* 16th ed. New York: McGraw Hill; 2005:2471–2490.)

published from 1988 to 1996 confirmed benefit for *H. influenzae* type b meningitis if dexamethasone was begun with or before intravenous antibiotics and suggested benefit for pneumococcal meningitis in children (10). In the European Dexamethasone in Adulthood Bacterial Meningitis Study of 301 adults with bacterial meningitis, 157 patients were randomized to receive dexamethasone and 144 patients were assigned to placebo 15 to 20 minutes before the first dose of an antimicrobial agent. There were 108 cases of pneumococcal meningitis. Within 14 days, five

(9%) of 58 patients with pneumococcal meningitis died in the dexamethasone group and 13 (26%) of 50 patients in the placebo group died (2). In addition to reducing mortality, dexamethasone was associated with a reduction in the number of patients who had an unfavorable outcome. Present recommendations are to initiate dexamethasone therapy (10 mg) before or with the first dose of antibiotics and continue dexamethasone, regardless of the bacteria causing meningitis, in a dose of 10 mg every 6 hours for 4 days (23).

FUNGAL MENINGITIS

Aging is associated with immune dysfunction, especially in cell-mediated immunity (25). This places older adults at risk for fungal meningitis. There are a number of fungi that can cause meningitis, the most common of which are *Cryptococcus neoformans*, *Histoplasma capsulatum*, and *Coccidioides immitis*. *Blastomyces dermatitidis*, *Candida* species, and *Sporothrix schenckii* may also be the causative organisms of meningitis, as may the rare fungi *Paracoccidioides brasiliensis*, *Chaetomium atrobrunneum*, *Cladophialophora bantiana*, *Pseudallescheria boydii*, and *Schizophyllum commune*.

Epidemiology in Older Adults

C. neoformans is an encapsulated yeast that is found worldwide in soil and in bird feces, particularly in pigeon droppings. Infection is acquired by inhaling cryptococcal organisms. Host resistance depends primarily on cell-mediated immunity. The loss of an efficient cell-mediated response by CD4 cells, cytotoxic lymphocytes, natural killer cells, and activated macrophages is the most important risk factor for cryptococcal meningitis. Humoral immunity also has an important role in the prevention of invasive disease by this fungus (6). The use of corticosteroids is a risk factor for cryptococcal meningitis, and many older adults are treated with prednisone for a variety of illnesses. *H. capsulatum* is a common, usually benign and self-limited fungal disease endemic in the midwestern United States and in Central and South America. Disseminated disease and CNS infection occurs primarily in individuals with impaired cell-mediated immunity. CNS infection is usually a subacute or chronic meningitis. Chronic steroid therapy is a risk factor for disseminated histoplasmosis. *C. immitis* is endemic to the southwestern United States, principally California, Arizona, and Texas, and also to Mexico and Central and South America. The fungus lives in the soil. Infection is acquired by inhaling airborne arthroconidia. Sixty percent of people who are infected with *C. immitis* have no symptoms or have an illness indistinguishable from an upper respiratory infection. There may also be signs and symptoms of a lower respiratory infection with fever, sweating, anorexia, weakness, arthralgias, cough, sputum production, and chest pain. The acute infection almost always resolves without specific therapy. If the acute pulmonary infection does not resolve, there may be a progressive pneumonia or chronic lung infection. Symptomatic extrapulmonary disease is more common in immunocompromised individuals, including those who are immunocompromised by aging (19). When *C. immitis* infects the CNS, it is usually in the form of a subacute meningitis.

Clinical Presentation

The majority of patients with fungal meningitis have fever and headache for 2 weeks or longer, a subacute meningitis syndrome. They may also have stiff neck, lethargy, and weight loss. As the disease progresses, patients develop cranial nerve palsies, cognitive difficulty, and eventually signs of increased ICP. Fungal meningitis may be associated with a history of or signs of pulmonary infection, and patients with coccidioidomycosis and cryptococcosis may also have skin lesions.

Diagnosis

The diagnosis of fungal meningitis is made by examination of the CSF (Table 26-3). The characteristic CSF abnormalities are a mononuclear or lymphocytic pleocytosis, an increased protein concentration, and a decreased glucose concentration. *C. immitis* is unique among the common fungal pathogens in that it may have a CSF eosinophilia. It is difficult to grow fungi in culture of CSF with the exception of *C. neoformans*. Since microscopy and culture of CSF are often negative, large volumes (>10 mL) of CSF should be cultured on at least three occasions to increase the yield for isolation of fungi. If fungi fail to grow in cultures obtained from CSF by lumbar puncture, high cervical or cisternal puncture should be performed.

Table 26-3. *Cerebrospinal Fluid (CSF) Analysis in Fungal Meningitis*

White blood cells	Mononuclear or lymphocytic pleocytosis
Glucose	<40 mg/dL
CSF:serum glucose ratio	<0.40
Protein	>50 mg/dL
India ink and fungal culture	Positive in 10% to 30% of cases
Cryptococcus neoformans	Cryptococcal polysaccharide antigen
Histoplasma capsulatum	histoplasma polysaccharide antigen
Coccidioides immitis	Complement fixation antibodies

The cryptococcal polysaccharide antigen test is a highly sensitive and specific test for cryptococcal meningitis. A reactive CSF cryptococcal antigen test establishes the diagnosis of cryptococcal meningitis. The typical neuroimaging abnormalities in cryptococcal meningitis are enhancement of the basilar meninges after the administration of gadolinium and progressive hydrocephalus (Fig. 26-3). The finding of progressive hydrocephalus in an older adult with fever and headache is highly suggestive of either fungal or tuberculous meningitis. The histoplasma polysaccharide antigen can be sent on CSF to make a diagnosis of histoplasma meningitis. Histoplasma polysaccharide antigen is reported to be positive in 40% of patients with histoplasma meningitis, but it may be falsely positive in coccidioidal meningitis (24). Complement fixation antibody titers should be sent on CSF to make a diagnosis of coccidioidal meningitis. The complement fixation antibody test on CSF is reported to have a specificity of 100% and a sensitivity of 75% in the setting of active disease. Measurement of antibodies against a 33-kd antigen from spherules of *C. immitis* in CSF is also a sensitive indicator of coccidioidal meningitis (6).

Treatment

Amphotericin B is the mainstay of therapy of fungal meningitis. The treatment of cryptococcal meningitis is divided into three stages. Therapy is initiated with a combination of amphotericin B 0.7 mg/kg/day plus flucytosine 100 mg/kg/day in four divided doses for 2 weeks. Flucytosine blood levels should be monitored and kept at 50 to 100 µg/mL. In patients with renal dysfunction, the liposomal form of amphotericin B (Ambisome) 5 mg/kg/day or amphotericin B lipid complex (ABLC) 5 mg/kg/day can be substituted for amphotericin B. After 2 weeks of induction therapy, patients who are responding to treatment can be switched to fluconazole 400 to 800 mg/day for 8 weeks. CSF should be recultured at the end of 10 weeks. If CSF fungal cultures are negative, the dose of fluconazole can be decreased to 200 mg/day. Fluconazole therapy is continued for 1 year (6). Meningitis due to *H. capsulatum* is treated with amphotericin B 0.7 to 1.0 mg/kg/day for at least 4 weeks and, often times, for as long as 12 weeks (until CSF fungal cultures are sterile). The addition of intrathecal amphotericin B (0.25 to 1.0 mg/dose every other day or twice weekly) may be required to eradicate the infection. After completing a course of amphotericin B, maintenance therapy with itraconazole 400 mg/day is initiated and continued for at least 6 months to 1 year. During that time, the CSF should be periodically re-examined for fungal smear and culture and histoplasma polysaccharide antigen. Initial therapy of *C. immitis* meningitis is either high-dose fluconazole (1,000 mg daily) as monotherapy or a combination of fluconazole and intrathecal amphotericin B (0.25 to 1.5 mg/dose three times per week) (5). Intrathecal amphotericin B is started at a dose of 0.1 mg/day and slowly increased depending on patient tolerance. The use of intrathecal amphotericin B may be associated with headache, fever, vomiting, and transient alterations in mental status. These symptoms may be lessened by adding 15 mg of hydrocortisone to the intrathecal mixture. Lifelong therapy with fluconazole 400 mg daily is recommended to prevent relapse of *C. immitis* meningitis. Patients who develop hydrocephalus during the course of fungal meningitis need a CSF diversion device. Shunts can be placed

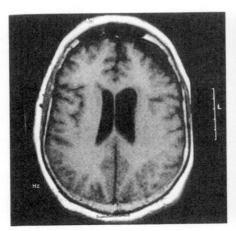 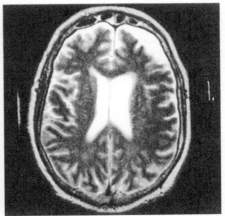

Figure 26-3. A. T1-weighted MRI scan and **B.** T2-weighted MRI scan in patient with cryptococcal meningitis demonstrating hydrocephalus, meningeal enhancement, and a subdural effusion.

Table 26-4. *Antimicrobial Therapy of Fungal Meningitis*

Fungus	Therapy
Cryptococcus neoformans	Induction therapy (for 2 weeks):
	Amphotericin B 0.7 mg/kg/day
	plus
	Flucytosine 100 mg/kg/day (in 4 divided doses)
	followed by
	Fluconazole 400–800 mg/day for 8–10 weeks
	or
	Itraconazole 400 mg/day for 8–10 weeks
	If CSF sterile: fluconazole 200 mg/day for 6 months–1 year
Histoplasma capsulatum	Amphotericin B 0.7–1.0 mg/kg/day for 4 weeks
	followed by
	Itraconazole 400 mg/day
Coccidioides immitis	Fluconazole 400–1,000 mg/day ± intrathecal amphotericin B
	(0.25–1.5 mg/dose)
	Fluconazole 400 mg/day for life
Treatment failure	Ambisome 4 mg/kg/day or amphotericin B lipid complex
	5 mg/kg/day
	or
	Intraventricular amphotericin B

in patients receiving antifungal therapy. Shunting procedures are a safe and effective therapy for hydrocephalus. Shunt placement in patients with acute infection will not disseminate cryptococcal infection into the peritoneum or bloodstream; in addition, shunting does not provide a nidus from which cryptococcal organisms are difficult to eradicate (13). A ventriculostomy can be used until CSF fungal cultures are sterile, and then the ventriculostomy is replaced by a ventriculoperitoneal shunt. The treatment of fungal meningitis is summarized in Table 26-4.

TUBERCULOUS MENINGITIS

Tuberculous meningitis is the result of endogenous reactivation of infection in caseous tuberculous foci adjacent to the subarachnoid space that developed during hematogenous spread of tubercle bacilli in the course of an earlier primary infection, usually pulmonary tuberculosis. Meningitis is the result of the discharge of bacilli and tuberculous antigens into the subarachnoid space.

Epidemiology in Older Adults

As stated above, tuberculous meningitis is the result of reactivation of infection in tuberculous foci that seeded the CNS during the course of an earlier primary infection. The majority of adults become infected with *Mycobacterium tuberculosis* when they inhale aerosolized droplet nuclei containing tubercle

bacilli. Not all infected persons have the same risk of developing pulmonary disease. An immunocompetent adult with untreated *M. tuberculosis* has a 5% to 10% lifetime risk of disease. The risk is greatest in the first 2 to 3 years after infection. Approximately 10% of immunocompetent persons with tuberculosis develop CNS disease (22). Risk factors for tuberculous meningitis include age, malnutrition, alcoholism, diabetes mellitus, chronic corticosteroid therapy, and HIV infection.

Clinical Presentation

In the older adult, in developed countries, tuberculous meningitis typically presents as a subacute or chronic meningitis characterized by fever, headache, night sweats, and malaise. As the disease progresses, the clinical course is complicated by seizure activity, stroke, progressive hydrocephalus, raised ICP, and eventually coma. The possibility of tuberculous meningitis should be *strongly considered* in the older adult with unrelenting headache, night sweats, a CSF lymphocytic pleocytosis with a mildly decreased glucose concentration (25 to 40 mg/dL), and progressive hydrocephalus by neuroimaging.

Diagnosis

The diagnosis of tuberculous meningitis is made by examination of the CSF. The characteristic CSF abnormalities are an elevated opening pressure, a lymphocytic pleocytosis (10 to 500 cells/mm³), a mildly decreased glucose concentration (25 to 40 mg/dL), and an elevated protein concentration. Spinal fluid should be examined by acid-fast stains and cultures and molecular diagnostic techniques for *M. tuberculosis* nucleic acid. The last tube of fluid collected at lumbar puncture is the best tube to send for acid-fast bacilli (AFB) smear. A pellicle may form in the CSF in tuberculous meningitis, or a cobweb-like clot may form on the surface of the fluid. Tubercle bacilli are best demonstrated in a smear of the clot or sediment. Positive smears are reported in 10% to 40% of cases. The growth of the organism is very slow, so cultures take weeks to be positive. Cultures are reported to be positive in 25% to 75% of cases of tuberculous meningitis, requiring 3 to 6 weeks for growth to be detectable (7,21). The transcription mediated amplification test that is Food and Drug Administration–approved for the detection of *M. tuberculosis* rRNA in sputum is now available on CSF (1).

In the absence of demonstrating the organism in smear or culture of CSF, the diagnosis of tuberculous meningitis is supported by finding a site of extrameningeal tuberculous infection. A chest radiograph should be obtained as part of the diagnostic evaluation of tuberculous meningitis. Radiographic evidence of pulmonary tuberculosis, specifically hilar adenopathy or an upper lobe infiltrate, is found in <50% of cases of tuberculous meningitis in adults. The Mantoux intradermal tuberculin skin test is helpful when positive. The test is interpreted 48 hours after placement and is considered positive if the amount of induration is >5 mm. The test may, however, be falsely negative even in the absence of immunosuppression and in association with a positive reaction to the common antigens used to determine anergy.

The most common neuroimaging abnormalities in tuberculous meningitis are hydrocephalus and leptomeningeal enhancement after contrast administration. In addition, there may be evidence of medium- or small-vessel infarction (Fig. 26-4), and tuberculomas may develop during therapy.

Treatment

Treatment of tuberculous meningitis in adults is initiated with a combination of isoniazid (300 mg/day), rifampin (10 mg/kg/day, up to 600 mg/day), and pyrazinamide (25 to 35 mg/kg/day) for 2 months, followed by isoniazid and rifampin for an additional 7 to 10 months of therapy. Pyridoxine in a dose of 50 mg daily is added to this regimen to avoid peripheral neuropathy due to isoniazid-induced pyridoxine deficiency. Monthly liver function studies should be obtained in adults receiving isoniazid and rifampin.

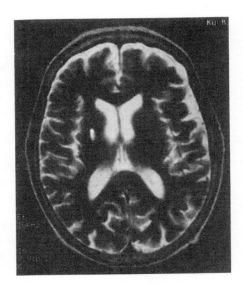

Figure 26-4. Cranial MRI scan in patient with tuberculous meningitis demonstrating right posterior limb internal capsule infarction.

The risk of hepatotoxicity from isoniazid is approximately 1%. This risk doubles with the addition of rifampin (7). In patients with a high probability of a drug-resistant strain of *M. tuberculosis*, therapy is initiated with a combination of isoniazid, rifampin, pyrazinamide, and either streptomycin (1 g daily by intramuscular injection) or ethambutol (15 to 25 mg/kg/day) for 2 months. This is followed by isoniazid and rifampin to complete a 9- to 18-month course of therapy. Patients at risk for drug-resistant strains of tuberculosis are those who have had inadequate treatment for pulmonary tuberculosis due to an irregular drug supply, inappropriate regimens, or poor compliance (12). The chief toxicity of ethambutol is optic neuritis, which occurs in as many as 3% of patients receiving 25 mg/kg/day but is very rare at a dose of 15 mg/kg/day (7). If ethambutol is required for long-term therapy because the organism is resistant to isoniazid, ethambutol is given in a dose of 25 mg/kg/day for 1 to 2 months and 15 mg/kg/day thereafter. Table 26-5 summarizes the antimicrobial therapy of tuberculous meningitis, including the adverse effect of antituberculous agents and the management of these complications.

The Infectious Disease Society of America recommends the use of corticosteroid therapy in patients with tuberculous meningitis (9). Corticosteroid therapy improves outcome of tuberculous meningitis (3). Dexamethasone 8 to 12 mg/day or the equivalent of prednisone is recommended, and corticosteroid therapy is tapered over 6 to 8 weeks (3).

Table 26-5. *Antimicrobial Therapy of Tuberculous Meningitis*

Antituberculous Agent	Adult Dose	Adverse Effect	Recommended Action
Isoniazid	300 mg/day single oral dose	Hepatotoxicity	Monthly LFT
		Peripheral neuropathy	Pyridoxine
Rifampin	10 mg/kg/day maximal daily dose—600 mg	Hepatotoxicity	Monthly LFT
		Turns urine orange brownish color	Warn patient this will happen
Pyrazinamide	25–35 mg/kg/day	Hepatotoxicity	Monthly LFT
		Hyperuricemia	Monitor uric acid
Streptomycin	1 g/day intramuscularly	Nephrotoxicity	Monthly creatinine; will need to decrease dose in renal insufficiency
		Vestibulotoxicity	Reassure patient this will improve after therapy
Ethambutol	15–20 mg/kg/day	Optic neuritis	Monthly eye examination

LFT liver function tests.

BRAIN ABSCESS

A brain abscess is a focal, suppurative process within the brain parenchyma.

EPIDEMIOLOGY IN OLDER ADULTS

A brain abscess in the older adult may be due to either bacteria or opportunistic pathogens such as *Toxoplasma gondii*, *Aspergillus* species, *Nocardia asteroides*, or mycobacterial or fungal species previously reviewed in this chapter. A brain abscess may also be due to *Taenia solium* (neurocysticercosis).

A bacterial brain abscess may develop from direct spread from a contiguous site of infection such as the paranasal sinuses, otitis media, mastoiditis, or dental infections. A brain abscess may follow head trauma or be a complication of a neurosurgical procedure. A brain abscess may be a complication of infective endocarditis or the hematogenous spread of bacteria from a pyogenic lung infection, the urinary tract, or an intra-abdominal infection. Table 26-6 lists the most likely etiologic organisms of a brain abscess based on predisposing or associated conditions.

CLINICAL PRESENTATION

The most common symptom of a brain abscess is a headache. The headache is often characterized as a constant, dull, aching sensation that is either hemicranial or generalized and refractory to analgesic therapy. Fever is present in only 50% of patients at the time of diagnosis, and the absence of fever should not exclude the diagnosis. New-onset focal or generalized seizure activity is a common presenting sign, as is a focal neurologic deficit. The latter predicts the location of the brain abscess. Hemiparesis is the most common localizing sign of a frontal lobe abscess. A temporal lobe abscess may present with a disturbance of language or an upper homonymous quadrantanopsia. A cerebellar abscess presents with nystagmus, difficulty with coordination, and ataxia. As the brain abscess evolves and is surrounded by edema, signs of increased ICP, including papilledema, nausea and vomiting, and drowsiness, develop. Meningismus is not present unless the abscess has ruptured into the ventricle or the infection has spread to the subarachnoid space.

DIAGNOSIS

The diagnosis of a brain abscess is made by CT or MRI. CT has the advantage of being easy to do in acutely ill patients, but MRI is better able to demonstrate the abscess in the early (cerebritis) stage and is superior to CT for identifying cerebellar abscesses. Neuroimaging studies should be obtained without and then with contrast. A brain abscess is hyperintense on diffusion-weighted MRI with low apparent diffusion coefficient values (16). The initial workup should also include a search for the primary site of infection. Sinusitis is well visualized on MRI. Blood cultures, an echocardiogram, a urinalysis and urine culture, and chest radiograph should be obtained. Approximately 90% of patients with a *Nocardia* brain abscess have pulmonary involvement (8). Serology should be sent to detect antibodies to *T. gondii*. The majority of patients with *Aspergillus* brain abscess have evidence of pulmonary disease on chest radiography.

The microbiologic diagnosis of a brain abscess is made by stain and culture of abscess material obtained by stereotactic needle aspiration.

TREATMENT

Antimicrobial therapy of a brain abscess is initially based on the source of infection and then modified when the results of stain and culture of abscess material are known

Table 26-6. *Etiologic Organisms of a Brain Abscess*

Predisposing Condition	Etiologic Organism
Paranasal sinusitis	Microaerophilic and anaerobic streptococci *Haemophilus* sp. *Bacteroides* sp. (non-*fragilis*) *Fusobacterium* sp.
Otitis media and mastoiditis	*Bacteroides* sp. (including *B. fragilis*) Streptococci *Pseudomonas aeruginosa* Enterobacteriaceae
Dental infections	Streptococci *Bacteroides fragilis*
Endocarditis	Viridans streptococci *S. aureus*
Pyogenic lung infection	*Streptococcus* sp. *Actinomyces* sp. *Fusobacterium* sp.
Urinary sepsis	Enterobacteriaceae Pseudomonaceae
Intra-abdominal source	*Streptococcus* sp. Enterobacteriaceae Anaerobes
Neurosurgical procedure	Staphylococci Enterobacteriaceae Pseudomonaceae
Immunocompromised	*Aspergillus* sp. (multiple abscesses) *Nocardia asteroides* (single abscess) *Toxoplasma gondii* (multiple abscesses) Mycobacteria *Cryptococcus neoformans* *Histoplasma capsulatum*

Adapted with permission from Calfee DP, Wispelwey B. Brain abscess. *Semin Neurol.* 200;20:353–360.

Table 26-7. *Antimicrobial Therapy of Brain Abscess*

Organism	Total Daily Adult Dose (dosing interval)
Streptococcus sp.	Penicillin G 20–24 million U/day (every 4 hours) or Cefotaxime 12 g/day (every 4 hours)
Bacteroides sp.	Metronidazole 2,000 mg/day (every 6 hours)
Fusobacterium sp.	Metronidazole 2,000 mg/day (every 6 hours)
Haemophilus sp.	Ceftriaxone 4 g/day (every 12 hours)
Pseudomonas aeruginosa	Ceftazidime 6 g/day (every 8 hours) or Meropenem 6 g/day (every 8 hours)
Staphylococci	
Methicillin-sensitive	Nafcillin 9–12 g/day (every 4 hours)
Methicillin-resistant	Vancomycin 30–45 mg/kg/day (every 8 hours)
Aspergillus sp.	Liposomal amphotericin B 5 mg/kg/day
Nocardia asteroides	Trimethoprim 15–20 mg/kg/day – Sulfamethoxazole 75–100 mg/kg/day
Toxoplasma gondii	Trimethoprim 15–20 mg/kg/day – Sulfamethoxazole 75–100 mg/kg/day

as well as antimicrobial susceptibility tests (Table 26-7). Prophylactic anticonvulsant therapy is recommended for at least 3 months after resolution of the abscess. The decision to discontinue anticonvulsant therapy is based on findings on electroencephalogram (EEG). If the EEG is abnormal, anticonvulsant therapy should be continued. If the EEG is normal, anticonvulsant therapy can be slowly withdrawn.

Steroids are not given routinely to patients with a brain abscess. Intravenous dexamethasone therapy (10 mg every 6 hours) is reserved for patients with mass effect due to brain abscess edema and increased cranial pressure. Serial CT or MRI scans should be obtained on a monthly or bimonthly basis to document resolution of the abscess (17).

INFECTIOUS ETIOLOGIES OF STROKE

Table 26-8 provides the recommended studies to be sent on CSF to rule out an infectious etiology of a stroke in the older adult. Bacterial and fungal etiologies of stroke are discussed under their own subsections in this chapter. Acute infection, such as bronchitis, may cause stroke by promoting a proinflammatory state resulting in thrombosis (4). Syphilitic meningovasculitis may be the etiology of a stroke in an older adult. The classic CSF abnormalities in syphilitic meningovasculitis are a lymphocytic pleocytosis, an elevated protein concentration, and a reactive CSF venereal disease research laboratory (VDRL) test. A reactive CSF VDRL confirms the diagnosis of neurosyphilis, except when the CSF is blood tinged. Blood in the CSF may give a false-positive CSF VDRL. A nonreactive CSF fluorescent treponemal antibody absorption test (FTA-ABS) or microhemagglutination–*Treponema pallidum* test (MHA-TP) excludes the diagnosis; however, a reactive CSF FTA-ABS or a reactive MHA-TP does not establish the diagnosis.

INFECTIOUS ETIOLOGIES OF DEMENTIA

Table 26-9 lists the CSF studies for infectious etiologies of dementia. In every patient with signs of dementia, there is hope that a reversible etiology can be detected and treated. In reality, however, there are few infectious etiologies of dementia. Patients with viral, fungal, or tuberculous meningitis may be confused, but a clinician would not mistake their confusion for dementia. Sporadic Creutzfeldt-Jakob disease and familial forms of prion diseases, such as Gerstmann-Straussler-Scheinker disease and fatal familial insomnia, are included in the differential diagnosis of dementia. Prions are infectious proteins that reproduce by stimulating the conversion of a normal protein (PrP^c) to a disease-causing isoform (PrP^s) (14). The sporadic form of Creutzfeldt-Jakob disease accounts for approximately 85% of all cases of prion diseases in humans (14). The cardinal manifestations of sporadic Creutzfeldt-Jakob disease are dementia, myoclonus, and ataxia. Diffusion-weighted MRI and fluid-attenuated inversion recovery (FLAIR) MRI show increased signal in the cortical ribbon and basal ganglia. Dementia and ataxia often precede the appearance of myoclonus, but once myoclonus is present, the classic EEG pattern of bisynchronous periodic sharp and slow-wave complexes is seen as well. The detection of the 14.3.3 protein in CSF has been suggested as a marker for prion disease; however, 14.3.3 has been detected in the CSF of patients with herpes simplex virus encephalitis, hypoxic encephalopathy, acute stroke, paraneoplastic disorders, and other conditions that induce acute neuronal damage (18). Gerstmann-Straussler-Scheinker disease presents initially with ataxia, and dementia develops later. Fatal familial insomnia presents with insomnia followed by dysautonomia. Dementia develops late in the course. A definitive diagnosis can only be made by brain biopsy. Currently, there is no specific treatment for prion diseases.

Table 26-8. *Cerebrospinal Fluid Studies for Infectious Etiologies of Stroke in the Older Adult*

1. Cell count
2. Glucose concentration
3. Gram stain, bacterial culture, and PCR
4. Latex agglutination
5. *Limulus* amebocyte lysate assay
6. VDRL
7. India ink and fungal culture
8. Acid-fast bacilli, *M. tuberculosis* culture, and *M. tuberculosis* rRNA

Table 26-9. *Cerebrospinal Fluid Studies for Infectious Etiologies of Dementia*

1. Cell count
2. Glucose concentration
3. Fungal smear and culture
4. Acid-fast smear, *M. tuberculosis* culture, and *M. tuberculosis* rRNA
5. Cryptococcal polysaccharide antigen
6. *Histoplasma* polysaccharide antigen
7. *Coccidioides immitis* complement fixation antibodies
8. 14.3.3 protein
9. VDRL

CONCLUSION

Every older adult with unrelenting headache should have CT or MRI scan followed by examination of the CSF. There are a number of tables in this chapter to guide the clinician in diagnostic studies on CSF. Similarly, every febrile older adult with a stroke should have CSF analysis to rule out an infectious etiology. Bacterial, fungal, and tuberculous meningitis are all treatable with antimicrobial agents, but delays in treatment lead to complications, including seizures, stroke, and hydrocephalus, that may not be reversible. Patients with fungal and tuberculous meningitis who develop hydrocephalus should have shunting procedures because untreated hydrocephalus is a major contributor to mortality in these diseases. The most important way to prevent pneumococcal meningitis in the older adult is by vaccination, and neurologists should routinely remind their patients to be certain they are revaccinated every 5 years.

REFERENCES

1. Centers for Disease Control and Prevention. Update: nucleic acid amplification tests for tuberculosis. *MMWR*. 2000;49:593–595.
2. de Gans J, van de Beek D. Dexamethasone in adults with bacterial meningitis. *N Engl J Med*. 2002;347:1549–1556.
3. Dooley DP, Carpenter JL, Rademacher S. Adjunctive corticosteroid therapy for tuberculosis: a critical reappraisal of the literature. *Clin Infect Dis*. 1997;25:872–887.
4. Elkind MSV, Cole JW. Do common infections cause stroke? *Semin Neurol*. 2006;26:88–99.
5. Galgiani JN, Ampel NM, Blair JE, et al. Treatment guidelines for coccidioidomycosis. *Clin Infect Dis*. 2005;41:1217–1223.
6. Gottfredsson M, Perfect JR. Fungal meningitis. *Semin Neurol*. 2000;20:307–322.
7. Leonard JM, Des Prez RM. Tuberculous meningitis. *Infect Dis Clin North Am*. 1990;4: 769–787.
8. Maccario M, Tortorano AM, Ponticelli C. Subcutaneous nodules and pneumonia in a kidney transplant recipient. *Nephrol Dial Transplant*. 1998;13:796–798.
9. McGowan JE, Chesney PJ, Crossley KB, et al. Guidelines for the use of systemic glucocorticosteroids in the management of selected infections. *J Infect Dis*. 1992;165:1–13.
10. McIntyre PB, Berkey CS, King SM, et al. Dexamethasone as adjunctive therapy in bacterial meningitis. *JAMA*. 1997;278:925–931.
11. National Committee for Clinical Laboratory Standards. *Performance Standards for Antimicrobial Susceptibility Testing*. Villanova, PA: National Committee for Laboratory Standards; 1994.
12. Pablos-Mendez A, Raviglione MC, Laszlo A, et al. Global surveillance for antituberculosis-drug resistance 1994–1997. *N Engl J Med*. 1998; 338:1641–1649.
13. Park MK, Hospenthal DR, Bennett JE. Treatment of hydrocephalus secondary to cryptococcal meningitis by use of shunting. *Clin Infect Dis*. 1999;28:629–633.
14. Prusiner SB. Shattuck lecture—neurodegenerative diseases and prions. *N Engl J Med*. 2001;344: 1516–1526.
15. Quagliarello VJ, Scheld WM. Treatment of bacterial meningitis. *N Engl J Med*. 1997;336: 708–716.
16. Reddy JS, Mishra AM, Behari S, et al. The role of diffusion-weighted imaging in the differential diagnosis of intracranial cystic mass lesions: a report of 147 lesions. *Surg Neurol*. 2006; 66:246.
17. Roos KL, Tyler KL. Meningitis, encephalitis, brain abscess, and empyema. In: Kasper DL, Braunwald E, Fauci AS, et al., eds. *Harrison's principles of internal medicine*. 16th ed. New York: McGraw Hill; 2005:2471–2490.
18. Sanchez-Juan P, Green A, Ladoganna A, et al. CSF tests in the differential diagnosis of Creutzfeldt-Jakob disease. *Neurology*. 2006;67: 637–643.
19. Stevens DA. Coccidioidomycosis. *N Engl J Med*. 1995;332:1077–1081.
20. Tauber MG, Moser B. Cytokines and chemokines in meningeal inflammation: biology and clinical implications. *Clin Infect Dis*. 1999; 28:1–12.
21. Traub M, Colchester ACF, Kingsley DPE, et al. Tuberculosis of the central nervous system. *Q J Med*. 1984;53:81–100.
22. Udani PM, Parekh UC, Dastur DK. Neurological and related syndromes in CNS tuberculosis: clinical features and pathogenesis. *J Neurol Sci*. 1971;14:341–357.
23. van de Beek D, de Gans J, Tunkel AR, et al. Community acquired bacterial meningitis in adults. *N Engl J Med*. 2006;354:44–53.
24. Wheat LJ, Kohler RB, Tewari RP, et al. Significance of *Histoplasma* antigen in the cerebrospinal fluid of patients with meningitis. *Arch Intern Med*. 1989;149:302–304.
25. Yoshikawa TT. Epidemiology and unique aspects of aging and infectious diseases. *Clin Infect Dis*. 2000;30:931–933.

SUGGESTED READINGS

Garcia-Monco JC. Central nervous system tuberculosis. *Neurol Clin.* 1999;17:737–759.

Gottfredsson M, Perfect JR. Fungal meningitis. *Semin Neurol.* 2000;20:307–322.

Johnson E, Mastrianni JA. Prion encephalopathies. In: Roos KL, ed. *Principles of neurologic infectious diseases.* New York: McGraw-Hill; 2005:307–326.

Roos KL. *Meningitis: 100 Maxims in Neurology.* New York: Arnold, London and Oxford University Press; 1996:1–208.

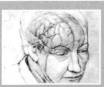

CHAPTER 27

Viral Illnesses in the Nervous System of the Elderly

Maria A. Nagel and John R. Corboy

In humans, morbidity and mortality caused by cancer, infection, and possibly autoimmunity increase with age. Viral infections of the nervous system contribute to this morbidity and mortality in both the community and in long-term care facilities. In 2004, persons 65 years and older comprised 36.3 million, or 12.4%, of the U.S. population. With the U.S. population 65 years and older continuing to rise to a projected 40 million in 2010 and 71.5 million in 2030 (www.aoa .gov/PROF/Statistics/profile/2005/4.asp), it is important to recognize the clinical features, diagnosis, treatment, complications, and sequelae of viral infections of the nervous system in this vulnerable patient population.

Viral diseases have several unique features in the elderly. First, infections can be more frequent and severe in this population. For West Nile virus infection, older age seems to be a main risk factor for severe meningoencephalitis and death; individuals older than 50 years have a 10-fold higher risk of developing neurologic symptoms, and the risk is 43 times higher in individuals older than 80 years (53). Second, different viral illnesses are more common in older individuals than in younger individuals, such as reactivation of varicella-zoster virus (VZV) to cause herpes zoster (shingles). Third, clinical presentation can differ, with the elderly patient presenting with atypical or fewer symptoms. Fourth, diagnostic procedures may have different yields, such as difficulty with lumbar puncture with degenerative spine disease. Fifth, treatment needs to take into account the higher incidence of adverse drug effects in this population and other comorbidities, such as renal failure. And finally, long-term sequelae of viral illnesses need to be recognized, such as the occurrence of post-polio syndrome (PPS) years after recovery from an initial acute attack of the poliomyelitis virus.

The increased susceptibility to infection in the elderly population is most likely multifactorial. Dysregulation of the immune system with ageing, or immunosenescence, is believed to be an important contributor to morbidity and mortality in the elderly. The mechanisms that underlie these age-related defects are broad and range from defects in the hematopoietic bone marrow to defects in peripheral lymphocyte migration, maturation, and function (28).

However, dysregulated T-cell function is believed to play a critical role because these cells are vital in mediating both cellular and humoral immunity. A number of factors have been associated with the decline of T-cell function with age including hematopoietic stem-cell defects; however, chronic involution of the thymus gland with resultant decreased output of naïve T cells is believed to be one of the major contributing factors to loss of immune function with age (29). Aside from immunosenescence, epidemiologic factors, such as exposures to infection in long-term health care facilities; malnutrition, which may result in decreased immune function (12); and comorbid conditions, such as diabetes and stroke, may also contribute to increased susceptibility to infections in the elderly.

Following is a discussion of the most common viral illnesses affecting the nervous system in the elderly including herpes zoster and postherpetic neuralgia (PHN) caused by VZV and PPS seen years after poliomyelitis virus infection.

VARICELLA-ZOSTER VIRUS AND NEUROLOGIC DISEASE

VZV is an exclusively human, double-stranded DNA alphaherpesvirus. Primary infection causes chickenpox (varicella), after which the virus becomes latent in cranial nerve ganglia, dorsal root ganglia, and autonomic ganglia along the entire neuraxis. Virus reactivation typically occurs in elderly, associated with an age-related decline in cell-mediated immunity, and in immunocompromised individuals. Multiple neurologic complications are seen with VZV reactivation. The most common are herpes zoster (shingles), which is characterized by pain and rash in one to three dermatomes, and PHN, which is pain that persists for >3 months and sometimes years after resolution of rash. Less frequently, VZV reactivation can cause vasculopathy, myelitis, progressive outer retinal necrosis, and zoster sine herpete (dermatomal pain without rash) (25).

HERPES ZOSTER

Herpes zoster affects some 600,000 to 900,000 mostly elderly or immunocompromised people in the United States each year (16,64). Its annual incidence is approximately 5 to 6.5 per 1,000 at age 60, increasing to 8 to 11 per 1,000 at age 70 (16).

Herpes zoster usually begins with a prodromal phase characterized by pain, itching, paresthesias (numbness/tingling), dysesthesias (unpleasant sensations), and/or sensitivity to touch (allodynia) in one to three dermatomes. A few days later, a unilateral maculopapular rash appears on the affected area, which then evolves into vesicles. These vesicles usually scab over in 10 days, after which the lesions are not contagious. Multiple dermatomes or a generalized infection are more likely to be involved in immunosuppressed patients, such as patients with a hematologic malignancy or iatrogenic immunosuppression. Rarely, the prodrome is not followed by typical zoster lesions (zoster sine herpete), making diagnosis difficult. In most patients, the disappearance of the skin lesions are accompanied by decreased pain, with complete resolution of pain within 4 to 6 weeks.

Herpes zoster can affect any level of the neuraxis, including cranial nerves, but is most frequently seen in thoracic dermatomes followed by lesions on the face, typically in the ophthalmic distribution of the trigeminal nerve [herpes zoster ophthalmicus (HZO)]. HZO is often accompanied by zoster keratitis, resulting in blindness if unrecognized and not treated. Thus, if visual symptoms are present in patients with ophthalmic distribution zoster, a slit-lamp examination by an ophthalmologist is imperative, especially if skin lesions extend to the medial side of the nose (Hutchinson sign). Herpes zoster can also affect the cranial nerve VII (geniculate) ganglion, causing weakness or paralysis of ipsilateral facial muscles with skin lesions in the external auditory canal/tympanic membrane (zoster oticus) and/or anterior two thirds of the tongue or hard palate. This peripheral facial weakness and zoster oticus constitutes the Ramsay Hunt syndrome [reviewed by Sweeney and Gilden (57)]. Additional cranial nerves may be involved, leading to tinnitus, hearing loss, nausea, vomiting, vertigo, and nystagmus. Less common presentations of herpes zoster include optic neuritis/neuropathy from optic nerve involvement (10,38); ophthalmoplegia from cranial nerves III, VI, and IV involvement (5,10,34,55); and osteonecrosis and spontaneous tooth exfoliation from involvement of the maxillary and mandibular distribution of the trigeminal nerve (22,37,63). Lower motor neuron–type weakness in the arm or leg may also follow cervical or lumbar distribution zoster, respectively [reviewed by Merchet and Gruener (40) and Yoleri et al. (68)]. Diaphragmatic weakness following cervical zoster (4) and abdominal muscle weakness, leading to abdominal herniation, following thoracic zoster (59) have also been reported.

Diagnosis of herpes zoster is straightforward based on the clinical presentation, characteristic rash, and pain/altered sensation. However, there are cases in which rash does not follow the prodrome (zoster sine herpete), making the diagnosis more challenging. Patients may only present with dermatomal distribution pain that does not cross the midline or unilateral facial or limb weakness. In these cases, a fourfold rise in serum antibody to VZV or the presence of VZV DNA in auricular skin, blood mononuclear cells, middle ear fluid, or saliva (20) may assist with diagnosis. Cerebrospinal fluid (CSF) can also be examined for the presence of VZV DNA and anti-VZV immunoglobulin (Ig) G antibody.

Treatment of herpes zoster is based on the patient's immune status and age; however, no universally accepted protocol exists. In immunocompetent individuals under age 50 years, analgesics (nonsteroidal anti-inflammatory agents, opioids) and topical treatments (calamine lotion, petroleum jelly, local anesthetic creams, occlusive bandages) are used to relieve pain (Fig. 27-1). Oral antivirals (acyclovir 800 mg five times a day for 10 days; famciclovir 500 mg orally three times daily; or valacyclovir 1,000 mg three times daily for 7 days) are not required but will speed the healing of rash and resolution of pain. These antivirals are generally well tolerated. Side effects include nausea, headache, diarrhea, and vomiting. It has also been reported that treatment of herpes zoster with 800 mg/day of oral acyclovir within 72 hours of rash onset may reduce the incidence of residual pain at 6 months by 46% in immunocompetent adults (32). Thus, in immunocompetent individuals over the age of 50, treatment with both analgesics and antivirals are recommended and are essential in patients with ophthalmic distribution zoster. Similarly, treatment of patients with the Ramsay Hunt syndrome within 7 days of onset appears to improve recovery (21,42). In addition to antivirals, prednisone (60 mg orally for 3 to 5 days) has also been used to reduce the inflammatory response, although double-blind, placebo-controlled studies to confirm additional efficacy are lacking. In immunocompromised patients, intravenous acyclovir, 10 mg/kg every 8 hours for 7 to 14 days, is recommended.

POSTHERPETIC NEURALGIA

The most common complication of herpes zoster is PHN, which is characterized by constant, severe, stabbing or burning, dysesthetic pain that persists for >3 months and sometimes years after resolution of the zoster skin lesions. As many as 1 million individuals are affected in the United States (8). The occurrence of PHN is closely associated with age. It is rare in patients younger than 50 years of age but is seen in up to 40% of patients with zoster who are older than 60 years (50). Other risk factors for PHN include severe pain during zoster and a prodrome of severe

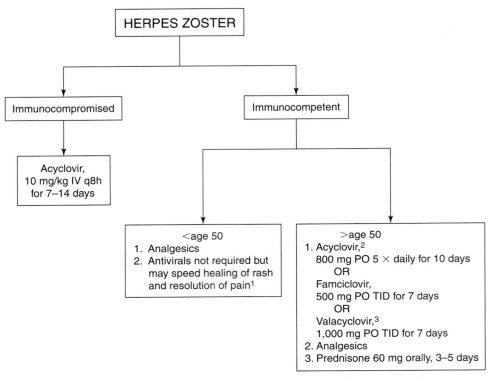

Figure 27-1. Treatment algorithm for herpes zoster.

[1]At any age, ophthalmic distribution zoster should be treated with oral antiviral agents with early referral to ophthalmology.
[2]Antivirals should be started within 3 days of rash.
[3]Valacyclovir is preferred due to higher bioavailability of active drug.

dermatomal pain prior to rash. Symptoms tend to improve over time, with less than 5% of patients still having pain at 1 year. However, during this period, pain can be quite debilitating, and the patient's quality of life can be severely affected, leading to depression. The cause of PHN is unknown, but two non–mutually exclusive theories have been proposed—that the excitability of ganglionic or spinal cord neurons is altered after zoster and that low-grade virus infection persists in ganglia despite resolution of the skin lesions (36,62).

Treatment of PHN is aimed at symptomatic pain relief with use of analgesics, including opiates and neuroleptic drugs, but no universal treatment exists. For topical treatment, lidocaine is administered as 5% patches, with up to three patches applied to the affected area at one time, for up to 12 hours within a 24-hour period (Fig. 27-2). As an alternative, capsaicin 0.075% can also be applied topically three to four times a day, but local skin irritation can limit its use. For systemic treatment of chronic pain, nonsteroidal anti-inflammatory drugs can be used in conjunction with neuroleptics and

other agents if pain is refractory. Gabapentin is widely used, with a starting dose of 300 mg daily and gradually titrating up as needed to a maximum of 3,600 mg/day (divided into three doses daily) (49,51). Pregabalin is given at 75 to 150 mg orally twice daily or 50 to 100 mg orally three times a day (150 to 300 mg/day). If minimal relief is obtained at 300 mg daily for 2 weeks, the dose can be increased to a maximum of 600 mg/day in two or three divided doses. Tricyclic antidepressants, including amitriptyline (10 to 25 mg orally at bedtime with a maximum dose of 150 to 200 mg/day), nortriptyline, and desipramine, lessen the pain of PHN. Newer anticonvulsants, such as topiramate, levetiracetam, lamotrigine, and oxcarbazepine are also being used. Oxycodone (controlled release, 10 to 40 mg orally every 12 hours) or controlled-release morphine sulfate can also be used (17). Levorphanol produces morphinelike analgesia at a dose of 2 mg orally every 6 to 8 hours as needed, with maximum doses of 6 to 12 mg daily (52). Combination treatment with morphine and gabapentin also decreases pain better than either drug alone or placebo (26).

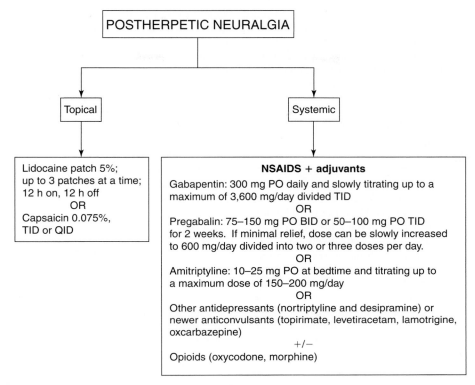

Figure 27-2. Treatment algorithm for postherpetic neuralgia.

Because chronic pain may reflect a low-grade viral ganglionitis, antiviral therapy has been used. Some studies indicate that oral acyclovir, famciclovir, or valacyclovir reduces the duration and severity of pain after zoster (7,31,61). In a recent prospective, open-label, phase I/II clinical trial in which 15 patients with moderate to severe PHN were treated with intravenous acyclovir for 2 weeks, followed by oral valacyclovir for 1 month, eight (53%) of 15 patients reported improvement of pain (46).

OTHER COMPLICATIONS OF VARICELLA-ZOSTER VIRUS REACTIVATION

Less frequently, reactivation of VZV can cause a vasculopathy. The most common presentation of VZV vasculopathy in the elderly is trigeminal distribution zoster followed days to weeks later by contralateral hemiplegia. Other patients present with combinations of headache, fever, mental status changes, and focal deficits from transient ischemic attacks, ischemic or hemorrhagic strokes, or aneurysms. However, the typical zoster rash and a CSF pleocytosis may not be present, and evaluating the CSF for both VZV DNA and anti-VZV IgG antibody would be needed to confirm the diagnosis (43). VZV reactivation can also cause a myelitis (24) or a progressive outer retinal

necrosis [reviewed by Austin (6)]. Diagnosis of these rare complications of VZV reactivation may again be complicated by the absence of rash; thus, spinal fluid, other body fluids, or tissue must be examined for the presence of VZV DNA and/or anti-VZV IgG antibody.

PREVENTION

A large-scale, placebo-controlled trial of prevention of shingles has been performed in immunocompetent adults aged 60 to 79 years using a modified version of the live, attenuated vaccine in use for primary prevention of VZV infection in children. Compared to those receiving placebo, treated patients had a 51% lower incidence of zoster, 67% reduction in PHN, and, among those who did develop zoster, less severity and mildly shorter duration of pain (45). The zoster vaccine was approved for use in the United States in 2006, but some questions about its use remain (35). These include cost-effectiveness, whether people aged 50 to 59 years should be vaccinated, the long-term effects of the vaccine in an older population who are not re-exposed to varicella due to a high rate of primary vaccination in the young, and how to protect immunocompromised patients. The vaccine is not licensed in immunocompromised states, but these are the patients most likely to develop herpes zoster. Surprisingly, despite the widespread use of the varicella vaccine, studies have reported that the incidence of herpes zoster has remained stable (33) or actually increased (67) since re-exposure to wild-type varicella has been postulated to have a protective effect (9,58).

ACUTE PARALYTIC POLIOMYELITIS AND THE POST-POLIO SYNDROME

Poliovirus (enteroviruses 1, 2, and 3) belongs to the RNA virus family Picornaviridae and is the cause of acute paralytic poliomyelitis. With the introduction of an effective polio vaccine in the mid-20th century, wild-type poliovirus has been virtually eliminated in the Western hemisphere, with new cases continuing to decline worldwide. In 1996, there were only 3,995 new cases of polio, predominantly occurring in Africa and southeast Asia, compared to 35,251 in 1988 (http://www.who.int/vaccines documents/DocsPDF/ww9705b.pdf). Despite the decline in cases of polio, we are now encountering the long-term sequelae of PPS as polio survivors age. It is important to recognize the features of PPS in the elderly (including new-onset weakness, fatigue, and pain) because they are nonspecific and can be often confused with other coexisting medical conditions.

ACUTE PARALYTIC POLIOMYELITIS

Acute paralytic poliomyelitis is characterized by flaccid paresis of the limbs, trunk, and bulbar musculature. Of individuals infected with poliovirus, 1% or less develop this neurologic syndrome (13). Infection begins by ingestion of the poliovirus, which then enters cells via the CD155 poliovirus cell receptor, which is a member of the Ig superfamily of proteins (39). Poliovirus then replicates in the oropharyngeal and intestinal mucosa. Virus is shed in the feces of infected individuals and is the primary mode of transmission. Virus replicates in the mucosa and then reaches the blood via lymph nodes to cause a transient viremia. Most infections end at this stage and present as sore throat, fever, and malaise.

Replication at extraneural sites including brown fat, reticuloendothelial tissues, and muscle increases the likelihood of virus entry to the central nervous system (CNS). Two non–mutually exclusive routes of poliovirus entry into the CNS have been proposed: (a) virus enters the CNS from blood, or (b) virus enters a peripheral nerve and is carried to the CNS by axonal transport. Upon virus entry into the CNS, virus replicates in motor neurons within the spinal cord (leading to the characteristic muscle paralysis), brainstem, and motor cortex. Skeletal muscle injury is

known to be a predisposing factor for poliomyelitis (provocation for poliomyelitis) and is believed to occur by stimulating retrograde axonal transport of poliovirus to the spinal cord, although the exact steps need to be elucidated. This provides a mechanism for selective eradication of a neuronal subpopulation, lower motor neurons (anterior horn cells) in the spinal cord, and bulbar nuclei.

It has been estimated that 50% of an individual's motor neurons can be partially or completely damaged during acute paralytic poliomyelitis, and yet a full clinical recovery can occur. In approximately 25% of individuals with a history of acute paralytic poliomyelitis, a chronic progressive illness characterized by lower motor neuron dysfunction develops years later (13). This syndrome, originally termed an "overuse phenomenon," was first reported by Raymond and Charcot in 1875 (48). They described a young man who had acute paralytic poliomyelitis at age 6 months who developed unilateral arm and leg weakness at age 19 years. Sporadic cases with similar descriptions of new, progressive weakness in patients with remote poliomyelitis continued to be reported, sometimes with associated upper motor neuron findings and suggestions of an association with amyotrophic lateral sclerosis (ALS). In 1972, Anderson et al. (3) described paralytic poliomyelitis survivors with diminished endurance caused by orthopaedic deformities and associated arthralgias and myalgias. That same year, Mulder et al. (41) described 32 patients with well-documented histories of acute paralytic poliomyelitis who, many years later, developed progressive weakness not attributable to orthopaedic deformities and distinguishable from ALS. A paucity of upper motor neuron findings and a slower rate of deterioration were seen in these patients. The observations of Anderson and Mulder were essential in the establishment of clinical criteria for PPS (13).

POST-POLIO SYNDROME

PPS is a clinical diagnosis and is characterized by a history of paralytic poliomyelitis; partial or complete recovery of neurologic function followed by a period of stability, usually several decades, and then persistent new muscle weakness or abnormal muscle fatigability with the exclusion of other causes of new symptoms (18). About 640,000 individuals in the United States have PPS (23), primarily affecting those surviving the last polio epidemic in the 1950s. The prevalence of PPS ranges from 15% to 80% of all patients with previous polio, depending on the criteria applied and the population studied (18). Higher age at onset of poliomyelitis appears to be inversely associated with PPS, and association with other chronic diseases suggest that chronic physical stress, particularly in weak motor units, can contribute to the disease (47). However, we still do not clearly know which individuals are at risk for deterioration (65).

In a subset of PPS patients, the symptoms are caused by musculoskeletal deformities, as described by Anderson et al. (3). Poliomyelitis survivors are predisposed to compression neuropathies and plexopathies from long-term use of wheelchairs, crutches, and braces. Pain, disuse atrophy, and diminished endurance can result from posture changes and joint deformities. These produce further deterioration and functional decline. Another subset of patients, sometimes overlapping with the first, will develop new weakness and atrophy, typically but not exclusively in previously involved limbs. This is a lower motor neuron disease characterized by progressive muscular atrophy (13). Specific symptoms relate to the region or regions affected. Bulbar involvement is frequent, even in patients lacking a history of bulbar involvement during acute poliomyelitis. This can lead to dysphagia or respiratory insufficiency, as in other motor neuron diseases. Sleep apnea can also occur. The origin of the sleep apnea may be central, obstructive, or a combination of these (14,30).

A variety of causes for PPS have been considered. Histopathologic and electrophysiologic data indicate that a chronic state of ongoing denervation and reinnervation exists in patients following acute paralytic poliomyelitis. It has been postulated that a combination of unaffected and affected but partially or fully recovered neurons coexists in the post-polio bulbar motor nuclei and spinal cord. Recovery results from two predominant mechanisms: (a) recovered function in the injured neurons and (b) reinnervation of denervated muscle fibers by remaining motor neurons. The latter process results in group typing on muscle biopsy and in large-amplitude, long-duration motor units on electromyelogram (EMG). Some neurons may be ineffective in maintaining sprouts to reinnervated fibers, leaving scattered denervated fibers. Others may succumb to premature cell death, leaving larger numbers of denervated fibers. When the balance of denervation outweighs reinnervation, weakness ensues (13). This progression in weakness is very slow. Some authors have shown that a statistical progression in weakness cannot be appreciated over a period of 3 years but can be seen after 10 years (13). A recent study using magnetic resonance spectroscopy suggests that metabolic alterations may cause an energy deficit in affected muscles, contributing to underlying muscle fatigue (54). Other contributing factors to PPS may be aging with motor neuron loss, overuse, and disuse.

Epidemiologic data suggest that age is not a direct factor in the development of PPS, but rather, it is the length of time following acute poliomyelitis. This finding detracts from normal aging and motor neuron senescence as a cause of PPS. High IgM GM-1 antiganglioside antibodies have been found in acute poliomyelitis and in PPS, but a causal role for these antibodies has not been established. Limited endomysial and spinal cord inflammation has also been reported. Antibody and polymerase chain reaction (PCR) studies have demonstrated evidence of persistent poliovirus infection in a minority of patients, leading to the hypothesis that persistent infection with mutated poliovirus may be the cause (13). However, it seems unlikely that ongoing viral replication and resultant cell death is the cause of PPS.

A specific diagnostic test is lacking. Nerve conduction studies and needle EMG should be performed to establish typical lower motor neuron involvement; to exclude other causes of symptoms and signs; to find concomitant nerve or muscle disorders, such as entrapments and neuropathies; and to assess the degree of motor neuron loss. Needle EMG changes are nonspecific. Fasciculation potentials and abnormal spontaneous activity (fibrillations and positive sharp waves) should be present, with superimposed changes of chronic denervation. These changes can be seen in all survivors of paralytic poliomyelitis, not simply those with PPS. The presence of abnormal spontaneous activity does not establish a diagnosis of PPS (13). Similar changes can also be seen in radiculopathies and in other motor neuron diseases. Single-fiber EMG demonstrates increased jitter, which is consistent with a disorder of neuromuscular junction transmission and endplate instability (13). The serum creatinine kinase may be mildly to moderately elevated, as in many motor neuron diseases. PPS is distinguished from ALS by the history of acute paralytic polio, the relative paucity of upper motor neuron findings, and the slow rate of progressive weakness.

There is no specific treatment for PPS, other than supportive care. The post-polio functional deterioration requires a multidisciplinary approach involving specific management of increasing impairment and enabling patients to cope with new disabilities. Clinical management of PPS centers on the following (18): (a) supervised, aerobic, isokinetic, and isometric muscular training for improvement of muscle weakness, fatigue, and pain, particularly training in a warm climate and doing nonswimming water exercises; however, excessive exercise should be avoided because this can exacerbate symptoms (1,2); (b) respiratory muscle training and early recognition of respiratory impairment with early introduction of noninvasive ventilatory aids to prevent or delay further respiratory decline; (c) group training and regular follow-up; (d) weight loss and use of properly fitted assistive devices (66); and (e) since many patients have significant anxiety associated with their symptoms, patient education and, sometimes, appropriate psychiatric treatment are an essential part of overall treatment.

No medication has been shown to be effective in the direct treatment of progressive weakness. Although initially promising, amantadine, acetyl cholinesterase inhibitors, and prednisone have been shown to be ineffective in the treatment of PPS (15,56,60). Modafinil does not appear to be effective in alleviating the symptoms of fatigue in PPS patients (11). A preliminary study using lamotrigine on 30 PPS patients indicated that lamotrigine may relieve PPS symptoms and may improve the life qualities of these patients (44). Recent studies suggest that intravenous Ig may improve pain in PPS patients but not muscle strength or fatigue (19,27). Larger studies are needed for the latter two treatments.

CONCLUSION

Overall, the elderly population is vulnerable to viral infections of the CNS, with many viral diseases producing more serious neurologic complications and sequelae. Specifically for this aging population, the neurologic complications of VZV reactivation (including herpes zoster and PHN) and PPS need to be recognized, and early treatment and supportive care need to be provided.

ACKNOWLEDGMENTS

Dr. Nagel is supported by National Institutes of Health training grant 5 T32 NS 007321.

REFERENCES

1. Agre JC. The role of exercise in the patient with post-polio syndrome. *Ann NY Acad Sci.* 1995; 753:321–334.
2. Agre JC, Rodriquez AA, Franke TM. Strength, endurance, and work capacity after muscle strengthening exercise in postpolio subjects. *Arch Phys Med Rehabil.* 1997;78:681–686.
3. Anderson AD, Levine SA, Gellert H. Loss of ambulatory ability in patients with old anterior poliomyelitis. *Lancet.* 1972;2:1061–1063.
4. Anderson JP, Keal EE. Cervical herpes zoster and diaphragmatic paralysis. *Br J Dis Chest.* 1969;63:222–226.
5. Archambault P, Wise JS, Rosen J, et al. Herpes zoster ophthalmoplegia. Report of six cases. *J Clin Neuroophthalmol.* 1988;8:185–193.
6. Austin RB. Progressive outer retinal necrosis syndrome: a comprehensive review of its clinical presentation, relationship to immune system status, and management. *Clin Eye Vis Care.* 2000;12:119–129.
7. Beutner KR, Friedman DJ, Forszpaniak C, et al. Valacyclovir compared with acyclovir for improved therapy for herpes zoster in immunocompetent adults. *Antimicrob Agents Chemother.* 1995;39: 1546–1553.
8. Bowsher D. The lifetime occurrence of herpes zoster and prevalence of post-herpetic neuralgia: a retrospective survey in an elderly population. *Eur J Pain.* 1999;3:335–342.
9. Brisson M, Gay NJ, Edmunds WJ, et al. Exposure to varicella boosts immunity to herpes-zoster: implications for mass vaccination against chickenpox. *Vaccine.* 2002;20:2500–2507.
10. Carroll WM, Mastaglia FL. Optic neuropathy and ophthalmoplegia in herpes zoster oticus. *Neurology.* 1979;29:726–729.
11. Chan KM, Strohschein FJ, Rydz D, et al. Randomized controlled trial of modafinil for the treatment of fatigue in postpolio patients. *Muscle Nerve.* 2006;33:138–141.
12. Chandra RK. Impact of nutritional status and nutrient supplements on immune responses and incidence of infection in older individuals. *Ageing Res Rev.* 2004;3:91–104.
13. Dalakas MC. The post-polio syndrome as an evoked clinical entity. Definition and clinical description. *Ann NY Acad Sci.* 1995;25:68–80.
14. Dean AC, Graham BA, Dalakas M, et al. Sleep apnea in patients with postpolio syndrome. *Ann Neurol.* 1998;43:661–664.
15. Dinsmore S, Dambrosia J, Dalakas MC. A double-blind, placebo-controlled trial of high-dose prednisone for the treatment of post-poliomyelitis syndrome. *Ann NY Acad Sci.* 1995; 753:303–313.
16. Donahue JG, Choo PW, Manson JE, et al. The incidence of herpes zoster. *Arch Intern Med.* 1995;155:1605–1609.
17. Dubinsky RM, Kabbani H, El-Chami Z, et al. Quality Standards Subcommittee of the American Academy of Neurology. Practice parameter: treatment of postherpetic neuralgia: an evidence-based report of the Quality Standards Subcommittee of the American Academy of Neurology. *Neurology.* 2004;63:959–965.
18. Farbu E, Gilhus NE, Barnes MP, et al. EFNS guideline on diagnosis and management of post-polio syndrome. Report of an EFNS task force. *Eur J Neurol.* 2006;13:795–801.
19. Farbu E, Rekand T, Vik-Mo E, et al. Post-polio syndrome patients treated with intravenous immunoglobulin: a double-blinded randomized controlled pilot study. *Eur J Neurol.* 2007; 14:60–65.
20. Furuta Y, Ohtani F, Aizawa H, et al. Varicella-zoster virus reactivation is an important cause of acute peripheral facial paralysis in children. *Pediatr Infect Dis J.* 2005;24:97–101.

21. Furuta Y, Ohtani F, Mesuda Y, et al. Early diagnosis of zoster sine herpete and antiviral therapy for the treatment of facial palsy. *Neurology*. 2000;55:708–710.

22. Garty BZ, Dinari G, Sarnat H, et al. Tooth exfoliation and osteonecrosis of the maxilla after trigeminal herpes zoster. *J Pediatr*. 1985;106: 71–73.

23. Gevirtz C. Managing postpolio syndrome pain. *Nursing*. 2006;36:17.

24. Gilden DH, Beinlich BR, Rubinstien EM, et al. Varicella-zoster virus myelitis: an expanding spectrum. *Neurology*. 1994;44:1818–1823.

25. Gilden DH, Kleinschmidt-DeMasters BK, LaGuardia JL, et al. Neurologic complications of the reactivation of varicella-zoster virus. *N Engl J Med*. 2000;342:635–645.

26. Gilron I, Bailey JM, Tu D, et al. Morphine, gabapentin, or their combination for neuropathic pain. *N Engl J Med*. 2005;352:1324–1334.

27. Gonzalez H, Sunnerhagen KS, Sjoberg I, et al. Intravenous immunoglobulin for post-polio syndrome: a randomised controlled trial. *Lancet Neurol*. 2006;5:493–500.

28. Gruver A, Hudson L, Sempowski G. Immunosenescence of ageing. *J Pathol*. 2007; 211:144–156.

29. Haynes BF, Markert ML, Sempowski GD, et al. The role of the thymus in immune reconstitution in aging, bone marrow transplantation, and HIV-1 infection. *Annu Rev Immunol*. 2000;18: 529–560.

30. Hsu AA, Staats BA. "Postpolio" sequelae and sleep-related disordered breathing. *Mayo Clin Proc*. 1998;73:216–224.

31. Huff JC. Antiviral treatment in chickenpox and herpes zoster. *J Am Acad Dermatol*. 1988;18: 204–206.

32. Jackson JL, Gibbons R, Meyer G, et al. The effect of treating herpes zoster with oral acyclovir in preventing postherpetic neuralgia. A meta-analysis. *Arch Intern Med* 1997;157:909–912.

33. Jumaan AO, Yu O, Jackson LA, et al. Herpes zoster incidence before and after declines in varicella incidence associated with varicella vaccination, 1992–2002. *J Infect Dis*. 2005;191: 1999–2001.

34. Karmon Y, Gadath N. Delayed oculomotor nerve palsy after bilateral cervical zoster in an immunocompetent patient. *Neurology*. 2005;65:170.

35. Kimberlin DW, Whitley RJ. Varicella-zoster vaccine for the prevention of herpes zoster. *N Eng J Med*. 2007;356:1338–1343.

36. Mahalingam R, Wellish M, Brucklier J, et al. Persistence of varicella-zoster virus DNA in elderly patients with postherpetic neuralgia. *J Neurovirol*. 1995;1:130–133.

37. Manz HJ, Canter HG, Melton J. Trigeminal herpes zoster causing mandibular osteonecrosis and spontaneous tooth exfoliation. *South Med J*. 1986;79:1026–1028.

38. Meenken C, van den Horn GJ, de Smet MD, et al. Optic neuritis heralding varicella zoster virus retinitis in a patient with acquired immunodeficiency syndrome. *Ann Neurol*. 1998;43:534–536.

39. Mendelsohn CL, Wimmer E, Racaneillo VR. Cellular receptor for poliovirus: molecular cloning, nucleotide sequence, and expression of a new member of the immunoglobulin superfamily. *Cell*. 1989;56:855–865.

40. Merchet MP, Gruener G. Segmental zoster paresis of limbs. *Electromyogr Clin Neurophysiol*. 1996;36:369–375.

41. Mulder DW, Rosenbaum RA, Layton DD. Late progression of poliomyelitis or forme fruste amyotrophic lateral sclerosis? *Mayo Clin Proc*. 1972;47:756–761.

42. Murakami S, Hato N, Horiuchi J, et al. Treatment of Ramsay Hunt syndrome with acyclovir-prednisone: significance of early diagnosis and treatment. *Ann Neurol*. 1997;41:353–357.

43. Nagel MA, Forghani B, Mahalingam R, et al. The value of detecting anti-VZV IgG antibody in CSF to diagnose VZV vasculopathy. *Neurology*. 2007;68:1069–1073.

44. On AY, Oncu J, Uludag B, et al. Effects of lamotrigine on the symptoms and life qualities of patients with post polio syndrome: a randomized, controlled study. *Neurorehabilitation*. 2005; 20:245–251.

45. Oxman MN, Levin MJ, Johnson GR, et al. A vaccine to prevent herpes zoster and postherpetic neuralgia in older adults. *N Engl J Med*. 2005;352:2271–2284.

46. Quan D, Hammack BN, Kittelson J, et al. Improvement of postherpetic neuralgia after treatment with intravenous acyclovir followed by oral valacyclovir. *Arch Neurol*. 2006;63:940–942.

47. Ragonese P, Fierro B, Salemi G, et al. Prevalence and risk factors of post-polio syndrome in a cohort of polio survivors. *J Neurol Sci*. 2005;236: 31–35.

48. Raymond M. Paralysie essentielle de l'enfance, atrophie musculaire consecutive. *Soc Biol*. 1875; 27:158.

49. Rice AS, Maton S. Gabapentin in postherpetic neuralgia: a randomised, double blind, placebo controlled study. Postperpetic Neuralgia Study Group. *Pain*. 2001;94:215–224.

50. Rogers RS III, Tindall JP. Herpes zoster in the elderly. *Postgrad Med*. 1971;50:153–157.

51. Rowbotham MC, Harden N, Stacey B, et al. Gabapentin for the treatment of postherpetic

neuralgia: a randomized controlled trial. *JAMA*. 1998;280:1837–1842.

52. Rowbotham MC, Manville NS, Ren J. Pilot tolerability and effectiveness study of levetiracetam for postherpetic neuralgia. *Neurology*. 2003;61: 866–867.

53. Sampathkumar P. West Nile virus: epidemiology, clinical presentation, diagnosis, and prevention. *Mayo Clin Proc*. 2003;78:1137–1143.

54. Sharma U, Kumar V, Wadhwa S, et al. In vivo (31)P MRS study of skeletal muscle metabolism in patients with postpolio residual paralysis. *Magn Reson Imaging*. 2007;25:244–249.

55. Sodhi PK, Goel JL. Presentations of cranial nerve involvement in two patients with herpes zoster ophthalmicus. *J Commun Dis*. 2001;33:130–135.

56. Stein DP, Dambrosia JM, Dalakas MC. A double-blind, placebo-controlled trial of amantadine for the treatment of fatigue in patients with the post-polio syndrome. *Ann NY Acad Sci*. 1995; 753:296–302.

57. Sweeney CJ, Gilden DH. Ramsay Hunt syndrome. *J Neurol Neurosurg Psychiatry*. 2001;71: 149–154.

58. Thomas SL, Wheeler JG, Hall AJ. Contacts with varicella or with children and protection against herpes zoster in adults: a case-control study. *Lancet*. 2002;360:678–682.

59. Tjandra J, Mansel RE. Segmental abdominal herpes zoster paresis. *Aust N Z J Surg*. 1986;56: 807–808.

60. Trojan DA, Colet JP, Shapiro S, et al. A multicenter, double-blinded trial of pyridostigmine in postpolio syndrome. *Neurology*. 1999;53:1225–1233.

61. Tyring S, Barbarash RA, Nahlik JE, et al. Famciclovir for the treatment of acute herpes zoster: effects on acute disease and postherpetic neuralgia. A randomized, double-blind, placebo-controlled trial. Collaborative Famciclovir Herpes Zoster Study Group. *Ann Intern Med*. 1995;123:89–96.

62. Vafai A, Wellish M, Gilden DH. Expression of varicella-zoster virus in blood mononuclear cells of patients with postherpetic neuralgia. *Proc Natl Acad Sci USA*. 1988;85:2767–2770.

63. Volvoikar P, Patil S, Dinkar A. Tooth exfoliation, osteonecrosis and neuralgia following herpes zoster of trigeminal nerve. *Indian J Dent Res*. 2002;13:11–14.

64. Wharton M. The epidemiology of varicella-zoster virus infections. *Infect Dis Clin North Am*. 1996;10:571–581.

65. Willen C, Thoren-Jonsson AL, Grimby G, et al. Disability in a 4-year follow-up study of people with post-polio syndrome. *J Rehabil Med*. 2007; 39:175–180.

66. Wise HH. Effective intervention strategies for management of impaired posture and fatigue with post-polio syndrome: a case report. *Physiother Theory Pract*. 2006;22:279–287.

67. Yih WK, Brooks DR, Lett SM, et al. The incidence of varicella and herpes zoster in Massachusetts as measured by the Behavioral Risk Factor Surveillance System (BRFSS) during a period of increasing varicella vaccine coverage, 1998-2003. *BMC Public Health*. 2005;5:68.

68. Yoleri O, Olmez N, Oztura I, et al. Segmental zoster paresis of the upper extremity: a case report. *Arch Phys Med Rehabil*. 2005;86:1492–1494.

PATIENT RESOURCE

Herpes Zoster and Postherpetic Neuralgia

National Institute of Neurological Disorders and Stroke–Shingles: http://www.ninds.nih.gov/disorders/shingles/detail_shingles.htm

VZV Research Foundation: http://www.vzvfoundation.org

National Foundation for the Treatment of Pain: http://www.paincare.org

American Chronic Pain Association (ACPA): http://www.theacpa.org

Post-Polio Syndrome

National Institute of Neurological Disorders and Stroke–Post-Polio Syndrome Information Page: http://www.ninds.nih.gov/disorders/post_polio/post_polio.htm

Post-Polio Health International: http://www.post-polio.org

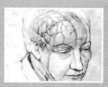

CHAPTER 28

Neuro-Oncology of the Elderly

Julie E. Hammack

Cancer is the second leading cause of death in persons over 65 years of age. In 2006, it was estimated that 782,482 Americans over 65 years of age were diagnosed with cancer and 397,640 persons in that age group died of the disease (53). With the shift in demographics to a larger percentage of elderly and with improved prevention and treatment of heart disease and stroke, elderly patients with cancer will become even more prevalent in the new century. As many as 20% to 25% of patients with systemic cancer harbor intracranial metastases at the time of death, and 5% of patients with systemic cancer develop epidural cord compression during the course of their illness. Applying these percentages to the statistics noted above indicates a very large number of patients presenting to their physicians with neurologic signs and symptoms directly related to their systemic malignancies.

Although primary CNS tumors currently account for <2% of all malignancies in the elderly, their frequency has increased steadily over the last three decades (25). The American Cancer Society estimates that 18,820 persons were diagnosed with primary CNS cancer in 2006 (patients >65 years old accounted for an estimated 35% of these cases) and 12,820 persons died from these tumors in that year (48% of those dying were 65 years or older) (53). Some studies have estimated the increase in incidence of primary brain tumors in patients over 65 years of age to be from 15% to 500% over the last 20 years (28,30,37). The increased incidence is particularly pronounced in the extreme elderly (≥85 years). The cause of this troubling increase is unclear. It may be caused, at least partially, by the widespread availability of sophisticated neuroimaging and increased access to specialized medical care for the elderly over the last 30 years. These advances alone, however, do not fully account for this trend. The incidence of primary malignant brain tumors started to rise even before the introduction of computed tomography (CT) scanning in the early 1970s, and the trend has continued to increase even since the 1980s, when CT scanning capability became standard in most medical facilities (65).

Neuro-oncology is the study of cancer's effects on the central and peripheral nervous system. This includes direct involvement of the nervous system by tumor and so-called "remote effects," which broadly include paraneoplastic disorders, cerebrovascular complications, infections, and toxic or metabolic disorders that can be secondary effects of cancer or its treatment. Table 28-1 lists the various categories of neurologic illness seen in patients with cancer.

This chapter focuses on the primary and metastatic tumors of the brain and spinal cord most commonly seen in the older adult. A section in this chapter outlines the well-described, although rare, paraneoplastic neurologic disorders.

CLASSIFICATION

Brain and spinal tumors can be broadly classified as either primary (tumor arising from cells of the brain and spinal cord or their coverings) or metastatic (tumor spread from other primary sites within the body). By definition, metastatic tumors are always malignant. Primary tumors can be benign or malignant, depending on the underlying histopathology. Overall, metastatic tumors are the most common brain tumors seen in elderly patients. However, in a patient presenting with a new, solitary brain neoplasm and no history of systemic cancer, a primary tumor is the more likely diagnosis.

Among primary brain tumors, most series suggest that meningioma is most common, followed by malignant (high-grade) glioma, pituitary adenoma, schwannoma (including acoustic neuroma), low-grade glioma, and primary central nervous system (CNS) lymphoma (PCNSL).

METASTATIC TUMORS

BRAIN METASTASES

Among older adults, metastatic tumors are more common than primary brain tumors, occurring in 20% to 25% of all patients dying of cancer, based on autopsy series (36,47,50). The incidence is less common in clinical series in which primarily symptomatic brain lesions will usually be included (56,64). Virtually any malignant systemic tumor can metastasize to the brain. Breast and lung cancers are the most common systemic tumors and, therefore, account for most brain metastases. Some less common malignancies have a special proclivity to metastasize to the brain. Thus, although melanoma accounts for only 4% of systemic tumors, it has accounted for as much as 10% of brain metastases, and as many as 40% of patients with melanoma were found to harbor brain metastases at autopsy (1).

Table 28-1. *Neurologic Illnesses in Patients with Cancer*

Direct tumor involvement	Infection
Brain or cord parenchymal metastases	*Listeria monocytogenes*
Meningeal metastases	*Cryptococcus neoformans*
Dural metastases	*Aspergillus fumigatus*
Epidural metastases	*Mucor*
Plexus metastases	Herpes zoster
Peripheral nerve metastases	JC virus
Toxic metabolic disorders	Cytomegalovirus
Liver or renal disease	Toxoplasmosis
Electrolyte disturbances (SIADH)	Adverse effects of therapy
Hypercalcemia	Radiation encephalopathy
Hypomagnesemia	Radiation myelopathy
Hypothyroidism	Radiation plexopathy/radiculopathy
Chemotherapy toxicity	Chemotherapy-induced encephalopathy
Opioid toxicity	Chemotherapy-induced neuropathy
Corticosteroid toxicity	Steroid psychosis
Vascular disorders	Steroid myopathy
Nonbacterial thrombotic endocarditis	Phantom limb syndrome
Disseminated intravascular coagulation	Postmastectomy pain syndrome
Hyperviscosity syndrome	Postthoracotomy syndrome
Thrombocytopenia	Paraneoplastic syndromes
Hypercoagulable state	Lambert-Eaton myasthenic syndrome
Dural sinus thrombosis	Myasthenia gravis
Tumor embolus	Paraneoplastic cerebellar degeneration
Tumor hemorrhage	Paraneoplastic limbic encephalitis
	Paraneoplastic sensory neuropathy
	Opsoclonus-myoclonus syndrome
	Polymyositis/dermatomyositis

SIADH, syndrome of inappropriate antidiuretic hormone.

Small-cell lung cancer is more than twice as likely to metastasize to the brain as other types of lung cancer.

Some evidence indicates that the incidence of metastatic brain tumors is increasing (47,50). This is likely caused by a combination of factors: (a) sophisticated neuroimaging allows diagnosis of brain metastases even at an asymptomatic stage; (b) improved treatment of the systemic cancer means that patients are living longer and have more opportunity to develop brain metastases; and (c) the CNS appears to be a "sanctuary" from the effects of chemotherapy, allowing brain metastases to grow, even when systemic tumor is controlled.

The pathogenesis is hematogenous tumor spread in most patients. In more than 50% of cases, the lesions are multiple. The "watershed" region of the cerebral hemispheres is the most likely site of metastases, and the corticomedullary junction is the most common point of origin (15). These pathologic data suggest that arterial tumor microemboli lodge in the distal capillary arcades of the cerebral arteries. Supratentorial metastases are distinctly more common than infratentorial (90% vs. 10%) in patients with breast and lung cancer. The metastases are more evenly divided between the supra- and infratentorial compartment in patients with colon cancer and uterine cancer. This suggests a possible role of metastasis via the Batson venous plexus, although some studies refute that hypothesis (15,42).

Clinical Presentation

Most brain metastases (80%) occur in patients in whom the diagnosis of systemic malignancy is already established. The clinical presentation varies considerably among individuals and largely depends on the location of the brain metastasis or metastases. In younger patients, the most common symptoms are headache and seizure. Among elderly patients, focal deficits (e.g., hemiparesis and aphasia) and cognitive changes are distinctly more common, perhaps because older brains have more atrophy and room to accommodate an expanding mass lesion. It is not clear why elderly patients are less likely to present with seizures. Perhaps the seizure threshold of the elderly brain is higher.

Not infrequently, elderly patients with brain metastases are misdiagnosed as having a "stroke." This is especially common in patients who do not have a previous diagnosis of a primary tumor or in those who present with very acute symptomatology. Focal seizure and tumor hemorrhage can both masquerade clinically as a stroke. The diagnosis usually is not difficult if a careful history is taken and neuroimaging is interpreted appropriately.

Diagnosis

A CT of the head with contrast is sufficient in most cases to make the diagnosis of brain metastases, although magnetic resonance imaging (MRI) of the head has become standard for diagnosis in most centers. CT is less expensive than MRI and easier to perform on a patient who is confused or uncooperative. In patients whose condition is deteriorating rapidly, CT is adequate to diagnose secondary conditions such as obstructive hydrocephalus and tumor hemorrhage. Extra care must be taken in elderly patients to ensure that their renal function is adequate to handle the iodinated contrast. Approximately 5% of patients will have an allergic reaction to the iodinated contrast dye, and the dye can precipitate focal seizures in as many as 10% of patients with brain metastases (2). MRI with contrast is more sensitive, particularly for small brain metastases. It is also more expensive and requires better patient cooperation.

Both CT and MRI demonstrate enhancing lesions, typically with central necrosis. Metastases are usually multiple, which can be better appreciated on MRI when the lesions are tiny. Typically in brain metastases, the lesions are well circumscribed and have a disproportionate amount of edema than expected for the size of the enhancing lesion (Fig. 28-1). These features may help distinguish them radiographically from primary brain tumors, which tend to be more diffuse and have a pattern of edema that more closely approximates the area of enhancement. A brain abscess may mimic the appearance of metastasis, although brain abscesses are rare unless the patient is immunocompromised.

In patients who have known metastatic systemic cancer, the diagnosis is generally made radiographically, and pathologic confirmation may not be required before treatment. The situation is more problematic in patients without a known systemic malignancy. If the radiographic picture is suggestive of metastatic tumor, a careful search for systemic malignancy should be undertaken. This begins with a thorough physical examination, followed by appropriate blood tests and imaging procedures [body CT, mammography, positron emission tomography (PET) scan]. Lung, breast, skin, renal, and gastrointestinal system are the most common sources of a primary malignancy in these cases. If no primary tumor can be found, then surgical biopsy or resection of one of the brain lesions is appropriate to make a diagnosis.

Treatment

Although the approach to treatment can vary, depending on the individual patient and type of malignancy, some interventions apply to all patients. Corticosteroids reduce peritumoral edema and can significantly reduce headache from raised intracranial pressure and may improve neurologic deficits produced by tumor mass effect. Approximately 30% to 40% of patients with brain metastases will have seizures at some point in their illness. This figure is higher among patients with hemorrhagic metastases and those with metastatic melanoma, in whom it is >50% (10). Any patient who has had a seizure should receive anticonvulsants, as should patients with metastatic melanoma. Otherwise, prophylactic anticonvulsants are best avoided because they interact with corticosteroids and various chemotherapy agents. Both phenytoin and carbamazepine can cause Stevens-Johnson syndrome,

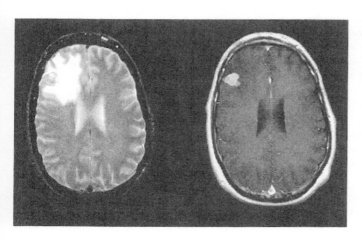

Figure 28-1. Brain metastasis. Axial MRI of the head: T2-weighted image (**left**) and T1-weighted image with gadolinium contrast (**right**). Note the large amount of edema compared to the lesion's size.

particularly in patients receiving whole-brain radiation therapy (WBRT) (16). Moreover, no significant reduction in the incidence of seizures has been seen in patients who received prophylactic anticonvulsants (20).

Surgery In patients with multiple lesions, surgery is limited to those who lack a known primary tumor. In this situation, biopsy without resection is appropriate to make a pathologic diagnosis. More extensive surgery is indicated in selected situations. For instance, in a patient with a large cerebellar metastasis obstructing the fourth ventricle, a resection of the offending metastasis may be life saving and allow the patient to tolerate WBRT without brain herniation. Data suggest that patients who have a surgically accessible solitary metastasis (as proved on enhanced MRI) and limited systemic cancer survive longer with less neurologic disability if they have resection of their metastasis (46,61). Surgery is a further consideration in patients with a recurrent metastasis after WBRT has been administered or in those with tumors that are known to be radiation resistant.

Radiation Therapy WBRT is the mainstay of treatment for most patients with brain metastases. It prolongs survival but is not considered curative. WBRT after resection of a solitary metastasis has been demonstrated to reduce the risk of CNS recurrence and neurologic death but did not improve survival overall when compared to patients receiving surgical resection alone (45). Most patients with brain metastases will die of progressive systemic cancer, not brain disease. The treatment is given to ports encompassing the whole brain, to a total dose of 2,000 to 3,000 cGy in 10 to 15 fractions. More accelerated radiation schedules may be appropriate in very frail patients with a short life expectancy. WBRT is usually well tolerated. Radiation-induced tumor swelling is best managed with corticosteroids. If they survive more than 6 to 12 months, elderly patients can be particularly susceptible to develop radiation encephalopathy. This is characterized by subcortical dementia with gait apraxia and urinary incontinence. CT and MRI demonstrate cortical atrophy, hydrocephalus ex vacuo, and diffuse white matter changes. More localized radiation, including gamma knife and stereotactic linear accelerator therapy, is probably best reserved for small recurrent brain metastases. The value of these latter therapies in the primary treatment of brain metastases remains to be clearly established.

Chemotherapy Most chemotherapy agents do not penetrate the blood–brain barrier well. Historically, chemotherapy agents have little efficacy in the treatment of most types of brain metastases. The recent development of chemotherapy agents that penetrate the blood–brain barrier, including temozolomide, topotecan, and signal transduction inhibitors, holds some promise in the treatment of brain metastases (11).

Prognosis

Once brain metastases have developed, the patient's cancer, with rare exception, has reached an incurable stage. Without treatment, life expectancy is usually less than 4 to 6 weeks, and most patients die from their neurologic disease in that setting. With radiation therapy, survival extends to a median of 3 to 6 months. Most treated patients will die of progressive systemic cancer, not of brain metastases. Long-term survival (>1 year) is exceedingly rare among elderly patients.

EPIDURAL CORD COMPRESSION

Tumor in the epidural space usually has spread from the adjacent vertebra. Vertebral metastases are common, occurring in 25% to 70% of patients with metastatic cancer. The thoracic spine is particularly susceptible because it makes up the largest bony mass of the spine. The solid tumors that most commonly metastasize to the vertebra are lung, breast, prostate, renal, and thyroid cancer. Myeloma is the most common hematopoietic tumor to produce epidural cord compression. Tumor can invade the epidural space through the intervertebral foramen, without direct invasion of bone. The latter mechanism is seen in lymphomas arising from the paraspinal lymph nodes. Clinical signs of epidural cord or cauda equina compression can develop in as many as 5% to 10% of patients with metastatic cancer (4).

Clinical Presentation

Pain, the most common initial symptom, is present in 95% of patients at presentation to the physician (24). The pain can derive from the bony vertebral involvement or from compression of spinal roots. Vertebral pain is usually sharp or dull, localized over the involved vertebra, and worse with activities that stress the spine, such as standing and twisting. Bone pain is typically worse at night. Radicular pain is sharp and lancinating and is distributed along the root's cutaneous dermatome. Radicular pain can also be worse with movement and with Valsalva maneuvers. Bone and radicular pain often precede neurologic deficits by weeks or months.

Neurologic deficits can develop acutely or subacutely and depend on the spinal level of involvement. Epidural tumor in the cervical and thoracic region will produce a myelopathy with spastic limb weakness, sensory level to pain and temperature, and loss of bowel, bladder, and sexual function. Lhermitte phenomenon may occur in patients with epidural tumors in the cervical or thoracic region. Compression of the thecal sac below L1 will produce a cauda equina syndrome with flaccid paraparesis, saddle distribution sensory loss, and loss of bowel, bladder, and sexual function. Epidural cord and cauda equina compression constitutes a neurologic emergency. Once neurologic function is lost, it may not be regained, despite appropriate treatment. Diagnosis and treatment, therefore, should proceed as quickly as possible.

Diagnosis

Although a plain X-ray study of the spine can identify the vertebral lesion in approximately 80% to 90% of patients with epidural tumor (48), it does not visualize the epidural space. MRI of the spine is superior in this regard and has largely replaced myelography, except for cases in which MRI cannot be performed (i.e., patients with cardiac pacemakers). MRI will demonstrate the level of vertebral and epidural involvement and confirm the presence of cord or cauda equina compression (Fig. 28-2). In addition to the spinal level of clinical interest, it is generally recommended that the entire spine be visualized with sagittal MRI views to rule out other levels of subclinical epidural involvement. As many as 30% of patients may have other levels of epidural involvement on MRI that are not suspected clinically (54).

Treatment

If epidural cord or cauda equina compression is clinically suspected, the patient should immediately be given high-dose intravenous corticosteroids. Dexamethasone

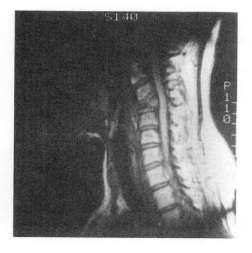

Figure 28-2. Epidural cord compression from vertebral metastasis (lung primary). Sagittal MRI of the cervical spine: T2-weighted image without contrast showing malignant involvement of C3 vertebra with compression fracture and extension of tumor into the epidural space with compression of the cord.

(100 mg) is the treatment of choice. This reduces tumor swelling and spinal cord edema. It may prevent neurologic deterioration while the patient is awaiting diagnostic procedures and more definitive treatment. Corticosteroids provide analgesia for bone-related pain. Opioid analgesia should be given concomitantly for patients with moderate to severe pain. Side effects of high-dose steroids include manic psychosis, insomnia, and hyperglycemia. Hiccoughs are extremely common. If dexamethasone is given as an intravenous bolus, 50% of patients will experience intense but short-lasting perineal burning (5). This effect is self-limited, but patients should be warned before the steroids are given as a bolus.

In patients with a histologically proved primary malignancy, emergent radiation therapy to the spine is the most appropriate treatment, in most instances. Generally, the treatment is given in 10 to 15 fractions to a maximum dose of 2,000 to 3,000 cGy. The radiation ports usually encompass two levels above and below the area of epidural tumor. Most patients should continue to receive corticosteroids during the radiation therapy on a tapering schedule. Surgical intervention may be appropriate in patients without a tumor diagnosis, those who have received previous radiation to the spine, and those with radiation-resistant tumors. Surgical procedures to remove epidural tumor are often extensive, requiring vertebral resection and spinal fusion. Not surprisingly, these aggressive procedures are often not appropriate for frail, elderly patients. Patients with recurrent or progressive epidural tumor in a previously radiated area may be candidates for a second course of radiation, if surgery is not feasible. In this instance, repeat radiation appears to carry a minimal risk of radiation myelopathy (55).

Prognosis

The presence of bony metastases implies advanced cancer, and most patients will die within 6 to 12 months of their systemic malignancy. The presence of epidural tumor will not usually hasten death unless the patient develops a complication of paralysis, such as deep venous thrombosis and pulmonary embolus, urosepsis from neurogenic bladder, or sepsis from decubitus ulcers. Timely diagnosis and treatment of epidural cord compression will reduce the likelihood that the patient will spend his or her remaining days wheelchair bound and dependent on others. If treatment is given before the development of severe neurologic dysfunction, the prognosis for neurologic recovery or maintenance of function is good. If treatment is not begun until after the patient is paraplegic and incontinent, then it is highly unlikely that steroids and radiation will bring recovery of function.

LEPTOMENINGEAL METASTASES

Leptomeningeal metastases are much less common than intraparenchymal brain and epidural cord metastases, but they still account for significant neurologic morbidity. Depending on the series cited, leptomeningeal metastases may be present in 4% to 10% of patients with solid tumors and 5% to 15% of patients with leukemia (12). The tumors that most commonly invade the leptomeninges are leukemia (particularly acute lymphoblastic leukemia), lymphoma, breast cancer, lung cancer, and melanoma. The incidence of leptomeningeal metastases has declined in leukemias and lymphomas, coincident with the use of "prophylactic" intrathecal chemotherapy and high-dose intravenous drug regimens that have good cerebrospinal fluid (CSF) penetration. Data suggest that the incidence of leptomeningeal cancer may be increasing in patients with solid tumors (e.g., breast and lung). The most likely reason for this is improved systemic chemotherapy, which allows patients to live longer but which does not penetrate the blood–brain barrier, allowing a sanctuary for tumor cells. The most likely mode of entry is hematogenous, although tumor cells can enter the CSF from intraparenchymal brain metastases adjacent to the pial or ependymal surface of the brain.

Clinical Presentation

Leptomeningeal tumor can involve the CNS at the supratentorial, posterior fossa, or spinal level and may involve all three levels simultaneously. Within the supratentorial compartment and posterior fossa, typical signs and symptoms include headache, cognitive decline, visual loss, diplopia, facial pain and anesthesia, dysarthria, hearing loss and tinnitus, dysphagia, and ataxia. Papilledema may be present, either as a result of hydrocephalus and raised intracranial pressure or from direct optic nerve infiltration. At the spinal level, multiple painful radiculopathies are common, occasionally with evidence of a myelopathy. The basal meninges of the brain and cauda equina are most commonly involved, presumably because gravity causes the cancer cells to settle in the most dependent CSF spaces.

Diagnosis

A contrasted MRI of the clinically involved area is the most useful imaging procedure. It often demonstrates diffuse or nodular linear enhancement of the basal meninges, surface of the spinal cord, and spinal roots (Fig. 28-3). Communicating hydrocephalus may be present, caused by obstruction of CSF egress in the basal meninges or arachnoid granulations. A normal contrast MRI of the head or spine does not exclude the diagnosis.

The definitive diagnostic procedure is examination of the CSF for malignant cells. Multiple lumbar punctures may be required to isolate malignant cells on cytologic examination (6,63). Virtually all patients will have some abnormality in the CSF, such as elevated opening pressure, elevated protein level, low glucose, elevated nucleated cell count, or CSF tumor marker (i.e., carcinoembryonic antigen) (12). If lymphoma is suspected, the CSF cytologic examination should include T- and B-cell surface markers to look for a monoclonal population of B cells, which is typical of lymphoma. CSF flow cytometry can be helpful diagnostically in this subset of patients. The lumbar puncture will help exclude other disorders (e.g., fungal and tubercular meningitis) and granulomatous diseases that can present in a similar fashion as leptomeningeal malignancy.

Treatment

Although spread of lymphoma and leukemia to the leptomeninges is a poor prognostic indicator, occasionally it is possible to clear the CSF of cancer cells with a combination of intra-CSF chemotherapy (methotrexate or cytarabine) and radiation therapy.

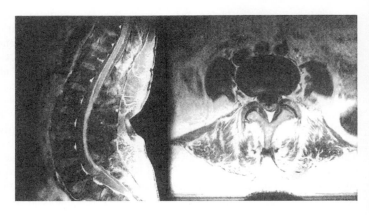

Figure 28-3. Leptomeningeal metastases (breast primary). Sagittal and axial MRI of the lumbar spine: T1-weighted images with gadolinium contrast demonstrating diffuse pial enhancement of the cord and enhancement and thickening of the lumbosacral roots.

Instead of intra-CSF therapy, some centers prefer to use high-dose intravenous methotrexate or cytarabine due to the excellent CNS penetration of these drugs. In patients with carcinoma, however, treatment of leptomeningeal involvement is considered palliative. Most patients with leptomeningeal carcinoma also have advanced systemic malignancy. Generally, it is appropriate to administer radiation therapy to the symptomatic areas only, in the hope of improving or maintaining neurologic function. Attempting to radiate the entire neuraxis will not rid the CSF of tumor cells and will produce significant myelosuppression. Some patients with leptomeningeal carcinoma may benefit from the addition of intra-CSF chemotherapy (methotrexate, cytarabine, or thiotepa) given either by lumbar puncture or Ommaya reservoir. Usually, this treatment is best reserved for patients with limited systemic cancer and good performance status.

Prognosis

When carcinoma spreads to the meninges, it portends a very poor prognosis. Without treatment, survival is usually <1 month (63). About one half of these patients die from complications of their neurologic illness, such as aspiration pneumonia and pulmonary embolus. The other half die from progression of their systemic cancer. Most patients with leptomeningeal carcinoma have extensive systemic tumor at the time the neurologic disease is diagnosed. Even with radiation or intra-CSF chemotherapy, the median survival is only 3 to 6 months from the onset of neurologic symptoms in most patients (6).

PARANEOPLASTIC NEUROLOGIC SYNDROMES

Paraneoplastic neurologic disease refers to disorders seen in association with systemic malignancy that are not caused by direct tumor involvement or by other toxic or metabolic, infectious, or vascular complications of cancer. Most of these disorders affect the central or peripheral nervous system in a specific clinical pattern and are believed to be of autoimmune origin. These are rare disorders that occur in <1% of patients with systemic cancer. It is important to rule out metastatic tumor and other neurologic complications of cancer before making the diagnosis of a paraneoplastic syndrome. It is important to include the possibility of paraneoplastic disease in the differential diagnosis of patients with cancer and neurologic disease and even to consider these disorders in patients without a history of cancer. As many as 60% of patients with paraneoplastic neurologic disease do not have a previous diagnosis of malignancy. In these patients, the neurologic syndrome heralds the diagnosis of cancer.

This section deals with the most common and best described paraneoplastic syndromes, including paraneoplastic cerebellar degeneration (PCD), paraneoplastic encephalomyelitis/paraneoplastic sensory neuronopathy (PEM/PSN), paraneoplastic opsoclonus-myoclonus (POM), and Lambert-Eaton myasthenic syndrome (LEMS). Much overlap exists between these syndromes, and many patients present with clinical features of two or more syndromes.

Most patients with these disorders have an identifiable antineuronal antibody specific to their paraneoplastic syndrome. In one disorder, LEMS, the antibody [anti-voltage gated calcium channel (VGCC)] is known to be pathogenic. In the other syndromes, the antibodies serve as a marker for the underlying tumor but have not been shown to produce the syndrome when transferred to laboratory animals. In each of these disorders, it is believed that the systemic tumor cell expresses an "onconeural antigen," which produces an immune response in the patient. This onconeural antigen shares similarities to antigens normally expressed by specific neural tissue. The host immune response (cell-mediated and humoral) then attacks both the tumor and the specific neural tissue that shares antigenic similarity. This theory is strengthened by the fact that patients' tumors often share antigenic similarities with neural tissue and by the frequent observation that patients with paraneoplastic neurologic disease often have limited or no metastatic disease and small primary tumors. The latter observation suggests that the immune response to tumor may be particularly strong in these patients.

PARANEOPLASTIC CEREBELLAR DEGENERATION

PCD is the best described and possibly the most common autoimmune paraneoplastic disorder. Clinically, it is characterized by the subacute onset of pancerebellar and brainstem signs and symptoms. Vertigo, nausea, gait and limb ataxia, dysarthria, nystagmus, and diplopia evolving over days or weeks are the most common clinical features. At the time of diagnosis, the patient is usually severely disabled and nonambulatory. Occasionally, PCD overlaps with some of the other paraneoplastic syndromes, and evidence of limbic encephalitis, LEMS, opsoclonus, and sensory neuronopathy may be present.

Most commonly seen in women, PCD is associated with breast, ovarian, uterine, and fallopian tube cancers. PCD is also seen in association with small-cell lung cancer, Hodgkin lymphoma, and a host of other malignancies (49). Pathologically, PCD is characterized by diffuse severe loss of Purkinje cells in the cerebellar cortex with associated astrocytic gliosis. Inflammatory changes are rarely seen but may be present in the meninges or deep cerebellar nuclei.

Diagnosis

Early in the course of the illness, CT and MRI of the head may be normal. These studies are essential to exclude other causes of cerebellar dysfunction, including tumor, abscess, infarct, and demyelinating disease. After several months, marked cerebellar atrophy is usually present in patients with PCD (Fig. 28-4). CSF is abnormal in 50% of patients showing nonspecific abnormalities, including lymphocytic pleocytosis and elevated protein (23).

The presence of antineuronal antibodies in the serum and CSF is extremely helpful in making the diagnosis of PCD. These antibodies are highly specific for the presence of an underlying tumor, but their absence does not exclude the possibility of a paraneoplastic cause. Anti-Yo (PCA-1 antibody) is found in the serum and CSF of patients with breast and gynecologic malignancies and PCD. This antibody is specific for the cytoplasm of the Purkinje cell and appears to bind to proteins that regulate DNA transcription and protein synthesis. Anti-Yo has been shown to react with patients' own tumors but not with similar tumors from patients without PCD (21). Anti-Hu (ANNA-1) is an antibody seen in patients with PCD and small-cell lung cancer (see below). Anti-Tr is an antibody reactive with Purkinje cell cytoplasm seen in some patients with Hodgkin's disease and PCD. CRMP-5 antibody is associated with a variety of paraneoplastic neurologic syndromes, including PCD, and is most closely linked to small-cell lung cancer. The aforementioned antibodies have not been shown to be pathogenic and should be considered as markers for their underlying tumors. They are extremely helpful, when present in the serum or CSF, in confirming the diagnosis of PCD and directing the search for the underlying malignancy if it is unknown.

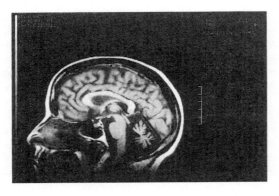

Figure 28-4. Paraneoplastic cerebellar degeneration. Sagittal MRI of the head: T1-weighted image without gadolinium demonstrating marked cerebellar atrophy.

If PCD is suspected, a complete search for underlying cancer is warranted. A complete medical history and physical examination are appropriate starting points. Investigations may include a CT of the chest, abdomen, and pelvis and, in women, a mammogram.

Treatment and Results

Unfortunately, no effective treatment currently exists for PCD. Immunosuppressive therapy with corticosteroids, plasma exchange, intravenous immunoglobulin (IVIG), and cyclophosphamide has been largely unsuccessful, although two studies report clinical stabilization or modest improvement with immunosuppressants (31,62). Occasionally, treating the underlying malignancy produces improvement, but this too is rare, perhaps because injury and death of Purkinje cells are rapid and probably completed by the time the diagnosis is made. Most patients are permanently and severely disabled by this syndrome and, thus, derive little benefit from the observation that their tumors are often less aggressive than expected (26).

PARANEOPLASTIC ENCEPHALOMYELITIS/PARANEOPLASTIC SENSORY NEURONOPATHY

PEM/PSN is a disorder that encompasses several syndromes affecting different areas of the nervous system, including the cerebellum, brainstem, cerebral hemispheres, spinal cord, and dorsal root ganglia. Pathologically, it is characterized by perivascular and parenchymal inflammation within multiple areas of the CNS. PEM/PSN is most commonly associated with lung carcinoma (particularly small cell) but has been reported with numerous other malignancies as well (22). As with PCD, the neurologic syndrome precedes the diagnosis of cancer in most patients (38).

The clinical manifestations depend on the area of involvement, and a given patient often develops signs and symptoms reflecting multifocal involvement of the nervous system. Limbic encephalopathy with subacute dementia, mood changes, and seizures is common, as is a pancerebellar syndrome, which can be clinically identical to that seen with PCD. Another clinical presentation is a rapidly ascending myelopathy with evidence of upper and lower motor neuron dysfunction, incontinence, and rising sensory level. Patients with dorsal root ganglionitis present with severe sensory ataxia, pseudoathetosis, painful paresthesias, and signs of autonomic dysfunction. A small percentage of patients with PEM/PSN will also develop LEMS.

Diagnosis

The results of neuroimaging are usually normal, although some patients have been reported to have nonspecific T2 signal abnormalities, with minimal or no enhancement within the temporal lobes, brainstem, or spinal cord. The CSF usually shows nonspecific inflammation with a lymphocytic pleocytosis and elevated protein level, but it may be normal. In patients with limbic encephalopathy, the electroencephalogram may show epileptiform changes, diffuse slowing, or both. Nerve conduction studies will show markedly reduced or absent sensory nerve action potentials in patients with PSN. Occasionally, reduction is seen in the compound muscle action potentials (CMAP) and evidence of denervation on needle examination.

The anti-Hu (ANNA-1) antibody is present in the serum and CSF of some patients with PEM/PSN. The antibody indicates that the patient likely harbors a bronchogenic carcinoma (usually small cell) (14). Anti-Yo, anti-Ri, anti-CRMP5, and anti-Ta are other antibodies that may be present in PEM/PSN, indicate underlying gynecologic, breast, lung, and testicular tumors, respectively. Many patients with PEM/PSN will not have serum or CSF antibodies, and their absence does not exclude the possibility of paraneoplastic disease.

A careful search for malignancy is required in any patient in whom PEM/PSN is suspected. If one of the specific antibodies is present, this will guide the search. If the patient is seronegative, a CT of the chest, abdomen, and pelvis is indicated in all patients. In men, a testicular ultrasound is advisable, and women should have a mammogram.

Treatment and Results

With most patients, the PEM/PSN disorder will progress rapidly over a period of weeks to the point of severe disability, and then stabilize. Some patients may die of complications of their neurologic illness such as aspiration and pulmonary embolus. Most patients will not respond to immunosuppressive therapy or plasmapheresis (58). Rarely, clinical improvement will occur if the underlying malignancy is discovered and treated. This seems to be particularly true in patients with PEM and testicular cancer.

PARANEOPLASTIC OPSOCLONUS-MYOCLONUS

POM, a rare but fascinating disorder, presumably is caused by autoimmune injury to the brainstem pause cells controlling conjugate ocular movement. Affected patients have spontaneous, chaotic, conjugate vertical and horizontal eye movements that are worse with fixation. These movements persist during sleep and eye closure. Cerebellar ataxia, myoclonus, and evidence of more diffuse CNS involvement may be present with dementia or altered sensorium. In adults, this syndrome is most commonly associated with small-cell lung cancer and breast cancer. Most patients develop the neurologic syndrome before the diagnosis of cancer.

As with other paraneoplastic syndromes, the neuroimaging and CSF examination are either normal or nonspecifically abnormal. Patients with small-cell lung cancer usually have anti-Hu antibody in the serum, CSF, or both, and patients with breast cancer are typically seropositive for anti-Ri. A careful search for malignancy is warranted because these patients seem more likely to improve neurologically with treatment of their cancers than other patients with paraneoplastic syndromes. As with other paraneoplastic syndromes, immunosuppressive therapy does not appear to be effective.

LAMBERT-EATON MYASTHENIC SYNDROME

LEMS is the only neurologic paraneoplastic disorder in which circulating antibodies have been demonstrated to produce clinical disease. The antibodies are directed against the VGCC on the presynaptic cholinergic nerve terminal. These calcium channels are involved in the release of acetylcholine at the neuromuscular junction, and their blockade results in muscle weakness that improves somewhat with repeated muscle contraction (facilitation). Acetylcholine release at other sites (muscarinic and nicotinic) in the peripheral nervous system is affected, resulting in autonomic dysfunction with dry eyes and mouth, incontinence, erectile dysfunction, postural hypotension, gastroparesis, and reduced sweating. LEMS is most closely associated with small-cell lung cancer, although only 50% to 60% of patients with LEMS harbor an underlying cancer.

The usual clinical presentation of LEMS is with proximal limb weakness, sometimes with myalgias and autonomic dysfunction. Ocular and pharyngeal weakness is relatively rare. The deep tendon reflexes are usually absent or markedly reduced.

Diagnosis

The diagnosis is confirmed with nerve conduction studies, which demonstrate low CMAP with low-frequency repetitive stimulation that repair with exercise and with rapid repetitive stimulation. Ninety percent will have anti-VGCC antibodies in the serum. The titer of the antibody does not correlate with disease severity. A careful search for bronchogenic carcinoma should be made in all patients with LEMS, particularly if they are or have been smokers.

Treatment and Results

The only paraneoplastic neurologic disorder that clearly responds to immunosuppressive treatment is LEMS. However, in patients who are found to have an underlying cancer, the first step in treatment is to treat the malignancy. Some patients will experience remission with treatment of their underlying cancer. Guanidine hydrochloride and 3, 4-diaminopyridine improve neuromuscular transmission by enhancing the release of acetylcholine. Pyridostigmine, an acetylcholinesterase inhibitor, is moderately helpful and can be used in conjunction with these medications. Immunosuppressive therapy, including IVIG, plasma exchange, corticosteroids, and azathioprine, may be used but should be reserved for patients who have not improved despite treatment of their malignancy. Most patients will have some persistence of signs and symptoms despite maximal treatment.

PRIMARY BRAIN TUMORS

As alluded to in the introduction to this chapter, primary brain tumors make up a small percentage of all cancer in the elderly. The incidence of malignant glioma and PCNSL has been steadily increasing over the last 20 years in the elderly for reasons that remain unclear. The most common primary brain tumors in the elderly are meningioma, glioma, vestibular schwannoma, pituitary adenoma, and PCNSL. This section focuses on meningioma, glioma, and CNS lymphoma because the management and prognosis of these tumors in elderly patients may differ from younger patients.

MENINGIOMA

Histologically, the most common primary brain tumor in the elderly is meningioma. Depending on the series cited, meningiomas account for as many as 50% of brain tumors diagnosed in the elderly (34). In autopsy series, this tumor was seen in as many as 1% to 2% of individuals (41,51). Meningiomas are more common in women by a factor of 3:1. Although they can occur at any age, they are most commonly diagnosed in the sixth and seventh decades of life.

Meningiomas derive from the arachnoid cap cells of the arachnoid granulations. They are most commonly seen along the cerebral convexities, along the falx cerebri, at the skull base, and in the thoracic spinal canal. Ten percent to 15% of patients may have multiple meningiomas. Although the cause of meningiomas is unknown, they are more common in patients with type 2 neurofibromatosis or breast cancer and those who have been exposed to cranial ionizing radiation (8). Seventy to 80% of meningiomas express progesterone receptors and, to a lesser extent, estrogen and androgen receptors. This feature may account for their preponderance in women and the increased incidence seen in women with a history of breast cancer. Vascular endothelial growth factor (VEGF), platelet-derived growth factor (PDGF), and epidermal growth factor (EGF) receptors may be expressed in some meningiomas. Meningiomas are almost always benign tumors. Atypical or "malignant" meningiomas account for <5% of cases (29).

Clinical Presentation

As many as one third of all meningiomas are asymptomatic at the time of their discovery (34). They are discovered when CT or MRI is performed for unrelated symptoms. In patients with symptomatic meningioma, headache, focal neurologic deficits, and seizure are the most common presenting signs and symptoms. As in the case of metastatic tumors, elderly patients may be less likely to present with signs of raised intracranial pressure and more likely to present with symptoms of cognitive decline and personality change. The classic bifrontal falcine or skull base meningioma commonly presents in this fashion. Because meningioma is a slow-growing tumor in most cases, the symptoms have often been present for many months before being diagnosed.

Diagnosis

CT and MRI are the most useful diagnostic procedures. Without contrast, CT often shows a calcified extra-axial, dural-based mass, with compression of the underlying brain, sometimes associated with peritumoral edema. With contrast, the tumor will enhance homogenously, and the presence of a "dural tail" of enhancement may be noted (Fig. 28-5). On noncontrast

Figure 28-5. Falcine meningioma. Axial and coronal MRI of the head: T1-weighted images with gadolinium contrast demonstrating a large, homogeneously enhancing mass arising from the falx with compression of adjacent brain. Note the enhancement of the adjacent dura on the coronal view (the dural "tail").

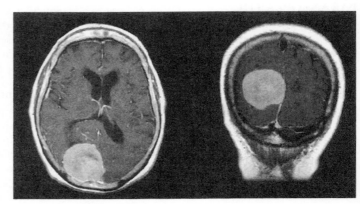

MRI, the tumor is relatively isointense with brain on T1- and T2-weighted images. With contrast, the tumor intensely and uniformly enhances and the aforementioned dural tail may be seen. MRI offers the advantage of visualizing the tumor in different planes and assessing the patency of any adjacent dural sinus, which meningiomas commonly invade and occlude. The tumor compresses but remains well demarcated from the underlying brain. Invasion of the underlying brain may suggest the presence of an atypical or malignant meningioma or an alternative diagnosis such as a dural metastasis from carcinoma or lymphoma.

Treatment

It is often best to observe small, asymptomatic tumors if serial CT or MRI of the head shows no evidence of tumor growth. This is particularly true in frail elderly patients where perioperative morbidity can be high (34), particularly in those with skull base lesions. In symptomatic meningiomas, surgical resection is the best treatment for patients with tumors of the convexity, anterior cranial fossa, anterior falx cerebri, foramen magnum, and spinal canal. In these areas, complete resection is often possible with low risk to the surrounding neural structures. In patients with tumors in the sphenoid wing, cavernous sinus, clivus, cerebellopontine angle, and posterior falx with involvement of the superior sagittal sinus, an attempt at an aggressive resection carries a high risk of cranial nerve deficits and brain injury. In these patients, either a less aggressive surgical approach or nonsurgical treatment may be indicated. It is important to keep in mind that elderly patients have a higher risk of surgical morbidity and mortality from medical complications than younger patients (3,17).

External-beam radiation therapy may be an alternative to surgery in some symptomatic patients, particularly in patients felt to be poor operative candidates either because of the location of the tumor or the patient's medical condition. Postoperative radiation may be required for cases in which a large amount of residual tumor remains or if the tumor recurs after surgery. Local control of tumor with radiation in these instances appears to be good (40,59). Adjuvant radiation therapy is indicated in patients with atypical or malignant meningiomas because the recurrence rate in these tumors is much higher. Radiosurgery with stereotactic linear accelerator or gamma knife appears to offer similar results, with less risk of radiation injury to the surrounding brain (33).

The role of chemotherapy in meningioma is not well defined. The antiprogestin, mifepristone (RU-486), has not yet been shown to be useful in the reatment of meningioma. Some preliminary evidence indicated that hydroxyurea, an inhibitor of DNA synthesis, may be a helpful adjuvant in the treatment of unresectable or recurrent meningioma, although these results have not been duplicated (39,57).

GLIOMA

Gliomas are tumors derived from the neuroglial cells: astrocytes, oligodendrocytes, and ependymal cells. A variety of classification systems exist, although these tumors are basically divided into low grade and high grade, depending on the presence of various histologic features, including pleomorphism, mitoses, necrosis, and vascular proliferation. Tumor cellular morphology and grading is important in predicting survival and selecting treatment. The factors most important in determining prognosis are patient age, tumor histology, and performance status. Extent of tumor resection can also be important prognostically, although primarily in younger patients. Of these factors, age appears to be paramount; patients >60 years of age generally fare worse than younger patients with the same tumor histology and performance status. In elderly patients, the most common glioma is a malignant glioma, including glioblastoma multiforme, anaplastic astrocytoma, anaplastic oligodendroglioma, and anaplastic mixed glioma. Glioblastoma, the most common form, carries the worst prognosis. Low-grade gliomas are rare in older patients. When they occur, their behavior is often more aggressive than that seen in younger patients.

The cause of glioma is unknown. An increased risk of glioma development is seen many years after receiving ionizing radiation to the head. Some evidence links large environmental exposures to electromagnetic fields and some chemicals to glioma (66). Some heritable syndromes have a higher risk of glioma, including Turcot's syndrome, Li-Fraumeni syndrome, and neurofibromatosis, although these usually present with brain tumors in younger adults. In most elderly patients, gliomas are entirely sporadic occurrences.

Clinical Presentation

Similar to metastatic tumors, the most common presenting symptoms of glioma in elderly patients are mental status changes, seizure, and focal neurologic deficits. Headache and other symptoms of raised intracranial pressure are distinctly less common than in younger patients but do occur. Elderly patients generally have some degree of brain atrophy and, thus, are better able to accommodate an expanding mass without early signs and symptoms of raised intracranial pressure. It is extremely common for the symptoms of glioma in the elderly to be initially mistaken for stroke or degenerative dementia.

Figure 28-6. Malignant glioma. Axial MRI of the head: T1-weighted image with gadolinium contrast and T2-weighted image. Note the large area of central necrosis, the enhancing rim, and the relatively small amount of surrounding edema.

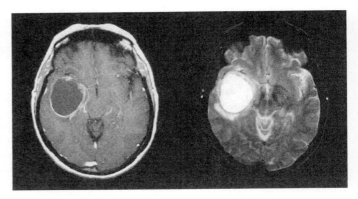

Diagnosis

The diagnostic studies of choice are CT or MRI of the head with contrast. Both will demonstrate edema and mass effect. Glioblastoma almost always enhances with contrast and typically has an area of central necrosis (Fig. 28-6). Low-grade gliomas are less likely to enhance. Unlike brain metastases, gliomas are usually solitary and have a more infiltrative appearance of the edema and contrast enhancement. Gliomas commonly spread along white matter tracts and may cross the corpus callosum.

A definitive diagnosis requires surgery. Although aggressive resection has been generally recommended in patients with both low- and high-grade glioma, the benefit in patients over 65 years of age is not clear (32). Certainly, in the extreme elderly (80+ years), aggressive resection is probably best replaced by a simple biopsy.

Treatment and Results

Biopsy is necessary to make a definitive diagnosis. As noted, more aggressive resection, which improves survival in younger patients (35), does not appear to do so in the elderly. Kelly and Hunt (32) noted that patients over 65 years of age who had aggressive resection of their malignant gliomas survived a mean of only 13 weeks longer than similar-aged patients who had only biopsy and similar postoperative therapy.

Radiation therapy is appropriate for most patients and does prolong survival to a modest degree. The standard therapy is 60 Gy of external-beam radiation in 30 to 33 fractions to encompass the postoperative tumor volume as seen on MRI or CT, with a margin of several centimeters. In elderly patients with malignant glioma and a poor performance status whose survival is expected to be particularly limited, a shortened course of radiation with larger fractions may be as effective (7). The incidence of radiation-induced leukoencephalopathy with cognitive changes is higher in elderly patients. However, because survival is limited in most elderly patients with GBM, this is not usually a major practical concern.

The response to chemotherapy in elderly patients is even more disappointing than the response to radiation therapy. Even in younger patients, only about 30% of patients will respond to chemotherapy, and the percentage is probably lower in elderly patients. Until recently, standard chemotherapy was with nitrosoureas (carmustine or lomustine). Since 2005, temozolomide has become the standard drug for treatment of high-grade glioma. This was based on the results of a phase III study comparing single-agent temozolomide with radiation followed by adjuvant temozolomide for 6 months to surgery and radiation alone in the treatment of glioblastoma multiforme. The median survival of patients receiving temozolomide was 2.4 months longer than patients receiving radiation alone. Temozolomide is an oral drug and is generally better tolerated than the nitrosoureas. Other drugs shown to have some activity against glioblastoma include procarbazine, cisplatin, irinotecan, and etoposide. A number of novel agents are currently under investigation for the treatment of malignant glioma (52). The most promising are drugs that target tumor growth factor receptors and their tyrosine kinase–based intracellular signaling pathways. Most malignant gliomas are dependent on growth factor stimulation for tumor growth and invasion. The most important growth factors in gliomas appear to be VEGF, EGF, and PDGF.

Even with aggressive surgery, radiation, and chemotherapy, malignant glioma is virtually always fatal. In patients over 65 years of age, median survival is 6 to 8 months, and very few longer term survivors are seen in this age group.

PRIMARY CENTRAL NERVOUS SYSTEM LYMPHOMA

Human immunodeficiency virus infection and chronic immunosuppression necessitated by organ transplantation, autoimmune disease, and cancer chemotherapy are factors that directly increase the risk of developing PCNSL, a relatively rare neoplasm. The incidence of this malignancy is on the rise, even in patients who are immunocompetent (18,65). In this latter group, advanced age appears to be the common factor. Most patients who are immunocompetent who develop PCNSL are 50 years of age or older. Latent Epstein-Barr infection is implicated as a cause of PCNSL in patients who are immunocompromised but not in those who are immunocompetent.

PCNSL is usually of B-cell origin and can develop anywhere within the CNS. The tumor is often multi-focal and has a proclivity to the periventricular white matter and basal ganglia. Leptomeningeal spread occurs in approximately 10% of patients, and as many as 10% to 20% of patients will have involvement of the vitreous humor of the eye (27).

Clinical Presentation

Progressive focal neurologic deficits and neuropsychiatric dysfunction are the most common presenting symptoms (60). Headache and seizures do occur but are less common, particularly in the elderly. In those with ocular involvement, visual obscuration, "floaters," or visual loss can occur; in those with leptomeningeal involvement, cranial neuropathies and spinal polyradiculopathies are common.

Diagnosis

In patients with PCNSL, head CT and MRI with contrast will demonstrate one or more homogeneously enhancing lesions, usually involving deep white matter or the basal ganglia (Fig. 28-7). The lesions tend to abut the ventricular surface. MRI is superior in defining the presence of leptomeningeal deposits and spinal cord involvement. PCNSL in patients who are immunocompromised often shows

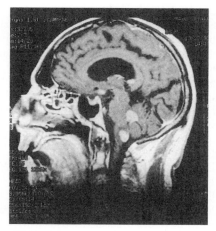

Figure 28-7. Primary central nervous system lymphoma. Sagittal MRI of the head: T1-weighted image with gadolinium contrast. Note the multiple enhancing lesions in the brainstem, fourth ventricle, corpus callosum, thalamus, and infundibulum.

central necrosis with ring enhancement. This imaging pattern is distinctly unusual in patients who are immunocompetent.

If PCNSL is suspected, MRI of the entire neuraxis is indicated for staging purposes. CSF examination, if it can be safely performed, may reveal lymphomatous involvement in 10% to 20% of patients. Obviously, lumbar puncture is contraindicated in those with significant supratentorial or posterior fossa mass effect and impending herniation. Slit lamp examination of the eyes is necessary for staging, and occasionally, vitreous aspiration and cytologic examination yield the diagnosis.

Approximately 4% of patients presenting with brain lymphoma will be found to have occult systemic lymphoma (43). These patients have metastatic systemic lymphoma and not PCNSL. To exclude this possibility, CT of the chest, abdomen, and pelvis; bone marrow examination; and, in men, testicular ultrasound are indicated as part of the staging process.

Assuming that no systemic disease is found, the vitreous is clear of cells, and CSF cytology is negative, diagnostic stereotactic biopsy of the brain lesion is indicated. Aggressive resection of PCNSL is not recommended. Extent of resection is not a prognostic variable, and attempts at resection often lead to disabling or fatal brain hemorrhage.

If PCNSL is suspected, it is best to avoid the preoperative use of corticosteroids, unless the patient is in imminent danger of herniation. Corticosteroids exert a tumor-lytic effect on lymphoma. Treatment with corticosteroids before biopsy can produce a rapid and dramatic tumor response and render the biopsy nondiagnostic. If the patient must receive corticosteroids, the biopsy should proceed as quickly as possible, assuming the targeted lesion is present on reimaging.

Pathologic examination of the tumor will usually reveal atypical lymphocytes in a perivascular location. Immunohistochemistry will reveal these to be monoclonal B cells, sometimes with reactive T cells intermixed. Epstein-Barr viral genome is commonly found within lymphoma cells in patients who are immunocompromised but not in the sporadic PCNSL found in those who are immunocompetent.

Treatment and Results

As in malignant glioma, age and performance status are important prognostic factors in patients with PCNSL. Historically, among patients older than 60 years, the median survival was <1 year, even with maximal therapy (13). Moreover, few long-term survivors were seen in this group of patients.

Previously, radiation was considered the primary therapy for PCNSL. More recently, chemotherapy has been found to have a clear role in treatment. The approach in patients who are immunocompetent is to treat with chemotherapy first and then proceed with WBRT at the time of tumor recurrence. High-dose intravenous methotrexate is now the standard of care in the initial treatment of PCNSL. Other standard drugs used in the treatment of systemic non-Hodgkin lymphoma are largely ineffective in treating PCNSL. High-dose methotrexate alone significantly prolonged survival with or without WBRT. The median survival in patients over age 60 was 32 months, and patients who received chemotherapy alone experienced less neurotoxicity than those who had received methotrexate followed by WBRT (19). The addition of WBRT in patients with a complete response to high-dose methotrexate did not prolong survival. Leptomeningeal spread is best treated either with high-dose intravenous methotrexate or intra-CSF methotrexate via Ommaya reservoir.

Although PCNSL often responds well to chemotherapy and/or radiation, it virtually always recurs. Treatment-related neurotoxicity is common in those patients who do survive for more than 1 year. Leuko-encephalopathy with subcortical dementia, gait apraxia, and incontinence is more common in elderly patients who have received WBRT than in younger patients who have received WBRT, with or without chemotherapy (9).

In frail elderly patients with very poor performance status, the expectations from treatment in PCNSL are limited. In these patients, it may be appropriate to advise supportive care only. Some benefit and little risk may be seen in giving pulse doses of corticosteroids (1 g intravenous methylprednisolone monthly) (44) to these patients at high risk of developing treatment-related toxicity from other modalities.

CONCLUSION

The diagnosis and care of elderly patients with primary and metastatic tumors of the nervous system and neurologic complications of systemic cancer are challenging. These disorders can present differently in elderly patients, and as with other neurologic disorders, elderly patients generally fare worse than their younger counterparts. Some cancer treatments are less effective or have greater toxicity in the elderly. The expanding numbers of older patients and the increasing incidence of brain tumors specific to this population require that the practicing neurologist be aware of the diagnostic and therapeutic issues unique to these patients.

REFERENCES

1. Amer MH, Al-Sarraf M, Baker LH, et al. Malignant melanoma and central nervous system metastases: incidence, diagnosis, treatment, and survival. *Cancer*. 1978;42:660–668.

2. Avrahami E, Weiss-Peretz J, Cohn DF. Epilepsy in patients with brain metastases triggered by intravenous contrast medium. *Clin Radiol*. 1989; 40:422–423.

3. Awad IA, Kalfas I, Hahn JF, et al. Intracranial meningiomas in the aged: surgical outcome in the era of computed tomography. *Neurosurgery*. 1989;24:557–560.

4. Bach F, Larsen BH, Rohde K, et al. Metastatic spinal cord compression. Occurrence, symptoms, clinical presentations and prognosis in 398 patients with spinal cord compression. *Acta Neurochir*. 1990;107:37–43.

5. Baharav E, Harpaz M, Mittelman M, et al. Dexamethasone-induced perineal irritation. *N Engl J Med*. 1986;314:515–516.

6. Balm M, Hammack J. Leptomeningeal carcinomatosis. Presenting features and prognostic factors. *Arch Neurol*. 1996;53:626–632.

7. Bauman GS, Gaspar LE, Fisher BJ, et al A prospective study of short-course radiotherapy in poor prognosis glioblastoma multiforme. *Int J Radiat Oncol Biol Phys*. 1994;29:835–839.

8. Black PM. Meningiomas. *Neurosurgery*. 1993; 32:643–657.

9. Blumenthal DT, DeAngelis LM. Aging and primary central nervous system neoplasms. *Neurol Clin North Am*. 1998;16:671–686.

10. Byrne TN, Cascino TL, Posner JB. Brain metastasis from melanoma. *J Neurooncol*. 1983;1: 313–317.

11. Cavaliere R, Schiff D. Cerebral metastases—a therapeutic update. *Nat Clin Pract Neurol*. 2006; 2:426–436.

12. Chamberlain M. Neoplastic meningitis. *Neurologist*. 2006;12:179–187.

13. Corry J, Smith JG, Wirth A, et al. Primary central nervous system lymphoma: age and performance status are more important than treatment modality. *Int J Radiat Oncol Biol Phys*. 1998; 41:615–620.

14. Dalmau J, Graus F, Rosenblum MK, et al. Anti-Hu-associated paraneoplastic encephalomyelitis/sensory neuronopathy. A clinical study of 71 patients. *Medicine*. 1992;71:59–72.

15. Delattre J-Y, Krol G, Thaler HT, et al. Distribution of brain metastases. *Arch Neurol*. 1988;45:741–744.

16. Delattre J-Y, Safai B, Posner JB. Erythema multiforme and Stevens-Johnson syndrome in patients receiving cranial irradiation and phenytoin. *Neurology*. 1988;38:194–198.

17. Djindjian M, Caron JP, Athayde AA, et al. Intracranial meningiomas in the elderly (over 70 years old): a retrospective study of 30 surgical cases. *Acta Neurochir*. 1988;90:121–123.

18. Eby NL, Grufferman S, Flannelly CM, et al. Increasing incidence of primary brain lymphoma in the US. *Cancer*. 1988;62:2461–2465.

19. Ferreri AJ, Abrey LE, Blay J-V, et al. Summary statement on primary central nervous system lymphomas from the Eighth International Conference on Malignant Lymphoma, Lugano, Switzerland, June 12 to 15, 2002. *J Clin Oncol*. 2003;21:2407–2414.

20. Forsyth PA, Weaver S, Fulton D, et al. Prophylactic anticonvulsants in patients with brain tumour. *Can J Neurol Sci*. 2003;30:106–112.

21. Furneaux HM, Rosenblum MK, Dalmau J, et al. Selective expression of Purkinje cell antigens in tumor tissue from patients with paraneoplastic cerebellar degeneration. *N Engl J Med*. 1990; 322:1844–1851.

22. Graus F, Keime-Guibert F, Rene R, et al. Anti-Hu-associated paraneoplastic encephalomyelitis: analysis of 200 patients. *Brain*. 2001;124: 1138–1148.

23. Hammack JE, Kimmel DW, O'Neill BP, et al. Paraneoplastic cerebellar degeneration: a clinical comparison of patients with and without Purkinje cell cytoplasmic antibodies. *Mayo Clin Proc*. 1990;65:1423–1431.

24. Helweg-Larsen S, Sorensen PS. Symptoms and signs in metastatic spinal cord compression: a study of progression from first symptom until diagnosis in 153 patients. *Eur J Cancer*. 1994; 30A:396–398.

25. Hess KR, Broglio KR, Bondy ML. Adult glioma incidence trends in the United States, 1977–2000. *Cancer*. 2004;101:2293–2299.

26. Hetzel DJ, Stanhope R, O'Neill BP, et al. Gynecologic cancer in patients with subacute cerebellar degeneration predicted by anti-Purkinje cell antibodies and limited in metastatic volume. *Mayo Clin Proc*. 1990;65:1558–1563.

27. Hochberg FH, Miller DH. Primary central nervous system lymphoma. *J Neurosurg*. 1988;68: 835–853.

28. Hoffman S, Propp JM, McCarthy BJ. Temporal trends in incidence of primary brain tumors in the United States, 1985–1999. *Neuro Oncol*. 2006;8:27–37.

29. Jaaskelainen J, Haltia M, Servo A. Atypical and anaplastic meningiomas: radiology, surgery, radiotherapy and outcome. *Surg Neurol*. 1986; 25:233–242.

30. Jukich PJ, McCarthy BJ, Surawicz TS, et al. Trends in incidence of primary brain tumors in the United States,1985–1994. *Neuro Oncol*. 2001;3:141–151.

31. Keime-Guibert F, Graus F, Fleury A, et al. Treatment of paraneoplastic neurological syndromes with antineuronal antibodies (anti-Hu, anti-Yo) with a combination of immunoglobulins, cyclophosphamide, and methylprednisolone. *J Neurol Neurosurg Psychiatry*. 2000;68:479–482.

32. Kelly PJ, Hunt C. The limited value of cytoreductive surgery in elderly patients with malignant gliomas. *Neurosurgery*. 1994;34:62–67.

33. Kondziolka D, Lunsford LD, Coffey RJ, et al. Stereotactic radiosurgery of meningiomas. *J Neurosurg*. 1991;74:552–559.

34. Kuratsu J, Ushio Y. Epidemiological study of primary intracranial tumors in elderly people. *J Neurol Neurosurg Psychiatry*. 1997;63:116–118.

35. Lacroix M, Abi-Said M, Fourney DR, et al. A multivariate analysis of 416 patients with glioblastoma multiforme: prognosis, extent of resection, and survival. *J Neurosurg*. 2001;95:190–198.

36. Lassman AB, DeAngelis LM. Brain metastases. *Neurol Clin*. 2003;21:1–23.

37. Lowry JK, Snyder JJ, Lowry PW. Brain tumors in the elderly. *Arch Neurol*. 1998;55:922–928.

38. Lucchinetti CF, Kimmel DW, Lennon VA. Paraneoplastic and oncologic profiles of patients seropositive for type 1 antineuronal nuclear autoantibodies. *Neurology*. 1998;50:652–657.

39. Mason WP, Gentili F, Macdonald DR, et al. Stabilization of disease progression by hydroxyurea in patients with recurrent or unresectable meningioma. *J Neurosurg*. 2002;97:341–346.

40. Mesic JB, Hanks GE, Doggett RL. The value of radiation therapy as an adjuvant to surgery in intracranial meningiomas. *Am J Clin Oncol*. 1986;9:337–340.

41. Nakasu S, Hirano A, Shimura T, et al. Incidental meningiomas in autopsy study. *Surg Neurol*. 1987;27:319–322.

42. O'Neill BP, Buckner JC, Coffey RJ, et al. Brain metastatic lesions. *Mayo Clin Proc*. 1994;69: 1062–1068.

43. O'Neill BP, Dinapoli RP, Kurtin PJ, et al. Occult systemic non-Hodgkin's lymphoma (NHL) in patients initially diagnosed as primary central nervous system lymphoma (PCNSL): how much staging is enough? *J Neurooncol*. 1995;25:67–71.

44. O'Neill BP, Haberman TM, Witzig TE, et al. Prevention of recurrence and prolonged survival in primary central nervous system lymphoma (PCNSL) patients treated with adjuvant high-dose methylprednisolone. *Med Oncol*. 1999;16: 211–215.

45. Patchell RA, Tibbs PA, Regine WF, et al. Postoperative radiotherapy in the treatment of single brain metastases to the brain. *JAMA*. 1998;280:1485–1489.

46. Patchell RA, Tibbs PA, Walsh JW, et al. A randomized trial of surgery in the treatment of

single metastases to the brain. *N Engl J Med.* 1990;322:494–500.

47. Pickren JW, Lopez G, Tsukada Y, et al. Brain metastases: an autopsy study. *Cancer Treat Symp.* 1983;2:295–313.

48. Portenoy RK, Galer BS, Salamon O, et al. Identification of epidural neoplasm: radiography and bone scintigraphy in the symptomatic and asymptomatic spine. *Cancer.* 1989;64:2207–2213.

49. Posner JB. *Paraneoplastic Syndromes. Neurologic Complications of Cancer. Contemporary Neurology Series.* Philadelphia: FA Davis; 1995.

50. Posner JB, Chernik NL. Intracranial metastases from systemic cancer. *Adv Neurol.* 1978;19:575–587.

51. Rausing A, Ybo W, Stenflo J. Intracranial meningioma. A population study of ten years. *Acta Neurol Scand.* 1970;46:102–110.

52. Reardon DA, Rich JN, Friedman HS, et al. Recent advances in the treatment of malignant astrocytoma. *J Clin Oncol.* 2006;24:1253–1265.

53. Ries LAG, Harkins D, Krapcho M, et al., eds. SEER cancer statistics review, 1975–2003, National Cancer Institute, Bethesda, MD. Available at: http: //seer.cancer. gov/csr/ 1975_2003/.

54. Schiff D, O'Neill BP, Wang CH, et al. Neuroimaging and treatment implications of patients with multiple epidural spinal metastases. *Cancer.* 1998;83:1593–1601.

55. Schiff D, Shaw EG, Cascino TL. Outcome after spinal reirradiation for malignant epidural spinal cord compression. *Ann Neurol.* 1995;37:583–589.

56. Schouten LJ, Rutten J, Huveneers HA, et al. Incidence of brain metastases in a cohort of patients with carcinoma of the breast, colon, kidney, and lung and melanoma. *Cancer.* 2002;94:2698–2705.

57. Schrell UM, Rittig MG, Anders M, et al. Hydroxyurea for treatment of unresectable and recurrent meningiomas. II. Decrease in the size of meningiomas in patients treated with hydroxyurea. *J Neurosurg.* 1997;86:840–844.

58. Sellevis Smitt P, Grefkens J, De Leeuw B, et al. Survival and outcome in 73 anti-Hu positive patients with paraneoplastic encephalomyelitis/sensory neuronopathy. *J Neurol.* 2002;249:745–753.

59. Taylor BW, Marcus RB, Friedman WA, et al. The meningioma controversy: postoperative radiation therapy. *Int J Radiat Oncol Biol Phys.* 1988;15:299–304.

60. Tomlinson FH, Kurtin PJ, Suman VJ, et al. Primary intracerebral malignant lymphoma: a clinicopathological study of 89 patients. *J Neurosurg.* 1995;82:558–566.

61. Vecht CJ, Haaxma-Reiche H, Noordijk EM, et al. Treatment of single brain metastasis: radiotherapy alone or combined with neurosurgery? *Ann Neurol.* 1993;3:583–590.

62. Vernino S, O'Neill BP, Marks RS, et al. Immunomodulatory treatment trial for paraneoplastic neurological disorders. *Neuro Oncol.* 2004;6:55–62.

63. Wasserstrom W, Glass JP, Posner JB. Diagnosis and treatment of leptomeningeal metastases from solid tumors: experience with 90 patients. *Cancer.* 1982;49:759–772.

64. Wen PY, Loeffler JS. Management of brain metastases. *Oncology (Williston Park).* 1999;13:941–954,957–961.

65. Werner MH, Phuphanich S, Lyman GH. The increasing incidence of malignant gliomas and primary central nervous system lymphoma in the elderly. *Cancer.* 1995;76:1634–1642.

66. Wrensch M, Bondy ML, Wiecke J, et al. Environmental risk factors for primary malignant brain tumors: a review. *J Neurooncol.* 1993;17:47–64.

WEBSITES

American Brain Tumor Association: http://www.abta.org/

National Cancer Institute: http://www.nci.nih.gov

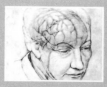

CHAPTER 29

Introduction: Neurologic Manifestations of Systemic Disease

Joseph I. Sirven

Although the practice of clinical neurology often appears as functioning as a separate and independent organ system, the nervous system does not operate in a vacuum. There are numerous relationships between the nervous system and other organ systems, some of which have been recently elucidated, that can lead to a multitude of neurologic manifestations of systemic disease. Indeed, there are several new neurologic problems that are now recognized as being secondary to primary pathology from other organ systems. This chapter surveys the common neurologic manifestations of systemic diseases that commonly occur in the older adult. The chapter will highlight the following organ systems: cardiac, pulmonary, gastrointestinal, endocrine, rheumatologic, immunologic/oncologic, and renal.

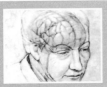

CHAPTER 29.1

Neurologic Manifestations of Systemic Disease: Cardiology and Pulmonary

Mayurkumar D. Bhakta

Although cardiovascular and pulmonary diseases greatly affect multiple organ systems, the neurologic manifestations are one of the most sensitive markers of pathologic disease. Within the cardiopulmonary-vascular system, neurologic changes can be seen every day by all levels of practitioners. These manifestations may be obvious or subtle, but all are important to recognize because they herald important disease states that may be treatable. This chapter will review the most common cardiac and pulmonary diseases that can cause neurologic sequelae.

CARDIAC DISEASES WITH NEUROLOGIC MANIFESTATIONS

The steadily aging population of the United States commonly suffers from some form of cardiac disease. Several of these common cardiac diseases can cause significant neurologic symptoms and possible disability. Cardiogenic embolism to the central nervous system (CNS) is associated with several conditions of the heart including atrial fibrillation (AF), myocardial infarction, cardiac valvular diseases, mitral annular calcification (MAC), mitral valve prolapse (MVP), cardiac valve replacement, left atrial myxoma, dilated cardiomyopathy, patent foramen ovale (PFO), and endocarditis. The results of embolisms can be varied, from transient ischemic attack (TIA) to large ischemic strokes, but their implications are important for both primary and secondary prevention of insults.

Systemic cardiogenic hypoperfusion commonly first manifests with CNS involvement in the form of delirium. Long periods of hypoperfusion, such as those involved with cardiac surgeries and cardiopulmonary bypass machines (CBPs), can also cause neurologic complications that are usually reversible. As the prevalence of coronary artery disease and valvular disease increases, so too will the incidence of cardiac surgeries and, therefore, neurologic involvement in the perioperative and operative period.

CARDIOEMBOLIC STROKE

The diagnosis of cardioembolic stroke is based on the identification of a potential cardiac source combined with the absence of other causes of stroke with variable consideration of neurologic features (25). It is important to identify cardioembolic stroke as a symptom of underlying cardiac disease. Recognition of the different etiologies of cardioembolic stroke will allow one to correctly risk stratify and properly administer the appropriate treatment because cardioembolic strokes may be preventable. There are a myriad of cardiac disease states that can lead to cardioembolic stroke. These include rhythm disorders (AF, atrial flutter, sick sinus syndrome), valvular disease (endocarditis, prosthetic cardiac valves, etc.), and structural abnormalities (cardiac tumors, PFO, atrial septal aneurysm).

Atrial Fibrillation

AF is the most common sustained cardiac arrhythmia, with estimations that >2 million Americans are currently afflicted (15). In population-based cohorts, 10% of all ischemic strokes are probably caused by AF, and the prevalence sharply increases with age. Nearly one third of patients older than 70 years of age with ischemic stroke have AF, and for those older than 75, AF is the leading cause of ischemic stroke (15). The main mechanism involved in AF-related cardioembolic disease is reduced contractility of the left atrial appendage, favoring stasis and thrombus formation (26). There are likely other underlying mechanisms of atrial thrombus formation given the low risk of stroke in patients with "lone AF" compared with "high-risk" groups in persistent AF, but these are yet to be identified.

The overall rate of ischemic stroke among patients with AF varies widely, ranging from 0.5% per year in patients with lone AF to 12% per year for patients with previous TIAs or strokes (15). Classifying patients with AF as low, moderate, or high risk of cardioembolism is paramount for primary prevention. A recent review of classification schemes identified the single most useful model and termed it the

Table 29-1. *CHADS Criteria*

Criteria	Description	Score
Congestive heart failure (CHF)	Recent history of CHF exacerbation	1
Hypertension	History of hypertension	1
Age	Age >75	1
Diabetes	History of either type 1 or type 2 diabetes	1
Stroke	Any history of prior cerebrovascular disease	2
Sum		6 or less

From Gage BG, Waterman AD, Shannon W, et al. Validation of clinical classification schemes for predicting stroke: results from the National Registry of Atrial Fibrillation. *JAMA.* 2001;285:2864–2870.

CHADS-2 score (Table 29-1) (18). In this model, the physician assigns 1 point each for the presence of congestive heart failure (CHF), hypertension, age of 75 years or older, and diabetes mellitus. In addition, the patient will be assigned 2 points for prior history of stroke or TIA. The sum of these points will then stratify the patients as being at a low, medium, or high risk. Patients with a score of 0 to 1 are low risk, with annual stroke risk being 1.9% to 2.8% per year, respectively. Intermediate risk is a score of 2 to 3 points, with annual risk being 4.0% to 5.9%. Any score from 4 to 6 is deemed to be high risk, with an annual stroke risk from 8.5% to 18.2%. Based on these scoring criteria, patients in the high-risk group should undergo anticoagulation with vitamin K antagonists, moderate-risk patients' anticoagulation should be individualized, and low-risk patients could possibly be managed with minimal anticoagulation alone in the form of aspirin.

For many years, patients in AF were cardioverted back to sinus rhythm and placed on antiarrhythmic medications for maintenance of the rhythm. The problem was the toxic effects of the antiarrhythmics on other organ systems. The Atrial Fibrillation Follow-Up Investigation of Rhythm Management (AFFIRM) trial compared mortality in patients who were cardioverted and maintained in sinus rhythm versus rate controlling with adequate anticoagulation. This multicenter study showed that there was no statistical difference in mortality or occurrence of stroke in either category, making rate control with adequate anticoagulation with warfarin a safe choice. The authors of the final publication also recommended anticoagulation in cardioverted patients based on risk stratification schemes.

For moderate- and high-risk patients per the CHADS-2 criteria, warfarin is the first-line therapy, with a target international normalized ratio (INR) of 2.0 to 3.0 (2). Patients who present with a stroke in AF should undergo a thorough evaluation to exclude ipsilateral severe atherosclerotic disease prior to initiation of therapy. If evaluation of stroke patients shows no further disease, anticoagulation with aspirin should be started immediately, and warfarin should be started as soon as the patient is medically stable and the cerebral edema from infarct has resolved (27).

Atrial Flutter

Atrial flutter is not as common of a persistent arrhythmia as AF, and there is no strong evidence to suggest its embolic potential. Studies that have looked at its embolic potential have been confounded by the presence of paroxysmal AF along with the atrial flutter (25). Recommendations in primary prevention of cardioembolic disease secondary to this rhythm are based more on the high prevalence of coexistent AF than the atrial flutter itself. Thus, warfarin adjusted to an INR 2.0 to 3.0 is the current recommendation.

Sick Sinus Syndrome

Sick sinus syndrome, also known as "tachy-brady syndrome," is characterized by fluctuations in heart rate that vary from pauses to tachycardia and possibly AF. The thromboembolic event rate in sick sinus syndrome is 5% to 10% per year (25). Atrial pacemaker insertion is associated with lower stroke rates but does not eliminate the need for anticoagulation. The need for anticoagulation is likely secondary to the high incidence of recurrent AF. The risk for stroke should be assessed as it would be for AF, and anticoagulation should be tailored as such.

Endocarditis

Infective endocarditis is defined as an infection of the heart valves (native and prosthetic), endothelial surfaces (myocardial and valvular structures), and implanted devices (pacemakers, etc.). This diagnosis should be suspected when patients present with acute onset of high fever, rigors, malaise, and new heart murmur. Headache and mental status changes are also common manifestations.

Embolization of vegetations (i.e., endocardial growths) is the second most frequent complication of endocarditis, with stroke being the commonly observed major consequence of the emboli. *Staphylococcus aureus* infection is associated with the highest stroke rate. The risk of embolization is higher with vegetations of the mitral valve than the aortic valve (3). Embolization tends to occur most commonly at

Table 29-2. *The Duke Criteria*

Major Criteria	Minor Criteria
Typical micro-organism isolated from two separate blood cultures, or micro-organism isolated from persistently positive blood cultures, or single positive blood culture for *Coxiella burnetii* (or phase 1 IgG antibody titer to *C. burnetii* >1:800) Evidence of endocardial involvement such as new valvular regurgitation, intracardiac mass, periannular abscess, or new dehiscence of prosthetic valve	Predisposition to infective endocarditis such as previous history of infective endocarditis, injective drug use, prosthetic heart valve, mitral valve prolapse, cyanotic congenital heart disease, or cardiac lesions creating turbulent flow Persistent fever Vascular phenomena (embolic disease) Immunologic phenomena such as Osler nodes, Roth spots, glomerulonephritis, etc. Microbiologic findings of atypical organisms (i.e., HACEK organisms)

HACEK, *Haemophilus* species, *Actinobacillus actinomycetemcomitans*, *Cardiobacterium hominis*, *Eikenella corrodens*, and *Kingella* species.
From Li JS, Sexton DJ, Mick N, et al. Proposed modifications to the Duke criteria for the diagnosis of infective endocarditis. *Clin Infect Dis.* 2000;30:633–638.

presentation or within 2 days of initiation of antibiotic therapy (12). Cerebral infarction due to emboli or mycotic aneurysm is the presenting sign of endocarditis in 14% of cases (29). The rate of embolic events decreases from 13 events per 1,000 patient days in the first week to <1.2 events per 1,000 patient days after 2 weeks of therapy with the appropriate antibiotic therapy (28). Given the rapid response to appropriate antibiotic therapy, anticoagulation is not necessary. If patients have mechanical valve endocarditis, anticoagulation should not be interrupted. The expected response to therapeutics requires prompt diagnosis of endocarditis when suspected. The most sensitive and specific method for diagnosing endocarditis was devised by Durak et al. (13) from Duke University Medical Center and is now known simply as the Duke Criteria. These criteria have been recently modified to increase sensitivity and specificity and have now become the standard of diagnosis (Table 29-2) (33).

Embolization of septic vegetation is not without its sequelae, especially in the CNS. Embolization to an arterial intraluminal space or to the vasa vasorum of the cerebral vessels can lead to mycotic aneurysms. These aneurysms carry the risk of rupture and intracranial and subarachnoid hemorrhage. The symptoms associated with a mycotic aneurysm are those associated with aneurysms and subarachnoid hemorrhages, namely meningeal irritation from either an acute or chronic leak into the CNS. Mycotic aneurysms account for 15% of all neurologic complications of endocarditis (39). If mycotic aneurysms are suspected, magnetic resonance imaging (MRI) is superior

to computed tomography (CT) for microabscess and aneurysm detection and should be used whenever possible.

Nonbacterial thrombotic endocarditis (NBTE) is caused by vegetations on the heart valves, without evidence of a causative infectious organism. This syndrome occurs more commonly in older individuals and is often associated with neoplasia, disseminated intravascular coagulation, or chronic illness. The primary neurologic complication of NBTE is embolism, which occurs in approximately 42% of cases (35). Diagnosis of NBTE is often difficult and involves a search for infectious causes first. Treatment is aimed at control of the underlying condition, and anticoagulation is recommended if embolization has occurred (51).

Myocardial Infarction

Cardioembolic stroke occurs in approximately 1% of hospitalized patients with myocardial infarction (8). The types of infarction that carry the highest risk of cardioembolism are transmural, apical, and anterolateral, with an increase in risk in patients with CHF or prior history of embolic stroke. The postulated mechanism is thrombus formation in the akinetic ventricle, followed by secondary embolism. Risk stratification of stroke during the acute phase of myocardial infarction includes both clinical and echocardiographic parameters (Table 29-3) (36). Anticoagulation with full-dose heparin followed by warfarin (INR = 2.0 to 3.0) for up to 3 months is recommended for patients who are at high risk (10). The long-term rate of ischemic stroke after myocardial infarction is 1% to 2% per year in the

Table 29-3. *Risk Factors for Nonhemorrhagic Stroke*

Baseline patient risk factors for nonhemorrhagic stroke following an acute myocardial infarction
Older age
Higher heart rate
History of stroke or transient ischemic attack
Diabetes
Previous angina
Hypertension

In-hospital characteristics associated with higher risk of nonhemorrhagic stroke following an acute myocardial infarction
Worse Killip class
Atrial fibrillation/flutter
Bypass surgery
Cardiac catheterization

From Mahaffey K, Granger CH, Sloan M, et al. Risk factors for in-hospital nonhemorrhagic stroke in patients with acute myocardial infarction treated with thrombolysis: results from GUSTO-1. *Circulation.* 1998;97:757–764.

absence of CHF, and aspirin therapy is advocated. No randomized trial comparing warfarin to aspirin in patients with CHF has been performed to determine the best treatment, but most cardiologists recommend warfarin treatment empirically (34).

Cardiac Valvular Disease

Mitral stenosis from rheumatic fever carries an increased risk of cardioembolic stroke, but no good estimates of absolute stroke rates are available. The risk increases at least 5% per year when associated with AF. Although evidence-based data are not available, warfarin therapy (INR = 2.0 to 3.0) for patients with rheumatic heart disease and AF has been recommended, with anticoagulation for patients without AF being less clear (24).

MVP is a common form of valvular disease present in approximately 6% of women and 4% of men (51). It is unclear as to whether MVP truly increases the risk of stroke. A recent study of stroke patients showed that the frequency of MVP (5%) is not increased when compared with control groups (5%) (19). In young patients with MVP, the coexistence of atrial septal aneurysm or PFO has confounded the identification of risk factors associated with stroke. Recommendations for primary prevention are therefore undefined. Patients who suffer a TIA with MVP and no other identifiable cause should be treated with aspirin, whereas those already on aspirin therapy with MVP who have a stroke or recurrent events should be anticoagulated with warfarin (51).

MAC is defined by calcification around the mitral valve and can be associated with mitral stenosis, regurgitation, and AF. Its incidence can be as high as 35% in older men (4). MAC is associated with an increased incidence of embolus, and some estimates indicate that the risk is double that of controls (6). The emboli appear to be composed mostly of fibrin but can also be comprised of calcium. Anticoagulation with warfarin is recommended for patients with MAC who also have evidence of embolization or concurrent AF (51).

Prosthetic heart valves carry a large risk of embolization. Patients who have a mechanical valve have permanent anticoagulation requirements (INR = 2.5 to 3.5), with antiplatelet therapy added to high-risk patients (24). Patients who are adequately anticoagulated have an approximate 2% to 4% per year embolism risk, with the percentage increased when the valve is in the mitral position. Bioprosthetic heart valves carry a considerably less annual risk (0.2% to 2.9%) of stroke, and antiplatelet therapy is often sufficient unless other risk factors are present (57).

Cardiac surgeries to cure the aforementioned valvular diseases are not without risk of TIA and stroke. In a series of 100 patients having valve procedures, 24 patients had focal deficits attributable to CNS involvement. Thirteen patients (54%) recovered completely in 2 months, and 22 (92%) recovered within 5 months, with the remaining patients having continued disability over 5 years (55). Recent studies have shown that stroke can occur in up to 2% to 5% of cardiac surgeries (52)

Atrial Myxoma and Cardiac Tumors

Atrial myxomas are the most common primary cardiac tumor, usually located at the fossa ovalis and visualized by transthoracic echocardiography. They cause approximately 1% of ischemic strokes in young patients (age ~50 years). The mechanism of insult is direct embolization of the tumor with frequent embolization to the retinal artery. Embolized tumor can continue to grow in the CNS, creating a mass effect or arterial aneurysms. Surgical excision is the treatment of choice, with the role of perioperative anticoagulation uncertain (20).

Less common are fibroelastomas, which are benign tumors located on the cardiac valves. There are several case reports of an association with cerebral emboli, but given that the incidence is so rare, a cause and effect relationship has yet to be established. Surgical excision without valve replacement is recommended (9)

Patent Foramen Ovale

PFO is the persistent connection of the right and left atrium via the foramen ovale, which usually closes within the first months of life. This is present in approximately 25% of the general population based on transesophageal echocardiographic imaging (25). Several case-controlled studies have highlighted an increased prevalence of PFO in younger patients with ischemic or cryptogenic strokes (7). The proposed mechanism of action was thrombus formation in the peripheral venous beds with embolization through the PFO, bypassing the pulmonary capillary beds. There have recently been studies that have shown evidence that PFO is not an increased independent risk factor for stroke. Hamann et al. (23) showed that, in patients with PFO-associated ischemic strokes, no venous source of emboli was present after investigation. Furthermore, in population-based prospective studies, Petty et al. (44) and Meissner et al. (38) showed that the presence of a PFO was not an independent risk factor for ischemic or cryptogenic stroke in the general population. It has also been shown that, in the majority of people, a right-to-left shunt requires Valsalva-like maneuvers to transiently raise right atrial pressures (23).

Based on the available information, patients with a PFO and ischemic strokes or TIA should undergo thorough evaluation for other stroke etiologies. The traditional method for detecting PFO has been transesophageal echocardiography. Even if no other source of embolism can be found, using the PFO as a foundation of diagnosis should be approached with skepticism. Antiplatelet therapy appears to be a sensible anticoagulation option given the aforementioned scenario. For patients with recurrent strokes with PFO and no other identifiable sources, a traditional option has been PFO surgical closure.

HYPOPERFUSION

The heart and the brain are interrelated in multiple aspects, but changes in vascular hemodynamics are some of the first to manifest if present. Cardiogenic hypoperfusion of the brain is common in bradycardia, tachycardia, and severe valvular disease. Hypoperfusion during cardiovascular surgeries should also be noted given the increasing incidence of cardiac disease in the aging world population.

Cardiogenic Hypoperfusion

Cardiogenic hypoperfusion states can lead to both reversible and irreversible damage to the CNS. It usually first manifests as delirium, presyncope, or syncope and can cause ischemia and possible infarct in areas of the CNS that are between vascular territories (watershed regions). These regions include the parieto-occipital and parietotemporal regions and the area around the central sulcus.

Bradycardia can cause CNS hypoperfusion from decreased cardiac output given the depressed stroke rate. Symptoms usually occur when the rate is so slow that the compensatory increase in stroke volume is inadequate to maintain blood pressure. Periods of ventricular asystole as short as 5 seconds can cause syncope (11). Multiple causes of bradycardia exist, with most being treatable. Medications such as beta-blockers, calcium channel blockers, digoxin, sympatholytics, and primary antiarrhythmics and other medications should always be questioned as the source of the problem. Inherent conduction problems such as ventricular bradycardia, sinus node disease, and second- or third-degree atrioventricular blocks should also be detected on standard electrocardiograms or Holter monitor testing.

Conversely, tachyarrhythmias can also cause a transient decrease in cardiac output. This occurs because the increased ventricular heart rate does not allow adequate diastolic time for filling, leading to a decrease in the stroke volume (as opposed to rate) and subsequent decrease in cardiac output. Ventricular tachyarrhythmias occur most frequently in patients with organic heart disease (e.g., coronary artery disease, previous myocardial infarction, etc.) or underlying myocardial dysfunction (e.g., hypertrophic cardiomyopathy). Unless associated with a bypass tract (i.e., Wolff-Parkinson-White), supraventricular arrhythmias, such as AF, rarely present with syncope, but rather present with palpitations and lightheadedness (11).

Structural abnormalities that decrease cardiac output from the heart can also cause CNS hypoperfusion. Valvular stenosis causes a physical impediment to cardiac output and can thus lead to decreased cerebral profusion. Mitral stenosis will present with symptoms of heart failure prior to symptoms of hypoperfusion. Aortic stenosis, however, can present with symptoms of lightheadedness and syncope secondary to poor cardiac output. The most common cause is congenital malformation with a bicuspid valve (54%), with the second most common cause being tricuspid valvular degeneration (45%) (50). Physical examination shows a crescendo-decrescendo murmur at the right upper sternal border and apex, a delayed carotid upstroke, and paradoxical splitting of the second heart sound. Diagnosis can be made with transthoracic echocardiography, and definitive treatment is surgical replacement.

Cardiac Surgery

As the population of the world begins to age, the incidence of cardiac disease that necessitates surgical interventions increases. Most cardiac surgical procedures require the heart to be in asystole and the vascular system to be placed on a CPB. The CPB connects the right atrium to the ascending aorta and provides a complete bypass of the pulmonary vascular beds and adequate oxygenation, volume output, and cerebrovascular pressures. The ultimate goal of CPB is to ensure adequate cerebral blood flow and to prevent emboli originating from the heart.

As discussed previously, the stroke risk during cardiac surgeries is 2% to 5%, with higher percentages occurring with increased age (52). The other major complication is diffuse encephalopathy, which is also called global hypoperfusion syndrome. The incidence of cardiac postoperative neurologic disorders varies widely because of the variability in the definitions of criteria and difficulty distinguishing it from anesthesia-related dysfunction. No studies have been done with a control group because no consensus of what would constitute a control group exists (42). Furthermore, the designs of studies to report neurologic dysfunction also have a large bearing on the outcome. Sotaniemi (54) showed that, in a study of 100 patients having valve replacement surgery, prospective neurologic examination revealed disorders in 37% of patients, whereas retrospective examinations did so in only 6%.

Estimations of the incidence of diffuse encephalopathy secondary to global hypoperfusion are difficult because of the aforementioned discussion. Furthermore, there tends to be a concentrated interest on reporting the "obvious" neurologic deficits because most subtle signs of encephalopathy are transient and resolve within days or weeks. To date, no reliable criteria are available for the clinical differentiation between patients with and without an organic background to explain the disturbances associated with the diffuse encephalopathy entity (56). There appears to be higher incidence of encephalopathy after coronary artery bypass grafting (CABG) versus valve replacements, which has been attributed to longer times on the CPB machines. Newman et al. (41) found that postoperative cognitive decline was prevalent (53%) at discharge in patients who underwent CABG and may persist for years postoperatively (42% at 5 years),

with older patients being at highest risk. There have not been studies done to see whether the cognitive decline was impending given the age of the patients or whether there is a direct relation to the surgery. The only known fact is that postoperative cognitive decline usually signals a continual decline to dementia in 5-year follow-up studies (41). Recently, there have been advances in cardiac surgeries that include off-pump bypass grafting that have shown satisfactory results and may alleviate many of the concerns when placing patients on CPB (40).

NEUROLOGIC MANIFESTATIONS OF PULMONARY DISEASE

Alterations in the pulmonary structure and vasculature due to disease usually lead to systemic manifestations secondary to alterations in gas exchange. These changes in the arterial blood gases cause an imbalance in the equilibrium that exists between the pulmonary and nervous systems. Changes in the oxygen and carbon dioxide concentrations, either acute or chronic, are quick to manifest with signs and symptoms that should be found on thorough neurologic examination and lead to further diagnosis and management.

The approach to this discussion should be based on the blood gas alterations seen with disease as opposed to the exhaustive lists of pulmonary diseases that cause these alterations. Mention will be made of the most common disease processes that lead to hypoxia, hypercapnia, and hypocapnia (Table 29-4).

HYPOXIA

Hypoxia is defined as a reduction in arterial oxygen tension (pO_2) below the normal range of 80 to 100 mm Hg. The value of reduction can be correlated to certain expected symptoms. A reduction of cerebral arterial oxygen tension to the range of 40 to 50 mm Hg can cause a deterioration of cognitive function.

Table 29-4. *Disease Processes That Lead to Hypoxia, Hypercapnia, and Hypocapnia*

Hypoxia	Hypercapnia	Hypocapnia
Asthma	Airway obstruction (COPD)	Salicylate toxicity
Pneumonia	Drugs (i.e., opioids, etc.)	Sepsis
Pulmonary embolism	Neuromuscular disease (i.e., Guillain-Barré, myasthenia gravis, botulism)	Acute pain
Interstitial lung disease	Structural disorder of the thorax	Hepatic encephalopathy
Shunt (i.e., atrial or ventricular septal defect, atelectasis, etc.)	Myxedema	Congestive heart failure
Pulmonary hypertension	Sleep apnea	Pulmonary embolism
Airway obstruction (COPD)	Obesity	

COPD, chronic obstructive pulmonary disease.

A reduction to <30 mm Hg leads to a loss of consciousness within 6 to 8 seconds (46). The effects of hypoxia are dependent on its severity, duration, and rate of onset. Acutely hypoxic patients will have different symptoms than chronically hypoxic patients (21).

Acute hypoxia occurs in processes such as pneumonia, pulmonary embolism, pneumothorax, bronchospasm, airway obstruction, and acute chronic obstructive pulmonary disease (COPD) exacerbations. A decrease in the blood oxygen tension in the range of 40 to 50 mm Hg causes delirium and decline of cognitive function, and 8 or more seconds below 30 mm Hg can lead to a loss of consciousness (46). Cells in the hippocampus and the Purkinje cells of the cerebellum die after 4 minutes of complete anoxia (31), and brain survival depends on maintaining a pO_2 of >20 to 22 mm Hg (49). Cerebral vasculature autoregulation of severe hypoxia leads to diffuse vasodilation, increased cerebral blood flow, and subsequent increased intracranial pressure. This increase in intracranial pressure is the likely cause of the symptoms seen with acute hypoxia (45). Recovery from acute hypoxia occurs with prompt restoration of oxygen to the vasculature. Consciousness will return within minutes, although stupor or confusion can persist for up to 2 minutes. Prognosis for anoxic encephalopathy depends on the duration, etiology, and severity and concurrent diseases (32).

Chronically depressed arterial oxygen tension occurs in disease processes such as COPD, pulmonary fibrosis, sleep apnea (obstructive, central, and mixed), and restrictive lung disease. Patients who suffer from these chronic symptoms usually also suffer from chronic hypercapnia, and therefore, it is difficult to associate symptoms specifically to an elevated carbon dioxide arterial tension (pCO_2) or decreased pO_2. Symptoms of chronic hypoxia include headaches, motor disturbances, and impaired cognition. Headaches related to chronic hypoventilation are usually frontal or occipital, aching and intense in nature, and maximal on awakening from sleep if associated with sleep apnea (discussed later). Associated physical findings include papilledema, tremor, and impaired consciousness. Electroencephalogram (EEG) findings include diffuse slowing with an abundance of theta and delta waves; alpha waves, if present, are also slow (5). In general, the changes are reversible, and permanent damage does not occur (21) because of compensatory mechanisms mediated through the renal, hematologic, and vascular mechanisms. Treatment is usually toward the underlying lung condition, and restoration of pO_2 levels to normal is paramount.

HYPERCAPNIA

Hypercapnia is defined by pCO_2 levels above the normal range of 37 to 43 mm Hg. Causes of hypercapnia are similar to the previous list of causes of chronic hypoxia, with the most frequent cause being COPD. Many of the symptoms and physical examination signs are also similar.

High levels of carbon dioxide in the bloodstream cause the arterial blood pH to fall below 7.35 and go into respiratory acidosis. This decrease in blood pH leads to a parallel decrease in cerebrospinal fluid (CSF) pH that is typically 0.10 lower than that of the arterial blood (21). This is secondary to the extreme diffusability of carbon dioxide across the blood–brain barrier. The CSF acidosis then possibly causes impairment of cerebral metabolism and other sequelae (47). In animal models, reversible breakdown of the blood–brain barrier can occur during periods of cerebral acidosis (17). These changes do not occur with metabolic acidosis because it is the carbon dioxide diffusing across the blood–brain barrier that causes these changes. Severe hypercapnia also leads to cerebral vasodilation and an increased CSF pressure much in the same way as severe hypoxia (45).

These physical changes in the brain can insidiously begin in patients as "forgetful, drowsy, somnolent, confused, anxious, disoriented, irritable, irrational, obstreperous, paranoid, psychotic, and psychopathic" (30). Early signs of hypercarbia include drowsiness, confusion, and forgetfulness, and higher levels can lead to coma. EEG changes are similar to those with metabolic encephalopathy. Severely elevated pCO_2 levels may warrant mechanical or positive pressure ventilation. Treatment with infused bicarbonate has no role because it does not diffuse across the blood–brain barrier and can worsen CSF acidosis (47). The optimal treatment would be reversal of the underlying pulmonary pathology and reversal of blood gases to normal levels.

HYPOCAPNIA

Hypocapnia is defined as a pCO_2 level below the normal range of 37 to 43 mm Hg. Isolated decreased pCO_2 leads to blood alkalosis, which causes cerebral vasoconstriction, leftward shift of the oxygen dissociation curve with reduced oxygen delivery, and reduction in plasma calcium and phosphate (53). Decreased carbon dioxide is usually secondary to hyperventilation, both voluntary and involuntary. Involuntary hyperventilation is most commonly secondary to salicylate toxicity, sepsis, acute pain, hepatic encephalopathy, CHF, and pulmonary embolism. Hyperventilation can also be secondary to brainstem strokes or tumors, encephalitis, Rett syndrome, Reye syndrome, malignant hyperthermia, and pyruvate dehydrogenase deficiency (14).

The increase in the arterial pH leads to a concomitant rise in the CSF pH secondary to the loss of carbon dioxide. Hypocapnia of longer than 3 hours in duration will be compensated in the CNS through loss of bicarbonate and increase in lactate (21). The decreased pCO_2 leads to cerebral vasoconstriction, which leads to decreased oxygen delivery to the brain. In the acute setting, each 1–mm Hg decrease in pCO_2 leads to a decrease of 2% in cerebral blood flow (48). These physiologic changes lead to symptoms of dizziness, unsteadiness, and blurred vision, followed by paresthesias of the upper and lower extremities.

CHRONIC OBSTRUCTIVE PULMONARY DISEASE

COPD deserves mention because it is a pulmonary disease state that usually presents with mixed gas imbalance. COPD occurs secondary to alterations in the lung parenchyma that lead to chronic hypoxia and hypercapnia. It is one of the most prevalent respiratory diseases and accounts for over half of all acute respiratory hospitalizations (43). These blood gas alterations lead to systemic effects of weight loss, skeletal muscle dysfunction, increase in risk of cardiovascular disease, and neurologic changes (1).

Mathur et al. (37) showed, via cerebral phosphorus-31 magnetic resonance spectroscopy, that the brain extensively uses the anaerobic pathway in patients with COPD. This implies that the COPD may lead to energy metabolism via a pathway that would produce lactate and further decreases CSF pCO_2. These alterations in the brain metabolism may explain the symptoms of agitation, confusion, and ultimately unconsciousness that occur with severe COPD. It may also be the explanation for the increased prevalence of depression in COPD and the reason why medications that change the chemical balance of the brain are successful tools for smoking cessation (58). One would also expect to see symptoms associated with chronic hypoxia and hypercarbia as discussed in their previous respective sections.

SLEEP APNEA

Sleep apnea is defined as the cessation of airflow during sleep and can be obstructive, central, or mixed. Obstructive sleep apnea (OSA) is the most common and is defined by oropharyngeal occlusion that halts airflow against continued respiratory inspiration. Central sleep apnea is a transient cessation of respiratory muscle drive from the CNS. Mixed sleep apneas have features of either OSA or central sleep apnea.

OSA is the most common sleep disorder seen in sleep clinics. It should be suspected in patients who are overweight, are middle-aged, have thick necks, and have a history of daytime somnolence. Neurologic manifestations include excessive daytime somnolence and headaches at night and upon awakening (16). Patients may also note unrefreshing sleep, cognitive delays, and chronic disorientation (8).

Unfortunately, the risk of cerebrovascular disease may also be increased in patients who suffer from OSA. Ferguson and Fleetham (16) found that 54% of male patients with strokes were chronic snorers with cognitive impairments proportional to the amount and severity of apneic episodes. Diagnosis can be made with overnight pulse oximetry or a formal sleep study. Treatment is based around augmenting the airflow and decreasing or eliminating the amount of obstruction. The first-line therapy should be the use of a continuous positive airway pressure (CPAP) machine to augment breathing at night. For those with obvious anatomic abnormalities and those who fail CPAP therapy, surgical procedures that fix the anatomic obstructions should be considered.

Central sleep apnea is usually a result of a primary CNS insult, such as medullary infarction, cervical spine surgery, encephalitis, and neuromuscular diseases. The disorder is felt to be secondary to alterations in the central chemoreceptor response to elevated pCO_2 levels. Mixed sleep apnea is usually the result of a primary neuromuscular disease such as amyotrophic lateral sclerosis (ALS), poliomyelitis, myasthenia gravis, and myotonic dystrophy. These diseases predispose these patients to increases in airway resistance and decreases in inspiratory muscle effort during rapid eye movement (REM) sleep (22). Presenting symptoms of both are similar to those of OSA, but there is less of an association with snoring. Treatment options are similar to those of OSA.

SUMMARY

The intricate relationship between the cardiopulmonary system and the CNS resides in a delicate equilibrium. Alterations in either of these systems can lead to neurologic manifestations, as discussed earlier. In the rare instances when the neurologic manifestations are the sentinel signs, it would be helpful for the neurologist to have a basic knowledge on how to work up the underlying disease.

REFERENCES

1. Agusti A. Systemic effects of chronic obstructive pulmonary disease. *Proc Am Thorac Soc.* 2005; 2:367–370.
2. Albers G, Amarenco P, Easton D, et al. Antithrombotic and thrombolytic therapy for ischemic stroke. *Chest.* 2001;119:300S–320S.
3. Anderson DJ, Goldstein LB, Wilkinson WE, et al. Stroke location, characterization, severity, and outcome in mitral vs aortic valve endocarditis. *Neurology.* 2003;61:1341–1346.
4. Aranow WS, Ahn C, Kronzon I. Prevalence of echocardiographic findings in 554 men and in

1,243 women aged >60 years in a long-term health facility. *Am J Cardiol*. 1997;79:379–380.

5. Austen FK, Carmichael MW, Adams RD. Neurologic manifestations of chronic pulmonary insufficiency. *N Engl J Med*. 1957;257:579–590.

6. Benjamin EJ, Plehn JF, D'Agostino RB, et al. Mitral annular calcification and risk of stroke in an elderly cohort. *N Engl J Med*. 1992;327:374–379.

7. Berthet K, Lavergne T, Cohen A, et al. Significant association of atrial abnormalities in young patients with ischemic stroke of unknown cause. *Stroke*. 2000;31:398–403.

8. Bradley T, Phillipson E. Sleep disorders. In: Murray J, Nadel J, eds. *Textbook of respiratory medicine*. 3rd ed. Philadelphia: WB Saunders; 2000:2153–2170.

9. Brown R, Khandheria B, Edwards W. Cardiac papillary fibroelastoma: a treatable cause of transient ischemic attack and ischemic stroke detected by transesophageal echocardiography. *Mayo Clin Proc*. 1995;70:863–868.

10. Cairns J, Theroux P, Lews D, et al. Antithrombotic agents in coronary artery disease. *Chest*, 2001;119:228S–252S.

11. Crawford M. *Current Diagnosis and Treatment in Cardiology*. 2nd ed. New York: McGraw-Hill; 2003.

12. Cunha BA, Gill MV, Lazar JM. Acute infective endocarditis. *Infect Dis Clin North Am*. 1996;10:811–834.

13. Durack DT, Lukes AS, Bright DK. New criteria for diagnosis of infective endocarditis: utilization of specific echocardiographic findings. Duke Endocarditis Service. *Am J Med*. 1994;96:200–209.

14. Evans R. Neurologic aspects of hyperventilation syndrome. *Semin Neurol*. 1995;15:115–125.

15. Feinberg WM, Blackshear JL, Alupacis A, et al. The prevalence of atrial fibrillation: analysis and implications. *Arch Intern Med*. 1995;155:469–473.

16. Ferguson K, Fleetham J. Sleep-related breathing disorders. 4. Consequences of sleep disordered breathing. *Thorax*. 1995;50:998–1004.

17. Fishman R. *Cerebrospinal Fluid in Disease of the Nervous System*. 2nd ed. Philadelphia: WB Saunders; 1992.

18. Gage BG, Waterman AD, Shannon W, et al. Validation of clinical classification schemes for predicting stroke: results from the National Registry of Atrial Fibrillation. *JAMA*. 2001;285:2864–2870.

19. Gilon D, Buonenno F, Jotte M, et al. Lack of an association between valve prolapse and stroke in young patients. *N Engl J Med*. 1999;341:8–13.

20. Giuliani ER, Gersh BJ, McGoon MD, et al., eds. *Mayo Clinic Practice of Cardiology*. 3rd ed. St. Louis: Mosby; 1996.

21. Griggs R, Sutton J. Neurologic manifestations of respiratory disease. In: Asbury A, McKhann G, McDonald WI, eds. *Disease of the nervous system: clinical neurobiology*. 2nd ed. Philadelphia: WB Saunders; 1992:1432–1441.

22. Guilleminault C, Robinson A. Central sleep apnea. *Neurol Clin*. 1996;14:611–628.

23. Hamann GF, Shatzer-Klotz D, Frohlig G, et al. Femoral injection of echo contrast medium may increase the sensitivity of testing for a patient foramen ovale. *Neurology*. 1998;50:1423–1428.

24. Hart RG. Intensity of anticoagulation to prevent stroke in patients with atrial fibrillation. *Ann Intern Med*. 1998;128:408.

25. Hart RG, Albers G, Koudstaal P. Cardioembolic stroke. In: Ginsberg M, Bogousslavsky J, eds. *Cerebrovascular disease: pathophysiology, diagnosis and management*. Vol 2. Malden, MA: Blackwell Science; 1998:1392–1429.

26. Hart RG, Halperin JL. Atrial fibrillation and stroke: concepts and controversies. *Stroke*. 2001;32:803–808.

27. Hart RG, Palacio S, Pearce LA. Atrial fibrillation, stroke, and acute antithrombotic therapy: analysis of randomized clinical trials. *Stroke*. 2002;33:2722–2727.

28. Heiro M, Nikoskelainen J, Engblom E, et al. Neurologic manifestations of infective endocarditis: a 17 year experience in a teaching hospital in Finland. *Arch Intern Med*. 2000;160:2781–2787.

29. Jones HR Jr, Siekaert RG. Neurological manifestations of infective endocarditis. Review of clinical and therapeutic challenges. *Brain*. 1989;112:1292–1315.

30. Kilburn K, Durham NC. Neurologic manifestations of respiratory failure. *Arch Intern Med*. 1965;116:409–415.

31. Levy DE, Brierly JB, Silverman DG. Brief hypoxia-ischemia initially damages cerebral neurons. *Arch Neurol*. 1975;32:450–456.

32. Levy DE, Caronna J, Burton S, et al. Predicting outcome from hypoxic ischemic coma. *JAMA*. 1985;253:1420–1426.

33. Li JS, Sexton DJ, Mick N, et al. Proposed modifications to the Duke criteria for the diagnosis of infective endocarditis. *Clin Infect Dis*. 2000;30:633–638.

34. Loh E, Sutton M, Wun CC, et al. Ventricular dysfunction and the risk of stroke after myocardial infarction. *N Engl J Med*. 1997;336:251–257.

35. Lopez JA, Ross RS, Fishbein MC, et al. Nonbacterial thrombotic endocarditis: a review. *Am Heart J*. 1987;113:773–784.

36. Mahaffey K, Granger CH, Sloan M, et al. Risk factors for in-hospital nonhemorrhagic stroke in patients with acute myocardial infarction treated with thrombolysis: results from GUSTO-1. *Circulation*. 1998;97:757–764.

37. Mathur R, Cox IJ, Oatridge A, et al. Cerebral bioenergetics in stable chronic obstructive pulmonary disease. *Am J Respir Crit Care Med*. 1999;160:1994–1999.

38. Meissner I, Khandheria BK, Heit JA, et al. Patent foramen ovale: innocent or guilty? Evidence from a prospective population-based study. *J Am Coll Cardiol*. 2006;47:440–445.

39. Mylonakis E, Calderwood SB. Infective endocarditis in adults. *N Engl J Med*. 2001;345:1318–1330.

40. Newman MA, Alvaraex JM, Kolybaba ML. Five year clinical follow up of patients who have had off pump coronary artery bypass grafting. *Heart Lung Circ*. 2003;12:157–162.

41. Newman MF, Kirchner J, Phillips-Bute B, et al. Longitudinal assessment of neurocognitive function after coronary artery bypass surgery. *N Engl J Med*. 2001:344:395–402.

42. Newman MF, Mathew JP, Grocott HP, et al. Central nervous system injury associated with cardiac surgery. *Lancet*. 2006;368:694–703.

43. Pearson MG, Littler J, Davies PD. An analysis of medical workload—evidence of patient to specialist mismatch. *J R Coll Physicians Lond*. 1994;28:230–234.

44. Petty GW, Khandheria BK, Meissner I, et al. Population-based study of the relationship between patent foramen ovale and cerebrovascular ischemia events. *Mayo Clin Proc*. 2006;81:602–608.

45. Phillipson EA. Disorders of ventilation. In Fauci A, Braunwald E, Isselbacher K, et al., eds. *Harrison's principles of internal medicine*. 14th ed. New York: McGraw-Hill; 1998:1476–1480.

46. Plum F, Posner JB. *Diagnosis of Stupor and Coma*. 3rd ed. Philadelphia: FA Davis; 1980:177–304.

47. Posner JB, Plum FL. Spinal fluid pH and neurologic symptoms in systemic acidosis. *N Engl J Med*. 1967;277:605–613.

48. Raichle ME, Posner JB, Plum FL. Cerebral blood flow during and after hyperventilation. *Arch Neurol*. 1970;23:394–403.

49. Refsum HE. Relationship between state of consciousness and arterial hypoxemia and hypercapnia in patients with pulmonary insufficiency breathing air. *Clin Sci*. 1963;25:3612.

50. Roberts WC, Ko JM. Relation of weights of operatively excised stenotic aortic valves to preoperative transvalvular peak systolic pressure gradients and to calculated aortic valve areas. *J Am Coll Cardiol*. 2004;44:1847–1855.

51. Salem DN, Levine HJ, Pauker SG, et al. Antithrombotic therapy in valvular heart disease. *Chest*. 1998;114:590–601.

52. Sila CA. Neurologic complications of vascular surgery. *Neurol Clin*. 1998;16:10–20.

53. Simon R. Breathing and the nervous system. In: Aminoff M, ed. *Neurology and general medicine: the neurological aspects of medical disorders*. New York: Churchill Livingstone; 1995:1–25.

54. Sotaniemi KA. Cerebral outcome after extracorporeal circulation. Comparison between prospective and retrospective aspects. *Arch Neurol*. 1983; 40:75–77.

55. Sotaniemi KA. Five-year neurological and EEG outcome after open-heart surgery. *J Neurol Neurosurg Psychiatry*. 1985;48:569–575.

56. Sotaniemi KA. Long term neurological outcome after cardiac operation. *Ann Thorac Surg*. 1995; 59:1336–1339.

57. Stein P, Alpert J, Bussey H, et al. Antithrombotic therapy in patients with mechanical and biological prosthetic heart valves. *Chest*. 2001;119: 220S–227S.

58. Wagena EJ, Huibers MJH, van Schayck CP. Antidepressants in the treatment of patients with COPD: possible associations between smoking cigarettes, COPD, and depression. *Thorax*. 2001;56:587–588.

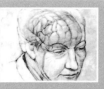

CHAPTER **2 9 . 2**

Neurologic Manifestations of Systemic Disease: GI and Endocrine

Vicki L. Shanker

GASTROINTESTINAL DISTURBANCE AND NEUROLOGIC DISEASE

Gastrointestinal dysfunction can often manifest as cerebral impairment in the older adult. Changes can be as subtle as short-term memory loss or difficulty with concentration. Often, these signs are the initial or only presentation of a gastrointestinal disturbance. To achieve a rapid diagnosis, it is valuable for the primary care physician to be alert and aware of these presentations. This chapter provides a brief overview of the major gastrointestinal disturbances associated with neurologic complications in the elderly.

HEPATIC ENCEPHALOPATHY

Hepatic encephalopathy is a neuropsychiatric syndrome that may occur secondary to hepatocellular failure. The development of hepatic encephalopathy is a poor prognostic sign associated with 1-year mortality rates close to 60%. Hepatitis, cirrhosis, and portosystemic shunting are common causes. The clinical presentation of hepatic encephalopathy has been categorized in the literature into four separate stages (Table 29-5).

The first stage is notable for subtle neuropsychiatric impairment and changes in the patient that may only be recognizable by close family and friends.

Symptoms include extreme mood disturbances, slurred speech, and mild confusion. A study of 148 pre–liver transplantation candidates reported significantly impaired immediate and delayed memory, attention, and executive functioning on neuropsychological testing (44). Intellectual function is initially preserved. Asterixis may be present on examination. This is a negative myoclonus where brief loss of tone can appear as hand flapping during wrist extension.

As the disease process continues, intellectual and motor functions are impaired, and basic activities of daily life become challenging. Consciousness may fluctuate. Signs on examination include hypotonia, hyporeflexia, and a positive Babinski sign. Comatose states dominate end-stage hepatic encephalopathy.

The pattern of encephalopathy described is similar to that seen in other metabolic disturbances. However, some signs have been identified as more specific to liver dysfunction. These include signs of parkinsonism such as tremor, monotonous speech, bradykinesia, and diminished facial expression (hypomimia). Increased muscle tone and dyskinesias may be seen as well (31).

Encephalopathic changes emerge over a period of days to weeks. In most patients, the disease does not develop past the first two stages. However, for patients in whom it does, the course is not necessarily unidirectional. The disease course can fluctuate

Table 29-5. *Hepatic Encephalopathy: Characteristics of Encephalopathic Stages*

Grade	Level of Consciousness	Personality/Behavioral Changes	Common Neurologic Signs
0	Alert	None	Absent
1	Alert; decreased attention	Mood changes Mild confusion Mild agitation	Subtle abnormalities best detected with psychometric studies
2	Lethargic	Overt personality changes Inappropriate behavior Fluctuating disorientation	Asterixis Hyperreflexia Loss of sphincter tone
3	Somnolent but arousable	Episodes of rage Persistent delirium	Asterixis Hyperreflexia Increased muscle tone
4	Comatose	Comatose	Decerebrate

Table 29-6. *Common Precipitators of Hepatic Encephalopathy*

Alcohol consumption
Benzodiazepine use
Dehydration
Electrolyte imbalances
Excessive protein intake
Gastrointestinal hemorrhage
Hepatoma/hepatocellular cancer
Hypotension
Infection
Placement of portosystemic shunt
Psychoactive drug use

between levels of impairment, or it can steadily worsen. Depending on the cause, the course of the disease can be acute, subacute, or chronic. A precipitating factor is often identified in an acute presentation but occurs variably in chronic forms (Table 29-6).

When the causative factor is identified and then eliminated or treated, resolution of the symptoms usually follows. In the absence of a precipitating event, prognosis is poor.

Diagnosis

Diagnosis is based primarily on history, physical examination, and a strong clinical suspicion. Hepatic encephalopathy is a diagnosis of exclusion, and potential confounders must be ruled out prior to its diagnosis. Predisposing factors of encephalopathy include an underlying infection, dehydration, electrolyte dysfunction, hypotension, gastrointestinal bleeding, and hepatocellular cancer. Additionally, excessive use of medications such as benzodiazepines, psychoactive drugs, or alcohol may produce an encephalopathy (16).

The workup focuses on evidence of hepatocellular insufficiency and mental impairment. Test results are consistent with, but not specific to, hepatic encephalopathy. Laboratory tests such as elevated liver function tests, increased prothrombin time, and raised ammonia levels may indicate hepatic dysfunction. Of note, ammonia levels are not always elevated with hepatic dysfunction. When ammonia levels are elevated, they do not consistently correlate with the degree of hepatic encephalopathy. Brain imaging is also nonspecific. Computed tomography (CT) is useful in these cases to rule out other considerations in the differential diagnosis. The main magnetic resonance imaging (MRI) findings reported in hepatic disease are symmetric pallidal hyperintensities in T1-weighted images. The nigral substance area and the dentate cerebellar nucleus may show similar abnormalities. Electroencephalograph (EEG) findings of triphasic waves are commonly found but are nonspecific.

A referral to a neuropsychologist is valuable in further assessment of mental dysfunction in hepatic encephalopathy.

Treatment

Treatment focuses largely on reduction of systemic ammonia and on inhibition of gamma-aminobutyric acid (GABA) receptor activation. Both have been identified as contributors to the pathophysiology of hepatic encephalopathy. Elevated ammonia levels augment GABA-mediated neurotransmission, increasing neuronal inhibition.

Nonabsorbable disaccharides (e.g., lactulose and lactitol) are used to osmotically remove ammonia from the body. They have traditionally been used as a first-line therapy based on the theory that the majority of ammonia production stems from colonic bacteria. The estimated daily dose ranges from 30 to 60 g. The dose is titrated to produce two to four soft acidic (pH <6) stools per day. In an acute episode, the recommended starting dose is 30 to 45 mL at 1- to 2-hour intervals until a laxative effect is observed. Elderly patients taking lactulose should be monitored closely for fluid and electrolyte loss with chronic use because they are more susceptible to neurologic impairment associated with dehydration and electrolyte loss than are younger patients.

Antibiotics have been used as a second-line approach. Neomycin (6 g/day) and metronidazole (800 mg/day), inhibitors of urease-producing bacteria, are used to reduce ammonia. In the geriatric population, serum concentrations of these medications tend to be elevated as total clearance is reduced. Thus, elderly patients are more likely to suffer from side effects, including ototoxicity, nephrotoxicity, and gastrointestinal disturbance. Rifaximin (1,200 mg/day) is a nonabsorbable alternative to neomycin and metronidazole. A small pilot study of patients with stage 2 hepatic encephalopathy compared the cost efficacy (via number of hospitalizations, medical treatments, and drug costs) in a group taking rifaximin versus a group taking lactulose (48). Researchers found that patients taking rifaximin required fewer hospitalizations and outpatient medical visits. They reported a significant cost efficacy of rifaximin over lactulose, begging further study of this drug. The question of an additive effect of lactulose with antibiotics is currently under investigation as well. Of note, studies of patients receiving antibiotics for liver disease have found that stool pH is increased, a sign that disaccharide-metabolizing bacteria are killed by the antibiotics as well (66). Absence of these bacteria reduces the effectiveness of lactulose.

Dietary protein restriction is another first-line approach to reducing intestinal production of ammonia. Patients are restricted to 20 g/day of protein. The dosage is increased by 10 g for 3 to 5 days until a tolerance threshold is reached. If tolerance is <1 g/kg, vegetable protein is recommended as the primary source of protein because of its high fiber content. Increased fiber intake aids in improved food motility through the gastrointestinal system, decreasing the opportunity for protein absorption.

Recently, researchers have begun to question the basis of evidence for the common usage of lactulose and protein restriction in the treatment of hepatic encephalopathy. Shawcross and Jalan (57) reviewed 22 randomized trials of lactulose and found insufficient evidence to recommend or refute its use. Use of lactulose was not found to significantly reduce mortality. With regard to dietary practices, a small trial of 20 patients with hepatic encephalopathy placed half of the participants on a normal protein diet and half on a restricted diet (14). There were no significant differences in disease course or in protein breakdown between these two groups. Studies such as these have suggested that research and, ultimately, clinical treatment may be redirected to a more systemic approach of ammonia reduction and elimination than currently understood and practiced.

Other current strategies for treatment of hepatic encephalopathy include the eradication of *Helicobacter pylori*, if present, because of its contribution to serum ammonia levels. Ornithine aspartate, an enzyme that converts ammonia to urea, is effective in serum ammonia reduction and can be taken orally. A recent trial found significant improvement in serum ammonia levels, EEG recordings, and mental status testing in a group taking oral ornithine aspartate (51). Benzoate or phenylacetate treatment reacts with glycine or glutamine, respectively, to increase metabolic conversion to form hippurate and phenacetylglutamine. Zinc is a necessary cofactor in two of the five enzymes in the urea cycle. Supplementation is recommended for those who are zinc deficient. Studies have explored the role of flumazenil, a benzodiazepine antagonist, in hepatic encephalopathy. Some have proposed that binding to the benzodiazepine receptor by substances not normally present in the brain plays an important role in hepatic encephalopathy. A Cochrane review (2) assessed the results of 13 randomized trials using flumazenil in the treatment of hepatic encephalopathy. It concluded that flumazenil had significant benefit in short-term improvement in patients with cirrhosis.

Liver transplantation is preferable to medical management in most patients with end-stage cirrhosis, regardless of age. However, other medical problems may limit the utility of this option. The surgical creation of portosystemic shunts, especially the transjugular intrahepatic portosystemic shunt, is a frequently used procedure in those awaiting transplantation.

However, patients >65 years of age are significantly more likely to develop hepatic encephalopathy after this procedure.

NUTRITIONAL AND VITAMIN DEFICIENCY

As the body ages, the efficiency of the gastrointestinal system to extract the necessary nutrients and vitamins from the diet can become impaired. External factors can further compound the risk of nutritional deficiency. For example, patients' medications may interfere with absorption, and patients' diets, especially individuals who are institutionalized, may be inadequate (12).

Vitamin B_{12} deficiency is a common problem in the elderly community. There are variable estimates of its prevalence, ranging from 12% of those living in the community to 30% to 40% of those in institutions (38,62). Some of this discrepancy is due to the variable criteria used to define vitamin B_{12} deficiency, with the lower limit of normal ranging from 150 pmol/L to 258 pmol/L. The peak age of neurologic presentations in vitamin B_{12} deficiency is estimated to occur between 60 and 70 years (52).

Gastric atrophy is among the most common changes in the aging gastrointestinal system. Estimates of atrophic gastritis in the geriatric population range from 11% to 50% (28,55). States of hypochlohydria or achlorhydria facilitate the atrophy of the stomach mucosa. *H. pylori* infection in the gut is the most frequent cause of atrophic gastritis, with an estimated 60% of the elderly infected. Pernicious anemia, another common source, is estimated to produce 15% to 50% of vitamin B_{12} deficiency cases in the elderly (3). Classic pernicious anemia is a chronic illness associated with lack of adequate intrinsic factor production secondary to inhibition of gastric parietal cells. Intrinsic factor is needed for the absorption of vitamin B_{12}.

There are several other etiologies that may contribute to vitamin B_{12} malabsorption. Bacterial overgrowth from lack of gastric acid production or chronic antibiotic use also produces nutritional malabsorption. Long-term ingestion of medications such as metformin, H_2 receptor antagonists, proton pump inhibitors, anticonvulsants, and colchicine may cause malabsorption. Other etiologies include a history of gastric surgery, chronic alcoholism, pancreatic exocrine failure, and Sjögren syndrome. Vitamin B_6, vitamin B_{12}, and folate are most notably affected by these changes.

The neurologic manifestations of vitamin B_{12} deficiency are well known and reported. Deficiency states may involve both the central and peripheral nervous system. Onset is often insidious. Nerve damage is usually due to demyelination. However, axonal degeneration and neuronal death can occur in more severe cases. Initial symptoms may be as subtle as lethargy or generalized weakness. The most common symptomatic presentation is burning or painful sensations in the distal extremities. The feet are usually affected prior to the hands. These symptoms are associated with polyneuritis. Cognitive symptoms may occur with or without peripheral involvement. Symptoms may range from mild irritability to depression, dementia, and psychosis. On rare occasions, there is optic nerve involvement, and patients may complain of visual loss.

The most frequent neurologic signs on examination are a diminished sense of vibration and proprioception in the legs due to involvement of the dorsal columns of the spinal cord. This may occur in conjunction with impaired distal cutaneous sensation. Sensory changes are usually in a stocking-glove distribution. Limb reflexes may vary. Subacute combined deficiency, a condition classically associated with vitamin B_{12} deficiency, involves both posterior columns and corticospinal tracts of the spinal cord. A spastic paraparesis is seen on examination. Involvement of the autonomic nervous system (ANS), including bowel, bladder, and sexual dysfunction, can be seen in some cases as well.

A suggested algorithm for evaluation of vitamin B_{12} deficiency is presented in Figure 29-1. When patients present with symptoms suggestive of vitamin B_{12} deficiency, a serum screen of vitamin B_{12} should be sent along with a complete blood cell count (CBC). Vitamin B_{12} levels <100 pmol/L warrant immediate therapy. When levels between 100 and 400 pmol/L are reported, additional serum tests should be sent (19). These include a homocysteine, methylmalonic acid, and holotranscobalamin (holo-TC) II assay. The former two are both in the pathway of vitamin B_{12} production, and elevated levels are suggestive of deficiency. Elevated homocysteine is a nonspecific finding because it is also involved in the pathway of folate production. Elevated methylmalonic acid is a more specific finding. Holo-TC contains biologically active vitamin B_{12} bound to transcobalamin II (TC II). TC II promotes vitamin B_{12} uptake by cells. Low serum holo-TC is considered the earliest and most sensitive marker for vitamin B_{12} deficiency (68). If additional tests confirm the presence of vitamin B_{12} deficiency, serologies for pernicious anemia should be performed. This includes an anti-intrinsic factor antibody, which has 50% sensitivity and 98% specificity, and an antigastric parietal cell antibody, which has 90% sensitivity and 50% specificity.

The Schilling test can be of assistance in identifying the source of vitamin B_{12} deficiency. The test is often separated into three separate stages. In the first phase of the test, the patient is given an oral dose of radiolabeled vitamin B_{12} followed by an intramuscular injection 2 hours later. The purpose of this is to saturate the body's vitamin B_{12} binding sites. The absorbed oral vitamin B_{12} cannot bind to the already saturated transcobalamin proteins and will be excreted in the urine by glomerular filtration. A percentage of the administered dose excreted in the urine over 24 hours is calculated. In patients with pernicious anemia or intestinal malabsorption, the urinary excretion is usually <6%, compared with the normal value, which is >9%. The second phase is performed in a manner similar to the first phase, with the exception that intrinsic factor is given with the oral dose of vitamin B_{12}. Pernicious anemia is suggested when the patient has an abnormal result in phase I followed by a normal test in phase II. When the Schilling test suggests pernicious anemia and anti-intrinsic factors are present, the diagnosis of pernicious anemia is virtually confirmed (specificity >99%). If the first two tests produce abnormal results, the patient is treated with 2 weeks of tetracycline for possible bacterial overgrowth. Phase III of the Schilling test is performed after a 2-week course of antibiotic. The test is the same as the second phase. If the test is normal, it can be deduced that bacterial overgrowth caused the vitamin deficiency. Of note, the test results can be normal in elderly patients with atrophic gastritis, despite deficiency, because these patients malabsorb only protein-bound vitamin B_{12}.

When vitamin B_{12} deficiency is suspected, the clinician should obtain a good history, including diet and medications. There are several options for supplementation of vitamin B_{12} once deficiency is identified. Traditionally, patients were given a 1,000 µg/day intramuscular (IM) injection for 1 week followed by a monthly 1,000 µg/day IM injection until the deficiency is corrected or for life. Recently, studies have argued that initial oral supplementation of 1,000 to 2,000 µg daily, followed by weekly and then monthly doses, is equally efficacious (37,63). Patients with confirmed pernicious anemia should be referred to a gastroenterologist. These patients should receive endoscopic surveillance every 3 to 5 years with multiple biopsies because of the association of pernicious anemia with gastric cancers including lymphoma, adenocarcinoma, and carcinoid tumors. Screens for other autoimmune conditions can be considered if symptomatically appropriate. Antibiotic treatment for *H. pylori* should be administered, if detected. The length and extent of neurologic recovery is correlated with the length and severity of disability prior to treatment. Older age may increase the risk of residual disability. Patients with suspected vitamin B_{12} deficiency should be cautioned against receiving nitric oxide during dental procedures because exposure may precipitate or rapidly advance current symptoms.

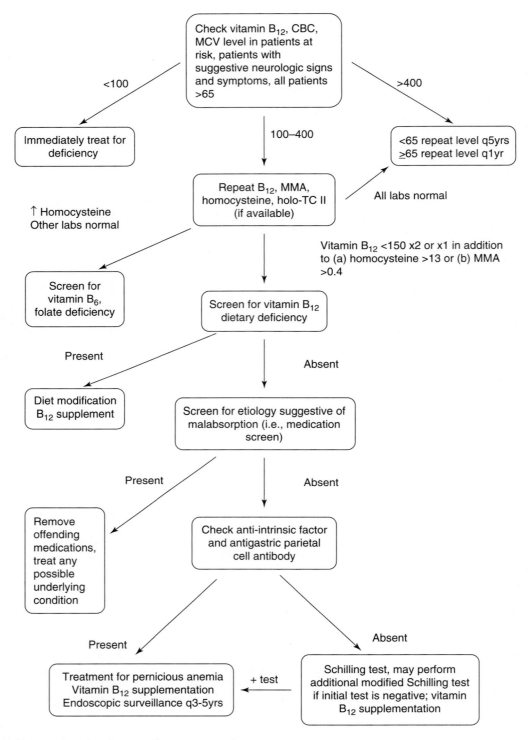

Figure 29-1. Algorithm chart: initial vitamin B_{12} evaluation.

Folate is found in leafy green vegetables and is supplemented in many foods. Despite this supplementation, evidence suggests that 30% of healthy older adults may continue to have deficiencies (15). Folate deficiency may be subtle and is not fully understood. The relationship of low folate states with depressive mood disorders is still under study. It is reported that patients with low levels of serum folate have poorer responses to antidepressant medication (29). When levels are low, folate supplementation is provided. There is no standard for the recommended dose used for supplementation. However, 0.8 mg/day taken over several months is usually sufficient to correct anemia (52). Treatment should continue for at least 6 months. Some treatment response should be seen by 3 months.

Precaution must be taken when using the mean corpuscular volume (MCV) value alone for screening or measuring treatment effects in patients with cobalamin or folate deficiency. Lack of adequate amounts of either vitamin impairs DNA synthesis, resulting in a megaloblastic anemia. A well-supplemented diet with folate may delay the identification of a vitamin B_{12} deficiency. Chronic treatment with folate or vitamin B_{12} supplementation may mask an emerging deficiency of the alternative vitamin, allowing neurologic damage to advance. This is why both cobalamin and folic acid should be assessed when symptoms are suggestive, regardless of CBC results.

Pyridoxine deficiency is reported to be present in as many as 32% of independent American elderly (40). Risk factors include older age, renal insufficiency, dialysis treatment, inflammatory disease, and chronic malnutrition. Certain medications may contribute to or provoke a pyridoxine deficiency. These include hydralazine, isoniazid, levodopa, D-penicillamine, and pyrazinamide. Unlike children, adults are better able to withstand low vitamin B_6 states and will often not display any clinical manifestations of insufficiency. Seizures in adults are rare. More common are slowly progressive sensory changes resulting in numbness, tingling, burning, or pain in the feet that may travel in a stocking-glove pattern to affect the hands as well, if left untreated. Examination may show impaired distal sensation, distal weakness, and decreased reflexes. Pyridoxine supplementation of 50 mg/day is sufficient for prevention and treatment of deficiency.

Folate, vitamin B_6, and vitamin B_{12} are all cofactors involved in homocysteine metabolism (59). Elevated levels of homocysteine are associated with increased risk of atherosclerotic disease and stroke (26,41). Hyperhomocysteinemia has been associated with late-onset mood disorder in the elderly as well (13). When elevated states of serum homocysteine are detected, it is important to screen and supplement the appropriate vitamins. Several studies have suggested that there is a relationship between elevated homocysteine levels and cognitive decline (10,21,46). Unfortunately, the current literature does not suggest that lowering homocysteine levels via B vitamin supplementation improves cognitive function (43).

Thiamine deficiency is rarely encountered, except in those with a history of alcoholism (24). Severe malnutrition and a history of gastrectomy are also risk factors (36). Minor contributions to thiamine deficiency include chronic dialysis therapy, chronic malabsorption syndromes such as celiac or tropical sprue, hyperthyroidism, chronic diarrhea, and diuretic therapy. Studies in Britain have found an incidence of thiamine deficiency in the elderly population ranging from 22% to 40% in an institutionalized population and from 8% to 31% in a noninstitutionalized population (64). Two disease states that can arise from thiamine deficiency are Wernicke-Korsakoff's psychosis and dry beriberi. The main characteristics of Wernicke's encephalopathy are mental status changes or global confusion, ophthalmoplegia, ataxia, and nystagmus. Korsakoff syndrome is a rare condition during which patients experience both anterograde and retrograde amnesia. Patients may confabulate to supplement their memory loss. Dry beriberi is a peripheral neuropathy usually identified by complaints of symmetric distal weakness, paresthesias, and pain. Hyporeflexia is usually seen on examination. The rate of symptomatic progression may vary from days to years.

Thiamine supplementation varies depending on the presentation and severity of symptoms. Patients suspected of peripheral neuropathy may start with 50 mg IM for several days followed by maintenance therapy of 2.5 to 5 mg/day. If a malabsorption syndrome is suspected, further workup is required, and higher doses may be needed. Wernicke's encephalopathy should be viewed as a medical emergency. Vital signs should be closely monitored, and patients should receive a CT scan of the brain to rule out other conditions on admission. A brain MRI may show increased intensity in the mammillary bodies and periaqueductal gray matter on T1-weighted images. Patients should be started on 100 mg of thiamine immediately. This can be given prior to or concurrently with intravenous (IV) glucose. Doses of 500 mg once to twice a day may be required during initial hospitalization. Patients should also receive IV magnesium because hypomagnesia is often concurrent with thiamine-deficient states, and thiamine replenishment is ineffective in low magnesium states. Once patients are able to resume a normal diet, they may begin maintenance doses of 100 mg/day. Patients with Wernicke's encephalopathy should be monitored for Korsakoff's syndrome and alcohol withdrawal. There is substantial morbidity and mortality associated with Wernicke's encephalopathy, and improvement after supplementation may not be seen for weeks to months.

Table 29-7. *Common Vitamin Deficiencies*

Nutritional Deficiency	Common Neurologic Presentations in the Elderly	Recommended Daily Intake in the Elderly	Recommended Treatment Doses
Vitamin B_6	Stocking-glove sensory loss Carpal tunnel syndrome	2.0–2.2 mg/day in men 1.6–2.0 mg/day women	50 mg daily
Vitamin B_{12}	Dementia Depression, apathy Stocking-glove sensory loss Subacute combined systemic degeneration	2.4 µg/day in men 2.4 µg/day in women	1000 µg/day IM for 1 week, followed by monthly IM injections (alternate schedules have been proposed)
Folate	Depression	400 µg/day	800 µg/day to 1 mg/day
Thiamine	Dry beriberi Wernicke's encephalopathy Korsakoff's syndrome	1.2 mg/day in men 1.1 mg/day in women	100 mg/day
Vitamin E	Peripheral neuropathy Spinocerebellar degeneration	15 mg/day from food or 22.5 IU/day	30–50 mg/day (usually 4–5 times RDA)

IM, intramuscular; RDA, Recommend Dietary Allowance.

There is no cure for Korsakoff syndrome, and treatment is supportive care.

Finally, patients with fat malabsorption are susceptible to developing vitamin E deficiency. Low levels of vitamin E have been associated with neuronal degeneration in the spinocerebellar tract, Clark columns, and the nuclei of Goll and Burdach, producing ataxia. There have also been several reports examining the relationship between vitamin E therapy for the prevention of neurodegenerative diseases. At this time, there are inconsistent data to support the relationship of Alzheimer's disease and vitamin E supplementation (18,39). Research to date has not shown a neuroprotective role of vitamin E in Parkinson's disease (58).

In summary, the elderly are susceptible to neurologic changes produced by underlying gastrointestinal disturbance. Table 29-7 summarizes the neurologic presentation, daily recommended allowances, and treatment of the most common vitamin deficiencies seen in the elderly. Most of these disturbances are reversible and often easily treated. Physicians with a heightened awareness of the various neurologic presentations may rapidly proceed to treatment of the underlying disorder, preventing further complications.

ENDOCRINE DISTURBANCE AND NEUROLOGIC DISEASE

Disturbances in the endocrine system often lead to metabolic imbalances and neurologic disease. Diabetes mellitus type 2, which is present in more than 14 million Americans, is the most prevalent of these imbalances in the elderly. This section addresses some of these changes and complications associated with diabetes as well as other endocrine disturbances in the elderly.

THYROID
Hypothyroidism

Hypothyroidism is a clinical syndrome produced by thyroid hormone deficiency. The prevalence of hypothyroidism in the elderly population has been estimated to be in the range of 0.9% to 17.5% (23,25). The incidence of hypothyroidism in women is greater than in men, at all ages.

Hashimoto thyroiditis is the most common cause of hypothyroidism in the elderly. Other causes include a history of radioactive iodine ablation therapy for Graves' disease, previous thyroidectomy, subacute thyroiditis, and use of drugs such as lithium and amiodarone (65).

Hypothyroidism often has an insidious onset in the elderly (27). Common clinical symptoms in the general population include depression, weight gain, hair loss, dry skin, cold intolerance, constipation, and muscle cramps. However, elderly patients often do not present with these classic symptoms. Instead, they may complain of anorexia and weight loss, incontinence, mental confusion, decreased mobility, and a recent history of falls. Frequently noted mental status changes include impaired concentration, word fluency, attention capabilities, and psychomotor function. Additionally, hypothyroidism can produce obstructive sleep apnea, myopathy, carpal tunnel syndrome, or cerebellar ataxia. Older patients, especially those with hypothermia, are more likely to develop myxedema coma (33).

On examination, patients often show impairment in learning, word fluency, attention, and tests of motor speed. Delayed relaxation of the ankle reflex, a common finding in hypothyroidism, is often difficult to observe in geriatric patients because many have diminished ankle reflexes as a normal change associated with aging. Decreased radial and biceps reflexes are more sensitive for this finding in the elderly.

Diagnostic evaluation of hypothyroidism should include laboratory measurements of thyroid-stimulating hormone (TSH), free thyroxine (T_4), and urinary triiodothyronine (T_3) (6). Elevated levels of TSH, in combination with depressed T_4 values, are characteristic of the disorder.

Many elderly patients will have TSH values between 10 and 20 μIU/L with a normal serum T_4. This subset of patients is diagnosed with subclinical hypothyroidism, most of whom are clinically asymptomatic. Prevalence estimates of subclinical hypothyroidism in the elderly have ranged from 7% to 17% of the ambulatory elderly population. Management of these patients is controversial. Some clinicians support treatment because approximately one fifth of the subclinical population will experience progression to overt hypothyroidism within 1 year of laboratory findings. Some recommend therapy in all patients with subclinical disease and thyroidal antibodies (11). Those who believe it is important to treat subclinical disease support regular testing of thyroid hormone and TSH levels to identify patients at risk. However, many physicians have questioned the benefit of hormone replacement in patients without overt clinical symptoms.

L-thyroxine is the standard medical treatment for hypothyroidism. The synthetic hormone has a long half-life and can convert to T_3 in vivo. In older patients, the recommended starting dose is 0.025 mg/day. The medication can be gradually titrated upward every 4 to 6 weeks, until laboratory values of TSH are within normal limits. Because clearance of T_4 is reduced in the elderly, it is not necessary to check TSH levels more than every 3 to 4 weeks. It is estimated that an effective dose of L-thyroxine in the elderly ranges between 0.075 and 0.125 mg/day.

Hyperthyroidism

The prevalence of hyperthyroidism in older persons is reported to range from 0.5% to 2.3% (4). Toxic multinodular goiter and Graves' disease are the most common causes of hyperthyroidism in the elderly (20). Patients taking thyroid hormone supplementation for an extended period of time may also develop hyperthyroidism in later years because of decreased metabolic clearance of thyroid hormone.

Common characteristics include heat intolerance, diaphoresis, palpitations, tremulousness, nervousness, restlessness, and weight loss. However, these symptoms are reported in only one fourth of all elderly patients with hyperthyroidism. Subtle complaints that

may warrant further workup in this population include chronic fatigue, emotional lability, muscle weakness, and wasting of the proximal muscles. Depression, lethargy, agitation, dementia, and confusion are common psychiatric manifestations. Failure to detect hyperthyroidism has serious implications because chronically elevated thyroid levels impact the cardiovascular system. Several studies have looked at the relationship between subclinical hyperthyroidism and cardiac disease in the elderly and found increased heart rates, increased prevalence of supraventricular arrhythmias, and increased rates of atrial fibrillation (8). Studies are currently exploring the role of subclinical hyperthyroidism in bone metabolism and fracture risk in the elderly.

Diagnosis can be confirmed with laboratory results of an elevated T_4 (or T_3 in cases where T_4 is normal) and a decreased TSH. Other findings may include an elevated alkaline phosphatase, mildly increased serum calcium, and decreased serum cholesterol.

Radioactive ablation is the recommended treatment for Graves' disease and is a preferred option in the elderly because of the operative risks associated with surgery. Medication therapy using antithyroid medications, such as propylthiouracil (PTU) and methimazole (MMI), is often considered for patients with nodular disease as well as subclinical hyperthyroidism. One study of elderly patients showed that use of antithyroid therapy restored patients with subclinical hyperthyroidism and atrial fibrillation back to sinus rhythm (22). Both commonly used antithyroid medications block the synthesis of T_4. PTU blocks the peripheral conversion of T_4 to T_3 as well. The dosage of PTU ranges from 200 to 400 mg/day. Common side effects of these medications include pruritus, urticaria, fever, arthralgias, and taste changes. Serious adverse effects include thrombocytopenia, hepatitis, agranulocytosis, cholestatic jaundice, and a lupus-like syndrome (42). MMI is administered at doses of 10 to 30 mg/day and is given once daily, improving compliance. Beta-blocker treatment is often used as adjunctive therapy in patients with arrhythmias. Medication therapy should proceed with caution because the elderly often have difficulty complying with these regimens and have an increased risk of toxicity.

Although treatment for overt hyperthyroidism is a clear necessity, the question arises when to treat subclinical disease. Guidelines recommend that endogenous cases of subclinical hyperthyroidism should be treated in patients older than 60 years of age when TSH is <0.1 mIU/L as well as in those at increased risk for heart disease and bone loss. Patients with subclinical disease who are followed should always be treated when symptoms suggestive of hyperthyroidism arise (60).

ADRENAL GLAND

The aging process is not associated with changes in cortisol production from the adrenal cortex. Both Cushing disease and adrenal insufficiency are rare in the elderly (67). However, because adrenal dysfunction is both a serious and often treatable condition, it should be considered in situations of unexplained hypotension or shocklike conditions. Neurologic complaints in those with excess cortisol include impotence and psychiatric problems. Screening for Cushing syndrome begins with a 24-hour collection of urine to test for urinary free cortisol. Levels higher than three to four times the normal values (150 g/dL) are suggestive of Cushing disease, although slightly lesser values may be inconclusive. Cushing syndrome can be confirmed with the dexamethasone suppression test (DST). The test is significant if, after receiving a 1-mg dose of oral dexamethasone given at 11:00 PM the previous evening, the fasting cortisol value is >5 µg/dL the following morning. Affective disorders and Alzheimer's disease can produce false-positive results in the overnight DST (45). It is hypothesized that this occurs as a result of glucocorticoid receptor downregulation in regions of the brain that usually inhibit glucocorticoid or cell loss (56). The 2-day, low-dose DST is a more sensitive test but more inconvenient.

A common cause of adrenal insufficiency in the elderly is hemorrhage in the adrenal glands (1). This is usually seen in those taking warfarin (Coumadin). Elderly patients with adrenal insufficiency may present with delirium or dementia. Serum cortisol response to a corticotropin analog is the standard test. The corticotropin stimulation test should not be done if acute adrenal collapse is suspected. In these instances, serum cortisol is measured, and the patient is rapidly administered hydrocortisone 100 mg IV, followed by a continuous infusion of hydrocortisone 10 mg/h IV until the cortisol level is normal. Imaging of the adrenal gland may indicate a metastatic, granulomatous, or atrophic process. Treatment is hydrocortisone maintenance doses of 20 mg in the morning and 10 mg at night. Dexamethasone and prednisone are favored alternative treatments because both drugs have longer half-lives and do not require biotransformation. Some patients will need mineralocorticoid treatment as well.

PARATHYROID

Hypoparathyroidism is a recognized cause of secondary parkinsonism. Physiologically, calcium channels are involved in dopaminergic regulation. When calcium levels are low, dopamine levels fall, and parkinsonian symptoms emerge. Treatment is aimed at resolution of the hypocalcemic state.

PANCREAS

Hyperglycemia

As the body ages, several changes occur that increase the risk of developing type 2 diabetes mellitus. The modifications include decreased glucose tolerance, increased adipose tissue, and increased insulin resistance. The age of the patient increases not only the risk of having type 2 diabetes mellitus but also the risk of developing complications from the disease. Neurologic complications of diabetes are more common than is often recognized by both the patient and the clinician, having an impact on both the central and peripheral nervous system. Increased awareness of these conditions allows for early detection, treatment, and prevention of progressive impairment.

The relationship between diabetes mellitus and stroke is well explored in the literature. It has been estimated that 20% to 22% of all strokes in the United States occur in patients with a history of diabetes (35). Studies have shown that diabetes is a risk factor for stroke as well as poststroke mortality (34). Strategies for intensive control of hyperglycemia have been successfully tested to decrease stroke risk. Current research is also exploring the role of diabetes mellitus in dementia. A review of 14 longitudinal population studies suggests a relationship of diabetes with both Alzheimer's and vascular dementia (9).

Diabetes is the most common cause of neuropathy in the Western hemisphere. Although only 15% of patients with diabetes present with symptoms and signs of neurologic deficits, it is estimated that half of all patients with diabetes mellitus manifest neuropathic symptoms or show nerve conduction abnormalities. One multicenter study estimated that 28.5% of the diabetic population has a neuropathy (69). Factors that increase the risk of developing a neuropathy include extended disease duration (12.5 to 13.5 years), age >50 years, and long-standing hyperglycemia secondary to poor diabetic control (61,69).

The underlying cause of both focal and multifocal diabetic neuropathy is thought to be ischemia to the vasa nervorum, the blood supply to the nerves. The most common neurologic presentation is a distal polyneuropathy that is primarily sensory in nature. Although most sensory changes in diabetic patients are painless, up to 10% of patients report unpleasant sensations and pain. Sensory complaints manifest themselves in many forms, including numbness and tingling, hyperesthesias, and dysesthesias. When patients complain of pain, it is often described as lightning stabs, shooting, prickling, aching, or burning. The pain often worsens at night. Sensory changes are most often localized bilaterally in the feet and lower legs. The hands are usually affected in more severe cases. The presenting pattern is identified as a stocking-glove pattern because of its classic distribution. Less commonly, the anterior chest and abdominal area can be involved as well.

Acute, painful neuropathy is a rare syndrome characterized by intense pain, predominantly in the distal lower extremities. The syndrome primarily appears in men who are diabetic. Patients complain of a burning sensation, with notable dysesthesias. Other symptoms include weight loss, depression, insomnia, and impotence. Sensory examination findings may be normal or show mild impairment in pain and temperature sensations. Motor examination findings may be significant for a mild foot weakness; however, normal examination results are not atypical. If nerve conduction study findings are abnormal, they will show decreased amplitude or absent sensory nerve action potentials. If a sural nerve biopsy is performed, axonal degeneration is noted (54). Chronic painful diabetes neuritis is termed when pain persists for more than 6 months. Electrodiagnostic studies show reduced nerve fiber density consistent with small nerve neuropathy. Patients with chronic pain often develop tolerance and addiction to pain medications (5).

Impairment of sensory function can have adverse effects. For example, patients with diabetes mellitus are more likely to have silent myocardial infarctions, delaying treatment. Additionally, distal sensory neuropathy decreases the patient's ability to detect foot trauma and increases the risk of infection and limb amputation (49). Older adults are especially susceptible to these risks. One English study found that 65% of diabetic amputees were older than 65 years of age (17).

Although symmetric polyneuropathy is the most common peripheral presentation in diabetics, there are several other possible patterns of disease distribution. Mononeuropathies and radiculopathies are seen, although much less frequently. Both tend to occur in older patients with undiagnosed or mild diabetes. Noncompressive focal and multifocal neuropathies can also occur. Although any cranial nerve can be affected, third- and sixth-nerve palsies are the most common (47). Isolated peripheral nerves can be affected as well. Femoral and sciatic nerves are most commonly involved in these cases. Diabetes increases susceptibility to compressive neuropathies, with carpal tunnel syndrome occurring in up to one third of all patients (32).

Thoracoabdominal neuropathy typically occurs in patients with long-standing diabetes. This truncal neuropathy, most often noted in patients over 50 years of age, is a condition in which the patient experiences hyperpathic pain on the chest in a T3 through T12 distribution. Half of these patients have significant weight loss. Electromyography may show denervation in the intercostal and abdominal muscles.

Diabetic amyotrophy, also termed lumbosacral radiculoplexus neuropathy, is distinctive because it mostly targets people over 50 years of age. The term describes a syndrome involving both sensory and motor impairment (53). Motor examination shows moderate to severe weakness and atrophy in the pelvifemoral muscles. Sensory abnormalities are described as aching or burning sensations in the back, hip, and thigh, with preserved sensation in these regions on physical examination. Both motor and sensory abnormalities have an asymmetric distribution. Onset can be acute or subacute. There may be unintentional weight loss from onset. Symptoms may progress for up to 6 months. Prognosis for recovery is good, with a reported 60% of patients showing good recovery within 1 to 2 years. Pulse corticosteroids (500 mg of prednisone weekly) may hasten recovery time. IV infusions of immunoglobulins (IVIG) and cyclophosphamide have been used for treatment as well because immunologic dysfunction is a proposed etiology of diabetic amyotrophy.

Chronic inflammatory demyelinating neuropathy (CIDP) is more common in patients with diabetes mellitus and is in the differential diagnosis for symptoms suggestive of diabetic amyotrophy. Diabetic patients are reportedly 11 times more likely to develop CIDP. Treatment with steroids, plasma exchange, and IVIG is the standard of care.

Glycemic control is important for secondary prevention of both central and peripheral neuropathies. When pain is a prominent feature, pain alleviation is the initial focus. The most common effective treatments include analgesics, tricyclic antidepressants, and antiepileptic medication (Table 29-8). Treatment should be started at subtherapeutic doses and slowly titrated to the lowest possible effective dose. Pain described as lancinating, burning, or dysesthestic may have better response to capsaicin and clonidine than alternative medications. Deep, dull, gnawing pain may respond better to tramadol, dextromethorphan, and antidepressants (5). However, in the elderly, problematic side effects often emerge (Table 29-8). Physical and occupational therapy have been shown to be effective in the relief of predominantly motor neuropathies.

Estimates indicate that 20% to 40% of patients with diabetes suffer from ANS dysfunction. The cardiovascular, gastrointestinal, and genitourinary systems are all at risk for damage (Table 29-9). One of the most detrimental effects of ANS impairment is the loss of a sympathetic response to hypoglycemic states. This loss usually occurs within the first 5 to 10 years after developing diabetes. Postural hypotension is especially common and problematic in the elderly because of an increased risk of falls. The elderly population is more likely to have complications from falls,

Table 29-8. *Common Medications Used in Painful Diabetic Neuropathy*

Classification	Common Drugs	Specific Issues Related to Older Populations
Analgesics (oral)	Ibuprofen Naproxen	The steady-state concentration of the medication can be doubled in the older population
Analgesics (topical)	Lidocaine patch	
Antiepileptic drugs (AEDs)	Carbamazepine Oxcarbazepine[a] Gabapentin[a] Pregabalin Topiramate[a]	Gabapentin and pregabalin are better tolerated in the elderly than alternative antiepileptics, although NNT is reportedly lower in older AEDs
Tricyclic antidepressants (TCA)	Nortriptyline[a] Desipramine Amitriptyline	Increased risk of toxicity in the elderly; blood levels should be monitored; although NNT is most favorable, elderly patients are more susceptible to anticholinergic side effects
Selective serotonin reuptake inhibitors and neuroepinephrine reuptake inhibitors		Caution in titration because elderly are at increased risk of side effects; avoid in patients with severe renal failure
Opioids	Oxycodone controlled release (CR) Morphine CR	Practice caution when increasing doses because elderly display increased bioavailability
Atypical opioids	Tramadol	Increased risk of CNS side effects in the elderly, including amnesia; adjustment of daily dose recommended for those >75 years old

CNS, central nervous system.
[a]Off label.

and thus, the presence of postural hypotension increases the morbidity and mortality rates of older patients. Some of the major ANS complaints and common presentations consistent with these dysfunctions are discussed in Table 29-9.

History and neurologic examination are usually sufficient for diagnosis. Additional tests can be useful for specific problems. If postural hypotension is suspected, the American Diabetes Association recommends a battery of five tests: heart rate changes; Valsalva maneuver during lying, standing, and deep breathing; and blood pressure measurements after standing and sustained hand grip (7).

Several strategies have emerged to help combat the effects of diabetes on the ANS. Postural hypotension can be treated with the use of elastic stockings, elevation of the head when lying down, increased fluid intake, and increased salt in the diet. Fludrocortisone, a medication that can increase plasma volume and arterial tone, is used in more severe cases.

Medications that increase the tone of the inferior esophageal sphincter and increase esophageal contraction have been used to improve gastric emptying in patients with gastroparesis. These medications include metoclopramide, cisapride, and domperidone. Although metoclopramide has been used successfully in younger populations, it can produce severe side effects including delirium, parkinsonism, sedation, and urinary retention. For this reason, it is usually avoided in treatment of geriatric populations. Some studies have reported that erythromycin is useful for improving gastric motility in patients with gastroparesis (30). Tetracycline has been found to be an effective treatment in some cases of diabetic diarrhea.

Patients with a neurogenic bladder should be advised to empty the bladder every 3 hours. In more severe cases, patients can be taught to perform manual abdominal compression with urination or to self-catheterize. Parasympathomimetics are sometimes helpful in treatment. Follow-up with a urologist should be encouraged in all cases of neurogenic bladder and sexual dysfunction.

Several studies have addressed the prevention of diabetic neuropathy. The only current conclusive statement is that good glycemic control translates into less frequent and less severe neuropathies (50). For this reason, maintenance of serum glucose should be closely monitored and kept as close to normal limits as possible.

Table 29-9. *Summary of Autonomic Nervous System Impairment*

Autonomic Nervous System Impairment	Neurologic Dysfunction	Common Symptoms/Signs
Cardiovascular	Postural hypotension	Light-headedness
		Weakness
		Impaired vision
	Impaired heart rate	Syncopal episodes
		Resting tachycardia
		Bradycardia
		Fixed heart rate
Gastrointestinal	Esophageal dysfunction	Epigastric discomfort
	Gastroparesis	Anorexia, nausea, vomiting, constipation
	Diarrhea	Watery; often nocturnal or postprandial
Genitourinary	Erectile dysfunction	Insidious onset seen in one third of diabetic men
	Neurogenic bladder	Increased urinary frequency followed by urinary retention and overflow incontinence
Other impairments	Thermoregulatory dysfunction	Distal anhydrosis, heat intolerance, gustatory sweating
	Pupillary constriction with impaired light response	
	Failure to respond to hypoglycemic states	Lethargy; increased risk of hypoglycemic coma

Hypoglycemia

Hypoglycemia is a significant problem in the elderly population suffering from diabetes. Missing the diagnosis can lead to severe consequences, including coma and death. Typically, the disease presents insidiously. Patients often appear confused and disoriented. They may complain of transient neurologic deficits, and their neurologic examination findings may fluctuate. The elderly are more susceptible to falls and hypothermia during these episodes. Diabetic medications should be closely monitored in these patients, and oral hypoglycemic agents should be stopped or maintained on the lowest possible dose.

CONCLUSION

It is important for the general physician to take into account that typical diseases often do not present typically in the older adult, especially in cases of endocrine dysfunction. Neurologic changes are often vastly different from those seen in a younger patient with the same disease. The classic signs or symptoms of a disease may not be evident on history or physical examination. Screening should be done often to prevent missing a diagnosis and delaying treatment. Failure to identify these diseases can lead to serious morbidity and mortality.

REFERENCES

1. Ackermann RJ. Adrenal disorders: know when to act and what tests to give. *Geriatrics.* 1994; 49:32–37.
2. Als-Nielsen B, Kjaegard LL, Gluud C. Benzodiazepine receptor antagonists for acute and chronic hepatic encephalopathy. *Cochrane Database Syst Rev.* 2001;4:CD002798.
3. Andres E et al, 2004.
4. Bagchi N, Brown TR, Parish RF. Thyroid dysfunction in adults over the age of 55 years. A study in an urban U.S. community. *Arch Intern Med.* 1990;150:785–787.
5. Bansal V, Kalita J, Misra UK. Diabetic neuropathy. *Postgrad Med J.* 2006;82:95–100.
6. Barzel US. Hypothyroidism. *Clin Geriatr Med.* 1995;11:239–249.
7. Belmin J, Valensi P. Diabetic neuropathy in elderly patients. *Drugs Aging.* 1996;8:416–429.

8. Biondi B, Palmieri E, Klain M, et al. Subclinical hyperthyroidism: clinical features and treatment options. *Eur J Endocrinol.* 2005;152:1–9.

9. Bissels GJ, Staekenberg S, Brunner E, et al. Risk of dementia in diabetes mellitus: a systemic review. *Lancet Neurol.* 2006;5:64–74.

10. Bottiglieri T, Laundy M, Crellin R, et al. Homocysteine, folate, methylation, and monoamine metabolism in depression. *J Neurol Neurosurg Psychiatry.* 2000;69:228–232.

11. Braverman LE. Subclinical hypothyroidism and hyperthyroidism in elderly subjects: should they be treated. *J Endocrinol Invest.* 1999;22:1–3.

12. Buchman A. Vitamin supplementation in the elderly: a critical evaluation. *Gastroenterologist.* 1996;4:262–265.

13. Chen CS, Tsai JC, Tsang HY, et al. Homocysteine levels, MTHFR C677T genotype, and MRI hyperintensities in late-onset major depressive disorder. *Am J Geriatr Psychiatry.* 2005;13:869–875.

14. Cordoba J, Lopez-Hellin J, Planas M, et al. Normal protein diet for episodic hepatic encephalopathy. *J Hepatol.* 2004;41:38–43.

15. D'Anci K, Roseberg I. Folate and brain function in the elderly. *Curr Opin Clin Nutr Metab Care.* 2004;7:659–664.

16. Dbouk N, McGuire BM. Hepatic encephalopathy: a review of its pathophysiology and treatment. *Curr Treat Options Gastroenterol.* 2006;9: 464–474.

17. Deerochanawong C, Home PD, Alberti KG. A survey of lower limb amputation in diabetic patients. *Diabet Med.* 1992;9:942–946.

18. DeLaGarza VW. Pharmacologic treatment of Alzheimer's disease: an update. *Am Fam Physician.* 2003;68:1365–1372.

19. Dharmajan et al, 2003.

20. Diez J. Hyperthyroidism in patients older than 55 years: an analysis of the etiology and management. *Gerontology.* 2003;49:316–323.

21. Elias MF, Sullivan LM, D'Agostino RB, et al. Homocysteine and cognitive performance in the Framingham offspring study: age is important. *Am J Epidemiol.* 2005;162:644–653.

22. Forfar JC, Feek CM, Miller HC, et al. Atrial fibrillation and isolated suppression of the pituitary thyroid axis. Response to specific antithyroid therapy. *Int J Cardiol.* 1981;1:43–48.

23. Griffen J. Review: hypothyroidism in the elderly. *Am J Med Sci.* 1990;299:344–345.

24. Griffiths LL, Brocklehurst JC, Sott DL, et al. Thiamine and ascorbic acid level in the elderly. *Gerontol Clin.* 1967;9:1–10.

25. Hansen J, Skovsted L, Siersbok-Nielsen K. Age dependent changes in iodine metabolism and thyroid function. *Acta Endocrinol.* 1975;79:60–65.

26. Homocysteine Studies Collaboration. Homocysteine and risk of ischemic heart disease and stroke: a meta-analysis. *JAMA.* 2002;288: 2015–2022.

27. Hurley DL, Gharib H. Detection and treatment of hypothyroidism and Graves' disease. *Geriatrics.* 1995;50:41–44.

28. Hurwitz A, Brady DA, Schaal E, et al. Gastric acidity in older adults. *JAMA.* 1997;278: 659–662.

29. Hutto BR. Folate and cobalamin in psychiatric illness. *Compr Psychiatry.* 1997;28:305–314.

30. Janssens J, Peters TL, Vantrappen G, et al. Improvement of gastric emptying in diabetic gastroparesis by erythromycin. *N Engl J Med.* 1990;322:1028–1031.

31. Jones EA, Weissenborn K. Neurology and the liver. *J Neurol Neurosurg Psychiatry.* 1997;63: 279–293.

32. Kelkar P. Diabetic neuropathy. *Semin Neurol.* 2005;25:168–173.

33. Khaira JS, Franklyn JA. Thyroid conditions in older patients. *Practitioner.* 1999;243:214–221.

34. Kissela B, Air E. Diabetes: impact on stroke risk and poststroke recovery. *Semin Neurol.* 2006;26: 100–107.

35. Kissela BM, Khoury J, Kleindorfer D, et al. Epidemiology of ischemic stroke in patients with diabetes: the greater Cincinnati/Northern Kentucky Stroke Study. *Diabetes Care.* 2005;28: 765–770.

36. Koike H, Misu K, Hattori N, et al. Postgastrectomy polyneuropathy with thiamine deficiency. *J Neurol Neurosurg Psychiatry.* 2001;71:357–362.

37. Kripke C. Is oral vitamin B_{12} as effective as intramuscular injection. *Am Fam Physician.* 2006;73:65.

38. Lindenbaum J, Rosenberg IH, Wilson PWF, et al. Prevalence of cobalamin deficiency in the Framingham elderly population. *Am J Clin Nutr.* 1994;60:2–11.

39. Luchsinger JA, Mayeaux R. Dietary factors and Alzheimer's disease. *Lancet Neurol.* 2004;3:579–587.

40. Manore MM, Vaughan LA, Carroll SS, et al. Plasma pyridoxal 58 phosphate concentration and dietary vitamin B-6 intake in free-living, low-income elderly people. *Am J Clin Nutr.* 1989;50: 339–345.

41. McCully KS. Homocysteine and vascular disease. *Nat Med.* 1996;2:386–389.

42. McKeon NJ. Hyperthyroidism. *Emerg Med Clin North Am.* 2005;23:669–685.

43. McMahon JA, Green TJ, Skeaff CM, et al. A controlled trial of homocysteine lowering and cognitive performance. *N Eng J Med.* 2006;354: 2764–2772.

44. Meyer T, Eshelman A, Abouljoud M. Neuropsychological changes in a large sample of liver transplant candidates. *Transplant Proc.* 2006;38: 3559–3560.

45. Miller AH, Sastry GS, Speranza AJ, et al. Lack of association between cortisol hypersecretion and nonsuppression on the DST in patients with Alzheimer's disease. *Am J Psychiatry.* 1994; 151:267–270.

46. Mooijaart SP, Gussekloo J, Frolich M, et al. Homocysteine, vitamin B-12, and folic acid and the risk of cognitive decline in old age: the Leiden 85-Plus study. *Am J Clin Nutr.* 2005; 82:866–871.

47. Moster ML. Neuro-ophthalmology of diabetes. *Curr Opin Ophthalmol.* 1999;10:376–381.

48. Neff GW, Kemmer N, Zacharias VC, et al. Analysis of hospitalizations comparing rifaximin versus lactulose in the management of hepatic encephalopathy. *Transplant Proc.* 2006;38: 3552–3555.

49. O'Connor PJ, Spann SJ, Woolf SH. Care of adults with type 2, diabetes mellitus. *J Fam Pract.* 1998;47:S13–S22.

50. Partanen J, Niskanen L, Lehtinen J, et al. Natural history of peripheral neuropathy in patients with non-insulin dependent diabetes mellitus. *N Engl J Med.* 1995;333:89–94.

51. Poo JL, Gongora J, Sanchez-Avila F, et al. Efficacy of oral L-ornithine-L-aspartate in cirrhotic patients with hyperammonemic hepatic encephalopathy. Results of a randomized, lactulose-controlled study. *Ann Hepatol.* 2006;5:281–288.

52. Reynolds E. Vitamin B_{12}, folic acid, and the nervous system. *Lancet Neurol.* 2006;5:949–960.

53. Riddle MC. Diabetic neuropathies in the elderly: management update. *Geriatrics.* 1990; 45:32–36.

54. Ross MA. Neuropathies associated with diabetes. *Med Clin North Am.* 1993;77:111–124.

55. Saltzman JR, Russell RM. The aging gut. Nutritional issues. *Gastroenterol Clin North Am.* 1998;27:309–324.

56. Sapolsky RM, Plotsky PM. Hypocortisolism and its possible neural base. *Biol Psychiatry.* 1990; 27:937–952.

57. Shawcross D, Jalan R. Dispelling myths in the treatment of hepatic encephalopathy. *Lancet.* 2005;365:431–433.

58. Shoulson I. DATATOP: a decade of neuroprotective inquiry. Parkinson's Study Group. Deprenyl and Tocopherol Antioxidative Therapy of Parkinsonism. *Ann Neurol.* 1988;44:S160–S166.

59. Stabler SP, Lindenbaum J, Allen RH. Vitamin B-12 deficiency in the elderly: current dilemmas. *Am J Clin Nutr.* 1997;66:741–749.

60. Surks MI, Ortiz E, Daniels GH, et al. Subclinical thyroid disease. Scientific review and guidelines for diagnosis and management. *JAMA.* 2004; 291:228–238.

61. Valensi P, Giroux C, Seeboth-Ghalayini B, et al. Diabetic peripheral neuropathy: effects of age duration of diabetes, glycemic control, and vascular factors. *J Diabetes Complications.* 1997;11: 27–34.

62. Van Asselt DZ, Blom HJ, Zuiderent R, et al. Clinical significance of low cobalamin levels in older hospital patients. *Neth J Med.* 2000; 57:41–49.

63. Vidall-Aaball J, Butler CC, Cannings-John R, et al. Oral vitamin B12 versus intramuscular vitamin B_{12} for vitamin B_{12} deficiency. *Cochrane Database Syst Rev.* 2005;20:CD004655.

64. Vir S, Love A. Thiamine status of institutionalized and noninstitutionalized aged. *Int J Vitam Nutr Res Suppl.* 1997;47:325–335.

65. Wallace K, Hofmann MT. Thyroid dysfunction: how to manage overt and subclinical disease in older patients. *Geriatrics.* 1998;53:32–41.

66. Weber FL Jr. Combination therapy with lactulose or lactitol and antibiotics. In: Conn HO, Bircher J, eds. *Hepatic encephalopathy: syndromes and therapies.* Bloomington, IL: Medi-Ed Press; 1994:285–297.

67. Winger JM, Hornick MD. Age-associated changes in the endocrine system. *Nurs Clin North Am.* 1996;31:827–844.

68. Wolters M, Strohe A, Hahn A. Cobalamin: a critical vitamin in the elderly. *Prev Med.* 2004;39: 1256–1266.

69. Young MJ, Boulton AJM, Macleod AF, et al. A multicentre study of the prevalence of diabetic peripheral neuropathy in the United Kingdom hospital clinical population. *Diabetolgia.* 1993;36:150–154.

SUGGESTED READINGS

Als-Nielsen B, Gluud L, Gluud C. Non-absorbable disaccharides for hepatic encephalopathy: systematic review of randomized trials. *BMJ.* 2004;328: 1046–1050.

Bansky G, Meier PJ, Riederer E, et al. Effects of the benzodiazepine receptor antagonist flumazenil in hepatic encephalopathy in humans. *Gastroenterology.* 1989;97:744–750.

Brenner RP. The electroencephalogram in altered states of consciousness. *Neurol Clin.* 1985;3:615–631.

Carmel R, Aurangzeb I, Ojan D. Associations of food-cobalamin malabsorption with ethnic origin, age, *Helicobacter pylori* infection, and serum markers of gastritis. *Am J Gastroenterol.* 2001;96:63–70.

Durson M, Caliskan M, Aluclu U, et al. The efficacy of flumazenil in subclinical to mild hepatic encephalopathic ambulatory patients. A prospective, randomized, double-blind, placebo-controlled study. *Swiss Med Wkly.* 2003;133:118–123.

Goulenok C, Bernard B, Cadranel JF, et al. Flumazenil vs. placebo in hepatic encephalopathy in patients with cirrhosis: a meta-analysis. *Aliment Pharmacol Ther.* 2002;16:361–372.

Grimm G, Ferenci P, Katzenshlager R, et al. Improvement of hepatic encephalopathy treatment with flumazenil. *Lancet.* 1988;2:1392–1394.

Grinblat J. Folate status in the aged. *Clin Geriatr Med.* 1985;1:711–728.

Krasinski SD, Russel RM, Samloff IM, et al. Fundic atrophic gastritis in an elderly population. Effect on hemoglobin and several serum nutritional indicators. *J Am Geriatr Soc.* 1986;34:800–806.

Nash TP. Treatment options in painful diabetic neuropathy. *Act Neurol Scand.* 1999;173(suppl):36–42.

Riordan SM, Williams R. Treatment of hepatic encephalopathy. *N Engl J Med.* 1997;337:473–479.

Samuels MH. Subclinical thyroid disease in the elderly. *Thyroid.* 1998;8:803–813.

United States Pharmacopeia. *United States Pharmacopeial Convention.* USPDI 19th ed. Taunton, MA: Micromedex Inc.; 1999.

WEBSITES

American Diabetes Organization: http://www.diabetes.org/

National Institutes of Health Senior Health Website: http://nihseniorhealth.gov/

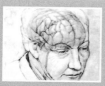

CHAPTER 29.3

Neurologic Manifestations of Systemic Disease: Disturbances of the Kidneys, Electrolytes, Water Balance, Rheumatology, Hematology/Oncology, Alcohol, and Iatrogenic Conditions

Kevin M. Biglan

NEUROLOGIC COMPLICATIONS OF RENAL DISEASE

Acute and chronic renal failure has a variety of deleterious effects on the nervous system. The mechanism of these effects is multifactorial and is due to a combination of uremia, disturbances of electrolytes and water balance, impaired drug metabolism, anemia, associated comorbid illness, and the effects of hemodialysis. The incidence of chronic renal failure increases with increasing age (12), and uremia accounts for 10% of delirium in the elderly (134).

ACUTE COMPLICATIONS OF RENAL FAILURE

Uremic Encephalopathy

Encephalopathy is common in acute renal failure. Given the increased risk of delirium in the elderly (67), encephalopathy is nearly universal in the older patient who develops an acute deterioration in renal function. Uremic encephalopathy is clinically similar to delirium from other metabolic derangements (179,180). Table 29-10 summarizes the clinical manifestations of this condition (30,179,180), with fatigue, apathy, difficulty with attention and concentration, and subtle motor signs predominating early. Later in the course, uremic encephalopathy can progress to coma and seizures (30,179,180). Symmetric upper motor neuron signs may also be seen.

The level of uremia correlates poorly with the degree of impairment, with the rapidity of renal deterioration being more important in the development of encephalopathy (30). Encephalopathy can occur not only in acute renal failure but also in the setting of decompensated chronic renal failure. Chronic renal failure can also predispose patients to delirium from other causes (67).

Table 29-10. *Manifestations of Uremic Encephalopathy*

Fatigue
Motor abnormalities: clumsiness, ataxia, paratonia, hyperreflexia, Babinski signs
Frontal lobe release signs
Delirium
Asterixis/myoclonus
Postural and kinetic tremor
Seizures

Computed tomography (CT) and magnetic resonance imaging (MRI) can reveal nonspecific changes but should be performed in all patients receiving hemodialysis secondary to the risk of spontaneous subdural hematomas (SDHs) (see Complications of Dialysis). Electroencephalography (EEG) can be useful in determining whether superimposed seizures are a contributing factor to a patient's confusion. In the absence of seizures, the EEG will show generalized slowing (30,179,180); however, spike and wave complexes can be seen in up to 14% of patients without clinical seizure activity (30).

Treatment of uremic encephalopathy entails correcting the underlying renal disease and, possibly, hemodialysis. Correction of an underlying anemia can further improve cognitive function in some patients (173). Seizures should be treated appropriately. Caution must be used with certain anticonvulsants (i.e., phenytoin and valproic acid) (11) because of reduced protein binding in renal failure secondary to hypoalbuminemia and a resultant increase in free levels of these drugs (179,180).

CHRONIC COMPLICATIONS OF RENAL FAILURE

Uremic Neuropathy

Neuropathy occurs in 60% to 100% of patients with chronic renal failure on hemodialysis (123). It is more common in older patients and men (30). It is a distal, symmetric, sensorimotor axonal polyneuropathy predominantly involving large fibers (30,123,180). Clinically, patients complain of paresthesias and distal motor weakness. Findings on physical examination are diminished or absent reflexes, muscle atrophy, and a stocking-glove sensory loss.

The severity and course are variable. Although mild cases may resolve or improve with dialysis, most cases are not appreciably influenced by dialysis (123). Successful renal transplantation is the only known cure and results in a dramatic improvement within days of transplantation (123).

Restless legs syndrome, a frequent accompaniment (212), is a condition characterized by abnormal sensations in the legs and arms accompanied by a desire to move the legs. Standing or walking relieves the symptoms, whereas rest exacerbates them. The symptoms are more severe in the evening or at night (221). Dopamine agonists (i.e., pramipexole or ropinirole) (165,212), given at night, are useful for ameliorating the symptoms.

Myopathy

Myopathy in renal failure is multifactorial secondary to cachexia, steroids, and water and electrolyte disturbances (74). Proximal muscle weakness and associated atrophy make up the clinical picture. Rarely, a fulminant painful myopathy associated with necrosis occurs (30). Neurophysiologic studies reveal a myopathic pattern, whereas muscle histology is nonspecific.

Cerebrovascular Disease

Cerebrovascular disease is a major cause of morbidity and mortality in patients with chronic renal failure, with a nearly 20% prevalence rate in one large series of chronic hemodialysis patients (41). Although this higher risk is likely associated with shared risk factors such as diabetes mellitus, hypertension, dyslipidemia, and smoking, chronic renal failure itself has been independently associated with an increased risk of stroke (1). As in the general population, increasing age is an important risk factor for stroke in this population. In addition, patients with chronic renal failure are at a higher risk for hemorrhagic stroke due to platelet dysfunction associated with uremia (53).

In general, the evaluation and management of stroke in patients with renal failure are the same as in other patients with stroke. Modifiable risk factors should be addressed in an attempt to prevent future strokes. Angiotensin-converting enzyme inhibitors or angiotensin II type 1 receptor blockers are recommended in diabetic kidney disease or nondiabetic kidney disease with significant proteinuria (210). Some controversy exists regarding the benefit of statins on stroke prevention in this population, however, and pending future statin studies are currently recommended (19). Anemia appears to be an important independent risk factor for stroke in renal failure, and erythropoietin injections may be considered as a preventive measure (1).

COMPLICATIONS OF DIALYSIS

Dialysis Disequilibrium Syndrome

The elderly are at high risk for developing dialysis disequilibrium syndrome, a rare but life-threatening complication of peritoneal dialysis or hemodialysis. Dialysis disequilibrium syndrome was more common prior to 1970 when patients were dialyzed more rapidly (30,179,180).

A wide variety of symptoms may be seen, from the mild (headaches, myalgias, and restlessness) to the severe (coma and seizures). Symptoms begin at the end of dialysis or shortly thereafter. Dialysis disequilibrium syndrome is the result of large osmotic gradients between the brain and plasma, resulting in large fluid shifts into the brain parenchyma (201). Clinically, this results in increased intracranial pressure and obtundation from cerebral edema (30,179,180).

Prevention is the key to managing this problem. Slow dialysis, every 1 to 2 days, and the use of osmotically active solutes have reduced the frequency of this complication.

Dementia

Impaired cognition is common in end-stage renal disease (129). A significantly higher percentage of patients on dialysis will have dementia compared with age-matched controls, with an annual incidence of 4.2% in elderly patients on dialysis (73,129). Although the cause is unclear, ischemic disease appears to play a prominent role (73,129). Also, cerebral atrophy is seen in patients with renal failure on dialysis, and the degree of atrophy correlates with duration of dialysis (118).

In addition, a specific syndrome of a progressive dementia has been associated with chronically dialyzed patients. It is commonly referred to as dialysis dementia, dialysis encephalopathy, or progressive myoclonic dialysis encephalopathy (162). Dialysis dementia is a progressive and potentially fatal disorder characterized by progressive cognitive decline (30). Disorders of speech—a slowness and hesitancy of speech and paraphasia—occur commonly and early in the course of this disorder (30,162). Some cases progress to an overt expressive aphasia, whereas others may represent an apraxia of speech (162). Myoclonus is ubiquitous, and ataxia and apraxia can occur. Changes in personality, with psychosis and hallucinations, occur in more advanced cases. Seizures occur late in as many as 60% to 100% of patients (30,162).

Frontal intermittent rhythmic delta activity is the most characteristic finding on EEG (30,162). Generalized slowing, triphasic waves, and spike and wave activity may also be seen on EEG (162). Neuroimaging and cerebrospinal fluid (CSF) examination are useful in ruling out other causes of the patient's deterioration (30).

Dialysis dementia has been linked to aluminum concentrations in dialysate water supply (48,136). The use of deionized water with low aluminum levels has nearly eliminated this condition (48). However, sporadic cases do occur and may be associated with aluminum-containing, phosphate-binding agents used in this population (30). Treatment consists of the use of aluminum-free water in the dialysate and aluminum chelating agents (desferrioxamine). Paradoxically, a period of clinical worsening may occur at the initiation of chelation therapy (30,102).

Subdural Hematoma

SDH can occur in 1% to 3% of patients receiving hemodialysis in the absence of trauma (30). The cause is multifactorial and likely reflects a combination of cerebral atrophy, large fluid shifts during dialysis, coagulopathies, and the use of anticoagulants during dialysis. Signs and symptoms include diminished level of consciousness, headache, and focal neurologic deficits. However, bilateral SDHs are common and can present with confusion, lethargy, and gait dysfunction. Therefore, a high index of suspicion must be maintained for this complication. All patients on dialysis who develop an alteration in mental status should have a CT scan to rule out the possibility of SDH. Conservative treatment, with close clinical follow-up, may be all that is needed in some patients; however, neurosurgical intervention may also be required.

NEUROLOGIC COMPLICATIONS OF DISTURBANCES OF ELECTROLYTES AND WATER BALANCE

DISTURBANCES OF SODIUM AND WATER BALANCE

Dehydration

Dehydration is the most common fluid disturbance in the elderly (132). Dehydration accounts for 1.5% of hospital admissions of the elderly and frequently complicates other illnesses (182). In addition, dehydration is a major risk factor for the development of delirium in the inpatient setting (109). Table 29-11 summarizes the major risk factors for dehydration in elderly nursing home patients (132).

Table 29-11. *Risk Factors for Dehydration*

Age >85 years
>4 chronic or acute diseases
>4 medications
Winter season
Assistance required with feeding
Immobility

Treatment of dehydration requires removing any offending drugs and hydration with isotonic saline until the patient is hemodynamically stable. Subsequently, 0.45% saline solution can be used until the water deficit is corrected. Caution must be used in using hypotonic solutions as they may precipitate hyponatremia.

Hyponatremia

In general, water balance is strictly maintained such that the serum sodium concentrations range between 138 and 142 mmol/L (125). Deficits in the ability of the kidney to dilute the urine, coupled with increased fluid intake, results in hyponatremia.

Neurologic complications of hyponatremia are dependent on the severity of the hyponatremia and the rate that it evolved and range from delirium to coma and seizures from cerebral edema (52,125). The decision to treat hyponatremia should be based on the presence of symptoms, severity and duration of hyponatremia, and the presence of hypovolemia (34).

When hyponatremia is known to have developed in <48 hours and the patient has neurologic symptoms, then rapid correction is warranted (125). This can be achieved by the infusion of hypertonic saline (3% NaCl) in combination with a loop diuretic (125). When the duration of hyponatremia is >48 hours or unknown and the patient has symptoms, it must be corrected with extreme caution to avoid central pontine myelinolysis (CPM) (125,131). The rate of sodium replacement should not exceed 1 to 2 mEq/L/h and not exceed 12 mEq/L in the first 24 hours or 18 mEq/L in the first 48 hours of treatment (206). Frequent monitoring of clinical and electrolyte status is needed in all patients undergoing treatment regardless of the rate of correction. Acute treatment should end when the patient's symptoms resolve, a serum sodium of 120 mEq/L is reached, or an increase of 20 mEq/L occurs. In patients with chronic hyponatremia and minimal or no neurologic symptoms, immediate treatment is not warranted, and conservative therapies such as fluid restriction can be instituted (217).

Hypernatremia

Hypernatremia is less common than hyponatremia; however, central nervous system (CNS) manifestations are frequently more prominent (125). Also, the elderly are more susceptible to hypernatremia than other age groups due to dehydration (18). Symptoms of delirium, with alterations in level of consciousness and seizures, can occur (52,125). Focal deficits may reflect subdural hemorrhage if the change in sodium levels occurred rapidly (10). In the most common setting, hypernatremia reflects a hypovolemic state, and treatment is as outlined for dehydration.

Central Pontine Myelinolysis

CPM is a catastrophic disorder associated with the rapid correction of hyponatremia. The term CPM is misleading because extrapontine white matter is frequently involved. Pathologically, extensive and symmetric white matter dysmyelination is out of proportion to neuronal loss. Clinical presentations vary, depending on the degree and location of myelinolysis, although more than 90% of patients will have the classic findings of spastic quadriparesis and pseudobulbar palsy. Prognosis varies from death to complete recovery. MRI of the brain reveals symmetric areas of T2 hyperintensity in the pontine and extrapontine white matter. Caution must be used in interpreting scans too early because the characteristic changes may delay the clinical presentation of CPM by 2 weeks (39,131).

The only treatment is prevention, and the hyponatremia must be corrected cautiously. However, CPM has been reported to develop despite safe correction of hyponatremia (131). Therefore, correcting the hyponatremia with the associated potential of myelinolysis must outweigh the risks of illness from hyponatremia.

DISTURBANCES OF POTASSIUM BALANCE

Hypokalemia

Hypokalemia is common in elderly patients admitted to the hospital (116). In its mildest forms, it is associated with myalgias and proximal muscle weakness; in severe cases, profound weakness, rhabdomyolysis, and tetany can occur (10). Rarely, this will occur acutely and be associated with thyrotoxicosis (3,216). Potassium replacement is effective in treating the symptoms (10).

Hyperkalemia

Hyperkalemia causes a profound, rapidly progressive, flaccid quadriplegia sparing the cranial nerve musculature (10,61). Paresthesias are sometimes seen. Drugs or renal failure are common causes (61). Mortality is related to cardiovascular complications (10). Aggressive reduction of the serum potassium results in resolution of the symptoms (61).

DISTURBANCES OF CALCIUM BALANCE

Hypocalcemia

Hypocalcemia is an abnormally low concentration of ionized calcium. It is usually the result of hypoparathyroidism (64,65) and is a well-recognized complication

of thyroid or parathyroid surgery (10). Tetany associated with perioral and limb paresthesia is the most common manifestation (10,65). Seizures and psychosis can also occur (10,52). The Chvostek sign (i.e., spasm of the facial muscles with percussion of the facial nerve) and Trousseau sign (i.e., spasm of the hand after inflation of a blood pressure cuff above the systolic blood pressure) are positive (64,65). Symptoms correct with calcium replacement (10).

Hypercalcemia

Hypercalcemia, which is more common than hypocalcemia, may be the result of hyperparathyroidism, malignancy, or drugs (64,65,95). Delirium can occur, but seizures are rare. Muscle weakness and fatigability are peripheral manifestations (10). Therapy is based on the underlying cause and clinical symptoms (95). Intravenous hydration, loop diuretics, glucocorticoids, and calcitonin can be used nonspecifically to reduce serum calcium levels while the underlying cause is being investigated (64,65).

DISTURBANCES OF MAGNESIUM BALANCE

Hypomagnesemia

Hypomagnesemia results from poor dietary intake or absorption or through increased magnesium loss via renal mechanisms (25). It is frequently associated with hypocalcemia, and the clinical symptoms are similar (10,25). Hypomagnesemia must always be suspected when a patient with hypocalcemia fails to respond to calcium replacement (10). Treatment with oral magnesium supplementation is usually sufficient.

Hypermagnesemia

Hypermagnesemia is rarely relevant clinically and is usually associated with renal failure (64,65). Somnolence, confusion, and weakness associated with reduced or absent reflexes are the neurologic manifestations (10). Treatment consists of dialysis in renal failure or intravenous administration of 100 to 200 mg of calcium (64,65).

NEUROLOGIC COMPLICATIONS OF CANCER

The incidence of cancer increases with age, putting the elderly at an increased risk for developing neurologic complications from cancer and its treatment. Besides routine chemotherapy, neurologic symptoms are the most common reason for hospitalization of individuals with known cancer (81). Neurologic disease in cancer occurs via four separate mechanisms: (a) metastatic involvement of brain parenchyma, meninges, or spinal cord; (b) direct extension into neural structures (e.g., lumbosacral plexus); (c) remote involvement (i.e., paraneoplastic syndromes); and (d) neurotoxic effects of cancer therapy (44,81,82,111). This section briefly discusses the first three mechanisms (see Chapter 28 for additional information on these topics), focusing primarily on the toxic effects of cancer therapy.

METASTATIC DISEASE

Metastasis can occur in any portion of the nervous system, although the brain is the most common region involved (44). Spinal cord involvement occurs through vertebral body metastasis and subsequent extension into the epidural space with cord compression (44). Less commonly, metastasis to the meninges can occur, presenting with symptoms of increased intracranial pressure, multiple cranial neuropathies, and multiple radiculopathies (44,87). Leptomeningeal metastases have a poor prognosis without aggressive therapy (87). Lung and breast cancers are the most common tumors to metastasize to the nervous system (44,87).

DIRECT INVASION

Pancoast tumors of the lung may extend into the brachial plexus, causing plexopathies that affect the muscles of the lower cord of the brachial plexus and Horner syndrome (115). Pelvic tumors can extend into the lumbosacral plexus (111,172). Finally, tumors of the nasopharynx can invade through the skull base, causing cranial neuropathies, pneumocephalus, and death (121,171). Treatment is dependent on tumor type and location.

PARANEOPLASTIC SYNDROMES

Neurologic paraneoplastic syndromes refer to signs and symptoms affecting nervous system tissue remote to the primary cancer and its metastases. Although these syndromes are common in specific cancers (e.g., myasthenia gravis and thymoma), they affect <1% of all cancer patients. However, they do have a significant impact on the patient's quality of life and can precede the cancer diagnosis in 50% of cases (155). Table 29-12 summarizes the well-characterized paraneoplastic syndromes and their associated antineuronal antibodies (46,155,175,185). The combination of CT scan and fluorodeoxyglucose (FDG) positron emission tomography (PET) is 100% sensitive at detecting tumors in patients with antineuronal antibodies and a paraneoplastic syndrome (133).

COMPLICATIONS OF CANCER TREATMENT
Chemotherapeutic Agents

Neurologic side effects of cancer treatments are common and frequently add to the confusion surrounding neurologic symptoms in these patients. Many chemotherapeutic agents have neurotoxic side effects (119).

Methotrexate

Intrathecal methotrexate (MTX) causes an acute meningeal reaction approximately 2 to 4 hours after administration. Meningismus, headache, nausea, lethargy, and spinal fluid pleocytosis are common (119). No long-term sequelae of this manifestation occur, and it resolves spontaneously in days (82,119). However, it may easily be confused with bacterial meningitis, which may result in delaying treatment.

Table 29-12. *Antineuronal Antibody and Associated Paraneoplastic Neurologic Syndromes*

Antibody	Syndrome	Tumor Types
Anti-Yo	Cerebellar degeneration	Ovary, breast, lung
Anti-Hu	Encephalomyelitis, sensory neuronopathy, autonomic dysfunction	SCL, neuroblastoma
Anti-Ri	Opsoclonus-myoclonus (adults), cerebellar degeneration	Breast, lung, gynecologic, bladder
Anti-CRMP5	Chorea, sensory neuropathy, cerebellar degeneration, encephalomyelitis	Breast, SCL
Anti-amphiphysin	Stiff-person syndrome	Breast
Anti-Ma1/Ma2	Limbic, brainstem encephalitis, cerebellar ataxia	Lung, testis
Anti-titin	Myasthenia gravis	Thymoma
Anti-GM1/MAG	AIDP/CIDP	Hodgkin, osteosclerotic myeloma
Anti-voltage-gated calcium channel (NMJ)	Lambert-Eaton myasthenic syndrome	SCL, prostate, cervix

SCL, small-cell lung; AIDP, acute inflammatory demyelinating polyneuropathy; CIDP, chronic inflammatory demyelinating polyneuropathy; NMJ, neuromuscular junction.

A subacute reaction to MTX can occur after multiple intrathecal injections (82). This reaction results in clinical signs of a spinal cord lesion with paraplegia and sensory level and bladder dysfunction. The condition gradually improves over days to months, and recovery is variable (119).

Encephalopathies associated with long-term MTX use have been identified independent of the method of delivery. Patients are confused, lethargic, and ataxic and may have seizures. A delayed leukoencephalopathy may also be seen months to years after treatment with intrathecal or intravenous MTX (68,82,119). This condition begins insidiously and progresses to dementia. It is much more common in older patients who also received whole-brain radiation (77).

Cytarabine

Cytarabine (AraC) can cause a reversible cerebellar syndrome peaking after 2 to 3 days of onset. Most patients recover completely after cessation of the drug. Age >50 years appears to be the greatest risk factor for this complication (176). AraC given intrathecally can cause a chemical meningitis and myelopathy similar to that seen with MTX (119).

Platinum

Platinum-based drugs (cisplatin and oxaliplatin) have long been associated with ototoxicity, causing symptoms of tinnitus and hearing loss (82,119). A distal symmetric, predominantly sensory axonal neuropathy is also seen (82,119). The neuropathy is dose dependent, and synergistic toxicity is seen with doxorubicin, vindesine, and etoposide (190). In addition, oxaliplatin causes an acute sensory neuropathy characterized by cold sensitivity, paresthesia, and pseudolaryngospasm that is rapidly reversible (88).

Vinca Alkaloids

The use of vinca alkaloids is limited due to their common neurotoxicities (82,119). Peripheral neuropathy occurs early in nearly all patients receiving vinca alkaloids (e.g., vincristine) (15,82,119). The neuropathy is a distal symmetric sensorimotor axonal polyneuropathy. Motor manifestations resolve with discontinuation of the drug, but sensory manifestations persist (82). Vincristine has been associated with an autonomic neuropathy that preferentially affects the gastrointestinal tract, causing constipation. Cranial neuropathies are also seen and must be distinguished from carcinomatous involvement of the meninges (82,119).

Hexamethylmelamine

Hexamethylmelamine causes a peripheral neuropathy similar to vincristine (82). It has also been associated with a wide variety of CNS effects, from parkinsonism to ataxia and seizures (119).

Fluorouracil

Fluorouracil can cause an acute cerebellar syndrome 2 weeks to 6 months into treatment (82,119). The incidence of this complication appears to be dose related (119). This syndrome is reversible with discontinuation of the drug; however, it rapidly recurs if the drug is reintroduced (82,119). Metastasis to the cerebellum constitutes the major differential diagnosis and must be ruled out if this condition occurs.

The combination of fluorouracil with levamisole has been associated with a multifocal inflammatory leukoencephalopathy. Symptoms begin within a few months of initiating treatment and are characterized by confusion and focal neurologic signs. MRI reveals multiple gadolinium-enhancing white matter lesions. Discontinuation of the drug and treatment with corticosteroids may result in improvement (176).

Taxanes

The taxanes (e.g., docetaxel and paclitaxel) are effective treatments against metastatic breast cancers, early breast cancer, and treatment-resistant ovarian cancers. The taxanes cause a distal, predominantly sensory axonal neuropathy (191).

RADIATION THERAPY

Radiation can have a negative impact on the nervous system by direct toxic effects of radiation on neural tissues or by damaging the vasculature that supplies neural tissue (49,57,153,169,187). Radiation-induced injury to the nervous system occurs when the neural tissue lies within the field of radiation. This can occur as incidental radiation (radiation to head and neck tumors with incidental brain radiation) or directly (whole-brain radiation for metastatic tumors).

Spinal Cord Injury

A transient myelopathy associated with incidental radiation to the spinal cord is the most common spinal cord complication of radiation treatments (57). Mild symptoms consisting of paresthesia and Lhermitte sign develop several months after treatment. Neurologic examination is usually unremarkable, and the symptoms resolve over 1 to 9 months (57).

A delayed progressive myelopathy is a more feared complication of radiation involving the spinal cord. The symptoms can occur as early as a few months after treatment or as long as 5 years after treatment (57). Paresthesia and anesthesia are the earliest manifestations, followed by disabling weakness and bladder dysfunction with the spinal cord level involved corresponding with the level radiated. A Brown-Sequard hemi-cord pattern may be seen (57,169). Neuroimaging is necessary to distinguish this condition from metastatic disease causing a compressive myelopathy.

An isolated lower motor neuron syndrome has been reported in individuals who have received spinal radiation. The lumbosacral spine is preferentially involved in this condition (209).

Cerebral Injury

Cerebral injury following therapeutic radiation is classified by the time of onset following treatment: acute, early delayed, and late. An acute reaction to brain radiation occurs within days of radiotherapy and manifests with headache, lethargy, and nausea. Prophylactic dexamethasone is recommended for individuals with a large tumor burden or who are receiving a large dose of radiation (57).

Early delayed encephalopathy is a self-limited complication occurring a few months after radiation and lasting several weeks before resolving (57). Headache and lethargy are the prominent symptoms. Neuroimaging may show worsening edema and be difficult to distinguish from tumor recurrence. Stereotactic biopsy may be necessary to rule out treatment failures. Dexamethasone may be beneficial.

Late cerebral injury is irreversible and can occur months to years after brain radiation (57). Dementia, seizures, headache, personality changes, and focal neurologic signs are common (49,57,187). Imaging may reveal focal abnormalities indistinguishable from tumor or diffuse abnormalities in the deep white matter and cerebral atrophy (49,57). DeAngelis et al. (49) recommend a trial of steroids and consideration of ventriculoperitoneal shunting.

Cerebrovascular disease of the intracranial and extracranial vessels is another cause of delayed cerebral injury associated with exposure of these vessels to therapeutic radiation. Transient ischemic attacks and strokes may develop secondary to radiation-induced accelerated atherosclerosis (57,153).

Peripheral Injury

Peripheral effects of radiation mainly include plexopathies associated with radiation of these structures (98). This condition may be difficult to distinguish from direct invasion of the plexus with tumor. Clinical and electrophysiologic myokymia may be more common in radiation injury than plexopathy from other causes (98). MRI of the plexus may be useful in identifying the cause.

NEUROLOGIC COMPLICATIONS OF HEMATOLOGIC ILLNESS

THROMBOTIC THROMBOCYTOPENIC PURPURA

Thrombotic thrombocytopenic purpura is a severe multisystem disease characterized by fever, thrombocytopenia, microangiopathic hemolytic anemia,

Table 29-13. *Differential Diagnosis of Thrombotic Thrombocytopenic Purpura in the Elderly*

Bacterial infections: *Shigella, Escherichia coli, Salmonella, Campylobacter jejuni, Yersinia, Pneumococcus*
Viral infections: coxsackie B, echovirus, influenza, Epstein-Barr virus, herpes simplex virus
Cancer: adenocarcinoma, lymphoma
Autoimmune disorders: antiphospholipid syndrome, scleroderma
Drugs: penicillin, sulfa, quinine, ticlopidine, cyclosporin, tacrolimus, chemotherapy
Bone marrow transplantation

neurologic symptoms, and impaired renal function (60). It tends to affect a younger population but can be seen in any age group. Table 29-13 reviews conditions affecting the elderly where thrombotic thrombocytopenic purpura is seen (60,80).

Neurologic complications can be secondary to ischemia in the small blood vessels or hemorrhage, resulting in permanent neurologic deficits. Transient and fluctuating neurologic signs without permanent deficits are more common. These can include headache, delirium, motor and sensory deficits, seizures, and even coma (60).

Plasma exchange is the mainstay of treatment but is not without risks (80). Corticosteroids, antiplatelet medications, and immunosuppressants may be necessary adjuncts in some cases. Splenectomy is reserved for patients who are refractory to other treatments (60).

DISSEMINATED INTRAVASCULAR COAGULATION

Disseminated intravascular coagulation (DIC) is a syndrome of widespread intravascular thrombosis followed by thrombocytopenia and hemorrhage. Multiple causes exist for DIC, including infection, trauma, cancer, and vascular diseases. Treatment is geared toward the underlying cause. Additionally, supportive care is frequently necessary. Fluid resuscitation, fresh frozen plasma, and platelet transfusions are useful. The neurologic complications are related to CNS ischemia (stroke) and hemorrhage (72).

NEUROLOGIC MANIFESTATIONS OF RHEUMATOLOGIC DISEASE AND SYSTEMIC VASCULITIDES

EPIDEMIOLOGY OF RHEUMATIC DISEASE IN THE ELDERLY

Spinal osteoarthritis and spondylosis are nearly universal consequences of aging. Other rheumatologic diseases are less common. Although most autoimmune rheumatologic diseases begin in young to middle adult-hood, they can also affect the older adult population. Notable exceptions include rheumatoid arthritis and giant cell arteritis, which increase in prevalence with age (186). This section will focus on the rheumatologic disorders primarily affecting the elderly. Table 29-14 provides information on the epidemiology of these disorders (17,33,56,100,113,126,154,163,181,186,195,199,204).

The incidence of neurologic complications of rheumatologic diseases varies from the exceedingly rare (e.g., the sensory neuronopathy of Sjögren's disease) (69,186) to the very common (e.g., headache in giant cell arteritis) (32). However, these neurologic complications may be the initial manifestation of the disease (90) and are frequently associated with high morbidity and mortality. For these reasons, this subgroup of disorders deserves special attention.

OSTEOARTHRITIS

Osteoarthritis is ubiquitous in the elderly and is a common cause of neurologic disease and disability. The most common complaint associated with osteoarthritis is pain. Low back pain is one of the most common reasons patients seek medical attention (186). Frank neurologic dysfunction secondary to radiculopathy, mononeuropathy, and myelopathy are common consequences of degenerative disease of the joints. Infrequently, osteoarthritis can impair cerebral blood flow, producing symptoms of cerebral ischemia (79).

Osteoarthritis is characterized by the slow, steady progression of articular pain. The pain worsens with use, is relieved with rest, and has little associated morning stiffness. Physical examination reveals a painful enlarged joint with a limited range of motion. Peripheral osteoarthropathy is rarely a cause of neurologic dysfunction. However, entrapment neuropathy at the carpal tunnel may be related to osteophyte formation and bony hypertrophy (55).

Osteoarthritis of the spine associated with spondylosis of the intervertebral disks is a much more common cause of neurologic morbidity. Spondylosis refers to the desiccation and degeneration of the intervertebral disk associated with aging or the combination of osteoarthritis of the intervertebral joints and degeneration of the intervertebral disks (186,213). The two conditions invariably coexist, and disk desiccation and loss of disk height associated with aging are likely causative factors in osteoarthritis of intervertebral joints (178).

Radiculopathy

Radiculopathies can result from two different mechanisms. Encroachment of the neural foramina by osteophytes and bony spurs is the most common cause of radiculopathy in the elderly. The foraminal narrowing usually remains quiescent until a minor trauma results in symptoms (213). Less common in the older population is acute disk herniation with resultant foraminal narrowing.

Clinically, radiculopathy is characterized by pain with radiation in a radicular pattern. Weakness and numbness in the distribution of the nerve root involved can also occur. Excessive mobility of the neck or back will exacerbate the symptoms, as will Valsalva maneuvers (213). In the cervical spine, the C6-7

Table 29-14. *Epidemiology of Rheumatic Diseases*

Disease	Prevalence (per 100,000)	Incidence (per million per year)	Female:Male Ratio	Age at Onset (years)	% with Neurologic Involvement
Rheumatoid arthritis	0.2–2.0	300	2–3:1	40–60	7–13 (excluding pain)
Systemic lupus erythematosus	0.0005–0.04	46–74	7–9:1	15–30	36
Systemic sclerosis	4×10^{-6}–0.007	6.3–18.7	3–15:1	30–50	6–40
Primary Sjögren			9:1	40–50	20
Sarcoidosis		40–100	3:2	20–40	5
Giant cell arteritis (age >50)	0.13–0.24	30–200	3:1	>60	10–40
Polyarteritis nodosa group	0.7–6.3	9	1:2	40–60	PAN/CSS = 50–75; MPA = 14–36
Wegener granulomatosis		4	1:2	30–45	22–54
Cryoglobulinemic vasculitis			2:1	50–65	40

PAN, polyarteritis nodosa; CSS, Churg-Strauss syndrome; MPA, microscopic polyangiitis.

Table 29-15. *Signs and Symptoms of Radiculopathy by Disk Level Affected*

Disc Level	Spinal Root	Muscles	Sensory Loss	Deep Tendon Reflexes
C2-3	C3	Levator scapulae	Lateral neck, lower occiput	None
C3-4	C4	Rhomboids, diaphragm	Lower neck	None
C4-5	C5	Deltoid	Lateral forearm	Biceps
C5-6	C6	Biceps	Thumb and index finger	Biceps/ brachioradialis
C6-7	C7	Triceps	3rd and 4th fingers	Triceps
C7-T1	C8	Intrinsic hand muscles	Medial forearm, 5th finger	Finger flexors

Disk Level	Spinal Root (medial disk)[a]	Muscles	Sensory Loss	Deep Tendon Reflexes
L2-3	L3	Hip flexors, quadriceps	Anterior thigh	Patellar
L3-4	L4	Quadriceps	Knee and medial leg	Patellar
L4-5	L5	Hip adductors, extensor great toe	Lateral leg, great toe	None
L5-S1	S1	Hip extension, plantar flexors	Lateral foot, sole of foot	Ankle jerk

[a]Lateral disc herniations may affect the nerve root above the disc level (e.g., the T12-L1 affects the T12 spinal root). Symptoms correspond to the spinal root affected.

followed by the C5-6 disk space is most commonly involved. In the lumbosacral spine the L4-5 and L5-S1 disks are usually involved (186). Table 29-15 outlines the clinical symptoms seen with radiculopathy by the nerve root involved (28,186).

A variety of examination maneuvers are useful in making the diagnosis of radiculopathy. In the Spurling maneuver, the head is extended and rotated toward the symptomatic side, resulting in reproduction of the radicular symptoms. The compression test entails pushing down on the head with resultant foraminal narrowing and exacerbation of symptoms. Abduction of the arm on the affected side results in pain diminishment in cervical radiculopathy (47). Lumbar radiculopathy can be similarly elicited. The straight leg-raising sign is positive if the patient reports pain radiating down the posterior aspect of the leg into the calf or foot when the hip is flexed >20 degrees while the knee is maintained in extension. A positive crossed straight leg-raising maneuver is more specific for radiculopathy but less sensitive. In this maneuver, pain is elicited in the opposite leg from the one raised (186).

Electrodiagnostic studies are useful in confirming suspected radiculopathy and in differentiating the role of other coexistent conditions (227). Plain radiographs of the cervical spine have a high false-positive rate in the elderly, frequently showing degenerative findings in asymptomatic individuals, and are not recommended in this population (150,213). Myelograms, CT scans,

or MRIs readily show the anatomic relationship of the spinal roots, intravertebral disks, and neural foramina. Each study has similar sensitivity and specificity (128), although MRI better reveals nerve root and cord compression (124). In addition, MRI can rule out more serious causes of radiculopathy in the elderly (e.g., metastatic cancer and epidural infections).

Although radiologic evaluation is important in the evaluation of possible radiculopathy, careful correlation of imaging results with patient history and physical examination findings is essential. When abnormal radiologic findings are seen in the absence of supportive historical, clinical, and electromyography (EMG) findings, other causes of the patient's symptoms must be sought.

The natural history of radiculopathy tends to be benign. Most individuals have complete or partial resolution of their symptoms (213). Therefore, conservative therapy is recommended initially. Medical therapy consists of nonsteroidal anti-inflammatory drugs (NSAIDs) (124,213). Caution should be exercised when using these agents in the elderly who are particularly susceptible to developing NSAID-associated peptic ulcers and hepatic and renal dysfunction (150,189). Soft collars can be useful in relieving pain. Exercise, initially under the guidance of a physical therapist, should be encouraged. Surgical decompression should be considered in an individual with disabling pain and weakness that persists for more than 3 months (213).

Spinal Stenosis

The degenerative changes of the spine that occur with aging can also cause progressive narrowing of the spinal canal (76,213). Symptoms arising from degenerative spinal stenosis occur at an average age of 73 years in women and at a slightly younger age in men (76). Narrowing of the cervical spinal canal causes myelopathy, whereas narrowing below the conus medullaris causes signs and symptoms of nerve root compression.

Unlike cervical radiculopathy, pain is not a common feature of cervical spinal stenosis. Symptoms are varied depending on the part of the cord involved and include weakness, clumsiness, anesthesia, paresthesia, balance and gait difficulties, urinary frequency, and incontinence (178,213). Upper motor neuron signs (i.e., spasticity, hyperreflexia, extensor plantar responses) predominate below the level of stenosis. Lower motor neuron signs (i.e., atrophy and hyporeflexia) may be seen at the level of stenosis because of involvement of the anterior horn cells and spinal roots. Lhermitte sign refers to an electric shock that radiates down the spine into the extremities with neck flexion (124,213). In the elderly, Lhermitte sign should prompt the search for a compressive lesion of the cervical spine.

Spinal stenosis of the lumbar spine causes compression of multiple nerve roots of the cauda equina. The condition progresses insidiously, usually beginning with low back pain. The classic signs and symptoms of cauda equina are outlined in Table 29-16 (28,76,93).

Pseudoclaudication, also known as "neurogenic claudication," occurs in 94% of patients with lumbar spinal stenosis (93). This condition refers to leg pain or paresthesia associated with walking or extension of the low back. Unlike true vascular claudication, it is relieved within minutes of resting or changing postures. Individuals with pseudoclaudication can walk long distances if bent at the waist and may bicycle without difficulties. This is in contrast to vascular claudication, where pain in the legs is elicited by any leg exercise (186). The straight leg-raising sign is uncommon, being positive in only 10% of patients (76,93).

Unlike radiculopathy, electrodiagnostic studies are less useful in the evaluation of spinal stenosis, although these studies can be useful in ruling out peripheral neuropathy or amyotrophic lateral sclerosis as a cause of the patient's symptoms. Although EMG can suggest or support the diagnosis of lumbar spinal stenosis, MRI is the study of choice (76). Plain radiographs, however, should not be ignored. Flexion and extension views of the spine can give valuable information about spine stability. CT imaging is not recommended, especially in the elderly. CT often misses multilevel disease and more ominous causes of stenosis (e.g., tumors, fractures, and infections). MRI is essential in the elderly to distinguish these causes of spinal stenosis from degenerative causes. CT myelography can be useful in individuals for whom MRI is contraindicated (76).

In general, spinal stenosis progresses in a stepwise manner over years. It begins insidiously with pain or intermittent paresthesia and can progress to a severely disabling condition (213). Patients with mild symptoms (i.e., those that do not interfere with daily function) have the best prognosis (213). In one study, two thirds of patients continued to have only mild impairment over 20 years with nonsurgical management (161).

Conservative therapy, focusing on education and a well-designed exercise program, can be useful in individuals with only mild impairment (213). Surgery is indicated when spinal stenosis interferes with performance of daily activities and quality of life or evolves over a short period of time (76,213). Patients need to be educated regarding the realistic outcomes of surgical decompression. Surgical treatment is aimed at preventing progressive disability and relieving symptoms of neurogenic claudication and gait impairment (76,93,163,213). Medical comorbidity has a negative impact on recovery after surgery, although older age is not a contraindication for surgery (76). In fact, when the history, physical examination, and MRI studies are consistent, surgery is an excellent option in this patient population (16).

RHEUMATOID ARTHRITIS

Rheumatoid arthritis is the second most common rheumatologic disorder, after osteoarthritis. Unlike most immune-mediated rheumatologic diseases, it has a predilection for an older population, and its incidence increases with age (186). It is a chronic, inflammatory, symmetric polyarthritis (36,186). It is a disease of the small joints of the hands and feet and, unlike osteoarthritis, is associated with morning

Table 29-16. *Signs and Symptoms of Cauda Equina Syndrome*

Symptoms	Signs
Early asymmetric radicular pain	Asymmetric sensory loss
Pain relieved with back flexion	Asymmetric weakness
Asymmetric numbness and paresthesia	Absent or decreased reflexes
Asymmetric weakness	
Late sphincter involvement	
Pseudoclaudication	

stiffness. It classically affects the metacarpopha-langeal, proximal interphalangeal, wrist, and metatar-sophalangeal joints (99). Extra-articular complications occur in 10% to 20% of patients, with neurologic complications being common (36).

Neurologic manifestations of rheumatoid arthritis are rarely, if ever, the presenting symptom, occurring late or in the presence of active articular or systemic disease. Carpal tunnel syndrome is the most common neurologic manifestation of rheumatoid arthritis. However, atlantoaxial subluxation with spinal cord compression at the C1-2 disk space is the most omi-nous cause of neurologic morbidity and mortality (36,56,91,150,186). Peripheral neuropathy (22,194, 202), myopathy (223), and, rarely, CNS involvement (110,140) have also been reported.

CERVICAL SUBLUXATION

Cervical subluxation is caused by chronic inflamma-tion of the synovial joints of the cervical spine, result-ing in weakening of the ligaments, cartilage, and bone of these joints (36,150). The destructive influence of this process results in intervertebral subluxation. The ligaments that maintain the odontoid process in posi-tion relative to the atlas bone and cranium are partic-ularly susceptible, and atlantoaxial subluxation is the most common abnormality of the cervical spine in rheumatoid arthritis (36,91,150,186). Radiographic evidence of cervical spine disease is seen in most patients (56,158); however, only 7% to 13% develop neurologic symptoms (56). Long disease duration, positive rheumatoid factor, male sex, and erosive peripheral joint disease increase the risk of developing this complication (36). The elderly are potentially at high risk as well because of the superimposition of spondylotic changes with rheumatoid changes in the neck (150).

Complaints referable to atlantoaxial subluxation can be vague or nonexistent (36). Neck pain and headache are nearly universal in individuals with rheumatoid arthritis and cervical spine disease (91, 186). When symptoms are present, they are similar to those described for cervical spinal stenosis from osteoarthritis. However, compression of the medulla or vertebral arteries may elicit complaints of paroxys-mal loss of consciousness, vertigo, dysarthria, balance difficulties, and visual disturbances (36,56).

Neurologic findings may be difficult to elicit in the patient with rheumatoid arthritis and cervical sublux-ation and often correlate poorly with radiographic findings (186). Although hyperreflexia is the most common neurologic finding in these patients (207), severe joint disease or peripheral neuropathy may mask hyperreflexia (56). In addition, the absence of neurologic findings is not necessarily predictive of a neurologic prognosis (56).

Despite the presence or lack of symptoms and signs, rheumatoid arthritis involvement of the cervical spine is life threatening. Mikulowski et al. (147) found 10 of 104 deaths associated with rheumatoid arthritis to be attributable to medullary compression secondary to severe atlantoaxial subluxation, and radiologic evi-dence of atlantoaxial subluxation was associated with an eightfold greater risk of death (184). Therefore, a high index of suspicion must be maintained to iden-tify those patients at risk for this complication.

Treatment decisions in rheumatoid cervical spine disease are complex and controversial (91). Studies are underway to evaluate the benefit of early surgery in this population (229). Individuals with neurologic deficits or intractable pain associated with cervical spine sub-luxation are candidates for surgical intervention (56,141). More challenging is identifying individuals at high risk for neurologic complications and death and avoiding unnecessary surgery in asymptomatic individ-uals. Figure 29-2 outlines a potential algorithm to assist in making these treatment decisions (26,56).

Entrapment Neuropathies

Peripheral nerve involvement is common in rheuma-toid arthritis, with entrapment neuropathies at the carpal tunnel and tarsal tunnel making up most of the peripheral nerve injuries (36). Carpal tunnel syndrome results from compression of the median nerve at the carpal tunnel in the wrist. Common clinical symptoms include nocturnal paresthesias in the first three digits of the hand, anesthesia in the median distribution of the hand, and, later, weakness of the abductor pollicis brevis. Tarsal tunnel syndrome results from compression of the posterior tibial nerve as it passes under the medial malleolus in the medial aspect of the ankle. Paresthesia and pain on the plantar sur-face of the foot are common symptoms. Conservative therapy with anti-inflammatory medications and wrist splints is frequently adequate. Surgical decompression can be considered in individuals who develop motor impairment (36).

Peripheral Neuropathy

Patients with rheumatoid arthritis may develop a diffuse peripheral neuropathy, the incidence of which appears to be associated with disease severity (36,186). Early studies evaluating outpatients suggest a low incidence of this complication (186). However, in one study that surveyed 70 patients with disease severe enough to require hospital admission, signs and symp-toms of a diffuse polyneuropathy were found in 64% (83). Two major types of peripheral neuropathy can be seen: a symmetric predominantly sensory neuropa-thy and a sensorimotor mononeuritis multiplex (36).

The predominantly sensory neuropathy is a distal symmetric neuropathy involving the small-fiber

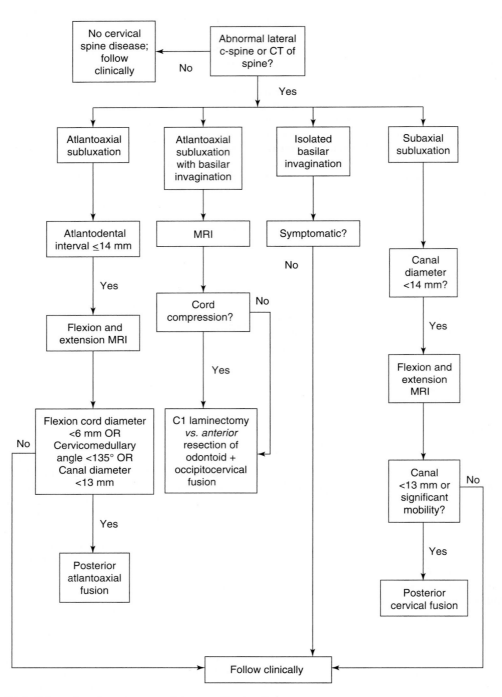

Figure 29-2. Diagnosis and management of rheumatoid spine disease.

sensory modalities of pain and temperature. Its onset is insidious, presenting with distal anesthesia and burning paresthesia (36). The prognosis in this condition is variable, with some individuals reporting spontaneous improvement and others remaining stable for years (186). In general, no specific treatment is warranted, although amitriptyline or gabapentin can be useful in alleviating the burning pain sometimes associated with this condition. It should be noted that gold therapy for rheumatoid arthritis has also been associated with a reversible neuropathy (23).

A mixed sensorimotor neuropathy is usually associated with a systemic vasculitis and presents as a mononeuritis multiplex (36,194,202). The appearance of mononeuritis multiplex often heralds a systemic vasculitis. It can present acutely and progress rapidly, distinguishing it from mononeuropathy secondary to entrapment. It is frequently associated with active rheumatoid arthritis, palpable purpura, skin ulcers, anemia, leukocytosis, high rheumatoid factor titers, hypocomplementemia, constitutional symptoms, ischemia in other organ systems, and proteinuria (36,194).

Prognosis in these patients is poor, with a 40% to 63% mortality rate (36,37). For fulminant cases, aggressive treatment is mandatory and consists of a combination of high-dose pulse steroids (methylprednisolone 1 g intravenous) and cyclophosphamide (0.5 g/m^2) (36). Plasmapheresis has been used in the past but has recently fallen out of favor because it lacks efficacy (43). Oral cyclophosphamide and prednisone have been advocated for less severe disease. Further treatment of systemic vasculitis is discussed in the section titled Systemic Vasculitides.

Myopathy

Although muscle weakness is a common complaint in rheumatoid arthritis, its cause is multifactorial. Disuse atrophy and drugs, especially steroids, have been implicated. Muscle enzyme levels are normal (36,186). Muscle biopsies show type II atrophy, without evidence of inflammation, necrosis, regeneration, or vasculitis (101).

Central Nervous System Involvement

CNS involvement in rheumatoid arthritis is extraordinarily rare. Isolated case reports have suggested that CNS vasculitis, meningitis, and rheumatoid nodule formation within the CNS can all occur (110,140,177).

SYSTEMIC LUPUS ERYTHEMATOSUS

Systemic lupus erythematosus is a disease primarily of young women (186,199) and is rarely, if ever, seen in the elderly.

SYSTEMIC SCLEROSIS

Systemic sclerosis, or scleroderma, is a rare disorder characterized by excessive fibrosis, microvascular disease, and autoimmune phenomena (186). Raynaud phenomenon is the most common presenting symptom, occurring in >90% of patients. Additional findings include characteristic fibrosis and thickening of the skin, symptoms of gastrointestinal dysmotility, abnormal pulmonary function, and an inflammatory arthritis and tenosynovitis (78,186). Antinuclear antibody (ANA) titers are frequently elevated (186). Peripheral nervous system (PNS) involvement in

the form of neuropathy and myopathy can be seen in upward of 40% of patients (17). CNS involvement is rare, although encephalopathy secondary to end-organ failure (e.g., renal crisis) can be seen (160,199).

The peak incidence of the disease occurs during the fourth and fifth decades (204). A 50% mortality rate is seen at 10 years (204); therefore, this disease is seen less common in an older population. Onset of the disease after 50 years of age is associated with a worse survival rate than in younger patients (204).

Peripheral Nervous System Involvement

Myopathy is the most common neurologic involvement in systemic sclerosis (17,78). An indolent chronic myopathy has been reported in 60% to 80% of patients (78). In this group, muscle enzyme levels may be normal or only mildly elevated, EMG findings are benign, and muscle biopsies show subtle histologic changes. A smaller but still substantial population will have evidence of an inflammatory myopathy (17,78,103). In these cases, marked elevation of muscle enzymes is seen (aldolase more so than creatinine kinase). EMG study shows low-amplitude polyphasic motor units. Muscle biopsy can be consistent with either a polymyositis or even inclusion body myositis (17,78). In the indolent and more benign form of myopathy, no specific treatment is necessary. More aggressive forms can be successfully treated with prednisone (60 mg/day) (17).

Peripheral nerve involvement is common and falls into three categories: polyneuropathy, cranial neuropathies (usually the trigeminal nerve), and entrapment neuropathies (usually the median nerve at the carpal tunnel) (17,78,149,199). The polyneuropathy associated with systemic sclerosis is an axonal mixed sensorimotor neuropathy (35). Frequently, the neuropathy is subclinical (149). Trigeminal neuropathy occurs in 4% of the patients (62) and begins with gradual sensory loss in a trigeminal distribution, sparing the motor portion of the nerve. Pain symptoms can be treated with medications used for neuropathic pain.

PRIMARY SJÖGREN SYNDROME

The diagnostic criteria for Sjögren syndrome are debated among rheumatologists (4,70). Using the strictest criteria, the diagnosis of Sjögren syndrome requires the presence of destruction of the exocrine portion of the lacrimal and salivary glands in association with evidence for a systemic autoimmune process (70,168). Applying these criteria, Sjögren syndrome is a rare disorder. However, with a more liberal criterion requiring only the presence of salivary and lacrimal gland dysfunction, it has an overall prevalence of 2% (5). Despite this controversy, it is likely that Sjögren syndrome is underrecognized in the elderly (4). Sjögren syndrome is often secondary to another rheumatic disease, such as rheumatoid arthritis; in this setting, the neurologic complications are as per the primary illness.

The hallmark of the disease is the presence of the "sicca syndrome," which includes xerophthalmia (dry eyes) and xerostomia (dry mouth). Xerophthalmia can be documented with the Schirmer test (186). Aging and drugs are common causes of the sicca syndrome (186); therefore, one must exercise caution in making the diagnosis of Sjögren syndrome in the elderly based on exocrine dysfunction alone. Evidence for autoimmunity is demonstrated by either showing a mononuclear infiltrate in a biopsy of the lacrimal or salivary glands or via the presence of autoantibodies in the sera of affected patients. ANA, anti-Ro (SS-A), and anti-La (SS-B) are the autoantibodies most commonly elevated in Sjögren syndrome (9,96).

Neurologic involvement is common, with a preference for the PNS (8,69,145). In fact, the original description of Sjögren syndrome included a patient with bilateral seventh nerve palsies (126). CNS manifestations were only recognized later (4); however, some reports suggest that the incidence of CNS involvement may be as high as 20% in some tertiary referral centers (7).

Peripheral Nervous System Involvement

A pure sensory neuronopathy is widely recognized as being associated with Sjögren syndrome (9,69). The cause is secondary to lymphocytic infiltration of the dorsal root ganglia (137). Dorsal column function (vibration and joint position sense) is preferentially affected. Trigeminal sensory neuropathies can coexist. A sensory neuropathy may be the first manifestation of Sjögren syndrome, even in the absence of more classic symptoms (69,152). Therefore, an evaluation for Sjögren syndrome should be pursued in any patient presenting with a pure sensory neuropathy. This condition can present subacutely (137) with asymmetric sensory loss and painful paresthesia. Treatment consists of the use of corticosteroids, but results have been equivocal (186).

Although sensory neuropathy is the classic PNS abnormality associated with Sjögren syndrome, a diverse group of disorders of the PNS can occur (152). Among those reported are mixed sensorimotor neuropathies (8,145), chronic relapsing inflammatory neuropathies (85), entrapment neuropathies (e.g., carpal tunnel syndrome) (8), autonomic neuropathy (152), cranial neuropathies (8,186), myopathies (5,92), and hypokalemic periodic paralysis (secondary to renal tubular acidosis) (42). A trigeminal sensory neuropathy, the prototypical cranial neuropathy encountered, can be unilateral or bilateral. Loss of sensation in the maxillary and mandibular distributions, with sparing of the orbital division, is common (186).

Central Nervous System Involvement

Sjögren syndrome has been associated with a wide variety of CNS manifestations from seizure and stroke to aseptic meningitis and myelitis (4,6,27,50). The most common clinical presentation is a relapsing-remitting CNS disease that is similar to multiple sclerosis. MRI examination of the brain may reveal areas of subcortical T2 hyperintensity that may be dismissed as ischemic disease from other causes in the elderly (4). CSF examination reveals a mild mononuclear pleocytosis, elevated protein, elevated immunoglobulin G (IgG) index, and oligoclonal banding (7). Rarely, CNS involvement can present as either a cortical or subcortical dementia. This dementia is potentially reversible with corticosteroid treatment, suggesting that Sjögren syndrome should be considered as a possible cause of reversible dementia (4).

No standardized therapeutic strategy exists for treating individuals with CNS manifestations of Sjögren syndrome. Therapy should be geared toward the subset of patients who develop cumulative neurologic impairment over time. The mainstay of treatment is the use of corticosteroids. Cyclophosphamide should be considered in those individuals who continue to deteriorate neurologically despite treatment with corticosteroids (50). Alexander (4) recommends intravenous pulse cyclophosphamide monthly for a minimum of 12 months in conjunction with oral corticosteroids for these patients.

SARCOIDOSIS

Sarcoidosis is a rare, multisystem, granulomatous disease of unknown cause. Lung is the most common organ system involved, affecting more than 90% of patients (114). The diagnosis is based on a compatible clinical presentation involving at least two distinct organ systems, with pathologic evidence of noncaseating granulomas, in the absence of evidence for other granulomatous diseases (e.g., mycobacterial or fungal disease) (114).

Sarcoidosis occurs in any ethnic group; however, in North America, it is 10 times more common in African-Americans. It affects predominantly young adults in their 20s and 30s; however, it can affect any age group. Neurologic involvement occurs in only 5% of all patients with sarcoidosis (205); however, when neurologic involvement does occur, it is the presenting manifestation of the illness in 50% of cases. In addition, neurologic involvement is associated with high morbidity and mortality rates and can be difficult to diagnose and treat (114).

As with many of the diseases discussed in this section, sarcoidosis can affect the entire neuraxis. Cranial nerve involvement is the most common neurologic manifestation (51,198,205). Other common features include meningitis, pituitary or hypothalamic dysfunction, polyneuropathy, and myopathy (38,51,164, 196,197,205). Seizures, strokelike episodes, and even intracranial mass lesions have all been reported (5,164,196,197).

Cranial Neuropathies

Cranial seventh nerve palsies occur in two thirds of individuals with neurosarcoidosis (198). It can be bilateral in up to one third of the cases (198). The presence of bilateral facial palsy must always raise the suspicion of a secondary cause, such as sarcoidosis. The optic nerve is commonly involved (51,164,198), presenting with decreased visual acuity and color vision, and may have restricted visual fields. Trigeminal and vestibulocochlear nerves may also be involved, and involvement can be bilateral (164,205).

Neuromuscular Involvement

Involvement of the peripheral nerves and muscle in sarcoidosis is common and varied (38,135,164,196, 205). Peripheral nerve involvement can have a variety of forms, from mononeuropathy to the Guillain-Barré syndrome (51,196,197). Asymptomatic involvement of muscle can occur in >50% of patients with sarcoidosis (51,135). In this circumstance, muscle biopsy reveals granulomas surrounded by normal tissue. Symptomatic myopathy associated with myalgias, proximal weakness, and elevated muscle enzymes occurs in a minority of patients but can be disabling (135).

Central Nervous System Involvement

Meningitis is a more common CNS complication of sarcoidosis (38,114,164). It preferentially involves the basal meninges and hypothalamus. It can result in hydrocephalus, increased intracranial pressure, and hypothalamic and pituitary dysfunction (51,164). Seizures may also occur and reflect granulomatous lesions of the cortex or intracranial mass lesions.

Diagnostic Evaluation

Neuroimaging reveals increased contrast uptake in the meninges. Spinal fluid analysis may reveal a mononuclear pleocytosis, elevated protein, and low glucose (114). Serum and CSF angiotensin-converting enzyme levels can be elevated, which is specific for sarcoidosis but relatively insensitive (164,195). Gallium scanning, on the other hand, is sensitive for the detection of extraneural sarcoid but nonspecific (208). However, the combination of uptake of gallium in the lacrimal and salivary glands (panda sign) with uptake in the hilar lymph nodes (lambda sign) is found almost exclusively in sarcoidosis (208).

Treatment

Most patients will respond in the short term to treatment with corticosteroids, although relatively high doses (40 to 80 mg/day of prednisone) are needed (114,196,197). The exact duration of treatment is not known. Johns and Michele (114) recommend starting with 40 mg/day of prednisone for 2 weeks and then gradually reducing the dose over 8 weeks. Patients are then maintained on 10 to 15 mg daily for 8 months, after which they are weaned gradually over 4 months until off the medications. Relapses occur in one third of individuals (195), requiring an increase in the prednisone dose. Occasionally, MTX, azathioprine, chlorambucil, thalidomide, and cyclosporine have been used successfully in steroid-resistant cases (196,197).

SYSTEMIC VASCULITIDES

The vasculitides are a group of disorders that share in common the histologic feature of inflammation directed against blood vessels (151). This inflammation can be secondary to one of the rheumatic diseases previously discussed, or the vascular inflammation can be the primary event. The nervous system is involved to varying degrees in all of the systemic vasculitides (151). The pathophysiology of neurologic involvement is primarily related to ischemia from occluded vessels or hemorrhage from weakened blood vessel walls (186).

Many of the systemic vasculitides affect the elderly. They are characterized by evidence of multiorgan disease, constitutional symptoms, multiple ischemic events in multiple vascular distributions, and a variety of organ-specific syndromes (186). This section reviews a few of the relatively more common systemic vasculitic syndromes that primarily involve the older population.

Temporal (Giant Cell) Arteritis

Temporal arteritis is a systemic granulomatous vasculitis of medium to large vessels, involving primarily branches of the carotid artery. It is a disease of the elderly, with >95% of cases occurring in those older than 50 years of age (186). Clinically, patients complain of headache, malaise, arthralgias, myalgias, scalp tenderness, and jaw claudication (120). Physical examination reveals a tender, indurated temporal artery with a diminished or absent pulse (120). Headache is the most frequent symptom, occurring in 70% to 90% of patients (200). Temporal arteritis should be suspected in all elderly patients with a new-onset headache or change in the pattern of a previous headache (200). Laboratory examination reveals an elevated erythrocyte sedimentation rate and an anemia of chronic disease (120). Table 29-17 summarizes the American College of Rheumatology criteria for diagnosing temporal arteritis (108). For a more detailed discussion of temporal arteritis, see Chapter 12.

Table 29-17. *American College of Rheumatology Criteria for the Diagnosis of Temporal Arteritis*[a]

Age ≥50 years old
New-onset localized headache
Decreased pulse or tenderness of the temporal artery
Erythrocyte sedimentation rate ≥50 mm/hour
Arterial biopsy showing a necrotizing arteritis or a
   granulomatous process

[a] The presence of three or more criteria has a specificity of 91% and a sensitivity of 93.5%.

Polyarteritis Nodosa Group

The polyarteritis nodosa (PAN) group is the prototypical systemic vasculitis (186). This group of disorders consists of PAN, Churg-Strauss syndrome, and microscopic polyangiitis (MPA) (90). These disorders are defined by symptoms of multiorgan involvement secondary to panarteritis of medium and small vessels (89,113). The absence of glomerulonephritis or vasculitic involvement of the small arterioles, venules, and capillary beds distinguishes PAN. Churg-Strauss syndrome is an eosinophilic inflammation of the respiratory tract associated with asthma. MPA affects the smallest vessels, and therefore, glomerulonephritis is common (86,113). Perinuclear antineutrophil cytoplasmic antibodies may be found in MPA and Churg-Strauss (86,113). This group of disorders occurs in all ages throughout adulthood, with the mean incidence in the fifth and sixth decades. Neurologic involvement occurs in all subtypes (113,199).

PNS involvement is the most common manifestation of these protean disorders (199). Mononeuritis multiplex is the classic pattern of peripheral nerve involvement. Almost any peripheral nerve can be involved; peroneal involvement is the most common, resulting in a foot drop (37). CNS involvement can occur in as many as 50% of cases and should not be overlooked because it is a leading cause of mortality in this population (199). CNS manifestations tend to occur late in the course of the disease in the setting of prominent systemic symptoms. CNS symptoms include ischemic events, hemorrhage, and encephalopathy.

Treatment entails aggressive immunosuppression. Generally, a combination of corticosteroids and cyclophosphamide is recommended. Intravenous pulse administration of methylprednisolone (15 mg/kg every 24 hours for 3 days) is used as initial treatment secondary to its rapid onset of effectiveness and relative safety (89). Following pulse corticosteroids, oral prednisone (1 mg/kg daily) is given and can later be tapered as the patient improves. The addition of cyclophosphamide given as an intravenous

pulse (0.6 g/m^2) monthly for 12 months further improves the prognosis (63,89), although evidence indicates that steroids are sufficient in a subset of patients (89). Other agents, such as azathioprine, MTX, intravenous immunoglobulin, mycophenolate mofetil, plasma exchange, rituximab, and tumor necrosis factor-alpha inhibitors can be offered to patients who are intolerant or unresponsive to cyclophosphamide (84,215).

Wegener Granulomatosis

Wegener granulomatosis is characterized by a granulomatous inflammation of the upper and lower respiratory tract associated with a focal glomerulonephritis and a systemic necrotizing vasculitis of small vessels (113). Most patients will have a central antineutrophil cytoplasmic antibody (86). Again, neurologic involvement is common (113,159).

Peripheral neuropathy, in the form of a mononeuritis multiplex, is the most common neurologic manifestation (159). Ischemic strokes and seizures are the most common CNS manifestations (20,159). Unique to Wegener granulomatosis is CNS involvement by direct invasion of granulomatous inflammatory tissue through the paranasal sinuses into the brain (199).

Treatment is similar to that outlined for PAN; however, recurrences can be more frequent (84,186).

Cryoglobulinemic Vasculitis

Cryoglobulinemic vasculitis is caused by the deposition of cryoglobulins in vessel walls and the subsequent inflammatory reaction this incites (113). Up to 90% of cases are associated with hepatitis C virus infection (127). The most common clinical manifestations are purpura, arthralgias, and glomerulonephritis (113,127). Polyneuropathy is commonly seen, and electrophysiologic evidence of neuropathy may be seen in 80% of patients (127).

Treatment for acute exacerbations or rapidly progressive cryoglobulinemic vasculitis is similar to that outlined for other systemic vasculitides. Maintenance treatment with interferon-alpha is suggested during clinical remission (127).

ALCOHOL AND THE NERVOUS SYSTEM

EPIDEMIOLOGY OF ALCOHOL USE IN THE ELDERLY

Recreational and problematic use of alcohol in the elderly is common. One study revealed that 62% of subjects between 60 and 94 years of age regularly drank alcohol (148). Thirteen percent of men and 2% of women were considered heavy drinkers (more than two drinks per day). Up to 16% of Americans over

Table 29-18. *Alcohol-Related Nervous System Disease*

Acute	Chronic
Altered mood	Wernicke's encephalopathy
Impaired cognition and judgment	Korsakoff's syndrome
Cerebellar dysfunction	Dementia
Ataxia	Cerebellar degeneration
Incoordination	Central pontine myelinolysis
Dysarthria	Neuropathy
Vestibular dysfunction	Myopathy
Nystagmus	Alcohol withdrawal syndrome
Impaired balance	Delirium tremens
Hypothermia	Seizures
Coma	
Seizures	

the age of 65 have an alcohol use disorder (146). Alcohol use also places a significant burden on the health care system. Of all hospitalizations in the elderly, 1% are directly related to alcohol use or an alcohol-related disease (2). An increase of 50% in the number of elderly alcoholics is believed to have occurred from 1970 to 2000 (13).

Neurologic sequelae of alcohol use are common. The alcohol-related neurologic disorders compromise a diverse group of illnesses that can affect every level of the nervous system, from cortex to muscle (Table 29-18). Alcoholic psychosis (i.e., alcoholic dementia, delirium, amnestic syndrome, and withdrawal hallucinosis) is the third most common alcohol-related admission diagnosis in the elderly (2). As the population continues to grow older and the number of elderly alcoholics increases, a dramatic increase can be expected in neurologic complications of alcohol use.

ACUTE EFFECTS OF ALCOHOL USE

Alcohol is a CNS depressant. Paradoxically, the initial effect of intoxication is excitation of the cortex. Slowing of motor and cognitive functioning soon follows as a result of direct toxic effects of alcohol on neurons. As serum alcohol levels increase, consciousness is progressively impaired, and coma can occur (193).

The elderly are particularly vulnerable to the effects of alcohol intoxication. The reduction in lean body mass in the elderly results in a relatively increased peak alcohol concentration for any given alcohol dose compared with younger individuals (183). Older adults are also particularly predisposed to falls. Alcohol intoxication impairs coordination and balance, slows motor

reaction, and can result in hypotension, greatly increasing the risk of falling (183). Individuals who chronically use alcohol can develop neuropathy, myopathy, and cerebellar degeneration, as well as impaired cognition and judgment, further increasing the risk of falling while intoxicated. This may account for the high incidence of fractures (13) and SDH in this population.

Rarely, acute alcohol intoxication can cause seizures (71). In the elderly population, symptomatic causes of seizures (e.g., SDH, strokes, or tumors) must be aggressively sought. More commonly, seizures are the result of alcohol withdrawal (58).

The treatment of acute alcohol intoxication is supportive, although the complications of chronic alcoholism should always be considered and treated accordingly. Patients should be observed, injuries resultant from intoxication should be treated, and fluid balance and a safe environment during recovery should be maintained (139).

CHRONIC EFFECTS OF ALCOHOL USE
Wernicke's Encephalopathy

Wernicke's encephalopathy is a potentially devastating and preventable disorder caused by thiamine deficiency (218). Most cases occur in alcoholic patients, although any malnourished individual is at increased risk. Thiamine deficiency in alcoholics is multifactorial and related to an inadequate diet, impaired gastrointestinal absorption, and impaired hepatic storage.

The classic clinical triad consists of encephalopathy or delirium, ophthalmoplegia, and ataxia. This classic triad is rarely seen or recognized clinically (97,211), and therefore, a high index of suspicion must be maintained to make the diagnosis. Oculomotor abnormalities are nearly universal (218) but can be subtle; they include nystagmus, adduction palsies, and conjugate gaze palsies. Gait ataxia occurs in approximately 87% of patients and results from cerebellar and vestibular injury (218). Autopsy studies looking at clinical symptoms retrospectively found the classic triad in only 10% of patients (97,211). Caine et al. (31) found that the presence of two of the following four signs was specific for the diagnosis: (a) dietary deficiencies, (b) oculomotor abnormalities, (c) cerebellar dysfunction, and (d) an altered mental state or mild memory impairment. MRI can aid in making the diagnosis, showing a high-intensity signal on T2 around the cerebral aqueduct and third ventricle (14,75).

Treatment Rapid and appropriate treatment is essential because patients can quickly progress through stupor to coma and even death (218). Treatment regimens for Wernicke's encephalopathy vary (105). Victor et al. (218) recommend immediate administration of 100 mg of intravenous thiamine per day for at least 5 days. Oral supplementation of thiamine should be continued thereafter. Treatment usually results in rapid resolution of oculomotor abnormalities, followed by improvement in ataxia and, lastly, improvement in mental function. Permanent sequelae are common, especially in alcoholics, and range from mild nystagmus to ataxia to the disabling amnestic disorder—Korsakoff's syndrome. Importantly, glucose should never be administered without concurrent thiamine in an alcoholic, confused, or potentially malnourished patient because this can unmask underlying thiamine deficiency and result in an acute Wernicke's encephalopathy (218,222).

Korsakoff's Syndrome

Of alcoholics recovering from Wernicke's encephalopathy, 80% will exhibit an amnestic disorder consistent with the Korsakoff's syndrome (218). Clinically, selective anterograde and retrograde memory loss with relative preservation of other cognitive functions characterizes the syndrome. Confabulation is common. Although the disorder is generally thought to reflect the sequelae of thiamine deficiency, it rarely occurs in patients without alcoholism recovering from Wernicke's encephalopathy (104). This suggests that the cause of Korsakoff's syndrome is multifactorial, including alcohol abuse, thiamine deficiency, and genetic predisposition (142). Pathologic and quantitative MRI studies of patients with Korsakoff's syndrome reveal damage to the anterior and midline thalamic nuclei, which correlates with memory impairment. Recovery is variable and independent of treatment, although alcohol abstinence and thiamine supplementation are recommended. Approximately 20% of patients will recover completely or nearly so (218).

Alcoholic Dementia

Dementias in the elderly alcoholic represent a wide spectrum of underlying diseases, from the aforementioned Korsakoff's syndrome to Alzheimer's disease. Neuropsychological tests show impairment in 50% to 70% of alcoholics, and these rates are probably higher in elderly alcoholics. Considerable debate occurs whether alcohol itself is neurotoxic or the dementia in alcoholics is secondary to other causes. Victor et al. (218) believe that the dementia seen in alcoholics is related solely to the Wernicke-Korsakoff's syndrome. They believe that this syndrome can contribute to broader cognitive deficits than the isolated memory disturbances commonly reported. The distinction is likely academic, and Oslin et al. (166) have proposed diagnostic criteria for alcoholic-related dementia that includes the Wernicke-Korsakoff's syndrome. An abbreviated list of criteria is found in Table 29-19.

In an elderly alcoholic, it is important not to attribute the cause of dementia solely to the toxic effects of alcohol. Searching for reversible causes of dementia is critical in the alcoholic patient. Nutritional deficits and vascular causes of dementia may be more common in these patients and should be aggressively sought. Neurodegenerative dementias, such as Alzheimer's disease, should also be identified because these dementias are more amenable to symptomatic therapy with acetylcholinesterase inhibitors. (See Chapter 21.3 for information on evaluating the patient with dementia.)

Treatment of alcohol-related dementia consists of alcohol abstinence and nutritional supplementation, particularly with thiamine. Naltrexone alone or as an adjunct to psychosocial intervention has been shown to assist in the treatment of alcohol dependence (130,167).

Cerebellar Degeneration

Isolated cerebellar degeneration secondary to Purkinje cell loss was first associated with alcohol use in 1959 (219). The prominent involvement of midline cerebellar structures (i.e., anterior and superior vermis) accounts for the clinical picture of gait ataxia, truncal titubation, and minimal appendicular involvement (218). The abnormalities seen grossly and pathologically are similar to those seen in Wernicke's encephalopathy, suggesting a common pathophysiology (138,219). The disorder tends to occur after years of alcohol use and is gradually progressive (138). The diagnosis is based on a history of chronic alcohol use, neurologic examination, and neuroimaging showing midline cerebellar atrophy (39). As expected,

Table 29-19. *Diagnostic Criteria for Alcohol Dementia*

Probable Alcohol Related Dementia	Features That Cast Doubt on the Diagnosis
Diagnosis of dementia associated with significant alcohol use	Presence of aphasia
Clinical or radiologic evidence of other alcohol-related end-organ or neurologic disease	Clinical evidence of neurologic focality (other than ataxia or neuropathy)
Improvement or stabilization of dementia after alcohol cessation	Radiologic evidence of infarction, subdural hematoma, or other focal brain disease

treatment requires alcohol cessation and nutritional supplementation. Physical therapy with gait training can improve gait and balance.

Central Pontine Myelinolysis

CPM is an acute neurologic disorder of cerebral white matter with potentially devastating effects. It is an iatrogenic condition associated with the rapid correction of hyponatremia. It is most commonly seen in alcoholics, which suggests some underlying predisposition in these patients (39). However, it can occur in any patient population and is discussed in detail under Neurologic Complications of Disturbances of Electrolytes and Water Balance.

Alcoholic Neuropathy

Polyneuropathy is common in alcoholic patients (40). More than half of all alcoholic patients in one study had clinical evidence of peripheral nerve injury (21). It is a sensory motor axonal polyneuropathy due to a combination of alcohol toxicity and nutritional deficits (228). Prognosis is variable, with some patients show improvement or stabilization in symptoms following alcohol cessation. Nutritional causes of peripheral neuropathy should be sought, particularly regarding the B vitamins (see Chapters 25 and 29.2).

Alcoholic Myopathy

Myopathy is an important cause of weakness in alcoholics. Approximately half of alcoholics are weak on physical examination, one third have complaints of muscle weakness and myalgias, and nearly half show evidence of myopathy on biopsy (214). In addition, elderly patients who abuse alcohol may be more likely to manifest symptoms of myopathy because muscle mass decreases with age (107).

Typically, onset is insidious and develops over weeks to months; however, an acute myopathy can occur in association with binge drinking. Patients develop acute weakness, pain, muscle tenderness, and muscle swelling. Muscle necrosis and myoglobinuria can occur. In the elderly patient, aggressive hydration, electrolyte determination, and cardiac monitoring are essential to prevent renal failure and cardiac arrhythmias (94). Ultimately, treatment for both acute and chronic myopathies entails alcohol abstinence. Recovery is gradual and can be complete (39).

Alcohol Withdrawal Syndrome

Despite its frequency, alcoholism is frequently missed in hospitalized elderly patients (24). Ten percent of elderly alcoholics admitted to the hospital develop delirium associated with alcohol withdrawal (66). Alcohol withdrawal should always be considered in the differential diagnosis of delirium in hospitalized elderly because alcohol withdrawal can be associated

Table 29-20. *Clinical Characteristics of Alcohol Withdrawal*

Tremor—rest, postural, and action
Nausea/vomiting
Delirium
Hallucinations/illusions
Agitation
Autonomic hyperactivity
Generalized tonic-clonic seizures

with serious morbidity and mortality (39). It is essential to recognize alcohol withdrawal in elderly patients and treat it aggressively and promptly.

Table 29-20 outlines the common characteristics of alcohol withdrawal. An irregular, fast, postural and kinetic tremor of the hands is the most common manifestation (156). Hallucinations, illusions, autonomic hyperactivity, nausea and vomiting, delirium, and tonic-clonic seizures are also seen (39,156). Delirium tremens, a condition characterized by severe confusion, agitation, insomnia, severe generalized tremor, hallucinations and delusions, and autonomic hyperactivity, is the most serious condition associated with alcohol withdrawal (39,156).

Figure 29-3 outlines two approaches to managing alcohol withdrawal. The fixed schedule regimen entails giving fixed doses of prophylactic medications around the clock to patients at risk for developing alcohol withdrawal. The symptom-triggered approach requires close monitoring of patients at risk and intervening when symptoms of alcohol withdrawal become apparent. Both approaches have been shown to be equally effective in reducing withdrawal symptoms; however, the symptom-triggered approach results in the administration of lower dosages of medication and a shorter duration of therapy (143). This is an especially important consideration in elderly patients, who are more sensitive to the sedative effects of benzodiazepines. It may be useful to use shorter acting agents in the elderly because long-acting agents can produce excessive sedation, confusion, and gait difficulties. Despite these considerations, longer acting agents are associated with smoother withdrawal and a lower risk of breakthrough symptoms and seizures (143).

Benzodiazepines should be used as first-line agents in managing withdrawal in all populations. In fact, monotherapy with benzodiazepines is usually sufficient to suppress withdrawal. The use of beta-blockers, carbamazepine, and neuroleptics has been studied in alcohol withdrawal, but these should not be used as first-line agents or as monotherapy. Beta-blockers should be reserved for patients with comorbid disease, particularly coronary artery disease, and significant

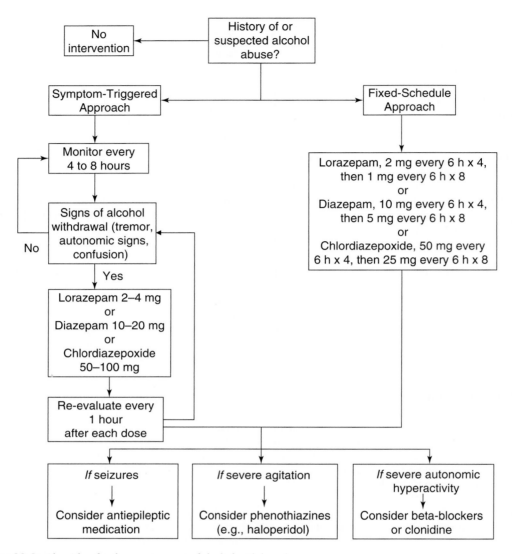

Figure 29-3. Algorithm for the management of alcohol withdrawal.

autonomic hyperactivity. Carbamazepine can be used in patients with seizures and has been shown to have some antiwithdrawal properties. In general, neuroleptic use should be avoided because they can precipitate seizures. However, these agents can be useful when dealing with a severely agitated and hallucinating patient. Finally, all patients with suspected alcohol abuse should be treated with thiamine supplementation (143).

IATROGENIC NEUROLOGIC COMPLICATIONS

Iatrogenic illness refers to the unintended deleterious consequences of medical diagnostic or therapeutic interventions. The remainder of this section reviews some common neurologic complications of medical interventions.

NEUROLOGIC COMPLICATIONS OF ORGAN TRANSPLANTATION
Complications of Immunosuppressive Medications

Cyclosporine Cyclosporine is a common immuno-suppressant agent used in transplantation (170). Neurologic complications occur in 15% to 40% of patients (117). Table 29-21 summarizes factors associated with an increased risk of neurologic side effects from cyclosporine (117,220).

Tremor is the most common neurologic complication, occurring early and diminishing over time

Table 29-21. *Risk Factors for Central Nervous System Toxicity from Cyclosporine*

Cranial radiation
Hypocholesterolemia
Hypomagnesemia
Beta-lactam antibiotic therapy
High-dose steroids
Hypertension
Uremia

(226). Delirium occurs in approximately 5% of patients (170). Lethargy, confusion, cortical blindness, and visual hallucinations characterize a distinct syndrome associated with reversible posterior leukoencephalopathy on neuroimaging (232). Another syndrome consists of cerebellar findings, focal weakness, and delirium. Focal or generalized seizures can occur and are associated with high serum levels of the drug (170).

Tacrolimus Tacrolimus has been associated with a wide variety of neurologic complications, with tremor and paresthesias being most common (29). Delirium is the most common serious complication, occurring in 16% of patients in one series (29). Other complications include coma, seizures, CPM, sleep disturbances, and nightmares (29,59,225). Reversible posterior leukoencephalopathy has been associated with tacrolimus (232). Most side effects are reversible with a reduction in the dose or elimination of the drug (170).

OKT3 Monoclonal Antibody OKT3 (muromonab) causes aseptic meningitis and acute encephalopathy. The meningitis occurs early after the drug is initiated, prompting an evaluation for an infectious cause. However, meningeal symptoms are self-limited and resolve within a few days and should not prompt discontinuation of the drug. The encephalopathy can be severe, with obtundation, myoclonus, and seizures. Similar to the meningitis, this condition is self-limited. However, it is slow to clear and can take weeks (170).

Corticosteroids Steroid myopathy is ubiquitous in individuals treated with chronic steroids. Clinically, patients have proximal muscle weakness that is most severe in the pelvic girdle. The myopathy resolves with discontinuation of the drug (170).

Steroid psychosis is a complex and variable constellation of clinical signs and symptoms (230). Depression, mania, anxiety, irritability, insomnia, restlessness, and fatigue can all be seen. The exact frequency of this complication is unknown, occurring in 2% to 57% of patients. Increasing age and steroid dosage are the strongest predictors of this complication. Withdrawal of the steroids can precipitate an acute worsening of symptoms. Prevention is the key to treatment. Using the lowest possible dose or every-other-day dosing can be useful. Valproic acid and carbamazepine can be useful as prophylactic agents. Neuroleptics and benzodiazepines are used to treat agitation and anxiety, respectively. Finally, when tapering steroids, a very slow taper is recommended.

Central Nervous System Infections
CNS infections may be the most common neurologic complication of transplantation (174). CNS infections are frequently life threatening, with mortality rates of 44% to 77% (45). Acute meningitis is usually caused by *Listeria monocytogenes*, whereas subacute and chronic meningitis are due to *Cryptococcus neoformans*, and focal brain infection is usually the result of *Aspergillus* infection (174). These infections account for 80% of CNS infections in this population (45). *Toxoplasma gondii* or *Nocardia asteroides* and polyoma J virus or other viruses causing progressive dementia are other important pathogens (170,174).

The familiar signs of CNS infection (fever, meningismus) are frequently lacking in these patients because of their use of strong immunosuppressant medications (170). Therefore, a high index of suspicion must be maintained to diagnose these infections.

Complications of the Specific Transplantation Procedure
Renal Transplantation Compression injuries of the femoral nerve or lateral femoral cutaneous nerve are common complications of renal transplantation surgery (170). Femoral nerve injury causes weakness of knee extension, with preservation of hip adduction. Sensory changes can occur along the anterolateral aspect of the leg or on the lateral aspect of the thigh. Caudal spinal cord ischemia may rarely occur (170).

Bone Marrow Transplantation The procedure for delivering the donor's bone marrow is benign and not associated with any neurologic sequelae. Although acute graft-versus-host disease (GVHD) is not associated with neurologic complications, chronic GVHD is fraught with a variety of autoimmune disorders affecting the nervous system, such as polymyositis and myasthenia gravis. Treatment consists of immune suppression (157).

Cardiac Transplantation Heart transplantation causes neurologic morbidity secondary to complications of cardiac bypass and the development of blood and air emboli. Up to 50% of patients show evidence of cerebral infarction or diffuse hypoxic-ischemic injury after transplantation (170). This increased risk of stroke continues after the surgery as a result of cardiac arrhythmias. Mechanical injuries to the brachial plexus also occur from the retraction of the chest wall during the surgery (170).

Liver Transplantation Of liver transplantation patients, 12% to 20% will experience neurologic complications, most during the first week following surgery (144). The most unusual of these is CPM (see Neurologic Complications of Disturbances of Electrolytes and Water Balance for a detailed description), which is found in 7% to 13% of patients at autopsy (144,170). In addition, encephalopathy is common, with the elderly being at the highest risk (144).

IATROGENIC COMPLICATIONS OF CRITICAL CARE
Delirium
Delirium is common in the hospitalized elderly, especially in the critical care setting (67). In these patients, the cause of the confusional state is often multifactorial. Iatrogenic influences, namely medications, play a large role (67). Table 29-22 summarizes the medications that can contribute to delirium in the critical care setting.

Critical Illness Polyneuropathy
Critical illness polyneuropathy is a common condition in critically ill patients, complicating 70% of coma-producing septic encephalopathies (231). It frequently becomes manifest as the patient begins to recover but is unable to be weaned from the ventilator (231,233). It is characterized by profound distal greater than proximal weakness and hypoareflexia (231,233). A facial diplegia can occur, although other cranial nerves are spared (233). Electrophysiologic studies reveal an axonal neuropathy with evidence of denervation (231,233). Treatment is supportive. Patients who survive their underlying illness have an excellent prognosis, although recovery can take many months. Proposed risk factors are summarized in Table 29-23 (224,231).

Table 29-22. *Drugs That May Contribute to Delirium*

Benzodiazepines	H$_2$ receptor antagonists
Barbiturates	Ciprofloxacin
Opioid narcotics	Digoxin
Antiemetics	Diphenhydramine
Anticonvulsants	Lidocaine

Table 29-23. *Risk Factors for the Development of Critical Illness Polyneuropathy*

Sepsis
Multiorgan failure
Corticosteroids
Nondepolarizing neuromuscular blocking agents
  (vecuronium, pancuronium)

Critical Illness Myopathy
Critical illness myopathy, an acute myopathy, occurs in intubated individuals receiving high-dose corticosteroids and vecuronium (231). Clinically, it is similar to the neuropathy previously discussed. Patients have a quadriparesis and difficulty weaning from the ventilator. Pathologic studies have revealed a loss of myosin filaments in the muscle (231).

MISCELLANEOUS NEUROLOGIC COMPLICATIONS OF MEDICATIONS
Medications Associated with Seizures
A variety of drugs have been implicated in causing seizures. Table 29-24 summarizes common medications associated with seizures (52,203).

Medications That Affect Neuromuscular Transmission
The list of drugs that affect neuromuscular transmission and, therefore, cause signs and symptoms of weakness is long. Most of these medications do not cause weakness in healthy patients. However, they can unmask evidence of a neuromuscular disease in asymptomatic patients and should be used cautiously in those with known neuromuscular

Table 29-24. *Drugs Associated with Seizures*

Phenothiazines
Atypical antipsychotics: clozapine
Tricyclic antidepressants associated
  with overdose
Bupropion
Selective serotonin reuptake inhibitors in combination
  with monoamine oxidase inhibitors or other
  serotonergic medications
Theophylline
Salicylate overdose
Chemotherapy: etoposide, ifosfamide, cisplatin
Antimicrobials: penicillin, metronidazole,
  isoniazid[a]
Benzodiazepine, barbiturate, or narcotic
  withdrawal

[a]Treat with vitamin B$_6$ replacement.

Table 29-25. *Drugs That May Impair Neuromuscular Transmission*

Aminoglycoside antibiotics
Miscellaneous antibiotics: penicillin, sulfa, tetracyclines, fluoroquinolones
Beta-blockers
Quinine/quinidine
Procainamide
Nondepolarizing neuromuscular blocking agents > polarizing
Phenothiazines
Chloroquine
D-penicillamine
Lidocaine/procaine, intravenously
Phenytoin

diseases (106). Only D-penicillamine, which is known to cause a myasthenic syndrome, should be absolutely avoided in patients with diseases of the neuromuscular junction (106). Table 29-25 summarizes the medications associated with impaired neuromuscular transmission (106).

Medications Associated with Movement Disorders

Drugs have been associated with every type of movement disorder. The elderly are particularly susceptible to neuroleptic-induced parkinsonism and tardive dyskinesia. Therefore, these drugs should be used cautiously in the elderly (112). Table 29-26 outlines the more common drug-induced movement disorders (54,112,122,188,192).

Table 29-26. *Drug-Induced Movement Disorders*

Phenomenology	Drugs	Phenomenology	Drugs
Tremor	Amphetamines	Myoclonus	Amphetamines
	Theophylline		Selective serotonin reuptake inhibitors
	Lithium		
	Valproic acid		Levodopa
	Levothroid		Dopamine agonists
	Tricyclic antidepressants	Parkinsonism	Neuroleptics
	Cyclosporine		Atypical antipsychotics
	Tacrolimus		Reserpine/tetrabenazine
	Levodopa		Methyldopa
Chorea	Dopamine agonists		Lithium
	Amantadine	Akathisia	Neuroleptics
	Phenytoin		Selective serotonin reuptake inhibitors
	Estrogen		
	Monoamine oxidase inhibitors		Tricyclic antidepressants
	Neuroleptics/neuroleptic-derived antiemetics[a]		Lithium
			Estrogens
Dystonia	Neuroleptics/neuroleptic-derived antiemetics	Restless legs syndrome	Neuroleptics
	Levodopa		Selective serotonin reuptake inhibitors
	Dopamine agonists		Phenytoin

[a]Chorea occurs as a component of the tardive dyskinesia syndrome and is a delayed complication of using this class of drugs.

REFERENCES

1. Abramson JL, Jurkovitz CT, Vaccarino V, et al. Chronic kidney disease, anemia, and incident stroke in a middle-aged, community-based population: the ARIC Study. *Kidney Int.* 2003;64: 610–615.
2. Adams WL, Yuan Z, Barboriak JJ, et al. Alcohol-related hospitalizations of elderly people. Prevalence and geographic variation in the United States. *JAMA.* 1993;270:1222–1225.
3. Akhter J, Wiede LG. Thyrotoxic periodic paralysis; a reversible cause of paralysis to remember. *S D J Med.* 1997;50:357–358.
4. Alexander E. Central nervous system disease in Sjögren's syndrome: new insights into immunopathogenesis. *Rheum Dis Clin North Am.* 1992;18:637–673.

5. Alexander EL. Neurologic disease in Sjögren's syndrome: mononuclear inflammatory vasculopathy affecting central/peripheral nervous system and muscle. A clinical review and update of immunopathogenesis. *Rheum Dis Clin North Am*. 1993;19:869–908.

6. Alexander EL, Alexander GE. Aseptic meningoencephalitis in primary Sjögren's syndrome. *Neurology*. 1983;33:593–598.

7. Alexander EL, Malinow K, Lejewski JF, et al. Primary Sjögren's syndrome with central nervous system disease mimicking multiple sclerosis. *Ann Intern Med*. 1986;104:323–330.

8. Alexander EL, Provost TT, Stevens MB, et al. Neurologic complications of primary Sjögren's syndrome. *Medicine*. 1982;61:247–257.

9. Alexander EL, Ranzenbach MR, Kumar AJ, et al. Anti-Ro(SS-A) autoantibodies in central nervous system disease associated with Sjögren's syndrome (CNS-SS): clinical, neuroimaging and angiographic correlates. *Neurology*. 1994;44:899–908.

10. Aminoff MJ. Neurologic complications of systemic disease in adults. In: Bradley WG, Daroff RB, Fenichel GM, et al., eds. *Neurology in clinical practice*. Boston: Butterworth-Heinemann; 2000:1029–1030.

11. Anderson GD. A mechanistic approach to antiepileptic drug interactions. *Ann Pharmacother*. 1998;32:554–563.

12. Andreoli TE, Evanoff GV, Ketel BL, et al. Chronic renal failure. In: Andreoli TE, Bennett JC, Carpenter CCJ, et al., eds. *Cecil's essentials of medicine*. Philadelphia: WB Saunders; 1993: 244–254.

13. Anonymous. Alcoholism in the elderly. Council on Scientific Affairs, American Medical Association. *JAMA*. 1996;275:797–801.

14. Antunez E, Estruch R, Cardenal C, et al. Usefulness of CT and MRI imaging in the diagnosis of acute Wernicke's encephalopathy. *AJR Am J Roentgenol*. 1998;171:1131–1137.

15. Argov Z, Mastaglia FL. Drug-induced peripheral neuropathies. *BMJ*. 1979;1:663–666.

16. Atlas SJ, Keller RB, Wu YA, et al. Long-term outcomes of surgical and nonsurgical management of lumbar spinal stenosis: 8 to 10 year results from the Maine Lumbar Spine Study. *Spine*. 2005;30:936–943.

17. Averbuch-Heller L, Steiner I, Abramsky O. Neurologic manifestations of progressive systemic sclerosis. *Arch Neurol*. 1992;49:1292–1295.

18. Ayus JC, Arieff AI. Abnormalities of water metabolism in the elderly. *Semin Nephrol*. 1996;16:277–288.

19. Baber U, Toto RD, de Lemos JA. Statins and cardiovascular risk reduction in patients with chronic kidney disease and end-stage renal failure. *Am Heart J*. 2007;153:471–477.

20. Bajema IM, Hagen EC, Weverling-Rijnsburger AW, et al. Cerebral involvement in two patients with Wegener's granulomatosis. *Clin Nephrol*. 1997;47:401–406.

21. Behse F, Buchthal F. Alcoholic neuropathy: clinical, electrophysiological, and biopsy findings. *Ann Neurol*. 1977;2:95–110.

22. Bekkelund SI, Torbergsen T, Husby G, et al. Myopathy and neuropathy in rheumatoid arthritis. A quantitative controlled electromyographic study. *J Rheumatol*. 1999;26:2348–2351.

23. Ben-Ami H, Pollack S, Nagachandran P, et al. Reversible pancreatitis, hepatitis, and peripheral polyneuropathy associated with parenteral gold therapy. *J Rheumatol*. 1999;26:2049–2050.

24. Beresford TP, Blow FC, Brower KJ, et al. Alcoholism and aging in the general hospital. *Psychosomatics*. 1988;29:61–72.

25. Berkelhammer C, Bear RA. A clinical approach to common electrolyte problems: 4. Hypomagnesemia. *Can Med Assoc J*. 1985;132:360–368.

26. Boden SD, Dodge LD, Bohlman HH, et al. Rheumatoid arthritis of the cervical spine. A long-term analysis with predictors of paralysis and recovery. *J Bone Joint Surg Am*. 1994;75: 1282–1297.

27. Bragoni M, Di Piero V, Priori R, et al. Sjögren's syndrome presenting as ischemic stroke. *Stroke*. 1994;25:2276–2279.

28. Brazis PW, Masdeu JC, Biller J. *Localization in Clinical Neurology*. 3rd ed. Boston: Little, Brown and Company; 1996.

29. Burkhalter EL, Starzl TE, Van Thiel DH. Severe neurological complications following orthotopic liver transplantation in patients receiving FK 506 and prednisone. *J Hepatol*. 1994;21:572–577.

30. Burn DJ, Bates D. Neurology and the kidney. *J Neurol Neurosurg Psychiatry*. 1998;65:810–821.

31. Caine D, Halliday GM, Kril JJ, et al. Operational criteria for the classification of chronic alcoholics: identification of Wernicke's encephalopathy. *J Neurol Neurosurg Psychiatry*. 1997;62:51–60.

32. Caselli RJ, Hunder GG. Giant cell (temporal) arteritis. *Neurol Clin*. 1997;15:893–902.

33. Caselli RJ, Hunder GG, Whisnant JP. Neurologic disease in biopsy-proven giant cell (temporal) arteritis. *Neurology*. 1988;38: 352–359.

34. Cawley MJ. Hyponatremia: current treatment strategies and the role of vasopressin antagonists. *Ann Pharmacother*. 2007;41:840–850.

35. Cerinic MM, Generini S, Pidnone A, et al. The nervous system in systemic sclerosis (scleroderma). *Rheum Dis Clin North Am*. 1996; 22:879–893.

36. Chang DJ, Paget SA. Neurologic complications of rheumatoid arthritis. *Rheum Dis Clin North Am.* 1993;19:955–973.

37. Chang RW, Bell CL, Hallett M. Clinical characteristics and prognosis of vasculitic mononeuropathy multiplex. *Arch Neurol.* 1984;41:618–621.

38. Chapelon C, Ziza JM, Piette JC, et al. Neurosarcoidosis: signs, course and treatment in 35 confirmed cases. *Medicine.* 1990;69:261–276.

39. Charness ME. Brain lesions in alcoholics. *Alcohol Clin Exp Res.* 1993;17:2–11.

40. Charness ME, Simon RP, Greenberg DA. Ethanol and the nervous system. *N Engl J Med.* 1989;321:442–454.

41. Cheung AK, Sarnak MJ, Yan G, et al. Atherosclerotic cardiovascular disease risks in chronic hemodialysis patients. *Kidney Int.* 2000;58:353–362.

42. Christensen KS. Hypokalemic paralysis in Sjögren's syndrome secondary to renal tubular acidosis. *Scand J Rheumatol.* 1985;14:58–60.

43. Clark WF, Rock GA, Buskard N, et al. Therapeutic plasma exchange: an update from the Canadian Apheresis Group. *Ann Intern Med.* 1999;131:453–462.

44. Clouston PD, DeAngelis LM, Posner JB. The spectrum of neurologic disease in patients with systemic cancer. *Ann Neurol.* 1992;31:268–273.

45. Conti DJ, Rubin RH. Infection of the central nervous system in organ transplant recipients. *Neurol Clin.* 1988;6:241–260.

46. Darnell RB, Posner JB. Paraneoplastic syndromes affecting the nervous system. *Semin Oncol.* 2006;33:270–298.

47. Davidson RI, Dunn EJ, Metzmaker JN. The shoulder abduction test in the diagnosis of radicular pain in cervical extradural compressive monoradiculopathies. *Spine.* 1981;6:441–446.

48. Davison AM, Walker GS, Oli H, et al. Water supply and aluminum concentration, dialysis dementia, and effect of reverse-osmosis water treatment. *Lancet.* 1982;2:785–787.

49. DeAngelis LM, Delattre JY, Posner JB. Radiation-induced dementia in patients cured of brain metastases. *Neurology.* 1989;39:789–796.

50. Delalande S, de Seze J, Fauchais AL, et al. Neurologic manifestations in primary Sjogren syndrome: a study of 82 patients. *Medicine.* 2004;83:280–291.

51. Delaney P. Neurologic manifestations in sarcoidosis: review of the literature, with a report of 23 cases. *Ann Intern Med.* 1977;87:336–345.

52. Delanty N, Vaughan CJ, French JA. Medical causes of seizures. *Lancet.* 1998;352:383–390.

53. DiMinno G, Martinez ML, McKean J, et al. Platelet dysfunction in uremia. Multifaceted defect partially corrected by dialysis. *Am J Med.* 1985;79:552–559.

54. Drake M. Restless legs with antiepileptic drug therapy. *Clin Neurol Neurosurg.* 1988;90:151–154.

55. Dray GJ, Jablon M. Clinical and radiologic features of primary osteoarthritis of the hand. *Hand Clin.* 1987;3:351–369.

56. Dreyer SJ, Boden SD. Natural history of rheumatoid arthritis of the cervical spine. *Clin Orthop.* 1999;366:98–106.

57. Dropcho EJ. Central nervous system injury by therapeutic irradiation. *Neurol Clin.* 1991;9:969–987.

58. Earnest MP, Yarnell PR. Seizure admissions to a city hospital: the role of alcohol. *Epilepsia.* 1976;17:387–393.

59. Eidelman BH, Abu-Elmagd K, Wilson J, et al. Neurologic complications of FK 506. *Transplant Proc.* 1991;23:3175–3178.

60. Eldor A. Thrombotic thrombocytopenic purpura: diagnosis, pathogenesis and modern therapy. *Baillieres Clin Haematol.* 1998;11:475–495.

61. Evers S, Engelien A, Karsch V, et al. Secondary hyperkalaemic paralysis. *J Neurol Neurosurg Psychiatry.* 1998;64:249–252.

62. Farrell DA, Medsger TA Jr. Trigeminal neuropathy in progressive systemic sclerosis. *Am J Med.* 1982;73:57–62.

63. Fauci AS, Katz P, Haynes BF, et al. Cyclophosphamide therapy of severe systemic necrotizing vasculitis. *N Engl J Med.* 1979;301:235–238.

64. Finkelstein JS, Mitlak BH, Slovik DM. Normal physiology of bone and bone minerals. In: Andreoli TE, Bennett JC, Carpenter CCJ, et al., eds. *Cecil's essentials of medicine.* Philadelphia: WB Saunders; 1993:530–538.

65. Finkelstein JS, Mitlak BH, Slovik DM. The parathyroid glands, hypercalcemia, and hypocalcemia. In: Andreoli TE, Bennett JC, Carpenter CCJ, et al., eds. *Cecil's essentials of medicine.* Philadelphia: WB Saunders; 1993:538–546.

66. Finlayson RE, Hurt RD, Davis LJ Jr., et al. Alcoholism in elderly persons: a study of the psychiatric and psychosocial features of 216 inpatients. *Mayo Clin Proc.* 1988;63:761–768.

67. Flacker JM, Marcantonio ER. Delirium in the elderly. Optimal management. *Drugs Aging.* 1998;13:119–130.

68. Fliessbach K, Urbach H, Hemlmstaedter C, et al. Cognitive performance and magnetic resonance imaging findings after high-dose systemic and intraventricular chemotherapy for primary central nervous system lymphoma. *Arch Neurol.* 2003;60:563–568.

69. Font J, Valls J, Cervera R, et al. Pure sensory neuropathy in patients with primary Sjögren's

syndrome: clinical, immunological, and electromyographic findings. *Ann Rheum Dis.* 1990;49:775–778.

70. Fox RI, Saito I. Criteria for the diagnosis of Sjögren's syndrome. *Rheum Dis Clin North Am.* 1994;20:391–407.

71. Freedland ES, McMicken DB. Alcohol-related seizures. Part 1: pathophysiology, differential diagnosis, and evaluation. *J Emerg Med.* 1993;11:463–473.

72. Frewin R, Henson A, Provan D. ABC of clinical haemotology: haemotological emergencies. *BMJ.* 1997;314:1333–1336.

73. Fukunishi I, Kitaoka T, Shirai T, et al. Psychiatric disorders among patients undergoing hemodialysis therapy. *Nephron.* 2002;91:344–347.

74. Galassi G, Ferrari S, Cobelli M, et al. Neuromuscular complications of kidney diseases. *Nephrol Dial Transplant.* 1998;13[Suppl 7]:41–47.

75. Gallucci M, Bozzao A, Splendiani A, et al. Wernicke encephalopathy: MR findings in five patients. *Am J Neuroradiol.* 1990;11:887–892.

76. Garfin SR, Herkowitz HN, Mirkovic S. Spinal stenosis. *Instr Course Lect.* 2000;49:361–374.

77. Gavrilovic IT, Hormigo A, Yahalom J, et al. Long-term follow-up of high-dose methotrexate-based therapy with and without whole brain irradiation for newly diagnosed primary CNS lymphoma. *J Clin Oncol.* 2006;24:4570–4574.

78. Generini S, Fiori G, Moggi P, et al. Systemic sclerosis. A clinical overview. *Adv Exp Med Biol.* 1999;455:73–83.

79. George B, Laurian C. Impairment of vertebral artery flow caused by extrinsic lesions. *Neurosurgery.* 1989;24:206–214.

80. George JN. Evaluation and management of patients with thrombotic thrombocytopenic purpura. *J Intensive Care Med.* 2007;22:82–91.

81. Gilbert MR, Grossman SA. Incidence and nature of neurologic problems in patients with solid tumors. *Am J Med.* 1986;81:951–954.

82. Goldberg ID, Bloomer WD, Dawson DM. Nervous system toxic effects of cancer therapy. *JAMA.* 1982;247:1437–1441.

83. Good AE, Christopher RP, Koepke GH. Peripheral neuropathy associated with rheumatoid arthritis: a clinical and electrodiagnostic study of 70 consecutive rheumatoid arthritis patients. *Ann Intern Med.* 1965;63:87–99.

84. Gorson KC. Vasculitic neuropathies: an update. *Neurologist.* 2007;13:12–19.

85. Gross M. Chronic relapsing inflammatory polyneuropathy complicating sicca syndrome. *J Neurol Neurosurg Psychiatry.* 1987;50:939–940.

86. Gross WL. Antineutrophil cytoplasmic autoantibody testing in vasculitides. *Rheum Dis Clin North Am.* 1995;21:987–1003.

87. Grossman SA, Krabak MJ. Leptomeningeal carcinomatosis. *Cancer Treat Rev.* 1999;25:103–119.

88. Grothey A. Clinical management of oxaliplatin-associated neurotoxicity. *Clin Colorectal Cancer.* 2005;5[Suppl 1]:S38–S46.

89. Guillevin L, Lhote F, Gayraud M, et al. Prognostic factors in polyarteritis nodosa and Churg-Strauss syndrome. A prospective study in 342 patients. *Medicine.* 1996;75:17–28.

90. Guillevin L, Lhote F, Gherardi R. Polyarteritis nodosa, microscopic polyangiitis, and Churg-Strauss syndrome: clinical aspects, neurologic manifestations, and treatment. *Neurol Clin.* 1997;15:865–866.

91. Gurley JP, Bell GR. The surgical management of patients with rheumatoid cervical spine disease. *Rheum Dis Clin North Am.* 1997;23:317–332.

92. Guttman L, Govindan S, Riggs JE, et al. Inclusion body myositis and Sjögren's syndrome. *Arch Neurol.* 1985;42:1021–1022.

93. Hall S, Bartleson JD, Onofrio BM, et al. Lumbar spinal stenosis. Clinical features, diagnostic procedures, and results of surgical treatment in 68 patients. *Ann Intern Med.* 1985;103:271–275.

94. Haller RG, Knochel JP. Skeletal muscle disease in alcoholism. *Med Clin North Am.* 1984;68:91–103.

95. Hanagan JR. Hypercalcemia in malignant disease. *Clin Ther.* 1982;5:102–112.

96. Harley JB, Alexander EL, Bias WB, et al. Anti-Ro (SS-A) and anti-La (SS-B) in patients with Sjögren's syndrome. *Arthritis Rheum.* 1986;29:196–206.

97. Harper C. The incidence of Wernicke's encephalopathy in Australia—a neuropathological study of 131 cases. *J Neurol Neurosurg Psychiatry.* 1983;46:593–598.

98. Harper CM, Thomas JE, Cascino TL, et al. Distinction between neoplastic and radiation-induced brachial plexopathy, with emphasis on the role of EMG. *Neurology.* 1989;39:502–506.

99. Harris ED Jr. Rheumatoid arthritis. Pathophysiology and implications for therapy. *N Engl J Med.* 1990;322:1277–1289.

100. Harris EN, Pierangeli S. Antiphospholipid antibodies and cerebral lupus. *Ann NY Acad Sci.* 1997;823:270–278.

101. Haslock DI, Wright V, Harriman DG. Neuromuscular disorders in rheumatoid arthritis. A motor-point muscle biopsy study. *Q J Med.* 1970;39:335–358.

102. Hernandez P, Johnson CA. Deferoxamine for aluminum toxicity in dialysis patients. *ANNA J*. 1990;17:224–228.

103. Hietaharju A, Jaaskelainen S, Kalimo H, et al. Peripheral neuromuscular manifestations in systemic sclerosis (scleroderma). *Muscle Nerve*. 1993;16:1204–1212.

104. Homewood J, Bond NW. Thiamin deficiency and Korsakoff's syndrome: failure to find memory impairments following nonalcoholic Wernicke's encephalopathy. *Alcohol*. 1999;19:75–84.

105. Hope LC, Cook CC, Thomson AD. A survey of the current clinical practice of psychiatrists and accident and emergency specialists in the United Kingdom concerning vitamin supplementation for chronic alcohol misusers. *Alcohol Alcohol*. 1999;34:862–867.

106. Howard JF Jr. Adverse drug effects on neuromuscular transmission. *Semin Neurol*. 1990; 10:89–102.

107. Hubbard BM, Squier MV. The physical ageing of the neuromuscular system. In: Tallis R, ed. *The clinical neurology of old age*. Oxford: John Wiley and Sons; 1989:3–26.

108. Hunder GG, Bloch DA, Michel BA, et al. The American College of Rheumatology 1990 criteria for the classification of giant cell arteritis. *Arthritis Rheum*. 1990;33:1122–1128.

109. Inouye SK. Prevention of delirium in hospitalized older patients: risk factors and targeted intervention strategies. *Ann Med*. 2000; 32:257–263.

110. Jackson CG, Chess RL, Ward JR. A case of rheumatoid nodule formation within the central nervous system and review of the literature. *J Rheumatol*. 1984;11:237–240.

111. Jaeckle KA, Young DF, Foley KM. The natural history of lumbosacral plexopathy in cancer. *Neurology*. 1985;35:8–15.

112. Jankovic J. Drug-induced and other orofacial-cervical dyskinesias. *Ann Intern Med*. 1981; 94:788–793.

113. Jennette JC, Falk RJ. Small-vessel vasculitis. *N Engl J Med*. 1997;337:1512–1523.

114. Johns CJ, Michele TM. The clinical management of sarcoidosis. A 50-year experience at the Johns Hopkins Hospital. *Medicine*. 1999; 78:65–111.

115. Jones DR, Detterbeck FC. Pancoast tumors of the lung. *Curr Opin Pulm Med*. 1998;4:191–197.

116. Judge TG. Hypokalaemia in the elderly. *Gerontol Clin*. 1968;10:102–107.

117. Kahan BD. Cyclosporine. *N Engl J Med*. 1989;321:1725–1738.

118. Kamata T, Hishida A, Takita T, et al. Morphologic abnormalities in the brain of chronically hemodialyzed patients without cerebrovascular disease. *Am J Nephrol*. 2000;20:27–31.

119. Kaplan RS, Wiernik PH. Neurotoxicity of antineoplastic drugs. *Semin Oncol*. 1982;9:103–130.

120. Keltner JL. Giant-cell arteritis. Signs and symptoms. *Ophthalmology*. 1982;89:1101–1110.

121. Kiu MC, Wan YL, Ng SH, et al. Pneumocephalus due to nasopharyngeal carcinoma: case report. *Neuroradiology*. 1996;38:70–72.

122. Kraus T, Schuld A, Pollmacher T. Periodic leg movements in sleep and restless legs syndrome probably caused by olanzapine. *J Clin Pharmacol*. 2000;19:478–479.

123. Krishnan AV, Kiernan MC. Uremic neuropathy: clinical features and new pathophysiological insights. *Muscle Nerve*. 2006;35:273–290.

124. Kriss TC, Kriss VM. Neck pain. Primary care work-up of acute and chronic symptoms. *Geriatrics*. 2000;55:47–48.

125. Kumar S, Berl T. Sodium. *Lancet*. 1998; 352:220–228.

126. Lafitte C. Neurological manifestations in Sjögren syndrome. *Arch Neurol*. 2000;57:411–413.

127. Lamprecht P, Gause A, Gross WL. Cryoglobulinemic vasculitis. *Arthritis Rheum*. 1999;42:2507–2516.

128. Larrson EM, Holtas S, Cronquist S, et al. Comparison of myelography, CT myelography and magnetic resonance imaging in cervical spondylosis and disk herniation. Pre- and postoperative findings. *Acta Radiol*. 1989;30: 233–239.

129. Lass P, Buscombe JR, Harber M, et al. Cognitive impairment in patients with renal failure is associated with multiple-infarct dementia. *Clin Nucl Med*. 1999;24:561–565.

130. Latt NC, Jurd S, Houseman J, et al. Naltrexone in alcohol dependence: a randomized controlled trial of effectiveness in a standard clinical setting. *Med J Aust*. 2002;176:530–534.

131. Laureno R, Karp B. Myelinolysis after correction of hyponatremia. *Ann Intern Med*. 1997;126:57–62.

132. Lavizzo-Mourey R, Johnson J, Stolley P. Risk factors for dehydration among elderly nursing home residents. *J Am Geriatr Soc*. 1988;36: 213–218.

133. Linke R, Schroeder M, Helmberger T, et al. Antibody-positive paraneoplastic neurologic syndromes. Value of CT and PET for tumor diagnosis. *Neurology*. 2004;63:282–286.

134. Lipowski ZJ. Acute confusional states (delirium) in the elderly. In: Albert ML, Knoefel JE, eds. *Clinical neurology of aging*. Oxford: Oxford University Press; 1994:347–362.

135. Lynch JP, Sharma OP, Baughman RP. Extrapulmonary sarcoidosis. *Semin Respir Infect.* 1998;13:229–254.

136. Mach JR, Korchik WP, Mahowald MW. Dialysis dementia. *Clin Geriatr Med.* 1988;4:853–867.

137. Malinow K, Yannakakis GD, Glusman SM, et al. Subacute sensory neuronopathy secondary to dorsal root ganglionitis in primary Sjögren's syndrome. *Ann Neurol.* 1986;20:535–537.

138. Mancall EL, McEntee WJ. Alterations of the cerebellar cortex in nutritional encephalopathy. *Neurology.* 1965;15:303–313.

139. Marco CA, Kelen GD. Acute intoxication. *Emerg Med Clin North Am.* 1990;8:731–748.

140. Markenson JA, McDougal JS, Tsairis P, et al. Rheumatoid meningitis: a localized immune process. *Ann Intern Med.* 1979;90:786–789.

141. Matsunaga S, Sakou T, Onishi T, et al. Prognosis of patients with upper cervical lesions caused by rheumatoid arthritis. *Spine.* 2003;28:1581–1587.

142. Matsushita S, Kato M, Muramatsu T, et al. Alcohol and aldehyde dehydrogenase genotypes in Korsakoff syndrome. *Alcohol Clin Exp Res.* 2000;24:337–340.

143. Mayo-Smith MF. Pharmacological management of alcohol withdrawal. A meta-analysis and evidence-based practice guideline. American Society of Addiction Medicine Working Group on Pharmacological Management of Alcohol Withdrawal. *JAMA.* 1997;278:144–151.

144. Mazariegos GV, Molmenti EP, Kramer DJ. Early complications after orthotopic liver transplantation. *Surg Clin North Am.* 1999;79:109–129.

145. Mellgren SI, Conn DL, Stevens JC, et al. Peripheral neuropathy in primary Sjögren's syndrome. *Neurology.* 1989;39:390–394.

146. Menninger JA. Assessment and treatment of alcoholism and substance-related disorders in the elderly. *Bull Menninger Clin.* 2002;66:166–183.

147. Mikulowski P, Wollheim FA, Rotmil P, et al. Sudden death in rheumatoid arthritis with atlanto-axial dislocation. *Acta Med Scand.* 1975;198:445–451.

148. Mirand AL, Welte JW. Alcohol consumption among the elderly in a general population, Erie County, New York. *Am J Public Health.* 1996;86:978–984.

149. Mondelli M, Romano C, Della P, et al. Electrophysiological evidence of "nerve entrapment syndromes" and subclinical peripheral neuropathy in progressive systemic sclerosis (scleroderma). *J Neurol.* 1995;242:185–194.

150. Monro P, Uttley D. Spinal cord and spinal root disease, secondary to diseases of the spine. In: Tallis R, ed. *The clinical neurology of old age.* Oxford: John Wiley and Sons; 1989:251–283.

151. Moore PM, Cupps TR. Neurological complications of vasculitis. *Ann Neurol.* 1983;14:155–167.

152. Mori K, Iijima M, Koike H, et al. The wide spectrum of clinical manifestations in Sjögren's syndrome-associated neuropathy. *Brain.* 2005;128:2480–2482.

153. Murros KE, Toole JF. The effect of radiation on carotid arteries. *Arch Neurol.* 1989;46:449–455.

154. Nakamura RM. Neuropsychiatric lupus. *Rheum Dis Clin North Am.* 1997;20:379–393.

155. Nath U, Grant R. Neurological paraneoplastic syndromes. *J Clin Pathol.* 1997;50:975–980.

156. Neiman J, Lang AE, Fornazzari L, et al. Movement disorders in alcoholism: a review. *Neurology.* 1990;40:741–746.

157. Nelson KR, McQuillen MP. Neurologic complications of graft-versus-host disease. *Neurol Clin.* 1988;6:389–403.

158. Neva MH, Kaarela K, Kauppi M. Prevalence of radiologic changes in the cervical spine—a cross sectional study after 20 years from presentation of rheumatoid arthritis. *J Rheumatol.* 2000;27:90–93.

159. Nishino H, Rubino FA, DeRemee RA, et al. Neurological involvement in Wegener's granulomatosis: an analysis of 324 consecutive patients at the Mayo Clinic. *Ann Neurol.* 1993;33:4–9.

160. Norton WL, Nardo JM. Vascular disease in progressive systemic sclerosis (scleroderma). *Ann Intern Med.* 1970;73:317–324.

161. Nurick S. The natural history and the results of surgical treatment of the spinal cord disorder associated with cervical spondylosis. *Brain.* 1972;95:101–108.

162. O'Hare JA, Callaghan NM, Murnaghan DJ. Dialysis encephalopathy. Clinical, electroencephalographic and interventional aspects. *Medicine.* 1983;62:129–141.

163. Okada K, Shirasaki N, Hayashi H, et al. Treatment of cervical spondylotic myelopathy by enlargement of the spinal canal anteriorly, followed by arthrodesis. *J Bone Joint Surg Am.* 1991;73:352–364.

164. Oksanen V. Neurosarcoidosis: clinical presentations and course in 50 patients. *Acta Neurol Scand* 1986;73:283–290.

165. Ondo W. Ropinirole for restless legs syndrome. *Mov Disord.* 1999;14:138–140.

166. Oslin D, Atkinson RM, Smith DM, et al. Alcohol related dementia: proposed clinical criteria. *Int J Geriatr Psychiatry.* 1998;13:203–212.

167. Oslin D, Liberto JG, O'Brien J, et al. Naltrexone as an adjunctive treatment for older patients with alcohol dependence. *Am J Geriatr Psychiatry.* 1997;5:324–332.

168. Oxholm P. Primary Sjögren's syndrome—clinical and laboratory markers of disease activity. *Semin Arthritis Rheum.* 1992;22:114–126.

169. Palmer JJ. Radiation myelopathy. *Brain.* 1972;95:109–122.

170. Patchell RA. Neurological complications of organ transplantation. *Ann Neurol.* 1994;36:688–703.

171. Peterson IM, Heim C. Inverted squamous papilloma with neuro-ophthalmic features. *J Clin Neuroophthalmol.* 1991;11:35–38.

172. Pettigrew LC, Glass JP, Maor M, et al. Diagnosis and treatment of lumbosacral plexopathy in patients with cancer. *Arch Neurol.* 1984;41:1282–1285.

173. Pickett JL, Theberge DC, Brown WS, et al. Normalizing hematocrit in dialysis patients improves brain function. *Am J Kidney Dis.* 1999;33:1122–1130.

174. Ponticelli C, Campise MR. Neurological complications in kidney transplant recipients. *J Nephrol.* 2005;18:521–528.

175. Posner JB. Paraneoplastic syndromes. In: Posner JB, ed. *Neurologic complications of cancer.* Philadelphia: FA Davis; 1995:353–385.

176. Posner JB. Side effects of chemotherapy. In: Posner JB, ed. *Neurologic complications of cancer.* Philadelphia: FA Davis; 1995.

177. Ramos M, Mandybur TI. Cerebral vasculitis in rheumatoid arthritis. *Arch Neurol.* 1975;32:271–275.

178. Rao R. Neck pain, cervical radiculopathy, and cervical myelopathy: pathophysiology, natural history, and clinical evaluation. *J Bone Joint Surg Am.* 2002;84:1871–1872.

179. Raskin NH, Fishman RA. Neurologic disorders in renal failure (first of two parts). *N Engl J Med.* 1976;294:143–148.

180. Raskin NH, Fishman RA. Neurologic disorders in renal failure (second of two parts). *N Engl J Med.* 1976;294:204–210.

181. Reich KA, Giansiracusa DF, Stongwater SL. Neurologic manifestations of giant cell arteritis. *Am J Med.* 1990;89:67–72.

182. Reyes-Ortiz CA. Dehydration, delirium and disability in elderly patients. *JAMA.* 1997;278:287–288.

183. Rigler SK. Alcoholism in the elderly. *Am Fam Physician.* 2000;61:1710–1716.

184. Riise T, Jacobsen BK, Gran JT. High mortality in patients with rheumatoid arthritis and atlantoaxial subluxation. *J Rheumatol.* 2001;28:2425–2429.

185. Ropper AH, Gorson KC. Neuropathies associated with paraproteinemia. *N Engl J Med.* 1998;338:1601–1607.

186. Rosenbaum RB, Campbell SM, Rosenbaum JT. *Clinical Neurology of Rheumatic Diseases.* Boston: Butterworth-Heinemann; 1996.

187. Rottenberg DA, Chernik NL, Deck MDF, et al. Cerebral necrosis following radiotherapy of extracranial neoplasms. *Ann Neurol.* 1977;1:339–357.

188. Sachdev P, Loneragran C. The present status of akathisia. *J Nerv Ment Dis.* 1991;179:381–389.

189. Sager DS, Bennett RM. Individualizing the risk/benefit ratio of NSAIDs in older patients. *Geriatrics.* 1992;47:24–31.

190. Sahenk Z. Toxic neuropathies. *Semin Neurol.* 1987;7:9–17.

191. Sahenk Z, Barohn R, New P, et al. Taxol neuropathy. Electrodiagnostic and sural nerve biopsy findings. *Arch Neurol.* 1994;51:726–729.

192. Sanz-Fuentenebro FJ, Huidobro A, Tejadas-Rivas A. Restless legs syndrome and paroxetine. *Acta Psychiatr Scand.* 1996;94:482–484.

193. Scheepers BD. Alcohol and the brain. *Br J Hosp Med.* 1997;57:548–551.

194. Schneider HA, Yonker RA, Katz P, et al. Rheumatoid vasculitis: experience with 13 patients and review of the literature. *Semin Arthritis Rheum.* 1985;14:280–286.

195. Scott TF. Neurosarcoidosis: progress and clinical aspects. *Neurology.* 1993;43:8–12.

196. Sharma OP. Neurosarcoidosis: a personal perspective based on the study of 37 patients. *Chest.* 1997;112:220–228.

197. Sharma OP. Treatment of sarcoidosis. If not corticosteroids, then what? *Pulm Perspect.* 1997;1:1–3.

198. Sharma OP, Sharma AM. Sarcoidosis of the nervous system. A clinical approach. *Arch Intern Med.* 1991;151:1317–1321.

199. Sigal LH. The neurologic presentation of vasculitic and rheumatologic syndromes. A review. *Medicine.* 1987;66:157–180.

200. Silberstein SD, Lipton RB, Goadsby PJ. *Headache in Clinical Practice.* 1st ed. Oxford: Isis Medical Media; 1998.

201. Silver SM, Sterns RH, Halperin ML. Brain swelling after dialysis: old urea or new osmoles? *Am J Kidney Dis.* 1996;28:1–13.

202. Sivri A, Guler-Uysal F. The electroneurophysiological evaluation of rheumatoid arthritis patients. *Clin Rheumatol.* 1998;17:416–418.

203. Snavely SR, Hodges GR. The neurotoxicity of antibacterial agents. *Ann Intern Med.* 1984;101:92–104.

204. Steen VD, Medsger TA Jr. Epidemiology and natural history of systemic sclerosis. *Rheum Dis Clin North Am.* 1990;16:1–11.

205. Stern BJ, Krumholz A, Johns C, et al. Sarcoidosis and its neurological manifestations. *Arch Neurol.* 1985;42:909–917.

206. Sterns RH, Cappuccio JD, Silver SM, et al. Neurologic sequelae after treatment of severe hyponatremia; a multicenter perspective. *J Am Soc Nephrol.* 1994;4:1522–1530.

207. Stevens JC, Cartlidge NE, Saunders M, et al. Atlanto-axial subluxation and cervical myelopathy in rheumatoid arthritis. *Q J Med.* 1971;40:391–408.

208. Sulavik SB, Spencer RP, Weed DA, et al. Recognition of distinctive patterns of gallium-67 distribution in sarcoidosis. *J Nucl Med.* 1990;31:1909–1914.

209. Tallaksen CM, Jetne V, Fossa S. Postradiation lower motor neuron syndrome—a case report and brief literature review. *Acta Oncol.* 1997;36:345–347.

210. Toto RD. Treatment of hypertension in chronic kidney disease. *Semin Nephrol.* 2005;25:435–439.

211. Torvik A, Lindboe CF, Rogde S. Brain lesions in alcoholics: a neuropathological study with clinical correlations. *J Neurol Sci.* 1982;56:233–248.

212. Trenkwalder C, Stiasny K, Pollmacher T, et al. L-dopa therapy of uremic and idiopathic restless legs syndrome: a double-blind, crossover trial. *Sleep.* 1995;18:681–688.

213. Truumees E, Herkowitz HN. Cervical spondylotic myelopathy and radiculopathy. *Instr Course Lect.* 2000;49:339–360.

214. Urbano-Marquez A, Estruch R, Navarro-Lopez F, et al. The effects of alcoholism on skeletal and cardiac muscle. *N Engl J Med.* 1989;320:409–415.

215. Uthman I. Pharmacological therapy of vasculitis: an update. *Curr Opin Pharmacol.* 2004;4:177–182.

216. van Dam GM, Reisman Y, van Wieringen K. Hypokalemic thyrotoxic periodic paralysis: case report and review of an Oriental syndrome. *Neth J Med.* 1996;49:90–97.

217. Verbalis JG. Disorders of body water homeostasis. *Best Pract Res Clin Endocrinol Metab.* 2003;17:471–503.

218. Victor M, Adams RD, Collins GH. *The Wernicke-Korsakoff Syndrome and Related Neurological Disorders due to Alcoholism and Malnutrition.* 2nd ed. Philadelphia: FA Davis; 1989.

219. Victor M, Adams RD, Mancall EL. A restricted form of cerebellar cortical degeneration occurring in alcoholic patients. *Arch Neurol.* 1959;71:579–688.

220. Walker RW, Brochstein JA. Neurologic complications of immunosuppressive agents. *Neurol Clin.* 1988;6:261–278.

221. Walters AS. Toward a better definition of the restless legs syndrome. The international restless legs syndrome study group. *Mov Disord.* 1995;10:634–642.

222. Watson AJ, Walker JF, Tomkin GH, et al. Acute Wernicke's encephalopathy precipitated by glucose loading. *Ir J Med Sci.* 1981;150:301–303.

223. Wegelius O, Pasternack A, Kuhlback B. Muscular involvement in rheumatoid arthritis. *Acta Rheumatol Scand.* 1969;15:257–261.

224. Wijdicks EFM, Litchy WJ, Harrison BA. The clinical spectrum of critical illness polyneuropathy. *Mayo Clin Proc.* 1994;69:955–959.

225. Wijdicks EFM, Wiesner RH, Dahlke LJ, et al. FK506-induced neurotoxicity in liver transplantation. *Ann Neurol.* 1994;35:498–501.

226. Wijdicks EFM, Wiesner RH, Krom RAF. Neurotoxicity in liver transplant recipients with cyclosporin immunosuppression. *Neurology.* 1995;45:1962–1964.

227. Wilbourn AJ, Aminoff MJ. AAEE minimonograph:32: the electrophysiologic examination in patients with radiculopathies. *Muscle Nerve.* 1988;11:1099–1114.

228. Wohrle JC, Spengos K, Steinke W, et al. Alcohol-related acute axonal polyneuropathy: a differential diagnosis of Guillain-Barré syndrome. *Arch Neurol.* 1998;55:1329–1334.

229. Wolfs JFC, Peul WC, Boers M, et al. Rationale and design of the Delphi Trial—I(RCT)2: international randomized clinical trial of rheumatoid craniocervical treatment, an intervention-prognostic trial comparing 'early' surgery with conservative treatment. *BMC Musculoskelet Disord.* 2006;7:1–12.

230. Wolkowitz OM, Reus VI, Canick J, et al. Glucocorticoid medication, memory and steroid psychosis in medical illness. *Ann NY Acad Sci.* 1997;823:81–96.

231. Young GB. Neurologic complications of systemic critical illness. *Neurol Crit Care.* 1995;13:645–658.

232. Zivkovic S. Neuroimaging and neurologic complications after organ transplantation. *J Neuroimaging.* 2007;17:110–123.

233. Zochodne DW, Bolton CF, Wells GA, et al. Critical illness polyneuropathy. A complication of sepsis and multiple organ failure. *Brain.* 1987;110:819–842.

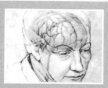

CHAPTER 30

Acute and Chronic Seizures in the Older Adult

Katherine H. Noe and Joseph I. Sirven

Epilepsy affects 1.5 to 3 million people of all ages in the United States annually. Although it is often mistakenly perceived as a childhood disorder, in fact, the most common time to develop seizures is after age 60. The prevalence of epilepsy in persons age 65 or older is twice that in young adults, and it continues to increase with age (Fig. 30-1) (27,28). Failure to recognize the increased prevalence of new-onset cases of epilepsy in the older adult may contribute to misdiagnoses. Furthermore, epilepsy in the elderly is distinct in its etiologies and presentation, which, along with increased medical comorbidity, adds to the difficulty in appropriate diagnosis and evaluation of seizures in the older adult compared to younger patients. Once recognized, the goals of seizure treatment in the elderly are the same as those for younger adults, namely to prevent future seizures and related injury and to maintain quality of life. In practice, however, epilepsy treatment in the older population presents unique challenges. Higher incidence of drug side effects, medication interactions, and altered pharmacokinetics are among areas of particular concern. Unfortunately, there is a dearth of evidence-based data regarding use of antiepileptic drugs (AEDs) in this group, and management of the older epilepsy

patient is often based on information extrapolated from younger patients without consideration for the unique problems and issues associated with a geriatric population. This review will discuss issues of diagnosis and treatment of epilepsy unique to the older age group.

EPIDEMIOLOGY

Seizures occur more frequently in the elderly, in part because they are often secondary to conditions more common in patients over age 60. These conditions include stroke, cerebral hemorrhage, tumor, and neurodegenerative diseases such as Alzheimer's dementia. Therefore, to gain a clear understanding of the incidence of seizure disorders in this age group, distinctions must be made between acute symptomatic seizures and epilepsy. Acute symptomatic seizures are those directly attributable to or provoked by an acute insult to the central nervous system (CNS) or by a systemic metabolic derangement. In contrast, epilepsy is a condition of repeated unprovoked seizures and is diagnosed only when two or more such seizures have occurred. Epilepsy can occur without a clear underlying etiology (idiopathic epilepsy) or from a chronic CNS lesion such as encephalomalacia from old stroke (remote symptomatic epilepsy). The evaluation and management of each of these seizure presentations will be discussed.

ACUTE SEIZURES

Acute symptomatic seizures are not uncommon in the elderly. In a population-based study from Rochester, Minnesota, the incidence was 82 per 100,000 person-years between the ages of 66 and 74, rising to 123 per 100,000 in those aged 75 or more (1). In elderly patients, about half of all acute symptomatic seizures are attributed to cerebrovascular disease (seizures occurring within 1 week of an ischemic or hemorrhagic stroke) (1,19,62). Other frequently cited etiologies included toxic/metabolic derangements, trauma, neoplastic disease, and medication or alcohol withdrawal (1,14,26,55). Disordered serum glucose, including hypoglycemia associated with insulin use and nonketotic hyperglycemia, is often a cause of seizures in diabetics (40,57). Hyponatremia, uremia,

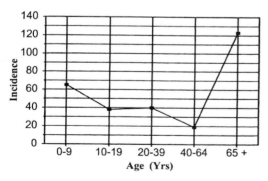

Figure 30-1. Age-specific average annual incidence of epilepsy per 100,000 population. (Adapted from Hauser WA, Annegers JF, Kurland LT. Incidence of epilepsy and unprovoked seizures in Rochester, Minnesota: 1935–1984. *Epilepsia.* 1993;34:453–468.)

and hypocalcemia are also well represented in the literature (37). Abrupt discontinuation of sedative and anxiolytic drugs is a prominent cause of seizures in this age group. All barbiturates and benzodiazepines present a risk of withdrawal seizures (44,67,76). Many commonly prescribed medications can also lower seizure threshold. Drugs such as antipsychotics, antidepressants, theophylline, antibiotics such as new-generation quinolones, and certain pain medications such as meperidine may lead to seizures (44,76). Over-the-counter herbal supplements such as ginkgo biloba may also have this effect (22,34). CNS infection is a relatively uncommon cause of acute seizures in the elderly patient in the United States but should be suspected in the setting of fever, meningeal signs, or immunosuppression. Acute symptomatic seizures are associated with increased 30-day mortality, with a case fatality in patients aged 65 or older of 30% to 40% (30). It is not yet known whether mortality reflects the severity of the underlying brain insult or an independent effect of seizure activity.

CHRONIC SEIZURES—EPILEPSY

The number of epilepsy cases also rises steadily after age 60 (Fig. 30-1). The annual incidence of epilepsy is 134 per 100,000 in those aged 65 years or older (27,28,36,38,55,66). The prevalence of chronic seizures may be even higher in the institutionalized elderly, with studies reporting 10% of nursing home residents with documented seizure activity and/or receiving AED therapy (17,35). Epilepsy in this age group is commonly related to remote CNS insults or to chronic progressive neurologic disease. In a population-based study from Rochester, Minnesota, major etiologies were cerebrovascular disease (33%), dementia (11.7%), neoplasm (4%), infection (0.6%), and trauma (1%) (Fig. 30-2) (26). In the remaining half of the patients, no definitive cause was identified (26). Similarly, in a Veterans Administration study of newly diagnosed epilepsy in patients aged 60 years and above, the most common etiology was stroke (43%), followed by arteriosclerosis (16%), unknown etiology (24%), and head trauma (7%) (54). The majority of older adults experience partial seizures, as would be predicted by the presence of underlying acquired etiologies. In persons with epilepsy aged 65 years or greater, 13% have simple partial seizures, 49% have complex partial seizures, and 29% have generalized or myoclonic seizures (27). This is in contrast with children, in whom the most prevalent seizure types are generalized (50%), with 11% having simple partial and 23% having complex partial events.

STATUS EPILEPTICUS

Status epilepticus (SE), which is defined as >30 minutes of continuous seizure activity or of intermittent seizures without return to consciousness, is also more common in older adults. The incidence of SE in the elderly is two to five times higher than in young adults (11,70). SE occurs not only in the setting of known seizure disorder, but it can also be the first presentation of epilepsy or a result of acute symptomatic derangements. In fact, 30% of all acute symptomatic seizures in older people present as SE (7). The elderly are not only more likely to develop SE, but are also more likely to die as a result. In a database of SE cases from Richmond, Virginia, the mortality rate for all adults was 26%, increasing to 38% after age 60 and to 50% after age 80 (11,12). Forty percent of SE cases in elderly are attributable to acute or chronic stroke (71). Although acute stroke is likely to contribute significantly to overall morbidity and mortality in these cases, the mortality of stroke with SE is three times greater than that seen with stroke alone (72). SE following anoxic brain injuries, such as is often seen after cardiopulmonary arrest, has a mortality rate close to 100% (71).

DIAGNOSTIC EVALUATION

One obstacle in the treatment of epilepsy in older adults is misdiagnosis. In a Veterans Administration study of new-onset epilepsy in elderly patients, seizure disorder was not seriously considered as a diagnosis at first evaluation in one fourth of the cases (52). Common misdiagnoses were syncope/blackout (46%), altered mental status (42%), and dementia (7%). Although it is relatively easy to recognize a classic generalized tonic-clonic seizure, older adults are more likely to experience partial seizures with clinical manifestations unique from those often seen in younger patients. One suggested reason is that the epileptic focus in older adults involves the frontal and parietal lobes rather than the temporal lobe (51). Thus, these patients are less likely to experience auras such as déjà vu and other symptoms classically associated with

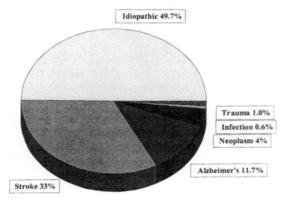

Figure 30-2. Etiology of epilepsy in the elderly.

temporal lobe epilepsy. Rather, these patients will complain of dizziness, posturing, paresthesias, and other symptoms related to frontal and parietal lobe function. Further confusion may arise in the elderly due to the increased presence of multiple comorbidities, polypharmacy, and, in some instances, difficulty obtaining the history due to underlying cognitive impairment. Lastly, the postictal period may last for days in the older adults, mimicking a delirium or dementia and further contributing to the difficulty in diagnosis.

Diagnosis requires a detailed and accurate history. Patients are often unaware of what has occurred, so obtaining an eyewitness account is invaluable. Syncope, transient ischemic attacks, transient global amnesia, and vertigo are common conditions at this age and can present similarly to seizures (68). Table 30-1 lists common discriminators of these events and seizures. Although these variables may be helpful, they remain nonspecific. Carefully detailed questions about the episodes and about epilepsy risk factors, including minor or major head trauma and concomitant medications, must be asked.

Further diagnostic testing is often needed to confirm or clarify the etiology of a seizure-like spell. Depending on the history evaluation of metabolic derangements, cardiac disease, cerebrovascular disorders, or vestibular dysfunction may be considered as appropriate. For epilepsy evaluation, electroencephalography (EEG) and neuroimaging are standard tests, the value and limitations of which are discussed further in the following sections.

ELECTROENCEPHALOGRAM

EEG is a cornerstone of seizure evaluation in all age groups. However, elderly patients are more likely to have nonspecific or nonepilepsy-related EEG changes, which can add to diagnostic errors in the unwary. Findings related to normal aging may include mild slowing or decreased amplitude of the background rhythms or intermittent slowing over the temporal head regions (33,46). EEG in this age group may also show benign patterns that are misinterpreted as epileptogenic by the inexperienced reader, such as small sharp spikes, wicket spikes, or subclinical rhythmic electrical discharges of adulthood (SREDA), the latter occurring exclusively in older adults (33,53, 56,73,74). To add to possible diagnostic confusion, truly epileptogenic findings, such as spikes or sharp waves, appear less commonly in the EEGs of elderly individuals with epilepsy than in those of young patients. Only 26% to 37% of older patients with epilepsy demonstrated epileptiform abnormalities on routine EEG (13,51). Thus, the absence of epileptiform abnormalities on an EEG should not exclude the diagnosis of seizures or epilepsy. When epileptogenic discharges are present, they are strongly suggestive of a seizure diagnosis; however, even this finding must be interpreted cautiously with the clinical history in mind. Epileptiform transients may be seen in patients with diseases other than epilepsy, such as dementia, stroke, neoplasms, and prion diseases (9,13,45). The "gold standard" of epilepsy diagnosis with EEG is the actual recording of a seizure. Therefore, when the diagnosis of seizures or epilepsy remains in question, prolonged inpatient video-EEG or ambulatory EEG monitoring should be strongly considered.

IMAGING

Imaging studies [magnetic resonance imaging (MRI) and computed tomography (CT)] should be performed as part of the initial evaluation of all older

Table 30-1. *Variables That Distinguish between Common Spells in the Elderly*

Variable	Seizure	Syncope	TIA	TGA	Vertigo
Warning/aura	Sometimes	Faint feeling	None	None	None
Duration	1–2 minutes	Seconds to minutes	Minutes to hours	Minutes to hours	Minutes to days
Effect of posture	None	Variable	None	None	Variable
Spell symptoms	Tonic-clonic movement but variable	Loss of tone/ brief clonic jerks	Deficits along a vascular pattern	Confusion/ amnesia	Nausea, ataxia, tinnitus
Incontinence	Variable	Variable	None	None	None
Heart rate	Increased	Irregular/ decreased	Variable	No effect	Variable
Postspell symptoms	Confusion, sleep	Alert	Alert	Alert	Alert
EEG during event	Epileptiform pattern	Diffuse slowing	Focal slowing	Rare slowing	No effect

TIA, transient ischemic attack; TGA, transient global amnesia; EEG, electroencephalography.

patients with epilepsy to identify and treat etiologies such as CNS hemorrhage, tumor, and abscess. MRI is the procedure of choice because it is superior to CT in detecting all pathologic processes except subarachnoid hemorrhage (77). CT is helpful in emergent situations or when MRI is contraindicated.

TREATMENT

WHEN SHOULD ANTIEPILEPTIC DRUGS BE INITIATED?

The main reason for prescribing AED therapy is to prevent further seizures. Related goals are preventing seizure-related morbidity and mortality and maintaining quality of life. For many elderly patients, critical issues are the continued ability to drive and maintain independent living. A single seizure with an obvious precipitating cause does not imply an underlying tendency toward seizure recurrence requiring AED treatment. For example, if an individual had seizures caused by a new medication or electrolyte disturbance, AEDs do not have to be initiated; rather, the offending medication is discontinued, or the underlying electrolyte imbalance is corrected. Patients found to have a history of two or more prior seizures are at high risk for future events and should be treated (29).

After a single idiopathic seizure, the decision to initiate treatment is based on an assessment of recurrence risk. Risk stratification is generally based on studies of younger adults because this issue has not been adequately evaluated in the elderly. Partial seizures, postictal paralysis, a family history of epilepsy, an EEG showing an epileptiform pattern, and an abnormal neurologic examination are all associated with a higher risk of recurrence in studies of younger adults (2,3,31). Age alone also may predict risk, with older patients more likely to have a seizure recurrence (31). This should not be construed to suggest that older patients should immediately be placed on AEDs after a first seizure. Rather, more investigation is needed to better identify those risk factors that are most likely to lead to seizure recurrence in this population. As a general guideline, any individual who has had a seizure and has a structural cortical lesion (i.e., tumor, encephalomalacia from a stroke or trauma) has a higher risk of seizure recurrence and would benefit from AEDs. Primary prophylaxis with AEDs for patients with new stroke or tumor is not routinely recommended (20,61).

CHOOSING A MEDICATION

The ideal AED for the elderly population would be highly effective but would avoid adverse side effects, drug interactions, complex dosing regimens, and undue expense. No perfect drug exists, and AED selection must therefore rely on careful consideration of what is best for a given individual. Effectiveness for seizure type, side effect profile, dosing regimen, medication interaction, and costs are among the important factors to consider. The great majority of elderly patients have partial seizures, for which all currently available AEDs with the exception of ethosuximide are potentially efficacious. In an evidence-based treatment guideline, the International League Against Epilepsy recommends lamotrigine and gabapentin as first-line agents for partial epilepsy in the elderly (21). Similarly, an expert consensus guideline based on a survey of leading U.S. epileptologists indicated that lamotrigine was recommended as treatment of choice for the older patient, followed by gabapentin or levetiracetam (32). For the rare older patient who has a primary generalized epilepsy, valproate, lamotrigine, topiramate, or levetiracetam would be appropriate choices (32). Table 30-2 summarizes all currently approved AEDs with side effect profiles and relative costs. The older AEDs, such as phenobarbital, phenytoin, valproate, and carbamazepine, continue to be highly prescribed. More than 50% of elderly patients on AEDs, both in the community and in nursing home populations, are prescribed phenytoin (35,50). However, newer and perhaps better choices are now available, with multiple agents introduced over the last decade. Table 30-3 outlines the potential advantages and disadvantages of the new AEDs compared with standard therapy in the older population.

SIDE EFFECTS

AEDs are one of the most common sources of adverse medication side effects in the elderly (24,25). In general, older and newer AEDs appear to have similar efficacy for partial seizures; however, the newer agents may offer advantages in side effect profile and tolerability. There are few clinical trials that compare new and old AEDs directly in elderly patients. The Veterans Administration Cooperative Study No. 428 compared carbamazepine, lamotrigine, and gabapentin for treatment of new-onset partial seizures in patients aged 60 or older in a randomized, prospective fashion (54). The study found similar efficacy for all three drugs; however, carbamazepine users were significantly more likely to experience adverse medication side effects resulting in early discontinuation. Another randomized, prospective study comparing lamotrigine with carbamazepine for newly diagnosed seizures in patients 65 and older in the United Kingdom also found carbamazepine users to be more than twice as likely to experience adverse side effects and related medication discontinuation (6). A pooled data analysis from this study plus 12 others confirmed the superior tolerability of lamotrigine versus carbamazepine and phenytoin in elderly patients (18). An

Table 30-2. *Current Antiepileptic Drugs Used in Elderly Patients*

Antiepileptic Drug	Drug Interactions	Common Adverse Effects	Cost
Carbamazepine	++	Diplopia, dizziness, idiosyncratic aplastic anemia, rash, hyponatremia, osteoporosis	$$
Felbamate	+++	Dizziness, headache, idiosyncratic hepatic failure or aplastic anemia, insomnia, weight loss	$$$
Gabapentin	+	Fatigue, transient GI distress	$$$
Lamotrigine	+	Dizziness, headache	$$$
Levetiracetam	+	Somnolence, coordination difficulties	$$$
Oxcarbazepine	++	Dizziness, diplopia, ataxia, hyponatremia	$$$
Phenobarbital	+++	Cognitive effects, respiratory depression, sedation	$
Phenytoin	+++	Ataxia, gingival hyperplasia, hirsutism, lymphadenopathy, nystagmus, osteoporosis	$
Pregabalin	+	Weight gain, sedation	$$$
Primidone	+++	Sedation, depression, dizziness	$
Tiagabine	++	GI distress, cognitive effects	$$$
Topiramate	++	Impaired memory, weight loss, word finding difficulty	$$$
Valproate	+++	Weight gain	$$
Zonisamide	++	Somnolence, dizziness, agitation, difficulty concentrating, weight loss	$$$

+/++/+++, least to most drug interactions; $/$$/$$$, least to most expensive; GI, gastrointestinal.

open-label study of levetiracetam as add-on therapy in patients over age 65 also found this to be a well-tolerated medication for this population (16). Common side effects of individual AEDs are summarized in Table 30-2.

DRUG INTERACTIONS

One of the more important considerations regarding choice of AED is drug interaction. According to the Centers for Medicare and Medicaid Services Current Beneficiary Survey in 2000 of community-dwelling elderly in the United States, the average number of filled prescriptions annually was 30, increasing to 40 or more in persons with at least three chronic medical conditions. In addition to concerns about compliance and expense, interactions resulting from multiple drug therapy can lead to significant adverse effects.

There are two broad types of drug interactions: pharmacokinetic and pharmacodynamic interactions. Pharmacokinetic drug interactions are defined as those interactions altering absorption, distribution, metabolism, or elimination. The most common pharmacokinetic drug interaction is an alteration in hepatic metabolism. Drugs that induce or inhibit hepatic metabolism of other drugs may either increase toxicity or reduce the effectiveness of other medications.

Among the AEDs, phenobarbital, primidone, phenytoin, and carbamazepine are inducers of cytochrome P450 enzymes, whereas valproate is an inhibitor (49). Therefore, these agents may be problematic for the older patient taking multiple drugs. Medications taken for other conditions may similarly cause adverse alterations in the metabolism of AEDs. For example, because macrolide antibiotics, such as erythromycin, inhibit hepatic enzyme induction, if erythromycin is used concomitantly with carbamazepine, carbamazepine toxicity can occur. For older patients on warfarin, its use in combination with a hepatic enzyme–inducing AED may result in decreased anticoagulant effect with potentially serious outcomes (49). Pharmacodynamic interactions are defined as interactions when medications have mechanisms of action that are either synergistic or antagonistic. For example, both benzodiazepines and barbiturates have an additive effect when combined because both affect the GABA^A binding site. Therefore, choosing an AED with a unique mechanism of action with limited hepatic metabolism may be most beneficial in the older patient. Thus, all of the new AEDs may be better choices for older adults with seizures. For a detailed discussion regarding AED drug interaction, the reader is referred to McLean (43).

Table 30-3. *Advantages and Disadvantages of Antiepileptic Drugs for Elderly Patients*

Antiepileptic Drug	Advantages	Disadvantages
Carbamazepine	Inexpensive Efficacy for partial seizures	Rash Bone disease Hyponatremia
Felbamate	Broad spectrum of coverage Efficacy for refractory seizures	Serious idiosyncratic side effects Expensive
Gabapentin	No drug interactions Renal excretion	Multiple daily doses Expensive
Lamotrigine	Broad spectrum of coverage Well tolerated Twice a day dosing	Slow to initiate Rash Expensive
Levetiracetam	Easy to initiate No drug interactions Renal excretion	Behavioral/mood problems Expensive
Oxcarbazepine	Well tolerated	Hyponatremia Expensive
Phenobarbital	Inexpensive Once-daily dosing Broad spectrum of coverage	Sedation Cognitive adverse effects Behavioral/mood problems Bone disease
Phenytoin	Inexpensive Once-daily dosing	Sedation Narrow therapeutic window Imbalance Bone disease
Pregabalin	No drug interactions	Weight gain Expensive
Topiramate	Broad spectrum of coverage Weight loss	Cognitive adverse effects Expensive
Tiagabine	Limited drug interactions	Multiple daily doses Cognitive adverse effects Expensive
Valproate	Broad spectrum of coverage	Weight gain Tremor Bone disease
Zonisamide	Well tolerated Once-daily dosing	Sedation Expensive

INITIATING AND MONITORING DRUG THERAPY

As with other medications in the elderly, when starting AEDs, it is good to follow the rule of "start low, go slow." Complex pharmacokinetic changes with aging such as altered gastrointestinal absorption, changes in serum protein binding, decreased hepatic metabolism, and renal clearance can all affect AED serum levels in ways that are complex and difficult to predict. Once AED therapy is established, adjustment of medication is primarily guided by clinical seizure control and side effects. Measuring AED concentrations can be of value in assessment of compliance and ascertaining toxicity. This monitoring of AED levels becomes even more important in the older population because older patients may have problems with memory, making compliance with a drug regimen difficult. The pharmacokinetic changes associated with advancing age of decreased drug clearance and reduced metabolism may contribute to toxicity, which may be prevented with a check of serum concentration (10). In an elderly nursing home population where compliance should be very high, serum levels of phenytoin varied two- to threefold over time in individual patients on stable oral doses of medication (4). It is important to remember that recommended serum level ranges for antiepileptic medications are based on younger patients and, therefore, may not be applicable to older patients. Older adults may be more sensitive to the sedative and cognitive effects of AEDs and may experience difficulties at lower than expected doses. For drugs such as phenytoin, older people may have a narrow therapeutic window, placing them at greater risk for toxicity. For highly protein-bound drugs, the lower protein binding seen in older age can result in a higher than expected free level of medication. Thus, serum concentrations of phenytoin, carbamazepine, and valproic acid should be monitored as total and free plasma concentrations. In contrast, the majority of the new AEDs are not highly protein bound and do not yet have defined serum concentrations. Thus, checking serum drug levels for the newer agents is not required and is generally not helpful in determining toxicity or therapeutic effect.

FALLS AND FRACTURES

Seizures can lead to falls and subsequent fractures (65,69), which can have profound consequences in an older individual's life, including loss of mobility, placement in a nursing home, or death. In a population-based study from the United Kingdom General Practice Research Database, persons with epilepsy had twice the fracture rate of the general population (63). Falling and fracture in elderly epilepsy patients is a complex issue, reflecting not only seizure-related trauma, but also the effect of AEDs on instability and bone health. Although older AEDs have often been associated with imbalance, second-generation drugs, with the exception of gabapentin and levetiracetam, have also been shown to carry this risk (58). AEDs that induce hepatic enzyme metabolism can contribute to development of osteoporosis via inactivation of vitamin D, leading to decreased calcium absorption (47). Both osteoporosis and osteopenia are significantly increased in patients chronically exposed to these drugs (15,48). For older patients at risk for the development of bone disease or in whom osteoporosis is already present, second-generation AEDs may again be a better choice. It is recommended to place all patients taking AEDs on prophylactic vitamin D and calcium supplementation and to follow serial bone density measurements.

NONMEDICATION THERAPIES

VAGUS NERVE STIMULATION

Vagus nerve stimulation (VNS) is a reasonable treatment option for medically refractory seizures in patients who are not candidates for traditional epilepsy surgery. In experienced surgical hands, the procedure has a low complication rate. Although usually done under general anesthesia, use of regional anesthesia is an option. There has been only one retrospective study looking at effectiveness of VNS in older adults, which found an average seizure reduction of 31% at 3 months, with 50% to 60% of patients achieving at least a 50% reduction by 1 year (60). No patients were seizure free. Adverse effects were found

to be few, consisting of hoarseness, coughing, and paresthesias. No clinically significant episodes of bradycardia were reported postoperatively. Additionally, there was a significant improvement in quality of life scores. Although the efficacy of VNS compares favorably to medications, it is almost always used as an adjunct rather than a replacement for AEDs. VNS is a contraindication for subsequent body magnetic resonance imaging and may complicate mammography; therefore, its use should be carefully considered in patients with a history of malignancy or other condition where serial imaging would be otherwise indicated.

EPILEPSY SURGERY

In about 30% to 40% of all epilepsy patients, seizures are not completely controlled by medical therapy. Epilepsy surgery is considered when disabling seizures continue despite appropriate AED therapy and when control of seizures would significantly improve quality of life. In particular, temporal lobectomy, the most common surgical procedure for epilepsy, has proliferated recently since its efficacy and safety have become well documented (64). In a randomized control trial of temporal lobectomy versus medical management for younger adults with refractory seizures, surgery was significantly more effective (58% vs. 8% seizure free at 1 year, respectively) and resulted in improved quality of life (75). Elderly patients are often not appropriate candidates for epilepsy surgery due to underlying medical comorbidities or to seizure etiology (e.g., a demented nursing home resident). Unfortunately, even older patients without these contraindications have traditionally not been considered surgical candidates due to concerns about the potential for increased age-related surgical complications and for possible decreased efficacy due to long-standing epilepsy duration. However, several retrospective studies have investigated surgical outcomes in selected patients over the age of 50 years and have found seizure-free outcomes to be similar to those of younger age groups without significant decline in memory function (5,8,23,39,42,59). Thus, although more studies are needed, older adults should not be excluded from surgical consideration based solely on age. Rather, exclusion criteria should be similar to those for younger patients, which would include lack of a definite epileptic focus or a seizure focus in an inoperable location such as the motor strip or areas of language and/or memory functioning. Although surgical complication rates in the previously mentioned studies were at acceptable levels, it is important to understand that these were highly selected candidates. Careful consideration of surgical risk and potential improvement in seizure control and overall quality of life must be made on an individual basis.

WHICH TREATMENT? MEDICATIONS VERSUS SURGERY

Figure 30-3 illustrates an algorithm for management of seizures in the older adult. Treatment is initiated after the second seizure. If seizures persist despite a trial of antiepileptic medication with documentation of a therapeutic level or adverse effects, then other AEDs are tried. Once three antiepileptic medications have been tried and seizures persist, then surgery should be considered. Surgery should only be pursued in individuals in whom there is likely to be an improvement in the quality of life or in a patient with injurious seizures. Thus, an older adult living in a nursing home with dementia and seizures would not

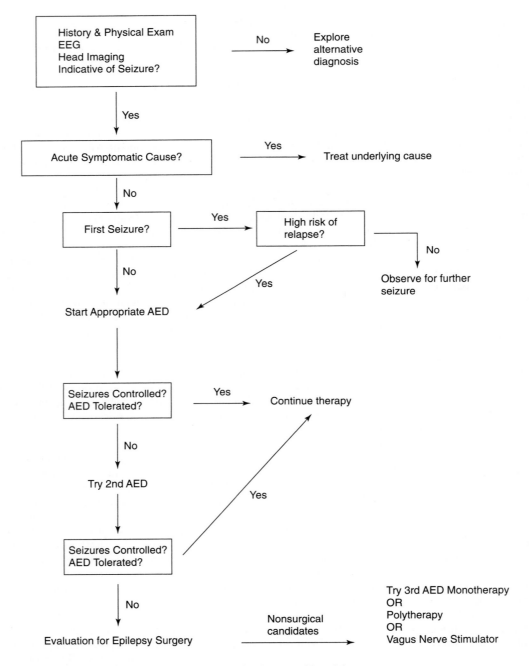

Figure 30-3. An algorithm for the treatment of epilepsy in older adults.

be an appropriate candidate for surgery. In sum, the benefits must outweigh the risks. If the patient is not a candidate for surgery or fails to respond to surgery, then VNS would be an appropriate option.

PSYCHOSOCIAL IMPLICATIONS OF SEIZURES IN OLDER PEOPLE

Seizures can impact the lives of older people in many ways. However, the study of quality of life issues in epilepsy remains largely neglected in this age group. In one survey of older adults with epilepsy living in the community, medication side effect (64%) and issues related to driving and transportation (64%) were by far the most commonly noted concerns (41). Although the specific laws vary from state to state, in general, having a seizure will result in revocation or suspension of driving privileges for a period of at least several months. Loss of driving privileges can be as devastating to older patients as it is to younger patients and may impact the ability to maintain independent living, especially if there is a lack of adequate public transportation. In the study by Martin et al. (41), 36% of those surveyed reported concerns related to embarrassment or social restrictions as a result of having epilepsy. Although the social stigma of epilepsy affects all age groups, it may be particularly heightened with elderly patients who come from a generation where seizures were often mistakenly considered a sign of mental illness, moral weakness, or even a cause for institutionalization. The common misperception that seizures are a condition of the young may contribute to a lack of acceptance of this diagnosis. Medical care providers should be aware of the psychosocial implications of a seizure diagnosis for elderly individuals and must recognize that these concerns can add to a patient's reluctance to accept diagnosis and treatment in some cases. Adequate counseling and education of patients and family members is a crucial component of care.

SUMMARY

Epilepsy in older people is a major public health problem with significant pathologic, psychosocial, and economic burdens on both individuals and society. With aging of the global population, epilepsy is likely to become even more prevalent over time. Yet, the impact of epilepsy and its new treatments have not been investigated as systematically in older patients as in younger ones. Future research into the pathophysiology of the aging brain and, in particular, its relation to epilepsy, as well as treatments of epilepsy in older people, is fundamental if we are to adequately treat the burgeoning aged population of the next century.

REFERENCES

1. Annegers JF, Hauser WA, Lee JR, et al. Incidence of acute symptomatic seizures in Rochester, Minnesota 1935–1984. *Epilepsia*. 1995;36:327–333.
2. Annegers JF, Shirts SB, Hauser WA, et al. Risk of seizure recurrence after an initial unprovoked seizure. *Epilepsia*. 1986;27:43–50.
3. Berg AT, Shinnar S. The risk of seizure recurrence following a first unprovoked seizure: a quantitative review. *Neurology*. 1991;41:965–972.
4. Birnbaum A, Hardie NA, Leppik IE, et al. Variability of total phenytoin serum concentrations within elderly nursing home residents. *Neurology*. 2003;60:555–559.
5. Boling W, Andermann F, Reutens D, et al. Surgery for temporal lobe epilepsy in older patients. *J Neurosurg*. 2001;95:242–248.
6. Brodie MJ, Overstall PW, Giorgi L, for the UK Lamotrigine Elderly Study Group. Multicentre, double-blind, randomized comparison between lamotrigine and carbamazepine in elderly patients with newly diagnosed epilepsy. *Epilepsy Res*. 1999;37:81–87.
7. Cascino GD, Hesdorffer D, Logroscino G, et al. Morbidity of nonfebrile status epilepticus in Rochester, Minnesota 1965–1984. *Epilepsia*. 1998;39:829–832.
8. Cascino GD, Sharbrough FW, Hirschorn KA, et al. Surgery for focal epilepsy in the older patient. *Neurology*. 1991;41:1415–1417.
9. Chatrian GE, Shaw CM, Leffman H. The significance of periodic lateralized epileptiform discharges in EEG. An electrographic, clinical, and pathological study. *Electroencephalogr Clin Neurophysiol*. 1964;17:177–193.
10. Cloyd JC, Lackner TE, Leppik IE. Antiepileptics in the elderly. Pharmacoepidemiology and pharmacokinetics. *Arch Fam Med*. 1994;3:589–598.
11. DeLorenzo RJ, Hauser WA, Towne AR, et al. A prospective population-based epidemiologic study of status epilepticus in Richmond, Virginia. *Neurology*. 1996;46:1029–1035.
12. DeLorenzo RJ, Pellock JM, Towne AR, et al. Epidemiology of status epilepticus. *J Clin Neurophysiol*. 1995;12:316–325.
13. Drury I, Beydoun A. Interictal epileptiform activity in elderly patients with epilepsy. *Electroencephalogr Clin Neurophysiol*. 1998;106:369–373.
14. Ettinger AB, Shinnar S. New-onset seizures in an elderly hospitalized population. *Neurology*. 1993;43:489–492.
15. Farhat G, Yamout B, Mikati A, et al. Effect of antiepileptic drugs on bone density in ambulatory patients. *Neurology*. 2002;58:1348–1353.

16. Ferrendelli JA, French J, Leppik I, et al. Use of levetiracetam in a population of patients aged 65 years and older: a subset analysis of the KEEPER trial. *Epilepsy Behav.* 2003;4:702–709.

17. Garrard J, Cloyd J, Gross C, et al. Factors associated with antiepileptic drug use among elderly nursing home residents. *J Gerontol A Biol Sci Med Sci.* 2000;55:384–392.

18. Giorgi L, Gomez G, O'Neill F, et al. The tolerability of lamotrigine in elderly patients with epilepsy. *Drugs Aging.* 2001;18:621–630.

19. Giroud M, Gras P, Fayolle H, Andre N, et al. Early seizures after acute stroke: a study of 1,640 cases. *Epilepsia.* 1994;35:959–964.

20. Glantz MJ, Cole BF, Forsyth PA, et al. Practice parameter: anticonvulsant prophylaxis in patients with newly diagnosed brain tumor: report of the Quality Standards Subcommittee of the American Academy of Neurology. *Neurology.* 2000;54:1886–1893.

21. Glauser T, Ben-Menachem E, Bourgeois B, et al. ILAE treatment guidelines: evidence-based analysis of antiepileptic drug efficacy and effectiveness as initial monotherapy for epileptic seizures and syndromes. *Epilepsia.* 2006;47:1094–1120.

22. Granger AS. Ginkgo biloba precipitating epileptic seizures. *Age Ageing.* 2001;30:523–525.

23. Grivas A, Schramm J, Kral T, et al. Surgical treatment for refractory temporal lobe epilepsy in the elderly: seizure outcome and neuropsychological sequels compared with a younger cohort. *Epilepsia.* 2006;47:1364–1372.

24. Gurwitz JH, Field TS, Avorn J, et al. Incidence and preventability of adverse drug events in nursing homes. *Am J Med.* 2000;109:87–94.

25. Gurwitz JH, Field TS, Harrold LR, et al. Incidence and preventability of adverse drug events among older patients in the ambulatory setting. *JAMA.* 2003;289:1107–1116.

26. Hauser WA. Epidemiology of seizures and epilepsy in the elderly. In: Rowan AJ, Ramsay ER, eds. *Epilepsy in the elderly.* Boston: Butterworth-Heinemann; 1997:7–18.

27. Hauser WA. Seizure disorders: the changes with age. *Epilepsia.* 1992;33:S6–S14.

28. Hauser WA, Annegers JF, Kurland LT. Incidence of epilepsy and unprovoked seizures in Rochester, Minnesota: 1935–1984. *Epilepsia.* 1993;34:453–468.

29. Hauser WA, Rich SS, Lee JR, et al. Risk of recurrent seizures after two unprovoked seizures. *N Engl J Med.* 1998;338:429–434.

30. Hesdorffer DC, D'Amelio M. Mortality in the first 30 days following incident acute symptomatic seizures. *Epilepsia.* 2005;46:S43–S45.

31. Hopkins A, Garman A, Clarke C. The first seizure in adult life: value of clinical features, electroencephalography and computerized tomographic scanning in prediction of seizure recurrence. *Lancet.* 1988;1:721–726.

32. Karceski S, Morrell MJ, Carpenter D. Treatment of epilepsy in adults: expert opinion, 2005. *Epilepsy Behav.* 2005;7:S1–S64.

33. Klass DW, Brenner RP. Electroencephalography of the elderly. *J Clin Neurophysiol.* 1995;12:116–131.

34. Kupiec T, Raj V. Fatal seizures due to potential herb-drug interactions with ginkgo biloba. *J Anal Toxicol.* 2005;29:755–758.

35. Lackner TE, Cloyd JC, Thomas LW, et al. Antiepileptic drug use in nursing home residents: effect of age, gender, and comedication on patterns of use. *Epilepsia.* 1998;39:1083–1087.

36. Loiseau J, Loiseau P, Duche B, et al. A survey of epileptic disorders in southwest France: seizures in elderly patients. *Ann Neurol.* 1990;27:233–237.

37. Loiseau P. Pathologic processes in the elderly and their association with seizures. In: Rowan AJ, Ramsey RE, eds. *Seizures and epilepsy in the elderly.* Boston: Butterworth-Heinemann; 1997:63–68.

38. Luhdorf K, Jensen LK, Plesner AM. Epilepsy in the elderly: incidence, social function, and disability. *Epilepsia.* 1989;30:389–399.

39. Malamut BL, Cloud B, Sirven JI, et al. Neuropsychological and psychosocial outcome after unilateral temporal lobectomy over age 45. *Neurology.* 1998;50[Suppl 4]:A202(abst).

40. Malouf R, Brust JCM. Hypoglycemia: causes, neurologic manifestations, and outcomes. *Ann Neurol.* 1985;17:421–430.

41. Martin R, Vogtle L, Gilliam F, et al. What are the concerns of older adults living with epilepsy? *Epilepsy Behav.* 2005;7:297–300.

42. McLachlan RS, Chovaz CJ, Blume WT, et al. Temporal lobectomy for intractable epilepsy in patients over age 45 years. *Neurology.* 1992;42:662–665.

43. McLean MJ. New antiepiletic medications: pharmacokinetic and mechanistic considerations in the treatment of seizures and epilepsy in the elderly. In: Rowan AJ, Ramsey RE, eds. *Seizures and epilepsy in the elderly.* Boston: Butterworth-Heinemann; 1997:239–307.

44. Messing RO, Closson RG, Simon RP. Drug-induced seizures: a 10-year experience. *Neurology.* 1984;34:1582–1586.

45. Muller HF, Kral VA. The EEG in advanced senile dementia. *J Am Geriatr Soc.* 1967;15:415–426.

46. Otomo E. Electroencephalography in old age: dominant alpha rhythm. *Electrencephalogr Clin Neurophysiol.* 1966;21:489–491.

47. Pack AM, Gidal B, Vasquez B. Bone disease associated with antiepileptic drugs. *Clev Clin J Med.* 2004;71:S42–S48.

48. Pack AM, Olarte LS, Morrell MJ, et al. Bone mineral density in an outpatient population

receiving enzyme inducing antiepileptic drugs. *Epilepsy Behav.* 2003;4:169–174.

49. Patsalos PN, Froscher W, Pisani F, et al. The importance of drug interactions in epilepsy therapy. *Epilepsia.* 2002;43:365–385.

50. Perucca E, Berlowitz D, Birnbaum A, et al. Pharmacological and clinical aspects of antiepileptic drug use in the elderly. *Epilepsy Res.* 2006;68S: S49–S63.

51. Ramsey RE, Pryor F. Epilepsy in the elderly. *Neurology.* 2000;55:S9–S14.

52. Ramsay RE, Rowan AJ, Pryor FM. Special considerations in treating the elderly patient with epilepsy. *Neurology.* 2004;62:S24–S29.

53. Roubicek J. The electroencephalogram in the middle aged and the elderly. *J Am Geriatr Soc.* 1977;25:145–152.

54. Rowan AJ, Ransay RE, Collins JF, et al. New onset geriatric epilepsy. A randomized study of gabapentin, lamotrigine, and carbamazepine. *Neurology.* 2005;64:1868–1873.

55. Sanders JWA, Hart YM, Johnson AL, et al. Natural General Practice Study of Epilepsy: newly diagnosed epileptic seizures in general population. *Lancet.* 1990;336:1267–1270.

56. Silverman AJ, Busse EW, Barnes RH. Studies in the process of aging: electroencephalographic findings in 400 elderly subjects. *Electroencephalogr Clin Neurophysiol.* 1955;7:67–77.

57. Singh BM, Gupta DR, Strobos RJ. Nonketotic hyperglycemia and epilepsia partialis continua. *Arch Neurol.* 1973;29:187–190.

58. Sirven JI, Fife TD, Wingerchuk DM, et al. Second generation antiepileptic drugs' impact on balance: a meta-analysis. *Mayo Clin Proc.* 2007;82:40–47.

59. Sirven JI, Malamut BL, O'Connor MJ, et al. Temporal lobectomy outcome in older versus younger adults. *Neurology.* 2000;54:2166–2170.

60. Sirven JI. VNS in the elderly group. Vagus nerve stimulation therapy for epilepsy in older adults. *Neurology.* 2000;54:1179–1182.

61. Sirven JI, Wingerchuk DM, Drazkowski JF, et al. Seizure prophylaxis in patients with brain tumors: a meta-analysis. *Mayo Clin Proc.* 2004;79:1489–1494.

62. So EL, Annegers JF, Hauser WA, et al. Population-based study of seizure disorders after cerebral infarction. *Neurology.* 1996;46:350–355.

63. Souverein P, Webb DJ, Petri H, et al. Incidence of fractures among epilepsy patients: a population based prospective cohort study in the general practice research database. *Epilepsia.* 2005;46:304–310.

64. Sperling MR, O'Connor MJ, Saykin AJ, et al. Temporal lobectomy for refractory epilepsy. *JAMA.* 1996;276:470–475.

65. Tallis R. Treatment of epilepsy in the elderly patient. In: Shorvon S, Dreifuss D, Fish D, et al., eds. *The treatment of epilepsy*. London: Blackwell Science Ltd.; 1996:227–237.

66. Tallis R, Hall G, Craig I, et al. How common are epileptic seizures in old age? *Age Ageing.* 1991;20:442–448.

67. Thomas P, Lebrun C, Chatel M. De novo absence status epilepticus as a benzodiazepine withdrawal syndrome. *Epilepsia.* 1993;34:355–358.

68. Tinuper P. The altered presentation of seizures in the elderly. In: Rowan AJ, Ramsey RE, eds. *Seizures and epilepsy in the elderly.* Boston: Butterworth-Heinemann; 1997:123–130.

69. Vestergaard P, Tigaran S, Rejnmark L, et al. Fracture risk in epilepsy. *Acta Neurol Scand.* 1999;99:269–275.

70. Vignatelli L, Tonon C, D'Allessandro R, et al. Incidence and short-term prognosis of status epilepticus in adults in Bologna, Italy. *Epilepsia.* 2003;44:964–968.

71. Waterhouse EJ, DeLorenzo RJ. Status epilepticus in older patients. Epidemiology and treatment options. *Drugs Aging.* 2001;18:133–142.

72. Waterhouse EJ, Vaughan JK, Barnes TY, et al. Synergistic effect of status epilepticus and ischemic brain injury on mortality. *Epilepsy Res.* 1998;29:175–183.

73. Westmoreland BF. Benign variants and patterns of uncertain clinical significance. In: Daly DD, Pedley TA, eds. *Current practice of clinical electroencephalography*. 2nd ed. New York: Raven Press; 1990:243–252.

74. Westmoreland BF, Klass DW. A distinctive rhythmic EEG discharge of adults. *Electroencephalogr Clin Neurophysiol.* 1981;51:186–191.

75. Wiebe S, Blume WT, Girvin JP, et al. A randomized controlled trial of surgery for temporal lobe epilepsy. *N Engl J Med.* 2001;345:311–318.

76. Zaccara G, Muscas GC, Messori A. Clinical features, pathogenesis and management of drug-induced seizures. *Drug Saf.* 1990;5:109–151.

77. Zimmerman R. Diagnostic methods II: imaging studies. In: Rowan AJ, Ramsay RE, eds. *Seizures and epilepsy in the elderly.* Boston: Butterworth-Heinemann; 1997:159–177.

SUGGESTED READING

Rowan AJ, Ramsay RE, eds. *Seizures and Epilepsy in the Elderly*. Boston: Butterworth-Heinemann; 1996.

WEBSITES

American Epilepsy Society: www.aesnet.org
Epilepsy Foundation of America: http://www.epilepsyfoundation.org/

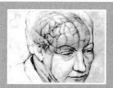

SECTION **IV**

PSYCHOSOCIAL ISSUES IN THE OLDER ADULT

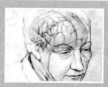

CHAPTER 31

Recognition and Management of Late Life Mood Disorders

James M. Ellison and Gary L. Gottlieb

Aging is not inevitably accompanied by a distur-bance of mood, yet depressive symptoms among elderly women and men are common and disabling. Most depressed elderly patients who seek treatment do so in a primary care setting, where detection is often poor and treatment is frequently inadequate. Individuals confined in long-term care facilities rely on primary care clinicians for treatment or referral to a mental health specialist, with the result that many go untreated. Elderly sufferers of depression or of mania, which is less prevalent, consume dispropor-tionately large amounts of medical health care resources (16,129) and die prematurely of medical causes (16,103) or suicide (27). For those who survive, the functional impairment associated with a mood dis-order can exhaust caregivers and tip the balance from independent living toward an early need for institu-tional care. Improved recognition and management of late life mood disorders can alleviate suffering, reduce functional impairment, decrease mortality, and spare caregivers a substantial burden. This chapter reviews the syndromes most frequently seen among the elderly, focusing on their clinical and epidemiologic characteristics and summarizing current approaches to management.

DIAGNOSIS OF LATE LIFE DEPRESSION

Depressive symptoms fall into several characteristic syndromes. The American Psychiatric Association's *Diagnostic and Statistical Manual of Mental Disorders, 4th Edition, Text Revision* (DSM) (7) defines major depressive episodes as requiring five or more core symptoms present during a 2-week period, not attrib-utable to the use of a substance or a medical illness. One of the symptoms must be depressed mood or loss of interest or pleasure, whereas others can be drawn from the following list: weight loss, insomnia or hypersomnia, psychomotor agitation or retardation, fatigue or loss of energy, worthlessness or guilt, dimin-ished concentration, and recurrent thoughts of death or suicide. Psychotic features such as delusions, hallu-cinations, or severe disturbance of motor function

(stupor or agitation) may also be present. Dysthymic disorder, a chronic but less florid depressive state, is diagnosed when depressed mood has been accompa-nied by two or more of the depressive symptoms listed earlier for an extended period of time (present more days than not for at least 2 years) (7). The presence of fewer, milder, or briefer symptoms is termed minor depression or subsyndromal depression.

In assessing elderly patients, the diagnosis of depression is made more challenging by muted or obscure expression of signs and symptoms. In con-trast with younger patients, the current cohort of depressed elderly often places less emphasis on a sad or depressed mood; instead, anger, irritability, anxiety, cognitive difficulties, or somatic concerns may be the focus of attention. Somatic symptoms associated with known medical illnesses affect most of the depressed elderly. Medically explainable symptoms are often mag-nified by the presence of depression and confounded by the presence of additional symptoms that are not medically explainable. Although psychological symp-toms of depression are present in most depressed elderly (113), their detection requires attentive inquiry. When cognitive impairment is prominent, mood symptoms are even less likely to be reported. Deterioration of function and interpersonal interactions may then provide the strongest clue to the presence of a mood disorder.

Among depressed elderly patients who present with prominent cognitive symptoms, the non-DSM diagnosis of dementia syndrome of depression (DSD) may be appropriate. Formerly termed *pseudodementia* because of the partial cognitive improvement associ-ated with successful resolution of other depressive symptoms, this syndrome can lead to an erroneous diagnosis of primary dementia, resulting in a missed opportunity to treat depression (52). Ample follow-up evidence now demonstrates that DSD, although responsive to antidepressant treatment in the short run, often presages the later appearance of a primary dementia (45,91). Features that help to differentiate DSD from a primary dementia include the more likely presence of an autonomous mood disorder, more rapid progression of symptoms, greater patient awareness of and complaint regarding cognitive symptoms, and previous history of a mood disorder. In addition to these features, on neuropsychological assessment, the patient may show poorer effort in attempting to perform tasks, greater intactness of recognition memory, better performance with prompting, and more variable performance on similarly difficult tasks (45).

DEMOGRAPHICS AND RISK FACTORS

Many clinicians and patients assume that mood disorders are more prevalent among the elderly than among young adults, given the recognized losses and stresses associated with aging, but epidemiologic data consistently contradict such an assertion. With the possible exception of the oldest old (144), evidence suggests that major depressive disorder is no more prevalent among the elderly than among younger adults (17). Data from the Epidemiologic Catchment Area studies estimated a 1-year prevalence among community-dwelling elderly of 2.7% for major depression (135). By contrast, subsyndromal depression affects a large number (8% to 15%) of community-dwelling elderly persons (17).

In contrast to the general population of community-dwelling elderly, specific subgroups have been shown to suffer a higher prevalence of depression. Borson et al. (19) detected major depression in 10% of an elderly population with chronic medical illnesses. In a primary care clinic setting, a prevalence of 5.6% was measured for major depression among the elderly patients, and an additional 7.9% had probable or masked depression (15). In long-term care facilities, the only mental disorder more common among the elderly than depression is dementia. The prevalence of major depression in nursing homes is estimated to be between 6% and 25%, with 30% to 50% of nursing home residents suffering subsyndromal symptoms (49). The annual rate of new cases of major depression in nursing homes is as high as 9.4%, and each year, an additional 7.4% develop new minor depressions (86).

Among the risk factors linked to late life depression, a higher prevalence is associated with female gender (17); lower levels of educational attainment; a history of childhood poverty, sexual assault, or parental separation or divorce; lower income and occupational attainments; widowhood or other unmarried states; lack of integration into a supportive social network; chronic financial or medical stresses; acute provoking events (34); and a history of heavy alcohol consumption (109). Neither race nor ethnicity appears to be an important risk factor for late life depression (76).

Depression and aging are themselves risk factors for suicide, an all too frequent complication of late life depression. The rate of completed suicide increases significantly with advancing age, notably among white men (70). Among the elderly, depression is strongly correlated with the risk of either suicide attempts (63,83) or completion (14,26,27). The increased prevalence of depression in various medical illnesses (e.g., multiple sclerosis, epilepsy, Huntington's disease, traumatic spinal lesions, cranial trauma, peptic ulcer disease, rheumatoid arthritis, cardiopulmonary diseases, renal disease requiring chronic hemodialysis, and chronic pain) may contribute to the increased suicide risk among patients with these illnesses (64).

DETECTION

Studies of service utilization indicate that the elderly with mood disorders are seriously undertreated. Most of the mentally ill elderly receive no services specifically for their psychiatric diagnoses. A recently published study of elderly patients treated in four primary care health maintenance organization (HMO) clinics, for example, found that only 7% of the depressed patients received treatment for depression in 1993, and only 11% to 22% of these patients saw a psychiatrist (130). In long-term care facilities, undertreatment is particularly common. As recently as 1985, the National Nursing Home Survey determined that <10% of the institutionalized elderly received services for their psychiatric diagnoses (37). Underrecognition and undertreatment are perpetuated by both provider and patient factors.

Primary care clinicians deliver most of the psychiatric care received by elderly adults. Although nearly 85% of older adults visit a primary care physician at least once a year, those with mood disorders frequently elude detection. Primary care clinicians may lack the time to thoroughly evaluate mood-related symptoms or the training and interest required for successful diagnosis and treatment. Psychotropic medications are frequently prescribed in primary care, but many of these medications are sedatives and hypnotics, rather than antidepressants (22). Unutzer et al. (128) raised the possibility that elderly patients receive different care from that provided to younger adults. They found that depressed patients older than 60 years of age receiving care from an HMO were less likely than younger depressed adults to receive adequate antidepressant doses within the first 90 days of treatment. The elderly patients were also less likely to have more than two primary care visits for depression within the first 12 weeks after a new antidepressant was prescribed or specialty mental health care within the first 6 months after the antidepressant prescription. Historically, the underprescribing of psychotherapy was highlighted by the observation that most older adults treated for a psychiatric diagnosis in primary care received only psychotropic drugs (22).

In addition to these provider factors, some patient factors interfere with effective treatment of depression in this population. Elderly patients may fail to recognize in themselves the symptoms of a depression. Shame may prevent them from divulging complaints perceived as stigmatizing. When psychiatric referral is offered, refusal appears to be common (132). The high cost of medications, despite some improvement in insurance coverage resulting from initiation of Medicare Part D, provides another powerful disincentive for accepting treatment. Even when treatment is begun, adherence to a treatment regimen is often limited. One to two thirds of the elderly do not comply or only partially comply with a prescribed medication regimen (124).

Detection of depression in the elderly can be facilitated by use of screening tools that are self-administered or rely on clinician assessments. Among the self-administered tools, the Beck Depression Inventory is validated in elderly patients. The clinician-administered Hamilton Depression Scale (HAM-D or HRSD) relies heavily on somatic symptoms, weakening its specificity in medically ill elderly patients. The Geriatric Depression Scale (GDS) is brief, easily administered, and focuses on depressive affects and cognitions. The Cornell Scale for Depression in Dementia (CSDD), which focuses on depressive behaviors, is suitable for rating of depressed patients with dementia but requires more time to administer because interviews with both the patient and the caregiver are required (2,10).

Depression must be differentiated from medical illnesses, especially those characterized by fatigue or apathy; from the effects of sedating or mood-altering medications and substances; and from other behavioral disturbances, including bereavement, anxiety disorders, or psychotic disorders. Many medical causes of depression can be detected by a limited evaluation. A minimal workup for depression in an elderly patient must include a comprehensive history, which may need to be supplemented or validated by another informant; review of relevant records and prior treatments; and a physical examination. A mental status examination with screening of cognitive functions [e.g., with the Mini-Mental State Examination (MMSE)] is also suggested. Research support has not established the optimal battery of laboratory tests for detection of medical conditions presenting with depressive symptoms, but the majority of relevant disorders are screened for with a panel that includes complete blood count, erythrocyte sedimentation rate, electrolytes, calcium, glucose, thyroid-stimulating hormone, renal and liver functions, and vitamin B_{12} and folate. An electrocardiogram is required before prescribing a tricyclic antidepressant to an older adult and establishes a useful baseline measure even for treatment with agents of lesser potential cardiotoxicity.

An imaging study, such as computed tomography (CT), magnetic resonance imaging (MRI), single photon emission computed tomography (SPECT), or positron emission tomography (PET), is of greatest diagnostic and prognostic value when cognitive symptoms accompany depressive symptoms. In many cases of depression in later life, an MRI will reveal subcortical white matter hyperintensities on fluid-attenuated inversion recovery (FLAIR) or T2-weighted images. Although these findings are not specific for depression, their presence in depressed individuals is associated with older age, later age at onset, and less frequent family history of mental illness (59). Various terms have evolved to describe late life depression with corticostriatal dysfunction manifested as executive dysfunction and often accompanied by greater risk of relapse, recurrence, and residual depressive symptoms (1). Vascular depression (5) and subcortical ischemic depression (60) focus on pathophysiology and etiology, whereas the clinical manifestations of depression with frontolimbic and frontostriatal dysfunction are alluded to in the syndromal designation of "depression-executive dysfunction syndrome" (3,4), a condition that can arise from vascular or nonvascular pathologies.

TREATMENT

PSYCHOTHERAPY

Although often neglected in the treatment of late life depression, several psychotherapeutic approaches have been shown to be effective treatment options for cognitively intact patients with mild to moderately severe nonpsychotic depression. Psychotherapy can be provided with or without antidepressant medication. A meta-analysis of studies found psychotherapeutic treatment to be more effective than placebo or no treatment (111). Interpersonal therapy (IPT), which was developed as a time-limited intervention for midlife depression, has been useful in treating older patients as well because it focuses on highly relevant issues including grief, loss, and role transitions (137). Cognitive-behavior therapy (CBT) provides another brief and effective approach and is aimed at helping patients identify and correct distorted thoughts that perpetuate depression while introducing more pleasurable activities into their lives (122). Psychodynamic group psychotherapy approaches have been evaluated in the elderly in comparison with cognitive behavioral approaches and found to be of similar efficacy (115), although a need exists for further studies to clarify the relative advantages of these different approaches. Other types of psychotherapy reported to be helpful have included reminiscence/life review, psychoeducation, and relaxation-meditation.

Individuals who are intolerant of medication and electroconvulsive therapy (ECT) or who prefer a psychosocial approach to treatment can be referred to a mental health specialist for a trial of psychotherapy in individual or group format. The presence of prominent family conflict, stressful life events, or poor social supports might be appropriate indications for inclusion of psychotherapy in a treatment plan (81). Psychotic or bipolar features, significant personality disorder symptoms, heightened suicidal risk, or substance abuse should, when possible, prompt the involvement of a mental health specialist to address the more complex and risky treatment courses associated with these attributes.

ANTIDEPRESSANT MEDICATION

Antidepressant treatment of late life depression, provided more frequently than psychotherapy, is the subject of several thorough and informative recent reviews (30,35,73,79,99,121). No specific agent or antidepressant class emerges as the clear preference, but medications are consistently shown superior to placebo treatment. Pharmacotherapy of late life depression is complicated by age-related pharmacodynamic and pharmacokinetic factors. In particular, the elderly show an increased sensitivity to anticholinergic and antidopaminergic side effects. These pharmacodynamic vulnerabilities are combined with the pharmacokinetic changes of delayed drug absorption, reduced oxidative metabolism, and diminished glomerular filtration and drug secretion. The net effects are slower attainment of steady-state kinetics, higher peak and steady-state serum drug levels, and, consequently, greater likelihood of adverse drug effects (145). Several of the newer antidepressants are inhibitors or substrates of the hepatic microsomal enzyme systems that interact also with commonly coadministered treatments for medical illnesses. Paroxetine, fluoxetine, and, to a lesser extent, sertraline inhibit the cytochrome P450 (CYP) 2D6 enzyme, potentially interfering with clearance of such coadministered medications as tricyclic antidepressants, selegiline, donepezil, dextromethorphan, codeine, meperidine, oxycodone, tramadol, encainide, flecainide, lidocaine, mexiletine, propafenone, metoprolol, propranolol, and timolol, among others. Nefazodone (infrequently prescribed following reports of rare but serious hepatic complications) and fluvoxamine are significant inhibitors of the CYP 3A4 enzyme, potentially interfering with clearance of several coadministered antidepressants, alprazolam, clonazepam, diazepam, midazolam, triazolam, buspirone, carbamazepine, lamotrigine, donepezil, acetaminophen, codeine, clarithromycin, erythromycin, ketoconazole, astemizole, tamoxifen, amiodarone, disopyramide, lidocaine, quinidine, calcium channel blockers, lovastatin, steroids,

caffeine, and omeprazole, among others. Fluvoxamine also inhibits the CYP IA2 enzyme, potentially limiting clearance of drugs including clozapine and warfarin (145).

Table 31-1 lists the antidepressants and their dosages for use in late life depression. Most clinicians now initiate treatment with one of the selective serotonin reuptake inhibitors (SSRIs) or other newer serotonergic or nonserotonergic agents, citing data that support claims of their equal efficacy, more tolerable side effect profiles (fewer anticholinergic, cardiac, and cognitive adverse effects, although greater adverse effects on gastrointestinal and sexual functions), lower discontinuation rates, and better overall effect on quality of life. The availability of several generic serotonergic antidepressants has diminished the cost advantage sometimes previously cited as a reason for prescribing a tricyclic antidepressant.

Among the serotonergic medications, fluoxetine was shown in a large multicenter placebo-controlled, double-blind trial to be well tolerated in a group of patients 60 years of age and older (125), although the percentage of patients rated on the HAM-D as responders to 20 mg/day after 6 weeks was somewhat low (36% vs. 27% with placebo). The remission rate was 21% for fluoxetine and 13% for placebo in the intent-to-treat analysis, and the discontinuation and adverse effects rates for fluoxetine and placebo were similar. A large open study in which elderly depressed patients received fluoxetine (20 mg/day) showed a remission rate of 35% in the intent-to-treat analysis (71). At higher doses (20 to 80 mg/day), the efficacy of fluoxetine was equivalent to that of doxepin and its side effects were better tolerated in a group of elderly depressed outpatients (29). A lower dosage of fluoxetine is not required in the elderly, although treatment can be initiated at 10 mg/day to reduce the risk of overwhelming the patient with initial side effects. The side effects of fluoxetine, similar to those of other serotonergic antidepressants, include nausea and other gastrointestinal symptoms, headache, altered sleep, and sexual dysfunction. Weight loss has been cited as a clinical concern in particular with fluoxetine, but Goldstein et al. (36) reported that this is associated with pretreatment high body mass index. Hyponatremia, although an uncommon complication of SSRI antidepressants, is believed to be more common among elderly patients.

In a double-blind comparison to fluoxetine (20 to 40 mg/day), sertraline (50 to 100 mg/day) produced a similar decrease in mean HAM-D score after 12 weeks in a group of outpatients with a mean age of 74 years. Sertraline was claimed superior on the basis of greater cognitive improvement on one of three administered tests, better improvement on the Physical Health and Psychological Health subscale of the Quality of Life Enjoyment and Satisfaction Questionnaire, and

Table 31-1. *Selected Antidepressants for Use in Late Life Depression*

Generic Name	Trade Name	Starting Dose/ Range (mg/day)	Treatment Dose/ Range (mg/day)	Notes
Tricyclic antidepressants (TCA)				
Nortriptyline	Pamelor Aventyl	10–25	25–100	TCA with least postural hypotension; follow plasma levels: therapeutic window 50–150 ng/mL
Desipramine	Norpramine	10–25	25–150	TCA with least anticholinergic effect
Selective serotonin reuptake inhibitors (SSRI)				
Fluoxetine	Prozac	10	10–40	Also available as oral solution
	Prozac Weekly	90 once weekly	90 once weekly	Initiate after establishment of daily dose regimen of 20 mg/day, waiting 1 week after last daily dose
Sertraline	Zoloft	25	50–200	Also available as oral solution
Paroxetine	Paxil	10	10–40	Possesses mild anticholinergic effects; also available as oral suspension
Citalopram	Celexa	10	10–40	Also available as oral solution
Escitalopram	Lexapro	10	10–20	Also available as oral solution
Fluvoxamine	Luvox	25	50–200	Sedation can be significant
Serotonin antagonist and reuptake inhibitors (SARI)				
Nefazodone	NA	50 bid	100–500 in divided doses	Often sedating; concern regarding hepatic effects
Trazodone	Desyrel	25–50	25–200	Dose range applies to trazodone's common use as a hypnotic agent; often coprescribed with another antidepressant
Serotonin norepinephrine reuptake inhibitors (SNRI)				
Venlafaxine	Effexor	25	50–225	Blood pressure elevation associated with higher dose range
	Effexor XR	37.5	50–225	
Duloxetine	Cymbalta	20	30–60	May have similar adverse effect profile to venlafaxine XR; may be beneficial in patients with selected pain syndromes
Norepinephrine dopamine reuptake inhibitors (NDRI)				
Bupropion	Wellbutrin	75	100–300	Contraindicated with eating disorders; extreme caution with seizure disorders or hepatic impairment
	Wellbutrin SR	75	100–300	
	Wellbutrin XL	150	150–300	
Noradrenergic and specific serotonergic antidepressant (NaSSA)				
Mirtazapine	Remeron	15	15–45	Can be sedating and appetite-increasing
Monoamine oxidase inhibitors (MAOI)				
Phenelzine	Nardil	15	15–45	Restrictions regarding diet and coadministered medications
Tranylcypromine	Parnate	10	10–40	
Selegiline skin patch	Emsam	6	6–12	Skin patch delivery mechanism; note that selective MAO inhibition allows greater dietary freedom at lowest dose, but drug-drug interactions may occur at all dose levels and caution regarding drug-food interactions is necessary >6 mg/day
Stimulants				
Methylphenidate	Ritalin	2.5	2.5–10 bid	Also available in slow-release preparations
Dextroamphetamine	Dextrostat, Dexedrine	2.5	2.5–10 bid	

NA, not applicable; bid, twice a day.

nonsignificant statistical trends toward a higher rate of remissions and a lower number of dropouts (31). Sertraline's linear kinetics (79), its lack of an active, long-acting metabolite, and its lesser inhibition of hepatic microsomal enzymes (101) are considered advantageous properties in treating the elderly. Treatment can be initiated at 25 or 50 mg/day in the elderly and titrated up to 100 to 150 mg/day.

The other SSRIs, too, have each been reported effective antidepressants in the elderly. Both sertraline and citalopram are characterized by a half-life appropriate for once-daily dosing, an absence of anticholinergic effects, and a minimum of drug-drug interactions. Their capacity to induce gastrointestinal side effects or sexual dysfunction appears on a par with the other selective serotonergic agents. In comparison with mianserin (30 to 60 mg/day), citalopram (20 to 40 mg/day) achieved similar rates of response in a group of elderly patients with and without dementia (44). Fluvoxamine has been compared with heterocyclic dothiepin, moclobemide, mianserin, and imipramine. Its efficacy has been reported as similar to these agents. Gastrointestinal side effects were the most common adverse effects, and cardiac effects were not significant (79). Paroxetine's anticholinergic properties, nonlinear kinetics, and association with discontinuation symptoms can be considered relative drawbacks to its use. Escitalopram, although generally similar to other SSRIs, remains a more costly option until it becomes available as a generic medication.

Venlafaxine is a blocker of norepinephrine, serotonin, and dopamine reuptake that lacks anticholinergic, antihistaminergic, and antiadrenergic side effects. One double-blind comparison study (65) and several open series (9,28,51,126,143) support its efficacy and safety in the elderly. The double-blind comparison was of venlafaxine (50 to 150 mg/day) with dothiepin (50 to 150 mg/day). Response to therapy was seen in 60% of each group, and discontinuation as a result of adverse reactions was low with both venlafaxine (7%) and dothiepin (8%). The side effect profile of venlafaxine is similar to that of SSRIs, and it shares with paroxetine a short elimination half-life and propensity for inducing discontinuation symptoms. In addition, it is known to increase diastolic blood pressure in some patients (101) but appeared not to increase it in old patients more than in young patients in an open trial that included both age groups (143). Treatment in the elderly can be initiated at 37.5 mg/day and titrated up to the appropriate dose, often in the range of 150 to 225 mg/day.

Duloxetine resembles venlafaxine in its mechanism of action as a serotonergic reuptake inhibitor with additional effects on the reuptake of norepinephrine and dopamine. In addition, it has been promoted as effective in reducing various neuropathic pain symptoms. One

secondary analysis of elderly subjects from two controlled studies found it to be more effective than placebo in patients aged 55 and older (77). A controlled study found 60 mg/day to be well tolerated and effective in reducing back pain and depression. Benefits were also demonstrated on ratings of verbal learning and memory (90).

Nefazodone, a serotonin reuptake blocker with 5-hydroxytryptamine-2 (5-HT$_2$) antagonism, has not been specifically studied in groups of elderly depressed patients. Its lack of alteration of sleep architecture may be an advantage (12), and some clinicians advocate its use because of anxiolytic effects, but safety concerns aroused by a report of three cases of subfulminant liver failure associated with nefazodone (11) have led to its relative abandonment. If nefazodone were to be prescribed to an elderly patient, it would be prudent to initiate treatment at half the usual starting dose for younger adults (i.e., 50 mg twice daily) and to be alert to the potential drug-drug interaction effects resulting from nefazodone's inhibition of the hepatic microsomal enzyme CYP 3A4, which would increase blood levels of several potentially coadministered medications (101).

Bupropion, a norepinephrine and dopamine reuptake inhibitor, is available in both immediate-release and slow-release formulations. A 7-week, double-blind, placebo-controlled comparison of immediate-release bupropion with imipramine in depressed patients ranging from 55 to 80 years of age showed significant superiority of bupropion over placebo and equivalent efficacy to imipramine. Bupropion's adverse effects were mild (21). A similar 4-week comparison also revealed bupropion to have a lower incidence of orthostatic hypotension than imipramine (42). Bupropion is associated with a small but significantly increased risk of seizures and should be avoided in patients who have a history of eating disorders or predisposing factors to seizures. The slow-release (SR) and extended-release (XL) forms may confer a greater degree of safety. Seizure risk is also decreased by administering the medication on a twice-daily regimen for the immediate-release form, with a daily dose of no more than 450 mg for immediate release or XL or 400 mg/day for SR and no single dose exceeding 200 mg. Bupropion was found to be safe in elderly patients with left ventricular impairment, ventricular arrhythmias, or conduction defects even at high doses (mean dose, 445 mg/day) in a follow-up study of 36 patients (97). Bupropion's mechanism of action, which may be noradrenergic/dopaminergic, raises the possibility that it would be anxiogenic, but this did not emerge as a problem in an SSRI/bupropion comparison. The SR form of bupropion (100 to 300 mg/day) was compared with paroxetine (10 to 40 mg/day) in a 6-week, randomized, double-blind comparison study among depressed elderly 60 years of age or older (134). Mean HAM-D and Hamilton Anxiety Rating Scale (HAM-A) scores decreased similarly with either drug, and the only significant difference among adverse events was the greater presence of somnolence and diarrhea in the paroxetine group. The elderly are predisposed to accumulate bupropion and its metabolites (118). Bupropion's side effects typically include headache, somnolence, insomnia, agitation, dizziness, diarrhea, dry mouth, and nausea. An unusual side effect reported in several elderly patients on bupropion was the tendency to fall backward (119).

Among currently available antidepressants, mirtazapine possesses a unique mechanism that joins antagonism of presynaptic noradrenergic alpha-2 presynaptic autoreceptors and heteroreceptors with antagonism of H_1, 5-HT_2, and 5-hydroxytryptamine-3 (5-HT_3) receptors. The resulting clinical effect is a depression-reducing increase in synaptic norepinephrine and serotonin levels, accompanied by sedation, appetite enhancement, and minimal nausea, a combination that might be anticipated to help anxious, insomniac, or anorexic elderly depressed patients. The two available controlled trials provide some support for mirtazapine's use in the elderly. A comparison of mirtazapine (15 to 45 mg/day) with amitriptyline (30 to 90 mg/day) in a 6-week, double-blind comparison among elderly depressed patients (60 to 85 years of age) yielded evidence of similar reduction of HAM-D and Montgomery Åsberg Depression Rating Scale (MADRS) scores but less improvement on the Clinical Global Impression–Global Improvement Scale and more cognitive disturbance (40). The incidence of anticholinergic effects in both groups was similar. A placebo-controlled, double-blind trial comparing mirtazapine (mean dose, 20.1 mg/day) with trazodone (mean dose, 151.1 mg/day) in outpatients above 55 years of age showed both to be more effective than placebo. A significantly higher incidence of appetite increase was reported with mirtazapine than with trazodone (24% vs. 6%, respectively), and both active treatments were frequently associated with dry mouth and somnolence. Mirtazapine treatment can be initiated at 15 mg at bedtime in the elderly and titrated cautiously to doses ranging between 30 and 45 mg/day. A lower initiation dose may be appropriate in some cases but appears to risk excessive sedation for others.

In a series of studies of late life depression, trazodone was shown effective. It was associated with fewer side effects than the tertiary amine tricyclics (107); however, its wide dosage range and capacity to cause orthostatic hypotension, priapism, sedation, confusion, and memory disturbances have relegated it to a subsidiary antidepressant role (101). It continues to be used frequently as a treatment for agitation in demented elderly patients (117) and as an aid for insomnia.

Although the tricyclic antidepressants are typically used only after failure of an SSRI, this is the result of their side effect profile (which is somewhat less tolerable) rather than a lesser degree of efficacy. An early comparison of fluoxetine with nortriptyline in melancholic elderly patients showed nortriptyline's efficacy to be superior, although the comparison was not carried out in parallel, double-blind groups (98). In comparisons with amitriptyline and doxepin, fluoxetine performed with similar efficacy and had fewer side effects (79). Comparisons of sertraline with amitriptyline and nortriptyline reported that sertraline produced similar improvements in depression and greater improvements in quality of life and cognitive performance with a lower rate of adverse effects (30,31,79), although nortriptyline dosing was not guided by use of serum levels. The SSRI paroxetine has been compared with the tricyclics doxepin, clomipramine, amitriptyline (79), and nortriptyline (74). In each of these reports, paroxetine was claimed to produce equal efficacy with similar or fewer adverse events. A double-blind comparison of citalopram (20 to 40 mg/day) with amitriptyline (50 to 100 mg/day) in elderly depressed patients showed equivalent antidepressant efficacy and fewer adverse effects (61).

Of the heterocyclic antidepressants comprising the tricyclic agents and the tetracyclic drug maprotiline, nortriptyline is the most extensively studied agent. Compared with other tricyclics, nortriptyline possesses significant anticholinergic properties but produces only limited orthostatic hypotension. Its use can be optimized by monitoring serum levels (99). A study of older patients with major depressive disorder in which the nortriptyline level was appropriately monitored showed a 60% remission rate in the intent-to-treat analysis. By the end of the fifth week, 89% of those who would achieve remission had done so (32). In a study that combined IPT with a therapeutic nortriptyline serum level, the intent-to-treat remission rate was even higher (78%), with only a 12% dropout rate (93). Roose and Suthers (99) caution that nortriptyline treatment is associated with significant anticholinergic effects, including an increase in heart rate.

Two studies attest to nortriptyline's usefulness in patients above 70 years of age. Katz et al. (50) treated 30 nursing home patients (mean age, 84 years) with placebo or nortriptyline (25 to 50 mg/day) and noted much improvement in 58.3% of the nortriptyline-treated patients but only in 9.1% of those on placebo. One third of patients dropped out because of side effects. Finkel et al. (31) treated 37 patients (mean age, 75 years) with nortriptyline and compared them with a similar group treated with sertraline. The response rate and measurements of quality of life were higher in the sertraline group, and those treated with sertraline were less likely to discontinue treatment for adverse effects (12.8% vs. 24.3% for nortriptyline). Monitoring of nortriptyline serum levels, not done in these studies, might possibly have improved nortriptyline's tolerability.

With the exception of desipramine, the use of which is supported by a small number of studies, the remaining heterocyclic antidepressants are less frequently recommended for use in the elderly. Desipramine, although associated with greater orthostatic hypotension than nortriptyline, remains a useful and effective agent. Both nortriptyline and desipramine are converted to toxic hydroxy-metabolites that require renal clearance—a factor of importance in the renally impaired patient (107). Use of heterocyclic antidepressants can be accompanied by side effects, including sedation, confusion, urinary retention, exacerbation of glaucoma, blurred vision, increase in heart rate, delayed ventricular conduction, dry mouth, constipation, fatigue, dizziness, atrial fibrillation, orthostatic hypotension, falls, and gait disturbance. Compared with the serotonergic agents, heterocyclic antidepressants are more dangerous in overdose. Their quinidine-like property of slowing cardiac conduction renders them undesirable for treatment of patients with bundle branch disease.

The currently available monoamine oxidase inhibitors, although found to be effective agents (107), have come to occupy a secondary role in the treatment of late life depression. Their associated side effects of orthostatic hypotension, anticholinergic-like properties, and need for careful monitoring of diet and other medications to avoid hypertensive interactions make them riskier drugs for use in the elderly when compared with newer agents (101). A newly available monoamine oxidase inhibitor antidepressant preparation, the selegiline skin patch, may be suitable for some elderly patients but has not been specifically studied yet in elderly cohorts.

Despite the frequency of their use, only limited controlled data are available to support the efficacy of stimulants as a depression monotherapy among the depressed elderly (108). Use of methylphenidate has been advocated on the basis of one controlled trial among medically ill, depressed geriatric patients (131) and other uncontrolled clinical series (13,43,46,88) that indicate significant response rates and limited adverse reactions. Factors that justify a stimulant trial for the treatment of depression typically include apathy or psychomotor retardation, concurrent medical illness, intolerance of standard antidepressants, and the need for a rapid response. Dextroamphetamine is considered similarly useful, although clinicians may avoid it because of concerns about misuse (75).

ELECTROCONVULSIVE THERAPY

ECT is a powerful and proven intervention in the treatment of late life depression. One California survey found its use in adults 65 years of age and older to be more than three times as frequent as among the general adult population (56). Despite the recent availability of newer and safer antidepressants, some elderly patients nonetheless fail to respond to medications as robustly as to ECT. Others fulfill alternative indications for the use of ECT, such as preference for that treatment modality, a history of prior good response to ECT, or need for a rapid clinical response because of acutely life-threatening illness or complications (8). No comparison has shown an antidepressant to have a response rate superior to that obtained with ECT, although the methodologies of such studies have been criticized (106). Not only response rates but also remission rates (asymptomatic state) are claimed to be superior with ECT (38). Delusions or psychomotor retardation are considered predictors of response to ECT (47). Prior medication resistance, but not increasing age, is considered a predictor of poorer response to ECT (106). Although the treatment is safe enough for use with frail elderly patients, an increased risk of complications is associated with factors such as increased intracranial pressure, unstable cardiac function, recent intracerebral hemorrhage, concurrent use of medications for medical conditions, or increased risk for undergoing anesthesia. Many patients know that ECT can adversely affect memory and resist the recommendation for this treatment on that basis, but memory effects are often mild and time-limited. Retrograde amnesia appears and clears rapidly after each seizure, whereas a longer lasting difficulty in retaining newly learned information often resolves within several weeks after ECT is concluded (106). ECT has been used successfully even among patients with concurrent dementia, although the likelihood of transient postictal confusion is heightened by pre-existing cognitive impairment (78).

Delusions, defined as fixed false beliefs, frequently occur concomitantly with late life depression (72). Treatment of delusional depression in younger adults appears to require coadministration of an antidepressant and an antipsychotic, but older patients have some difficulty tolerating antipsychotics' side effects. Evidence of the efficacy of ECT in treating delusional depression, combined with the frequency of intolerance of adequate combined pharmacotherapy in elderly patients, makes ECT a reasonable early choice in treating this syndrome. In younger patients, the newer antipsychotic, olanzapine, has already been shown to be effective in both prospective (55) and retrospective studies (102). Controlled studies of olanzapine and the other atypical antipsychotics may, in time, add evidential support to their use in treating late life delusional depression.

TREATMENT-RESISTANT DEPRESSION

For patients who have shown no response to an antidepressant trial of adequate dosage and duration, a switch to a different antidepressant is recommended. No consistent evidence supports the notion that switching to a different class of antidepressants will produce a result superior to a within-class switch, but some clinicians prefer to involve an additional or different mechanism of action when switching from an ineffective antidepressant. The apathetic SSRI nonresponder may improve on bupropion, for example, or the anxious/insomniac SSRI nonresponder may benefit from a switch to mirtazapine.

For partial responders, several augmenting or coprescribing approaches have been advocated. Lithium augmentation, although not supported by all studies, is often successful at blood levels between 0.4 and 0.8 mmol/L (47). Bupropion has safely been used in medically frail elderly patients as an augmenter to serotonergic agents (114). Triiodothyronine at doses sufficient to lower thyroid-stimulating hormone (TSH) to the lower quartile of the normal reference range has proved helpful for younger populations with resistant depression [for example, see Nierenberg et al. (82)], but this approach has not been systematically explored in the elderly. Stimulants such as methylphenidate, dextroamphetamine, or modafinil are added to antidepressants by some clinicians, and the addition of methylphenidate has been reported to accelerate and improve response to citalopram in a group of elderly depressives (62). Atypical antipsychotic medications, several of which appear to be appropriate antidepressant augmenters in younger adults, lack controlled trials in the elderly, although aripiprazole was shown an effective augmenter of SSRIs in a small open study (104). Growing concerns about the medical consequences of atypical antipsychotic use make it imperative that further data on their benefits and risks be obtained before their routine use is espoused enthusiastically. In postmenopausal depressed elderly women, Schneider et al. (110) demonstrated an augmenting effect when estrogen replacement therapy (ERT) was added to fluoxetine (20 mg/day), but concern about adverse medical consequences of ERT has largely curtailed the use of this intervention. In one report, a brief pulse of dexamethasone aided treatment of two elderly patients with resistant depression (18).

TREATMENT OF DEPRESSION IN DEMENTED PATIENTS

Depressive disorders are estimated to affect a mean of 19% of patients with Alzheimer's disease (138), and depressive symptoms affect up to 63% (123). The prevalence of depression among patients who have vascular dementia may be even higher than among those with Alzheimer's disease (80). The GDS remains a valid and reliable instrument in patients with MMSE scores as low as 15 (69), and other instruments, too, may be useful in patients with mild to moderate dementia (48). Caregivers of demented patients tend to report more depressive symptoms than are detected on clinical interviews, a phenomenon that could reflect the increased variability of mood and other depressive symptoms in demented patients, leading to overreporting by caregivers and underrecognition by clinicians (48). Apathy, passivity, decreased initiative, and poor concentration are often symptoms associated with dementia and are, therefore, less specific than mood symptoms themselves in diagnosing depression in demented patients.

In several placebo-controlled antidepressant trials, significant benefits were seen with antidepressant treatment of depressed demented patients. Clomipramine, sertraline, citalopram, and moclobemide are the most evidence-based antidepressants at this time for treating depression in dementia (84,100,123). Whichever agent is chosen, a heightened vulnerability to adverse medication effects would be expected in demented patients.

PROGNOSIS AND MAINTENANCE TREATMENT

Although the rate of response to treatment of depression in the elderly was high in a study that involved well-monitored and adequate treatment, 90% of the patients placed on placebo maintenance after successful treatment experienced a recurrence of depression (94). Because adequate treatment of late life depression is the exception rather than the rule, the actual prognosis for depressed elderly patients, therefore, would seem to be poor under naturalistic conditions. Data consistent with the bleaker appraisal come from a meta-analysis of outcomes for elderly subjects in the community and primary care, which indicated that, after 24 months, only one third of the subjects were well, whereas one third were depressed, and 21% had died (25). It has become clear that late life depression contributes to excess mortality, not merely from suicide but also by increasing the mortality associated with some medical illnesses. In a recent longitudinal, 4-year study of 2,847 men and women aged 55 to 85 years, the presence of major depression increased by threefold the risk of cardiac death, whereas the presence of minor depression was associated with a risk increase approximately half as large (87). Similarly, depression can increase the risk for cerebrovascular disease (58) and the mortality rate following a cerebrovascular accident (39).

Maintenance pharmacotherapy and psychotherapy have been shown in several studies to reduce the risk of recurrence. In one large cohort, the Pittsburgh study, a group of recovered late life depressed patients was randomized to one of three treatment conditions and followed for 3 years. The patients who received combined IPT and maintenance nortriptyline (80 to 120 ng/mL) did best, with a recurrence rate of only 20%. Patients who received nortriptyline without IPT did less well, with a recurrence rate of 43%, which was less than half the recurrence rate among placebo subjects (94). A subsequent report on this study indicated that patients maintained on a higher plasma level of nortriptyline (80 to 120 ng/mL) experienced more constipation but fewer residual depressive symptoms than patients maintained on a lower level (40 to 60 ng/mL) of nortriptyline (95). Although some patients with milder baseline levels of depression and excellent remission during acute and continuation therapy stages did well on maintenance IPT alone, a high baseline level of depression (HAM-D ≥ 20) was a strong predictor of relapse (120). Full-dose antidepressant maintenance has gained further support from the report by Flint and Rifat (33) of the efficacy of full-dose antidepressant medication, supplemented in some cases with adjunctive lithium, in a 4-year follow-up study of patients 60 years of age and older that showed a 70% cumulative probability of remaining well without recurrence during that period. More recent maintenance studies have demonstrated efficacy with citalopram (53) or paroxetine (92) in reducing recurrence following successful treatment of a late life depressive episode.

BIPOLAR DISORDER IN LATE LIFE

Compared with accumulating knowledge about late life depression, much less is understood about the characteristics of bipolar disorder in the elderly. A bipolar disorder diagnosis requires current or past manic or hypomanic symptomatology. The diagnosis of a manic episode requires the presence of at least three of the following symptoms in addition to an elevated mood or at least four of the symptoms in addition to an irritable mood: grandiosity, decreased need for sleep, pressure to keep talking, flight of ideas, distractibility, increased activity, or excessive involvement in potentially risky pleasurable pursuits (e.g., inappropriate spending or sexual behavior) (7). Current or previous hypomanic or manic behavior determines a bipolar diagnosis even when the predominant presenting clinical picture is depressive. The individual with both manic and depressive episodes is diagnosed as bipolar I, whereas a syndrome of hypomanic and depressive episodes is termed bipolar II (7).

Bipolar depression, which is diagnosed when depressive symptoms occur with concurrent or prior manic or hypomanic symptoms, is often treated with antidepressants. Increasingly, this is regarded as a hazardous approach because accumulating evidence indicates that such treatment is associated with induction of manic episodes, increased cycling, development of treatment resistance, and ineffective prophylaxis of subsequent episodes (6,89,133). Mood-stabilizing medications and their dosages are presented in Table 31-2. Lithium salts, although they have received less attention in elderly populations (20), remain a first-line agent. An oft-cited but very small study in younger adults suggested that bupropion, in comparison with desipramine, was less frequently associated with induction of manic episodes during 1 year of prospective follow-up (105). Also, in younger populations, quetiapine and olanzapine/fluoxetine have been demonstrated to be effective acute therapies for bipolar depression. Studies in the elderly are needed.

Mania is uncommon among community-dwelling elderly, with approximately 0.1% of individuals above 65 years of age meeting diagnostic criteria for bipolar disorder type I and 0.7% meeting criteria for bipolar disorder type II (135,136). This group, nonetheless, constitutes 5% to 19% of the elderly who seek treatment for mood disorders (140). In long-term care facilities, the prevalence of bipolar disorders may be as high as 9.0% (24). As a group, elderly patients with bipolar disorder show more severe symptoms, greater impairment in community-living skills, increased use of mental health services (psychiatric partial hospitalization or hospitalization, skills training services, or case management services), and greater cognitive impairment than a comparison group with unipolar depression (16). In addition, greater frequency of episodes has been demonstrated in the bipolar elderly (24).

Mania with first onset in late life has been a matter of particular interest because late onset is associated with an increased presence of medical (including metabolic, infectious, and neoplastic disorders), neurologic (including vascular lesions, brain injury, and degenerative disorders), or medication-related causes (including antidepressant treatment, steroids, and sympathomimetics). Furthermore, late-onset mania is characterized by a lower rate of bipolar family history, a possibly increased vulnerability to relapse, and a mortality rate even higher than that among the elderly who are depressed (24,57,112,140). An increase in the number of subcortical hyperintensities on MRI has been demonstrated in a group of late-onset manic patients (67).

TREATMENT

Guidelines for the treatment of mania in the elderly derive from uncontrolled studies and extrapolation from findings in younger adults. Acute treatment of

Table 31-2. *Selected Mood Stabilizers for Use in Late Life Mood Disorders*

Generic Name	Trade Name	Starting Dose/ Range (mg/day)	Treatment Dose/ Range (mg/day)	Notes
Lithium salts				
Lithium carbonate	Eskalith	300	300–1,500	Follow blood level; target therapeutic
Lithium controlled release	Lithobid Eskalith CR	450	450–1,800	range for bipolar disorder is 0.4–1.0 mEq/L; target level unclear for depression augmentation
Lithium citrate	N/A	150	300–1,500	
Anticonvulsants				
Divalproex sodium	Depakote	250	250–2,000	Enterically coated, less gastrointestinal intolerance; therapeutic level usually within blood level range of 50–100 µg/mL
Valproic acid	Depakene	250	250–2,000	Therapeutic level usually within blood level range of 50–100 µg/mL
Carbamazepine	Tegretol	100	200–1,000	Cytochrome P450 enzyme inducer; therapeutic level usually within blood level range of 4–12 µg/mL
Lamotrigine	Lamictal	12.5	25–200	Slow titration is required to minimize risk of adverse reaction (Stevens-Johnson syndrome)
Gabapentin	Neurontin	100	200–2,000	Not shown to be effective in treating bipolar disorder

mania in younger adults often employs antipsychotic agents, particularly when concurrent psychotic symptoms are present, but these may be more problematic in older adults because of the increased likelihood of adverse effects, including orthostatic hypotension, sedation, and extrapyramidal symptoms, including tardive dyskinesia. The atypical antipsychotics, which are associated with fewer extrapyramidal symptoms, merit further exploration in the acute treatment of late life mania. They have not been specifically studied in the elderly with bipolar disorder, but in younger patient groups, clozapine, risperidone, olanzapine, quetiapine, aripiprazole, and ziprasidone have each been shown to be beneficial (41,127). Based on recent data, all of the atypical antipsychotics carry boxed warnings about the increased risk for adverse effects, including increased mortality in patients with dementia-related psychosis. It may be appropriate to extrapolate these risks to nondemented elderly patients, many of whom share cardiovascular and cerebrovascular medical risk factors with demented patients. Information about the antipsychotic agents for use in late life mood disorders is presented in Table 31-3.

Lithium salts and divalproex are regarded as first-line agents in treating geriatric acute mania (141,142). Available as lithium carbonate or as the liquid lithium citrate, lithium salts have not been studied in the

elderly under double-blind conditions but are supported by open trial results. In the elderly, lithium salts are known to be toxic at lower levels than in younger adults, justifying use of levels as low as 0.4 to 0.8 mEq/L (20). The presence of cognitive impairment or pre-existing tremor further increases the likelihood of a toxic reaction. The side effects of lithium include polyuria, tremor, mental slowing and memory difficulties, sinus node dysfunction, peripheral edema, hypothyroidism or nontoxic goiter, and a worsening of arthritis, nausea, diarrhea, and acne or psoriasis. Lithium's serum level can be raised by many nonsteroidal anti-inflammatory drugs and by thiazide diuretics. In the elderly, reduced renal clearance or hepatic metabolism can increase the serum levels of lithium or divalproex sodium, respectively (67).

Divalproex, an anticonvulsant shown to be effective in treating acute mania in younger adults, is modestly effective and well tolerated in elderly manic patients (68,96,142). Among a mixed-age population studied retrospectively, lithium-refractory patients and those with neurologic abnormalities were a particularly responsive group for treatment with valproic acid (116). In addition, younger patients with mixed states (concurrent depressive and manic symptoms) respond better to valproic acid than to lithium (20). Valproic acid is an inhibitor of CYP enzymes, which

Table 31-3. *Selected Antipsychotic Agents for Use in Late Life Mood Disorders*

Generic Name	Trade Name	Starting Dose/ Range (mg/day)	Treatment Dose/ Range (mg/day)	Notes
Typical antipsychotic agents [a]				
Haloperidol	Haldol	0.5	0.25–5	Available also as liquid, IM injection, IV injection
	Haldol decanoate	12.5 IM q 14–28 days	25–100 IM q 28 days	
Perphenazine	Trilafon	2	4–32	Available also as liquid, IM injection
Fluphenazine	Prolixin	0.5	0.5–5	Available also as liquid, IM injection
	Prolixin decanoate	12.5 mg IM q 7–14 days	12.5–50 mg IM q 14–21 days	Depot injection
Atypical antipsychotic agents				
Risperidone	Risperdal	0.25	0.5–3	Available also as oral concentrate, disintegrating oral tablet, or long-acting depot IM injectable solution
Olanzapine	Zyprexa	2.5	2.5–10	Available also as disintegrating oral tablet or short-acting IM injectable solution
Quetiapine	Seroquel	25	50–500	Low in EPS
Ziprasidone	Geodon	20	20–60 bid	Monitoring of QTc suggested; available also as short-acting IM injectable solution
Aripiprazole	Abilify	5	5–30	Available also as oral solution, orally disintegrating tablet, or short-acting IM injectable solution
Clozapine	Clozaril	6.25	25–200	Anticholinergic, low in EPS
Paliperidone	Invega	Awaiting further data in elderly		

IM, intramuscular; IV, intravenous; q, every; bid, twice a day; EPS, extrapyramidal symptoms; QTC, corrected QT interval.
[a] High potency agents are generally preferred, so low potency drugs are not included in this list.

can increase the levels of many coadministered drugs. Sedation, weight gain, nausea, transient hair loss, hyperammonemia, and rare severe reactions (aplastic anemia, pancreatitis, and hepatic failure) have been associated with treatment (20,67).

Other anticonvulsants have been used in elderly bipolar patients but as yet without support from controlled studies. Carbamazepine is considered problematic because of its side effects and drug interactions. Among several newer anticonvulsants that have aroused interest, lamotrigine in particular has gathered support for use as a maintenance treatment in younger adults with bipolar depression (23). No studies yet attest to its efficacy and safety in the treatment of specific cohorts of elderly bipolar subjects.

As with depression, ECT remains an important intervention in the acute treatment of late life bipolar episodes, whether depressive or manic, especially in those patients who are resistant to medication or who require a rapid symptomatic resolution. Most

responders can then be switched to pharmacotherapeutic maintenance. The combination of ECT with lithium, which has been associated with confusional reactions, is to be avoided (141).

Regarding maintenance treatment and prevention of subsequent episodes of mania or depression in bipolar elderly, little information is available (139). Valproic acid and lithium, which were demonstrated to be effective in younger populations, are commonly used in the elderly as well. Maintenance ECT is an option for patients whose depressive or manic bipolar symptoms respond poorly to maintenance medication regimens (66,127).

SUMMARY

As our population of elderly continues to grow, the importance of recognizing and properly treating the mood disorders of late life will continue to increase. Detection, differential diagnosis, aggressive and comprehensive treatment, maintenance therapy, and vigorous follow-up are necessary to achieve success in the management of late life disorders. Optimal treatment will benefit patients and their families by reducing a major source of morbidity in late life and deferring the need for caregiver support. Society's benefit, moreover, will be apparent in patients' increased productivity, sustained autonomy, and lesser use of health care resources.

REFERENCES

1. Alexopoulos GS. The vascular depression hypothesis: 10 years later. *Biol Psychiatry*. 2006; 60:1304–1305.

2. Alexopoulos GS, Abrams RC, Young RC, et al. Cornell Scale for Depression in Dementia. *Biol Psychiatry*. 1988;23:271–284.

3. Alexopoulos GS, Kiosses DN, Klimstra S, et al. Clinical presentation of the "depression-executive dysfunction syndrome" of late life. *Am J Geriatr Psychiatry*. 2002;10:98–102.

4. Alexopoulos GS, Meyers BS, Young RC, et al. Executive dysfunction and long-term outcomes of geriatric depression. *Arch Gen Psychiatry*. 2000;57:285–290.

5. Alexopoulos GS, Meyers BS, Young RC, et al. 'Vascular depression' hypothesis. *Arch Gen Psychiatry*. 1997;54:915–922.

6. Altshuler LI, Post RM, Leverich GS, et al. Antidepressant-induced mania and cycle acceleration: a controversy revisited. *Am J Psychiatry*. 1995;152:1130–1138.

7. American Psychiatric Association. *Diagnostic and Statistical Manual of Mental Disorders*, *Text Revision*. 4th ed. Washington, DC: American Psychiatric Association; 2000.

8. American Psychiatric Association (APA Task Force on ECT). *The Practice of Electroconvulsive Therapy: Recommendations for Treatment, Training, and Privileging*. Washington, DC: American Psychiatric Press; 1990.

9. Amore M, Ricci M, Zanardi R, et al. Long-term treatment of geropsychiatric depressed patients with venlafaxine. *J Affect Disord*. 1997;46: 293–296.

10. Applegate WB, Blass JP, Williams TF. Instruments for the functional assessment of older patients. *N Engl J Med*. 1990;322:1207–1214.

11. Aranda-Michel J, Koehler A, Bejarano PA, et al. Nefazodone-induced liver failure: report of three cases. *Ann Intern Med*. 1999;130:285–288.

12. Armitage R, Rush AJ, Trivedi M, et al. The effects of nefazodone on sleep architecture in depression. *Neuropsychopharmacology*. 1994;10:123–127.

13. Askinazi C, Weintraub RJ, Karamouz N. Elderly depressed females as a possible subgroup

of patients responsive to methylphenidate. *J Clin Psychiatry*. 1986;47:467–469.

14. Barraclough BM. Suicide in the elderly. *Br J Psychiatry*. 1971;6(suppl):87–97.

15. Barrett JE, Barrett JA, Oxman TE, et al. The prevalence of psychiatric disorders in a primary care practice. *Arch Gen Psychiatry*. 1988;45: 1100–1106.

16. Bartels SJ, Forester B, Miles KM, et al. Mental health service use by elderly patients with bipolar disorder and unipolar major depression. *Am J Geriatr Psychiatry*. 2000;8:160–166.

17. Blazer DG. Epidemiology of late-life depression. In: Schneider LS, Reynolds CF 3rd, Lebowitz BD, et al., eds. *Diagnosis and treatment of depression in late life*. Washington, DC: American Psychiatric Press; 1994:9–19.

18. Bodani M, Sheehan B, Philpot M. The use of dexamethasone in elderly patients with antidepressant-resistant depressive illness. *J Psychopharmacol*. 1999;13:196–197.

19. Borson S, Bames RA, Kukull WA, et al. Symptomatic depression in elderly medical outpatients. I. Prevalence, demography, and health service utilization. *J Am Geriatr Soc*. 1986;34: 341–347.

20. Bowden CL. Anticonvulsants in bipolar elderly. In: Nelson JC, ed. *Geriatric psychopharmacology*. New York: Marcel Dekker; 1998:285–299.

21. Branconnier RJ, Cole JO, Ghazvinian S, et al. Clinical pharmacology of bupropion and imipramine in elderly depressives. *J Clin Psychiatry*. 1983;44:130–133.

22. Burns BJ, Taube CA. Mental health services in general medical care and in nursing homes. In: Fogel BS, Furino A, Gottlieb GL, eds. *Mental health policy for older Americans: protecting minds at risk*. Washington, DC: American Psychiatric Press; 1990:63–83.

23. Calabrese JR, Bowden CL, Sachs GS, et al. A double-blind placebo-controlled study of lamotrigine monotherapy in outpatients with bipolar I depression. *J Clin Psychiatry*. 1999;60: 79–88.

24. Chen ST, Altshuler LL, Spar JE. Bipolar disorder in late life: a review. *J Geriatr Psychiatry Neurol*. 1998;11:29–35.

25. Cole MG, Bellavance F, Mansour A. Prognosis of depression in elderly community and primary care populations: a systematic review and meta-analysis. *Am J Psychiatry*. 1999;156:1182–1189.

26. Conwell Y. Suicide in the elderly patients. In: Schneider LS, Reynolds III CF, Lebowitz BD, et al., eds. *Diagnosis and treatment of depression in late life*. Washington, DC: American Psychiatric Press; 1994:397–418.

27. Conwell Y, Duberstein PR, Cox C, et al. Relationships of age and axis I diagnoses in victims of completed suicide: a psychological autopsy study. *Am J Psychiatry*. 1996;153: 1001–1008.

28. Diereck M. An open-label evaluation of the long-term safety of oral venlafaxine in depressed elderly patients. *Ann Clin Psychiatry*. 1996;8: 169–178.

29. Feighner JP, Cohn JB. Double-blind comparative trials of fluoxetine and doxepin in geriatric patients with major depressive disorder. *J Clin Psychiatry*. 1985;46:20–25.

30. Finkel SI. Efficacy and tolerability of antidepressant therapy in the old-old. *J Clin Psychiatry*. 1996;57[Suppl 5]:23–28.

31. Finkel SI, Richter EM, Clary CM, et al. Comparative efficacy of sertraline vs. fluoxetine in patients age 70 or over with major depression. *Am J Geriatr Psychiatry*. 1999;7:221–227.

32. Flint AJ, Rifat SL. The effect of sequential antidepressant treatment on geriatric depression. *J Affect Disord*. 1996;36:95–105.

33. Flint AJ, Rifat SL. Maintenance treatment for recurrent depression in late life. *Am J Geriatr Psychiatry*. 2000;8:112–116.

34. George LK. Social factors and depression in late life. In: Schneider LS, Reynolds CF 3rd, Lebowitz BD, et al., eds. *Diagnosis and treatment of depression in late life*. Washington, DC: American Psychiatric Press; 1994:131–153.

35. Gerson S, Belin TR, Kaufman A, et al. Pharmacological and psychological treatments for depressed older patients: a meta-analysis and overview of recent findings. *Harvard Rev Psychiatry*. 1999;7:1–28.

36. Goldstein DJ, Hamilton SH, Masica DN, et al. Fluoxetine in medically stable, depressed geriatric patients: effects on weight. *J Clin Psychopharmacol*. 1997;17:365–369.

37. Gottlieb GL. Barriers to care for older adults with depression. In: Schneider LS, Reynolds CF 3rd, Lebowitz BD, et al., eds. *Diagnosis and treatment of depression in late life*. Washington, DC: American Psychiatric Press; 1994:377–396.

38. Hamilton M. The effect of treatment on the melancholias (depression). *Br J Psychiatry*. 1982; 140:223–230.

39. House A, Knapp P, Bamford J, et al. Mortality at 12 and 24 months after stroke may be associated with depressive symptoms at 1 month. *Stroke*. 2001;32:696–701.

40. Hoyberg OJ, Maragakis B, Mullin J, et al. A double-blind multicentre comparison of mirtazapine and amitriptyline in elderly depressed patients. *Acta Psychiatr Scand*. 1996;93:184–190.

41. Jarema M. Atypical antipsychotics in the treatment of mood disorders. *Curr Opin Psychiatry*. 2007;20:23–29.

42. Kane JM, Cole K, Sarantakos S, et al. Safety and efficacy of bupropion in elderly patients: preliminary observations. *J Clin Psychiatry*. 1983;44: 134–136.

43. Kaplitz SE. Withdrawn, apathetic geriatric patients responsive to methylphenidate. *J Am Geriatr Soc*. 1975;23:271–276.

44. Karlsson L, Godderis J, Augusto De Mendonca Lima C, et al. A randomised, double-blind comparison of the efficacy and safety of citalopram compared to mianserin in elderly, depressed patients with or without mild to moderate dementia. *Int J Geriatr Psychiatry*. 2000;15: 295–305.

45. Kaszniak AW, Christenson GD. Differential diagnosis of dementia and depression. In: Storandt M, VandenBos GR, eds. *Neuropsychological assessment of dementia and depression in older adults: a clinician's guide*. Washington, DC: American Psychological Association; 1997:81–117.

46. Katon W, Raskind M. Treatment of depression in the medically ill elderly with methylphenidate. *Am J Psychiatry*. 1980;137:963–965.

47. Katona CLE. The management of depression in old age. In: *Depression in old age*. Chichester, United Kingdom: John Wiley and Sons; 1994: 93–121.

48. Katz IR. Diagnosis and treatment of depression in patients with Alzheimer's disease and other dementias. *J Clin Psychiatry*. 1998;59[Suppl 9]: 38–44.

49. Katz IR, Parmelee PA. Depression in elderly patients in residential care settings. In: Schneider LS, Reynolds CF 3rd, Lebowitz BD, et al., eds. *Diagnosis and treatment of depression in late life*. Washington, DC: American Psychiatric Press; 1994:437–461.

50. Katz IR, Simpson GM, Curlik SM, et al. Pharmacologic treatment of major depression for elderly patients in residential care settings. *J Clin Psychiatry*. 1990;51[Suppl 7]: 41–47.

51. Khan A, Rudolph R, Baumel B, et al. Venlafaxine in depressed geriatric outpatients: an open label clinical study. *Psychopharmacol Bull*. 1995;31: 753–788.

52. Kiloh LG. Pseudo-dementia. *Acta Psychiatr Scand*. 1961;37:336–351.

53. Klysner R, Bent-Hansen J, Hansen HL, et al. Efficacy of citalopram in the prevention of recurrent depression in elderly patients: placebo-controlled study of maintenance therapy. *Br J Psychiatry*. 2002;181:29–35.

54. Koenig HG, Meador KG, Cohen HJ, et al. Depression in elderly hospitalized patients with medical illness. *Arch Intern Med*. 1988;148:1929–1936.

55. Konig F, von Hippel C, Petersdorff T, et al. First experiences in combination therapy using olanzapine with SSRIs (citalopram, paroxetine) in delusional depression. *Neuropsychobiology*. 2001;43:170–174.

56. Kramer BA. Use of ECT in California, 1977–1983. *Am J Psychiatry*. 1985;142:1190–1192.

57. Krauthammer C, Klerman GL. Secondary mania: manic syndromes associated with antecedent physical illness or drugs. *Arch Gen Psychiatry*. 1978;35:1333–1339.

58. Krishnan KRR. Depression as a contributing factor in cerebrovascular disease. *Am Heart J*. 2000;140[Suppl 4]:70–76.

59. Krishnan KRR, Hays JC, Blazer DG. MRI-defined vascular depression. *Am J Psychiatry*. 1997;154:497–501.

60. Krishnan KRR, Taylor WD, McQuaid DRE, et al. Clinical characteristics of magnetic resonance imaging-defined subcortical ischemic depression. *Biol Psychiatry*. 2004;55:390–397.

61. Kyle CJ, Peterson BE, Overo KF. Comparison of the tolerability and efficacy of citalopram and amitriptyline in elderly depressed patients treated in general practice. *Depress Anxiety*. 1998;8:147–153.

62. Lavretsky H, Park S, Siddarth P, et al. Methylphenidate-enhanced antidepressant response to citalopram in the elderly: a double-blind, placebo-controlled pilot trial. *Am J Geriatr Psychiatry*. 2006;14:181–185.

63. Lyness JM, Conwell Y, Nelson JC. Suicide attempts in elderly psychiatric inpatients. *J Am Geriatr Soc*. 1992;40:320–324.

64. Mackenzie TB, Popkin MK. Suicide in the medical patient. *Int J Psychiatry Med*. 1987;17:3–22.

65. Mahapatra SN, Hackett D. A randomised, double-blind, parallel-group comparison of venlafaxine and dothiepin in geriatric patients with major depression. *Int J Clin Pract*. 1997;51:209–213.

66. McDonald WM. Epidemiology, etiology, and treatment of geriatric mania. *J Clin Psychiatry*. 2000;61[Suppl 13]:3–11.

67. McDonald WM, Nemeroff CB. The diagnosis and treatment of mania in the elderly. *Bull Menninger Clin*. 1996;60:174–196.

68. McFarland BH, Miller MR, Straurnflord AA. Valproate use in the older manic patient. *J Clin Psychiatry*. 1990;51:479–481.

69. McGivney SA, Mulvihill M, Taylor B. Validating the GDS depression screen in the nursing home. *J Am Geriatr Soc*. 1994;42:490–492.

70. McIntosh JL, Santos JF, Hubbard RW, et al. *Elder Suicide: Research, Theory and Treatment*. Washington, DC: American Psychological Association; 1994.

71. Mesters P, Cosyns P, Dejaiffe G, et al. Assessment of quality of life in the treatment of major depressive disorder with fluoxetine, 20 mg, in ambulatory patients aged over 60 years. *Int Clin Psychoharmacol*. 1993;8:337–340.

72. Meyers BS, Greenberg R. Late-life delusional depression. *J Affect Disord*. 1986;11:133–137.

73. Mottram P, Wilson K, Strobl J. Antidepressants for depressed elderly. *Cochrane Database Syst Rev*. 2006;1:CD003491.

74. Mulsant BH, Pollock BG, Nebes RD, et al. A double-blind randomized comparison of nortriptyline and paroxetine in the treatment of late-life depression: 6-week outcome. *J Clin Psychiatry*. 1999;60[Suppl 20]:16–20.

75. Murray GB, Cassem E. Use of stimulants in depressed patients with medical illness. In: Nelson JC, ed. *Geriatric psychopharmacology*. New York: Marcel Dekker; 1998:245–257.

76. Myers JK, Weissman MM, Tischler GL, et al. Six-month prevalence of psychiatric disorders in three communities. *Arch Gen Psychiatry*. 1984;41:959–970.

77. Nelson JC, Wohlreich MM, Mallinckrodt CH, et al. Duloxetine for the treatment of major depressive disorder in older patients. *Am J Geriatr Psychiatry*. 2005;13:227–235.

78. Nelson JP, Rosenberg DR. ECT treatment of demented elderly patients with major depression: a retrospective study of efficacy and safety. *Convuls Ther*. 1991;7:157–165.

79. Newhouse PA. Use of serotonin selective reuptake inhibitors in geriatric depression. *J Clin Psychiatry*. 1996;57[Suppl 5]:12–22.

80. Newman SC. The prevalence of depression in Alzheimer's disease and vascular dementia in a population sample. *J Affect Disord*. 1999;52:169–176.

81. Niederehe GT. Psychosocial therapies with depressed older adults. In: Schneider LS, Reynolds CF 3rd, Lebowitz BD, et al., eds. *Diagnosis and treatment of depression in late life*. Washington, DC: American Psychiatric Press; 1994:293–315.

82. Nierenberg AA, Fava M, Trivedi MH, et al. A comparison of lithium and T(3) augmentation following two failed medication treatments for depression: a STAR*D report. *Am J Psychiatry*. 2006;163:1519–1530.

83. Nieto E, Vieta E, Lazaro L, et al. Serious suicide attempts in the elderly. *Psychopathology*. 1992;25:183–188.

84. Nyth AL, Gottfries CG, Lyby K, et al. A controlled multicenter clinical study of citalopram and placebo in elderly depressed patients with and without concomitant dementia. *Acta Psychiatr Scand.* 1992;86:138–145.

85. Oslin DW, Streim JE, Katz IR, et al. Heuristic comparison of sertraline with nortriptyline for the treatment of depression in frail elderly patients. *Am J Geriatr Psychiatry.* 2000;8: 141–149.

86. Parmelee PA, Katz IR, Lawton MP. Incidence of depression in long term care settings. *J Gerontol.* 1992;47:MI89–MI96.

87. Penninx BWJH, Beekman ATF, Honig A, et al. Depression and cardiac mortality. Results from a community-based longitudinal study. *Arch Gen Psychiatry.* 2001;58:221–227.

88. Pickett P, Masand P, Murray GB. Psychostimulant treatment of geriatric depressive disorders secondary to medical illness. *J Geriatr Psychiatry Neurol.* 1990;3:146–151.

89. Quitkin FM, Kane JM, Rifkin A, et al. Lithium and imipramine in the prophylaxis of unipolar and bipolar III depression: a prospective, placebo-controlled comparison. *Psychopharmacol Bull.* 1981;17:142–144.

90. Raskin J, Wiltse CG, Siegal A, et al. Efficacy of duloxetine on cognition, depression, and pain in elderly patients with major depressive disorder: an 8-week, double-blind, placebo-controlled trial. *Am J Psychiatry.* 2007;164:900–909.

91. Reifler BV. A case of mistaken identity: pseudo-dementia is really predementia. *J Am Geriatr Soc.* 2000;48:593–594.

92. Reynolds CF 3rd, Dew MA, Pollock BG, et al. Maintenance treatment of major depression in old age. *N Engl J Med.* 2006;354:1130–1138.

93. Reynolds CF 3rd, Frank E, Kupfer D. Treatment outcome in recurrent major depression: a post hoc comparison of elderly ("young old") and midlife patients. *Am J Psychiatry.* 1996;153: 1288–1292.

94. Reynolds CF 3rd, Frank E, Perel JM, et al. Nortriptyline and interpersonal psychotherapy as maintenance therapies for recurrent major depression: a randomized controlled trial in patients older than 59 years. *JAMA.* 1999;281: 39–45.

95. Reynolds CF 3rd, Perel JM, Frank E, et al. Three-year outcomes of maintenance nortriptyline treatment in late-life depression: a study of two fixed plasma levels. *Am J Psychiatry.* 1999;156:1177–1181.

96. Risinger RC, Risby ED, Risch SC. Safety and efficacy of divalproex sodium in elderly bipolar patients. *J Clin Psychiatry.* 1994;55:215.

97. Roose SP, Dalack GW, Glassman AH, et al. Cardiovascular effects of bupropion in depressed patients with heart disease. *Am J Psychiatry.* 1991;148:512–516.

98. Roose SP, Glassman AH, Attia E, et al. Comparative efficacy of selective serotonin reuptake inhibitors and tricyclics in the treatment of melancholia. *Am J Psychiatry.* 1994;151: 1735–1739.

99. Roose SP, Suthers KM. Antidepressant response in late-life depression. *J Clin Psychiatry.* 1998; 59[Suppl 10]:4–8.

100. Roth M, Mountjoy CQ, Amrein R. Moclobemide in elderly patients with cognitive decline and depression: an international double-blind, placebo-controlled trial. *Br J Psychiatry.* 1996;168:149–157.

101. Rothschild AJ. The diagnosis and treatment of late-life depression. *J Clin Psychiatry.* 1996;57:[Suppl 5]:5–11.

102. Rothschild AJ, Bates KS, Boehringer KL, et al. Olanzapine response in psychotic depression. *J Clin Psychiatry.* 1999;60:116–118.

103. Rovner BW. Depression and increased risk of mortality in the nursing home patient. *Am J Med.* 1993;94:19S–22S.

104. Rutherford B, Sneed J, Miyazaki M, et al. An open trial of aripiprazole augmentation for SSRI non-remitters with late-life depression. *Int J Geriatr Psychiatry.* 2007;22:986–991.

105. Sachs GS, Lafter B, Stoll AL, et al. A double-blind trial of bupropion versus desipramine for bipolar depression. *J Clin Psychiatry.* 1994;55:391–393.

106. Sackeim HA. Use of electroconvulsive therapy in late-life depression. In: Schneider LS, Reynolds CF 3rd, Lebowitz BD, et al., eds. *Diagnosis and treatment of depression in late life.* Washington, DC: American Psychiatric Press; 1994:259–277.

107. Salzman C. Pharmacological treatment of depression in elderly patients. In: Schneider LS, Reynolds CF 3rd, Lebowitz BD, et al., eds. *Diagnosis and treatment of depression in late life.* Washington, DC: American Psychiatric Press; 1994:181–244.

108. Satel SL, Nelson JC. Stimulants in the treatment of depression: a critical overview. *J Clin Psychiatry.* 1989;50:241–249.

109. Saunders PA, Copeland JR, Dewey ME, et al. Heavy drinking as a risk factor for depression and dementia in elderly men. Findings from the Liverpool longitudinal community study. *Br J Psychiatry.* 1991;159:213–216.

110. Schneider LS, Small GW, Hamilton SH, et al. Estrogen replacement and response to fluoxetine in a multicenter geriatric depression trial. *Am J Geriatr Psychiatry.* 1997;5:97–106.

111. Scogin F, McElreath L. Efficacy of psychosocial treatments for geriatric depression: a quantitative review. *J Consult Clin Psychol.* 1994;62:69–74.

112. Shulman KI, Tohen M. Unipolar mania reconsidered: evidence from an elderly cohort. *Br J Psychiatry.* 1994;164:547–549.

113. Simon GE, VonKorff M, Piccinelli M, et al. An international study of the relation between somatic symptoms and depression. *N Engl J Med.* 1999;341:1329–1335.

114. Spier SA. Use of bupropion with SRIs and venlafaxine. *Depress Anxiety.* 1998;7:73–75.

115. Steuer JL, Mintz J, Hammen CL, et al: Cognitive-behavioral and psychodynamic group psychotherapy in treatment of geriatric depression. *J Consult Clin Psychol.* 1984;52:180–189.

116. Stoll AL, Banov M, Kolbrener M, et al. Neurologic factors predict a favorable valproate response in bipolar and schizoaffective disorders. *J Clin Psychopharmacology.* 1994;14:311–313.

117. Sultzer DL, Gray KF, Gunay I, et al. A double-blind comparison of trazodone and haloperidol for treatment of agitation in patients with dementia. *Am J Geriatr Psychiatry.* 1997;5:60–69.

118. Sweet RA, Pollock BG, Kirshner M, et al. Pharmacokinetics of single- and multiple-dose bupropion in elderly patients with depression. *J Clin Pharmacol.* 1995;35:876–884.

119. Szuba MP, Leuchter AF. Falling backward in two elderly patients taking bupropion. *J Clin Psychiatry.* 1992;53:157–159.

120. Taylor MP, Reynolds CF 3rd, Frank E, et al. Which elderly depressed patients remain well on maintenance interpersonal psychotherapy alone? Report from the Pittsburgh study of maintenance therapies in late-life depression. *Depress Anxiety.* 1999;10:55–60.

121. Taylor WD, Doraiswamy PM. A systematic review of antidepressant placebo-controlled trials for geriatric depression: limitations of current data and directions for the future. *Neuropsychopharmacology.* 2004;29:2285–2299.

122. Thompson LW. Cognitive-behavioral therapy and treatment for late-life depression. *J Clin Psychiatry.* 1996;57[Suppl 5]:29–37.

123. Thompson S, Herrmann N, Rapoport MJ, et al. Efficacy and safety of antidepressants for treatment of depression in Alzheimer's disease: a metaanalysis. *Can J Psychiatry.* 2007;52:248–255.

124. Tideiksaar R. Drug noncompliance in the elderly. *Hosp Physician.* 1984;20:92–93, 96–98, 101.

125. Tollefson GD, Holman SL. Analysis of the Hamilton Depression Rating Scale factors from a double-blind, placebo-controlled trial of fluoxetine in geriatric major depression. *Int Clin Psychopharmacology.* 1993;8:253–259.

126. Tsolaki M, Fountoulakis KN, Nakopoulou E, et al. The effect of antidepressant pharmacotherapy with venlafaxine in geriatric depression. *Int J Geriatr Psychopharmacol.* 2000;2:83–85.

127. Umapathy C, Mulsant BH, Pollock BG. Bipolar disorder in the elderly. *Psychiatric Ann.* 2000; 30:473–480.

128. Unutzer J, Katon W, Russo J, et al. Patterns of care for depressed older adults in a large-staff model HMO. *Am J Geriatr Psychiatry.* 1999;7: 235–243.

129. Unutzer J, Patric DL, Simon G, et al. Depressive symptoms and the cost of health services in HMO patients aged 65 years and older. A 4-year prospective study. *JAMA.* 1997;277: 1618–1623.

130. Unutzer J, Simon G, Belin TR, et al. Care for depression in HMO patients aged 65 and older. *J Am Geriatr Soc.* 2000;48:871–878.

131. Wallace AE, Kofoed LL, West AN. Double-blind, placebo-controlled trial of methylphenidate in older, depressed, medically ill patients. *Am J Psychiatry.* 1995;152:929–931.

132. Waxman HM, Carner EA, Klein M. Underutilization of mental health professionals by community elderly. *Gerontologist.* 1984;24: 23–30.

133. Wehr TA, Sack DA, Rosenthal NE, et al. Rapid cycling affective disorder: contributing factors and treatment responses in 51 patients. *Am J Psychiatry.* 1988;145:179–184.

134. Weihs KL, Settle EC, Batey SR, et al. Bupropion sustained release versus paroxetine for the treatment of depression in the elderly. *J Clin Psychiatry.* 2000;61:196–202.

135. Weissman MM, Bruce NEL, Leaf PF, et al. Affective disorders. In: Robbins LN, Regier DA, eds. *Psychiatric disorders in America.* New York: Free Press; 1991:53–80.

136. Weissman MM, Leaf PJ, Tischler GL, et al. Affective disorders in five United States communities. *Psychol Med.* 1988;18:141–153.

137. Weissman MM, Markowitz JC. Interpersonal psychotherapy. Current status. *Arch Gen Psychiatry.* 1994;51:599–606.

138. Wragg RE, Jeste D. Overview of depression and psychosis in Alzheimer's disease. *Am J Psychiatry.* 1989;146:577–587.

139. Young RC. Bipolar mood disorders in the elderly. *Psychiatr Clin North Am.* 1997;20: 121–136.

140. Young RC. Geriatric mania. *Clin Geriatr Med.* 1992;8:387–399.

141. Young RC. Use of lithium in bipolar disorder. In: Nelson JC, ed. *Geriatric psychopharmacology.* New York: Marcel Dekker; 1998:259–272.

142. Young RC, Gyulai L, Mulsant BH, et al. Pharmacotherapy of bipolar disorder in old age. Review and recommendations. *Am J Geriatr Psychiatry*. 2004;12:342–357.

143. Zimmer B, Kant R, Zeiler D, et al. Antidepressant efficacy and cardiovascular safety of venlafaxine in young vs old patients with comorbid medical disorders. *Int J Psychiatry Med*. 1997;27:353–364.

144. Zonderman AB, Costa PT. The absence of increased levels of depression in older adults: evidence from a national representative study. Paper presented at the annual meeting of the American Psychological Association, San Francisco, CA, 1991; cited in Blazer DG. Epidemiology of late-life depression. In: Schneider LS, Reynolds CF 3rd, Lebowitz BD, et al., eds. *Diagnosis and treatment of depression in late life*. Washington, DC: American Psychiatric Press; 1994:9–19.

145. Zubenko, GS, Sunderland T. Geriatric psychopharmacology. Why does age matter? *Harvard Rev Psychiatry*. 2000;7:311–333.

SUGGESTED READINGS

Katona CLE. *Depression in Old Age*. Chichester, United Kingdom: John Wiley and Sons; 1994.

Kennedy GJ, ed. *Suicide and Depression in Late Life*. New York: John Wiley and Sons; 1996.

Nelson JC, ed. *Geriatric Psychopharmacology*. New York: Marcel Dekker; 1998.

Salzman C, ed. *Clinical Geriatric Psychopharmacology*. 3rd ed. Baltimore: Williams & Wilkins; 1998.

Schneider LS, Reynolds CF 3rd, Lebowitz BD, et al., eds. *Diagnosis and Treatment of Depression in Late Life*. Washington, DC: American Psychiatric Press; 1994.

WEBSITES OF INTEREST FOR PATIENT SUPPORT

National Depressive & Manic-Depressive Association (educational materials and supportive peer groups for patients and their support systems): http://www.ndmda.org/

Dr. Ivan Goldberg's Depression Central (information for clinicians, patients, and their support systems): http://www.psycom.net/depression.central.html

Dr. Peter Brigham's "The Psychopharmacology of Bipolar Disorder" (current therapeutic information): http://home.comcast.net/~pmbrig/BP_pharm.html

National Alliance on Mental Illness (information about mental illness and about advocacy for the mentally ill): http://www.nami.org/

American Foundation for Suicide Prevention (support groups for bereaved survivors of others' suicides): http://www.afsp.org/

Depression Caregiver Support (message board offering support and interaction for caregivers): http://www.members.tripod.com/garyicare/

National Association of Geriatric Care Managers (locate a professional care manager in your area): http://www.caremanager.org/

CHAPTER 32

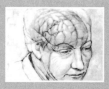

Medically Unexplained Symptoms in Older Adults

Jennifer J. Bortz

Neurologists routinely assess patients with symptoms for which medical causes are unknown, and psychiatric illness is ultimately suspected. Among first-time referrals for neurologic consultation, Fink et al. (21) documented at least one medically unexplained symptom in 63% of male and 59% of female patients. More than one third of these patients fulfilled International Classification of Diseases 10th Revision (ICD-10) criteria for somatoform disorder. Similarly high prevalence rates were documented according to the fourth edition of the *Diagnostic and Statistical Manual of Mental Disorders* (DSM-IV) criteria. In primary and secondary care settings, symptoms not adequately explained by a known medical condition account for 25% to 50% of clinical presentations. Advancing age adds yet another dimension of complexity to the evaluation of medically unexplained symptoms; dynamic changes in physical, neurochemical, metabolic, emotional, and behavioral functioning may be virtually inseparable.

Late-life psychiatric disorders are a common and complex source of excess functional disability. The prevalence of severe depressive symptoms in individuals aged 65 to 79 years is approximately 15%. More than 20% of persons aged 80 years and older have similarly severe manifestations of depression (50). In a collaborative study conducted under the auspices of the World Health Organization (WHO), somatization was deemed common across cultures and associated with "significant (health) problems and disability" (26). Health anxiety and related psychiatric concomitants in older adults are associated with considerable adversity, including increased medical utilization, longer duration of inpatient hospitalization, diminished quality of life, and decline in functional independence. Somatic symptoms also predict poorer outcomes on older patients' ratings of overall health, quality of life, restrictions in physical and social activity *independent* of depression, and physical health status. Among patients presenting in primary care settings, Smith (66) found a ninefold increase in health care utilization expenditures among older patients with concomitant somatization. Costs to patients, as well as to their families, are likely inestimable.

This chapter begins with an overview of classification schemes used in the differential diagnosis of somatoform disorders followed by a brief epidemiology review. Biologic, psychological, and psychosocial mechanisms are then discussed as inseparable sources of somatization in older adults. Theoretical bases of unconscious symptom production are described and further exemplified in discussions of psychogenic nonepileptic seizures (PNES), tremor, and gait disturbance. A discussion of common treatment barriers and therapeutic approaches of benefit to older adults concludes this chapter.

CLASSIFICATION SCHEMES

The third edition of the *Diagnostic and Statistical Manual of Mental Disorders* (DSM-III) first introduced somatoform disorders as a provisional diagnostic category in 1980. The subsequent and current edition, DSM-IV, replaced the concept of neurosis with multiple new diagnoses that could not be explained by a general medical condition or clearly associated with depression or anxiety. Specifically, DSM-IV omitted "organic" rule-out differentials in recognition of both known and highly suspected biologic substrates of primary psychiatric disorders (67). The phrase "due to a general medical disorder" appears in its place. The classification "Mental Disorders Due to a General Medical Condition" is also new to this edition. Such revisions were intended to underscore the physical versus mental distinction as an anachronistic perspective in modern medicine. The fifth edition of this classification is due to be published in 2012. One of the most widely debated revisions is the diagnostic category of somatization disorders. Major criticisms and proposed solutions to related shortcomings of DSM-IV follow a brief description of the existing framework.

Within the diagnostic classification of somatoform disorders, the DSM-IV delineates seven categorical entities: Conversion Disorder, Hypochondriasis, Somatization Disorder, Pain Disorder, Undifferentiated Somatoform Disorder, Body Dysmorphic Disorder, and Somatoform Disorder Not Otherwise Specified.

Table 32-1. *Diagnostic Criteria for Conversion Disorder*

A. One or more symptoms or deficits affecting voluntary motor or sensory function that suggest a neurologic or other general medical condition.

B. Psychological factors are judged to be associated with the symptom or deficit because the initiation or exacerbation of the symptom or deficit is preceded by conflicts or other stressors.

C. The symptom or deficit is not intentionally produced or feigned (as in factitious disorder or malingering).

D. The symptom or deficit cannot, after appropriate investigation, be fully explained by a general medical condition, or by the direct effects of a substance, or as a culturally sanctioned behavior or experience.

E. The symptom or deficit causes clinically significant distress or impairment in social, occupational, or other important areas of functioning or warrants medical evaluation.

F. The symptom or deficit is not limited to pain or sexual dysfunction, does not occur exclusively during the course of somatization disorder, and is not better accounted for by another mental disorder.

From American Psychiatric Association. *Diagnostic and Statistical Manual of Mental Disorders*. 4th ed. Washington, DC; 1994, with permission.

The unifying trait of disorders falling within the somatoform classification is that patients present for evaluation of somatic complaints for which a physical cause is not the primary etiology. By definition, a physiologic cause has either been ruled out or is *independently* unable to explain symptom severity, frequency, and/or associated degree of functional disability.

The defining feature of somatization is that covert psychological factors are presumed to play a major role in symptom production. Importantly, this role is not feigned or otherwise consciously produced. Such symptoms fall within the distinct categories of Factitious Disorders or Malingering, which will not be addressed in this chapter. DSM-IV criteria for somatoform disorders most commonly seen in older adults are presented in Tables 32-1 through 32-4.

DSM-IV is under considerable scrutiny regarding its restrictive classification of unexplained medical illness, as well as falling short in its attempt to improve understanding of these disorders, facilitate research, and enhance clinical care (11,45,70). It has been

Table 32-2. *Diagnostic Criteria for Hypochondriasis*

A. Preoccupation with fears of having, or the idea that one has, a serious disease based on the person's misinterpretation of bodily symptoms.

B. The preoccupation persists despite appropriate medical evaluation and reassurance.

C. The belief in criterion A is not of delusional intensity (as in delusional disorder, somatic type) and is not restricted to a circumscribed concern about appearance (as in body dysmorphic disorder).

D. The preoccupation causes clinically significant distress or impairment in social, occupational, or other important areas of functioning.

E. The duration of the disturbance is at least 6 months.

F. The preoccupation is not better accounted for by generalized anxiety or another somatoform disorder.

From American Psychiatric Association. *Diagnostic and Statistical Manula of Mental Disorders*. 4th ed. Washington, DC; 1994, with permission.

Table 32-3. *Diagnostic Criteria for Pain Disorder*

A. Pain in one or more anatomic sites is the predominant focus of the clinical presentation and is of sufficient severity to warrant clinical attention.

B. The pain causes clinically significant distress or impairment in social, occupational, or other important areas of functioning.

C. Psychological factors are judged to have an important role in the onset, severity, exacerbation, or maintenance of the pain.

D. The symptom or deficit is not intentionally produced or feigned (as in factitious disorder or malingering).

E. The pain is not better accounted for by a mood, anxiety, or psychotic disorder and does not meet criteria for dyspareunia.

From American Psychiatric Association. *Diagnostic and Statistical Manual of Mental Disorders*. 4th ed. Washington, DC; 1994, with permission.

Table 32-4. *Diagnostic Criteria for Somatization Disorder*

A. A history of many physical complaints beginning before age 30 years that occur over a period of several years and result in treatment being sought or significant impairment in social, occupational, or other important areas of functioning

B. Each of the following criteria must have been met, with individual symptoms occurring at any time during the course of the disturbance:
   1. Four pain symptoms: a history of pain related to at least four different sites or functions (e.g., head, abdomen, back joints, extremities, chest, rectum, during menstruation, during sexual intercourse, or during urination)
   2. Two gastrointestinal symptoms: a history of at least two gastrointestinal symptoms other than pain (e.g., nausea, bloating, vomiting other than during pregnancy, diarrhea, or intolerance of several different foods)
   3. One sexual symptom: a history of at least one sexual or reproductive symptom other than pain (e.g., sexual indifference, erectile or ejaculatory dysfunction, irregular menses, excessive menstrual bleeding, vomiting throughout pregnancy)
   4. One pseudoneurologic symptom: a history of at least one symptom or deficit suggesting a neurologic or localized weakness, difficulty swallowing or lump in throat, aphonia, urinary retention, hallucinations, loss of touch or pain sensation, double vision, blindness, deafness, seizures, dissociative symptoms such as amnesia, or loss of consciousness rather than fainting)

C. Either (1) or (2):
   1. After appropriate investigation, each of the symptoms in Criterion B cannot be fully explained by a known general medical condition or the direct effects of a substance (e.g., a drug of abuse, a medication)
   2. When there is a related general medical condition, the physical complaints or resulting social or occupational impairment are in excess of what would be expected from the history, physical examination, or laboratory findings

D. The symptoms are not intentionally produced or feigned (as in factitious disorder or malingering)

From American Psychiatric Association. *Diagnostic and Statistical Manual of Mental Disorders*. 4th ed. Washington, DC; 1994, with permission.

argued that the empirical foundation for the current classification is limited, as is its discriminative validity in separating somatization from mood and anxiety disorders. Many patients seen in primary care settings do not meet the symptom threshold required for major diagnostic classification, yet clearly present with excess symptom production and functional impairment (29). In one study of 191 consecutive patients seen in family practice settings, the majority of patients either met criteria for somatization disorder not otherwise specified (NOS) or undifferentiated somatization disorder (29.93% and 27.3%, respectively). The prevalence of major DSM-IV somatoform diagnoses, in contrast, was relatively small and ranged between 1.0% and 8.1% (20). Thus, although somatization as a symptom is common, relatively few patients actually meet diagnostic criteria for major classification. In addition, patients may be diagnosed with an Axis I psychiatric disorder and Axis III medical condition when both diagnoses refer to the same presentation. As described by Strassnig et al. (70), "the current system—with the 'medical' and 'psychiatric' specialties investigating essentially the same phenomena from different perspectives not only clearly reflects a persisting 'mind-body' distinction, but also at worst creates oxymoronic diagnostic labeling of patients."

In anticipation of DSM-V publication, debates regarding revisions of existing classification schemes have increasingly escalated. Initiatives intended to summarize existing knowledge and bring together diverging classification proposals on somatoform disorders include the Conceptual Issues in Somatoform and Similar Disorders (CISSD) project, expert meetings of the American Psychiatric Association (APA), and the WHO on Somatic Presentation on Psychiatric Disorders. Among many proposals are those advocating for abridged diagnostic criteria intended to simplify diagnostic classification as multisymptomatic or monosymptomatic somatization, with pain disorder assigned to the latter classification. Others advocate for abolition of the somatization category all together and, in its place, would position somatic symptoms on Axis III as functional somatic symptoms and syndromes. In this framework, hypochondriasis would be renamed as "health anxiety disorder" subsumed within the anxiety disorders spectrum, and only dissociative and conversion symptoms would remain on Axis I. Ultimately, a consensus has emerged regarding the need for improvement of the existing classification scheme. The extent to which DSM-V will facilitate better understanding of psychological distress and its relationship to physical illness, in addition to its ability to advance clinical care and research in older adults, will undoubtedly be key measures of success within our rapidly aging population.

EPIDEMIOLOGY

As highlighted in the foregoing discussion, estimates regarding the overall prevalence of somatoform disorders vary widely due to differences in diagnostic criteria, as well as sample characteristics, and even to discrepancies in determining what is considered a medical disease and what is not. In primary care settings, the prevalence of somatoform disorders was estimated to be between 22% and 58% (20). Community surveys have shown an "exaggerated concern about health" in approximately 10% of older adults (9). Somatization is recognized not only as the presence of somatic symptoms without a known or sole physiologic cause, but it also entails complaints made to a health professional, taking medications, or making significant lifestyle alterations due to symptom burden (54).

Current literature provides conflicting information regarding demographic characteristics of late-life somatization; whereas some researchers report that gender, education, age, depression, socioeconomic status, and social activity covary with somatization symptoms, other studies show no relationship with gender, ethnicity, situational stress, recent bereavement, retirement, or physical disability (4,48). In terms of age-related factors, Pribor et al. (54) found no age-related differences in symptom frequency, number of surgeries, medical hospitalizations, or psychiatric hospitalizations in their study of 353 women meeting DSM-IV criteria for somatization disorder. Only 10% of their sample, however, was over the age of 65. Sheehan and Banerjee (64) underscore the difficulty of estimating the prevalence of late-life somatization in this population due to discrepancies in defining clinical populations, sampling procedures, and diversity of measurement instruments.

MECHANISMS OF SOMATIZATION IN OLDER ADULTS

BIOLOGIC FOUNDATIONS

Neurologic, genetic, and biochemical links to somatization and other psychiatric conditions are advancing at a rapid pace. A recent Medline search yielded 9,284 articles identified with the keywords "psychiatric" and "imaging or neuroimaging" or "genetic or genomic." Approximately 60% of these articles (i.e., 5,672) were published since the year 2000.

Functional neuroimaging studies have documented metabolic correlates of conversion symptoms, including selective decreases in frontal and subcortical circuits subserving motor control in patients with

hysterical paralysis, metabolic decreases in somatosensory cortices in patients with medically unexplained anesthesia, and decreases in visual cortex in patients with psychogenic blindness [see review by Vuilleumier (72)]. In one such study, Vuilleumier et al. (73) assessed functional unilateral sensorimotor loss via single photon emission computed tomography (SPECT) in seven patients with actively symptomatic hemiplegia. Imaging studies were repeated 2 to 4 months after deficit resolution. Results showed consistent hyperperfusion in thalamus and basal ganglia in the contralateral hemisphere, which are findings consistent with known pathophysiology of the organic equivalent. Moreover, perfusion abnormalities were absent at follow-up, when symptoms associated with unilateral hemiparesis had fully abated (73). Such parallel changes in cerebral perfusion suggest shared neuroanatomic pathways between symptoms of organic and functional origin. Similar techniques have greatly enhanced our understanding of structural and functional correlates of major depression, anxiety, and thought disorders at various ages and levels of chronicity [see reviews by Moresco et al. (49) and Parsey and Mann (51)].

Genetic predispositions for somatization symptoms have also been identified. Up to half of the stable variance in self-report of somatization symptoms was attributed to genetic factors in the absence of familial-environmental effects in the "Virginia 30,000" twin-family sample (36). More recently, Saito et al. (62) reviewed studies of familial aggregation, twins, candidate gene association, and pharmacogenomics in an attempt to understand genetic underpinnings of irritable bowel syndrome (IBS). Overall, modest support for a genetic basis of IBS was derived from familial and twin studies, with stronger associations found for pharmacogenomic factors. Bienvenu et al. (8) found a higher incidence of somatoform disorders in family members of people with hypochondriasis or other "obsessive-compulsive spectrum disorders" compared to first-degree relatives of case-control probands. Major confounding factors in familial association studies include exposure to similar environments and reporting bias due to increased familial awareness of target symptoms. The potential for genomic advances to better our understanding of the role of genetics in the pathophysiology and clinical manifestation of psychogenic disorders is considerable. However, the literature continues to support, particularly with regard to treatment initiatives, the importance of psychological and psychosocial dynamics that underlie and promote emotional distress in older adults.

PSYCHOLOGICAL FOUNDATIONS

Illness is an inextricable part of aging; excess functional disability is not. Thus, adequate assessment and treatment of somatization spectrum disorders require fundamental knowledge of psychological mechanisms within the broader perspective of illness behavior.

A growing body of research has emerged regarding *"abnormal illness behavior,"* a term that encompasses a variety of symptom presentations in which excessive concern about illness predominates and extensive evaluation and medical treatment is sought (53). Although this term applies to complaints associated with well-defined medical conditions, it has primarily been ascribed to disorders or symptoms not explained by primary medical conditions. As further described by Kirmayer and Looper (38), illness behavior reflects important dimensions of somatization that include sociocultural perspectives, developmental processes, and physiologic mechanisms. Specific psychological dimensions of illness behavior entail cognitive, perceptual, and behavioral aspects of a patient's response to symptoms or disease expressed as heightened somatic sensitivity, symptom attribution, catastrophizing, and denial.

A majority of patients with medically unexplained symptoms exhibits high sensitivity to somatic symptoms, including increased intensity and duration of pain or other bodily sensations, higher levels of subjective stress, and sheer number of symptoms relative to healthy and patient controls. Somatizing patients also show a greater tendency to attribute common physical symptoms to major illness and to more serious pathology. Such symptoms are then further amplified via catastrophic thoughts and rumination.

Catastrophizing refers to the generation of unrealistic and excessive fears regarding health status and outcome, such as when the individual maintains a focus on low-incident side effects or adverse events leading to disastrous, although improbable, outcomes. Relatedly, somatizing patients excessively worry about symptoms or conditions in a pathologic manner that induces negative affect, anxiety, and heightened autonomic arousal. Hypervigilance to signs and sensations may occur in a manner that promotes "somatosensory amplification," which, in turn, is reinforced through a confirmatory bias that maintains this closed-loop system. A major advantage of cognitive-behavioral models of somatization is that they facilitate interventions specifically targeting dysfunctional and unrealistic thoughts and beliefs.

At the other extreme of the cognitive continuum are forms of unconscious symptom production associated with *minimization* of illness, or denial, long considered the primary mechanism underlying conversion disorders. Based on the early works of Briquet, Charcot, Freud, Breuer, and Janet, somatization is understood to reflect painful psychological turmoil translated into a more acceptable and concrete (i.e., physical) form.

". . . In hysteria the unbearable idea is rendered innocuous by the quantity of excitation attached to it being transmitted into some bodily form of expression . . . conversion may be either total or partial, and it proceeds along the line of the motor or sensory innervation that is more or less intimately related to the traumatic experience." Freud (22)

Sadavoy (61) provides a useful theoretical understanding of psychiatric disorders in the context of developmental changes in late life. According to this conceptualization, as impulse and action-oriented defenses diminish with normal aging, other responses to affective states become increasingly evident. Expression of these inner states, in turn, often mimics symptoms associated with Axis I disorders. The expression of distress is further tied to unique personality traits, characterologic adjustment, and external stressors. A list of stress reactions commonly occurring in late life is presented in Table 32-5. Thus, personality structure and both internal and external stressors are considered to mediate excess symptom production in older adults.

Relatedly, major authors in the field have emphasized the contribution of interpersonal and psychosocial factors to late-life somatization. Symptom perception models maintain that attention and related cognitive resources once directed toward others become progressively drawn inward (25,38), promoting a greater awareness of, and focus upon, bodily functioning. Selective attention thus serves to amplify patients'

Table 32-5. *Stress Reactions in Late Life*

Stresses	Psychological Reactions
Social status and friendship pattern changes	Impotence, lost self-esteem, lost productivity
Physical change; beauty, strength	Narcissistic assault
Illness/infirmity	Dependency conflicts
Cognitive decline	Ego deficits/impaired affect control
Sexual decline	Shame
Bereavement	Abandonment conflicts
Economic stress	Uncertainty/lost control
Loss of stature (e.g., retirement)	Impotence, lost self-esteem, lost productivity
Relocation to institution	Forced intimacy/separation anxiety
Awareness of mortality	Death anxiety
Social status and friendship pattern changes	Separation/individuation
Family changes (e.g., parenting roles)	Dominance and intimacy conflicts

From Sadavoy J. *Handbook of Counseling and Psychotherapy with Older Adults.* New York: John Wiley & Sons; 1999, with permission.

awareness and sensitivity to changes in physical status, which, in turn, facilitates symptom reporting. Research on symptom reporting in conditions of bodily focused and distracted attention for hypochondriacal patients (27) and panic patients (39) indicates that heightened somatic awareness contributes to higher reports of perceived symptoms and sensations. Difficulty meeting personal and social expectations (9) and perceived inadequacies in social or personal domains are also hypothesized to underlie such functional complaints.

In summary, somatization in older adults is facilitated by a combination of biologic, psychological, and psychosocial mechanisms. Such factors interact in some weighted measure that is individual specific to produce excess functional, physical, and emotional disability.

In the next section, we review theoretic considerations and common presentations of conversion in patients presenting with neurologic complaints.

COMMON FORMS OF NEUROLOGIC CONVERSION DISORDERS

PSYCHOGENIC SEIZURE DISORDERS

In any clinical setting, separating PNES from true epileptic seizures is a difficult, time- and resource-consuming endeavor. The degree of sign and symptom overlap with true epilepsy is considerable because PNES can mimic virtually any type of seizure disorder. Furthermore, a significant number of patients with nonepileptic seizure (NES) have concomitant histories of neurologic insult, including seizures and other nonspecific electroencephalogram (EEG) abnormalities (41). Inpatient 24-hour video-EEG monitoring is required to establish the diagnosis of psychogenic seizures with relative confidence. In this setting, PNES is diagnosed when all other causes of events have been ruled out and when patients' typical events occur, either spontaneously or via placebo induction, during the course of normal EEG recordings. The likelihood of seizures that can escape scalp EEG detection, specifically ictal discharges arising from areas deep within the brain, must also be considered unlikely in arriving at a diagnosis of PNES.

The highest incidence of new-onset seizures is now among individuals over the age of 60 years—a figure twice that in patients 40 to 59 years of age and six to 10 times higher among those 75 years and older relative to younger populations (56). Approximately one third of seizures in this population are idiopathic. Cerebrovascular disease accounts for 30% to 50% of new-onset seizures in older adults. Approximately 16% are associated with tumor (16). The incidence of

PNES in late life is unknown but is an extremely common differential among admissions to tertiary care epilepsy centers. Up to 40% of patients admitted for diagnostic workup of intractable seizures to comprehensive epilepsy centers are found to have psychiatric imitators of epilepsy (23). In younger populations, established risk factors of PNES include a history of childhood sexual and/or physical abuse and female gender. Links between trauma histories and conversion are well documented. However, a small number of studies suggests that there may be important distinctions in older versus younger PNES cohorts.

Two recent studies identified clinical features and potential risk factors of late-onset psychogenic seizures. In an 8-year retrospective chart review, PNES was diagnosed in one third (13 of 59) of patients 60 years or older via inpatient video-EEG monitoring studies (34). Motor activity was reported as the primary symptom in 62% of patients, and more than two thirds of patients did not evidence a loss of responsiveness. A majority of patients were diagnosed with somatoform disorders, although additional information regarding trauma history or more specific aspects of the diagnosis was not available per medical record review.

Recently, Behrouz et al. (7) documented first-onset PNES in nine (9.6%) of 94 patients aged 60 years and older admitted for long-term video-EEG monitoring studies. Generalized motor events occurred in four patients (44%), unresponsiveness occurred in five patients (56%), and complex and varied presentations were present in two patients, with episodes ranging from mild tremor to intense verbal outbursts. Duncan et al. (15) compared early versus late onset of PNES events in patients over and under age 55. Unlike younger counterparts, late-onset PNES occurred more frequently in males, in greater association with severe physical problems, and in the context of a higher number of health-related trauma experiences. Patients with psychogenic events beginning after age 55 also reported markedly fewer incidents of antecedent sexual abuse (one vs. 78 patients, or 4% vs. 32%) and were found to have better baseline levels of mental health. Although not empirically verified, these factors suggest better treatment efficacy and prognosis of treating PNES in older adults as well as the possibility of prevention in high-risk patients with significant health-related anxiety or trauma.

Psychogenic movement disorders (PMDs) similarly mimic almost any behavioral symptom associated with central or peripheral motor symptoms, including tremor, balance and gait disturbance, myoclonus, dystonias, dyskinesias, and tics. Tremor, gait disturbance, and postural instability are common in older adults, and as such, their psychogenic counterparts are discussed in greater detail in the following sections.

PSYCHOGENIC MOVEMENT DISORDERS

In a recent commentary, the current chairman of the National Institute of Neurological Disorders and Stroke (NINDS), National Institutes of Health, Human Motor Control section, deemed PMDs a "crisis for neurology" (28). Support for this claim stems from evidence that: (a) a significant number of patients present with medically unexplained movement disorders; (b) the diagnosis is difficult and, at times, elusive; (c) the pathophysiology is unknown; (d) treatment options, overall, are poorly defined; and (e) prognosis is guarded since patients are often resistant to both diagnosis and therapeutic intervention.

The incidence of PMDs is estimated at 1% to 9% in the general population and may be as high as 15% in specialized movement disorder clinics. The diagnosis of PMD is largely dependent on exclusion of all alternative organic etiologies as well as ruling in nonneurologic signs and symptoms. Problems related to diagnostic classification have emerged as well. The system of Fahn and Williams (18), as described in the following section, continues to be a useful means of identifying the degree of diagnostic certainty ascribed to various types of motor conversion disorders. Further obscuring diagnostic clarity is the fact that 10% to 15% of patients with PMDs have concomitant primary movement disorders.

Tremor

The diagnosis of psychogenic tremor is based on exclusion of all other etiologies as well as the presence of atypical clinical presentations (14). A typical features include a complex mixture of resting, postural and action features marked by a fluctuating course, spontaneous remission, and/or changing characteristics. Psychogenic tremor is typically associated with abrupt onset, abrupt remission, or both. Amplitude is often diminished during periods of distraction. Entrainment during motor coordination tasks and presence of the coactivation sign (i.e., resistance to passive movement in testing for rigidity) are common markers of functionality. Psychogenic tremor may also appear in the contralateral limb upon forced restraint of the involved limb.

In the largest longitudinal study of patients with psychogenic tremor to date, Jankovic et al. (32) followed 228 patients for an average of 3.4 years (±2.8 years after initial evaluation), of whom 25% (n = 127) were diagnosed with psychogenic tremor. Seventy-two percent of patients were female, and average age at initial evaluation was 43.7 ± 14.1 years. Patients' clinical presentation was characterized by abrupt onset in 78.7% of the cohort, distractibility in 72.4% of the cohort, and variability in amplitude and frequency in 62.2% of the cohort. Approximately one third of patients had intermittent and inconsistent symptoms (35.4% and 29.9%, respectively). Variable direction

was documented in 17.3% of cases. A majority of patients identified a precipitating event preceding tremor onset, including personal life stress (33.9%), trauma (23.6%), major illness (13.4%), surgery (9.4%), and reaction to medical treatment/procedure (8.7%). Evidence of secondary gain was noted in approximately one third of patients; however, the authors specifically do not address the potential contribution of established, coexisting movement disorders (e.g., dystonia in 39% of patients) to those factors, particularly maintaining disability status and dependence on compensation. Two thirds of patients were diagnosed with a concomitant psychiatric disorder, most commonly depression (56.7%). Finally, 56% of psychogenic tremor patients reported improvement at study completion. Unfortunately, the vast majority of patients (31.9%) were said to benefit from the vagaries of "physicians' prescribed treatment." A slim minority attributed improvement to the elimination of stressors, medication, or stress-intervention therapies despite identifying such factors as common precipitants.

Kim et al. (37) conducted a 10-year retrospective medical chart and videotape review in a cross-sectional study that similarly attempted to identify clinical characteristics of psychogenic tremor. Patients were classified according to Fahn and Williams' (18) categories of diagnostic certainty: (a) documented, (b) clinically established, (c) probable, and (d) possible. *Documented* classification required symptom improvement with psychotherapy, suggestion, or placebo or evidence of symptom remission when left alone. Patients considered to be *clinically established* evidenced movements that were inconsistent or incongruent with organic tremor, in the context of (a) other definite psychogenic neurologic signs, (b) multiple somatizations, or (c) obvious psychiatric disturbance. These two groups were merged to form the *clinically definite* group. Less stringent criteria were present in the probable and possible categories, and both of these diagnostic groups were subsequently excluded from the study.

A total of 46 female and 24 male patients fulfilled *clinically definite* criteria. Disappearance or marked suppression of tremor when concentrating on other motor or mental tasks occurred in 80% of patients. In 88% of patients, variability in frequency, direction, amplitude, or site of tremor was evidenced. Thirty-nine percent of patients had other concomitant PMDs: 48% had psychogenic myoclonus, 41% had dystonia, 7% had parkinsonism, and 22% had movements that were so unusual that they could not be classified. Seven patients (10%) had more than one concomitant PMD. The authors conclude that psychogenic tremor can be differentiated from neurologic tremor on the basis of characteristic clinical and historical features and not solely on the basis of exclusion. They acknowledge, however, that the diagnosis often requires extended or repeated observation. As with other conversion symptoms, a concomitant neurologic disorder may be present. In such cases, separating neurologic from psychogenic tremor may be an extremely difficult if not impossible task.

Although beyond the scope of this review, advances in ancillary technologies hold promise in improving the diagnostic and classification accuracy of psychogenic tremor. This includes use of highly complex computer-based statistical algorithms, devices such as accelerometry and electromyography (EMG) to prospectively record and measure variability in tremor frequency and functional imaging of striatal dopamine integrity (44,46,52,55,74).

Gait and Balance Disorders

Gait and balance disorders are of considerable concern in older adults due to an increased risk of falls and related complications, including death. In 2003, 13,700 deaths due to falls and 1.8 million fall-related injuries requiring emergency department treatment occurred in individuals aged 65 years and older. Between 1993 and 2003, the rate of age-adjusted deaths due to falls increased significantly for both men and women (45.3% and 59.5% higher, respectively). Consistently higher rates have been documented in men versus women (31.8 vs. 19.5 per 100,000, respectively). Falls account for the majority of hip fractures, which often lead to long-term functional impairment and/or admission to extended-care facilities (69). The risk of falls and associated morbidity due to psychogenic gait and balance disorders is unknown.

The published incidence of psychogenic gait in neurology patients ranges from 3.3% to over 10% in large academic centers (12,47,71). Characteristics of psychogenic gait include abrupt buckling of the knees, swaying with eyes closed, foot-dragging in the absence of leg circumduction, hyperreflexia, and psychogenic Romberg and Babinski signs. Rapid postural adjustment is often preserved in psychogenic gait disturbance. Inability to turn or walk when leg movements are preserved while lying down is a well-documented sign of conversion, termed *astasia-abasia*. However, ataxia due to central cerebellar lesions and frontal gait disorders may manifest a similar dissociation (33).

Fear of falling (FOF) may also mimic gait and balance disorders, particularly in individuals with Parkinson's disease (PD). Adkin et al. (1) found increased FOF to be associated with greater postural instability in nondemented PD patients compared with age-matched controls. Symptoms associated with FOF include exaggerated impairment in stance and gait, "sliding" steps, and excessive grasping at furniture or walls, with onset often occurring after a fall. FOF has been shown to affect spatial and temporal gait parameters in older adults, including decreased spread, shorter stride length, increased stride width, and double limb support time (10). Excess functional disability due to FOF may lead to significant restrictions in physical activity, social interaction, and emotional well-being. As in other motor conversion disorders, improvement of gait and balance dysfunction may occur with distraction (42).

TREATMENT

Treatment of unexplained medical illness begins with the fundamental conviction that medical care, first and foremost, serves to alleviate excess suffering. Emotional distress exacerbates the majority of symptoms and disease processes, whether explicitly or implicitly identified as a primary complaint. Such symptoms increase functional disability and diminish overall quality of life and thus require consideration equal to that of well-defined medical conditions. In this age cohort, however, formidable barriers to therapeutic delivery and efficacy exist, including (a) adequate detection of psychiatric issues contributing to symptom production, (b) formulation of viable treatment recommendations that can be adequately implemented by physicians and related health care providers, and (c) facilitating patients' willingness to pursue treatment. Because most older adults are seen in primary care settings, basic screening and knowledge of treatment options for management of illness behavior begin in this setting and are core competencies for such providers.

This chapter concludes with brief reviews regarding basic assessment, opportunities, and options in treating late-life somatization.

ASSESSMENT

As reviewed earlier in this chapter, medically unexplained physical symptoms are common but underrecognized and undertreated. Depression, stress, and related underpinnings of somatization are often not disclosed on interview, even when care providers directly inquire about patients' emotional status. Resistance in acknowledging or disclosing issues associated with emotional distress occurs in the context of widespread misunderstanding and stigma about psychiatric issues in general. Thus, both deliberate and unconscious masking of psychological distress by more socially acceptable complaints of physical illness and disability contribute to underdetection of abnormal illness behavior, particularly among older adults. Constraints of clinical time and resources further add to diagnostic difficulties in geriatric patients who inherently have more extensive medical and psychosocial histories.

Screening tests are often useful in highlighting patient perceptions and sensitivities in need of further assessment or clarification. Medical and psychosocial domains central to identifying individual-specific stressors include current health status, medical conditions affecting close friends and family, caregiving roles, personal and situational losses (e.g., deaths, retirement, relocation), change in financial status, and available social support.

Several instruments have been developed to assess broad dimensions of excess illness behavior. Such measures are relatively brief and easily administered. Most provide cutoff scores or normative ranges that separate normal from abnormal values derived from controlled clinical studies. Qualitative information, gathered from review of individual items or statements endorsed by patients, often provides further insight into unique areas of concern. Thus, although an aggregate score may not exceed a given cutoff for significance, endorsement of statements like "Most of the time I feel blue" or "The future seems hopeless to me" allows the clinician to further inquire into how such experiences affect daily functioning. The danger in any screening instrument, however, is that it necessarily assesses a sample of behavior or attitudes from otherwise broad domains, and results may be easily misinterpreted as over- or underrepresenting illness behavior. Another limitation is that most instruments have not been validated with older adults. However, these instruments may be extremely useful in expanding the scope of clinical interviews to include domains related to illness behavior. A list of common screening tests for somatization appears in Table 32-6.

TREATMENT FORMULATION AND INTERVENTION

From such descriptive categories, a number of therapeutic recommendations may emerge targeting individual-specific psychosocial stressors, worries,

Table 32-6. *Screening Tests for Somatization and Related Disorders*

Test	Reference
Brief Symptom Inventory (BSI)	Derogatis and Melisaratos (13)
Geriatric Depression Scale (GDS)	Sheikh et al. (65)
Health Anxiety Inventory (HAI)	Salkovskis et al. (63)
Illness Attitudes Scale (IAS)	Kellner (35)
Screening for Somatoform Symptoms (SOMS-7)	Rief and Hiller (59)
Somatosensory Amplification Scale (SAS)	Barsky et al. (6)
Whiteley 7-Item Scale	Fink et al. (19)
Primary Care Evaluation of Mental Disorders (PRIME-MD)	Spitzer et al. (67)

support system deficiencies, and activity levels. Vegetative symptoms of distress, such as sleep or appetite disturbance, or changes in mental, physical, and social activity level may be highly amenable to basic behavioral interventions (e.g., sleep hygiene education, nutrition/dietary consultation, prescribed exercise) and may incidentally improve mood and somatic symptoms. Pharmacologic intervention may be useful in cases where depression or anxiety appear prominent. However, somatizing patients also tend to be at higher risk of medication tolerance and dependence. These issues are particularly concerning because these issues, in addition to polypharmacy, are major problems in treating older adults, regardless of the indication or setting. Moreover, it is important to recognize that symptom substitution is particularly common in patients with unexplained medical illness; although it is possible to successfully treat most target symptoms, the likelihood that other refractory symptoms will emerge or worsen is high if underlying causes are not addressed. For these reasons, pharmacologic treatment, when clearly indicated, should ideally be combined with psychological approaches to symptom reduction. Two levels of intervention are described below: interventions designed to be implemented by general practitioners and interventions intended to be referred to behavioral health specialists for therapeutic intervention.

A key foundation for treating medically unexplained symptoms is educating patients in the fundamentals of biologic mechanisms of stress and health consequences that are specific, concrete, and relevant to presenting complaints. Providing basic statistics, such as those listed in Table 32-7, serves to validate the impact of stress on health as well as normalize the problem by highlighting how common and damaging stress can be. This groundwork may then lead to further education regarding physiologic reactions (i.e., sympathetic and parasympathetic nervous system mechanisms) that may exacerbate illness behavior or arise de novo. A basic understanding of stress mechanisms further allows for "legitimizing" of symptoms as well as better acceptance of treatment recommendations intended to gradually diminish, rather than categorically cure, troublesome symptoms. Overall, patient education, as delivered by referring physicians and extenders, is essential in forming a foundation for therapeutic intervention.

Once patients have a basic understanding of how stress can produce or exacerbate many "physical" symptoms, therapeutic interventions can be introduced. To this end, brief educational programs have been developed to train primary care physicians in fundamental procedures intended to decrease somatization behavior. Most have centered upon teaching different ways to understand and/or realistically interpret functional symptoms and are introduced through cognitive

Table 32-7. *Health-Related Effects of Stress*

- 43% of all adults suffer adverse health effects from stress.[a]
- 75% to 90% of all doctors office visits are for stress-related complaints.[a]
- Stress is linked to six of the leading causes of death: heart disease, cancer, lung ailments, accidents, cirrhosis of the liver, and suicide.[a]
- Stress of family caregiving for persons with dementia has been shown to impact a person's immune system for up to 3 years *after* their caregiving ends, thus increasing their chances of developing a chronic illness themselves.[b]
- Family caregivers who provide care 36 or more hours weekly are more likely than noncaregivers to experience symptoms of depression or anxiety. For spouses, the rate is six times higher; for those caring for a parent, the rate is twice as high.[c]
- Older adult spouse caregivers with a history of chronic illness themselves who are experiencing caregiving–related stress have a 63% higher mortality rate than their non–caregiving peers.[d]
- Family caregivers experiencing extreme stress have been shown to age prematurely. This level of stress can take as much as 10 years off a family caregiver's life.[e]

---

[a] Kiffer JF. *APA Survey*. Cleveland: Department of Health Psychology and Applied Psychophysiology, The Cleveland Clinic Foundation; 2004.

[b] Kiecolt-Glaser JK, Preacher KJ, MacCallum RC, et al. Chronic stress and age-related increases in the proinflammatory cytokine IL-6. *Proc Natl Acad Sci U S A.* 2003;100:9090–9095.

[c] Cannuscio CC, Jones C, Kawachi I, et al. Reverberations of family illness: a longitudinal assessment of informal caregiving and mental health status in the Nurses' Health Study. *Am J Public Health.* 2002;92:1305–1311.

[d] Shultz et al. (1999).

[e] Epel ES, Blackburn EH, Lin J, et al. Accelerated telomere shortening in response to life stress. *Proc Natl Acad Sci U S A.* 2004;101:17312–17315.

restructuring models. Larisch et al. (40) conducted a randomized, controlled study of 42 general practitioners who either applied training in reattribution techniques or provided nonspecific psychosocial primary care to 127 patients with medically unexplained symptoms. Initial results were encouraging. Reductions in physical symptoms, depression, and anxiety and improvement in physical functioning at 3 months postintervention were documented among patients receiving reattribution training. However, at the 6-month follow-up, only reductions in physical symptoms remained significant. The authors concluded that the effect of reattribution techniques were "small and limited to physical symptoms" (40). Other studies of general practitioner–initiated reattribution training, in which the goal is to normalize interpretation of symptoms and modify beliefs about causes, have met with limited success, as have other brief treatments including reflecting interviews and various communication techniques (2,57). Overall, the literature appears to support the conclusions of a recent Cochran Database review, in which summary findings documented little evidence supporting the efficacy of psychosocial interventions by general practitioners (31).

One reason for limited success of physician-initiated treatment is that unexplained medical illness tends to present as more chronic and complex conditions that are not amenable to brief or unskilled treatment intervention. This is not unlike other major medical problems in which patients require outside referrals for specialty care and more extensive treatment

regimens than can reasonably be implemented within the context of a general medical practice.

Cognitive-behavioral therapy (CBT) has been found to successfully reduce a variety of somatization behaviors [see reviews by Allen et al. (3) and Looper et al. (43)]. CBT is based on affecting behavior change by targeting maladaptive and negative thoughts, beliefs, and attitudes. CBT has been shown to be effective for a variety of conditions, particularly anxiety and depression, and may be useful in patients with unexplained medical illness. In one such study, Barsky and Ahern (5) conducted a randomized controlled trial comparing 102 patients assigned to individualized CBT targeting hypochondriacal thinking and beliefs with 85 patients assigned to medical treatment-as-usual. At the 12-month follow-up, CBT patients showed lower levels of hypochondriacal symptoms, attitudes, and beliefs and health-related anxiety as well as diminished social role dysfunction relative to the no-treatment controls. Similarly, Escobar et al. (17) conducted a randomized controlled trial of CBT that compared 84 patients with somatization disorder who underwent a 10-session, individually administered CBT regimen plus psychiatric consultation intervention with patients receiving psychiatric consultation alone. Results showed significant improvement in self-reported function and somatic symptoms as well as a greater decrease in health care costs at the 15-month follow-up. CBT has also been found to be effective in the treatment of late-life depression and anxiety disorders (24,30,68), chronic low back pain (58), and insomnia (60). Unfortunately, 50% to 90% of patients with medically unexplained symptoms do not complete mental health referrals (17). Recent studies also support the notion that the efficacy of CBT interventions may be diminished in older adult patients with compromised executive system (i.e., frontal lobe) functioning, underscoring the need to fully assess and consider cognitive competency in any form of educational or behavioral intervention.

Overall, the usefulness of primary care interventions appears best suited to patients with new-onset and/or mild somatization problems or patients who fully refuse referral for specialty care. Patients with complex, medically refractory symptoms should be referred to psychiatrists, psychologists, or other specialty providers in the same manner that other medical specialists are called upon to care for patients with disorders that fall within unique areas of expertise.

SUMMARY AND CONCLUSIONS

Recognition of unexplained medical illness in late life presents numerous clinical challenges, including those created by strict adherence to formal diagnostic criteria. Mechanisms of illness behavior are understood to include a combination of biologic, psychological, and social factors—each increasing in complexity with advancing age. As reviewed earlier, hallmark symptoms of seizure, movement, and balance disorders may present as primary conversion or other forms of somatization. Risks of misdiagnosis or failure to treat potentially reversible causes of excess functional disability in older adults are considerable.

Awareness of unique treatment barriers affecting older adults, the persistence of ageism, and consequences of not treating unexplained medical illness provides a basis for moving forward in both diagnostic and treatment arenas. Gains have been made, with increasing numbers of primary care physicians exerting greater effort in diagnosis and treatment planning. However, sizable gaps remain between adequate detection and treatment of abnormal illness behavior in this growing and uniquely vulnerable population. Interventions that combine patient education with graduated and multidisciplinary implementation of individual-specific therapeutic strategies, such as CBT and other forms of cognitive reattribution approaches, appear promising but await evidence-based confirmation of efficacy with older adults.

REFERENCES

1. Adkin et al., 2003.
2. Aiarzaguena, 2007.
3. Allen et al., 2001.
4. Barsky AJ. The diagnosis and management of hypochondriacal concerns in the elderly. *J Geriatr Psychiatry*. 1992;25:129–141.
5. Barsky and Ahern, 2004.
6. Barsky et al., 1990.
7. Behrouz R, Heriaud L, Benbadis SR. Late-onset psychogenic nonepileptic seizures. *Rev Neurobiol*. 2007;81:129–151.
8. Bienvenu OJ, Samuels JF, Riddle MA, et al. The relationship of obsessive-compulsive disorder to possible spectrum disorders: results from a family study. *Biol Psychiatry*. 2000;48:287–293.
9. Blazer D. Geriatric psychiatry. In: Hales R, Yudofsky S, eds. *The American Psychiatric Press textbook of psychiatry*. Washington, DC: American Psychiatric Press; 1996.
10. Chamberlin et al., 2005.
11. Creed F. Can DSM-V facilitate productive research into the somatoform disorders? *J Psychosom Res*. 2006;60:331–334.
12. Daniel, 2004.
13. Derogatis LR, Melisaratos N. The Brief Symptom Inventory: an introductory report. *Psychol Med*. 1983;13:595–605.
14. Deuschl G, Bain P, Brin M. Consensus statement of the Movement Disorder Society on Tremor. Ad Hoc Scientific Committee. *Move Disord*. 1998;13:2–23.
15. Duncan R, Oto M, Martin E, et al. Late onset psychogenic nonepileptic attacks. *Neurology*. 2006; 66:1644–1647.
16. Eisenschenk S, Gilmore R. Adult-onset seizures: clinical solutions to a challenging patient workup. *Geriatrics*. 1999;54:18–28.
17. Escobar, 2006.
18. Fahn S, Williams DT. Psychogenic dystonia. *Adv Neurol*. 1988;50:431–455.
19. Fink P, Ewald H, Jensen J, et al. Screening for somatization and hypochondriasis in primary care and neurological in-patients: a seven-item scale for hypochondriasis and somatization *J Psychosom Res*. 1999:46:261–273.
20. Fink P, Sorensen L, Engberg M, et al. Somatization in primary care: prevalence, health care utilization, and general practitioner recognition. *Psychosomatics*. 1999;40:330–338.
21. Fink P, Steen Hansen M, Sondergaard L. Somatoform disorders among first-time referrals to a neurology service. *Psychosomatics*. 2005;46:540–548.
22. Freud S. The defense neuro-psychoses. In: *Collected papers*. Volume 1. London: Hogarth; 1953:59–75.
23. Gates and Mercer, 1995.
24. Gorenstein, 2007.
25. Gottlieb GL. Hypochondriasis: a psychosomatic problem in the elderly. *Adv Psychosom Med*. 1989; 19:67–84.

26. Gureje O, Simon GE, Ustun TB, et al. Somatization in cross cultural perspective: a World Health Organization study in primary care. *Am J Psychiatry*. 1997;154:989–995.

27. Haenen AM, Schmidt AJ, Schoenmakers M, et al. Suggestibility in hypochondriacal patients and healthy control subjects: an experimental case-control study. *Psychosomatics*. 1997;38:543–547.

28. Hallett M. Psychogenic movement disorders: a crisis for neurology. *Curr Neurol Neurosci Rep*. 2006;6:269–271.

29. Hiller W, Rief W, Fichter MM. Further evidence for a broader concept of somatization disorder using the somatic symptom index. *Psychosomatics*. 1995;36:285–294.

30. Hollen, 2005.

31. Huibers MJH, Beurskens AJHM, Bleijenberg G, et al. *Psychosocial Interventions Delivered by General Practitioners. The Cochran Collaboration*. 2007. New York: John Wiley & Sons; 2007.

32. Jankovic J, Vuong KD, Thomas M. Psychogenic tremor: long-term outcome. *CNS Spectr*. 2006; 11:501–508.

33. Keane JR. Hysterical gait disorders: 60 cases. *Neurology*. 1989;39:586–589.

34. Kellinghaus C, Loddenkember T, Dinner DS, et al. Non-epileptic seizures of the elderly. *J Neurol*. 2004;251:704–709.

35. Kellner R., 1987.

36. Kendler KS, Walters EE, Truett KR, et al. A twin-family study of self-report symptoms of panic-phobia and somatization. *Behav Genet*. 1995;25: 499–515.

37. Kim YJ, Pakiam SI, Lang AE. Historical and clinical features of psychogenic tremor: a review of 70 cases. *Can J Neurol Sci*. 1999;26:190–195.

38. Kirmayer LJ, Looper KJ. Abnormal illness behaviour: physiological, psychological and social dimensions of coping with distress. *Curr Opin Psychiatry*. 2006;19:54–60.

39. Kroeze S, van den Hout M, Haenen MA, et al. Symptom reporting and interoceptive attention in panic patients. *Percept Mot Skills*. 1996;82: 1019–1026.

40. Larisch et al., 2004.

41. Lelliot and Fenwick, 1991.

42. Lempert, Brandt, Dieterich, & Huppert, 1991.

43. Looper et al., 2002.

44. Marti et al., 2006.

45. Mayou R, Kirmayer LJ, Simon G, et al. Somatoform disorders: time for a new approach in DSM-V. *Am J Psychiatry*. 2005;162:847–855.

46. McAuley J, Rothwell J. Identification of psychogenic, dystonic, and other organic tremors by a coherence entrainment test. *Mov Disord*. 2004; 19:253–267.

47. Miyasaki JM, Sa DS, Galvez-Jimenez N, et al. Psychogenic movement disorders. *Can J Neurol Sci*. 2003;30:S94–S100.

48. Monopoli A, Vaccaro A. Depression, hypochondriasis, and demographic variables in a non-institutionalized elderly sample. *Clin Geropsychol*. 1998;19:75–79.

49. Moresco RM, Matarrese M, Fazio F. PET and SPET molecular imaging: focus on serotonin system. *Curr Top Med Chem*. 2006;6:2027–2034.

50. Older Americans, 2005.

51. Parsey RV, Mann JJ. Applications of positron emission tomography in psychiatry. *Semin Nucl Med*. 2003;33:129–135.

52. Piboolnurak P, Rothey N, Ahmed A, et al. Psychogenic tremor disorders identified using tree-based statistical algorithms and quantitative tremor analysis. *Mov Disord*. 2005;20:1543–1549.

53. Pilowsky I. From conversion hysteria to somatisation to abnormal illness behaviour? *J Psychosom Res*. 1996;40:345–350.

54. Pribor EF, Smith DS, Yutzy SH. Somatization disorder in elderly patients. *Am J Geriatr Psychiatry*. 1994;2:109–117.

55. Raethjen J, Kopper F, Govindan RB, et al. Two different pathogenetic mechanisms in psychogenic tremor. *Neurology*. 2004;63:812–815.

56. Ramsay RE, Macias FM, Rowan AJ. Diagnosing epilepsy in the elderly. *Int Epilepsy Behav*. 2006; 8:649–650.

57. Rasmussen, 2006.

58. Reid et al., 2003.

59. Rief W, Hiller W, 2003.

60. Rybarczyk et al., 2005.

61. Sadavoy J. Integrated psychotherapy for the elderly. *Can J Psychiatry*. 1994;39:19–26.

62. Saito YA, Petersen GM, Locke GR 3rd, et al. The genetics of irritable bowel syndrome. *Clin Gastroenterol Hepatol*. 2005;3:1057–1065.

63. Salkovskis PM, Rimes KA, Warwick HM, et al. The Health Anxiety Inventory: development and validation of scales for the measurement of health anxiety and hypochondriasis. *Psychol Med*. 2002;32:843–853.

64. Sheehan B, Banerjee S. Review: somatization in the elderly. *Int J Geriatr Psychiatry*. 1999;14:1044–1049.

65. Sheikh RL, Yesavage JA. Geriatric Depression Scale (GDS). Recent evidence and development of a shorter version. *Clin Gerontologist*. 1986;5:165–173.

66. Smith GR. The course of somatization and its effects on utilization of health care resources. *Psychosomatics*. 1994;35:263–267.

67. Spitzer RL, Williams JB, Kroenke K, et al. Utility of a new procedure for diagnosing mental disorders in primary care. The PRIME-MD 1000 study. *JAMA*. 1994;14:1749–1756.

68. Stanley et al., 2003.

69. Stevens JA, Corso PS, Finkelstein EA, et al. The costs of fatal and non-fatal falls among older adults. *Inj Prev.* 2006;12:290–295.

70. Strassnig M, Stowell KR, First MB, et al. General medical and psychiatric perspectives on somatoform disorders: separated by an uncommon language. *Curr Opin Psychiatry.* 2006;19:194–200.

71. Sudarsky L. Psychogenic gait disorders. *Semin Neurol.* 2006;26:351–356.

72. Vuilleumier P. Hysterical conversion and brain function. *Prog Brain Res.* 2005;150:309–329.

73. Vuilleumier P, Chicherio C, Assal F, et al. Functional neuroanatomical correlates of hysterical sensorimotor loss. *Brain.* 2001;124:1077–1090.

74. Zeuner KE, Shoge RO, Goldstein SR, et al. Accelerometry to distinguish psychogenic from essential or parkinsonian tremor. *Neurology.* 2003;61:548–550.

SUGGESTED READING

Alexopoulous GS. Geriatric depression reaches maturity. *Int J Geriatr Psychiatry.* 1992;7:305–362.

American Psychiatric Association. *Diagnostic and Statistical Manual of Mental Disorders.* 4th ed. Washington, DC: American Psychiatric Association; 1994.

American Psychological Association. *What Practitioners Should Know about Working with Older Adults.* Washington, DC: American Psychiatric Association; 1997.

Bassett SS, Folstein MF. Memory complaint, memory performance, and psychiatric diagnosis: a community study. *J Geriatr Psychiatry Neurol.* 1993;6:105–111.

Bortz JJ, O'Brien KP. Psychotherapy with older adults: theoretical issues, empirical findings, and clinical applications. In: Nussbaum PD, ed. *Handbook of neuropsychology and aging.* New York: Plenum Press; 1995.

Conwell Y, Rotenberg M, Caine ED. Completed suicide at age 50 and over. *J Am Geriatr Soc.* 1990;38:640–644.

Engle-Friedman M, Bootzin RR, Hazelwood L, et al. An evaluation of behavioral treatments for insomnia in the older adult. *J Clin Psychol.* 1992;48:77–90.

Evyapan D, Kumral E. Pontine anosognosia for hemiplegia. *Neurology.* 1999;53:647–649.

Friedman L, Bliwise DL, Yesavage JA, et al. A preliminary study comparing sleep restriction and relaxation treatments for insomnia in older adults. *J Gerontol.* 1991;46:P1–P8.

Gaig C, Marti MJ, Tolosa E, et al. 123I-Ioflupane SPECT in the diagnosis of suspected psychogenic Parkinsonism. *Mov Disord.* 2006;21:1994–1998.

Haas LJ, Spendlove DC, Silver MP, et al. Psychopathology and emotional distress among older high-utilizing health maintenance organization patients. *J Geropsychol.* 1999;54A:M577–M582.

Kroenke K, Spitzer RL, deGruy FV, et al. Multisomatoform disorder: an alternative to undifferentiated somatoform disorder for the somatizing patient in primary care. *Arch Gen Psychiatry.* 1997;54:352–358.

Kroenke K, Spitzer RL, deGruy FV, et al. A symptom checklist to screen for somatoform disorders in primary care. *Psychosomatics.* 1998;39:263–272.

LaRue A. *Aging and Neuropsychological Assessment.* New York: Plenum; 1992.

Little JT, Reynolds CF, Dew MA, et al. How common is resistance to treatment in recurrent, nonpsychotic geriatric depression? *Am J Psychiatry.* 1998;155:1035–1038.

Livingston G, Manela M, Katona C. Cost of community care for older people. *Br J Psychiatry.* 1997;171:56–59.

Mendez MF. Huntington's disease: update and review of neuropsychiatric aspects. *Int J Psychiatry Med.* 1994;24:189–208.

Murray CJL, Lopez AD, eds. The global burden of disease and injury series, volume 1: a comprehensive assessment of mortality and disability from diseases, injuries, and risk factors in 1990 and projected to 2020. NIH Publication No. 01-4586. Cambridge, MA: Harvard School of Public Health on behalf of the World Health Organization and the World Bank, Harvard University Press; 1996.

Reynolds CF, Frank E, Perel JM, et al. Nortriptyline and interpersonal psychotherapy as maintenance therapies for recurrent major depression: a randomized controlled trial in patients older than 59 years. *JAMA.* 1999;281:39–45.

Rogers WH, Wells KB, Meredith LS, et al. Outcomes for adult outpatients with depression under prepaid or fee-for-service financing. *Arch Gen Psychiatry.* 1993;50:517–525.

Starkstein SE, Federoff JP, Price TR, et al. Apathy following cerebrovascular lesions. *Stroke.* 1993;24:1625–1630.

Stewart SH, Watt MC. Illness Attitudes Scale dimensions and their associations with anxiety-related constructs in a nonclinical sample. *Behav Res Ther.* 2000;38:83–99.

Stuss DT, Gow CA, Hetherington CR. "No longer Gage": frontal lobe dysfunction and emotional changes. *J Consult Clin Psychol.* 1992;60:349–359.

Waxman HM. Community mental health care for the elderly-a look at the obstacles. *Public Health Rep.* 1986;101:294–300.

Williams DT, Ford B, Fahn S. Phenomenology and psychopathology related to psychogenic movement disorders. *Adv Neurol.* 1995;65:231–257.

Yesavage JA, Brink TL, Rose TL, et al. Development and validation of a geriatric depression scale: a preliminary report. *J Psychiatric Res.* 1983;17:37–49.

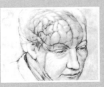

CHAPTER 33

Long-Term Care Options for the Aging

Deborah W. Frazer

THE DEFINITION OF LONG-TERM CARE

Long-term care refers to all residential and health services required to support individuals with chronic disease or disability. In contrast, acute care refers to health services provided for a limited period of time, generally until a specific health condition has resolved. Acute care is usually provided in hospitals or outpatient physician offices. It is generally paid for by private or public health insurance, such as Medicare. Long-term care can be provided in a variety of settings, including nursing homes, assisted living facilities, or private homes. No single payment system is widely used for long-term care.

THE NEED FOR LONG-TERM CARE

The well-documented aging of the U.S. population is attended by two demographic corollaries: dramatic increase in the number of individuals with physical disabilities and those with mental disabilities such as Alzheimer's disease. These impairments are chronic and may be progressive as well.

The number of Americans 65 years of age and older is projected to increase from 12.4% of the population in 2003 to 20% of the population in 2030 (7). Americans 85 years of age and older, who are the heaviest users of long-term care, are the fastest growing segment of the population. The over 85 age group is expected to increase by 43% from 2005 to 2020 (7).

With advancing age comes increased physical frailty and dependence. The average nursing home resident is a woman in her 80s with some cognitive impairment and needing help with four of five activities of daily living (ADL), such as bathing, eating, dressing, transferring, and toileting. Alzheimer's disease and other dementias are associated with increasing age. With the neurologic losses of dementia come further declines in functional abilities. The total number of Americans in need of long-term care is expected to rise from 13 million in 2000 to 27 million in 2050, representing an increase of over 100%. This is largely driven by the increasing number of elderly in need of long-term care, which will rise from 8 million in 2000 to 19 million in 2050, an increase of over 130% (2). With these projections for an aging population with attendant physical and mental disability, it is clear why

health care experts refer to long-term care as "the looming crisis" (1). Federal and state governments are making efforts to educate the public about the need to prepare for long-term care choices and financing, but the complexity and need for individualization of choices makes that effort daunting. As a starting point, physicians and other professionals can refer elders and their families to the Medicare Website on long-term care (www.medicare.gov/LongTermCare/Static/Home.asp). Here, they will find basic information about types of long-term care, as well as general information about choices and finances. An interactive "Long-Term Care Planning Tool" may be an intriguing way for Web-savvy elders and/or their families to begin the discussion. At another government Website (www.longtermcare.gov/LTC/Main_Site/index.aspx), one can order a free "Own Your Own Future Planning Kit." However, these general tools will not solve the specific dilemmas of individual elders and their families. Therefore, it is incumbent upon physicians and other professionals to be generally knowledgeable about long-term care, as well as knowing local opportunities, resources, and options.

A BRIEF HISTORY OF LONG-TERM CARE

What did our grandparents do for long-term care? Why won't that work for us and our patients?

First, our grandparents did not have the same life expectancy. In 1940, the survival rate from age 65 to age 90 was 7%; in the year 2000, that rate has more than tripled to 26% (3). Only recently do most people face the prospect of an extended old age, probably with one or more chronic disabilities.

Second, for those in earlier generations who did live into their seventh, eighth, or ninth decades of life, immediate and extended families were usually available for care giving. In years past, women typically worked at home, providing homemaking and care giving for children, elders, and other dependent family members. With the growth of women in the paid labor force, the increased mobility of U.S. families, and the rising rate of divorce, family-based long-term care has been strained (4).

Third, earlier versions of long-term care did include care sites that are used today, but they have been transformed. Many counties in the United States developed county homes or poor houses for the sick or disabled indigent. Similarly, churches and synagogues sponsored homes for the aged that contained a mix of skilled nursing and personal care services. Although many of these government and faith-sponsored "homes" still exist today, they have undergone radical changes to keep pace with funding and regulatory changes.

The three historical sources of long-term care—family, faith-sponsored, and government—persist today. However, these sources alone are unlikely to be able to meet the rapidly increasing demand for long-term care services in the future.

THE RISE AND FALL OF NURSING HOMES AS THE LONG-TERM CARE SITE OF CHOICE

When the Social Security Act was passed in the 1930s, no agreement existed on a national health care system. In the 1960s, in a partial move toward national health care, Congress passed legislation mandating government sponsorship of Medicare (acute health care for the elderly) and Medicaid (acute health care for the poor). Medicaid dollars (a mix of federal and state monies) also were designated for use by indigent nursing home residents.

The latter usage of Medicaid funds quickly became a major public health care expenditure. Nursing homes, as the only government-paid site for long-term care, grew rapidly. Middle-class families learned to "spend down" an elder's resources to become eligible for an "MA" (Medicaid) bed. The state and federal governments watched with alarm as every bed certified by Medicaid was quickly filled, with no end to demand in sight. A nursing home industry arose, with for-profit and publicly traded companies joining an area previously dominated by faith organizations and county governments. By the 1980s, many states imposed a moratorium on new nursing home bed construction, and a lengthy Certificate of Need process was required to obtain authorization to build new nursing homes. At the same time that demand for publicly funded nursing home beds was skyrocketing, a crisis was looming in the quality of care being provided. A landmark report from the Institute of Medicine in 1985 detailed the ominous conditions that existed in many nursing homes and prompted the Nursing Home Reform Act contained in the Omnibus Budget Reconciliation Acts of 1987, 1989, and 1990. These reforms required greatly increased regulation and monitoring of nursing homes, which, in turn, increased costs.

By the early 1990s, with the demographic press of an aging population and crises in costs and quality in nursing homes, conditions were ripe to develop new alternatives for long-term care.

LOOKING FOR OPTIONS: GROWTH OF THE "CONTINUUM OF CARE"

The term "continuum of care" refers to the expansion of options for elder care sites. Rather than having to choose between "staying in my own home" or "being put in a nursing home," families and providers began to recognize that more options were possible (Table 33-1). Figure 33-1 portrays the relationship of frailty to the options for long-term care.

HOME CARE

A variety of services are now available to support elders in their own homes. These are collectively referred to as Home and Community-Based Services (HCBS). Skilled services are prescribed by a physician and provided by licensed health care professionals. These can include medication monitoring, wound or catheter care, health education for the elder or family member, rehabilitation services, medical social work, nutritional assessment and counseling, and respiratory services.

In addition to these professional services, a variety of home support or homemaker services are available, including help with ADL (e.g., bathing, dressing, eating, toileting) or instrumental activities of daily living (IADL) (e.g., housekeeping, laundry, shopping, transportation). These activities can be performed by home health aides or homemakers who may or may not be state certified. They may work for public agencies, such as an Area Agency on Aging, or a private, for-profit or nonprofit agency. Elders or their families can also hire a home caregiver directly. The range of in-home elder caregivers is analogous to the range of in-home child caregivers, where families are often confused by differing titles (e.g., nanny, mother's helper, sitter), training, certifications, costs, and supervision.

Unlike in-home child care, home care for elders at times is paid for by public funds. Medicare may pay for prescribed care for a limited period of time following a hospitalization. Medicaid, the state program for low-income individuals, will pay for home care in some states under some conditions (e.g., as an alternative to nursing home care). Some long-term care insurance policies pay for some aspects of home care, but coverage varies widely from policy to policy. Frequently, home care is paid for directly by the elder or family. Extensive home care services can cost as much as nursing home charges.

A recent development to help elders pay for care services while remaining in their homes is the reverse mortgage, now available through many banks. Many elders, having been in their homes for decades, find

Table 33-1. *Long-Term Care (LTC) Options: A Summary of Characteristics*

	Home Care	Family Care	Independent Living Community	Assisted-Living Community	Skilled Nursing Home	Continuing Care Retirement Community
Cost	Modest, if covered by insurance; expensive, if not	Modest	Somewhat more than living at home	Expensive; paid privately	Expensive; can be covered by third party	Expensive; paid privately
Health insurance coverage	Yes	No	No	No	Yes, for acute conditions	Yes, but only for acute conditions
Medical coverage	Yes	No	No	No	Yes, for acute conditions	Yes, but only for acute conditions
Medical assistance coverage	Yes	No	No	Experimentally, in one or two states	Yes	Generally not
Long-term care insurance coverage	Usually	No	No	Sometimes	Yes, with limits	Sometimes
Independence	Yes	No	Yes	Yes	No	Usually
Privacy	Yes	No	Usually	Usually	No	Usually
Flexibility to move	Yes	Yes	Yes	Yes	Not usually	Not usually
Lifetime security	No	Yes, if it is working out and resources are available	No	Not usually	Usually	Yes
Extensive nursing care	No	No	No	No	Yes	Yes
Federal regulations	Yes, under Medicare	No	No	No	Yes	Yes
24-hour nursing supervision	No	No	No	A few have	Yes	Yes, in the Healthcare section

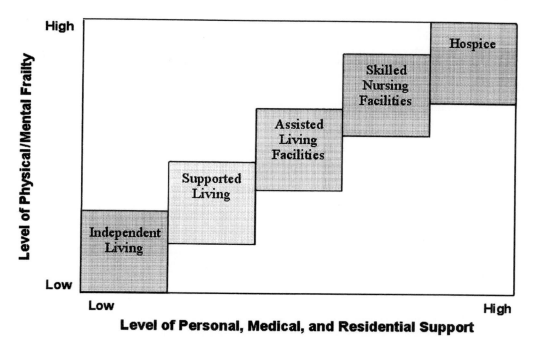

Figure 33-1. Continuum of long-term care.

themselves "house poor" (i.e., living in highly appreciated housing from which they get no financial benefit, yet for which they pay high property taxes). The reverse mortgage is one way to address the needs of elders in this situation. In essence, the bank takes ownership (but not possession) of the elder's home, paying the elder a monthly mortgage fee, and allowing the elder to remain in the home. This boosts the elder's income, thus allowing the elder to benefit from appreciation in the home's value. This solution is attractive to those who wish to stay in their homes but need extra money to pay for services.

Another recent development in home care is the concept of life care at home. Available only in selected geographic areas and paid for privately, this arrangement guarantees an individual or couple lifetime care, as much as possible in the elders' home. Typically, the elders are required to be in good physical and mental condition when entering the program. An entrance fee is charged and monthly fees begin immediately, even though no services may be necessary. Additional fees may be necessary as services are required in later years. Care is coordinated through a care manager, who conducts regular assessments and care plans. In essence, life care at home is a variant of long-term care insurance. Elders often find that it provides peace of mind, and they enjoy the ongoing relationship with the care manager.

Elders and their families must be selective about home care providers. These are people who will be in

the elder's private home, perhaps unsupervised. They may have access to everything from jewelry or cash to bank accounts and credit cards. Frail elders are vulnerable to psychological or physical abuse by caregivers. In the case of an elder who is physically or cognitively impaired, it is especially important to hire and monitor a competent and trustworthy caregiver. Help with referrals and selection is often provided through physicians, social workers, the local Area Agency on Aging, or a private geriatric care manager. Some referral sources, such as the Area Agency on Aging, cannot recommend a specific agency but can delete an agency from their list in cases of significant complaints about an agency.

Physicians can provide a great service to elders and their families by helping them with home care decisions. Having a psychologist, social worker, or geriatric care manager as part of the office team (as staff or consultants) facilitates a seamless referral process for the elder and family and helps the physician attend to the psychosocial aspects of care that are so intertwined with medical conditions. Such ancillary staff or consultants can do the extensive research necessary to identify high-quality local providers of home care services and to match providers with the needs and financial resources of a physician's patients.

The elder and/or family (ideally, in conjunction with a professional) need to consider the following points regarding potential providers: how long they have been in business; how employees are selected, trained, and supervised; how they develop a plan or care; if and how care is documented; fees, billing, and funding sources; emergency procedures; complaint procedures; and references.

FAMILY CARE

Moving in with a sibling, daughter, or son is another variation on home care. The elder leaves his or her own home (and thus realizes the appreciated value of the home) and joins a relative's household. Savings are achieved by combining households, and many of the nonprofessional care services (ADL and IADL) can be provided by family members. Loneliness, a major problem of widowed or homebound elders, is alleviated. The chief disadvantages of this arrangement are loss of independence, autonomy, and privacy for elder and family and the additional caregiver burden that may be placed on family members. To reduce the burden on families, any of the home care services mentioned earlier can also be provided in the family member's home.

Families often quickly move to family care arrangements because of the financial benefits, family tradition, and psychological factors such as love, obligation, or guilt. Although it is a satisfying arrangement for many families, it can very stressful for others. Families should be encouraged to have extensive discussions before reaching a decision, with all members present and perhaps with a physician, social worker, or religious counselor facilitating the discussion. Especially in the case of a caregiving child, discussion should include how other siblings will concretely support the designated caregiving sibling, both emotionally and financially. The caregiving child should not underestimate the stress this arrangement can place on a busy household, especially in cases where a spouse and teenage children are at home. A trial period is strongly advised.

RESPITE CARE

Respite care is the term used for an elder's short-term stay in an institutional setting (nursing home or assisted living) to provide respite for the caregiver. Perhaps the caregiver is a spouse who must have surgery or a middle-aged daughter who wants to vacation with her husband and children. Respite stays, typically 1 to 2 weeks, are paid privately. If taken in a pleasant, well-appointed assisted living facility, it can feel like a vacation for the elder. A nursing home respite stay would only be advisable for someone who needs skilled nursing services while the caregiver is away. Otherwise, it is more likely to feel institutional to the elder.

Some states provide respite care funds to family caregivers, recognizing the significant care giving work that these families are doing and everyone's need for some time away. A local Area Agency on Aging will have information about public respite care funding.

INDEPENDENT LIVING COMMUNITIES

Independent living communities are facilities for older adults who do not need significant medical or personal care support but who wish to live in a community designed for older adults. These are sometimes called "active adult communities" or "retirement communities."

Independent living communities include apartments, condominiums, and single-family housing. They may be urban, suburban, or rural, and communities are available across the economic spectrum. The additional services that a community provides will reflect its location and the socioeconomic status of its members. Among the typical services are security (ranging from a security guard to a "gated" community), organized activities (trips, outings, in-house gatherings, classes, and clubs), exercise opportunities (tennis, golf, exercise equipment, or classes), and meal plans (often consisting of one meal per day in a restaurant-style dining center).

Most independent living communities are rental arrangements, although in some versions, the members purchase their homes. Participation in these communities is typically on a private-pay basis, although some subsidized "senior housing" is available.

It should be noted that many elders enjoy living in unofficial independent living communities; these are usually apartment buildings with a high proportion of elderly residents. In gerontology, these are known as "naturally occurring retirement communities," or NORCs. Residents tend to watch out for each other and provide informal support to those who need temporary or modest amounts of assistance.

Independent living communities are often a transitional phase as elders seek freedom from the burdens of home ownership but do not yet need health or personal care services. It is important to help elders and their families plan beyond this phase—to think through the options should more medical or personal care become necessary.

ADULT DAY CENTERS

Adult day centers provide a service variously referred to as Adult Day Center, Adult Care Center, Adult Day Health Center, or Adult Day Care Center. What all these have in common is that they provide a place for elders to congregate during the day. The hours and services vary widely. All provide at least one meal (lunch), whereas some provide breakfast, snacks, and supper. All provide social and creative activities onsite; some may provide outings and trips offsite as well. A key differentiator is the extent to which the site provides professional health care services, such as skilled nursing, rehabilitation, medical social services, or medication management. Most have a nurse available. Some centers provide personal care, even including showers, nail care, and hairdressing. Many centers provide transportation.

The schedule of hours and days also varies widely, from as few as 4 hours per day to as many as 12 hours per day and from a few days per week to 7 days. Some centers are targeted more to cognitively impaired individuals, whereas others are targeted to individuals with physical challenges.

An adult day center provides a safe, social environment for elders. It can be an excellent adjunct or alternative to in-home care. Family members providing care may want their loved one to attend an outside program, especially if the family member works during the day. If the family member is not working outside the home, the adult day center can provide some hours each week of respite from the demands of care giving. Typically, adult day centers are paid privately, although Medicare or other insurance may pay for some skilled professional services if the individual qualifies for the service.

PACE PROGRAMS

The acronym PACE stands for "Program of All-inclusive Care for the Elderly." At this writing, these programs are federally subsidized demonstration programs that have shown a high degree of success in delivering quality care to frail elders while maintaining them in their home settings at a lower cost to taxpayers than nursing home placement.

The core feature of the PACE program is an adult day center that provides extensive direct services, as well as case management. Every participant enrolled in a PACE program is assigned to a case manager who coordinates all medical and social services, both at the site and at home. The case manager is responsible for cost management as well. The target group for PACE programs includes elders who are frail enough to be nursing home eligible but who wish to be, and can be, maintained at home with extensive and well-coordinated services.

If medical, quality of life, and financial outcomes continue for these programs, it is likely that they will continue to expand, at least in urban low-income areas.

ASSISTED LIVING COMMUNITIES

Assisted living communities vary widely from state to state because they are regulated at the state level (vs. nursing homes, which are regulated at the federal level) (6). In most states, the definition includes a residential facility that provides personal care as needed for ADL and other supportive services (e.g., transportation). Typically, residents do not need extensive skilled medical care for an extended period of time. Some states (e.g., New Jersey and Florida) are permitting higher levels of nursing care to occur in assisted living settings. Many assisted living facilities have special units for individuals with Alzheimer's disease or related dementias. These units are often

"secured" (locked) to prevent harm from wandering. Ideally, they should also provide higher staffing ratios and extensive activity or recreational programming.

The broad concept of assisted living includes group homes, personal care or boarding homes, and sheltered care homes. Sponsors of these facilities include churches, other nonprofit agencies, local governmental agencies, and for-profit companies. Assisted living communities experienced phenomenal growth in the 1990s. Most of the expansion occurred in for-profit chains (perhaps even to the point of overexpansion, as indicated by some Chapter 11 filings). These companies brought in many concepts from the hospitality and hotel industry to serve individuals who formerly were served by the health care sector through nursing homes. Planners are hopeful that the expansion of assisted living choices will encourage individuals and families to use private pay dollars to purchase more consumer-oriented, hospitality residential services when only personal assistance is required. This establishes a continuum, so that nursing homes are used for skilled nursing and medical care, serving a more medically acute population. The assisted living facilities would be primarily paid privately, whereas public funds would be available for skilled nursing home care. Some states are experimenting with some use of public funds to support assisted living.

Monthly fees in assisted living facilities can range from about $1,500 to as much as $6,000, depending on size, location, and the extent of services and amenities. A minimal amount of personal care (1/2 to 1 hour daily) and two meals per day are usually included in a basic fee. More expensive services include continence management, medication management, and full meal service. At the highest end, assisted living communities may provide spa services, private dining facilities, limousine service to cultural events, libraries, and even an "open bar" during cocktail hour. The amount, level, and type of skilled nursing care that is available or permitted varies by state regulation and by facility.

SKILLED NURSING FACILITIES

Skilled nursing facilities (SNFs) are also known as nursing homes or convalescent centers. SNFs provide professional nursing care under the direction of a physician. The medical and nursing care is usually more intense than that provided in an assisted living facility but less than that provided in a hospital. Much of the type of care that was only done in hospitals 10 or 15 years ago is now done in SNFs, such as respiratory and catheter care, intravenous antibiotics, and rehabilitation services. Nursing homes can be used for short-term stays for respite, transitional care between hospital and home, or rehabilitation. They also are used for long-term care, including end-of-life care.

Nursing home costs can range from $4,000 to $8,000 per month. It often comes as a shock to individuals and families that Medicare may not cover these costs. Medical eligibility and financing for SNF care are complicated. For example, shorter stays may be covered by Medicare (for up to 90 days) but only if the individual has a qualifying hospital stay before SNF admission. Private health insurance may cover some or all of a short-term stay. However, neither Medicare nor private health insurance ever covers long-term care. Parts of a long-term stay may be covered by long-term care insurance. Indigent individuals are generally covered, if they meet the eligibility requirements, by the Medical Assistance program. Many people enter nursing homes paying with private funds and then switch to Medical Assistance when their personal funds are depleted. Individuals and their families should seek professional assistance to navigate the complexity of nursing home financing. Hospital social workers, Area Agencies on Aging, eldercare lawyers, and financial planners provide this type of financial counseling.

HOSPICE

Hospice care is reserved for those near the end of life, usually defined as within 6 months. Originally, and most typically, hospice was used for cancer patients. It is also used for patients with terminal acquired immunodeficiency syndrome (AIDS) and various other end-stage diseases. Hospice is provided as a Medicare benefit, under strict regulation. Until recently, it required that patients forego aggressive medical treatment to prolong life in exchange for services designed to improve the quality of the end of life. Such services could be provided at home, in a hospice-specific facility, or within a nursing home. The services usually include home health aides, chaplaincy, social services, professional nursing, and pain management.

Although the number of recipients of hospice care has increased, the average length of stay has declined. This is attributed to physician confusion about the requirements of the program and resulting hesitance to refer to it until an individual is very close to death. The Centers for Medicare and Medicaid Services is now encouraging physicians not to wait until a week or two before death to refer to hospice and is experimenting with allowing access to medical treatments that may slow or even halt their disease (5).

CONTINUING CARE RETIREMENT COMMUNITIES

Continuing care retirement communities (CCRCs) offer the entire continuum of care (independent living, assisted living, and skilled nursing) in one location. They provide companionship and freedom from the burdens of homeownership in the independent living section, accompanied by the security of guaranteed lifetime care, on a financially predictable basis. It is a lifetime contract for a residence, cleaning and maintenance, recreational opportunities, meals, personal care, and skilled nursing care. Thus, CCRCs are the financial equivalent to merging residential costs and long-term care insurance. CCRCs are all privately paid, often requiring a substantial entrance fee (roughly equivalent to the cost of one's house), followed by lifelong monthly fees. They primarily serve middle to upper income individuals and couples.

The CCRCs can have extended waiting lists, sometimes as much as 8 years. They typically require that elders be well enough to enter the independent living section. This extended time in independent living allows people to form important new friendships and explore the recreational and volunteer opportunities that are available. Many older adults report that CCRCs feel something like a college campus, and indeed, some are located adjacent to college campuses.

This type of facility is an option that requires significant advance planning. Because of the legal and financial complexity of the contracts, it is always important to discuss this option (and specific contracts) with a lawyer, accountant, or financial planner.

FACTORS TO CONSIDER WHEN CHOOSING AMONG RESIDENTIAL CARE OPTIONS

Many factors need to be considered when choosing a long-term care option, including preferences of the individual, couple, and family; current and predicted costs; matching care needs to provider capabilities; quality of care; and matching personal lifestyles to the environment of care (Fig. 33-2).

Preferences of the Individual, Couple, and Family

The first and perhaps most important preference is for geographic location. This decision can be complex and raise many sensitive issues in the family. Are mom and dad choosing to be near one child rather than another? Are they going to Florida and expecting all the children to come as needed, despite the children's own family and job responsibilities? Do they really know what it will feel like to leave their friends, community, and house of worship? Are they committing to an irreversible decision? How convenient is the nursing home or assisted living community to the home or workplace of the primary caregiving child? As with any other residential decision, the first thing to consider is location, location, location!

A second and related decision is the decision to "stay in my own home" versus "moving to a new place." Most elders express a wish to "die in my own home"; however, most will, in fact, die in a hospital or SNF. For those who choose to stay in their homes, it is

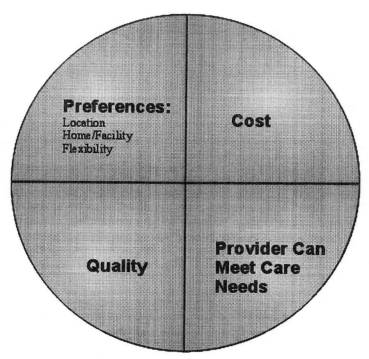

Figure 33-2. Factors to consider when choosing long-term care.

important to go over the costs, the potential burden to children, and the risks of being home alone. Many elders are happy at home until one member of a couple dies, leaving the remaining spouse grieving and lonely. Additionally, in many communities, the ability to drive a car is critical to maintain a comfortable quality of life: How will dad get along when he can no longer drive? On the positive side, staying at home can be the best way to maintain dignity, privacy, and autonomy to the end of life. As always in long-term care, it is critical to discuss—in detail—preferences for end-of-life care with the family physician and to execute the proper living will and durable power of attorney documents to ensure that those preferences are respected. These legal documents can include "do not hospitalize" provisions that make it more likely that the older adult's wishes to "die in my own home" are respected.

As mentioned, it is important when discussing preferences to include the issue of "burden to others." Elders frequently cite that they do not want to be a burden to their children, but if the issues are not discussed openly among all family members, the elder may not understand correctly what feels burdensome to a child and what does not. Likewise, elders typically want to stay as independent as possible but may not fully understand how different decisions would affect independence. Facilitating an open conversation about burden among family members is an excellent contribution the physician, nurse, or social worker can make.

Long-term care facilities and services are provided in the United States by for-profit, not-for-profit, religious, and governmental organizations. Examples are seen of excellent care and poor care in each ownership category, but elders should consider whether type of ownership is an important issue for them.

Finally, elders and their families should determine their preferences for commitment and security versus flexibility. For example, many assisted living facilities operate on a monthly rental agreement, with only 30 days notice required to leave (or to be asked to leave). At the other extreme are CCRCs, which can require more than a $100,000 entrance fee that is not refundable after a 1- or 2-year period. The individual's tolerance for risk or desire for security should be a factor in decision making, as well as the relative predictability of the health or disease status of the person.

Current and Expected Costs

Although no one has a crystal ball, physicians can be of great help to elders and their families in thinking through what future costs might be. For example, if a family member develops Alzheimer's disease at a relatively young age and has no comorbid conditions, the expected length of care giving can exceed 10 years, with the final few years likely to require extensive personal care. Helping the family to envision gradually increasing personal care, at home or in a facility or both, is useful for them. On the other hand, an uncontrolled diabetic with high blood pressure and significant complications of the diabetes is likely to need skilled nursing care within a relatively short time frame but is not likely to need care for the extended years that a well-controlled diabetic might. Having a rough estimate of the length of expected care giving can help families with financial planning.

Understanding the type of care that will likely be needed also helps families with financial planning. If skilled care is likely, as in the case with a diabetic, then it is more likely to be covered by third-party payers, at least for a limited time. If, however, the care is likely to be companion or personal care, it will not be covered except by certain long-term care insurance policies. Encourage families to explore exactly what type of coverage they have and how it may or may not cover the expected care.

If an extended nursing home stay seems likely at some point in the future (even the distant future), the physician should encourage the elder and family to seek legal and financial planning advice about asset management, insurance coverage, and ways to reduce the risk of impoverishment.

Matching Care Need to Provider Capabilities

The most difficult type of long-term care to understand correctly is assisted living. The definition varies so widely that consumers are hard pressed to understand whether this residential option will serve their or their parents' care needs. Consumers need answers to many questions about the facility and assistance provided by personnel, including the following:

Does the facility provide assistance with all ADL?
Is help available for toileting, including an every 2-hour continence management program?
Will they help with transferring from wheelchair to bed?
Will they help with IADL, such as transportation and shopping?
Are persons available to provide safe and professional financial management, such as bill paying and mail management?
Will they supervise medications or actually administer them for a confused elder?
Are the people administering medications and other assistance with health care needs (e.g., insulin shots, eye drops, skin care) licensed and trained to deliver this care?
If an elder should need temporary skilled nursing care, can it be provided within the assisted living facility?
As skilled care needs increase, how would the facility handle it?
At what point do care needs exceed the assisted living facility's ability to meet them?

Quality of Care

Quality of care and maintaining quality of life are difficult to define and measure. Generally, elders and families should look for long-term care that maintains the highest level of independence, dignity, and respect; offers opportunities for intellectual, social, physical, and spiritual stimulation (but also the option to retreat from those); and fosters warm and caring interpersonal relationships among residents and between residents and staff. Happy and satisfied staff who are direct caregivers are often a marker of good-quality care. Asking current residents whether they feel the above criteria are met is a good starting point for assessing quality.

Matching Personal Lifestyle to Environment of Care

In some ways, matching personal lifestyle to care environment is similar to the points raised earlier but is closer to the concept of finding the right match between the personality of the elder and the personality of the environment of care. Has this elder always been reclusive, private, and suspicious or anxious around others? If so, an intensely social environment of care (e.g., a semiprivate room in a skilled nursing center) could be extremely stressful. Has this elder always been an extrovert who loves people, parties, and social occasions? Then being alone in a private home could be extremely stressful.

Another factor in finding the right fit between person and environment is the extent to which an individual only wants to be with others like himself or herself—with shared history, values, interests, food preferences, religious commitments, and so forth. Some elders prefer this type of homogeneous setting, whereas others thrive in a more religiously, culturally, racially, and socioeconomically diverse setting.

The final match characteristic goes back to location, location, location, but in terms of the personality of the location. Thought is especially needed when an elder is moving to be near a caregiving child as to whether the move entails switching from an urban, suburban, or rural setting to a different setting. Equally important are regional differences found among the country's many diverse areas. Deeply ingrained regional styles can cause a distressing feeling of "not fitting in," especially when a frail elder does not have much reserve capacity to learn and adapt the new ways.

CONCLUSION

The United States currently has no system of long-term care. A fragmented patchwork of care is available, which, in some cases, can provide what our elders and families need and can afford. Until a comprehensive, accessible, coordinated system of long-term care is available, it is incumbent on all professionals, and most especially the physicians who are guiding patient care, to understand and help families to understand what options are available to them.

REFERENCES

1. American Health Care Association. *The Looming Crisis: Long Term Health Care*. Washington, DC: American Health Care Association; 2000.
2. Assistant Secretary for Planning and Evaluation, U.S. Department of Health and Human Services. *Report to Congress: The Future Supply of Long-Term Care Workers in Relation to the Aging Baby Boom Generation*. Washington, DC: U.S. Department of Health and Human Services; 2003.
3. Cutler NE. Middle age and long-term care: the two meanings of "middle." Conference presentation, "Long Term Care at the Crossroads," Center for Advocacy for the Rights and Interests of the Elderly. Philadelphia, September 2000.
4. Frazer DW. Family disruption: understanding and treating the effects of dementia onset and nursing home placement. In: Duffy M, ed. *Handbook of counseling and psychotherapy with older adults*. New York: John Wiley & Sons; 1999.
5. Gage B, Miller SC, Mor V, et al. *Synthesis and Analysis of Medicare's Hospice Benefit: Executive Summary and Recommendations*. Washington, DC: Assistant Secretary for Planning and Evaluation, U.S. Department of Health and Human Services; 2000.
6. General Accounting Office. *Assisted Living: Quality-of-Care and Consumer Protection Issues in Four States*. Washington, DC: General Accounting Office; 1999.
7. He W, Sengupta M, Velkoff VA, et al. *U.S. Bureau of the Census, Current Population Reports, P23-29, 65+ in the United States: 2005*. Washington, DC: U.S. Government Printing Office; 2005.

SUGGESTED READINGS

American Association of Homes and Services for the Aging. Choosing a quality nursing home. Washington, DC: American Association of Homes and Services for the Aging; 2000.

American Association of Homes and Services for the Aging. *Continuing Care Retirement Communities: A Guidebook for Consumers*. Washington, DC: American Association of Homes and Services for the Aging Publications.

Centers for Medicare and Medicaid Services, Department of Health and Human Services. *Your Guide to Choosing a Nursing Home*. Washington, DC: Centers for Medicare and Medicaid Services, Department of Health and Human Services; 2004.

WEBSITES

American Association of Homes and Services for the Aging: http://www.aahsa.org/

American Association of Retired Persons: http://www.aarp.org/

Assistant Secretary for Planning and Evaluation: http://aspe.hhs.gov/

Assisted Living Federation of America: http://www.alfa.org

Administration on Aging: http://www.aoa.dhhs.gov/

Center for Medicare and Medicaid Services (formerly HCFA): http://www.cms.hhs.gov/

Family Caregiver Alliance: http://www.caregiver.org

Hospice Foundation of America: http://www.hospicefoundation.org/

Medicare for Consumers: http://www.medicare.gov/

National Alliance for Caregiving: http://www.caregiving.org/

National Clearinghouse for Long-Term Care: http://www.longtermcare.gov/LTC/Main_Site/index.aspx

National Family Caregivers: http://nfcacares.org/

National Hospice and Palliative Care Organization: http://www.nhpco.org/

U.S. Department of Health and Human Services/Healthfinder: http://www.healthfinder.gov/

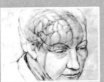

CHAPTER 34

Ethical Legal Issues in the Care of Older Patients with Neurologic Illnesses

Bryan D. James and Jason H.T. Karlawish

The care of elderly patients with neurologic illnesses includes managing a number of medical problems that include substantial ethical and legal issues. These issues are the result of morbidities caused by these illnesses. Neurodegenerative dementias typically impair a patient's ability to make a decision. Other people, such as their caregivers, must decide for them. Other neurologic illnesses such as epilepsy may not primarily affect a patient's cognition, but they do have a significant impact on the patient's ability to perform important tasks such as driving. Finally, in many chronic and progressive illnesses (e.g., amyotrophic lateral sclerosis), cures are not available. Hence, clinicians must have the skills to address matters of death and dying and discuss quality of life.

Unlike the other issues in this book that a physician addresses by applying the principles of medical science, ethical and legal issues require a physician to apply the principles of moral theory. Key principles are respect for autonomy (allowing a competent patient to voluntarily choose care), beneficence (minimizing interventions' risks and maximizing their benefits), and justice (treating equal people in an equal manner). At first inspection, applying these principles may seem to be matters of having a good character and knowing a good lawyer. But, as important as those matters are, a clinician needs to have skills similar to those used to diagnose and treat the diseases that raise these ethical and legal issues. These skills will allow the clinician to identify ethical and legal issues, categorize them, and find efficient ways to address them. The failure to master these skills can have a significant impact on the quality of patient care.

This chapter focuses on five key issues that physicians encounter in the care of elderly patients with neurologic illnesses. These are (a) competency and decision-making capacity; (b) advance care planning; (c) common challenges in end-of-life decision making, including terminal sedation and assisted suicide; (d) driving; and (e) elder abuse. The general structure of this chapter is to address the nature and scope of each issue and provide practical steps to identify and address it.

COMPETENCY AND DECISION-MAKING CAPACITY: THE FOUNDATION OF EFFECTIVE DECISION MAKING

The concepts of *competency and decision-making capacity* are the foundations of effective decision making. A physician should respect the choices made by competent patients and seek out a surrogate to make choices for those who are not competent. These concepts are operationalized in the practice of informed consent. This section presents definitions of the concepts and outlines techniques to assess them and to make decisions when a patient is not competent. It also presents other models for decision making.

SCOPE OF THE PROBLEM

Many neurologic illnesses have an impact on cognition. The neurodegenerative dementias (e.g., Alzheimer's disease) are common causes of impairments. For example, among patients with mild to moderate Alzheimer's disease, fully 95% of them cannot adequately understand the information needed to make a treatment decision (45). This impairment can have a dramatic impact on the patient's ability to make a competent treatment choice.

WHEN SHOULD A PHYSICIAN ASSESS DECISION-MAKING CAPACITY AND COMPETENCY?

All adults are competent until shown otherwise. Several clinical situations are seen when it is prudent to assess a patient's decision-making capacity and competency. In general, these are situations when the patient faces choices that involve significant risks or uncertain benefits or when the patient refuses a low-risk and high-benefit intervention. For example, in the situation of a patient who accepts a low-risk intervention, such as aspirin therapy for a transient ischemic attack, the physician would have little reason to carefully assess the patient's decision-making capacity. In contrast, the use of warfarin for this same problem should warrant a more careful assessment of the patient's decision-making capacity. This should be done regardless of the patient's decision to accept or decline the drug. In all of these conditions, the issue is not that the physician has reversed the assumption that the patient is competent. The issue is assuring that the physician has adequately taught the patient the key facts and engaged in a meaningful dialogue about the pros and cons of the physician's recommendation.

THE CONCEPTS OF COMPETENCY AND DECISION-MAKING CAPACITY

Decision-making capacity and competency are distinct concepts. Decision-making capacity describes a person's ability to understand, appreciate, and rationally manipulate information (4). It is an individual quality akin to qualities such as intelligence, mood, or weight. In this way, decision-making capacity is a quality that can be measured just as intelligence is measured using tools such as the Wechsler Adult Intelligence Scale or weight is measured using a scale calibrated in kilograms. In contrast, competency is a judgment about a person. Competent describes a person whose abilities to understand, appreciate, and rationally manipulate information are adequate to make a choice, given the risks, benefits, and alternatives of the decision (4).

HOW TO ASSESS COMPETENCY AND DECISION-MAKING CAPACITY

To assess decision-making capacity, it is important to assess a patient's ability to understand, appreciate, and rationally manipulate the key information about a decision. Table 34-1 summarizes these abilities, with definitions and standard phrases to assess them. *Understanding* describes a patient's ability to know the meaning of the information. Assess this by asking the patient to say back in his or her own words the information disclosed. For example, ask a patient, "Can you tell me in your own words what are the reasons for having the spinal tap?" Because understanding requires cognitive skills that include short-term memory and language, disease that impairs these cognitive functions can impair a patient's ability to understand.

Appreciation describes a patient's ability to recognize that the information applies to him or her. Assess this by asking the patient to set aside a decision and answer whether the patient thinks the facts apply to him or her. For example, ask a patient, "You may or may not want to have the spinal tap, we'll talk about that more in a minute. For now, I'd like to ask you about the risks and benefits of the procedure. Do you think that the spinal tap can benefit you?" Later, ask the patient, "Do you think that the spinal tap can harm you?" Then, ask a question to assess whether the patient thinks that he or she has the disease or problem under treatment. In all of these questions,

Table 34-1. *The Elements of Decision-Making Capacity—Their Definitions and Standard Ways to Assess Them*

Understanding: the ability to state the meaning of the relevant information (risks, benefits, indications, diagnosis, and options of care).
> *Sample question to assess understanding:* "Can you tell me in your own words what I just said about. . . .?"

Appreciation: the patient's ability to recognize that the information applies to him or her.
> *Sample question to assess appreciation of treatment:* "Regardless of what your choice is, do you think that it is possible the medication can benefit you?" "Regardless of what your choice is, do you think that it is possible the medication can harm you?"
> *Sample question to assess appreciation of diagnosis:* "Can you tell me in your own words what you see as your medical problem?"

Rationally manipulating information: the abilities to compare information and infer consequences of choices.
> *Sample question to assess comparative reasoning:* "How is taking the medicine better than not taking it?"
> *Sample question to assess consequential reasoning:* "How might taking the medicine affect your everyday activities?"

the issue is whether the patient acknowledges that the information applies to him or her personally. Diseases can impair insight and judgment (e.g., a delusional disorder seen in schizophrenia, or Lewy body or frontal dementias) and can impair a patient's ability to appreciate information.

Rationally manipulating information describes two capacities: *comparative* and *consequential reasoning.* Comparative reasoning describes a person's ability to examine options head-to-head. For example, ask the patient, "Can you tell me how not having the spinal tap is better than having it?" Consequential reasoning describes a person's ability to infer outcomes of the various options faced. For example, ask the patient, "What are some ways that having the spinal tap might affect your daily activities?"

The sample questions above are analogous to the questions a physician uses to assess a patient's chief complaint, such as headache or memory loss. In a clinical encounter, the issue of headache is raised. Physicians have concepts they want to assess, such as vascular headache, migraine, and so on. To do this, the physician has a set of well-rehearsed probe questions. Based on the patient's answers to these questions, the physician generates an assessment of the likelihood that the patient's headache is vascular, a migraine, or from some other cause. In the assessment of some complaints (e.g., depression), these questions can be standardized to the degree that they are collected into a scale. For example, the 15- or 30-item Geriatric Depression Scale asks a series of questions such as, "Are you basically satisfied with your life?" (79). The patient's scores on each question are added up to generate an overall score of depressive symptoms. Although a score is not determinative of depression, the greater the patient's score is, the more likely that the patient has depression.

In the case of decision-making capacity, measure the patient's ability to understand, appreciate, and rationally manipulate information. Ask standard questions and then assess the adequacy of the patient's answers. Efforts are made to correct deficiencies. After each answer, score the patient's performance (poor, good, or excellent). The sum of these scores is then used to substantiate an assessment of how well the patient performs on each of the measures of decision-making capacity.

In addition to assessing these capacities, include an assessment of the patient's cognition and affect. These data are particularly useful because they will help to explain why deficits exist in a patient's decision-making capacity. Hence, assessing competency has not only an ethical warrant but also a clinical one. It may be the initial clue that a patient suffers from a clinically significant disorder in affect or cognition.

All adults are competent unless shown otherwise. Use data that describe a patient's decision-making capacity and the risks and benefits of the decision at hand to judge whether the patient is not competent. For example, a patient with mild Alzheimer's disease faces the decision of whether to enroll in a clinical trial. In conversation, a physician may find that the patient appreciates the information and can reason about how the clinical trial will affect daily life but has considerable difficulty understanding all of the information and comparing options. In such a case, the judgment of whether the patient is competent will rely on the degree of the impairments in understanding and comparative reasoning. For example, the patient may not understand that the project is research and includes random assignment to drug or placebo. The physician must judge whether this misunderstanding, in the context of the risks and potential benefits of the research, means that the patient is not competent.

OTHER MODELS FOR DECISION MAKING

Competency and decision-making capacity are foundations of the principle of respect for autonomy. They derive from theories of rational decision making that

are operationalized in the doctrine of informed consent. In other words, they assume that people do and should "weigh the risks and benefits" before making a voluntary decision. Many patients do engage in this kind of decision making, and a physician should regard it as a key model to guide the role of doctor as teacher. However, a physician needs to respect that patients may not adhere to this same model.

Patients use other models for making decisions about clinical care and research. Chief among these models are decisions based on trust in other persons (e.g., family or physician) or trust in institutions (e.g., a university or pharmaceutical company) (24,47). In a trust-based model, the person will cede the task of assessing the information or even making the decision to another person such as a family member or physician. This other person is identified as *entrusted*. Although this model does differ from one that features rationally weighing information, it fits within the principle of respect for autonomy. It is reasonable for a person to cede authority to another, provided that the decision to do so is voluntary and informed.

For a model based on trust to function ethically, the physician needs to recognize factors that can undermine trust. *Conflict of interest*, chief among these factors, is the term that describes a condition of two or more relationships that possess inherently contradictory commitments or obligations. For example, a physician who owns a for-profit testing facility and also prescribes testing at that facility is in a conflict of interest. Such a conflict can undermine or even negate the patient's trust. A physician has an obligation to disclose or even avoid the conflict.

ADVANCE CARE PLANNING

Advance care planning describes a competent person's preferences for future medical care. The physician's role in providing diagnosis and prognosis warrants a role in assisting the patient in this planning. Planning can take two forms: conversations that lead to considered plans or structured documents called "advance directives."

ADVANCE DIRECTIVES

An *advance directive* is a set of instructions indicating a competent person's preferences for future medical care. It is used to guide health care professionals in the event that the person should become unable to communicate personal wishes or incompetent to participate in medical decision making. In general, an advance directive addresses ethically problematic decisions involving life-sustaining treatment for patients who are terminally ill or near death. Advance directives are intended to preserve patient autonomy by ensuring that patients are able to direct their future medical treatment and to help physicians avoid ethical dilemmas in treating incompetent patients.

Two kinds of advance directives exist: a living will and a durable power of attorney (DPA). *Living wills* are documents that instruct physicians proactively regarding the initiation, continuation or discontinuation, or withholding or withdrawal of particular forms of life-sustaining medical treatment (25). A *DPA* for health care is a document that designates a person (also known as an "agent," "surrogate," "proxy," or "attorney-in-fact") to make medical decisions on a person's behalf should that person become unable to do so. A DPA allows for greater flexibility than a living will because the agent can make decisions, should certain circumstances arise. Authorities, such as the American Bar Association, recommend that a patient have both a living will and a DPA (63). Additionally, a patient's oral statements in conversations with relatives, friends, and health care providers are also recognized ethically and, in some states also legally, as advance directives, provided they are properly charted in the medical record. Table 34-2 lists a few good World Wide Web resources for more information on advance directives.

The authority of an advance directive has been tested by court cases including a Supreme Court decision (25). All 50 states and the District of Columbia have laws recognizing the use of advance directives. Each state has a form based on the specifics of its laws. These legally binding documents take effect only when medical decisions must be made and the physician finds that the patient is not capable of making them. In some instances, the physician must also judge that the patient is in a terminal condition. A person can revoke or change the advance directive at any time. A physician who morally objects to a patient's advance directive may choose not to comply but must facilitate the patient's transfer to another physician. The *Patient Self-Determination Act (PSDA)*

Table 34-2. *Web Resources on Advance Directives*

American Association of Retired Persons (AARP)
   http://www.aarp.org/programs/advdir/home.html
Your choice in dying (can download state-
   specific advance directive forms) *http://www.
   yourchoiceindying.com*
Medline Plus: Death and Dying (links to many good
   sites) *http://www.nlm.nih.gov/medlineplus/
   deathanddying.html*
US Living Wills Registry *www.uslivingwillregistry.com*
An organized set of links to living will (advance
   directive) web pages. *http://www.mindspring.com/
   ~scottr/Will.html*

---

is a federal law requiring health care facilities that receive Medicaid and Medicare funds to inform patients of their rights to execute advance directives. The requirements are to ask patients at admission if they have previously executed an advance directive, provide information about advance directives to patients and their proxies, and inform patients of their rights to execute advance directives if they wish (25,65).

Although the law has attempted to make information on advance directives more accessible to patients, few patients actually complete one (20,27,39). Approximately 3% to 14% of the general adult population and 10% to 12% of hospitalized patients and nursing home residents have advance directives (28). Rates of completion are higher among older patients and patients in poorer health than among patients who are relatively young and healthy (29,50). Ethnic and cultural factors can also influence completion rates. Whites and Asians are more likely to complete advance directives than are blacks and Hispanics (51,62,65). Education has also been shown to be an independent predictor of completion (65,67).

A number of factors responsible for the low rate of completion of advance directives have been examined, including misconceptions of the role of clinicians or family members in end-of-life decisions and the perception that directives do not accomplish the goal of patient autonomy (28,69). The latter concern may be justified because physicians are often unaware that a patient has an advance directive (28) or are careless about following a patient's wishes (30). Furthermore, studies suggest that advance directives have little effect on resuscitation decisions (69,70), use of medical treatments in general (28,64), or costs (64,68,69). The ineffectiveness of advance directives is a major problem. If patients are to be encouraged to complete advance directives, they must be respected at the time they are intended to take effect.

Perhaps the greatest barrier to completion or following an advance directive is the lack of physician communication with patients. Although the PSDA mandates that advance directives must be discussed with patients, many physicians express concerns that these discussions take too much time or lead to patient suspicion that maximal care will not be provided (62,65). However, studies have shown that the latter concern may be unwarranted, as most patients surveyed expressed desires to have such discussions (18,40,62). Concerns also exist that living wills are not specific enough to deal with certain clinical questions (19,55,70). A further concern is that an advance directive is ineffectual because physicians may not consider a patient "absolutely, hopelessly ill" during periods of diminished capacity, thus not executing the patient's directive (69). For advance directives to serve their purpose in preserving patient autonomy after losing competency and decreasing problematic clinical decision making, physicians must educate patients about completing directives and attempt to better understand their patient's preferences for the use of life-sustaining treatment.

PHYSICIAN-PATIENT COMMUNICATION ABOUT ADVANCE CARE

Documents that describe advance care plans are only as useful as the degree to which the people who will use them understand, appreciate, and reason through what the document says. In short, the documents do not obviate the need for communication between physicians and patients about patient values and goals. Such communication can occur during the physician-patient conversation about treatment decisions. If a patient has a serious chronic illness (e.g., amyotrophic lateral sclerosis), the physician should obtain explicit instructions about treatments that are likely to be needed in the future (21). Aside from such likely scenarios, the focus of advance care communication should not simply be specific treatment decisions. In advance care conversations, physicians often discuss the easiest scenarios; few patients would wish to be kept alive if they were permanently unconscious with no hope of recovery, whereas most patients would desire aggressive treatment in a reversible situation (73). But such conversation will not be useful when more complex end-of-life decisions arise.

To adequately assure that the physician's future actions respect the patient's autonomy, advance care conversations must go beyond preferences for specific treatment options and elicit the patient's deeper values and goals. Patients asked about their goals for advance care planning list influencing what interventions are done to them as only one of their goals. They also identify the goals of preparing for death, gaining a sense of control, strengthening relationships, and relieving burdens on others (46,66). Once the patient's values and goals are clarified, specific decisions can be easier to make. It is important for the physician not to hide behind technical aspects and avoid eliciting the patient's emotions. Patients' emotions and concerns are important when exploring their goals.

How can physicians explore patients' goals? The same technique they use in everyday clinical encounters can facilitate discussions about future care. In particular, open-ended questions and follow-up questions that incorporate the patient's own words are listed in Table 34-3 (21,41).

Four important points can guide the physician-patient discussion. First, explicitly ask the patient about uncertainty. Patients often state that they would

only want life-sustaining treatment if it will help them. This attitude is completely rational but does not take into account the reality that physicians are often uncertain about the outcome. Patients should be asked about such situations with questions such as, "What if we are not sure whether we will be able to get you off the breathing machine?" (21). Second, ask whether reversibility of the condition would alter the patient's views. For example, if the patient states that he or she would never want to be placed on a ventilator, ask, "What if we could get you off in a short period of time?" (21). Also ask whether the patient would want any treatment at all in "states worse than death" (21). Controversial treatments such as artificial nutrition and hydration should be discussed here. Third, clarify what the patient means when using potentially vague and loaded terms such as "vegetable" or "quality of life" (21). Finally, it is important to make sure throughout advance care planning that you and your patient are communicating effectively. Do not dominate the conversation; spend as much time listening as talking. In short, many of the same principles described earlier in the section on assessing competency and decision-making capacity apply here. The principle to good communication is "ensuring that the patient *understands* the implications of his or her stated preferences and that the doctor *understands* the patient's values (emphasis ours)" (21). Do everything possible to establish trust that everything possible will be done to meet the patient's goals and continue to respect the patient's autonomy.

Table 34-3. *Useful Questions to Prompt a Discussion about End-of-Life Care*

[a]1. What concerns you most about your illness?
[a]2. How is treatment going for you (your family)?
[a]3. As you think about your illness, what is the best and the worst that might happen?
[a]4. What has been most difficult about this illness for you?
[a]5. What are your hopes (your expectations, your fears) for the future?
[a]6. As you think about the future, what is most important to you (what matters most to you)?
[b]7. Are there any situations in which you would not think life was worth living?
[b]8. What makes life worth living?

[a]Lo B, Quill T, Tulsky J. Discussing palliative care with patients. *Ann Intern Med.* 1999;130:744–749, with permission.
[b]Fischer GS, Arnold RM, Tulsky JA. Talking to the older adult about advance directives. *Clin Geriatr Med.* 2000;16:239–254, with permission.

Advance care planning is extremely important in the goal to respect the patient's autonomy and control over his or her future care. Studies have shown that most patients with chronic and fatal disease can express their preferences for life-extending or ameliorative care, and for most of these patients, these preferences remained stable over the course of their disease (1). Education and advance care planning can give patients self-control over their future care should they no longer be able to express these preferences. This is particularly important because medical decisions are not simply driven by patient preferences but also by the preferences of their health care providers and the options available from the system in which they receive care (57). Hence, the physician must proactively elicit the patient's values.

COMMON CHALLENGES IN END-OF-LIFE DECISION MAKING

Discussions with patients and their families can be high-octane, emotionally charged events that address deeply personal issues and values. The steps and questions described earlier are designed to provide the physician with structure so that the conversations reach a conclusion and have focus. In the course of these conversations, ethically charged concepts and judgments may be used. These include distinctions between *withdrawing* versus *withholding* treatment, *extraordinary* versus *ordinary* treatment, requests for physician-assisted suicide or terminal sedation, and surrogate decision making. It is important for physicians to know where medical ethics and the law stand on these potentially controversial topics.

WITHDRAWING VERSUS WITHHOLDING TREATMENT

Physicians will often face the decision to withhold or withdraw treatment from a patient at the end of life. Many physicians feel justified in withholding treatments they have never started but have reservations about withdrawing treatments they have already initiated. The withholding or withdrawing distinction draws heavily on the distinction between omission (not performing an action) and commission (performing an action) (7). Not starting a procedure can be seen as abstaining from subjecting the patient to an overly invasive intervention. On the other hand, withdrawing a treatment that has already been started can be psychologically difficult, and this discomfort stems mostly from a sense of responsibility for action to bring about the patient's death. The act of withdrawing can also be seen as an act of abandonment or breach of expectations or

promises. Although such a distinction is psychologically understandable, moral philosophers and the law view the distinction between withdrawing and withholding as untenable (6,7,49).

In the first place, the distinction between withholding as an omission and withdrawing as a commission is ambiguous. Withdrawing can happen through an omission such as not putting the infusion into a feeding tube, and withholding the next stage of treatment can be viewed as stopping treatment (i.e., withdrawing) (6). More importantly, both starting and stopping treatment can be justified, depending on the circumstances; both can *cause* the death of a patient, and both can *allow* the patient to die.

Crimes and moral wrongs can be committed by both omission and commission. The morality and legality do not and should not rest on the distinction, but rather on the obligation the physician has to act in accordance with the patient's interests and wishes in the particular situation (6). Adherence to the distinction can have unfortunate influences on patient care. It can lead to *overtreatment* when treatment is continued past the point where it is beneficial or desirable to the patient, and it can lead to *undertreatment* if patients and families worry about being trapped by treatment that once begun cannot be stopped (49). Therefore, the distinction is morally suspect and can cause dangerous situations for patients. Treatment can always be permissibly withdrawn if it can be permissibly withheld.

ORDINARY VERSUS EXTRAORDINARY TREATMENT

Another distinction that has been invoked in care for patients at the end of life is that of ordinary versus extraordinary treatment. This distinction has its origins in Catholic moral theology and has become a widely used tenet in medical decision making (6,7,49). The historical rule has been that ordinary treatments cannot legitimately be forgone, whereas extraordinary treatments can. Patient refusal of ordinary treatment has long been considered suicide, whereas refusal of extraordinary treatments has been accepted. In the same manner, physicians and families do not commit homicide by withdrawing or withholding extraordinary treatment. However, the main problem with this distinction is that no clear definition of the two terms is available, and no meaningful difference is seen between them.

Ordinary has often been taken to mean "usual" or "customary," and extraordinary has been seen as meaning "unusual" or "uncustomary." This interpretation is difficult to apply in an age where the standard of care is constantly and rapidly changing. Furthermore, the customary treatment for a disease may not be appropriate for every patient. Whether the customary means of treatment should be applied depends on the particular patient's wishes and conditions as a whole (6,49). Other proposed criteria for the distinction include whether the treatment is simple or complex, natural or artificial, noninvasive or highly invasive, inexpensive or expensive, and routine or heroic (6). These criteria are highly subjective, and they also do not capture certain deeper moral considerations. For example, if a complex treatment is available and in accordance with the patient's wishes and interests, why should it be morally distinguished from a simple treatment?

The distinction between ordinary versus extraordinary treatment misses the morally relevant issue in medical decision making, which is the balance of benefits and burdens of any particular treatment when applied to a particular patient in a particular case. All treatments in any of the above scenarios can be beneficial or burdensome, depending on the particulars. Thus, the distinction between ordinary and extraordinary collapses into the balance between benefits and burdens for the patient (6,7,49). This should be the focus of discussion with patients or their surrogates, using the steps and techniques described in the previous two sections.

PHYSICIAN-ASSISTED SUICIDE AND TERMINAL SEDATION

Strong arguments occur on both sides of the controversial debates over physician-assisted suicide and terminal sedation. Assisted suicide is "the practice of providing a competent patient with a prescription for medication for the patient to use with the primary intention of ending his or her own life" (48). Oregon is the only state in the nation to have legalized this practice. In the first year of implementation, 23 persons received prescriptions for lethal medications, and 15 of them died after taking the medications (11). In contrast, terminal sedation is within the law of all states (76,77). The term terminal sedation describes "the use of high doses of sedatives to relieve extremes of physical distress" (58). The focus of this section is on how to discuss these options for palliative care with the patient. Other references provide the techniques to perform these practices (58).

A discussion begins when the physician and the patient or surrogate accept that the patient is terminally ill. In providing assisted suicide, the patient must also possess decision-making capacity sufficient to be competent. A desire to escape interminable suffering is not necessarily irrational, and thus, the traditional medical view that the desire to end one's life is a sign of depression must be carefully examined in these circumstances (72). The elements of informed consent must be present according to the steps described

in the first section of this chapter. Assess that the decision maker understands, appreciates, and reasons through the risks, benefits, and likely outcomes of assisted suicide, terminal sedation, and alternatives such as palliative care and voluntary cessation of eating and drinking (72). It is expected that these are emotional discussions.

Tulsky et al. (72) describe useful phrases and probes to structure these discussions. Attend to the emotions of the patient and family through emphatic listening and asking appropriate open-ended questions. The emotions and values of the patient are very important because the core issue is deep suffering. Allow patients to share their thoughts and feelings fully. When a patient seems to be asking for assistance in dying, it is appropriate to address the request directly. For example, "I hear you saying that you might consider hastening your death. How were you hoping that I might be able to help you?" If the patient is more vague about the request, a response might be, "You've referred several times to wishing it were all over. Although you haven't quite said it, it sounds like you're thinking that there are alternatives to dying naturally. Can you share with me what you're thinking in that regard?" All alternatives to suicide such as palliative treatment and what can be reasonably expected from it should be discussed.

If the patient continues to request assisted suicide, physicians must assess their own values and beliefs about this practice. Physicians who are willing to participate may respond, "As you know, the law allows me to prescribe medications that you could use to end your life. There are situations in which I may be willing to do this to relieve your suffering. Let's talk more about this option." Physicians who are not willing to participate must let the patient know that the law allows such an option but they are personally unable to participate.

If a physician is comfortable in providing terminal sedation or cessation of eating and drinking, he or she can raise these options, which are legal even in states where assisted suicide is illegal. If a physician considers all such activities unacceptable, a response could be, "My own conscience does not allow me to do that. I am sure that other physicians in our community would consider that possibility with you." A physician who is not willing to participate in assisted suicide must avoid any sense of abandonment.

SURROGATE DECISION MAKING

A patient may not possess adequate decision-making capacity to participate in an informed consent or advance care planning. This is especially likely at the end of life when conditions such as delirium can impair cognitive function and is certainly common in the care of patients with neurodegenerative dementias. In these instances, the physician needs to turn to others known as *surrogates*. In general, surrogates are family members who have either acted informally as decision makers or are authorized in a DPA. Many of the same steps and techniques described earlier for assessing decision-making capacity and discussing end-of-life care apply to surrogates as they do to patients. However, some unique issues are seen.

When deciding for others, the patient's preferences, to the extent that they are known, and the patient's dignity and quality of life should guide the surrogate in making decisions. Using patient preferences is called a "substituted judgment." However, in many cases, preferences are unknown or, because of significant changes in the patient's health and well-being, they are not relevant to the decision at hand. In these circumstances, the focus is on the patient's dignity and quality of life; in other words, the patient's best interests (36).

An additional challenge of surrogate decision making is that the surrogate often has other roles, such as being the patient's caregiver, and has values and emotions that can influence decision making. These roles, values, and emotions have two implications. First, the surrogate may have an understanding of the patient's illness that significantly differs from the physician's understanding. To practice effective decision making, the physician needs to know this understanding. Before a decision is made, the physician should prompt the surrogate to narrate how he or she understands the patient's current situation. A useful open-ended question is, "I know I've cared for your Mom for many years, but a lot has happened. What's your understanding of how she got to this point and what's wrong?" The second implication of these roles, values, and emotions is that a caregiver's distress (or burden) and depression can have an impact on how that person assesses the patient's quality of life (42) and the value placed on disease course extension (35). Hence, screen the surrogate for distress and depression and, when appropriate, address these issues.

DRIVING LIMITATION AND CESSATION

The assessment of the older adult's ability to drive safely is an important issue for neurologists because many neurologic illnesses lead to an increased likelihood of sensory, motor, and cognitive deficits that can have an impact on the ability to drive. Although the law recognizes driving as a privilege and not a right, the ability to drive is an expression of liberty and independence and provides a sense of self-esteem and control over one's everyday life. Most older Americans rely on the automobile as their primary means of transportation (32). Driving cessation often leads to decreased quality

of life, loss of control, increased loneliness and isolation, and depression (44). However, physicians do have a duty to protect their patients' lives and maintain public safety. A physician must balance the autonomy and quality of life of their patient with the safety of their patient and society. Hence, a recommendation to limit or cease driving should be based on relevant criteria such as tests of functional competency.

As the population of Western countries ages, the percentage of older drivers is increasing (9,53). Although older adults drive less than younger adults and, thus, account for fewer crashes, they are involved in a disproportionate number of crashes per mile driven (32,53,78). Additionally, older drivers suffer higher rates of injury and fatality in a crash than other age groups because of increasing fragility (56).

Many relevant factors lead to this increased accident rate for older drivers, including an increased likelihood of visual and hearing deficits, as well as declines in motor and cognitive functions (13,15,23,26,44,52, 56,59–61,74). Many central nervous system–active medications commonly used by the elderly can affect driving ability (9,56). Coexisting medical conditions prevalent in the elderly (e.g., seizure disorders, stroke, dementia, or Parkinson's disease) can also affect driving ability (9,10,52,61).

The condition that has received the most attention in studies of decreased driving ability in the elderly is dementia. Dementing illnesses can result in cognitive and behavioral changes that can impair the ability to drive. These changes include memory problems, visuospatial deficits, increased reaction time, impaired judgment, and attentional deficits (15). Most notably, selective attention and perceptual-motor reaction time have been shown to lead to mistakes at intersections, at traffic signals, or in changing lanes (15). Of note, however, although drivers with later stages of Alzheimer's disease may pose a significant safety problem (43), drivers with early dementia display driving impairment comparable to that tolerated in other segments of the driving population (16,17,31). Competency to drive is an expression of particular functional abilities and cannot be inferred automatically from a diagnosis of dementia (15,16,22,54,71).

Physicians cannot rely on age and diagnoses alone to assess a patient's ability to drive. Instead, they must assess the patient's driving history, specific functional abilities, and the significant risk factors listed earlier in making this determination. First, a history focusing on the driving task should be obtained from knowledgeable informants such as caregivers, family, or friends. The history should focus on new problems with driving such as "accidents, violations, near-misses, failure to yield, driving too slow, and routinely getting lost" (10,15,54). Also, recognize environmental factors that relate to injury risk such as driving frequency, distance, and patterns (difficult areas, congested hours, and nighttime are especially dangerous) and the type of vehicle driven (10,56). To assess functional status, a focus on new activities of daily living (ADL) dependencies can reveal a breakdown in skills that had been overlearned and intact. These dependencies can reflect a decline in several areas of cognition and are more important than memory loss as indirect evidence for impaired driving skills (10,54). The Mini-Mental Status Examination can also be indirect evidence if it reveals deficiencies in visuospatial skills and attention (10,26,44,54,56). Tests of the driver's vision and motor function may reveal potential problems with the driving task (56). If the patient has any medical conditions or is on any medications that can affect driving ability, be aware of the potential for driving safety problems and, at the very least, bring these to the attention of the driver. Alcohol use is, of course, another significant risk factor and should be assessed.

If the presence of a driving-impaired condition is confirmed, perform another level of assessment to determine the patient's ability to drive. Gather more information about the condition or refer the patient to other professionals who can better determine the patient's ability to drive (56). Occupational therapists can perform formal driving screens that include tests of perception, cognition, reaction time, and on-the-road evaluation (10,54,56). Furthermore, many states have laws requiring physicians to report patients with certain medical conditions that can impair driving ability to the department of transportation (56). An extreme example is a California law requiring that all cases of dementia be reported (8). Physicians should be familiar with their state's laws on reporting, some of which are listed in Table 34-4. If reported, the patient will participate in a more complete evaluation.

There are a number of ways to manage a patient's impaired ability to drive. Driving cessation is not the only option and should only be considered for patients with significant and unmanageable impairments. The first step is to eliminate the conditions responsible for problems with driving, whether this be reducing medications, eliminating alcohol consumption, managing medical problems, or maximizing vision and hearing (54). Environmental and behavioral patterns may also need to be changed, such as limiting driving frequency, driving on slower roadways, daytime driving, adapting the vehicle, or using another passenger as a navigator, depending on the specific problem (10,54). Viable alternatives to driving (e.g., public transportation services) should also be discussed. The physician's decision to stop or restrict driving should be discussed openly with the patient and caregiver and appropriately documented.

Table 34-4. *Reporting Requirements by State*

States that **require** physicians to report health conditions that are hazardous to driving to licensing agencies:
> Pennsylvania, New Jersey, Delaware, Georgia, Nevada, Oregon, California (requires reporting of dementia)

Immunity: In all seven states, reporting physicians have immunity from litigation.

States that **permit** physician reporting:
> Connecticut, Florida, Illinois, Maryland, Minnesota, Oklahoma, Rhode Island, Utah, North Dakota, Ohio

Immunity: All states *except* North Dakota and Ohio grant immunity to reporting physicians.

Other jurisdictions allow physician reporting only after the patient has refused to report himself or herself.

From National Highway Traffic Administration. *Safe Mobility for Older People Notebook.* Washington, DC: US Department of Transportation; 1999.

ELDER ABUSE

Elder abuse, first described in the medical literature in 1975, is a recent domestic violence issue to gain public attention (37,38). Between 1 and 2 million, or 10%, of Americans over 65 years of age are the victims of abuse every year. Among these, nearly half (4%) may be victims of moderate to severe abuse (14,37). This represents an increase of about 100,000 cases per year since 1981 (14). Furthermore, this abuse is frequent and recurring in up to 80% of cases (14). Unfortunately, only one of 14 cases of elder abuse is reported (5,33). These figures indicate that elder abuse is a significant threat to the health and well-being of elderly Americans and that physicians need to have the skills to identify, report, and intervene in situations of elder abuse. It is particularly important that physicians have these skills because most elderly persons are likely to have some encounter with a physician and most states require reporting of suspected abuse.

The increase in the prevalence of elder abuse has been attributed to a number of factors, most notably the vast growth of the elderly population (37), a longer life expectancy, and a change in family structure (14). Despite this increase in prevalence, abuse of the elderly is difficult to quantify because of the many barriers to its identification and reporting. Both the victim and the abuser tend to downplay the seriousness of the abuse, and health professionals often do not accurately diagnose abuse because of disbelief, fear of accusation, or lack of awareness of the extent of the problem (14). One of the largest obstacles to reliable research on the issue is the variation in terminology and lack of one accepted definition of elder abuse.

A review of 21 studies on elder abuse found 34 terms to describe elderly abuse (37). This variation has made it difficult to compare and compile the data from different studies. However, all discussions of elder abuse share certain key elements and general descriptions of abuse types. The definition of elder abuse according to the American Medical Association (AMA) is "an act or omission which results in harm or threatened harm to the health and welfare of an elderly person" (3). Most authors accept four basic categories of such acts or omissions. *Physical abuse* includes hitting, grabbing, pushing, and other acts that cause bodily injury. Some physical abuse definitions include sexual abuse and nonconsensual intimate contact, but some authors list this as a separate category. *Psychological abuse*, also called "emotional and verbal abuse," includes verbal and nonverbal insults, humiliation, infantilization, and threats (37). Financial or material abuse includes theft, misappropriation of funds, and coercion (changing a will or deed) (37). Neglect is the failure of the caregiver to provide appropriate care, usually in assistance with ADL (37). Other recognized categories are self-neglect, which is conducted by the patient who threatens his or her own health or safety (37); violation of personal rights (34); abandonment (2); and even miscellaneous (37). A consensus on definitions and terms is needed to compare studies and findings.

Most risk factors for elder abuse deal with the social environment that the elder and abusive caregiver are placed within, such as stress, isolation, a family history of violence, and especially dependency. The dependence of the caregiver on the elder for financial and emotional support and the dependency of the elder on the caregiver for functional help with daily living are major sources of tension. Caregivers who are psychologically and emotionally unstable and abusing substances are at high risk of abusing those in their care.

The detection and assessment of elder abuse are difficult because, unlike most medical problems, patients and their caregivers are unlikely to report the problem spontaneously (14). The AMA recommends that physicians routinely ask geriatric patients about abuse, even if signs are absent (5). To identify abuse, look for certain observations that are indicative of abuse. These include delays between an injury or illness and the seeking of medical attention, frequent visits to the emergency room (despite a health plan), and presentation of a functionally impaired patient without a caregiver (38). If a screen suggests abuse, this should be followed by a detailed history. Both the patient and caregiver should be interviewed together and separately. Hence, these questions can be integrated into a routine clinical encounter where a portion of the time is spent with the patient alone. Questions to elicit information about abuse include: "Are you afraid of anyone at home?" "Has anyone tried to harm you in any way?" "Have you been forced to use your money in a way you didn't want to?" (37).

It is important that these interviews avoid confrontation and express empathy and understanding (37,38). Physicians need to have easily applicable skills to assess for caregiver stress, a common risk factor for abuse. A useful method is to ask about the presence of potentially stressful events (e.g., whether a patient with dementia repeats the same question over and over again). If this screen shows that the event occurs, the appropriate follow-up question is to determine how much distress the event causes. For example, "How bothersome is that?" The more bother that the caregiver reports for these events, the more stress he or she is experiencing. This assessment should be accompanied with a screen for depressive symptoms because clear links are seen between the distress (or burden) of care giving and the incidence and severity of depressive symptoms (12,75).

A physical examination may reveal injury indicative of abuse (37,38). If possible, a home assessment by a health professional can uncover important indicators of abuse (14). Finally, a physician should be familiar with the patient's social and financial resources, which can help in identifying a source of stress and conflict, suggest possible exploitation, and is important if an intervention is needed (38).

If abuse is confirmed, the physician must intervene to stop the abusive situation. Physicians must know their state's laws on reporting elder abuse. Every state has such laws, and 46 states as well as the District of Columbia require mandatory reporting of abuse. Colorado, New York, Wisconsin, and Illinois have voluntary reporting laws (34). The goal of intervention is to provide the patient with a more enjoyable and fulfilling life (37). This is accomplished by ensuring the safety of the elderly patient while respecting the patient's autonomy (37,38). The focus should be preservation of the family and not the *rescue* of victims (37). Ideally, a multidisciplinary team of caretakers from the medical, social service, mental health, and legal professions should be utilized (14). Interventions should be tailored to the specific situation. If the elderly person is in immediate danger, hospitalization may be justified (37,38). If a high burden of chronic disease is the cause of stress for the caregiver, home care or respite services may be appropriate (38). If psychopathologic factors in the abuser are the cause of the problem, alternative living arrangements should be considered (38). Supportive counseling and psychotherapy may be necessary for the abusive caregiver (14). When a competent patient insists on remaining in the abusive environment, the physician should emphasize the patient's other options and offer whatever interventions the patient will accept. For noncompetent patients, the court may need to appoint a guardian or conservator. If interventions do not stop the abuse, long-term care may be necessary.

CONCLUSION

The care of elderly patients with neurologic illnesses includes managing a number of medical problems that have substantial ethical and legal issues. This chapter focused on common issues that arise in the course of the doctor-patient relationship. In this intimate and largely private relationship, the physician has substantial power and responsibility. The steps and techniques described in this chapter allow a physician to properly exercise this power and responsibility. Specifically, they place the principles of beneficence, respect for autonomy, and justice in balance. This is especially important when addressing tough issues such as withdrawing treatment, providing terminal sedation, or reporting a case of elder abuse or driving impairment. The goal of this chapter is not to proscribe outcomes but to define methods so that all affected can accept the outcome and the process that led to the outcome.

REFERENCES

1. Albert SM, Murphy PL, Bene MLD, et al. A prospective study of preferences and actual treatment choices in ALS. *Neurology*. 1999;53:278–283.
2. American College of Physicians. Management of elder abuse and neglect. *Ann Emerg Med*. 1998; 31:149–150.
3. American Medical Association. *Model Elderly Abuse Reporting Act*. Chicago: American Medical Association; 1985.
4. Appelbaum PS, Grisso T. Assessing patients' capacities to consent to treatment. *N Engl J Med*. 1988;319:1635–1638.
5. Aravanis S, Adelman R, Breckman R, et al. *Diagnostic and Treatment Guidelines on Elder Abuse and Neglect*. Chicago: American Medical Association; 1992.
6. Beauchamp TL, Childress JF. *Principles of Biomedical Ethics*. 4th ed. New York: Oxford University Press; 1994.
7. Bok S. Death and dying: euthanasia and sustaining life: ethical views. In: Reich WT, ed. *Encyclopedia of bioethics*. Vol. I. New York: Free Press; 1978: 268–278.
8. California Health & Safety Code § 103900 (West, 2000)
9. Carr D. The older adult driver. *Am Fam Physician*. 2000;61:141–146, 148.
10. Carr D, Schmader K, Bergman C, et al. A multidisciplinary approach in the evaluation of demented drivers referred to geriatric assessment centers. *J Am Geriatr Soc*. 1991;39:1132–1136.
11. Chin AE, Hedberg K, Higginson GK, et al. Legalized physician-assisted suicide in Oregon. The first year's experience. *N Engl J Med*. 1999;340:577–583.
12. Clyburn LD, Stones MJ, Hadjistavropoulos T, et al. Predicting caregiver burden and depression in Alzheimer's disease. *J Gerontol B Psychol Sci Soc Sci*. 2000;55B:S2–S13.
13. Colsher PL, Wallace RB. Geriatric assessment and driver functioning. *Clin Geriatr Med*. 1993; 9:365–375.
14. Council on Scientific Affairs. Elder abuse and neglect. *JAMA*. 1987;257:966–971.
15. Donnelly RE, Karlinsky H. The impact of Alzheimer's disease on driving ability: a review. *J Geriatr Psychiatry Neurol*. 1990;3:67–72.
16. Drachman DA, Swearer JM. Driving and Alzheimer's disease: the risk of crashes. *Neurology*. 1993;43:2448–2456.
17. Dubinsky RM, Stein AC, Lyons K. Practice parameter: risk of driving and Alzheimer's disease (an evidence-based review). *Neurology*. 2000;54: 2205–2211.
18. Edinger W, Smucker D. Outpatient's attitudes regarding advance directives. *J Fam Pract*. 1992;35:650–653.
19. Eisendrath S, Jonsen A. The living will: help or hindrance? *JAMA*. 1983;249:2054–2058.
20. Emanuel L, Barry M, Stoeckle J, et al. Advance directives for medical care: a case for greater use. *N Engl J Med*. 1991;324:889–895.
21. Fischer GS, Arnold RM, Tulsky JA. Talking to the older adult about advance directives. *Clin Geriatr Med*. 2000;16:239–254.
22. Fitten LJ, Perryman KM, Wilkinson CJ, et al. Alzheimer's and vascular dementias and driving. *JAMA*. 1995;273:1360–1365.
23. Foley DJ, Wallace RB, Eberhard J. Risk factors for motor vehicle crashes among older drivers in rural community. *J Am Geriatr Soc*. 1995;43: 776–781.
24. Fost NC. A surrogate system for informed consent. *JAMA*. 1975;233:800–803.
25. Furrow BR, Johnson SH, Jost TS, et al. *Health Law. Cases, Materials, and Problems*. American Casebook Series. St. Paul: West Publishing Co.; 1991.
26. Gallo JJ, Rebok GW, Lesikar SE. The driving habits of adults aged 60 years and older. *J Am Geriatr Soc*. 1999;47:335–341.
27. Gamble E, McDonald P, Lichstein P. Knowledge, attitudes and behavior of elderly persons regarding

living wills. *Arch Intern Med.* 1991;151: 277–280.

28. Goodman M, Tarnoff M, Slotman GJ. Effect of advance directives on the management of elderly critically ill patients. *Crit Care Med.* 1998;26: 701–704.

29. Gordon NP, Shade SB. Advance directives are more likely among seniors asked about end-of-life preferences. *Arch Intern Med.* 1999;159: 701–704.

30. Gregor J, Dunn D. Implementation of the Patient Self-Determination Act in a community hospital. *N Engl J Med.* 1995;92:438–442.

31. Hunt L, Morris JC, Edwards D, et al. Driving performance in persons with mild senile dementia of the Alzheimer's type. *J Am Geriatr Soc.* 1993;41:747–753.

32. Jette AM, Branch LG. A ten-year follow-up of driving patterns among the community-dwelling elders. *Hum Factors.* 1992;34:25–31.

33. Jones J, Dougherty J, Scheble D, et al. Emergency department protocol for the diagnosis and evaluation of geriatric abuse. *Ann Emerg Med.* 1988;17: 1006–1015.

34. Jones JS, Veenstra TR, Seamon JP, et al. Elder mistreatment: national survey of emergency physicians. *Ann Emerg Med.* 1997;30:473–479.

35. Karlawish JHT, Klocinski J, Merz JF, et al. Caregivers' preferences for the treatment of patients with Alzheimer's disease. *Neurology.* 2000;55:1008–1014.

36. Karlawish JHT, Quill T, Meier DE. A consensus-based approach to practicing palliative care for patients who lack decision-making capacity. *Ann Intern Med.* 1999;130:835–840.

37. Kleinschmidt KC. Elder abuse: a review. *Ann Emerg Med.* 1997;30:463–472.

38. Lachs MS, Pillemer K. Abuse and neglect of elderly persons. *N Engl J Med.* 1995;332: 437–443.

39. LaPuma J, Orentichler D, Moss R. Advance directives on admission: clinical implications and analysis of the Patient Self-determination Act of 1990. *JAMA.* 1991;266:402–405.

40. Lo B, McLeod G, Saika G. Patient attitudes to discussing life-sustaining treatment. *Arch Intern Med.* 1986;146:1613–1615.

41. Lo B, Quill T, Tulsky J. Discussing palliative care with patients. *Ann Intern Med.* 1999;130:744–749.

42. Logsdon RG, Gibbons LE, McCurry SM, et al. Quality of life in Alzheimer's disease: patient and caregiver reports. *J Mental Health Aging.* 1999;5: 21–32.

43. Lucas-Blaustein MJ, Filipp L, Dungan C, et al. Driving in patients with dementia. *J Am Geriatr Soc.* 1988;36:1087–1091.

44. Marattoli RA, Leon CFMd, Glass TA, et al. Driving cessation and increased depressive symptoms: prospective evidence from the New Haven EPESE. *J Am Geriatr Soc.* 1997;45:202–206.

45. Marson DC, Ingram KK, Cody HA, et al. Assessing the competency of patients with Alzheimer's disease under different legal standards. *Arch Neurol.* 1995; 52:949–954.

46. Martin D, Thiel E, Singer P. A new model of advance care planning: observations from people with HIV. *Arch Intern Med.* 1999;159:86–92.

47. McKneally MF, Martin DK. An entrustment model of consent for surgical treatment of life-threatening illness: perspective of patients requiring esophagectomy. *J Thorac Cadiovasc Surg.* 2000;120: 264–269.

48. Meier DE, Emmons C-A, Wallenstein S, et al. A national survey of physician-assisted suicide and euthanasia in the United States. *N Engl J Med.* 1998;338:1193–1201.

49. Meisel A. Legal myths about terminating life support. *Arch Intern Med.* 1991;151:1497–1502.

50. Miles S, Koepp R, Weber E. Advance end-of-life treatment planning: a research review. *Arch Intern Med.* 1996;156:1062–1068.

51. Morrison SR, Zayas LH, Mulvihill M, et al. Barriers to completion of health care proxies: an examination of ethnic differences. *Arch Intern Med.* 1998;158:2493–2497.

52. National Highway Traffic Safety Administration. *Safe Mobility for Older People Notebook.* Washington, DC: US Department of Transportation; 1999.

53. National Highway Traffic Safety Administration. *Traffic Safety Facts 1999. Older Population.* Available at: http://www.nhtsa.dot.gov/people/ncsa/pdf/ Older99.pdf. Accessed November 15, 2000.

54. Odenheimer GL. Dementia and the older driver. *Clin Geriatr Med.* 1993;9:349–364.

55. Pantilat SZ, Alpers A, Wachter RM. A new doctor in the house: ethical issues in hospitalist systems. *JAMA.* 1999;282:171–174.

56. Pasupathy S, Lavizzo-Mourey R. The older driver. In: Forciea MA, Lavizzo-Mourey R, Schwab EP, eds. *Geriatric secrets.* 2nd ed. Philadelphia: Hanley and Belfus; 2000:115–120.

57. Pritchard RS, Fisher ES, Teno JM, et al. Influence of patient preferences and local health system characteristics on the place of death. *J Am Geriatr Soc.* 1998;46:1242–1250.

58. Quill TE, Byock IR. Responding to intractable terminal suffering: the role of terminal sedation and voluntary refusal of foods and fluids. *Ann Intern Med.* 2000;132:408–414.

59. Retchin SM, Cox J, Fox M, et al. Performance-based measurement among elderly drivers and nondrivers. *J Am Geriatr Soc.* 1988;36:813–819.

60. Reuben DB. Assessment of older drivers. *Clin Geriatr Med.* 1993;9:449–459.
61. Reuben DB, Silliman RA, Traines M. The aging driver: medicine, policy, and ethics. *J Am Geriatr Soc.* 1988;36:1135–1142.
62. Rubin SM, Strull WM, Fialkow MF, et al. Increasing the completion of the durable power of attorney for health care: a randomized, controlled trial. *JAMA.* 1994;271:209–212.
63. Sabatino CP. 10 Legal myths about advance directives. In: *Clearinghouse review: ABA Commission on Legal Problems of the Elderly.* Chicago: National Center on Poverty Law; 1994:653–657.
64. Schneiderman L, Kronick R, Kaplan R. Effects of offering advance directives on medical treatments and costs. *Ann Intern Med.* 1992;117:599–606.
65. Silverman HJ, Truma P, Schaeffer MH, et al. Implementation of the Patient Self-Determination Act in a hospital setting: an initial evaluation. *Arch Intern Med.* 1995;155:502–510.
66. Singer P, Martin D, Lavery J, et al. Reconceptualizing advance care planning for a patient's perspective. *Arch Intern Med.* 1998;158:879–884.
67. Stelter K, Elliott B, Bruno C. Living will completion in older adults. *Arch Intern Med.* 1992;152:954–959.
68. Teno J, Lynn J, Connors A Jr, et al. The illusion of end-of-life resource savings with advance directives. *J Am Geriatr Soc.* 1997;45:513–518.
69. Teno J, Lynn J, Phillips R, et al. Do formal advance directives affect resuscitations decisions

and the use of resources for seriously ill patients? *J Clin Ethics.* 1994;5:23–30.
70. Teno J, Lynn J, Wegner N, et al. Advance directives for seriously ill hospitalized patients: effectiveness with the patient self-determination act and the SUPPORT intervention. *J Am Geriatr Soc.* 1997;45:500–507.
71. Trobe JD, Waller PF, Cook-Flannagan CA, et al. Crashes and violations among drivers with Alzheimer's disease. *Arch Neurol.* 1996;53:411–416.
72. Tulsky JA, Ciampa R, Rosen EJ. Responding to legal requests for physician-assisted suicide. *Ann Intern Med.* 2000;132:494–499.
73. Tulsky JA, Fischer GS, Rose MR, et al. Opening the black box: how do physicians communicate about advance directives? *Ann Intern Med.* 1998;129:441–449.
74. Underwood M. The older driver: clinical assessment and injury prevention. *Arch Intern Med.* 1992;152:735–740.
75. Vitaliano PP, Russo J, Young HM, et al. The screen for caregiver burden. *Gerontologist.* 1991; 31:76–83.
76. *Vacco v Quill,* 117 S. Ct. 2293 (1997).
77. *Washington v Glucksberg,* 117 S. Ct. 2258 (1997).
78. Williams AF, Carsten O. Driver age and crash involvement. *Am J Public Health.* 1989;79:326–327.
79. Yesavage J, Brink T, Rose T, et al. Development and validation of a geriatric depression screening scale: a preliminary report. *J Psychiatr Res.* 1982–1983;17:37–49.

CHAPTER 35

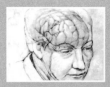

Driving in the Elderly with Medical Conditions

Joseph F. Drazkowski

The act of driving a motor vehicle is a privilege and not a right, and driving is regulated by statutes in all 50 states in the United States and most countries around the world. Obtaining one's license as a young adult is often considered to be a rite of passage toward independence. However, the loss of one's license is associated with a loss of independence, especially in the elderly. The elderly, particularly in the United States, require mobility for many basic activities including doctor visits and grocery shopping.

Driving is a common activity in the United States, as highlighted in the most recent figures from the Federal Bureau of Transportation Statistics (5). Unfortunately, driving is also associated with morbidity and mortality from accidents. There were 42,643 motorists killed in the United States in 2003, with 2,889,000 people injured in 6,328,000 motor vehicle crashes during 2,880,000 million miles driven.

The ability to operate a motor vehicle safely depends on multiple factors and requires the operator to interact and react to multiple stimuli within the driving environment (9). These factors include traditional motor and sensory skills as well as a certain level of cognitive integrity. Most of the primary senses impact the ability to drive and are highlighted in Table 35-1.

As our population ages, the ability to drive and remain independent will likely gain more importance and scrutiny. It is estimated that, in 2000, 13% of the population was comprised of drivers over 65 years of age and accounted for 18% of all traffic fatalities (34). It is estimated that 60% to 95% of so-called excess fatalities in the elderly due to car crashes result from

Table 35-1. *Factors That Influence the Ability to Drive*

Poor motor skills
Sensory deficits
Visual impairment/loss
Slowed reaction time
Cognitive deficits
Hearing loss
Loss of a limb
Mood/psychiatric disturbances

physical fragility (18). Car crashes can be life-changing events for the driver, passengers, and any victims. Car crashes involving medically impaired drivers and producing significant death and injury are often sensational in that they make "good copy" for the media (29,32). Reporting on these crashes or medical conditions in the popular press often introduces negative stigmatization of many medical conditions (7). Such reporting has consequences and can potentially influence public policy, opinion, and law. As a result of such recently reported crashes attributed to medical conditions, the Arizona legislature is considering whether to require physicians to report any patient who has a medical condition that could affect driving to a newly created medical review board for driving.

In the past, drivers less than 19 years of age were the most dangerous on the road. Young people crash at a higher rate for a number of reasons, with inexperience often cited as the most common reason (36). Although elderly drivers generally do not have issues of inexperience leading to car crashes, drivers over the age of 85 years have a higher crash rate than teenagers. Drivers past the age of 70 are particularly involved in certain types of crashes, including so-called angle, overtaking, and intersection crashes. The same older driver group is less involved in rear-end collisions (21). The reasons for this higher crash rate are many, but declining physical abilities are often cited to be a major contributor (22,25,37). Studies of elderly drivers with common medical and neurologic conditions often are limited by their design. Current studies of most drivers, the elderly included, are retrospective and uncontrolled in design.

The licensing process for private, noncommercial driving is generally codified by law in the individual states in the United States or countries in Europe. Driving restrictions related to various medical conditions are sometimes specifically mentioned in the law, whereas at other times, a more general restriction about any medical condition that could potentially impair driving is the standard. However, driving in persons with epilepsy (PWE) is specifically restricted in most jurisdictions (15). The restrictions are quite variable, with the seizure-free interval ranging from 3 to 12 months in the United States and the median restriction being 6 months (15). The European Union has suggested a 12-month restriction in member nations with a 6-month restriction for a first time unprovoked seizure for private vehicle operators (11). For commercial drivers, the laws are much more restrictive, especially for those who drive interstate. The Federal Department of Transportation sets the regulations for interstate driving, which are generally administered and enforced by individual states. Consequently, the regulations for interstate commercial drivers are essentially uniform across the country. Intrastate driving is regulated by individual states, and laws governing driving are more variable.

Applying for a license requires an applicant to testify that he or she is medically fit to drive. Once a license is obtained, the renewal period is variable for private vehicle operators. An example of this is in Arizona, where the time period to renew one's license can be more than 20 years (10). Much can change in this lengthy time period; operators are required to self-report any change in medical condition that may impair driving and undergo a medical review that determines one's fitness to drive. The variability of state laws basically requires that the individual practitioner be familiar with individual state requirements where they practice.

Currently, there are six states that require medical practitioners to report a patient who has epilepsy to the driving authority (Table 35-2). Some states require reporting specifically for epilepsy, whereas others use the standard of altered consciousness. The American Academy of Neurology, American Epilepsy Society, and a recent European consensus conference all oppose mandatory physician reporting for epilepsy patients, citing an interference with the doctor-patient relationship (17). Patients will be reluctant to report a worsening of their medical condition to their physician if they know they will be reported to the authorities. Most states allow the health care provider to report the patient if necessary. California specifically requires the reporting of several other medical conditions that might impair driving, but epilepsy remains the most restricted medical condition when it comes to driving. A recent attempt to repeal mandatory reporting in California made it through the legislature and was vetoed by the governor.

Medical conditions account for a small percentage of all car crashes (9). The fatality rate for epilepsy-related

Table 35-2. *States That Require Reporting of Seizures*

California	New Jersey
Nevada	Pennsylvania
Oregon	Delaware

crashes is higher than for other medical conditions (27), but the number of crashes related to epilepsy remains comparable to other medical conditions such as diabetes, heart disease, and even psychiatric conditions (9). If one groups alcohol-related crashes with "medically" related crashes, they account for about 40% of fatalities and about 7% of all crashes (9). One recent analysis of medically related auto accidents in Arizona showed that crashes related to epilepsy were more likely to be single-vehicle crashes (75%) with a trend toward more injuries when compared with other medically related crashes. All drivers had valid licenses to drive, and crashes occurred in both urban and rural settings. The average estimated speed at the time of the crash was lower than the posted limit, and weather was not found to be a factor in any of the crashes (9).

DRIVING AND EPILEPSY IN THE ELDERLY

The population in the United States is aging, and people older than 65 years represent the highest incidence of new-onset epilepsy. As in other age groups, the etiologies vary, with the highest known etiology being cerebrovascular disease and the most common seizure type being complex partial (13). Epilepsy in the elderly may be considered to be milder than in younger people, often responding to a low dose of a single antiepileptic drug (AED) (30). Side effects of AEDs in the elderly deserve consideration given the higher incidence of comorbid medical conditions. AEDs can affect even the most healthy of individuals in untoward ways. Older AEDs have well-known effects that may potentially affect driving. Affects of AEDs on vision, memory, balance, and coordination have been described (28). Although seizures are usually brief in duration, the affects of AEDs can be profound and persistent, making the ability to drive safely more questionable. The prevalence of epilepsy in the elderly is 1.5%, which is about two times the normal rate. Fifty percent of new-onset epilepsy cases are in the elderly, and 10% of nursing home patients are on an AED (8).

There have been several studies over the years that have evaluated the incidence of accidents with PWE drivers. In a study of 20,000 London bus drivers over 11 years, eight crashes were due to seizure (24). It is uncertain how many drivers in this study had epilepsy. In a survey of 10,000 fatal car crashes, 5,000 were alcohol related, six were caused by cardiac death, and one was due to a seizure (31). Beaussart et al. (4) showed that only 50% of seizures that occurred behind the wheel led to a crash. Of all medically related crashes, 19% were due to seizures according to Waller (33).

In general, the principles of driving in PWEs are similar to younger people. Driving is highly restricted and regulated when the seizures are not in control. Syncope is a much more common disorder in the elderly than epilepsy (16). If a cause of syncope can be identified and corrected, such as placing a pacemaker, one could potentially drive safely. If the syncope is due to a diabetic autonomic neuropathy, effective treatment may be more challenging. Altered consciousness impairs driving regardless of whether it is due to an arrhythmia or seizure. One should consider treating syncope similarly to seizure when considering driving restrictions.

DRIVING AND ALZHEIMER'S DISEASE

Alzheimer's disease (AD) is currently the most common cause of dementia in the United States. AD is often thought of as disease that produces memory loss. Although the disease indeed does include this problem, there are other features of the disease that may potentially impact the ability of the person with AD to drive safely. Comorbid features of AD that may affect driving are listed in Table 35-3. The effect of AD on driving goes beyond memory impairment and getting lost while going out for a drive. We have all heard the story of an elderly person with AD going out for a drive, getting lost, and being found hundreds of miles away from home. These stories are concerning because they can potentially affect public safety. A tragic example of this is the incident of an AD patient with poor visual-spatial skills and motor control running his car through a farmer's market killing 10 people after mistaking the accelerator pedal for the brake pedal.

Tragically, these events are often sensational in that they get reported in the popular press. The challenge is to prevent such events from happening. Predicting their occurrence is difficult. The American Academy of Neurology (AAN) has developed a practice parameter to help practitioners, patients, and families determine when the person with AD should stop driving. Potentially impaired AD drivers can be tested using the Clinical Dementia Rating (CDR)

Table 35-3. *Features of AD That May Affect Driving*

Motor impairment (apraxia, bradykinesia)
Visual impairment (asimultanagnosia)
Cognitive impairment
   Memory (getting lost)
   Visual-spatial skills
   Attention/multitasking skills
   Judgment
Other sensory impairment

scale, which evaluates the abilities of a patient and reports from observers regarding activities of daily living. The higher the score is, the more impaired the person with AD. The guidelines suggest that a CDR of 0.5 impacts driving to a moderate degree but warrants repeat observation and evaluation at 6-month intervals. The time spent between a CDR of 0.5 and 1 is correlated with a 2.3-fold increase in crashes compared with controls. The relative risk of a crash with a CDR of 0.5 is 5.6, and with a CDR of 1.0, it rises to 12. When the patient has a CDR score of 1 or higher, it is suggested that the patient in question should not drive because they have an eightfold increase in crashes (1).

After making the diagnosis of AD, taking away the ability to drive is potentially problematic. Fifty percent of patients do not stop driving for 3 years after getting the diagnosis (6). Recalling that poor judgment is part of the disease, it has been shown that people with AD continue to drive even after having shown difficulty with driving (19). What about testing the person with AD to determine driving ability? Depending on the study, 41% to 63% of patients with mild AD fail a road test (12,14). Using driving simulators has the potential to screen and determine whether a particular driver with AD is safe (26), but the complex nature of these machines has limited their widespread application.

PARKINSON'S DISEASE AND DRIVING

Parkinson's disease (PD) is another common disease of the elderly. PD has cardinal features of bradykinesia, rest tremor, gait instability, and rigidity. Any of these features could affect driving. As the disease advances, other features of the disease, some of which could be due to medications, may impair driving. These include the development of dyskinesias, cognitive impairment, and so-called micro-sleeps. Generally, as the disease progresses, driving performance worsens. Zesiewicz et al. (38) showed that, as patients advance on the United Parkinson's Disease Rating Scale from 1 to 4, their likelihood of crashing is ensured by the time they reach stage 4. This study also showed that the patient with PD does not reduce total miles driven and has a higher crash rate than age-matched controls.

STROKES AND DRIVING

Stroke, like other prominent diseases of the elderly, can be devastating with regard to driving. We are all familiar with the common motor disabilities associated with the occurrence of stroke. In severe cases when the motor system is profoundly affected, such as with a dominant hemisphere hemiplegia, it is generally apparent that one should not drive with such deficits. The stroke can also affect cognitive functions similar to the degenerative diseases discussed earlier. Even if the stroke is less severe but involves either a loss of vision or double vision, the safe operation of a motor vehicle could still be in doubt. For example, a hemianopsia could disqualify driving; however, monocular vision affecting depth perception may be allowed. Judgment, balance, and coordination may also be affected and may impact safe driving in a similar manner to the degenerative diseases listed earlier. Applying lessons learned from degenerative diseases should be used to assess driving in the stroke patient. Because most stroke patients have a unique clinical picture, one should appropriately individualize counseling about driving. Consider using a specialized adaptive driving program often administered by physical therapy and rehabilitation departments that evaluates classroom and "on the road" skills. This type of evaluation has the advantage of placing the person in a real-world situation with evaluators who have specialized expertise and objectivity in driving evaluations.

OLD AGE

When we are teenagers, many of us look forward to getting our driver's license and becoming more independent. This time of inexperience and youthful exuberance leads to a higher crash and fatality rate, especially in drivers under 25 years old. Car crashes in this age group are the leading cause of death. As we pass into middle age, the annual mileage driven increases, and the crash and fatality rates decrease to the point of this age group becoming the safest drivers on the road. As we get older, our driving mileage decreases, and the crash rate begins to climb. Drivers older than 85 years of age have the highest crash rate of all drivers on the road, despite driving the fewest miles per year (23) (Table 35-4).

BREAKING THE NEWS

Once the diagnosis of a disease process that affects driving has been made, the patient must be told that they cannot drive. Breaking the news to the patient and family is often challenging. Restriction of driving in

Table 35-4. *Incidence of Motor Vehicle Accidents (MVA) by Age Group*

Age Group	Incidence
16–19 years	28.6 MVA/million
40–45 years	3.7 MVA/million (13,000 miles/year)
80–85 years	15.1 MVA/million (2,600 miles/year)
>85 years	38.6 MVA/million

the elderly has potentially multiple ramifications for the patient and family. The Older Drivers Project and the American Medical Association have compiled a guide using available scientific data that can assist health care providers to recognize and counsel patients and families on this subject (3,35). If the patient is living alone, taking away the driving privilege leads to reduced independence and self-esteem. The loss of mobility often leads to decreased participation in activity and quality of life due to a sense of isolation. Increased burden is placed on the family if they suddenly have to transport the patient; if the condition is bad enough, the patient may have to move out of the home and into supervised care. Depression is a possibility as a result of taking the keys away (20).

Considering these issues, the discussion with patients and families can be optimized by ensuring privacy and committing to a long-term relationship. Try to explain the disease process and generally the progression if appropriate. Look at the situation and individualize the restriction as appropriate. Consider easing into the restriction by limiting night driving and freeway driving. As necessary, stress to the patients the consequences of injuring themselves or others if involved in a crash. Explain the local regulations, and help them fill out any forms as necessary. Explain that there is a possibility that if they continue to drive illegally and a crash occurs that their insurance company may not cover the losses. If a disagreement ensues, consider sending patients for a second opinion, an independent adaptive driving evaluation, or a road test through the state. In the end, if there is continued driving, despite appropriate counseling, one may need to report the situation to driving authorities as recommended by the American Medical Association (2).

SUMMARY

Driving and the restriction of driving have special implications for the elderly and their families. Health care practitioners should carefully consider common medical conditions that affect the elderly and their ability to drive. The restriction of driving represents a transition for the family and patient alike. As health care providers, we should provide the patient with the best medical advice and advocate for the patient when possible. We should be familiar with the local driving regulations, fill out any forms from the driving authorities, and educate the patient and family about how the patient's disease impacts the ability to drive. Understand that driving is an important issue to most patients; consider scheduling extra time to discuss and answer questions, be patient, and, when necessary, use appropriate resources.

REFERENCES

1. American Academy of Neurology. Guidelines for driving and Alzheimer's disease. Available at: http://www.aan.com. Accessed February 20, 2007.
2. American Medical Association. Drivers and medical conditions: reporting unsafe drivers is appropriate. Available at: http://safety.transportation.org/htmlguides/old_drvr/assets/app10.pdf. Accessed February 20, 2007.
3. American Medical Association. Older driver safety. Available at: http://www.ama-assn.org/ama/pub/category/8925.html. Accessed February 19, 2007.
4. Beaussart M, Beaussart-Defaye J, Lamiaux JM, et al. Epileptic drivers—a study of 1,089 patients. *Med Law*. 1997;16:295–306.
5. Bureau of Transportation Statistics. National transportation statistics 2005. Available at: http://www.bts.gov/publications/national_transportation_statistics/2005/. Accessed October 11, 2007.
6. Carr DB. Motor vehicle crashes and drivers with dementia Alzheimer's type. *Alzheimer's Dis Assoc Disord*. 1997;11[Suppl 1]:38–41.
7. Caspermeyer JJ, Sylvester EJ, Drazkowski JF, et al. Evaluation of stigmatizing language and medical errors in neurology coverage by US newspapers. *Mayo Clin Proc*. 2006;81:300–306.
8. Cloyd JC, Lackner TE, Leppik IE. Antiepileptics in the elderly. Pharmacoepidemiology and pharmacokinetics. *Arch Fam Med*. 1994;3:589–598.
9. Drazkowski JF, Fisher RS, Sirven JI, et al. Seizure-related motor vehicle crashes in Arizona before and after reducing the driving restriction from 12 to 3 months. *Mayo Clin Proc*. 2003;78: 819–825.
10. Driver licenses; physician mandatory reporting. Arizona House Bill #2761. Introduced February 15, 2007 to Licensing. Available at: http://www.azleg.gov/DocumentsForBill.asp?Bill_Number=2761. Accessed February 16, 2007.
11. Epilepsy and driving in Europe. A report of the second European working group on epilepsy and driving. ec.europa.eu/transport/roadsafety/behavior/doc/epilepsy_and_driving_in_europe_final_report_v2_en.pdf. Final report 04/03/05
12. Fox GK, Bowden SC, Bashford GM, et al. Alzheimer's disease and driving: prediction and assessment of driving performance. *J Am Geriatr Soc*. 1997;45:949–953.
13. Hauser WA. Seizure disorders: the changes with age. *Epilepsia*. 1992;33:S6–S14.
14. Hunt LA, Murphy CF, Carr D, et al. Reliability of the Washington University Road Test. A performance-based assessment for drivers with dementia of the Alzheimer's type. *Arch Neurol*. 1997;54:707–712.
15. Krauss GL, Ampaw L, Krumholz A. Individual state driving restrictions for people with epilepsy in the US. *Neurology*. 2001;57:1780–1785.
16. Krumholz A. Syncope. In: Fisher RS, ed. *Imitators of epilepsy*. New York: Demos Publications; 1994:91–109.
17. Lee W, Wolfe T, Shreeve S. Reporting epileptic drivers to licensing authorities is unnecessary and counterproductive. *Ann Emerg Med*. 2002;39: 656–659.
18. Li G, Braver ER, Chen LH. Fragility versus excessive crash involvement as determinants of high death rates per vehicle-mile of travel among older drivers. *Accid Anal Prev*. 2003;35:227–235.
19. Logsdon RG, Teri L, Larson EB. Driving and Alzheimer's disease. *J Gen Intern Med*. 1992;7: 583–588.
20. Marottoli RA, Mendes de Leon CF, Glass TA, et al. Driving cessation and increased depressive symptoms: prospective evidence from the New Haven EPESE. Established Populations for Epidemiologic Studies of the Elderly. *J Am Geriatr Soc*. 1997;45:202–206.
21. Mayhew DR, Simpson HM, Ferguson SA. Collisions involving senior drivers: high-risk conditions and locations. *Traffic Injury Prev*. 2006; 7:117–124.
22. McGwin G Jr., Sims RV, Pulley L, et al. Relations among chronic medical conditions, medications, and automobile crashes in the elderly: a population-based case-control study. *Am J Epidemiol*. 2000; 152:424–431.
23. National Highway Traffic Safety Administration. Crash and safety facts 2002. Available at: http://64.233.167.104/search?q=cache:51BAa4atA9AJ:www-nrd.nhtsa.dot.gov/pdf/nrd-30/NCSA/TSF2002/2002alcfacts.pdf+nhtsa+car+crash+statistics&hl=en&ct=clnk&cd=2&gl=us.
24. Norman LG. Medical aspects of road safety. *Lancet*. 1960;1:989–994.
25. Owsley C, Stalvey BT, Wells J, et al. Visual risk factors for crash involvement in older drivers with cataract. *Arch Ophthalmol*. 2001;119:881–887.
26. Rizzo M, Reinach S, McGehee D, et al. Simulated car crashes and crash predictors in drivers with Alzheimer's disease. *Arch Neurol*. 1997; 54:545–551.
27. Sheth SG, Krauss G, Krumholz A, et al. Mortality in epilepsy: driving fatalities vs other causes of death in patients with epilepsy. *Neurology*. 2004; 63:1002–1007.
28. Sirven JI, Fife TD, Wingerchuk DM, et al. Second-generation antiepileptic drugs' impact on balance: a meta-analysis. *Mayo Clin Proc*. 2007;82: 40–47.
29. Spano J. A driver's swath of death. *Los Angeles Times*. September 13, 2006:A1.

30. Stephen LJ, Kelly K, Mohanraj R, et al. Pharmacological outcomes in older people with newly diagnosed epilepsy. *Epilepsy Behav*. 2006;8:434–437.

31. van der Lugt PJ. Traffic accidents caused by epilepsy. *Epilepsia*. 1975;16:747–751.

32. Villa J. Burned police officer takes stand in cabby's trial. *The Arizona Republic*. February 22, 2002:A1.

33. Waller JA. Medical impairment and highway crashes. *JAMA*. 1969;208:2293–2296.

34. Wang CC, Carr DB, Older Drivers Project. Older driver safety: a report from the Older Drivers Project. *J Am Geriatr Soc*. 2004;52:143–149.

35. Wang CC, Kosinski CJ, Schwartzberg JG, et al. *Physician's Guide to Assessing and Counseling Older Drivers*. Washington, DC: National Highway Traffic Safety Administration; 2003.

36. Williams AF, Ferguson SA. Rationale for graduated licensing and the risks it should address. *Inj Prev*. 2002;8[Suppl 2]:ii9–ii14.

37. Young T, Shahar E, Nieto FJ, et al. Predictors of sleep-disordered breathing in community-dwelling adults: the Sleep Heart Health Study. *Arch Intern Med*. 2002;162:893–900.

38. Zesiewicz TA, Cimino CR, Malek AR, et al. Driving safety in Parkinson's disease. *Neurology*. 2002;59:1787–1788.

APPENDIX

RESOURCES

Although this list represents a comprehensive guide to organizations that address the clinical care needs of older people, it is not a resource of all social service agencies and organizations assisting older citizens. If you have questions that do not specifically relate to one of the following organizations, please contact your state or area agency on aging as listed by the Administration on Aging (AOA). These agencies provide information on, and refer callers to, local services for senior citizens. To locate state and area agencies on aging, visit the AOA Website at http://www.aoa.gov or call the Elder-care Locator service (1-800-677-1116) operated by the National Association of Area Agencies on Aging.

NOTE: The organizations on this list are arranged in categories in the following order:

General Aging
End-of-Life Issues
Education
Legal Issues and Elder Abuse
Resources on Specific Health Problems:
  Cancer
  Diabetes
  Digestive Problems
  Head and Neck Problems
  Hearing Problems
  Heart and Circulation Problems
  Joint, Muscle, and Bone Problems
  Lung and Breathing Problems
  Memory and Thinking Problems
  Neurologic Problems
  Nutritional Concerns
  Pain
  Psychological Problems
  Sexuality and Sexual Concerns
  Sight Problems
  Skin Problems
  Urinary Problems

GENERAL AGING

Administration on Aging
330 Independence Avenue, SW
Washington, DC 20201
Tel: (202) 619-0724
Fax: (202) 401-7620

Website: http://www.aoa.gov
E-mail: aoainfo@aoa.gov

Agency for Health Care Policy and Research
Clinical Practice Guidelines
Government Printing Office
Superintendent of Documents
Washington, DC 20402
Tel: (202) 512-1800
Online retrieval: http://www.ahcpr.gov

Aging Network Services
440 East-West Highway
Bethesda, MD 20814
Tel: (301) 657-4329
Fax: (301) 657-3250
Website: http://www.agingnets.com
E-mail: ans@agingnets.com

Alliance for Aging Research
2021 K Street, NW, Suite 305
Washington, DC 20006
Tel: (202) 293-2856
Fax: (202) 785-8574
Website: www.agingresearch.org

American Academy of Home Care Physicians
P. O. Box 1037
Edgewood, MD 21040
Tel: (410) 676-7966
Fax: (410) 676-7980
Website: www.aahcp.org
E-mail: aahcp@mindspring.com

American Association of Homes & Services for the Aging
901 E Street, NW, Suite 500
Washington, DC 20004-2011
Tel: (202) 783-2242
Fax: (202) 783-2255
Website: www.aahsa.org
E-mail: info@aahsa.org

American Association of Retired Persons
601 E Street, NW
Washington, DC 20049
Tel: (800) 424-3410
Website: www.aarp.org
E-mail: member@aarp.org

American College of Health Care Administrators
1800 Diagonal Road, Suite 355
Alexandria, VA 22314
Tel: (703) 549-5822
Fax: (703) 739-7901
Toll free: (888) 888-ACHCA (2-2422)
Website: www.achca.org
E-mail: info@achca.org

American Federation for Aging Research
1414 Avenue of the Americas
New York, NY 10019
Tel: (212) 752-2327
Fax: (212) 832-2298
Website: www.afar.org
E-mail: amfedaging@aol.com

American Geriatrics Society
The Empire State Building
350 Fifth Avenue, Suite 801
New York, NY 10118
Tel: (212) 308-1414
Fax: (212) 832-8646
Website: www.americangeriatrics.org
E-mail: info.amger@americangeriatrics.org

American Health Care Association
1201 L Street, NW
Washington, DC 20005
Tel: (202) 842-4444
Fax: (202) 842-3860
Toll free for publications only: (800) 321-0343
Website: www.ahca.org

American Hospital Association
1 North Franklin
Chicago, IL 60606
Tel: (312) 422-3000
Fax: (312) 422-4796
Website: www.aha.org

American Medical Directors Association
10480 Patuxent Parkway, Suite 760
Columbia, MD 21044
Tel: (410) 740-9743
Toll free: (800) 876-2632
Fax: (410) 740-4572
Website: www.amda.com

American Occupational Therapy Association
P. O. Box 31220
Bethesda, MD 20824-1220
Tel: (301) 652-2682
Fax: (301) 652-7711
Website: www.aota.org

American Red Cross
Attn: Public Inquiry Office
431 18th Street, NW
Washington, DC 20006

Tel: (202) 639-3520
Website: www.redcross.org

American Senior Fitness Association
P. O. Box 2575
New Smyrna Beach, FL 32170
Tel: (904) 423-6634
Fax: (904) 427-0613
Website: www.seniorfitness.net
E-mail: sfa@ucnsb.net

American Seniors Housing Association
1850 M Street, NW, Suite 540
Washington, DC 20036
Tel: (202) 974-2300
Fax: (202) 775-0112
Website: www.nmhc.org
E-mail: info@nmhc.org

American Social Health Association
Hotlines under the auspices of the ASHA
CDC National AIDS Hotline (English)—Toll free:
   (800) 342-AIDS
CDC National AIDS Hotline (Spanish)—Toll free:
   (800) 344-7432
CDC National AIDS Hotline—TTY Toll free:
   (800) 243-7889
CDC National STD Hotline —Toll free: (800)
   227-8922
CDC National Immunization Information
   Hotline—Toll free: (800) 232-2522
Website: www.ashastd.org

American Society on Aging
822 Market Street, Suite 511
San Francisco, CA 94103-1824
Tel: (415) 974-9600
Fax: (415) 974-0300
Website: www.asaging.org
E-mail: info@asaging.org

American Society of Consultant Pharmacists
1321 Duke Street
Alexandria, VA 22314-3516
Tel: (703) 739-1300
Fax: (703) 739-1321
Toll free: (800) 355-2727
Toll free fax: (800) 707-ASCP
Fast fax: (800) 220-1321
Website: www.ascp.com
E-mail: info@ascp.com

Assisted Living Federation of America
10300 Eaton Place, Suite 400
Fairfax, VA 22030
Tel: (703) 691-8100
Fax: (703) 691-8106
Website: www.alfa.org
E-mail: info@alfa.org

B'nai B'rith
1640 Rhode Island Avenue, NW
Washington, DC 20036-3278
Tel: (202) 857-6600
Fax: (202) 857-1099
Toll free: (888) 388-4224
Website: www.bnaibrith.org
Senior Housing
Tel: (202) 857-6581
Fax: (202) 857-0980
E-mail: senior@bnaibrith.org

Catholic Charities
1731 King Street, Suite 200
Alexandria, VA 22314
Tel: (703) 549-1390
Fax: (703) 549-1656
Website: www.catholiccharitiesusa.org

CDC National Prevention Information Network
For information on HIV, AIDS, STD, TB
P. O. Box 6003
Rockville, MD 20849-6003
Tel: (301) 562-1098
Toll free: (800) 458-5231
Toll free fax: (888) 282-7681
Toll free TTY: (800) 243-7012
Website: www.cdcnpin.org
E-mail: info@cdcnpin.org

Children of Aging Parents
1609 Woodbourne Road, Suite 302-A
Levittown, PA 19057
Tel: (215) 945-6900
Fax: (215) 945-8720
Toll free information/referral: (800) 227-7294
Website: www.caps4caregivers.org

Commission on Accreditation for Rehabilitation Facilities (CARF)
4891 East Grant Road
Tucson, AZ 85712
Tel: (520) 325-1044
Fax: (520) 318-1129
Website: www.carf.org

Department of Veteran Affairs
Office of Public Affairs
810 Vermont Avenue, NW
Washington, DC 20420
Tel: (202) 273-5700
Fax: (202) 273-6705
Website: www.va.gov

Disabled American Veterans
807 Maine Avenue, SW
Washington, DC 20024
Tel: (202) 554-3501
Fax: (202) 554-3581
Website: www.dav.org

Family Caregivers Alliance
69 Market Street
Suite 600
San Francisco, CA 94104
Tel: (415) 434-3388
Fax: (415) 434-3508
Website: www.caregiver.org
E-mail: info@caregiver.org

Gerontological Society of America
1030 15th Street, NW, Suite 250
Washington, DC 20005
Tel: (202) 842-1275
Fax: (202) 842-1150
Website: www.geron.org

Healthcare Information and Management Systems Society
230 East Ohio Street, Suite 500
Chicago, IL 60611-3269
Tel: (312) 664-4467
Fax: (312) 664-6143
Website: www.himss.org

Interfaith Caregivers Alliance
One West Armour Boulevard, Suite 202
Kansas City, MO 64111
Tel: (816) 931-5442
Fax: (816) 931-5202
Website: www.interfaithcaregivers.org
E-mail: info@interfaithcaregivers.org

Joint Commission on Accreditation of Healthcare Organizations (JCAHO)
One Renaissance Boulevard
Oakbrook Terrace, IL 60181
Tel: (630) 792-5000
Fax: (630) 792-5005
Website: www.jcaho.org

Medicare Hotline
Toll free English and Spanish: (800) MEDICARE (633-4227)
Website: www.medicare.gov

National Adult Day Services Association
409 Third Street, SW
Washington, DC 20024
Tel: (202) 479-6682
Fax: (202) 479-0735
Website: www.ncoa.org/nadsa
E-mail: nadsa@ncoa.org

National Aging Information Center (NAIC)
(A Service of the Administration on Aging)
330 Independence Avenue, SW, Room 4656
Washington, DC 20201
Tel: (202) 619-7501
TTY: (202) 401-7575
Fax: (202) 401-7620

Website: http://www.aoa.gov/naic
E-mail: naic@aoa.gov

National Asian Pacific Center on Aging
Melbourne Tower, Suite 914
1511 Third Avenue
Seattle, WA 98101
Tel: (206) 624-1221
Fax: (206) 624-1023
Website: www.napca.com

National Association of Area Agencies on Aging
927 15th Street, NW, 6th Floor
Washington, DC 20005
Tel: (202) 296-8130
Fax: (202) 296-8134
Website: www.n4a.org
E-mail: rseay@n4a.org
Toll free eldercare locator: Operated as a cooperative partnership of the Administration on Aging, the National Association of Area Agencies on Aging, and the National Association of State Units on Aging: (800) 677-1116.

National Association of Directors of Nursing Administration
10999 Reed Hartman Highway, Suite 233
Cincinnati, OH 45242
Tel: (513) 791-3679
Fax: (513) 791-3699
Toll free: (800) 222-0539
Website: www.nadona.org
E-mail: info@nadona.org

National Association for Home Care
228 7th Street, SE
Washington, DC 20003
Tel: (202) 547-7424
Fax: (202) 547-3540
Website: http://www.nahc.org

National Association of Professional Geriatric Care Managers
1604 North Country Club Road
Tucson, AZ 85716
Tel: (520) 881-8008
Fax: (520) 325-7925
Website: www.caremanager.org

National Association for the Support of Long Term Care
1321 Duke Street, Suite 304
Alexandria, VA 22314
Tel: (703) 549-8500
Fax: (703) 549-8342
Website: www.NASL.org

National Caucus and Center on Black Aged, Inc.
1424 K Street, NW
Washington, DC 20005

Tel: (202) 637-8400
Fax: (202) 327-0895
Website: www.ncba-aged.org
E-mail: ncba@aol.com

National Citizens' Coalition for Nursing Home Reform
1424 16th Street, NW, Suite 202
Washington, DC 20036-2211
Tel: (202) 332-2275
Fax: (202) 332-2949
Website: www.nccnhr.org
E-mail: nccnhrl@nccnhr.org

National Council on the Aging
409 3rd Street, SW
Washington, DC 20024
Tel: (202) 479-1200
Fax: (202) 479-0735
Website: www.ncoa.org
E-mail: info@ncoa.org

National Council on Patient Information and Education
4915 Saint Elmo Avenue, Suite 505
Bethesda, MD 20814-6053
Tel: (301) 656-8565
Fax: (301) 656-4464
Website: www.talkaboutrx.org
E-mail: ncpie@erols.com

National Family Caregivers Association
10400 Connecticut Avenue, #500
Kensington, MD 20895-3944
Tel: (301) 942-6430
Fax: (301) 942-2302
Toll free: (800) 896-3650
Website: www.nfcacares.org
E-mail: info@nfcacares.org

National Health Information Center
P. O. Box 1133
Washington, DC 20013-1133
Tel: (301) 565-4167
Toll free: (800) 336-4797
Fax: (301) 884-4256
Website: www.health.gov/nhic
E-mail: nhicinfo@health.org

National Indian Council on Aging
10501 Montgomery Boulevard NE, Suite 210
Albuquerque, NM 87111-3846
Tel: (505) 292-2001
Fax: (505) 292-1922
Website: www.nicoa.org
E-mail: dave@nicoa.org

National Institute on Aging
Building 31, Room 5C27
31 Center Drive, MCS 2292
Bethesda, MD 20892-2292

Tel: (301) 496-1752
Fax: (301) 496-1072
Website: www.nih.gov/nia

National Institute on Aging Information Clearinghouse
P. O. Box 8057
Gaithersburg, MD 20898-8057
Toll free: (800) 222-2225

National Institute on Disability and Rehabilitation Research ABLEDATA
8630 Fenton Street, Suite 930
Silver Spring, MD 20910
Tel: (301) 608-8998
Fax: (301) 608-8958
Toll free: (800) 227-0216
Website: www.abledata.com
E-mail: adaigle@macroint.com

National Rehabilitation Information Center
1010 Wayne Avenue, Suite 800
Silver Spring, MD 20910
Toll free: (800) 346-2742
Fax: (301) 562-2401
Website: www.naric.com/naric

National Subacute Care Association
7315 Wisconsin Avenue, Suite 424E
Bethesda, MD 20814
Tel: (301) 961-8680
Fax: (301) 961-8681
Website: www.nsca.net
E-mail: nsca@tiac.net

Projecto Ayuda
1452 West Temple Street, Suite 100
Los Angeles, CA 90026
Tel: (213) 487-1922
Fax: (213) 202-5905

United Seniors Health Cooperative
1331 H Street, NW
Washington, DC 20005
Tel: (202) 393-6222
Fax: (202) 783-0588
Website: www.ushc-online.org

Visiting Nurse Associations of America
11 Beacon Street, Suite 910
Boston, MA 02108
Tel: (617) 523-4042
Fax: (617) 227-4843
Website: www.vnaa.org

Well Spouse Foundation
610 Lexington Avenue, Suite 208
New York City, NY 10022
Tel: (212) 644-1241
Fax: (212) 644-1338
Toll free: (800) 838-0879

Website: www.wellspouse.org
E-mail: wellspouse@aol.com

END-OF-LIFE ISSUES

Americans for Better Care of the Dying
2175 K Street, NW, Suite 820
Washington, DC 20037
Tel: (202) 530-9864
Fax: (202) 467-2271
Website: www.abcd-caring.org
E-mail: caring@erols.org

Center to Improve Care of the Dying
Rand Corporation
Tel: (703) 413-1100

Choice in Dying, Inc.
1035 30th Street, NW
Washington, DC 20007
Tel: (202) 338-9790
Fax: (202) 338-0242
Toll free: (800) 989-WILL (9455)
Website: www.choices.org

Compassion in Dying
6312 SW Capital Highway, PMB 415
Portland, OR 97201
Tel: (503) 221-9556
Fax: (503) 228-9160
Website: www.compassionindying.org
E-mail: info@compassionindying.org

GriefNet
Website: www.griefnet.org

Hospice Association of America
228 Seventh Street, SE
Washington, DC 20003
Tel: (202) 546-4759
Fax: (202) 547-9559
Website: www.hospice-america.org

Hospice Education Institute
190 Westbrook Road
Essex, CT 06426-1510
Tel: (860) 767-1620
Fax: (860) 767-2746
Toll free for publications: (800) 331-1620
Hospice link referral service—Toll free: (800) 331-1620
Website: www.hospiceworld.org
E-mail: hospiceall@aol.com

Hospice Foundation of America
2001 S Street, NW, Suite 300
Washington, DC 20009
Tel: (202) 638-5419
Toll free: (800) 854-3402
Fax: (202) 638-5312

Website: www.hospicefoundation.org
E-mail: hfa@hospicefoundation.org

The Last Acts Campaign
Barksdale Ballard & Co.
1951 Kidwell Drive, Suite 205
Vienna, VA 22182
Tel: (703) 827-8771
Fax: (703) 827-0782
Website: www.lastacts.org

Life with Dignity
1744 Riggs Place, NW, Suite 300
Washington, DC 20009
Tel: (202) 986-0118
Website: http://members.aol.com/lwdfdn
E-mail: lwdfdn@aol.com

National Hospice and Palliative Care Organization
1700 Diagonal Road, Suite 300
Alexandria, VA 22314
Tel: (703) 837-1500
Website: www.nhpco.org
E-mail: info@nhpca.org

EDUCATION

Association for Gerontology in Higher Education
1030 15th Street, NW, Suite 240
Washington, DC 20005-1503
Tel: (202) 289-9806
Fax: (202) 289-9824
Website: www.aghe.org

Association of American Medical Colleges
2450 N Street, NW
Washington, DC 20037-1126
Tel: (202) 828-0400
Fax: (202) 828-1125
Website: www.aamc.org

LEGAL ISSUES AND ELDER ABUSE

Legal Services for the Elderly
130 West 42nd Street, 17th Floor
New York, NY 10036
Tel: (212) 391-0120
Fax: (212) 719-1939
E-mail: hn4923@handsnet.org

National Academy of Elder Law Attorneys
1604 North Country Club Road
Tucson, AZ 85716
Tel: (520) 881-4005
Fax: (520) 325-7925
Website: www.naela.org
E-mail: info@naela.com

National Association of State Units on Aging
1225 I Street, Suite 725
Washington, DC 20005

Tel: (202) 898-2578
Fax: (202) 898-2583
Website: www.nasua.org
E-mail: info@nasua.org

National Center on Elder Abuse
A consortium of the following six partners with NASUA, the lead agency:
National Association of State Units on Aging (NASUA)
Commission on Legal Problems of the Elderly of the American Bar Association (ABA)
The Clearinghouse on Abuse and Neglect of the Elderly of the University of Delaware (CANE)
The San Francisco Consortium for Elder Abuse Prevention of the Goldman Institute on Aging (GIOA)
The National Association of Adult Protective Services Administrators (NAAPSA)
The National Committee to Prevent Elder Abuse (NCPEA)

National Clearinghouse on Elder Abuse
Literature
University of Delaware
College of Human Resources, Education and Public Policy
Department of Consumer Studies
211 Allison Annex
Newark, DE 19716
Tel: (302) 831-3525
Fax: (302) 831-6081

National Committee for Prevention of Elder Abuse
Research
Institute on Aging
UMASS Memorial Health Care
119 Belmont Street
Worcester, MA 01605
Tel: (508) 334-6166
Fax: (508) 334-6906
Website: www.preventelderabuse.org

National Senior Citizens Law Center
1101 14th Street, NW, Suite 400
Washington, DC 20005
Tel: (202) 289-6976
Fax: (202) 289-7224
Website: www.nsclc.org

RESOURCES ON SPECIFIC HEALTH PROBLEMS

CANCER

American Cancer Society, Inc.
National Headquarters
1599 Clifton Road, NE

Atlanta, GA 30329
Tel: (404) 320-3333
Fax: (404) 329-5787
Toll free National Cancer Information Center:
  (800) 227-2345
Website: www.cancer.org

National Cancer Institute
Public Inquiries Office
Building 31, Room 10A31
31 Center Drive, MSC 2580
Bethesda, MD 20892-2580
Tel: (301) 435-3848
Toll free: (800) 4-CANCER(422-6237)
Website: www.nci.nih.gov

DIABETES

American Diabetes Association
Attn: Customer Service
1701 North Beauregard Street
Alexandria, VA 22311
Tel: (703) 549-1500
Fax: (703) 549-6995
Toll free: (800) DIABETES (232-3472)
Website: www.diabetes.org
E-mail: customerservice@diabetes.org

National Diabetes Information Clearinghouse
1 Information Way
Bethesda, MD 20892-3560
Tel: (301) 654-3327
Fax: (301) 907-8906
Website: diabetes.niddk.nih.gov
E-mail: ndic@info.niddk.nih.gov

DIGESTIVE PROBLEMS

American Liver Foundation
75 Maiden Lane, Suite 603
New York, NY 10038
Toll free: (800) GO LIVER (465-4837)
Website: www.liverfoundation.org
E-mail: webmail@liverfoundation.org

**National Digestive Disease Information
  Clearinghouse**
2 Information Way
Bethesda, MD 20892-2480
Tel: (301) 654-3810
Website: www.digestive.niddk.nih.gov
E-mail: nddic@info.niddk.nih.gov

United Ostomy Association
19772 MacArthur Boulevard, Suite 200
Irvine, CA 92612-2405
Tel: (949) 660-8624
Fax: (949) 660-9262
Toll free: (800) 826-0826
Website: www.uoa.org
E-mail: info@uoa.org

HEAD AND NECK PROBLEMS

**American Academy of Otolaryngology-Head
  and Neck Surgery, Inc.**
1 Prince Street
Alexandria, VA 22314-3357
Tel: (703) 836-4444
Fax: (703) 683-5100
TTY: (703) 519-1585
Website: www.entnet.org

American Council for Headache Education
19 Mantua Road
Mt. Royal, NJ 08061
Tel: (856) 423-0258
Toll free: (800) 255-ACHE (2243)
Fax: (856) 423-0082
Website: www.achenet.org

American Dental Association
211 East Chicago Avenue
Chicago, IL 60611
Tel: (312) 440-2500
Fax: (312) 440-2800
Website: www.ada.org

National Headache Foundation
428 West St. James Place, 2nd Floor
Chicago, IL 60614-1750
Tel: (773) 388-6399
Toll free: (888) NHF-5552
Fax: (773) 525-7357
Website: www.headaches.org
E-mail: info@headaches.org

**National Institute of Dental & Craniofacial
  Research**
National Institute of Health
Bethesda, MD 20892-2190
Tel: (301) 496-4261
Fax: (301) 496-9988
Website: www.nidcr.nih.gov
E-mail: nidcrinfo@mail.nih.gov

HEARING PROBLEMS

American Tinnitus Association
P. O. Box 5
Portland, OR 97207-0005
Tel: (503) 248-9985
Fax: (503) 248-0024
Toll free: (800) 634-8978
Website: www.ata.org
E-mail: tinnitus@ata.org

Better Hearing Institute
515 King Street
Suite 420
Alexandria, VA 22314
Toll free: (800) EARWELL (327-9355)
Fax: (703) 750-9302

Website: www.betterhearing.org
E-mail: mail@betterhearing.org

International Hearing Society
16880 Middlebelt Road, Suite 4
Livonia, MI 48154
Tel: (734) 522-7200
Fax: (734) 522-0200
Toll free hearing aid helpline: (800) 521-5247
Website: www.hearingihs.org

National Institute on Deafness and Other Communication Disorders
National Institute of Health
31 Center Drive, MSC 2320
Bethesda, MD 20892-2320
Tel: (301) 496-7243
Fax: (301) 402-0018
Toll free NIDCD Information Clearinghouse: (800) 241-1044
Website: www.nidcd.nih.gov
E-mail: webmaster@ms.nidcd.nih.gov

Self Help for Hard of Hearing People
7910 Woodmont Avenue, Suite 1200
Bethesda, MD 20814
Tel: (301) 657-2248
Fax: (301) 913-9413
TTY: (301) 657-2249
Website: www.shhh.org
E-mail: national@shhh.org

HEART AND CIRCULATION PROBLEMS

American Association of Cardiovascular and Pulmonary Rehabilitation
7600 Terrace Avenue, Suite 203
Middleton, WI 53562
Tel: (608) 831-6989
Fax: (608) 831-5485
Website: www.aacvpr.org
E-mail: accvpr@tmahq.com

American Heart Association
7272 Greenville Avenue
Dallas, TX 75231
Tel: (214) 373-6300
Toll free: (800) 242-8721
Website: www.americanheart.org
AHA's Stroke Connection: (800) 553-6321

Courage Stroke Network
3915 Golden Valley Road
Golden Valley, MN 55422
Tel: (763) 520-0520
Fax: (763) 520-0577

National Heart, Lung and Blood Institute
Office of Prevention, Education and Control
31 Center Drive, MSC 2480
Bethesda, MD 20892-2480

Tel: (301) 496-5437
Fax: (301) 402-2405
Website: www.nhlbi.nih.gov
E-mail: nhlbiinfo@rover.nhlbi.nih.gov

National Institute of Neurological Disorders and Stroke
NIH Neurological Institute
P. O. Box 5801
Bethesda, MD 20824
Toll free: (800) 352-9424
Website: www.ninds.nih.gov

National Stroke Association
9707 E. Easter Lane
Englewood, CO 80112
Tel: (303) 649-9299
Fax: (303) 649-1328
Toll free: (800) STROKES (787-6537)
Website: www.stroke.org

JOINT, MUSCLE, AND BONE PROBLEMS

American Academy of Orthopedic Surgeons
6300 North River Road
Rosemont, IL 60018-4262
Tel: (847) 823-7186
Toll free: (800) 346-AAOS (2267)
Fax: (847) 823-8125
Website: www.aaos.org
E-mail: custserv@aaos.org

American Podiatric Medical Association
9312 Old Georgetown Road
Bethesda, MD 20814
Tel: (301) 571-9200
Fax: (301) 530-2752
Toll free for patient education literature only: (800) FOOT-CARE
Website: www.apma.org
E-mail: askapma@apma.org

Arthritis Foundation
1330 West Peachtree Street
Atlanta, GA 30309
Tel: (404) 872-7100
Toll free information: (800) 283-7800
Fax: (404) 872-0457
Website: www.arthritis.org
E-mail: help@arthritis.org

Lupus Foundation of America
1300 Piccard Drive, Suite 200
Rockville, MD 20850-4303
Tel: (301) 670-9292
Toll free for information packet: English (800) 558-0121; Spanish (800) 558-0231
Fax: (301) 670-9486
Website: www.lupus.org

**National Arthritis and Musculoskeletal
and Skin Diseases Information
Clearinghouse**
National Institutes of Health
1 AMS Circle
Bethesda, MD 20892-3675
Tel: (301) 495-4484
Toll free: (877) 22-NIAMS (64267)
Fax: (301) 718-6366
Website: www.nih.gov/niams
E-mail: via Website

National Osteoporosis Foundation
1232 22nd Street, NW
Washington, DC 20037-1292
Tel: (202) 223-2226
Fax: (202) 223-2237
Toll free information: (800) 223-9994
Website: www.nof.org
E-mail: customerservice@nof.org

LUNG AND BREATHING PROBLEMS

**American Association of Cardiovascular and
Pulmonary Rehabilitation**
7600 Terrace Avenue, Suite 203
Middleton, WI 53562
Tel: (608) 831-6989
Fax: (608) 831-5485
Website: www.aacvpr.org
E-mail: accvpr@tmahq.com

American Lung Association
1740 Broadway
New York, NY 10019
Tel: (212) 315-8700
Fax: (212) 265-5642
Toll free: (800) LUNG-USA (800-586-4872)
Website: www.lungusa.org
E-mail: info@lungusa.org

National Heart, Lung and Blood Institute
Office of Prevention, Education and Control
31 Center Drive, MSC 2480
Bethesda, MD 20892-2480
Tel: (301) 496-5437
Fax: (301) 402-2405
Website: www.nhlbi.nih.gov
E-mail: nhlbiinfo@rover.nhlbi.nih.gov

MEMORY AND THINKING PROBLEMS

Alzheimer's Association
919 North Michigan Avenue, Suite 1100
Chicago, IL 60611-1676
Tel: (312) 335-8700
TTY: (312) 335-8882
Fax: (312) 335-1110
Toll free information: (800) 272-3900
Website: http://www.alz.org

E-mail: info@alz.org
Safe Return Program—identification tags, medical
alert bracelets: (888) 572-8566

**Alzheimer's Disease Education and Referral
Center**
P. O. Box 8250
Silver Spring, MD 20907-8250
Tel: (301) 495-3311
Fax: (301) 495-3334
Toll free information service: (800) 438-4380
Website: www.alzheimers.org
E-mail: adear@alzheimers.org

NEUROLOGIC PROBLEMS

American Academy of Neurology
1080 Montreal Avenue
St. Paul, MN 55116
Tel: (651) 695-1940
Fax: (651) 695-2791
Website: www.aan.com
E-mail: web@aan.com

American Parkinson's Disease Association
1250 Hylan Boulevard, Suite 4B
Staten Island, NY 10305-1946
Tel: (718) 981-8001
Toll free information hotline: (800) 223-2732
Fax: (718) 981-4399
Website: www.apdaparkinson.org
E-mail: info@apdaparkinson.org

Epilepsy Foundation of America
4351 Garden City Drive
Landover, MD 20785
Tel: (301) 459-3700
Toll free info & referral: (800) 332-1000
Fax: (301) 577-2684
Website: www.efa.org

Huntington's Disease Society of America
158 West 29th Street, 7th Floor
New York, NY 10001
Tel: (212) 242-1968
Fax: (212) 239-3430
Toll free hotline: (800) 345-4372
Website: www.hdsa.org
E-mail: hdsainfo@hdsa.org

**National Institute of Neurological Disorders
and Stroke**
NIH Neurological Institute
P. O. Box 5801
Bethesda, MD 20824
Toll free: (800) 352-9424
Website: www.ninds.nih.gov
(For other stroke information, see Heart and
Circulation Problems)

Parkinson's Disease Foundation
William Black Medical Building
Columbia-Presbyterian Medical Center
710 West 168th Street
New York, NY 10032
Tel: (212) 923-4700
Toll free: (800) 457-6676
Fax: (212) 923-4778
Website: www.pdf.org
E-mail: info@pdf.org

NUTRITIONAL CONCERNS

Food and Nutrition Information Center
U.S. Department of Agriculture
National Agriculture Library Building
10301 Baltimore Avenue, Room 304
Beltsville, MD 20705-2351
Tel: (301) 504-5719
Fax: (301) 504-6409
Website: http://www.nal.usda.gov/fnic
E-mail: fnic@nal.usda.gov

Meals on Wheels Association of America
1414 Prince Street, Suite 202
Alexandria, VA 22314
Tel: (703) 548-5558
Fax: (703) 548-8024
Website: www.mowaa.org

PAIN

American Chronic Pain Association
P. O. Box 850
Rocklin, CA 95677
Tel: (916) 632-0922
Fax: (916) 632-3208
Website: www.theacpa.org
E-mail: acpa@pacbell.net

American Geriatrics Society
The Empire State Building
350 Fifth Avenue, Suite 801
New York, NY 10118
Tel: (212) 308-1414
Fax: (212) 832-8646
Website: www.americangeriatrics.org
E-mail: info.amger@americangeriatrics.org

American Pain Society
4700 West Lake Avenue
Glenview, IL 60025
Tel: (847) 375-4715
Fax: (847) 375-7777
Website: www.ampainsoc.org
E-mail: info@ampainsoc.org

City of Hope Pain Resource Center
City of Hope National Medical Center
Department of Nursing Research & Education
1500 East Duarte Road

Duarte, CA 91010
Tel: (626) 359-8111, ext. 3829
Website: mayday.coh.org
E-mail: bferrell@coh.org

National Chronic Pain Outreach Association
P. O. Box 274
Millboro, VA 24460-9606
Tel: (540) 862-9437
Fax: (540) 862-9485
Website: http://www.chronicpain.org
E-mail: ncpoa@cfw.com

PSYCHOLOGICAL PROBLEMS

American Association of Geriatric Psychiatry
7910 Woodmont Avenue, Suite 1050
Bethesda, MD 20814-3004
Tel: (301) 654-7850
Fax: (301) 654-4137
Website: www.aagpgpa.org
E-mail: main@aagpgpa.org

National Alliance for the Mentally Ill
Colonial Place Three
2107 Wilson Boulevard, Suite 300
Arlington, VA 22201-3042
Tel: (703) 524-7600
Fax: (703) 524-9094
Toll free: (800) 950-6264
Website: www.nami.org

National Institute of Mental Health Information Resources & Inquiries
6001 Executive Boulevard, Room 8184,
   MSC 9663
Bethesda, MD 20892-9663
Tel: (301) 443-4513
Fax: (301) 443-5158
Website: www.nimh.nih.gov
E-mail: nimhinfo@nih.gov

National Mental Health Association
Information Center
1021 Prince Street
Alexandria, VA 22314-2971
Tel: (703) 684-7722
Fax: (703) 684-5968
Toll free information: (800) 969-NMHA (6642)
Website: www.nmha.org

SEXUALITY AND SEXUAL CONCERNS

American College of Obstetricians and Gynecologists
P. O. Box 96920
Washington, DC 20090-6920
Tel: (202) 863-2518
Fax: (202) 484-1595
Website: www.acog.com
E-mail: resources@acog.org

American Urological Association
1120 North Charles Street
Baltimore, MD 21201
Tel: (410) 727-1100
Fax: (410) 223-4370
Website: www.auanet.org
E-mail: aua@auanet.org

**Sexuality Information and Education Council
of the United States**
130 West 42nd Street, Suite 350
New York, NY 10036
Tel: (212) 819-9770
Fax: (212) 819-9776
Website: www.siecus.org
E-mail: siecus@siecus.org

SIGHT PROBLEMS

American Academy of Ophthalmology
P. O. Box 7424
San Francisco, CA 94120
Tel: (415) 561-8500
Fax: (415) 561-8533
Toll free: (800) 222-3937
Website: www.eyenet.org
E-mail: comm.@aao.org

American Foundation for the Blind
11 Penn Plaza, Suite 300
New York, NY 10001
Tel: (212) 502-7600
Toll free: (800) AFB LINE (232-5463)
Fax: (212) 502-7777
Website: www.afb.org
E-mail: afbinfo@afb.net

American Optometric Association
243 North Lindbergh Boulevard
St. Louis, MO 61341
Tel: (314) 991-4100
Fax: (314) 991-4101
Toll free: (800) 365-2219
Website: http://www.aoanet.org

Better Vision Institute
1655 North Fort Meyer Drive, Suite 200
Arlington, VA 22209
Tel: (703) 243-1508
Toll free: (800) 642-3253
Fax: (703) 243-1537
Website: www.visionsite.org
E-mail: vca@visionsite.org

Foundation for Glaucoma Research
200 Pine Street, Suite 200
San Francisco, CA 94104
Tel: (415) 986-3162
Fax: (415) 986-3763
Website: www.glaucoma.org

National Eye Institute
Information Office
2020 Vision Place
Bethesda, MD 20892-3655
Tel: (301) 496-5248
Fax: (301) 402-1065
Website: www.nei.nih.gov
E-mail: 2020@nei.nih.gov

Prevent Blindness America
500 East Remington Road
Schaumberg, IL 60173
Tel: (847) 843-2020
Fax: (847) 843-8458
Toll free: (800) 331-2020
Website: http://www.preventblindness.org
E-mail: info@preventblindness.org

SKIN PROBLEMS

American Academy of Dermatology
930 North Meacham Road
Schaumberg, IL 60173
Tel: (847) 330-0230
Toll free: (888) 462-DERM (3376)
Fax: (847) 330-0050
Website: www.aad.org

**American Academy of Facial Plastic
and Reconstructive Surgery**
310 South Henry Street
Alexandria, VA 22314
Tel: (703) 299-9291
Fax: (703) 299-8898
(800) 332-FACE
Website: www.aafprs.org
E-mail: info@aafprs.org

**American Social Health Association Herpes
Resource Center**
P. O. Box 13827
Research Triangle Park, NC 27709
Tel: (919) 361-8400
Fax: (919) 361-8425
Website: http://www.ashastd.org
E-mail: phidra@ashastd.org

**National Arthritis and Musculoskeletal and Skin
Diseases Information Clearinghouse**
National Institutes of Health
1 AMS Circle
Bethesda, MD 20892-3675
Tel: (301) 495-4484
Toll free: (877) 22-NIAMS (64267)
Fax: (301) 718-6366
Website: www.nih.gov/niams
E-mail: via Website

The Skin Cancer Foundation
P. O. Box 561
New York, NY 10156

Tel: (212) 725-5176
Toll free: (800) SKIN-490 (754-6490)
Fax: (212) 725-5751
Website: www.skincancer.org
E-mail: info@skincancer.org

URINARY PROBLEMS

National Association for Continence (NAFC)
P. O. Box 8310
Spartanburg, SC 29305-8310
Tel: (864) 579-7900
Toll free: (800) BLADDER (252-3337)
Fax: (864) 579-7902
Website: www.nafc.org

**National Kidney and Urologic Diseases
Information Clearinghouse**
3 Information Way
Bethesda, MD 20892-3560
Tel: (301) 654-4415
Fax: (301) 907-8906

Website: www.niddk.nih.gov
E-mail: ndic@info.niddk.nih.gov

National Kidney Foundation
30 East 33rd Street, Suite 1100
New York, NY 10016
Tel: (212) 889-2210
Toll free: (800) 622-9010
Fax: (212) 689-9261
Website: www.kidney,org
E-mail: info@kidney.org

The Simon Foundation for Continence
P. O. Box 835
Wilmette, IL 60091
Tel: (847) 864-3913
Toll free: (800) 23-SIMON (237-4666)
Fax: (847) 864-9758
Website: www.simonfoundation.org
E-mail: simoninfo@simonfoundation.org

INDEX

Page numbers followed by *t* indicate table, page numbers in bold indicate algorithms.